T0297080

SELF-ASSESSMENT QUESTIONS FOR CLINICAL MOLECULAR GENETICS

SELF ASSESSMENT QUESTIONS FOR CLINICAL
PHARMACOKINETICS

SELF-ASSESSMENT QUESTIONS FOR CLINICAL MOLECULAR GENETICS

HAIYING MENG

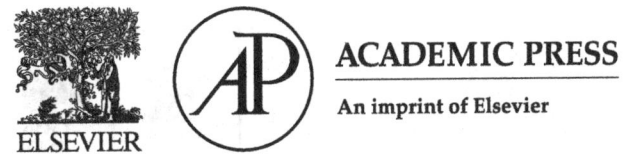

ACADEMIC PRESS
An imprint of Elsevier

ELSEVIER

Academic Press is an imprint of Elsevier
125 London Wall, London EC2Y 5AS, United Kingdom
525 B Street, Suite 1650, San Diego, CA 92101, United States
50 Hampshire Street, 5th Floor, Cambridge, MA 02139, United States
The Boulevard, Langford Lane, Kidlington, Oxford OX5 1GB, United Kingdom

Notices
Knowledge and best practice in this field are constantly changing. As new research and experience broaden our understanding, changes in research methods, professional practices, or medical treatment may become necessary.

Practitioners and researchers must always rely on their own experience and knowledge in evaluating and using any information, methods, compounds, or experiments described herein. In using such information or methods they should be mindful of their own safety and the safety of others, including parties for whom they have a professional responsibility.

To the fullest extent of the law, neither the Publisher nor the authors, contributors, or editors, assume any liability for any injury and/or damage to persons or property as a matter of products liability, negligence or otherwise, or from any use or operation of any methods, products, instructions, or ideas contained in the material herein.

British Library Cataloguing-in-Publication Data
A catalogue record for this book is available from the British Library

Library of Congress Cataloging-in-Publication Data
A catalog record for this book is available from the Library of Congress

ISBN: 978-0-12-809967-4

For Information on all Academic Press publications
visit our website at https://www.elsevier.com/books-and-journals

Publisher: Stacy Masucci
Acquisition Editor: Tari K. Broderick
Editorial Project Manager: Tracy I. Tufaga
Production Project Manager: Poulouse Joseph
Cover Designer: Victoria Pearson

Typeset by MPS Limited, Chennai, India

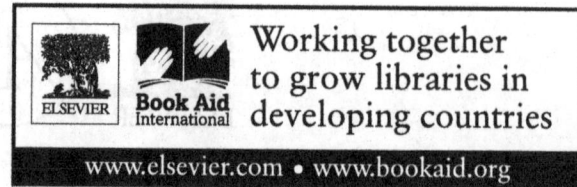

Working together
to grow libraries in
developing countries

www.elsevier.com • www.bookaid.org

Dedication

I dedicate this work to my parents (Yalan Chen - 陈雅兰 and Xianyi Meng - 孟宪义), who have always encouraged me to love others and to reach my full potential.

Contents

About the Author

Haiying Meng, M.D. and Ph.D., FACMG, is a clinical molecular geneticist and cytogeneticist and is currently affiliated with Quest Diagnostics Nichols Institute. She came to United States with M.D. and Ph.D. degrees. After postdoctoral training in Yale University, she 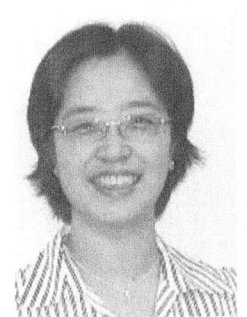 learned clinical molecular genetics and cytogenetic at Cincinnati Children's Hospital as a clinical fellow. In 5 years of practice, she worked on more than 20,000 cases. She loves her job, but considers the traffic around DC suburban area as waste of time. She enjoys teaching, and wrote this book to help others. Currently she lives in Chantilly, Virginia with her husband, their two children, and a family pet.

Preface

Genetics and Genomics are a relatively young science compared to others in medicine. In 1991, the Executive Committee of the American Board of Medical Specialties (ABMS) and the Assembly of the ABMS approved the application of the American Board of Medical Genetics and Genomics (ABMGG) to be a new board of the ABMS. Independently, the Council on Medical Education of the American Medical Association approved the application in the same year. Since then, 743 individuals have been certified in clinical molecular genetics and genomics by ABMGG (as of 2018). In 1995, the Association for Molecular Pathology (AMP) was formed to provide further structure and leadership to the emerging field of molecular diagnostics, especially in infectious diseases and acquired genetic changes in neoplasms. Certification in molecular genetic pathology is a joint function of ABMGG and the American Board of Pathology (ABP).

Clinical molecular genetics laboratory practice has become especially important during the past decade, with an unpredictable future since we have entered the "genomic era" with breakthroughs in the genomic technologies and database curation. The growing role of genomics in health care, for patient diagnoses, treatment and disease prevention thrives with the global effort of personalized medicine. Meanwhile, we are facing challenges of the new model of health systems (Fig. 1), insurance policies, and bioinformatics.

As a clinical molecular genetics practitioner or a practitioner in training, there are much broader requirements than just technical expertise. I randomly copied and pasted the following job description for a clinical molecular laboratory director position: "Demonstrate leadership qualities within and beyond the practice setting as a hospital representative. Maintain a work environment to enhance physician/staff satisfaction and retention. Support community outreach activities to educate patients and providers, or promote hospital activities. Participate in the development and implementation of clinical care models that promote efficient use of resources and optimal quality. Provide education and oversight of residents or service. Ensure regulatory compliance of AABB, CAP, FDA, OSHA, DPH, TJC, CLIA,

CMS. Ensure quality laboratory services for all aspects of test performance (pre-analytic, analytic, and post-analytic)." The clear message from this description is that it takes a lot more to be a clinical molecular geneticist than the fellowship and PhD training. Clinical molecular practice is a subject with relationships with other branches of medicine that are not easily untangled. No matter what career path leads us to this fellowship, we always have our strengths, as well as some underdeveloped areas that need to be strengthened.

In this book, I hope to present clinical molecular genetics from a practical point of view. It includes 14 chapters. They are General Molecular Genetic Knowledge; Regulations from Oversight Agencies; Molecular Genetic Nomenclature; Disorders of

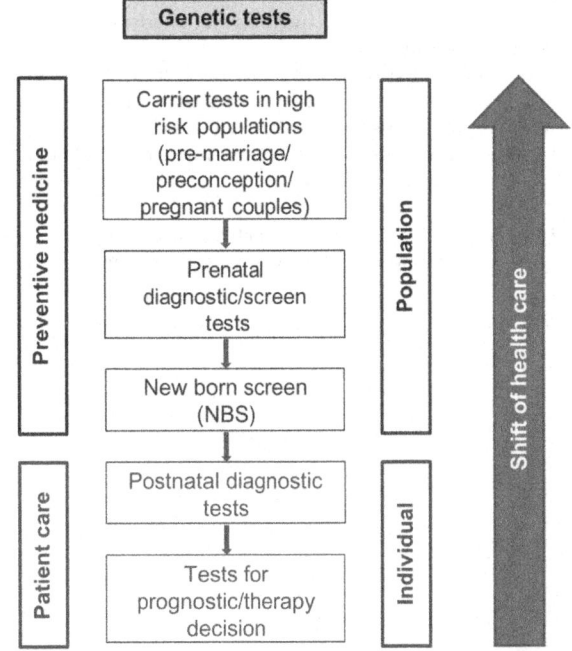

FIGURE 1 This figure illustrates the shift of health care from patient-care–oriented to preventive-case–oriented. This shift fundamentally affects the clinical laboratory genetics practice, which is enabled by advanced medical technologies and bioinformatics. Meanwhile, it is also complicated by existing medical practices, insurance policies, among other things.[1]

Unstable Repeat Sequences; Cystic Fibrosis; Nonneoplastic Hematological Disorders; Oncology—Constitutional; Oncology—Acquired; Lysosomal Storage Disorders; Neuromuscular Disorders; Prenatal, Newborn Screen, and Metabolic Disorders; Other Common Genetic Syndromes; Pharmacogenetics; and Genetic Counseling—Introduction.

There is much more beyond what is covered in this book that we learn from day-to-day practice. I hope we may encourage each other, and constantly learn from the genetic research with a humble heart "on the integrity of both individual genetics providers and the profession as a whole. Ensuring public trust mandates that genetics providers' actions are in the best interests of patients and clients, that they set and maintain standards of competence and integrity, and that they provide expert advice to society on how genetic knowledge is to be applied to healthcare" (http://www.abmgg.org). And finally, I take this opportunity to remind us that the Hippocratic Oath is for all practitioners of medicine including us:

> I swear to fulfill, to the best of my ability and judgment, this covenant...
>
> I will respect the hard-won scientific gains of those physicians in whose steps I walk, and gladly share such knowledge as is mine with those who are to follow.
>
> I will apply, for the benefit of the sick, all measures which are required, avoiding those twin traps of overtreatment and therapeutic nihilism.
>
> I will remember that there is art to medicine as well as science, and that warmth, sympathy, and understanding may outweigh the surgeon's knife or the chemist's drug.
>
> I will not be ashamed to say "I know not," nor will I fail to call in my colleagues when the skills of another are needed for a patient's recovery.
>
> I will respect the privacy of my patients, for their problems are not disclosed to me that the world may know. Most

especially must I tread with care in matters of life and death. Above all, I must not play at God.

> I will remember that I do not treat a fever chart, a cancerous growth, but a sick human being, whose illness may affect the person's family and economic stability. My responsibility includes these related problems, if I am to care adequately for the sick.
>
> I will prevent disease whenever I can, for prevention is preferable to cure.
>
> I will remember that I remain a member of society, with special obligations to all my fellow human beings, those sounds of mind and body as well as the infirm.
>
> If I do not violate this oath, may I enjoy life and art, respected while I live and remembered with affection thereafter. May I always act so as to preserve the finest traditions of my calling and may I long experience the joy of healing those who seek my help.

Reference

1. Meng H, Xu W. Clinical molecular genetic laboratory practice, where we stand in 2018. *J Mol Genet Med* 2018;**12**:368 Available from: https://doi.org/10.4172/1747-0862.1000368.

Further Reading

- American Board of Medical Genetics and Genomics <http://abmgg.org/>
- Association for Molecular Pathology <https://www.amp.org/>
- American Board of Pathology <https://www.abpath.org/>
- College of American Pathologies
- Certification in Molecular Pathology in the United States (Training and Education Committee, the Association for Molecular Pathology). *J Mol Diagn* 2002;**4**(4):181–4 [PMC1907356].
- Certification in Molecular Pathology in the United States: an update from the Association for Molecular Pathology Training and Education Committee. *J Mol Diagn* 2012;**14**(6):541–9 [PMID: 22925695].

Acknowledgments

This book could not have been written without the help of many people, and I would like to take an opportunity to thank my husband, Leiling Chen, our two children, Luke Chen and Joshua Chen, for their support, without which this book neither could nor would have been written. I also wish to thank Drs. Wenbo Xu (Department of Molecular Genetics, True Health Diagnostics, VA) and Sung-Hee Oh (Department of Pathology, Baystate Health Center, MA) for proofreading some of the chapters, Mrs. Cheryl L Bissaillon (Department of Pathology, Baystate Health Center, MA; FMR1 and others) and Dr. Marilyn Li (the Division of Genomic Diagnostics and Director of Cancer Genomic Diagnostics at Children's Hospital of Philadelphia; Figures 1-24 and 1-25) for providing images for figures. My sincere appreaciation goes to my colleagues at Cincinnati Children's Hosptical at Ohio, Dayton Children's Hospital at Ohio, Baystate Health Center at masachusett, and Quest Diagnostics at Virginia for accompany me on this journey of clinical moelcular genetic practice. Finally, I'd like to thank the staff at ELSEVIER Publisher for their dedication and patience in this five years.

CHAPTER

1

General Molecular Genetic Knowledge

Clinical laboratories use molecular genetic techniques to analyze DNA, RNA, or proteins for diagnosis, risk assessment, possible prognosis, progress monitoring, and prospective therapy treatments. In the 1980s, clinical laboratories primarily used the molecular genetic techniques to analyze variants for diagnosis. The earliest assays were targeted to a few disorders such as sickle cell disease and cystic fibrosis. These early molecular diagnoses often involved indirect mutation detection through linkage analyses, which is extremely labor-intensive and required large samples of peripheral-blood from patients.

In 1986, Mullis et al. discovered the polymerase chain reaction (PCR), which revolutionized molecular diagnosis. Assays in use previously were quickly modified to incorporate the use of PCR-amplified DNA.[1] During the 1990s, the identification of more genes in the human genome and the invention of Sanger sequencing led to the emergence of a distinct field of molecular and genomic laboratory medicine. PCR-Sanger became the most common technique for the analysis of many genetic disorders in clinical molecular laboratories. In 2003, the near completion of the Human Genome Project exponentially heightened the importance of molecular genetics in laboratory medicine. The 1000 Genome Project accumulated genetic information from the general population for variations in classification.

Nowadays, next-generation sequencing (NGS) incorporated with automated large-scale sequence analysis appears to be more and more essential for the diagnosis of many genetic disorders in clinical molecular laboratories. The growing role of bioinformatics brought the advanced mathematical and computing approach into clinical molecular genetic practice. The discovery of circulating cell-free DNA (cfDNA) revolutionized prenatal genetic testing and tumor screening/monitoring. Clinical molecular genetic practice offers the prospect of personalized medicine.

As the title of this chapter suggests, we are going to review basic genetic knowledge through the most commonly used assays in clinical molecular genetic laboratories, including NGS, from a historical point of view. It seems to be boring for professionals. Hopefully, it will refresh some memories for the following chapters.

QUESTIONS

1. A pediatric geneticist saw a 12-month-old boy for tetralogy of Fallot, cleft palate and lip, recurrent infection, and developmental delay. Since the American College of Medical Genetics and Genomics (ACMGG) recommends chromosome microarray analysis (CMA) as the first-tier clinical diagnostic test for individuals with developmental disabilities or congenital anomalies, the geneticist ordered CMA for this patient. Which one of the following specimens has highest quality of DNA, and most suitable for CMA?
   A. 1 mL of blood in a green top tube
   B. 1 mL of blood in a purple (lavender) top tube
   C. 1 mL of saliva
   D. 0.5–1 cm diameter of a dried blood spot
   E. 10 mm^2 of formalin-fixed tissue
2. A courier picked up a whole-blood sample (EDTA, lavender) from an outreach blood-draw station for *BCR/ABL1* quantitative testing at the main hospital. Which one of the following conditions is preferred for the transportation of this sample?
   A. Ambient
   B. On ice packs
   C. In dry ice
   D. None of above
3. A courier picked up a whole-blood sample (lavender) from an outreach blood-draw station for *JAK2* V617F quantitative testing at the main hospital. Which one of the following conditions is preferred for the transportation of this sample?

Self-assessment Questions for Clinical Molecular Genetics.
DOI: https://doi.org/10.1016/B978-0-12-809967-4.00001-6

   A. Ambient
   B. On ice packs
   C. In dry ice
   D. None of the above

4. A technologist in a clinical molecular genetic laboratory extracted nucleic acid from a peripheral-blood sample for *BCR-ABL1* quantitative testing. Which one of the following conditions is preferred for storage of the extracted nucleic acid before the test is performed?
   A. Ambient
   B. Refrigerated (4°C)
   C. − 20°C
   D. None of the above

5. A technologist in a clinical molecular genetic laboratory extracted nucleic acid from a peripheral-blood sample for *JAK2* V617F quantitative testing. Which one of the following conditions is preferred for storage of the extracted nucleic acid before the test is performed?
   A. Ambient
   B. Refrigerated (4°C)
   C. − 20°C
   D. − 80°C
   E. None of the above

6. As a clinical molecular laboratory director, you led a continue education session for the technologists about quality control for PCR reaction. At the end of the presentation, a junior technologist asked how to tell whether a PCR result is false negative. In which one of the following situations would the results on the tested specimens be considered as false negative for amplification?
   A. The positive control is negative.
   B. The positive control is positive.
   C. The negative control is positive.
   D. The negative control is negative.

7. As a clinical molecular laboratory director, you led a continue education session for the technologists about quality control for PCR reaction. At the end of the presentation, a junior technologist asked how to tell if a PCR result is false positive. In which one of the following situations would the results on the tested specimens be considered as false positive for amplification?
   A. The positive control is negative.
   B. The positive control is positive.
   C. The negative control is positive.
   D. The negative control is negative.

8. A 6-year-old boy was brought to a genetics clinic by his parents for tremor and epilepsy. The doctor ordered a G-banded chromosome karyotype analysis. Which one of the following would be the preferred specimen for this test?

   A. Bone-marrow sample in a sodium heparin tube (green top)
   B. Bone-marrow sample in an EDTA tube (lavender top)
   C. Cerebral spinal fluid (CSF) sample
   D. Peripheral blood in a sodium heparin tube (green top)
   E. Peripheral blood in an EDTA tube (lavender top)
   F. None of the above

9. A 6-year-old boy was brought to a genetics clinic by his parents for tremor and epilepsy. The doctor ordered a chromosome microarray analysis. Which one of the following specimens would be the preferred sample for this test?
   A. Bone-marrow sample in a sodium heparin tube (green top)
   B. Bone-marrow sample in an EDTA tube (lavender top)
   C. Cerebral spinal fluid (CSF) sample
   D. Peripheral blood in a sodium heparin tube (green top)
   E. Peripheral blood in an EDTA tube (lavender top)
   F. None of the above

10. A molecular geneticist has been working for a start-up private clinical laboratory for 2 months. He has been writing policies while working on validations. Which one of the following conditions would be most appropriate for his laboratory to store DNA specimens for 2 years after clinical testing?[2]
   A. Ambient
   B. Refrigerated (4°C)
   C. − 20°C
   D. − 80°C
   E. None of the above

11. A molecular geneticist has been working for a start-up private clinical laboratory for 2 months. He has been writing policies while working on validations. Which one of the following conditions would be most appropriate for his laboratory to store RNA specimens for 2 years after clinical testing?
   A. Ambient
   B. Refrigerated (4°C)
   C. − 20°C
   D. − 80°C
   E. None of the above

12. A molecular scientist in a clinical laboratory bought reagents to validate an assay for fragile X syndrome with PCR and Southern blot methods. The restriction enzymes came in today. How should he store the enzymes?
   A. Room temperature
   B. Refrigerator
   C. Frost free freezer

D. Nondefrost freezer
E. Dry ice
F. None of the above

13. A technologist in a clinical molecular genetic laboratory is responsible for DNA extraction for this week. He uses a NanoDrop (spectrophotometer) to determine the quantity of DNA specimens after extraction. He tested specimens for OD230, OD260, and OD280. Which one of the following absorbance reads is for nucleic acid?[3]
   A. OD230
   B. OD260
   C. OD280
   D. All of the above
   E. None of the above

14. A technologist in a clinical molecular genetic laboratory is responsible for DNA extraction for this week. He uses a NanoDrop (spectrophotometer) to determine the quantity of DNA specimens after extraction. He tested specimens for OD230, OD260, and OD280. Which one of the following absorbance reads is for protein?[3]
   A. OD230
   B. OD260
   C. OD280
   D. All of the above
   E. None of the above

15. A technologist in a clinical molecular genetic laboratory is responsible for DNA extraction for this week. He uses a NanoDrop (spectrophotometer) to determine the quantity of DNA specimens after extraction. He tested specimens for OD230, OD260, and OD280. Which one of the following absorbance reads is for the contamination of carbohydrates, phenols, peptides, and aromatic compounds introduced during DNA extraction?[3]
   A. OD230
   B. OD260
   C. OD280
   D. All of the above
   E. None of the above

16. A technologist in a clinical molecular genetic laboratory uses a spectrophotometer to determine the quantity of DNAs after extraction. He tests specimens for both OD230, OD260, and OD280. The ratio of OD260/OD280 was 1.3. Which one of the following statements is most appropriate?[3]
   A. This ratio of OD260/280 indicates unacceptable protein contamination.
   B. This ratio of OD260/280 indicates unacceptable RNA contamination.
   C. This ratio of OD260/280 indicates unacceptable aromatic compounds contamination.
   D. All of the above.
   E. None of the above.

17. A technologist in a clinical molecular genetic laboratory used a spectrophotometer to determine the quantity of a DNA sample. He tested for OD230, OD260, and OD280. The ratio of OD260/OD230 was 1.3. Which one of the following statements is most appropriate?[3,4]
   A. This ratio of OD260/230 indicates unacceptable protein contamination.
   B. This ratio of OD260/230 indicates unacceptable RNA contamination.
   C. This ratio of OD260/230 indicates unacceptable aromatic compound contamination.
   D. All of the above.
   E. None of the above.

18. A technologist in a clinical molecular genetic laboratory used a spectrophotometer to determine the quantity of a DNA sample. The absorbance reading at 260 nm from $100\times$ dilution is 0.12. What is the DNA concentration?[3,4]
   A. 600 μg/μL
   B. 600 μg/mL
   C. 480 μg/μL
   D. 480 μg/mL
   E. 4.8 μg/mL

19. A technologist in a clinical molecular genetic laboratory used a spectrophotometer to determine the quantity of an RNA sample. The absorbance reading at 260 nm from $100\times$ dilution is 0.12. What is the RNA concentration?[3,4]
   A. 600 μg/μL
   B. 600 μg/mL
   C. 480 μg/μL
   D. 480 μg/mL
   E. 4.8 μg/mL

20. A technologist in a clinical molecular genetic laboratory used a spectrophotometer to determine the quantity/quality of five DNA samples. The absorbance readings at 230, 260, and 280 nm were recorded in the following table:

Sample	OD260	OD280	OD230
1	0.48	0.23	0.48
2	0.3	0.16	0.16
3	0.25	0.22	0.03
4	0.16	0.09	0.09
5	0.2	0.12	0.15

Which one of the above samples is contaminated with a high level of protein?[3,4]

A. 1
B. 2
C. 3
D. 4
E. 5

21. A technologist in a clinical molecular genetic laboratory used a spectrophotometer to determine the quantity/quality of five DNA samples. The absorbance reading at 230, 260, and 280 nm were recorded in the following table:

Sample	OD260	OD280	OD230
1	0.48	0.23	0.48
2	0.3	0.16	0.16
3	0.25	0.22	0.03
4	0.16	0.09	0.09
5	0.2	0.12	0.15

Which one of the above samples is contaminated with high level of aromatic compounds during DNA extraction?[3,4]

A. 1
B. 2
C. 3
D. 4
E. 5

22. Which one of the following RNA sequences inhibits gene expression in vivo?[4]

A. hnRNA (heterogeneous nuclear RNA)
B. miRNA (microRNA)
C. mRNA (messenger RNA)
D. rRNA (ribosomal RNA)
E. siRNA (small interfering RNA)
F. tRNA (transfer RNA)
G. None of the above

23. Which one of the following nucleotides does not present in vivo?[4]

A. Circulating nucleic acids
B. hnRNA
C. microRNA
D. rRNA
E. siRNA
F. tRNA
G. None of the above

24. The genetic code consists of 64 triplets of nucleotides. These triplets are called "codons." With three exceptions, each codon encodes for 1 of the 20 amino acids used in the synthesis of proteins. There is some redundancy in the code. Most of the amino acids are encoded by more than one codon. Which one of the following types of nucleotide contains genetic codons, which may be translated into an amino acid sequence?[4]

A. microRNA
B. mRNA
C. rRNA
D. siRNA
E. tRNA
F. None of the above

25. Noninvasive prenatal screening (NIPS) that uses cell-free DNA from the plasma of pregnant women offers tremendous potential as a screening method for fetal aneuploidy. In 2011, cell-free DNA (cfDNA) analysis became clinically available, and the American College of Obstetricians and Gynecologists (ACOG) and the Society for Maternal–Fetal Medicine recommended it as a screening option for women at increased risk of fetal aneuploidy. This population was defined as women 35 years or older, fetuses with ultrasonographic findings indicative of an increased risk of aneuploidy, women with a history of trisomy-affected offspring, a parent carrying a balanced Robertsonian translocation with an increased risk of trisomy 13 or trisomy 21, and women with positive first-trimester or second-trimester screening test results. Which one of the factors affects the fetal fraction of the cfDNA in the maternal blood more than others?[5-8]

A. Fetal anomalies
B. Maternal age
C. Maternal weight
D. Not sure
E. None of the above

26. Which one of the following fluorescence dyes may be used to quantify RNA?[4]

A. DABA (3,5-diaminobenzoic acid)
B. Hoechst 33258
C. PicoGreen
D. OliGreen
E. SybrGreen II

27. A scientist plans to develop a PCR-RFLP (restriction fragment length polymorphism) assay for hereditary hemochromatosis (HH) in a clinical molecular laboratory. Which type of genetic marker will he target in this assay?

A. Copy-number variants (CNVs)
B. Short tandem repeats (STRs)
C. Single-nucleotide polymorphisms (SNPs)
D. Variable-number tandem repeat (VNTR)
E. None of the above

28. A scientist plans to validate a chromosome microarray assay. Which one of following methods for DNA extraction will yield higher-quality DNA than others for chromosome microarray analysis?[4]

A. Chelex (ion-exchange resin) extraction
B. Whatman FTA (Flinders Technology Associates) paper (collection, storage, and isolation)
C. Organic (phenol–chloroform) extraction
D. Promega Maxwell system
E. Qiagen silica-exchange resin
F. None of the above

29. A scientist plans to develop a Sanger sequencing–based assay for Gaucher disease in a clinical molecular laboratory. Which one of following methods may he use to purify the PCR products for sequencing?[4]
A. Agarose gel
B. Ethanol or isopropanol precipitation
C. ExoSAP-IT (exonuclease I and shrimp alkaline phosphatase)
D. Filter column
E. All of the above
F. None of the above

30. A scientist plans to develop a Sanger sequencing–based assay for Gaucher disease in a clinical molecular laboratory. Which one of following methods may NOT be used to purify the PCR products for sequencing?[4]
A. Agarose gel
B. Ethanol or isopropanol precipitation
C. ExoSAP-IT (exonuclease I and shrimp alkaline phosphatase)
D. Filter minicolumn
E. SpeedVac
F. None of the above

31. A scientist planned to develop a Sanger sequencing–based assay for Gaucher disease in a clinical molecular laboratory. Which one of following methods is most cost-effective for purification of PCR products without switching tubes?[4]
A. Agarose gel
B. Ethanol or isopropanol precipitation
C. ExoSAP-IT (exonuclease I and shrimp alkaline phosphatase)
D. Filter minicolumn
E. SpeedVac
F. All of the above
G. None of the above

32. A scientist planned to develop a Sanger sequencing–based assay for Gaucher disease in a clinical molecular laboratory. Which one of following PCR purification methods has the lowest yield?[4]
A. Agarose gel
B. Ethanol or isopropanol precipitation
C. ExoSAP-IT (exonuclease I and shrimp alkaline phosphatase)
D. Filter minicolumn
E. SpeedVac
F. Not sure

33. If an assay with forward allele-specific oligonucleotide (ASO) probes is designed to detect pathogenic variants in the CFTR gene for cystic fibrosis, which mismatch pairs should be avoided when designing the probes, according to the ACMG Standards and Guidelines for Clinical Genetics Laboratories?[9]
A. G:T and G:A
B. C:T and C:A
C. T:C and T:G
D. A:C and A:G
E. None of the above

34. Both forward allele-specific oligonucleotide (ASO) probes and reverse dot-blot hybridization (RDB) may be used to detect pathogenic variants in the CFTR gene for cystic fibrosis. Which one of the following descriptions is NOT for RDB, according to the ACMG Standards and Guidelines for Clinical Genetics Laboratories?[9]
A. It uses multiplex PCR reaction.
B. PCR products are labeled.
C. PCR products are spotted onto replicate filters (dot blots).
D. Probes are bound to nylon membranes.
E. PCR products are hybridized to the probes.

35. A clinical molecular laboratory used reverse dot blot hybridization (RDB) to detect pathogenic variants in the CFTR gene for cystic fibrosis. How should the laboratory store the probe-spotted membranes, according to the ACMG Standards and Guidelines for Clinical Genetics Laboratories?[9]
A. 4°C refrigerator, and dark
B. 4°C refrigerator
C. −20°C freezer, and dark
D. −20°C freezer
E. Room temperature, and dark
F. Room temperature

36. What do forward allele-specific oligonucleotide (ASO), reverse dot blot hybridization (RDB), oligonucleotide ligation assay (OLA), and fluorescence resonance energy transfer (FRET) have in common, according to the ACMG Standards and Guidelines for Clinical Genetics Laboratories?[9]
A. Probes are designed for the different alleles.
B. PCR products are labeled.
C. Primers are designed for the different alleles.
D. Probes are bound to nylon membranes.
E. Probes are labeled.
F. All of the above.
G. None of the above.

37. Which one of the following techniques is relatively higher throughput and more accurate in detection of pathogenic variants in the CFTR gene than others, according to the ACMG Standards and Guidelines for Clinical Genetics Laboratories?[9]

A. Forward allele-specific oligonucleotide (ASO)
B. Reverse dot blot hybridization (RDB)
C. Amplification refractory mutation system (ARMS)
D. Oligonucleotide ligation assay (OLA)
E. Sanger sequencing

38. Dr. Z, a director of a molecular pathology laboratory, planned to validate an oligonucleotide ligation assay (OLA) to detect carriers of cystic fibrosis. How many probes will Dr. Z use for each pathogenic variant in the *CFTR* gene, according to the ACMG Standards and Guidelines for Clinical Genetics Laboratories?[9]
   A. 1
   B. 2
   C. 3
   D. 4
   E. Not sure
   F. None of the above

39. A director of a molecular pathology laboratory plans to validate an oligonucleotide ligation assay (OLA) to detect carriers of cystic fibrosis. How many tubes of reactions should be tested for each pathogenic variant, according to the ACMG Standards and Guidelines for Clinical Genetics Laboratories?[9]
   A. 1
   B. 2
   C. 3
   D. 4
   E. Not sure
   F. None of the above

40. Dr. Z, a director of a molecular pathology laboratory, plans to validate a fluorescence resonance energy transfer (FRET) assay to detect carriers of cystic fibrosis. How many probes will Dr. Z use for each pathogenic variant in the *CFTR* gene, according to the ACMG Standards and Guidelines for Clinical Genetics Laboratories?[9]
   A. 1
   B. 2
   C. 3
   D. 4
   E. Not sure
   F. None of the above

41. A director of a clinical molecular genetic laboratory plans to validate a TaqMan assay for quantitative *JAK2* V617F variant analysis to assist in the diagnosis of myeloid proliferative neoplasms (MPNs). How many probes will this assay use in each well, according to the ACMG Standards and Guidelines for Clinical Genetics Laboratories?
   A. 1
   B. 2
   C. 3
   D. 4

E. Not sure
F. None of the above

42. A clinical molecular genetic laboratory uses dHPLC (denaturing high-performance liquid chromatography) to detect pathogenic variants in the *TP53* gene for Li–Fraumeni syndrome followed by sequencing to confirm identified variants. Which one of the following is the sequence of elution by the column, according to the ACMG Standards and Guidelines for Clinical Genetics Laboratories?[9]
   A. Homoduplex, heteroduplex, followed by single-stranded fragments
   B. Single-stranded fragments, heteroduplex, followed by homoduplex
   C. Single-stranded fragments, homoduplex, followed by heteroduplex
   D. Homoduplex, single-stranded fragments, followed by heteroduplex
   E. Heteroduplex, homoduplex, followed by single-stranded fragments

43. A clinical molecular genetic laboratory evaluates a dHPLC (denaturing High Performance Liquid Chromatography) assay to detect pathogenic variants in the *CFTR* gene for cystic fibrosis. Which one of the following statements is appropriate, according to the ACMG Standards and Guidelines for Clinical Genetics Laboratories?[9]
   A. dHPLC can be used for fragments up to 1000 bp.
   B. dHPLC is more sensitive for the detection of pathogenic variants than Sanger sequencing.
   C. The dHPLC assay may be used as a diagnostic test.
   D. dHPLC is more sensitive for the detection of heterozygotes than homozygotes.
   E. None of the above.

44. Dr. Z, a director of a molecular pathology laboratory, plans to use short tandem repeat (STR) markers for linkage analysis to help a four-generation family (108 members) with a rare familial congenital cardiovascular disease. Which one of the following STRs tends to be more noticeable for stutter artifact?[9]
   A. Mononucleotide repeats
   B. Trinucleotide repeats
   C. Pentanucleotide repeats
   D. None of the above

45. Which one of the following assays may be used to detect heterozygous deletions or duplications of exons, genes, or chromosomes?
   A. Single-stranded conformation polymorphism
   B. Heteroduplex analysis
   C. Denaturing gradient-gel electrophoresis
   D. Multiplex ligation-dependent probe amplification (MLPA)
   E. None of the above

46. Which one of the following diseases is NOT commonly caused by heterozygous deletions or duplications of exons, genes or chromosomes?[9]
    A. Alpha thalassemia
    B. Charcot—Marie—Tooth type 1
    C. Duchenne muscular dystrophy
    D. Spinal muscular atrophy
    E. Xeroderma pigmentosum
    F. All of the above
    G. None of the above

47. Dr. Z, a director of a molecular pathology laboratory, plans to validate a quantitative real time RT-PCR assay for the *BCR-ABL1* fusion gene. And he plans to accept bone marrow, peripheral blood, and lymph node for this test. Which one of the following specimen handlings is the most appropriate for this test, according to the ACMG Standards and Guidelines for Clinical Genetics Laboratories?[9]
    A. Bone marrow, blood, and solid tissues should be frozen for transportation to keep RNAs stable.
    B. Bone marrow and blood should be frozen, but solid tissues should be transported to the lab on wet ice.
    C. Bone marrow and blood should not be frozen, but solid tissues should be transported to the lab on dry ice.
    D. Bone marrow, blood, and solid tissues should be transported to the lab on wet ice.
    E. All of the above.
    F. None of the above.

48. A scientist planned to develop a Sanger sequencing—based test for Gaucher disease in a clinical molecular genetic laboratory. There is no FDA-cleared/approved assay available. He downloaded the genetic sequence of the *GBA* gene and was ready to design the primers for PCR reaction. How many base pairs are usual for the primers for both the specificity and efficiency?[4]
    A. 6 bp
    B. 25 bp
    C. 40 bp
    D. 60 bp
    E. None of the above

49. A scientist planned to develop a Sanger sequencing—based test for Gaucher disease in a clinical molecular genetic laboratory. There is no FDA-cleared/approved assay available. He designed and ordered the primers. Which one of the following is the correct order for each cycle of PCR reaction?[4]
    A. Annealing → denaturation → extension
    B. Annealing → extension → denaturation
    C. Denaturation → annealing → extension
    D. Denaturation → extension → annealing
    E. None of the above

50. A scientist planned to develop a Sanger sequencing—based test for Gaucher disease in a clinical molecular genetic laboratory. There is no FDA-cleared/approved assay available. He designed and ordered the primers. After the first try on the PCR reaction with both positive and negative samples, he found that most amplicons worked well. But one amplicon showed only a very weak band for the PCR product, but a strong band for primer dimer. Which one of the following most likely is the reason for the primer dimer band in this amplicon?
    A. Complementarity in the primer sequences
    B. High GC content in the primer sequences
    C. High primer concentration
    D. Low annealing temperature
    E. None of the above

51. A scientist planned to develop a Sanger sequencing—based test for Gaucher disease in a clinical molecular genetic laboratory. There is no FDA-cleared/approved assay available. He designed and ordered the primers. After the first try on the PCR reaction with both positive and negative samples, he found that most exons/amplicons worked well. However, one exon/amplicon showed a lot of nonspecific PCR products. Which one of the following could result in nonspecific PCR products?
    A. High primer concentration
    B. Low annealing temperature
    C. Pseudogenes
    D. All of the above
    E. None of the above

52. A scientist planned to develop a Sanger sequencing—based assay for Gaucher disease in a clinical molecular genetic laboratory. There is no FDA-cleared/approved assay available. He designed and ordered the primers. After the first try on the PCR reaction with both positive and negative samples, he found that most exons/amplicons worked well. However, one exon/amplicon showed a lot of nonspecific PCR products. What could he do to reduce the nonspecific PCR products in the amplicon?
    A. Decrease the primer concentration
    B. Increase the annealing temperature
    C. Redesign the primers to avoid pseudogenes
    D. All of the above
    E. None of the above

53. A scientist planned to develop a Sanger sequencing—based assay for Gaucher disease in a clinical molecular genetic laboratory. There is no

FDA-cleared/approved assay available. He
designed and ordered the primers. Which one of
the following efforts could be a part of quality
control for PCR contamination?[4]
  A. A nontemplate control
  B. A reagent blank control
  C. A separate area for PCR setup
  D. Fewer PCR cycles
  E. All of the above
  F. None of the above
54. Theoretically how many copies of a targeted
    sequence could be made after a PCR reaction
    with 30 cycles?[4]
  A. 2^{30}
  B. 2^{30-1}
  C. 30^{2+1}
  D. 2^{30+1}
  E. 2×30
  F. None of the above
55. A technologist in a clinical molecular genetic
    laboratory is responsible for fragile X testing this
    week. This laboratory uses PCR and Southern blot
    for this test. The amplicon size of the PCR products
    is about 100–500 bp. Which one of the following
    agarose gels will she use to resolve the fragments?[4]
  A. 0.1%
  B. 0.5%
  C. 1%
  D. 2%
  E. 4%
56. A technologist in a clinical molecular genetic
    laboratory is responsible for fragile X testing this
    week. This laboratory uses PCR and Southern
    blot for this test. The DNA fragment size of the
    Southern blot is expected be between 2000 and
    8000 bp. Which one of the following agarose gels
    will he use to resolve the fragments?[4]
  A. 0.1%
  B. 0.5%
  C. 1%
  D. 2%
  E. 4%
57. A technologist in a clinical molecular genetic
    laboratory is responsible for fragile X testing
    this week. This laboratory uses PCR and
    Southern blot for this test. She sets up an
    agarose gel to check the PCR products before
    capillary electrophoresis (see figure below). "M"
    stands for the molecular weight size marker
    for electrophoresis (100, 200, 300, 400 bp, etc.).
    Which one of the following specimens has the
    biggest PCR products?
  A. A
  B. B
  C. C

  D. D
  E. E
  F. F

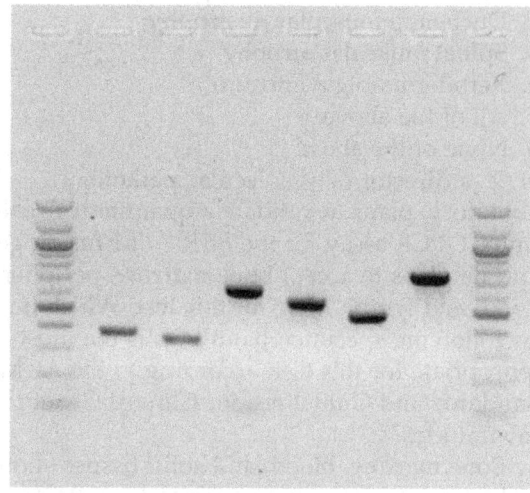

58. A technologist in a clinical molecular genetic
    laboratory is responsible for fragile X testing this
    week. This laboratory uses PCR and Southern
    blot for this test. He sets up an agarose gel to
    check on the products before capillary
    electrophoresis (see figure below). "M" stands for
    molecular weight size marker for electrophoresis
    (100, 200, 300, 400 bp, etc.). Which one of the
    following specimens has the smallest PCR
    products?
  A. A
  B. B
  C. C
  D. D
  E. E
  F. F

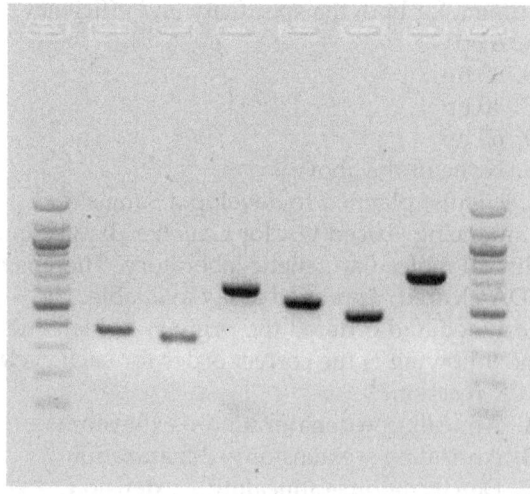

59. A technologist in a clinical molecular genetic laboratory tested two samples (A and B) for hereditary hemochromatosis with PCR-RFLP this week. The results are shown in the figure below. "M" stands for molecular weight marker (100, 200, 300, 400 bp, etc.), "C" for a homozygous control for p.C282Y, "D" for a compound heterozygous control for p.C282Y and p.H63D, and "E" for a no-template control (negative control). The top part of the gel shows the results for p.C282Y, and the bottom part for p.H63D. What is the genotype result of sample A?
  A. Wild type/wild type
  B. p.H63D/wild type
  C. p.H63D/p.H63D
  D. p.H63D/p.C282Y
  E. p.C282Y/wild type
  F. p.C282Y/p.C282Y
  G. None of the above

hereditary hemochromatosis with PCR-RFLP this week. The results are shown in the figure below. "M" stands for molecular weight marker (100, 200, 300, 400 bp, etc.), "C" for a homozygous control for p.C282Y, "D" for a compound heterozygous control for p.C282Y and p.H63D, and "E" for a no-template control (negative control). The top part of the gel shows the results for p.C282Y, and the bottom part for p.H63D. What is the genotype result for sample B?
  A. Wild type/wild type
  B. p.H63D/wild type
  C. p.H63D/p.H63D
  D. p.H63D/p.C282Y
  E. p.C282Y/wild type
  F. p.C282Y/p.C282Y
  G. None of the above

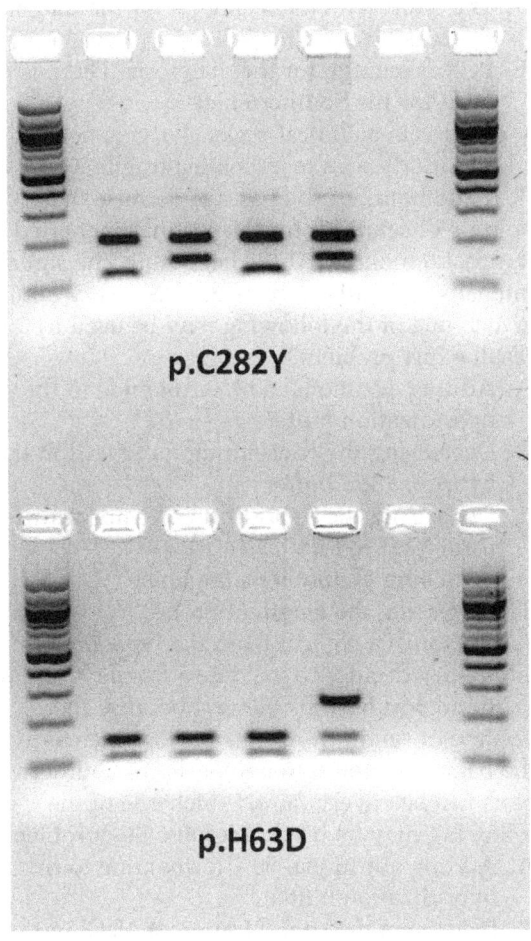

60. A technologist in a clinical molecular genetic laboratory tested two samples (A and B) for

61. A scientist initiated a project to develop a new assay for high-throughput genomic DNA analysis in a clinical molecular genetic laboratory. Which one of the following methods is the most sensitive for DNA detection as compared with the others?

A. Ethidium bromide
B. FAM fluorophore
C. Isotopic P^{32}
D. Luciferase
E. Silver stain
F. None of the above

62. A technologist in a clinical molecular genetic laboratory is responsible for fragile X testing this week. This laboratory uses PCR and the Southern blot for this test. Which one of the following statements is true about PCR and the Southern blot?[10]
    A. The analyzable DNA fragments for PCR are usually smaller than the ones for the Southern blot.
    B. PCR may detect the methylation status of the allele(s), while the Southern blot cannot.
    C. The Southern blot is less labor-intensive than PCR.
    D. The Southern blot is enough for the diagnosis. There is no need for PCR.
    E. PCR is enough for the diagnosis. There is no need for the Southern blot.

63. A director in a clinical molecular genetic laboratory decides to validate a fragile X test with PCR and Southern blot assays because the volume of send-out for this test has increased in the past 6 months. At the beginning, the signal intensity of Southern blots has been very faint. Which one of the following may be used to resolve this problem?[4]
    A. Adding additional 50% formamide to the hybridization buffer
    B. Decreasing the concentration of NaCl in the hybridization buffer
    C. Decreasing the hybridization temperature from 75°C to 65°C
    D. Switching to another company
    E. Increasing the length of probe

64. A director in a clinical molecular genetic laboratory decides to validate a fragile X test with PCR and Southern blot assays because the volume of send-out for this test has increased. At the beginning the signal intensity of Southern blots has been very faint. Which one of the following may be used to resolve this problem?[4]
    A. Adding additional 50% formamide to the hybridization buffer
    B. Increasing the concentration of NaCl in the hybridization buffer
    C. Increasing the hybridization temperature from 65°C to 75°C
    D. Switching to another company
    E. Increasing the length of probe

65. A director in a clinical molecular genetic laboratory decides to validate a fragile X test with

PCR and Southern blot assays because the volume of send-out for this test has increased. At the beginning, the signal intensity of Southern blots has been very faint. Which one of the following may be used to resolve this problem?[4]
    A. Decreasing formamide in the hybridization buffer from 50% to 20%
    B. Decreasing the concentration of NaCl in the hybridization buffer
    C. Increasing the hybridization temperature from 65°C to 75°C
    D. Switching to another company
    E. Increasing the length of probe

66. A scientist in a clinical molecular genetic laboratory works on designing primers for an assay. Which one of the following primers has highest T_m as compared with the others?[4]
    A. AGTCTGGGACGGCGCGGCAATCGCA
    B. TCAAAAATCGAATATTTGCTTATCTA
    C. AGTTAAGCATAGAATTTGCCATTCTGTT
    D. CATTGAGATATCGAAATTTGATGAT AATTA
    E. GTATTTATGTATTTTTAGCAACGCAAA

67. A scientist in a clinical molecular genetic laboratory found an old Sanger sequencing film in a storage room (see the figure below). Which one of the following DNA sequences is the correct read of this film?[4]
    A. ACGTTCATGGGCATATTGCCAG
    B. CTGGCAATATGCCCATGAACGT
    C. GACCGTTATACGGGTACTTGCA
    D. TGCAAGTACCCGTATAACGGTC
    E. None of the above

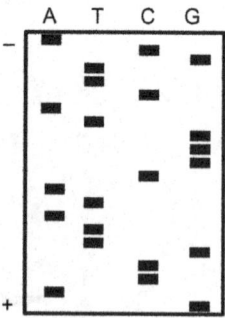

68. A scientist reviews Sanger sequencing results for Gaucher disease in a clinical molecular laboratory. A chromatograph of one of the exons from both directions is shown in figure below. Which nucleotide does the "C" in the middle mutate to?[4]
    A. A
    B. C/A
    C. T
    D. C/T
    E. Not clear

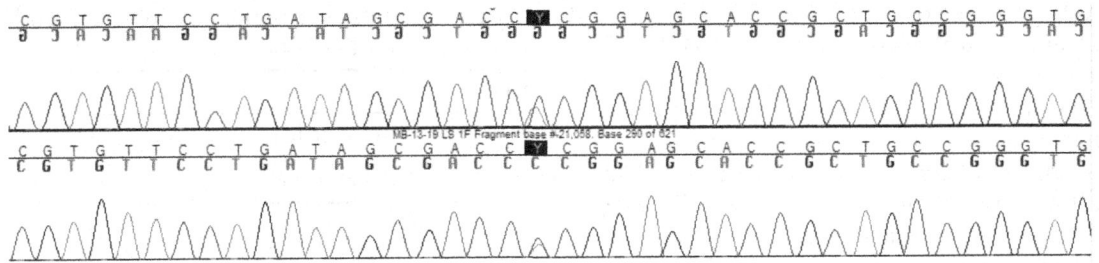

69. A scientist reviews Sanger sequencing results for Gaucher disease in a clinical molecular laboratory. A chromatograph of one of the exons from both directions is shown in figure below. AC in the reference sequence of the cDNA is mutated to a heterozygous T at position 268 in a sample from a patient. Which one of the following variants does the patient NOT have, according to this chromatograph?[4]
A. Silent
B. Missense
C. Nonsense
D. Frameshift
E. Splice site

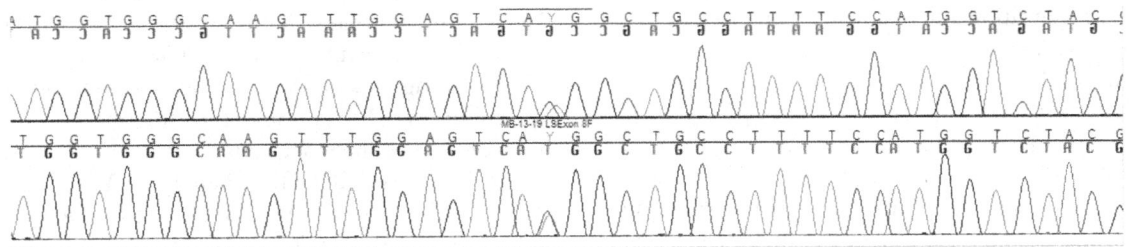

70. A scientist reviews Sanger sequencing results for Tay–Sachs disease in a clinical molecular laboratory. A chromatograph of one of the exons from one direction is shown in the figure below. Which one of the following may explain the results?
A. Nonspecific PCR reaction
B. Indels
C. DNA cross-contamination
D. All of the above
E. None of the above

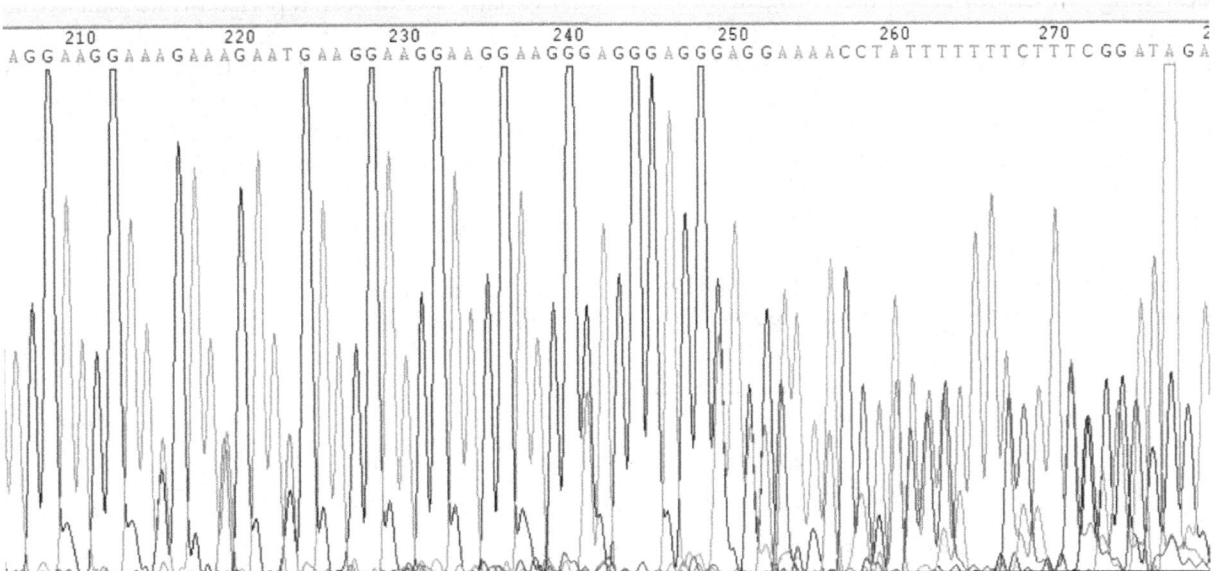

71. Long QT syndrome (LQTS) is a cardiac electrophysiological disorder, characterized by QT prolongation and T-wave abnormalities on the ECG and the ventricular tachycardia torsade de pointes (TdP). In some instances, TdP degenerates to ventricular fibrillation and causes aborted cardiac arrest (if the individual undergoes defibrillation) or sudden death. Approximately 20% of families meeting clinical diagnostic criteria for LQTS do not have detectable pathogenic variants in 1 of the 15 genes associated with LQTS. Approximately 50% of individuals have a pathogenic variant in 1 of the 15 genes. This is an example of:

  A. Allelic heterogeneity
  B. Locus heterogeneity
  C. Pleiotropy
  D. Epistasis
  E. Haplotype

72. Which one of the following sequences is most likely to be a recognition site of a restriction enzyme?

  A. GAAGAA
  B. GAAAAG
  C. GAATTC
  D. GAACTTC
  E. GAACTT

73. A clinical genetic laboratory scientist worked on designing primers for one of the oncogenes. She had a hard time designing the forward primer for exon 3. Which one of the following primers most likely will not work?

  A. 5′ Gc/tCACCACGCTCTTCTGTCT
  B. 5′ GCCACCACg/aCTCTTCTGTCT
  C. 5′ GCCACCACGCTCTTCTGTCt/c
  D. All of the above
  E. None of the above

74. A clinical genetic laboratory scientist worked on designing primers for one of the oncogenes. He had a hard time designing the forward primer for exon 3. Which one of the following primers potentially could be better than others?[4]

  A. 5′ Gc/tCACCACGCTCTTCTGTCT
  B. 5′ GACGGCACACCACACCTCt/c
  C. 5′ AAGGGGGACAGCATCCCCCC
  D. 5′ CCTCGGACGCCCACCCACCGG
  E. 5′ AAAAAAACGACCATTTAT

75. A clinical genetic laboratory scientist worked on designing primers for one of the oncogenes. The potential primer regions in introns 2 and 3 for exon 3 are listed below.

Intron 2	Intron 3
5′ GTACCACGCTCTTCTGTCT …	GAACCGAAGCGTACAGTCGCC
3′ CATGGTGCGAGAAGACAGA …	CTTGGCTTCGCATGTCAGCGG

Which one of the following pairs may be primers for exon 3 of the oncogene?[4]

  A. GTACCACGCTCTTCTGTCT and GAACCGAAGCGTACAGTCGCC
  B. GTACCACGCTCTTCTGTCT and CTTGGCTTCGCATGTCAGCGG
  C. GTACCACGCTCTTCTGTCT and GGCGACTGTACGCTTCGGTTC
  D. CATGGTGCGAGAAGACAGA and GAACCGAAGCGTACAGTCGCC
  E. CATGGTGCGAGAAGACAGA and CTTGGCTTCGCATGTCAGCGG

76. A clinical genetic laboratory scientist worked on designing primers for RT-PCR. She was visually checking candidate sequences. Which one of the following RNAs underlines the reverse complementary sequence?

  A. 5′ CGACGUUGUAAGUUCAAACGACGGCC AGUGUUGUAGUGAACGUCAUGG 3′
  B. 5′ CGACGUUGUAAGUUCAAACGACGGCC AGUGUUGUAGAACGUCAUGG 3′
  C. 5′ CGACGUUGUAAGUUCAAACGACGGCC AGUGUUGUAGAACGUCAUGG 3′
  D. None of the above

77. A reference sequence in the table below is mutated to … cag GGA GCC AAT CTT GCT AGC CCT AGA TTT GGT TCT **t**tt … tag GAC in a Caucasian patient. The gene is an OMIM disease gene, which is related to an autosomal dominant disease. The variant has not been reported in any patients, and it is not found in the parents of the patient. However, in the 1000 Genome Project this variant was found in 10% of the North African population, but not in any other populations. Which one of the following classifications is most appropriate?[11,12]

  A. Benign
  B. Likely benign
  C. Unknown clinical significance
  D. Likely pathogenic
  E. Pathogenic

	Exon 3												Exon 4
	26	27	28	29	30	31	32	33	34	35	36		37
	Gly	Ala	Asn	Leu	Ala	Ser	Pro	Arg	Phe	Gly	Ser		Asp
…cag	GGA	GCC	AAT	CTT	GCT	AGC	CCT	AGA	TTT	GGT	TCT	**g**tt…tag	GAC
	76	79	82	85	88	91	94	97	100	103	106		109

78. There is a 2-bp deletion in the following reference sequence so that the sequence is mutated to ... cag GGA GCC AAT CTT GC**T** **C** CCT AGA TTT GGT TCT gtt ... tag GAC in a Caucasian patient. The gene is an OMIM disease gene, which is related to an autosomal dominant disease. The variant has not been reported in any patients It is found neither in the parents of the patient, nor in general populations. Which one of the following classifications is most appropriate?[11,12]
   A. Benign
   B. Likely benign
   C. Unknown clinical significance
   D. Likely pathogenic
   E. Pathogenic

Exon 3												Exon 4
26	27	28	29	30	31	32	33	34	35	36		37
Gly	Ala	Asn	Leu	Ala	Ser	Pro	Arg	Phe	Gly	Ser		Asp
...cag GGA	GCC	AAT	CTT	GC**T**	**AGC**	CCT	AGA	TTT	GGT	TCT	gtt ... tag	GAC
76	79	82	85	88	91	94	97	100	103	106		109

79. A reference sequence in the table below is the last exon of a gene, which is mutated to ... cag GGA GCC AAT CTT GCT AGC CCT AGA TTT GGT T**G**G gtt gta gca ... in a Caucasian patient. The gene is an OMIM disease, which is related to an autosomal dominant disease gene. The variant has not been reported in any patients. It is found neither in the parents of the patient nor in general populations. Which one of the following most likely describes this variant?
   A. Frameshift mutation
   B. Missense
   C. Nonsense
   D. Splice-site mutation
   E. Nonstop mutation

Exon 11										
111	112	113	114	115	116	117	118	119	120	
Gly	Ala	Asn	Leu	Ala	Ser	Pro	Arg	Phe	Gly	
... cag GGA	GCC	AAT	CTT	GCT	AGC	CCT	AGA	TTT	GGT	TAG	gtt tga gca ...
333	336	339	342	345	348	351	354	357	360	363

80. A reference sequence in the table below is the last exon of a gene, which is mutated to ... cag GGA GCC AAT CTT GCT AGC CCT AGA TTT GGT T**G**G gtt gta gca ... in a Caucasian patient. The gene is an OMIM disease, which is related to an autosomal dominant disease gene. The variant has not been reported in any patients. It is found neither in the parents of the patient nor in the general population. Which one of the following classifications does this variant most likely fit in?[11,12]
   A. Benign
   B. Likely benign
   C. Unknown clinical significance
   D. Likely pathogenic
   E. Pathogenic

Exon 11										
111	112	113	114	115	116	117	118	119	120	
Gly	Ala	Asn	Leu	Ala	Ser	Pro	Arg	Phe	Gly	
... cag GGA	GCC	AAT	CTT	GCT	AGC	CCT	AGA	TTT	GGT	TAG	gtt tga gca ...
333	336	339	342	345	348	351	354	357	360	363

81. A molecular geneticist has been working for a start-up private clinical laboratory for 2 months. He has been validating assays in addition to writing policies for this company. Which chemical would be most appropriate for him to use to prevent nucleic acid samples from degrading during gel electrophoresis?
   A. DNase-free reagents
   B. RNase-free reagents
   C. EDTA in the reagents
   D. Heparin in the reagents
   E. None of the above

82. Which one of the following is NOT a stop codon?
   A. TAA
   B. TAG
   C. TGA
   D. TGG
   E. None of the above

83. Which one of the following codons is NOT a stop codon?
   A. TAA
   B. TAT
   C. TAG
   D. TGA
   E. All of the above
   F. None of the above

84. Which one of the following codons is a stop codon?
   A. TAG
   B. TAT
   C. TTG
   D. TGT

85. Which one of the following codons is a stop codon?
   A. TAC
   B. TAT
   C. TGA
   D. TGT
   E. All of the above
   F. None of the above

86. Which one of the following is the start codon?
   A. ATC
   B. ATG
   C. TAG
   D. TGA
   E. None of the above

87. A reference sequence in the table below is mutated to ... cag ATG GCC AAT CTT GCT AGC CCT AGA TTT GGT TCT ttt ... tag GAC in a Caucasian patient. The gene is an OMIM disease, which is related to an autosomal dominant disease. The variant has not been reported in any patients. It is found neither in the parents of the patient nor in the general population. Which one of the following descriptions of this variant is most accurate?
   A. Frameshift mutation
   B. Missense
   C. Nonsense
   D. Splice-site mutation
   E. Nonstop mutation

Exon 3												Exon 4
26	27	28	29	30	31	32	33	34	35	36		37
Gly	Ala	Asn	Leu	Ala	Ser	Pro	Arg	Phe	Gly	Ser		Asp
... cag	GGA	GCC	AAT	CTT	GCT	AGC	CCT	AGA	TTT	GGT	TCT	gtt ... tag	GAC
	76	79	82	85	88	91	94	97	100	103	106		109

88. A clinical genetics laboratory director plans to validate a high-resolution melting analysis (HSMA) assay for the COL4A5 gene to assist in the diagnosis of Alport syndrome. Which one of the following specimens will most likely show a positive result with this assay?[4]
   A. A peripheral-blood specimen from a mutation-positive patient
   B. A peripheral-blood specimen from a mutation-positive patient mixed with a wild-type control in a 1:1 ratio
   C. A peripheral-blood specimen from a wild-type control
   D. A control specimen without a template
   E. None of the above

89. A genetics counselor meets with a new patient in her clinic. She draws the pedigree for the patient (see the figure below: the arrow indicates the patient). Which one of the following most likely explains why the proband's mother does NOT have symptoms of this disorder?[13]

A. Clinical heterogeneity
B. De novo mutation in the proband
C. Nonpenetrance
D. Variable expression
E. X-inactivation

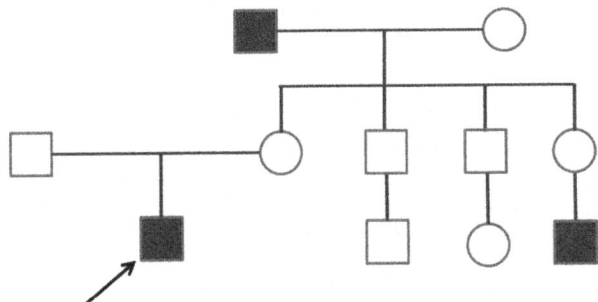

90. A genetics counselor meets with a new patient in her clinic. She draws the pedigree for the patient (see the figure below; the arrow indicates the patient). Which one of the following most likely explains why the proband's mother does NOT have symptoms of this disorder?[13]
A. Clinical heterogeneity
B. De novo mutation in the proband
C. Reduced penetrance
D. Variable expression
E. X inactivation

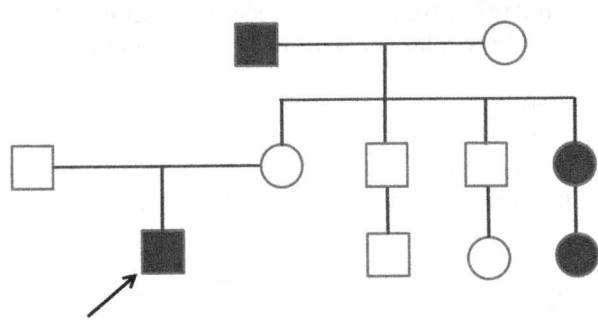

91. A technologist in a clinical molecular genetics laboratory tested a peripheral-blood specimen for BCR-ABL1 with a quantitative assay. Which of the following nucleotides would be extracted from the specimen for the test?
A. cDNA
B. gDNA
C. mRNA
D. tRNA
E. None of the above

92. A technologist in a clinical molecular genetic laboratory tested one specimen for BCR-ABL1 with a quantitative assay after 1:100 dilution. In which direction would the fluorescence curve be shifted if the sample was not diluted?
A. Toward the left
B. Toward the right
C. Upward
D. Downward
E. None of the above

93. A technologist in a clinical molecular genetic laboratory tested five specimens for BCR-ABL1 with a quantitative assay yesterday. The results are shown in the figure below. Which one of the samples has highest concentration of BCR-ABL1?
A. A
B. B
C. C
D. D
E. None of the above

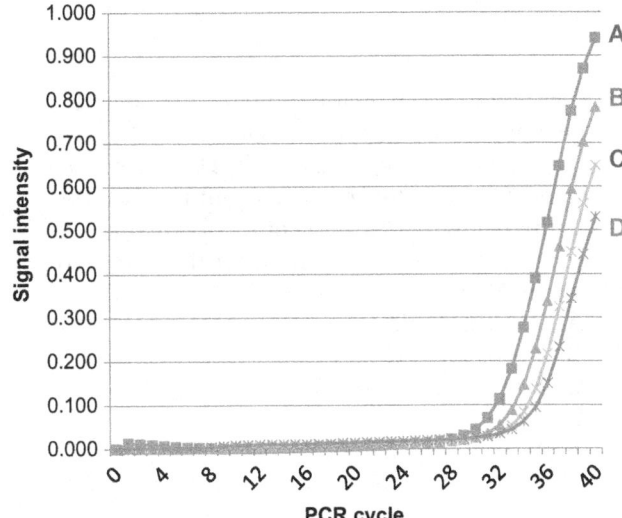

94. A technologist in a clinical molecular genetic laboratory was responsible for BCR-ABL1 quantitative testing this month. She generated a standard curve for the concurrent run. Which panel in the following figure is most likely the right one for the standard curve?[4]
A. A
B. B
C. C
D. D
E. None of the above

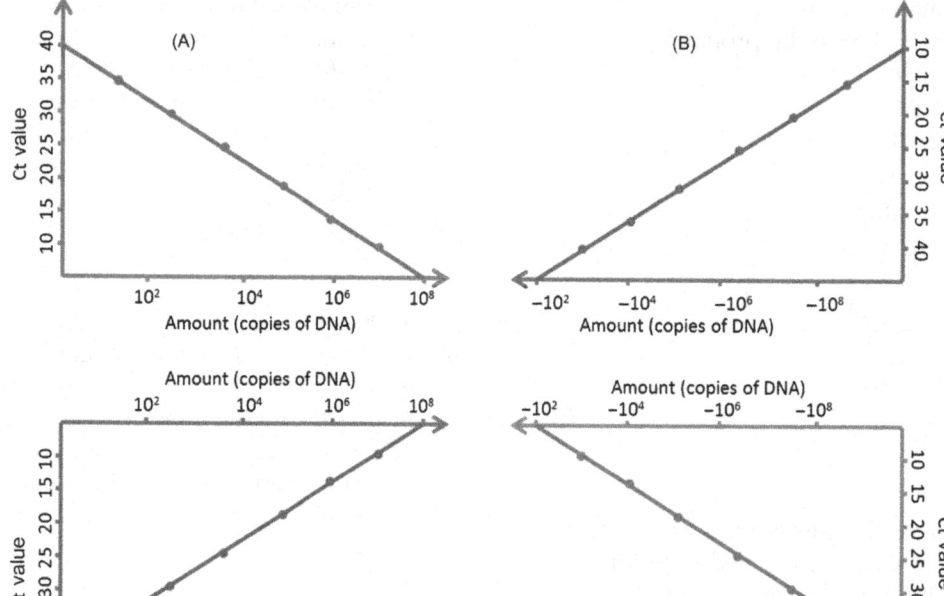

95. A technologist in a clinical molecular genetic laboratory was responsible for *BCR-ABL1* quantitative testing this month. He generated a standard curve for the concurrent run (see the figure below). Which one of the following equations is most likely right for this standard curve?[4]

  A. $Y = 3.32X - 20$
  B. $Y = 3.32X + 20$
  C. $Y = -3.32X - 20$
  D. $Y = -3.32X + 20$
  E. None of the above

96. A technologist in a clinical molecular genetic laboratory was responsible for *BCR-ABL1* quantitative testing this month. She generated standard curves for all 4 weeks (see figure). Which one of the following curves is the most efficient?[4]

  A. A
  B. B
  C. C
  D. D
  E. None of the above

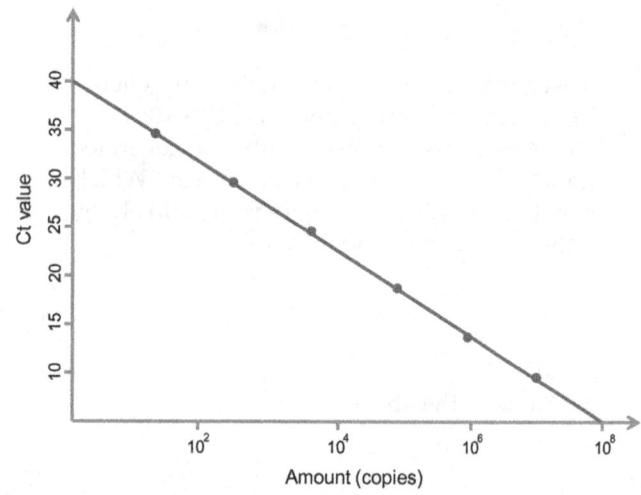

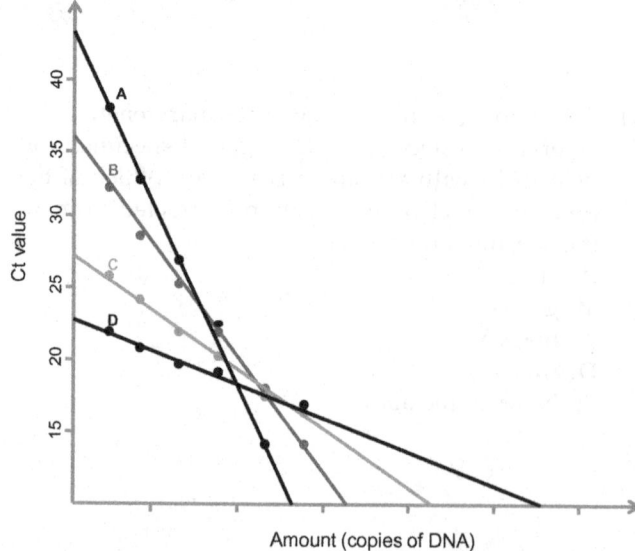

97. A technologist in a clinical molecular genetic laboratory tested five samples for *BCR-ABL1* with a quantitative TaqMan assay yesterday. Which one of the following components in the TaqMan reagents is fluorescence-labeled for signal detection?[4]

    A. Probe(s)

    B. Primer(s)

    C. dNTPs

    D. ddNTPs

    E. None of the above

98. A technologist in a clinical molecular genetic laboratory tested five samples for *BCR-ABL1* with a quantitative TaqMan assay yesterday. Which activity of Taq polymerase does the TaqMan assay use to release the fluorescence signal from the quencher?[4]

    A. $3'-5'$ endonuclease

    B. $5'-3'$ endonuclease

    C. Taq A overhang

    D. $3'-5'$ exonuclease

    E. $5'-3'$ exonuclease

99. A scientist in a clinical molecular genetic laboratory worked on developing an assay for the *BRAF* V600E (c.1799T > A) variant. She planned to use a TaqMan SNP genotyping assay for V600E developed by Applied Biosystems (ABI). She purchased three positive control samples for the validation. They were homozygous c.1799T > A (V600E), heterozygous c.1799T > A (V600E), and heterozygous c.1798_1799GT > AA (V600K). Which one of the following genotyping results would be for one of the positive controls, heterozygous 1798_1799GT > AA(V600K), with this TaqMan assay?[4]

    A. Homozygous, wild-type

    B. Homozygous, V600E

    C. Homozygous, V600K

    D. Heterozygous, V600K

    E. None of the above

100. BJ came to a genetics clinic because both his mother and maternal grandfather have a late-onset autosomal dominant disease. The deleterious variant was not identified in the family by sequencing all exons and 40-bp introns at the intron–exon boundary in the causative gene. A tetranucleotide repeat in the intron 2 of the gene was tested in all the family members shown in figure below. Four alleles of the tetranucleotide repeat were identified in the family. Which one of the following statements is most appropriate?

    A. BJ is at a decreased risk for the disease.

    B. BJ is at an increased risk for the disease.

    C. BJ will not have the disease, but his maternal aunt will have it.

    D. It is hard to determine.

    E. This result indicates nonpaternity/maternity issues.

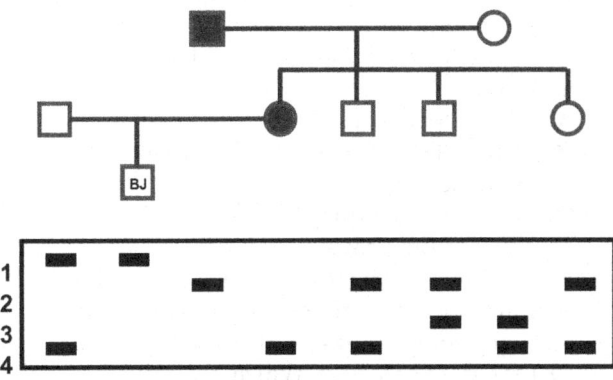

101. BJ came to a genetics clinic because both his mother and maternal grandfather have a late-onset autosomal dominant disease. The deleterious variant was not identified in the family by sequencing all exons and 40-bp introns at the intron–exon boundary in the causative gene. A tetranucleotide repeat in the intron 2 of the gene was tested in all the family members (see figure below). Four alleles of the tetranucleotide repeat were identified in the family. Which one of the following genotypes does BJ most likely have for this tetranucleotide repeat?

    A. 1/1

    B. 1/deletion

    C. 1/2

    D. 1/3

    E. 1/4

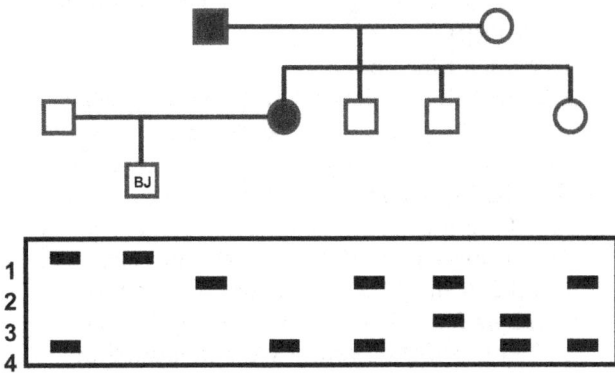

102. A four-generation family has three members with a late-onset autosomal dominant disease. The disease-causing mutation was not identified in this family by sequencing all exons and 40-bp introns at the boundary of exons of the gene. A tetranucleotide repeat in the intron 2 of the gene was tested in all the family members for linkage analysis. Which one of the following assays would be most commonly used for microsatellite analysis in clinical laboratories nowadays?
    A. Allelic-specific PCR
    B. PCR and fluorescence capillary electrophoresis
    C. PCR and RFLP
    D. TaqMan genotyping assay
    E. None of the above

103. A principle investigator proposed to conduct a genomewide association study (GWAS) on coronary artery disease with 10,000 cases and 10,000 controls in 2013. Which one of the following genetic markers would be the most appropriate for this study?[14]
    A. RFLPs
    B. SNPs
    C. STRs
    D. VNTRs
    E. None of the above

104. A laboratory core facility in an academic institute offers genome-wide association studies to principal investigators. Which one of the following would be more appropriate for GWAS studies than the others?[14]
    A. Identifying causative gene(s) for Smith—Magenis syndrome
    B. Identifying causative gene(s)/mutation(s) for Crohn disease
    C. Identifying causative mutation(s) for autosomal recessive hearing loss in a pedigree
    D. Identifying causative mutation(s) for myoclonic epilepsy with ragged red fibers (MERRF)
    E. None of the above

105. All four children of a healthy couple have an autosomal recessive disease (see the figure below). The deleterious variant was not identified in the family by sequencing all exons and 40-bp introns at the intron—exon boundary in the causative gene. A tetranucleotide repeat in intron 2 of the gene was tested in all family members for linkage analysis. Four alleles of the tetranucleotide repeat were identified in the family. Which one of the following ratios most likely represents the odds that the tetranucleotide repeat is not in linkage with the disease gene?[4]

A. 1:16
B. 1:32
C. 1:64
D. 1:128
E. 1:256

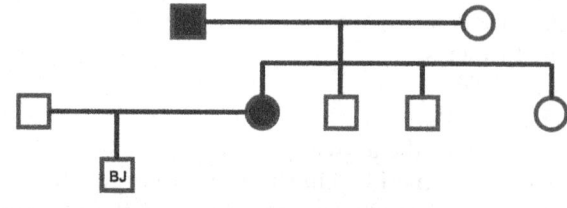

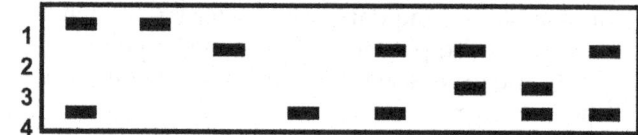

106. All three children of a healthy couple have an autosomal recessive disease (see the figure below). The deleterious variant was not identified in the family by sequencing all exons and 40-bp introns at the intron—exon boundary in the causative gene. A tetranucleotide repeat in intron 2 of the gene was tested in all family members for linkage analysis. Four alleles of the tetranucleotide repeat were identified in the family. Which one of the following ratios most likely represents the odds that the tetranucleotide repeat is not in linkage with the disease gene?[4]
    A. 1:16
    B. 1:32
    C. 1:64
    D. 1:128
    E. 1:256

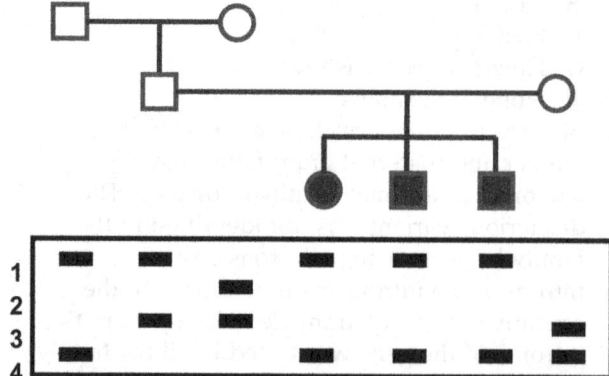

107. Age-related macular degeneration (AMD) with both genetic and environmental influences is the leading cause of severe and irreversible vision loss in the Western world. There is no effective treatment for all types of AMD. There is evidence

that smoking is a risk factor for AMD. Which one of the following genetic terms is the best to describe this phenomenon?[4,13]

A. Variable expression
B. Genetic heterogeneity
C. Pleiotropy
D. Incomplete penetrance
E. Dominant-negative

108. Age-related macular degeneration (AMD) is a late-onset complex disease with both genetic and environmental influences. It is a deterioration or breakdown of the eye's macula, which may result in blurred or no vision in the center of the visual field. There is no effective treatment for all types of AMD. A researcher studied the effect of smoking to AMD (see the table below). Which one of the following options is most likely odds that AMD is associated with smoking status?[15]

A. 1.29
B. 3
C. 3.86
D. 7
E. 9

	AMD patient	Healthy individual
Smoker	30	70
Nonsmoker	10	90

109. Age-related macular degeneration (AMD) is a late-onset complex disease with both genetic and environmental influences. It is a deterioration or breakdown of the eye's macula, which may result in blurred or no vision in the center of the visual field. There is no effective treatment for all types of AMD. A researcher studied the effect of smoking to AMD (see the table below). Which one of the following options most likely is the relative risk for AMD with smoking status?[16]

A. 1.29
B. 3
C. 3.86
D. 7
E. 9

	AMD patient	Healthy individual
Smoker	30	70
Nonsmoker	10	90

110. Osteogenesis imperfecta (OI) is caused by pathogenic variants in either the COL1A1 or COL1A2 gene that encodes the chains of type I procollagen. Fibrillar collagens are the major structural proteins of connective tissue, which are

used to build triple helices of preprocollagen. The triple helices of preprocollagen, sometimes homotrimers or heterotrimers, are assembled into closely packed cross-linked arrays to form rigid fibrils. The mutant collagen polypeptides caused by pathogenic variants in the COL1A1 or COL1A2 genes associate with normal chains, which disrupt the formation of the triple helix. This can reduce the yield of functional collagen to below 50%. Which one of the following describes the phenomenon?[13]

A. Dominant-negative variable expression
B. Genetic heterogeneity
C. Incomplete penetrance
D. Pleiotropy
E. Variable expression

111. Charcot–Marie–Tooth (CMT) disease is a group of progressive disorders that affect the peripheral nerves and result in loss of sensation and wasting (atrophy) of muscles in the feet, legs, and hands. There are several types of CMT disease. Within the various types of CMT disease, subtypes such as CMT1A, CMT1B, CMT2A, CMT4A, and CMTX1 are distinguished by the specific gene that is altered. Which one of the following describes this phenomenon in a genetic term?[13]

A. Dominant-negative
B. Genetic heterogeneity
C. Incomplete penetrance
D. Pleiotropy
E. Variable expression

112. CHARGE syndrome is an autosomal dominant condition with multiple congenital malformations caused by pathogenic variants in the CHD7 gene in the majority of individuals tested. The acronym CHARGE stands for coloboma, heart defects, atresia of the choanae, retardation of growth and development, genital abnormalities, and ear anomalies. The CHD7 gene is ubiquitously expressed in many fetal and adult tissues. Haploinsufficiency of the CHD7 gene leads all the symptoms in different organs and systems for CHARGE. Which one of the following describes this phenomenon in a genetic term?[13]

A. Dominant-negative
B. Genetic heterogeneity
C. Incomplete penetrance
D. Pleiotropy
E. Variable expression

113. Wiskott–Aldrich syndrome (WAS) is an X-linked disorder with immunodeficiency and a reduced ability to form blood clots. A scientist developed a Sanger sequencing assay for WAS in a start-up private clinical molecular genetic laboratory. In

the report templates, he wrote the limitations of this assay. Which one of the following is NOT one of the limitations of Sanger sequencing?[4]
  A. Large deletion/duplication
  B. Nonsense mutation
  C. Polymononucleotide stretches in the amplicon
  D. Polymorphism in the primer region
  E. Tissue mosaicism

114. Hypertrophic cardiomyopathy (HCM) is one of the most common monogenic autosomal dominant cardiovascular diseases. It often goes undiagnosed because many people with the disease have few, if any, symptoms and can lead normal lives with no significant problems. However, in a small number of people with HCM, the thickened heart muscle can cause shortness of breath, chest pain, or problems in the heart's electrical system, resulting in life-threatening arrhythmias. HCM is caused by

pathogenic variants in approximately 20 genes encoding proteins of the cardiac sarcomere. Which one of the following describes this genetic phenomenon most accurately?[13]
  A. Allelic heterogeneity
  B. Genetic heterogeneity
  C. Incomplete penetrance
  D. Locus heterogeneity
  E. Variable expression

115. A physician referred BJ (the arrow points to him in the pedigree below) to a genetics clinic to rule out a genetic etiology for hearing loss. Which one of the following types of genetic diseases may BJ have, based on the pedigree?[13]
  A. Autosomal dominant
  B. Autosomal recessive
  C. X-linked dominant
  D. X-linked recessive
  E. Mitochondrial inherited

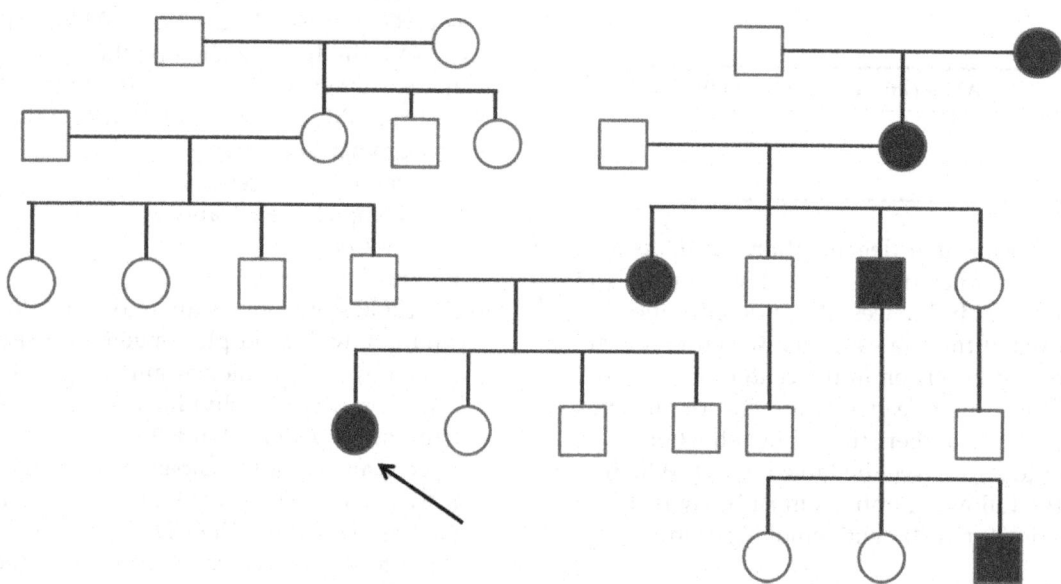

116. A physician referred BJ (the arrow points to him in the pedigree below) to a genetics clinic to rule out a genetic etiology for hearing loss. Which one of the following types of genetic diseases may BJ have, based on the pedigree?[13]

  A. Autosomal dominant
  B. Autosomal recessive
  C. X-linked dominant
  D. X-linked recessive
  E. Mitochondrial inherited

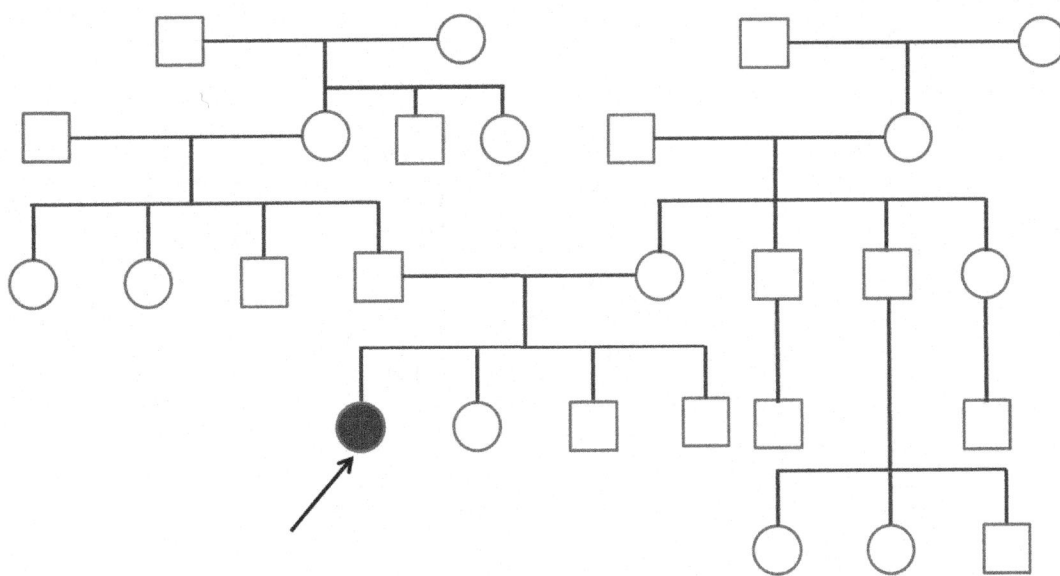

117. A physician referred BJ (the arrow points to him in the pedigree below) to a genetics clinic to rule out a genetic etiology for hearing loss. Which one of the following types of genetic diseases may BJ have, based on the pedigree?[13]

    A. Autosomal dominant
    B. Autosomal recessive
    C. X-linked dominant
    D. X-linked recessive
    E. Mitochondrial inherited

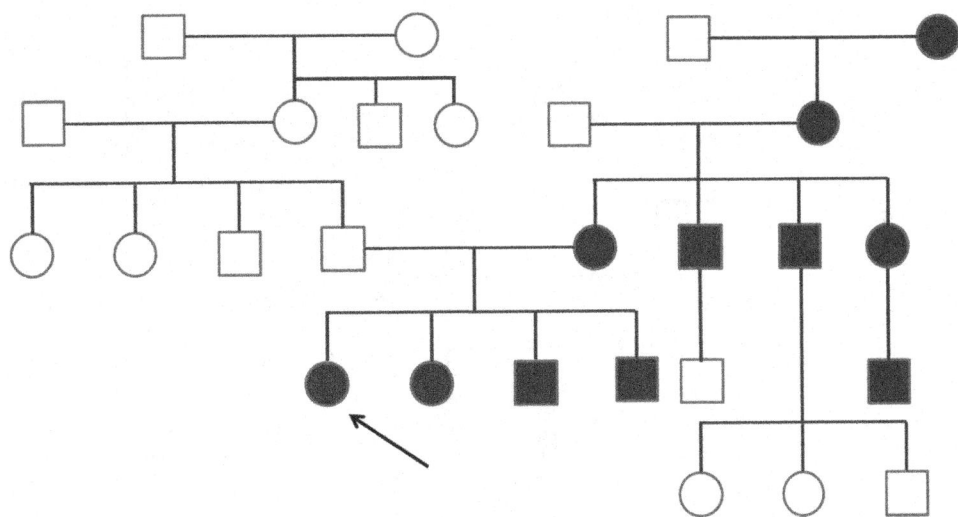

118. A physician referred BJ (the arrow points to him in the pedigree in figure below) to a genetics clinic to rule out a genetic etiology for hearing loss. Which one of the following types of genetic diseases may BJ have, based on the pedigree?

    A. Autosomal dominant
    B. Autosomal recessive
    C. X-linked dominant
    D. X-linked recessive
    E. Mitochondrial inherited

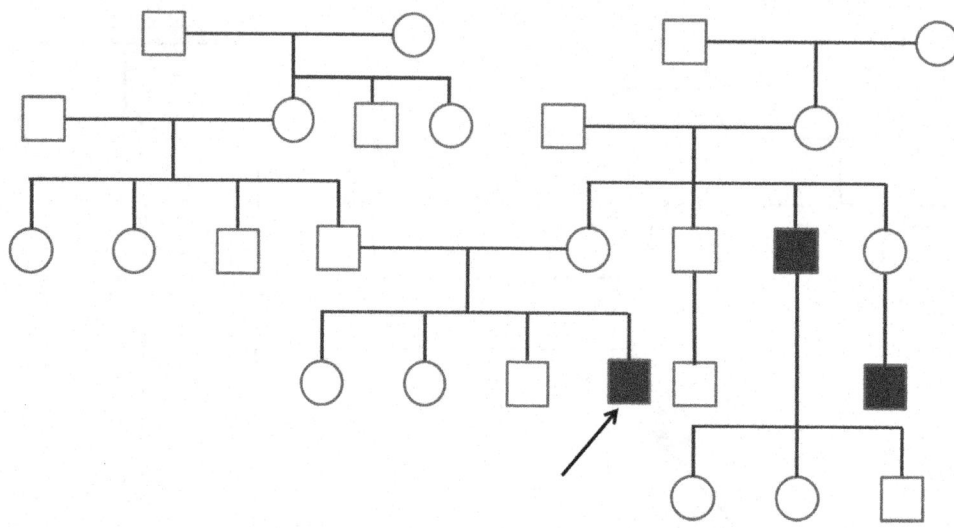

119. A physician referred BJ (the arrow points to him in the pedigree in figure below) to a genetics clinic to rule out a genetic etiology for hearing loss. Which one of the following types of genetic diseases may BJ have, based on the pedigree?[13]

    A. Autosomal dominant
    B. Autosomal recessive
    C. X-linked dominant
    D. X-linked recessive
    E. Mitochondrial inherited

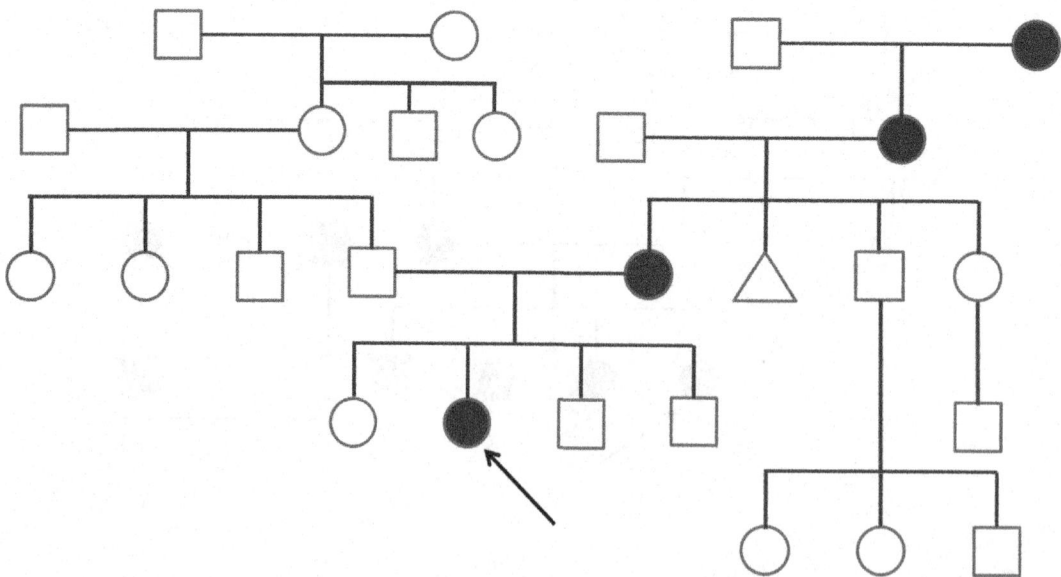

120. BJ (the arrow points to him in the pedigree in figure below) came to a genetics clinic because he had a family history of a disease. Which one of the following types of genetic diseases may BJ have, based on the pedigree?[13]

    A. Autosomal dominant
    B. Autosomal recessive
    C. X-linked dominant
    D. X-linked recessive
    E. Mitochondrial inherited

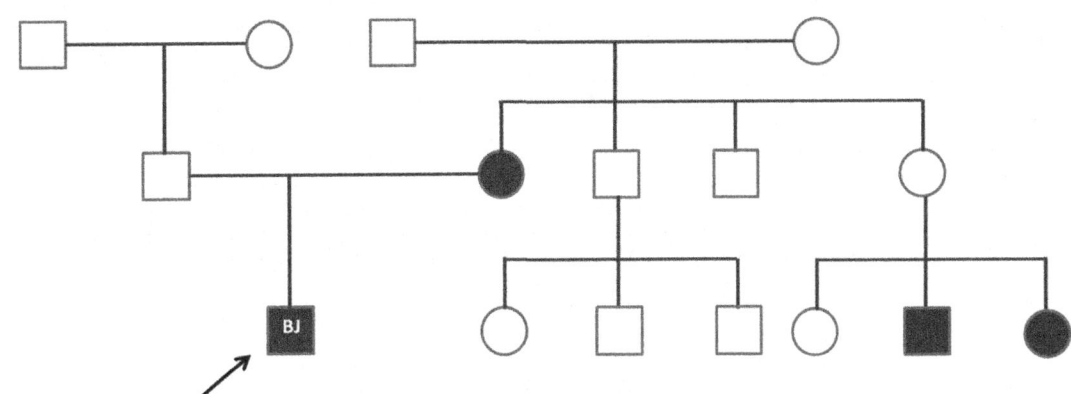

121. BJ (the arrow points to her in the pedigree in figure below) was a 2-day-old girl in a neonatal intensive-care unit (NICU) for severe hypotonia. A medical geneticist was called for consultation. Which one of the following genetic diseases does BJ most likely have?[13]

A. Achondroplasia
B. Fragile X syndrome
C. Krabbe disease
D. Mitochondrial encephalomyopathy, lactic acidosis, and stroke-like episodes (MELAS)
E. Prader–Willi syndrome
F. X-linked adrenoleukodystrophy

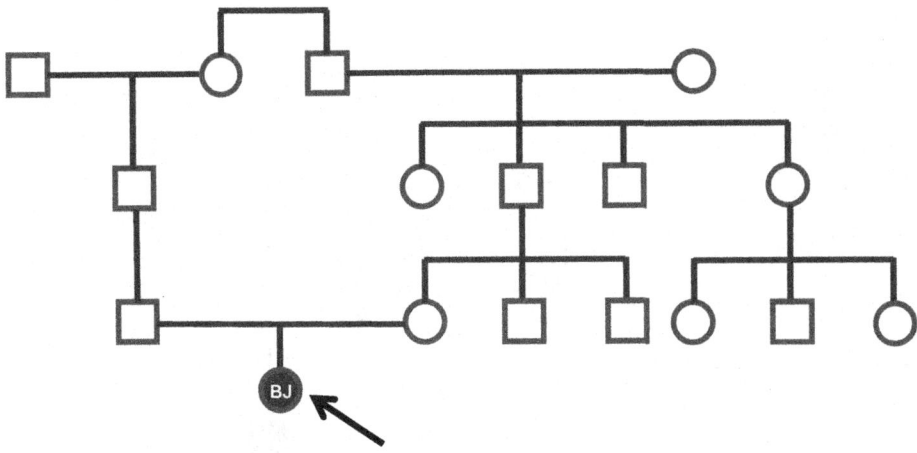

122. BJ (the arrow points to her in the pedigree below) was a 2-day-old girl in a neonatal intensive-care unit (NICU) for severe hypotonia. A medical geneticist was called for consultation. Which one of the following genetic disorders does BJ most likely have?[13]

A. Achondroplasia
B. Fragile X syndrome
C. Krabbe disease
D. Mitochondrial Encephalomyopathy Lactic Acidosis and Stroke like Episodes (MELAS)
E. Prader–Willi syndrome
F. X-linked adrenoleukodystrophy

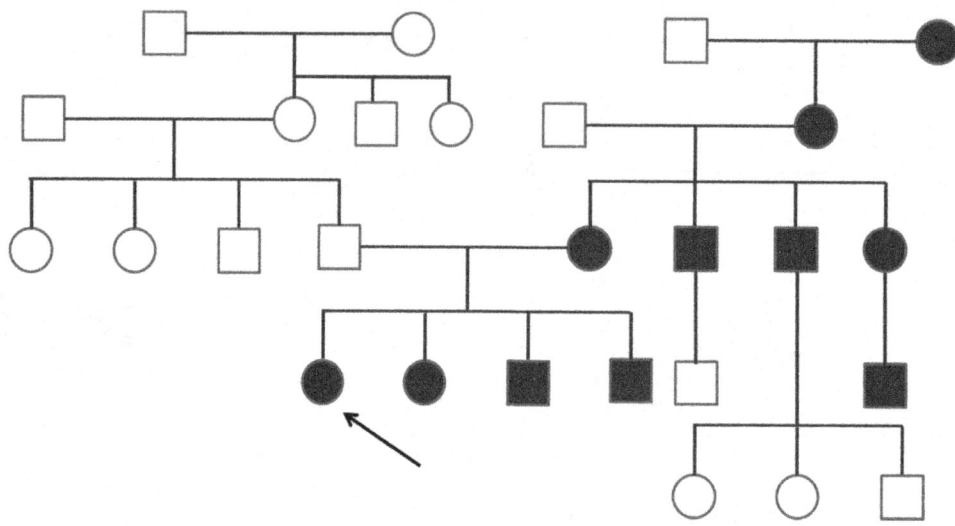

123. BJ (the arrow points to her in the pedigree below) was a 2-day-old girl in a neonatal intensive-care unit (NICU) for severe hypotonia. A medical geneticist was called for consultation. Which one of the following genetic diseases does BJ most likely have?[13]

  A. Achondroplasia

  B. Fragile X syndrome
  C. Krabbe disease
  D. Mitochondrial Encephalomyopathy Lactic Acidosis and Stroke like Episodes (MELAS)
  E. Prader–Willi syndrome
  F. X-linked adrenoleukodystrophy

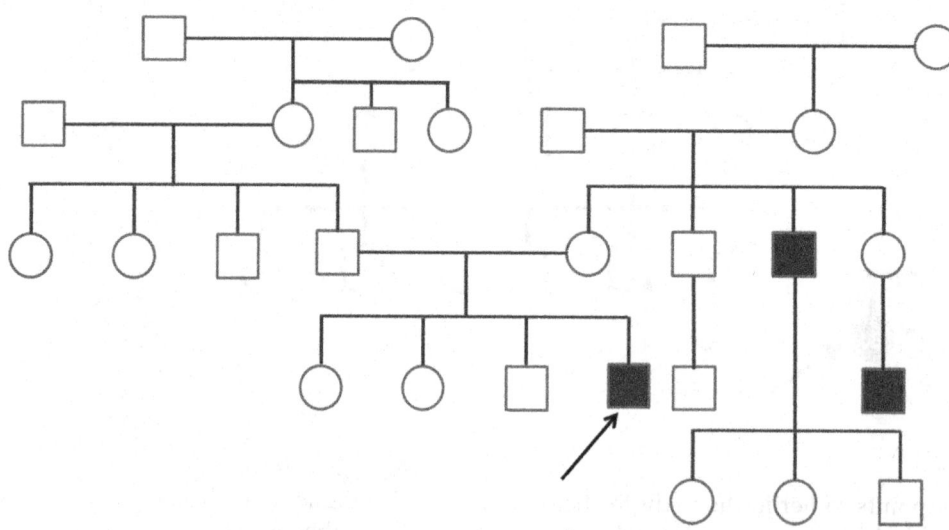

124. An 18-year-old male, BJ, was referred to a genetics clinic for myoclonic epilepsy. His family history was remarkable for his mother and two cousins with similar symptoms. Physical examination showed that he had generalized muscle wasting and weakness, myoclonus, and ataxia. Results of a muscle biopsy identified abnormal mitochondria and ragged-red fibers.

Which one of the following explains why the maternal aunt does not have symptoms of the disease?[13]

  A. Allelic heterogeneity
  B. Locus heterogeneity
  C. Heteroplasmy
  D. Variable expression
  E. Incomplete penetrance

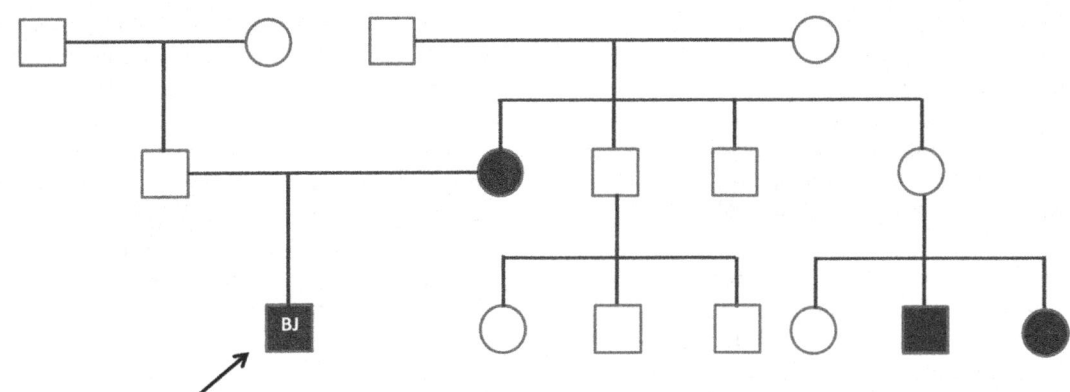

125. An 18-year-old male, BJ, was referred to a genetics clinic for mitochondrial myoclonic epilepsy. Which one of the following descriptions regarding mtDNA is NOT correct?[13]
  A. Each cell contains multiple mitochondria.
  B. Each mitochondrion contains multiple mtDNAs.
  C. The proportion of mutant mtDNA can be variable throughout a person's life.
  D. The risk to children of affected males is 0%.
  E. The risk to children of affected females is 50%.
  F. The mutation rate of mtDNA is 10-fold higher than nuclear DNA.

126. An 18-year-old male, BJ, was referred to a genetics clinic for mitochondrial myoclonic epilepsy. Which one of the following descriptions regarding mtDNA is correct?[13]
  A. Each cell has one mitochondrion.
  B. Each mitochondrion has one copy of a mitochondrial genome.
  C. Mitochondrial genomes encode all the genes for the electron transport chain.
  D. Mitochondrial genomes are protected by histones.
  E. There are no introns in the mitochondrial genome.
  F. None of the above.

127. Susceptibility to coronary artery disease (CAD) is claimed to be 40%–60% inherited, but until recently, genetic risk factors predisposing to CAD have been elusive. A principal investigator uses linkage analysis to study CAD. LOD scores (Z) of a polymorphism on 15q were analyzed. The data from five families are shown below, where $\theta = 0.05$:

Family	1	2	3	4	5
Z	1.41	0.51	−0.69	1.12	−0.21

Which one of the following is the LOD score of the five families together?[4]
  A. 0.12
  B. 2.14
  C. 3.94
  D. 3.04
  E. None of the above

128. Susceptibility to coronary artery disease (CAD) is claimed to be 40%–60% inherited, but until recently genetic risk factors predisposing to CAD have been elusive. A principle investigator uses linkage analysis to study for CAD. LOD scores (Z) of a polymorphism on 15q are shown in the following table:

θ	0.00	0.01	0.05	0.10	0.15	0.20	0.25
Z	−∞	5	6	4.2	3	2.1	1.5

What is the genetic distance between the marker and the disease at the peak LOD?[4]
  A. 5 cM
  B. 0.5 M
  C. 0.5 cM
  D. 0.05 cM
  E. None of the above

129. Pathogenic variants in the *BRCA1* and *BRCA2* genes may account for 5%–10% of all breast cancers. Most people who develop breast cancer have no family history of the disease. A principal investigator used linkage analysis to study a four-generation family for *BRCA1*- and *BRCA2*-negative breast cancers. A SNP was found to have an odds ratio of 10,000 favoring linkage. What would be the LOD score of this SNP marker?[4]
  A. 2
  B. 3
  C. 4
  D. 1000

E. 10,000

F. 100,000

G. None of the above

130. An 18-year-old male, BJ, was referred to a genetics clinic for mitochondrial myoclonic epilepsy. Which one of the following characteristics does mitochondrial DNA NOT have?

A. Heteroplasmy describes a mixture of mutant and normal mtDNA in one sample.

B. The mitochondrial genome is much smaller than the nuclear genome.

C. Sperm usually don't carry mitochondrial genomes.

D. The mutation rate of the mitochondrial genome is 10-fold greater than that of the nuclear genome.

E. There are multiple copies of mitochondrial genomes in one cell.

F. None of the above.

131. A certain molecular screening test can identify 90% of those with a disease and 20% of those without the disease. The frequency of the disease is 1/100 in a population. What is the positive predictive value of the test in this population?

A. <5%

B. 12%

C. 83%

D. 99%

E. None of the above

132. A certain molecular screening test can identify 80% of those with a disease and 30% of those without the disease. The frequency of the disease is 1/100 in a population. What is the negative predictive value of the test in this population?

A. <5%

B. 12%

C. 78%

D. 99%

E. None of the above

133. Prader–Willi and Angelman syndromes are two clinically distinct disorders associated with multiple anomalies and mental retardation. They involve genes that are located in the same region in the genome and are characterized by genetic imprinting. A laboratory scientist plans to develop an assay for Prader–Willi/Angelman syndromes. Which one of the following epigenetic mechanisms is altered in patients with Prader–Willi/Angelman syndromes?[13]

A. Histone modification

B. Methylation

C. miRNA

D. siRNA

E. None of the above

134. Prader–Willi and Angelman syndromes are two clinically distinct disorders associated with multiple anomalies and mental retardation. They involve genes that are located in the same region in the genome and are characterized by genetic imprinting. A laboratory scientist plans to develop a methylation assay for Prader–Willi/Angelman syndromes. Which region in the human genome usually is the target for a methylation study?[4]

A. Promoter

B. Exon

C. Intron

D. 5′ UTR

E. 3′ UTR

135. Prader–Willi and Angelman syndromes are two clinically distinct disorders associated with multiple anomalies and mental retardation. They involve genes that are located in the same region in the genome and are characterized by genetic imprinting. A laboratory scientist plans to develop a methylation assay for Prader–Willi/Angelman syndromes. For what location should he design the primer?[13]

A. Promoter region of NIPA1

B. Promoter region of NIPA2

C. Promoter region of SNRPN

D. Promoter region of UBE3A

E. None of the above

136. Prader–Willi and Angelman syndromes are two clinically distinct disorders associated with multiple anomalies and mental retardation. They involve genes that are located in the same region in the genome and are characterized by genetic imprinting. A laboratory scientist plans to develop a methylation assay for Prader–Willi/Angelman syndromes. Which one of the following statements regarding methylation study is NOT correct?[4]

A. Methylated C residues spontaneously deaminate to form T residues over time.

B. Methylation means covalently adding −CH3 at the 5′ end of the cytosine ring by methyltransferases.

C. Methylation study may be used to analyze X-chromosome inactivation.

D. Methylation usually happens in the noncoding regions of the genome.

E. Treatment of DNA with sodium bisulfite converts methylcytosine residues to uracil.

137. Which one of the following epigenetic modifications would increase expression of a gene?[4]

A. Methylation of cytosine bases 5′ to the gene

B. Histone acetylation close to the gene

C. MicroRNAs complementary to the gene transcript

D. siRNAs complementary to the gene transcript

E. None of the above

138. Prader—Willi syndrome (PWS) and Angelman syndrome (AS) are clinically distinct neurodevelopmental genetic disorders that map to 15q11-q13. The primary phenotypes are attributable to loss of expression of imprinted genes within this region, which can arise by means of a number of mechanisms. The most sensitive single approach to diagnosing both PWS and AS is to study methylation patterns within 15q11-q13. A laboratory scientist plans to develop a methylation assay for Prader—Willi/Angelman syndromes. Which one of the following statements regarding methylation study with sodium bisulfite is correct?[4]

A. It converts C to T.

B. It converts C to A.

C. It converts C to G.

D. It converts C to U.

E. None of the above.

139. A laboratory scientist plans to develop a methylation assay for Prader—Willi/Angelman syndromes. Which one of the following statements regarding bisulfite treatment for methylation study is correct?[4,13]

A. Bisulfite converts an unmethylated cytosine to uracil in mRNA.

B. Bisulfite converts a methylated cytosine to uracil in mRNA.

C. Bisulfite converts an unmethylated cytosine to uracil in DNA.

D. Bisulfite converts a methylated cytosine to uracil in DNA.

E. None of the above.

140. A laboratory scientist plans to develop a methylation assay for Prader—Willi/Angelman syndromes. Which one of the following contributes to the technical difficulties of sodium bisulfite—mediated methylation study?[4]

A. 5-Hydroxymethylcytosine

B. Degradation of DNA during bisulfite treatment

C. Incomplete conversion

D. Fragmentation

E. All of the above

141. A laboratory scientist plans to develop a methylation assay for Prader—Willi/Angelman syndromes. Which one of the following methods may NOT be used as a downstream method for sodium bisulfite—mediated methylation study?

A. Bisulfite-specific PCR (BSP)

B. Chromosome microarray

C. High-resolution melting analysis

D. Methylation-specific restriction digestion

E. Pyrosequencing

F. Sanger sequencing

142. In glioblastoma, the most malignant intrinsic brain tumor entity in adults, the promoter methylation status of the gene encoding for the repair enzyme O^6-methylguanine-DNA methyltransferase (MGMT) indicates increased efficacy of current standard of care, which is concomitant and adjuvant chemoradiotherapy with the alkylating agent temozolomide. In the elderly, MGMT promoter methylation status has recently been introduced to be a predictive biomarker that can be used for stratification of treatment regimens. A laboratory scientist planned to develop a methylation assay for MGMT to guide the treatment for glioblastoma. If the unmethylated DNA sequence is 5′ TCT CGA CGT TCG TAG GTC CTC GCG CAC TCC TCC GAA AAC GAA ACG, which would the methylated sequence be after sodium bisulfite treatment?[4,13]

A. 5′ TCT CGA CGT TCG TAG GTC CTC GCG CAC TCC TCC GAA AAC GAA ACG

B. 5′ TCT TGA TGT TTG TAG GTC CTT GTG CAC TCC TCC GAA AAT GAA ATG

C. 5′ TTT TGA TGT TTG TAG GTT TTT GTG TAT TTT TTT GAA AAT GAA ATG

D. 5′ TTT CGA CGT TCG TAG GTT TTC GCG TAT TTT TTC GAA AAT GAA ACG

E. None of the above

143. A laboratory scientist planned to develop a methylation assay for MGMT to guide the treatment for glioblastoma. If the unmethylated DNA sequence is 5′ TCT CGA CGT TCG TAG GTC CTC GCG CAC TCC TCC GAA AAC GAA ACG, which would the unmethylated sequence be after sodium bisulfite treatment?[4,13]

A. 5′ TCT CGA CGT TCG TAG GTC CTC GCG CAC TCC TCC GAA AAC GAA ACG

B. 5′ TCT TGA TGT TTG TAG GTC CTT GTG CAC TCC TCC GAA AAT GAA ATG

C. 5′ TTT TGA TGT TTG TAG GTT TTT GTG TAT TTT TTT GAA AAT GAA ATG

D. 5′ TTT CGA CGT TCG TAG GTT TTC GCG TAT TTT TTC GAA AAT GAA ACG

E. None of the above

144. A laboratory scientist planned to develop a methylation assay for Prader—Willi/Angelman syndromes. The untreated DNA sequence is 5′ tgcgcggccgcagaggcaggctggcgcg. After sodium bisulfite treatment, which one of the following could be the primer for the methylated allele?[4,13]

A. 5′ cacaccaacctacctctacaaccacaca

B. 5′ cgcgccaacctacctctacgaccgcgca

C. 5′ agcgcggccgcagaggcaggcaggcgcg

D. 5′ tgcgcggtcgtagaggtaggttggcgcg

E. 5′ tgtgtggttgtagaggtaggttggtgtg

F. None of the above

145. A laboratory scientist planned to develop a methylation assay for Prader–Willi/Angelman syndromes. The untreated DNA sequence is 5′ tgcgcggccgcagaggcaggctggcgcg. After sodium bisulfite treatment, which one of the following could be the primer for the unmethylated allele?

 A. 5′ cacaccaacctacctctacaaccacaca

 B. 5′ cgcgccaacctacctctacgaccgcgca

 C. 5′ tgcgcggtcgtagaggtaggttggcgcg

 D. 5′ tgtgtggttgtagaggtaggttggtgtg

 E. 5′ tgcgcggccgctgtggctggctggcgcg

 F. None of the above

146. A pathologist requested *MGMT* methylation study for an formalin-fixed, paraffin-embedded (FFPE) specimen. On the requisition, the indication for the test was glioblastoma. Pyrosequencing was the method for *MGMT* methylation study in this clinical molecular laboratory. Which one of the following reagents is fluorescently labeled in pyrosequencing reaction?[4]

 A. One of the primers

 B. dNTP

 C. ddNTP

 D. Any one of above

 E. None of the above

147. Which one of the sequencing reactions is NOT based on the "sequencing by synthesis" principle?[4]

 A. Illumina genomic DNA sequencing

 B. Pyrosequencing

 C. Roche 454 sequencing

 D. Sanger sequencing

 E. None of the above

148. A pathologist requested *MGMT* methylation study for an formalin-fixed, paraffin-embedded (FFPE) specimen. On the requisition, the indication for the test was glioblastoma. Pyrosequencing was the method for *MGMT* methylation study in this clinical molecular laboratory. Which one of the following pyrosequencing results is correct, according to the figure below?[4]

 A. GCAGCT

 B. GCAGGCCT

 C. GCTAGCT

 D. GCTAGGCCT

 E. None of the above

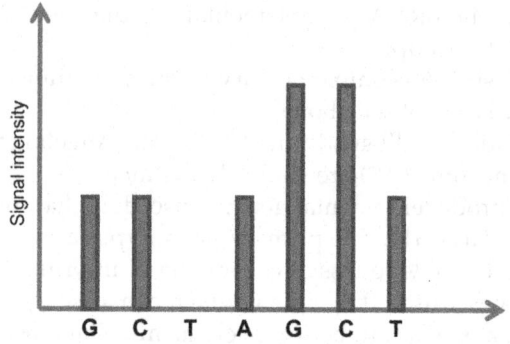

149. Fragile X syndrome is characterized by a range of developmental problems, including learning disabilities and cognitive impairment resulting from pathogenic variants in the *FMR1* gene on chromosome X. Usually, males are more severely affected by this disorder than females. A technologist runs fragile X testing with PCR and Southern blot techniques in a clinical molecular genetic laboratory. The most appropriate order for Southern blotting is:[4]

 1 = Denaturing the fragments

 2 = Developing the film

 3 = Digesting the DNA sample

 4 = Performing gel electrophoresis

 5 = Hybridizing with the DNA probe(s)

 6 = Transferring to a nitrocellulose membrane

 A. 1, 2, 3, 4, 5, 6

 B. 1, 2, 3, 5, 6, 4

 C. 3, 4, 1, 6, 5, 2

 D. 3, 4, 6, 1, 5, 2

 E. None of the above

150. A technologist works on fragile X testing with PCR and Southern blotting in a clinical molecular genetic laboratory. Which one of the following is NOT an advantage of Southern blotting over PCR?[17]

 A. It can be used as a technique for forensic "DNA fingerprints."

 B. It effectively detects a nonamplifiable sequencing, such as a high GC region including CGG repeats.

 C. It effectively detects a specific long DNA sequence.

 D. It is cheaper than PCR.

 E. None of the above.

151. Carriers of sickle cell anemia have greater resistance to *Plasmodium falciparum* malaria than individuals who have two normal copies of the beta-globin gene. When a carrier's red blood cells are invaded by the malaria parasite, the cells sickle and are destroyed. In these populations,

Hardy—Weinberg equilibrium is disturbed for the beta-globin gene because of sickle cell anemia. This disturbance of genetic inheritance in populations is referred to as:

A. Genetic drift
B. Heterozygote advantage
C. Negative selection
D. Phenocopy
E. Positive selection
F. None of the above

152. Fragile X syndrome results from pathogenic variants in the *FMR1* gene on chromosome X. A technologist works on fragile X testing with PCR and Southern blotting in a clinical molecular genetic laboratory. For Southern blotting, he used a restriction enzyme to distinguish methylated alleles from the nonmethylated ones. Which one of the following descriptions regarding restriction enzymes is correct?

A. Restriction enzymes always cut within the recognition size.
B. Restriction enzymes usually cut a mirror-like palindromic double-stranded DNA sequence.
C. Restriction enzymes usually cut a mirror-like palindromic single-stranded DNA sequence.
D. Restriction enzymes usually cut an inverted repeat mirror-like palindromic single-stranded DNA sequence.
E. Restriction enzymes usually cut an inverted repeat palindromic double-stranded DNA sequence.
F. None of the above.

153. Fragile X syndrome is characterized by a range of developmental problems, including learning disabilities and cognitive impairment. Usually males are more severely affected by this disorder than females. A technologist works on fragile X testing with PCR and Southern blotting in a clinical molecular genetic laboratory. For Southern blots, he used a restriction enzyme to distinguish methylated alleles from the nonmethylated ones. Which one of the following DNA sequences most likely is a restriction enzyme recognition site (from 5′−3′)?

A. CAGCAG
B. GTAATG
C. GAATTG
D. GATATC
E. GTCAC
F. None of the above

154. In the Ashkenazi Jewish population from Eastern European, it has been estimated that one in three individuals is a carrier of one of several genetic conditions. These diseases include Tay—Sachs disease, Canavan, Niemann—Pick, Gaucher, familial dysautonomia, Bloom syndrome, Fanconi anemia, cystic fibrosis, and mucolipidosis IV. Why are these genetic diseases are so common in Ashkenazi Jewish people?

A. Founder effect
B. Heterozygote advantage
C. Negative selection
D. Phenocopy
E. Positive selection
F. None of the above

155. Hartnup disease is an autosomal recessive condition caused by reduced neutral amino acid absorption from the intestine and reabsorption from the kidney, leading to low levels of blood tryptophan. Pellagra, the niacin deficiency disease, is clinically similar to Hartnup disease. Which one of the following genetic terms may be used to describe the similar clinical presentation between Hartnup disease and niacin deficiency?

A. Founder effect
B. Heterozygote advantage
C. Negative selection
D. Phenocopy
E. Positive selection
F. None of the above

156. An 18-year-old male, BJ, was referred to a genetics clinic for mitochondrial myoclonic epilepsy. Which one of the following statements regarding mtDNA is correct?[4,13]

A. Pathogenic variants in mtDNA is less likely to be pathogenic than nuclear DNA.
B. The most common symptom caused by pathogenic variants in mtDNA is myopathy.
C. The mtDNA follows Mendelian inheritance.
D. The total number of mtDNA molecules per human cell is approximately 50—100.
E. A mitochondrial genome encodes 11 protein-coding genes.
F. None of the above.

157. The cell cycle is the series of events that take place in a cell leading to division and duplication of its DNA to produce two daughter cells. Which one of the following is the correct order of the cell cycle?[4,13]

A. G0→G1→G2→S→Mitosis
B. G0→G1→S→G2→Mitosis
C. G0→G1→Mitosis→G2→S
D. G0→S→G1→G2→Mitosis
E. G0→S→G1→Mitosis→G2
F. None of the above

158. A recently graduated PhD has been trained in a clinical genetic laboratory to interpret next generation sequencing (NGS) data. Which one of the pathogenic variants in the sequences below is most likely to be benign if this is the beginning of exon 1 of a gene?[11]
   A. Change from AT**G** GCG CAT to AT**C** GCG CAT
   B. Change from ATG **G**CG CAT to ATG **A**CG CAT
   C. Change from ATG GC**G** CAT to ATG GC**A** CAT
   D. Change from ATG GCG **C**AT to ATG GCG **C**GT
   E. None of the above

159. Duchenne muscular dystrophy (DMD) is an X-linked form of muscular dystrophy, affecting around 1 in 3600 boys, which results in muscle degeneration and premature death. Deletions of exons, especially exon 50, of *DMD* account for approximately 60%−70% of pathogenic variants in individuals with DMD. Which one of the following molecular genetic tests will NOT be suitable for this kind of deletion?[13]
   A. Chromosomal microarray (CMA)
   B. Multiplex ligation-dependent probe amplification (MLPA)
   C. Quantitative PCR
   D. Sanger sequencing
   E. None of the above

160. The hemolytic disease of the fetus and newborn (HDFN) is caused by alloimmunization of the mother through exposure to fetal red blood cells. Anti-Rh accounts for the majority of HDFN. Which one of the following statements about the RH genes is correct?[4]
   A. *RHC*, *RHD*, and *RHE* alleles are inherited as haplotypes in eight possible combinations.
   B. The *RHD* pseudogene is the most common type of RHD-negative blood type.
   C. The offspring of an *RHD*-positive female is at risk for HDFN.
   D. Anti-RhD is the most common type of the HDFN.
   E. All of the above.
   F. None of the above.

161. Ninety-one percent of the African American population is RHD-positive. What percent of the population are homozygous and heterozygous for RHD?[13]
   A. 49% DD and 42% Dd
   B. 63% DD and 28% Dd
   C. 70% DD and 21% Dd

   D. 75% DD and 16% Dd
   E. 80% DD and 11% Dd

162. Which one of the following statements is correct regarding the Knudson, or multiple-hit, hypothesis?[18−20]
   A. The Knudson hypothesis applies to tumors caused by both proto-oncogenes and tumor suppressor genes.
   B. The Knudson hypothesis applies to both hereditary and acquired cancers.
   C. The Knudson hypothesis was proved to be wrong.
   D. The Knudson hypothesis was confirmed to be correct by chromothripsis.
   E. None of the above.

163. Which one of the following tumors may NOT be explained by Knudson hypothesis?[18,19]
   A. Colorectal cancer due to familial polyposis
   B. Li−Fraumeni syndrome
   C. Multiple endocrine neoplasia type 2 (MEN2)
   D. Retinoblastoma
   E. Wilms tumor
   F. None of the above

164. Which one of the following tumors may NOT be explained by the Knudson hypothesis?[18,19]
   A. Breast/ovarian cancer due to *BRCA1/BRCA2*
   B. Lynch syndrome
   C. Noonan syndrome
   D. Retinoblastoma
   E. von Hippel−Lindau syndrome
   F. None of the above

165. In genetics, a centimorgan (cM) is a unit for measuring genetic linkage, which is defined as the distance between genetic markers for which the expected average number of intervening chromosomal crossovers (recombination) in a single generation is 0.01. On average, to how many base pairs does 1 cM approximately correspond in the human genome?[21]
   A. 1000
   B. 10,000
   C. 100,000
   D. 1,000,000
   E. 10,000,000

166. In genetics, a cM is a unit for measuring genetic linkage, which is defined as the distance between genetic markers for which the expected average number of intervening chromosomal crossovers (recombination) in a single generation is 0.01. On average, 1 cM corresponds to approximately 1 million base pairs in the human genome. What is the genetic length of the human genome for a female?[21]

A. 8800 cM
B. 5400 cM
C. 4400 cM
D. 3700 cM
E. 2700 cM

167. In genetics, a centimorgan (cM) is a unit for measuring genetic linkage, which is defined as the distance between genetic markers for which the expected average number of intervening chromosomal crossovers (recombination) in a single generation is 0.01. On average, 1 cM corresponds to approximately 1 million base pairs in humans. What is the genetic length of human genome for male?[21]
   A. 8500 cM
   B. 5400 cM
   C. 4400 cM
   D. 3700 cM
   E. 2700 cM

168. In genetics, a centimorgan (cM) is a unit for measuring genetic linkage, which is defined as the distance between genetic markers for which the expected average number of intervening chromosomal crossovers (recombination) in a single generation is 0.01. On average, 1 cM corresponds to approximately 1 million base pairs in humans. What is the sex-average genetic length of the human genome?[21]
   A. 8500 cM
   B. 5400 cM
   C. 4400 cM
   D. 3700 cM
   E. 2700 cM

169. A clinical genetics laboratory has been evaluating the utility of exome sequencing for patients with constitutional genetic diseases. Exome sequencing usually covers:
   A. 10 Mb
   B. 20 Mb
   C. 30 Mb
   D. 40 Mb
   E. 50 Mb
   F. 100 Mb

170. A clinical genetics laboratory has been evaluating the utility of exome sequencing for patients with constitutional genetic diseases. What percentage of the genome does exome sequencing usually cover?
   A. 0.1%
   B. 1%
   C. 5%
   D. 10%
   E. 20%
   F. 30%

171. The International Human Genome Sequencing Consortium published the first draft of the human genome sequence in the journal *Nature* in February 2001, with the sequence of the entire genome's 3 billion base pairs.[22] A startling finding of this first draft was that the number of human genes appeared to be significantly fewer than previous estimates, which ranged from 50,000 genes to as many as 140,000. The full sequence was completed and published in April 2003. Which one of the following sequencing techniques was used for the Human Genome Project?
   A. Illumina DNA sequencing by synthesis
   B. Iron Torrent DNA sequencing
   C. Pyrosequencing
   D. Roche 454 sequencing
   E. Sanger sequencing
   F. SOLiD DNA sequencing
   G. All of the above
   H. None of the above

172. Gaucher disease is a rare genetic disorder characterized by the deposition of glucocerebroside in cells of the macrophage—monocyte system. The disorder results from the deficiency of the enzyme glucocerebroside. Pathogenic variants in the *GBA* gene cause Gaucher disease. A scientist planned to develop a Sanger sequencing–based test for Gaucher disease in a clinical molecular laboratory. Which one of the following orders is correct for Sanger sequencing?[4,13]
   A. DNA extraction→PCR amplification→DNA dilution→sequencing reaction→capillary electrophoresis
   B. DNA extraction→PCR amplification→DNA purification→capillary electrophoresis
   C. DNA extraction→PCR amplification→gel electrophoresis→DNA purification→sequencing reaction→capillary electrophoresis
   D. DNA extraction→PCR amplification→DNA purification→gel electrophoresis→DNA purification→capillary electrophoresis
   E. None of the above

173. A pathologist requested *MGMT* methylation study for a formalin-fixed, paraffin-embedded (*n*FFPE) specimen. On the requisition form, the indication for the test was glioblastoma. Pyrosequencing was the method for *MGMT* methylation study in this laboratory. Which one of the following orders is correct for pyrosequencing?[4,13]
   A. DNA extraction→PCR amplification→DNA purification/template

preparation→pyrosequencing
reaction→capillary electrophoresis
B. DNA extraction→PCR amplification→DNA purification/template preparation→pyrosequencing reaction
C. DNA extraction→PCR amplification→DNA purification/template preparation→capillary electrophoresis
D. DNA extraction→PCR amplification→gel electrophoresis→DNA purification→pyrosequencing reaction
E. None of the above

174. A scientist plans to develop a molecular assay for engraftment monitoring after bone-marrow transplantation. Which one of the following genetic variants is the most appropriate marker for engraftment monitoring?[4]
A. Copy number variants
B. Epigenetic makers
C. SNPs
D. STRs
E. VNTRs
F. Mitochondrial DNA
G. None of the above

175. A laboratory scientist plans to develop a molecular assay for maternal-cell contamination (MCC) tests for product-of-conception (POC) and prenatal samples. Which one of the following genetic variants is the most appropriate marker for MCC testing?[4]
A. Copy number variants
B. Epigenetic makers
C. SNPs
D. STRs
E. VNTRs
F. Mitochondrial DNA
G. None of the above

176. A forensic scientist received bone samples potentially belonging to the last Russian royal family, who were executed in 1918. Living members of the family, including Prince Philip, donated their DNA for confirmation of the relationship. Prince Philip is the great nephew of the last queen. Which one of the following genetic markers is the most appropriate marker to confirm whether the bones belong to the Russian royal family?[4]
A. Copy number variants
B. Epigenetic makers
C. SNPs
D. STRs
E. VNTRs
F. Mitochondrial DNA
G. None of the above

177. Canavan disease (CD) is a progressive neurodegenerative disorder, caused by aspartoacylase deficiency. The prevalence of CD in the Ashkenazi Jewish population is estimated to be approximately 1 in 10,000. More than 50 pathogenic variants in the *ASPA* gene associated with CD have been described. Two pathogenic variants, c.854A > C(p. 285A) and c.693C > A (p.Y231X) account for 97.4% of Ashkenazi Jewish CD alleles. The c.914C > A(p.A305E) accounts for 1% of Ashkenazi Jewish pathogenic variants. The c.433-2A > G accounts for an additional 0.5% of Ashkenazi Jewish pathogenic variants. What is the clinical sensitivity of an assay for all four pathogenic variants to detect Ashkenazi Jewish couples who are at risk of giving birth to CD patients, given that the analytical sensitivity is 100%?
A. 100%
B. 99%
C. 98%
D. 97%
E. 96%
F. 95%

178. Cystic fibrosis (CF) is an inherited disorder that causes severe damage to the lungs and digestive system. A laboratory scientist planned to develop a molecular assay to screen for carriers of CF. During the validation he found that 90 of 100 positive samples showed positive results, while 20 of 100 negative samples showed positive results. What is the analytical sensitivity of this assay?
A. 53%
B. 67%
C. 80%
D. 85%
E. 90%
F. 96%
G. None of the above

179. Tay–Sachs disease is a rare autosomal recessive genetic disorder characterized by a progressive deterioration of nerve cells and of mental and physical abilities that begins around 7 months of age and usually results in death by the age of 4. Ashkenazi Jews and French Canadians have a high incidence of Tay–Sachs disease. A laboratory scientist planned to develop a molecular assay to screen for carriers of Tay–Sachs disease. During the validation he found that 90 of 100 positive samples showed positive results while 20 of 100 negative samples showed positive results. What is the analytical specificity of this assay?
A. 53%
B. 67%

C. 80%
D. 85%
E. 90%
F. 96%
G. None of the above

180. A laboratory scientist planned to develop a molecular assay to screen for carriers of Canavan disease (CD) in the Ashkenazi Jewish population. During the validation he that found 90 of 100 positive samples showed positive results, while 20 of 100 negative samples showed positive results. What is the analytical accuracy of this assay?
A. 53%
B. 67%
C. 80%
D. 85%
E. 90%
F. 96%
G. None of the above

181. Niemann–Pick disease (NPD) is a group of inherited severe metabolic conditions in which lipids collect in the lysosomes in cells of the spleen, liver, and brain. Ashkenazi Jews have a high incidence of NPD. A laboratory scientist planned to develop a molecular assay to screen for carriers of NPD. During the validation he found that 90 of 100 positive samples showed positive results, while 20 of 100 negative samples showed positive results. What is the positive predict value of this assay if the prevalence of NPD is not taken into the consideration?
A. 80%
B. 82%
C. 85%
D. 88%
E. 90%
F. 96%
G. None of the above

182. Fanconi anemia (FA) is caused by changes that are responsible for copying and repairing DNA in cells. These changes result in a high incidence of breaks in an individual's chromosomes. Fanconi anemia is characterized by reduced production of all types of blood cells. While many serious problems are associated with this disorder, the most difficult is an increased risk for cancer. There are various forms of Fanconi anemia that can occur in individuals from any ethnic background. There are at least 15 genes currently known to cause this disorder—one specific form, Fanconi anemia group C, is the most common found in Ashkenazi Jews. A laboratory scientist planned to develop a molecular assay to screen for carriers of FA group C in the Ashkenazi Jewish population. During the validation he found that 90 of 100 positive samples showed positive results, while 20 of 100 negative samples showed positive results. What is the negative predict value of this assay if the prevalence of FA is not taken into the consideration?
A. 80%
B. 82%
C. 85%
D. 88%
E. 90%
F. 96%
G. None of the above

183. Mucolipidosis IV (MLIV) is an autosomal recessive neurodegenerative lysosomal storage disorder. The carrier frequency in the Ashkenazi Jewish population is about 1 in 127. Two pathogenic variants, IVS3-2A > G and del6.4kb, in the *MCOLN1* gene account for approximately 95% of the Ashkenazi Jewish pathogenic variants. What is the clinical negative predict value for detecting carriers of MLIV in Ashkenazi Jewish population when only the two pathogenic variants were tested (assuming that the analytic sensitivity and specificity are 100%)?
A. 1269/1270
B. 2520/2521
C. 1/2520
D. 1/1270
E. 1/127

184. Which one of the following techniques did a clinical molecular geneticist use to analyze a bone marrow specimen for recurrent pathogenic variants in myelodysplastic/myeloproliferative neoplasms (MDS/MPN) according to the figure below?[4,23]
A. Illumina DNA sequencing by synthesis
B. Multiplex ligation-dependent probe amplification (MLPA)
C. Pyrosequencing
D. Sanger sequencing
E. STR fragment-size analysis by capillary electrophoresis
F. None of the above

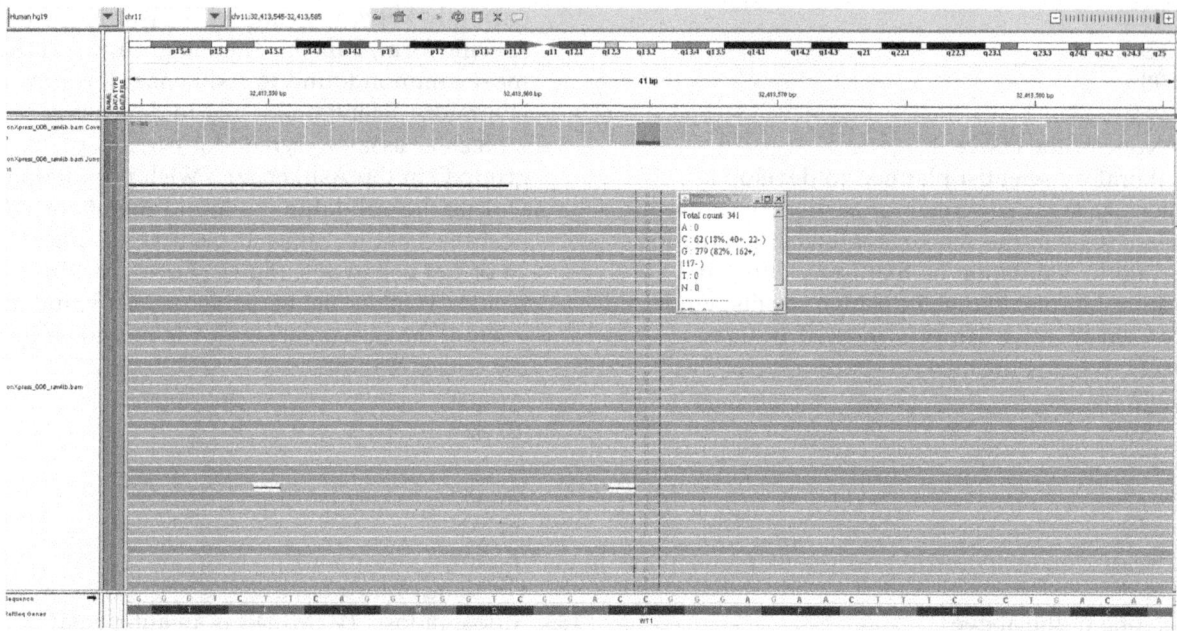

Source: From CAP annual conference, Edappallath S, DiGiuseppe J, Meng H, Chang F, Liu L, Li MM, Johari V. Mixed Phenotype Acute Leukemia, T/Myeloid: Bilineal or Unilineal?: (Poster No. 179).

185. A clinical molecular geneticist used an NGS assay to analyze bone marrow for recurrent pathogenic variants in MDS/MPN. What was the reading depth of this run for this specimen at the targeted region shown in the figure below?

    A. 41
    B. 62
    C. 279
    D. 341
    E. Unclear

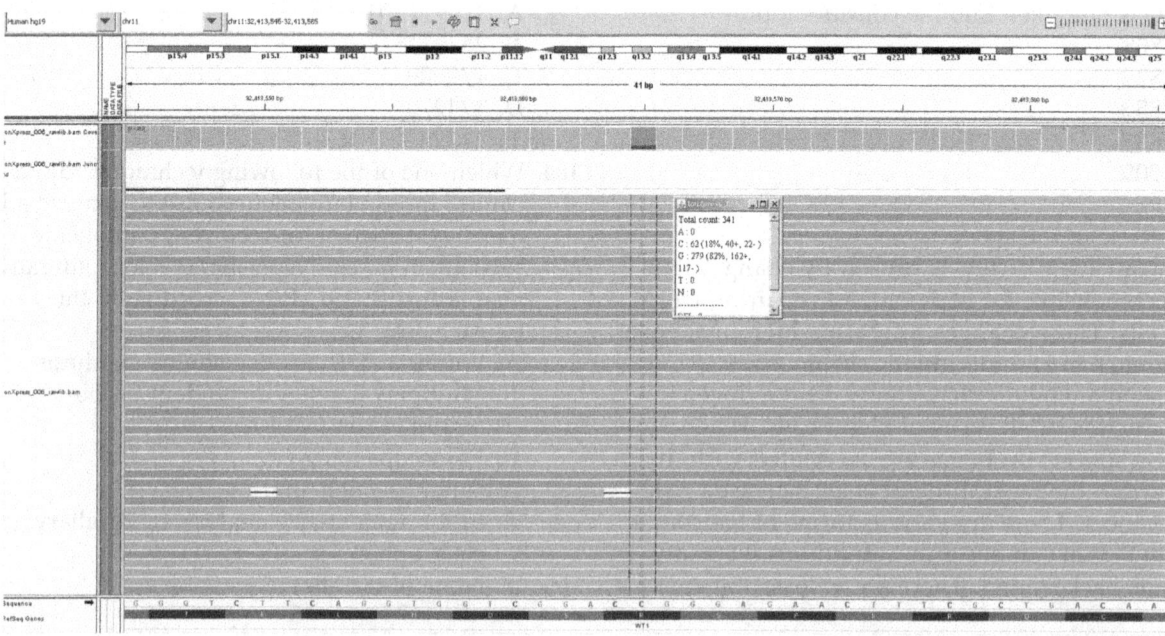

Source: From CAP annual conference, Edappallath S, DiGiuseppe J, Meng H, Chang F, Liu L, Li MM, Johari V. Mixed Phenotype Acute Leukemia, T/Myeloid: Bilineal or Unilineal?: (Poster No. 179).

186. A clinical molecular geneticist used a next generation sequencing (NGS) assay to analyze bone marrow for recurrent pathogenic variants in myelodysplastic/myeloproliferative neoplasms (MDS/MPN). What was the coverage of this region, according to the figure below?

A. 41
B. 62
C. 279
D. 341
E. Unclear

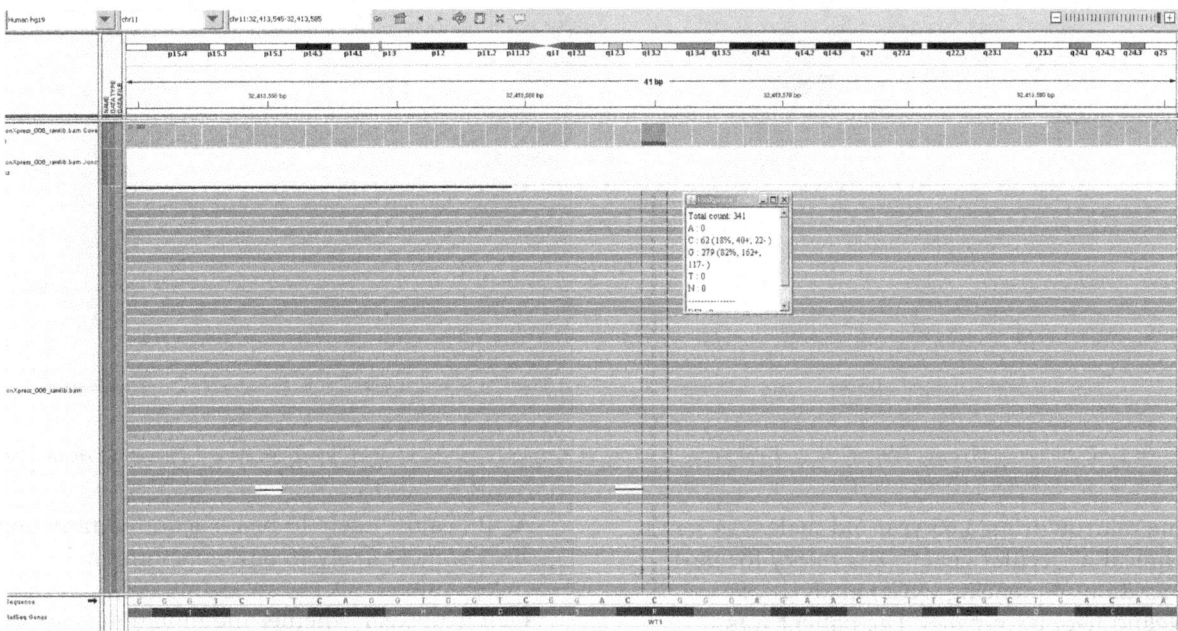

Source: From CAP annual conference, Edappallath S, DiGiuseppe J, Meng H, Chang F, Liu L, Li MM, Johari V. Mixed Phenotype Acute Leukemia, T/Myeloid: Bilineal or Unilineal?: (Poster No. 179).

187. A clinical molecular geneticist used a next generation assay (MPN) to analyze bone marrow from a 65-year-old female for myelodysplastic/myeloproliferative neoplasms (MDS/MPN). The result discovered a pathogenic finding in the *WT1* (Wilms tumor 1) gene. Which one of the following statements is NOT appropriate, according to the figure?

A. The reading depth in this specimen was enough to detect acquired abnormalities.

B. This result indicated the patient had a constitutional mutation for Wilms tumor, which predisposed the patient to other neoplasms.

C. The molecular geneticist used Genome Reference Consortium GRCh37 as the reference sequence for this analysis.

D. The molecular geneticist found a C:G mutation in *WT1* on 11p13.

E. None of the above

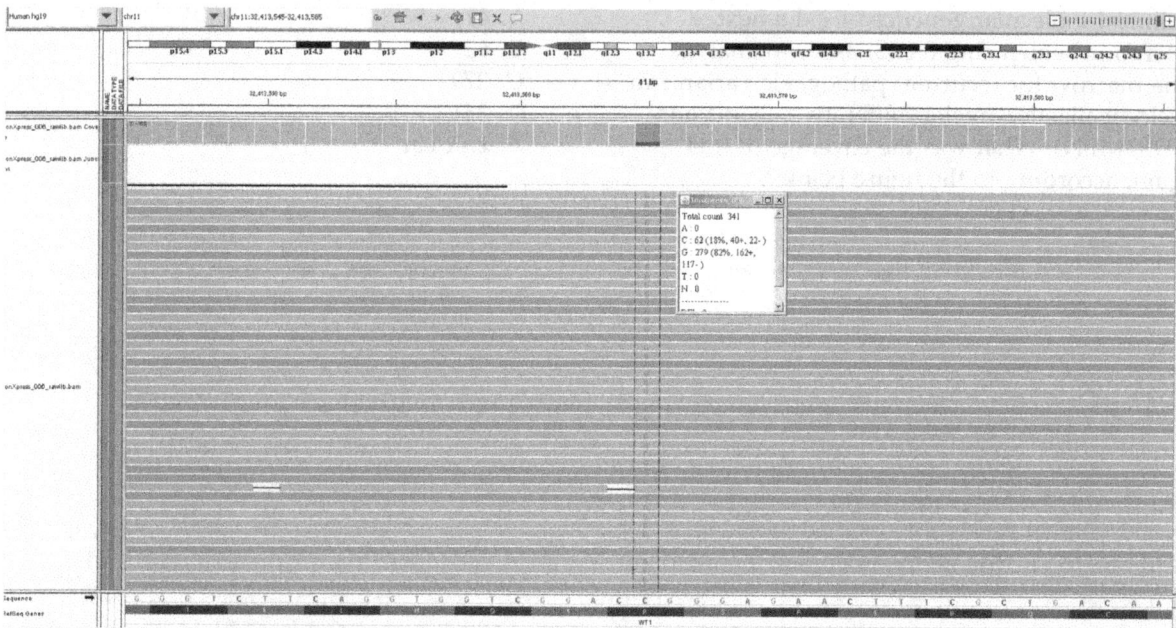

Source: From CAP annual conference, Edappallath S, DiGiuseppe J, Meng H, Chang F, Liu L, Li MM, Johari V. Mixed Phenotype Acute Leukemia, T/Myeloid: Bilineal or Unilineal?: (Poster No. 179).

188. Bone marrow from a 65-year-old male was sent to a clinical molecular genetic laboratory for next generation sequencing (NGS) analysis of a myeloid neoplasm panel. The patient was diagnosed with acute myeloid leukemia (AML) morphologically with the same specimen. The molecular result discovered a pathogenic in/del in the *FLT3* gene. Which one of the following interpretations would be most appropriate, according to the figure?

A. It is most likely to be an acquired mutation.
B. It is most likely to be a constitutional mutation.
C. It is unclear whether the mutation is acquired or constitutional. Testing of a peripheral-blood sample is recommended.
D. All of the above.
E. None of the above.

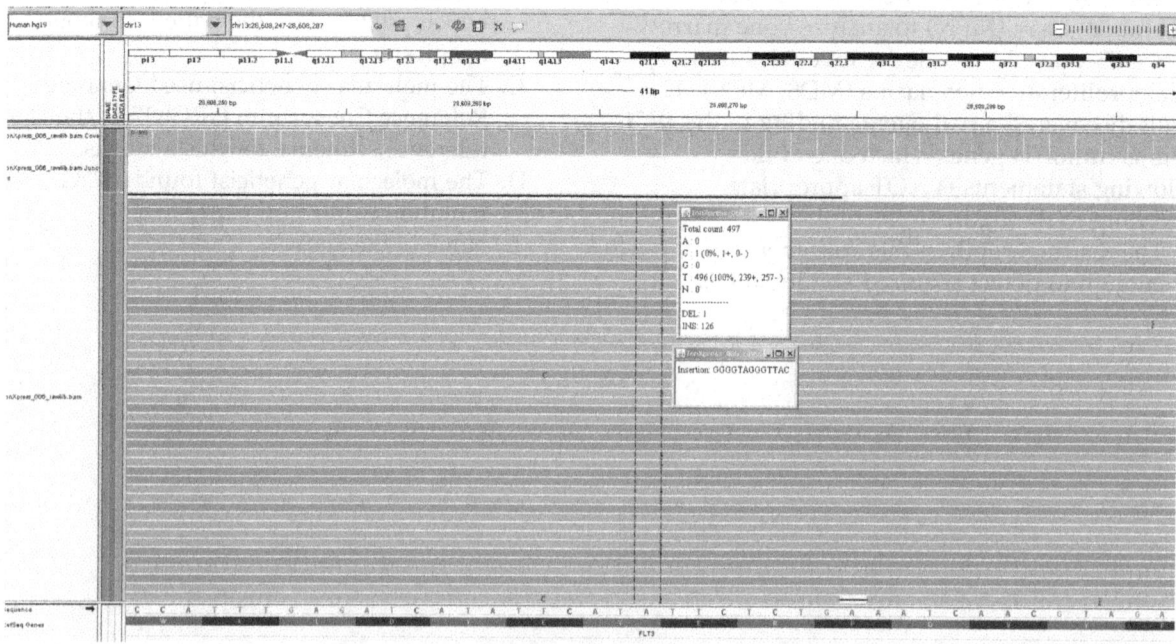

Source: From CAP annual conference, Edappallath S, DiGiuseppe J, Meng H, Chang F, Liu L, Li MM, Johari V. Mixed Phenotype Acute Leukemia, T/Myeloid: Bilineal or Unilineal?: (Poster No. 179).

189. Which one of the next-generation sequencing (NGS) methods is technologically similar to pyrosequencing?
    A. Illumina DNA sequencing by synthesis
    B. Iron Torrent DNA sequencing
    C. Roche 454 sequencing
    D. SOLiD DNA sequencing
    E. All of the above
    F. None of the above

190. Which one of the next-generation sequencing (NGS) methods is NOT based on the sequencing-by-synthesis method?
    A. Illumina DNA sequencing by synthesis
    B. Iron Torrent DNA sequencing
    C. Roche 454 sequencing
    D. SOLiD DNA sequencing
    E. All of the above
    F. None of the above

191. A director has been evaluating the clinical utility of next-generation sequencing (NGS) in a clinical molecular laboratory. Which one of the following NGS methods produces a shorter reading length than others?
    A. Illumina DNA sequencing by synthesis
    B. Pyrosequencing
    C. Roche 454 sequencing
    D. Sanger sequencing
    E. None of the above

192. A director has been evaluating the clinical utility of next-generation sequencing (NGS) in a clinical molecular laboratory. Which one of the following NGS methods produces the shortest reading length?
    A. Iron Torrent DNA sequencing
    B. Pyrosequencing
    C. Roche 454 sequencing
    D. Sanger sequencing
    E. None of the above

193. Which one of the following sequencing methods has the highest accuracy?
    A. Illumina DNA sequencing by synthesis
    B. Iron Torrent DNA sequencing
    C. Roche 454 sequencing
    D. Sanger sequencing
    E. SOLiD DNA sequencing
    F. None of the above

194. Which one of the following is the first step for next-generation sequencing (NGS) assays?[4]
    A. Bioinformatics
    B. Emulsion PCR or "Polony" PCR
    C. Library preparation
    D. Sanger confirmation
    E. None of the above

195. A clinical molecular geneticist plans to develop a next-generation sequencing (NGS) panel in a laboratory. Which one of the following parameters would he use to monitor the accuracy of the detections to decrease the false positive findings?[4]
    A. Reading deeps
    B. Location of the variant in the fragments
    C. Ratio of the forward to reverse reading
    D. All of the above
    E. None of the above

ANSWERS

1. **B**. Whole blood is a common specimen source for nucleic acid testing. *Whole blood often yields a very high quality and ample quantity of nucleic acid for testing, as compared with saliva, dried blood spots, and fixed tissue.* The impact of anticoagulants on downstream analysis must be considered before collecting specimens. *For DNA-based analyses, ethylenediaminetetraacetic acid (EDTA, purple/lavender-top tube) or acid–citrate–dextrose (ACD, yellow-top tube) are the most common anticoagulants.* Both chelate metal ion, such as magnesium (Mg^{2+}) are added to inhibit DNase and RNase activity in order to preserve DNA/RNA in the specimens. ACD is useful when prolonged shipping may be involved. Sodium heparin (green-top tube) has the advantage over EDTA of not affecting levels of most ions, which is good for keeping cells alive for cytogenetic analysis. However, heparin may interfere with nucleic acid testing and some immunoassays. Dried blood spots, formalin-fixed anatomic samples, swabs, and saliva usually do not yield high-quality DNA. Chromosome microarray analysis may work with formalin-fixed samples, but it is preferable to do the analysis with high-quality DNA extracted from a whole-blood sample.

    Therefore, 1 mL of blood in a purple (lavender) top tube has the highest-quality DNA and is the most suitable for CMA.

2. **B**. Chronic myeloid leukemia (CML) is a clonal hematologic stem-cell malignancy. In greater than 90% of cases, there is a Philadelphia chromosome (Ph) from a reciprocal translocation between the long arms of chromosomes 9 and 22, or t(9;22)(q34;q11). The molecular consequence of the Ph is the physical juxtapositioning of sequences from the *BCR* gene on chromosome 22 adjacent to sequences from the *ABL1* gene on chromosome 9 encoding a nonreceptor tyrosine kinase. Targeted inhibition of *BCR-ABL1* with tyrosine kinase inhibitors (imatinib, dasatinib, nilotinib) is the standard treatment for CML (and Ph + ALL).

By measuring *BCR-ABL1* RNA levels using a sensitive real-time fluorescent PCR method, the presence of leukemic cells may be detected at a very low level. A relative ratio of *BCR-ABL1* RNA to reference-gene RNA is used to report the quantity of hybrid *BCR-ABL1* genes.

Since RNA is fragile, usually the peripheral blood or bone marrow for *BCR-ABL1* molecular test is requested to be sent to the laboratory within 24 h. *The sample should be refrigerated until transportation and should be transported on ice packs (DO NOT freeze the sample).*

Therefore, the preferred transportation condition for this sample is on ice packs for an RNA-based assay like *BCR-ABL1*.

3. **A**. Chronic myeloproliferative neoplasms (MPNs) are clonal hematopoietic stem-cell malignancies characterized by excessive production of blood cells. Essential thrombocythemia (ET), myelofibrosis (MF), and polycythemia vera (PV) are the three most common *BCR-ABL1*—negative MPNs and are associated with thrombosis and hemorrhage, splenomegaly, and the risk of transformation to acute myeloid leukemia. Diagnostic criteria for polycythemia vera (PV), essential thrombocythemia (ET), and idiopathic myelofibrosis (MF) adopted by the World Health Organization (WHO) include identification of a clonal marker, with a specific recommendation to test for the *JAK2* V617F variant in exon 14. *JAK2* V617F is a gain-of-function mutation that leads to clonal proliferation. It is present in about 95% of PV cases and about half of ET and MF cases. Peripheral-blood and bone-marrow specimens usually are collected for *JAK2* molecular tests.

The specimens should be delivered to lab at ambient temperature. If there is a delay of more than 24 h in delivery, refrigerate the sample (DO NOT FREEZE).

Therefore, the preferred transportation condition for this sample is ambient for a DNA-based assay like *JAK2* V617F.

4. **C**. This is an RNA-based assay. By measuring *BCR-ABL1* RNA levels using a sensitive real-time fluorescence PCR method, the presence of leukemic cells may be detected at a very low level. A relative ratio of *BCR-ABL1* RNA to reference-gene RNA is used to report the quantity of hybrid *BCR-ABL1* gene. *Since RNA is fragile, the extracted RNA should be frozen before the test is performed.*

Therefore, the preferred storage condition for RNA is −20°C before the test is performed.

5. **B**. Peripheral-blood and bone-marrow specimens usually are collected for *JAK2* molecular tests. The specimens should be delivered to labs at ambient temperature. If there is a delay of more than 24 h in delivery, refrigerate the sample (DO NOT FREEZE). *The extracted DNA should be kept refrigerated at 4°C before the test is performed.*

Therefore, the preferred storage condition for DNA is refrigerated (4°C) before the test is performed.

6. **A**. Positive and negative controls are always included in each PCR run for quality control. *If the positive control shows a negative result, it indicates that the PCR reaction may have failed, which leads to false negative results on the tested specimens.*

Therefore, if a positive control showed a negative result, the PCR reaction on the tested specimens may be considered as false negative for amplification.

7. **C**. Positive and negative controls are always included in each PCR run for quality control. *If the negative control shows a positive result, it indicates that the PCR reaction may take place when there are no templates, which leads to false positive results on the tested specimens, so-called DNA contamination.*

Therefore, if a negative control showed a positive result, the PCR reaction on the tested specimens may be considered as false positive for amplification.

8. **D**. *The patient may have a constitutional genetic condition, which may be detected with a peripheral-blood sample collected by venipuncture.* It is much easier to obtain a peripheral-blood sample than to perform a lumbar puncture to obtain cerebroal spinal fluid (CSF), or a bone-marrow tap for bone-marrow sample. EDTA in the tube (lavender-top tube) may protect DNA in the peripheral-blood sample from degradation by chelating Mg^{2+} ions, which is the key component to active DNase and RNase. Mg^{2+} ions are also the key component to active DNA/RNA polymerase for PCR reaction. During the DNA/RNA extraction procedure, ethanol (EtOH) precipitation steps usually result in the majority of EDTA being removed. If EDTA becomes an issue for in vitro amplification of whole unfractionated blood, it can be overcome with addition of extra $MgCl_2$. However, many blood specimens in EDTA do not grow.

Sodium heparin (green-top tube) is the preferred anticoagulator for G-banded chromosome studies. It prevents blood from coagulating but can be copurified with the nucleic acids, depending upon the preparation method used. Heparin is a well-known inhibitor of PCR and preferably should be avoided if the blood sample will be used for PCR analysis.

Therefore, peripheral blood in a sodium heparin tube (green top) would be preferred for G-banded chromosome karyotype analysis.

9. **E.** In this case, the chromosome microarray analysis (CMA) is ordered for a constitutional condition. *A peripheral-blood sample is the most convenient and preferred sample type.* Since CMA is a molecular-based test, DNA will be usually used for the analysis. *An EDTA tube (lavender top) is the preferred container for the blood samples, since EDTA in the tube may protect DNA in the peripheral-blood sample from degradation by chelating Mg^{2+} ions, which is the key component to active DNase and RNase.* Mg^{2+} ions are also the key component to active DNA/RNA polymerase for PCR reaction. During the DNA/RNA extraction procedure, EtOH precipitation steps usually result in the majority of the EDTA being removed.

Sodium heparin (green top) is the preferred anticoagulator for G-banded chromosome studies. It prevents blood from coagulating but can be copurified with the nucleic acids, depending upon the preparation method used. Heparin is a well-known inhibitor of PCR and preferably should be avoided if the blood sample will be used for PCR analysis. It can be digested with heparinase, but that is not worth the effort.

Therefore, peripheral blood in an EDTA tube (lavender top) would be preferred for G-banded chromosome karyotype analysis.

10. **D.** Recommendations by the DNA Bank Network and International Society for Biological and Environmental (ISBER, http://www.isber.org/) highlight that *long-term storage of DNA samples in buffer should be carried out at $-80°C$ or below.*

Therefore, the preferred the long-term storage temperature for DNA specimens is $-80°C$.

11. **D.** As specified by International Society for Biological and Environmental (ISBER, http://www.isber.org/), *long-term storage of purified RNA (tRNA, mRNA, miRNA, siRNA) is at its most stable when stored at $-80°C$,* with storage at $-20°C$ being acceptable for the short term.

Therefore, the preferred the long-term storage temperature for RNA specimens is $-80°C$.

12. **D.** *It is recommended by most manufacturers to store restriction enzymes at $-20°C$.* Enzymes usually are stored in buffered with high concentration of glycerol and remain liquid at temperatures down to $-35°C$. If these enzymes are stored at colder temperatures (e.g., in the presence of dry ice) the products will freeze. Proteins subjected to repeated freeze/thaw cycles may lose activity.

Therefore, it is better to store the restriction enzyme in a nondefrost freezer.

13. **B.** There are several ways to quantify nucleic acid concentrations. If the solution is pure, one can use a spectrophotometer to measure the amount of ultraviolet radiation absorbed by the bases. *Nucleic acids absorb light at 260 nm through the adenine residues.*

Therefore, the OD260 value is used to calculate DNA concentration.

14. **C.** There are several ways to quantify nucleic acid concentrations. If the solution is pure, one can use a spectrophotometer to measure the amount of ultraviolet radiation absorbed by the bases. Nucleic acids absorb light at 260 nm through the adenine residues. *Protein absorbs light at 280 nm through the aromatic tryptophan and tyrosine residues.*

Therefore, the OD280 value is used to calculate protein concentration. Protein contamination is measured by OD260/OD280.

15. **A.** There are several ways to quantify nucleic acid concentrations. If the solution is pure, one can use a spectrophotometer to measure the amount of ultraviolet radiation absorbed by the bases. Nucleic acids absorb light at 260 nm through the adenine residues. Protein absorbs light at 280 nm through the aromatic tryptophan and tyrosine residues. *EDTA, carbohydrates, and phenol all have absorbances near 230 nm.*

Therefore, the OD260/OD230 ratio shows the contamination of carbohydrates, phenols, peptides, aromatic compounds.

16. **A.** The OD260 value is used to calculate DNA concentration. An OD260 of 1 gives a concentration dsDNA of 50 ng/μL. Protein contamination is measured by OD260/OD280. A 260/280 ratio of approximately 1.8 is generally accepted as "pure" for DNA; a ratio of approximately 2.0 is generally accepted as "pure" for RNA. RNA will typically have a higher 260/280 ratio owing to the higher ratio of uracil (260/280: 4.00) compared to that of thymine (260/280: 1.47). *The value becomes smaller when protein contamination increases.*

Therefore, a ratio of 1.3 for OD260/OD280 indicates unacceptable protein contamination.

17. **C.** ssDNA, dsDNA, RNA, proteins and other carbohydrates absorb light in the range of 230–280 nm. The quantity of DNA can be measured at 260 nm. An OD260 of 1 means a dsDNA concentration of 50, 33 ng/μL of ssDNA, 20–30 ng/μL of oligonucleotide, and 40 ng/μL of RNA. The OD260/OD230 ratio shows the contamination of carbohydrates, phenols, peptides, and aromatic compounds. Expected 260/230 values are commonly in the range of 2.0–2.2. *If the ratio is appreciably lower than expected, it may indicate the presence of contaminants, which absorb at 230 nm.*

Therefore, a ratio of 1.3 for OD260/OD230 indicates unacceptable aromatic compound contamination.

18. **B**. A spectrophotometer may be used to measure the amount of ultraviolet radiation absorbed by the bases. Nucleic acids absorb light at 260 nm through the adenine residues. *Using the absorbance unit at 260 nm is equivalent to 50 g/L (or 50 µg/mL) of dsDNA and 40 µg/mL of RNA.* To determine the concentration, multiply the spectrophotometer reading in absorbance units by the appropriate conversion factor.

Therefore, in this case it is
$0.12 \times 50 \times 100 = 600$ g/L (or 600 µg/mL).

19. **D**. A spectrophotometer may be used to measure the amount of ultraviolet radiation absorbed by the bases. Nucleic acids absorb light at 260 nm through the adenine residues. *Using the absorbance unit at 260 nm is equivalent to 50 g/L (50 ng/µL, or 50 µg/mL) of double-stranded DNA and 40 µg/mL of RNA.* To determine concentration, multiply the spectrophotometer reading in absorbance units by the appropriate conversion factor.

Therefore, in this case it is
$0.12 \times 40 \times 100 = 480$ g/L (or 480 µg/mL).

20. **C**. Nucleic acids absorb light at 260 nm through the adenine residues. Protein absorbs light at 280 nm through the aromatic tryptophan and tyrosine residues. This measure is not highly accurate. However, general ranges indicate at least the presence of protein contaminants. The absorbance of the nucleic acid at 260 nm should be 1.6–2.00 times more than the absorbance at 280 nm. *If the 260 nm/280 nm ratio is less than 1.6, the nucleic acid preparation may be contaminated with unacceptable amounts of protein and not of sufficient purity for use.* Such a sample can be improved by column purification, reprecipitating the nucleic acid, or repeating the protein removal step of the isolation procedure. A DNA solution with an OD260/OD280 ratio higher than 2.0 may be contaminated with RNA. Some procedures for DNA analysis are not affected by contaminating RNA, in which case the DNA is still suitable for use.

Therefore, sample 3 is contaminated with a high level of protein (OD260/280 = 0.25/0.22 = 1.14).

21. **A**. Nucleic acids only absorb light that has a wavelength of 260 nm. Organic contaminants like phenol and other aromatic compounds (TRIzol), and some reagents used in RNA extraction absorb light of a 230-nm wavelength. *Samples with a low 260/230 (below about 1.8) have a significant presence of these organic contaminants* that may interfere with other downstream processes like RT-PCR or

chromosome microarray, which results in substantially less optimal results.

Therefore, sample 1 is contaminated with a high level of aromatic compounds (OD260/230 = 0.48/0.48 = 1.00).

22. **B**. *In vivo microRNA inhibits RNA expression.* MicroRNAs (or miRNAs) are a novel class of small, noncoding endogenous single-stranded RNAs (approximately 22 bp) that regulate gene expression by directing their target mRNAs for degradation or translational repression. MicroRNAs resemble the small interfering RNAs (siRNAs) of the RNA interference (RNAi) pathway, except miRNAs derive from regions of RNA transcripts that fold back on themselves to form short hairpins, whereas siRNAs derive from longer regions of double-stranded RNA. The human genome may encode over 1000 miRNAs and appear to target about 60% of the genes in human.

In vitro, siRNA inhibits RNA expression. Small interfering RNA (siRNA) is a synthetic double stranded RNA (approximately 20–25 bp in length with 3′ overhang) designed to specifically target a particular mRNA for degradation. Heterogeneous nuclear RNA (hnRNA), also called precursor mRNA (pre-mRNA), is an immature single strand of messenger ribonucleic acid (mRNA). Pre-mRNA is synthesized from a DNA template in the cell nucleus by transcription. Pre-mRNAs include both exons and introns. After splicing to remove the introns and adding 5′ cap of 7-methylguanosine and a poly-A tail, hnRNA is processed into mRNA. Mature mRNA is exported out of the nucleus and eventually translated into a protein, which is a process accomplished in conjunction with ribosomes. Transfer ribonucleic acid (tRNA) is a type of RNA molecule that helps decode an mRNA sequence into a protein. The tRNA molecule has a distinctive folded structure with three hairpin loops that form the shape of a three-leafed clover. One of these hairpin loops contains a sequence called the "anticodon," which can recognize and decode an mRNA codon. Each tRNA has its corresponding amino acid attached to its end. When a tRNA recognizes and binds to its corresponding codon in the ribosome, the tRNA transfers the appropriate amino acid to the end of the growing amino acid chain. Then the tRNAs and ribosome continue to decode the mRNA molecule until the entire sequence is translated into a protein. Ribosomal ribonucleic acid (rRNA) is the RNA component of the ribosome and is essential for protein synthesis in all living organisms.

Therefore, microRNA inhibits gene expression in vivo.

23. E. *In vitro Small interfering RNA (siRNA) inhibits RNA expression.* Small interfering RNA (siRNA) is a synthetic double-stranded RNA (approximately 20–25 bp in length with 3′ overhang) designed to specifically target a particular mRNA for degradation. siRNA functions by causing mRNA to be broken down after transcription. In principle, any gene can be knocked down by a synthetic siRNA with a complementary sequence; siRNAs are an important tool for validating gene function and drug targeting in the postgenomic era.

The term *circulating nucleic acids (CNAs)* refers to segments of DNA or RNA found in the bloodstream. Most of the DNA and RNA in the body are located within cells, but a small amount of nucleic acids can also be found circulating freely in the blood. These DNA, RNA, and small RNA molecules are thought to come from dying cells that release their contents into the blood as they breakdown. CNAs offer a noninvasive approach to a wide range of diagnostics of clinical disorders that will allow the basic information necessary not only for use in predictive medicine but also for direct use in acute medicine. Further free CNAs offer unique opportunities for early diagnosis of clinical conditions (e.g., early cancer detection).

In vivo microRNA inhibits RNA expression. MicroRNAs (or miRNAs) are a novel class of small, noncoding endogenous single-stranded RNAs (approximately 22 bp) that regulate gene expression by directing their target mRNAs for degradation or translational repression. Heterogeneous nuclear RNA (hnRNA), also called precursor mRNA (pre-mRNA), is an immature single strand of messenger ribonucleic acid (mRNA). Pre-mRNA is synthesized from a DNA template in the cell nucleus by transcription. Pre-mRNAs include both exons and introns. After splicing to remove the introns and adding 5′ cap of 7-methylguanosine and a poly-A tail, hnRNA is processed into mRNA. Mature mRNA is exported out of the nucleus and eventually translated into a protein, which is a process accomplished in conjunction with ribosomes. Transfer ribonucleic acid (tRNA) is a type of RNA molecule that helps decode an mRNA sequence into a protein. The tRNA molecule has a distinctive folded structure with three hairpin loops that form the shape of a three-leafed clover. One of these hairpin loops contains a sequence called the "anticodon," which can recognize and decode an mRNA codon. Each

tRNA has its corresponding amino acid attached to its end. When a tRNA recognizes and binds to its corresponding codon in the ribosome, the tRNA transfers the appropriate amino acid to the end of the growing amino acid chain. Then the tRNAs and ribosome continue to decode the mRNA molecule until the entire sequence is translated into a protein. Ribosomal ribonucleic acid (rRNA) is the RNA component of the ribosome and is essential for protein synthesis in all living organisms.

Therefore, siRNA does not present in vivo.

24. B. Messenger RNA (mRNA) is synthesized complementary and antiparallel to the template strand (anticodons) of DNA, so *the resulting mRNA consists of codons corresponding to those in the coding strand of DNA.* The anticodons of tRNA adapt each three-base mRNA codon to the corresponding amino acid. Therefore, mRNA contains genetic codons for amino acid sequence.

Heterogeneous nuclear RNA (hnRNA), also called precursor mRNA ("pre-mRNA"), is an immature single strand of messenger ribonucleic acid (mRNA). Pre-mRNA is synthesized from a DNA template in the cell nucleus by transcription. Pre-mRNAs include both exons and introns. After splicing to remove the introns, and adding 5′ cap of 7-methylguanosine and a poly-A tail, hnRNA is processed into mRNA. Mature mRNA is exported out of the nucleus and eventually translated into a protein, which is a process accomplished in conjunction with ribosomes.

Transfer ribonucleic acid (tRNA) is a type of RNA molecule that helps decode an mRNA sequence into a protein. The tRNA molecule has a distinctive folded structure with three hairpin loops that form the shape of a three-leafed clover. One of these hairpin loops contains a sequence called the "anticodon," which can recognize and decode an mRNA codon. Each tRNA has its corresponding amino acid attached to its end. When a tRNA recognizes and binds to its corresponding codon in the ribosome, the tRNA transfers the appropriate amino acid to the end of the growing amino acid chain. Then the tRNAs and ribosome continue to decode the mRNA molecule until the entire sequence is translated into a protein. Ribosomal ribonucleic acid (rRNA) is the RNA component of the ribosome and is essential for protein synthesis in all living organisms.

MicroRNAs (or miRNAs) are a novel class of small, noncoding endogenous single-stranded RNAs (approximately 22 bp) that regulate gene expression by directing their target mRNAs for degradation or translational repression. Small interfering RNA (siRNA) is a synthetic double-stranded RNA (approximately 20–25 bp in length with 3' overhang) designed to specifically target a particular mRNA for degradation.[4]

Therefore, mRNA contains genetic codons, which may be translated into an amino acid sequence.

25. C. The fetal fraction, the amount of the cell-free DNA (cfDNA) in the maternal blood that is of fetal origin, is essential for accurate test results. Some laboratories require a fetal fraction of at least 4% for a reportable result. Other laboratories, however, do not measure or report the fetal fraction. The fetal fraction typically increases with advancing gestational age. Lower amounts of fetal DNA can be caused by a number of factors, including maternal weight and mosaicism. *As maternal weight increases, fetal fraction DNA in maternal plasma decreases.* According to the data from Ariosa (https://www.harmonytestusa.com/), the average fetal fraction for a woman who weighs 45 kg (99 lb) is 18%, but that drops to 4% for women weighing 150 kg (330 lb). For patients weighing more than 250 lb, 10% or more may have a fetal fraction of less than 4%. Mosaicism may also play a role in fetal fraction. However, mosaicism is not common.

Therefore, maternal weight is the most important factor for fetal fraction of cell-free DNA in maternal blood.

26. E. *RNA may be measured in solution using SybrGreen II RNA gel stain.* However, SybrGreen II is not specific to RNA and will bind and fluoresce with double-stranded DNA as well.

3,5-Diaminobenzoic acid (DABA) combined with alpha methylene aldehydes (deoxyribose) to yield a fluorescent product. In early ages, it was used to measure DNA concentration. Hoeschst 33258 is a DNA-specific dye used more recently. This dye combines with adenine–thymine (A–T) base pairs in the minor groove of the DNA double helix and is thus specific for intact double-stranded DNA. However, the binding specificity for A–T residues complicates measurements of DNA that have unusually high or low GC (G: guanine; C: cytosin) content. PicoGreen binds to double-stranded DNA, then releases brighter fluorescence Like Hoeschst 33258. Single-stranded DNA and RNA do not bind to PicoGreen. OliGreen is designed to bind to short pieces of single-stranded DNA. OliGreen will not fluoresce when bound to double-stranded DNA or RNA.

Therefore, SybrGreen II may be used to quantify RNA.

27. C. Hereditary hemochromatosis (HH) is an autosomal recessive disorder characterized by enhanced intestinal absorption of dietary iron. The major pathogenic variant associated with HH is the c.845G > A(p.Cys282Tyr) in the *HFE* gene that occurs in approximately 80% of HH cases. In addition, a high proportion of the remaining patients are compound heterozygous for the p.Cys282Tyr and the common c.187C > G(p.His63Asp) alteration. A third pathogenic variant may also be assessed, which is the substitution of cysteine for serine at amino acid position 65, c.193A > T(p.Ser65Cys). *Restriction-fragment–length polymorphism (RFLP) is a relatively old technique to exploit single-nucleotide polymorphisms (SNPs) in DNA sequences if the SNPs are located in a restriction enzyme recognition site.* p.Cys282Tyr may be detected with Rsa 1, and p.His63Asp is detected with Mbo I.

Therefore, single nucleotide polymorphisms (SNPs) will be the target of the PCR-RFLP assay for hereditary hemochromatosis (HH).

28. C. Chromosome microarray usually requires high-quality genomic DNA. *Organic (phenol–chloroform) extraction may purify DNA from detergents, proteins, salts, and reagents used during the cell-lysis step, and yields relatively pure, high-molecular-weight DNA.* However, it is time consuming, requires sample to be transferred to multiple tubes, and involves use of hazardous and smelly chemicals.

Chelex 100 is molecular biology grade resin from BioRad. It ensures the complete removal of PCR inhibitors, contaminating metal ions that catalyze the digestion of DNA. It confers an advantage for PCR-based typing methods because it removes inhibitors of PCR and can be done in a single tube, which reduces the potential for laboratory-induced contamination and sample switching. However, the DNA extracted by Chelex 100 is not purified; a lot of salt and proteins from the cells remain in the supernatant. Whatman FTA paper is a unique matrix for the rapid preparation and ambient storage of DNA from whole blood and other biological samples. It is useful for both storage and extraction. The DNA extracted with FTA paper is good enough for PCR reaction, but the quality and the quantity of the DNA are limited. The Promega Maxwell DNA extraction system and the Qiagen column are quick methods for DNA extraction, which produce quality enough for PCR, but not so well for genomewide copy number analysis with a chromosome microarray.

Therefore, organic (phenol–chloroform) extraction will yield higher-quality DNA for chromosome microarray analysis than the others choices listed.

29. E. *All the methods listed may be used for DNA purification.* The ExoSAP protocol is the simplest way to clean-up PCR products before sequencing. The exonuclease I removes leftover primers, while the shrimp alkaline phosphatase removes any remaining dNTPs. The nice thing about this method is that one do not need to pipette PCR products out of their original PCR tubes, which minimizes the potential for PCR contamination of the lab and equipment. Gel purification allows one to isolate and purify DNA fragments based on size, but the yield is relatively low. Following electrophoresis, individuals can cut DNA bands out of the agarose gel and purify the DNA samples. This is a commonly used technique for molecular cloning, such as PCR-based or restriction enzyme–based cloning. Ethanol/isopropanol precipitation is a commonly used technique for concentrating and desalting nucleic acid (DNA or RNA) preparations in aqueous solution. Salt and ethanol/isopropanol decrease the solubility of DNA/RNA, which forces the precipitation of nucleic acids out of solution. The quality of DNA is very good after precipitation, but it takes a relatively long time. Filtration/affinity column may separate DNA fragments from protein and salt in the solution.

Therefore, agarose gel, ethanol or isopropanol precipitation, ExoSAP-IT, and filter column may all be used to purify the PCR products for Sanger sequencing.

30. E. SpeedVac is a device used in chemical and biochemical laboratories for the efficient and gentle evaporation of solvents from many samples at the same time and from samples contained in microtiter plates. *It can be used to concentrate DNA samples but not to purify DNA.*

The ExoSAP protocol is the simplest way to clean up PCR products before sequencing. The exonuclease I removes leftover primers, while the shrimp alkaline phosphatase removes any remaining dNTPs. The nice thing about this method is that one does not need to pipette PCR products out of their original PCR tubes, which minimizes the potential for PCR contamination of the lab and equipment. Gel purification allows one stop for isolation and purification of DNA fragments based on size, but the yield is relatively low. Following electrophoresis, individuals can cut DNA bands out of the agarose gel and purify the DNA samples. This is a commonly used technique for molecular cloning, such as PCR-based or restriction enzyme–based cloning. Ethanol/isopropanol precipitation is a commonly used technique for concentrating and desalting nucleic acid (DNA or RNA) preparations in

aqueous solution. Salt and ethanol/isopropanol decrease the solubility of DNA/RNA, which forces the precipitation of nucleic acids out of solution. The quality of DNA is very good after precipitation, but it takes a relatively long time. A filtration/affinity column may separate DNA fragments from protein and salt in the solution.

Therefore, SpeedVac may NOT be used to purify the PCR products for Sanger sequencing.

31. C. All the methods listed may be used for DNA purification except SpeedVac. The *ExoSAP protocol is the simplest (most cost-effective) way to clean up PCR products before sequencing.* The exonuclease I removes leftover primers, while the shrimp alkaline phosphatase removes any remaining dNTPs. The nice thing about this method is that one does not need to pipette PCR products out of their original PCR tubes, which minimizes the potential for PCR contamination of the lab and equipment.

Gel purification allows one to isolate and purify DNA fragments based on size, but the yield is relative low. Following electrophoresis, individuals can cut DNA bands out of the agarose gel and purify the DNA samples. This is a commonly used technique for molecular cloning, such as PCR-based or restriction enzyme–based cloning. Ethanol/isopropanol precipitation is a commonly used technique for concentrating and desalting nucleic acid (DNA or RNA) preparations in aqueous solution. Salt and ethanol/isopropanol decrease the solubility of DNA/RNA, which forces the precipitation of nucleic acids out of solution. The quality of DNA is very good after precipitation, but it takes a relatively long time. A filtration/affinity column may separate DNA fragments from protein and salt in the solution.

SpeedVac can be used to concentrate DNA samples but not to purify DNA.

Therefore, ExoSAP is the most cost-effective for purification of PCR products without switching tubes.

32. A. All the methods listed may be used for DNA purification except SpeedVac. *Gel purification allows one to isolate and purify DNA fragments based on size, but the yield is relative low.* Following electrophoresis, individuals can cut DNA bands out of the agarose gel and purify the DNA samples. This is a commonly used technique for molecular cloning, such as PCR-based or restriction enzyme–based cloning.

The ExoSAP protocol is the simplest (most cost-effective) way to clean up PCR products before sequencing. The exonuclease I removes leftover primers, while the shrimp alkaline phosphatase removes any remaining dNTPs. The nice thing about this method is that one does not need to pipette PCR products out of their original PCR tubes, which minimizes the potential for PCR contamination of the lab and equipment. Ethanol/isopropanol precipitation is a commonly used technique for concentrating and desalting nucleic acid (DNA or RNA) preparations in aqueous solution. Salt and ethanol/isopropanol decrease the solubility of DNA/RNA, which forces the precipitation of nucleic acids out of solution. The quality of DNA is very good after precipitation, but it takes a relatively long time. A filtration/affinity column may separate DNA fragments from protein and salt in the solution.

SpeedVac can be used to concentrate DNA samples but not to purify DNA.

Therefore, agarose gel has the lowest yield as a PCR purification method.

33. **A**. According to the CAP ACMG Standards and Guidelines for Clinical Genetics Laboratories, 2008 Edition, G8.1, "Design and Labeling of ASO Probes: ASOs for the normal and mutant sequence pair should be derived from the same DNA strand. *Since G:T and G:A mismatches are less destabilizing during hybridization reactions, it is important to avoid a G:T or G:A mismatch between the mutant oligonucleotide and the normal template.* ASO probes are labeled for radioactive or chemiluminescence detection. If radioactively labeled, the laboratory determines the need for purification and quantification prior to use."

Therefore, G:T or G:A mismatches should be avoided for an assay with forward allele-specific oligonucleotide (ASO) probes, according to the ACMG Standards and Guidelines for Clinical Genetics Laboratories.

34. **C**. According to the CAP ACMG Standards and Guidelines for Clinical Genetics Laboratories, 2008 Edition, G8.1 and G8.2, "The forward allele-specific oligonucleotide (ASO) method is based upon hybridization of a labeled oligonucleotide probe containing either wild-type sequence or known mutant sequence to the target, patient DNA. Generally, PCR products from multiplex PCR reactions of patient DNAs are manually or robotically spotted onto replicate filters (dot blots) and then hybridized to labeled ASOs under specific conditions."

In G8.2 "An alternative approach to ASO is reverse dot-blot (RDB) hybridization. In this method, the roles of the oligonucleotide probe and the target amplified DNA are reversed. *Probe pairs, complementary to mutant and normal DNA sequences, are bound to nylon membranes in the form of dots or*

slots. DNA that has been amplified in multiplex reaction(s) and labeled using end-labeled primers or internal incorporation of biotinylated dUTP, is hybridized to the membrane."

Therefore, PCR products are spotted onto replicate filters (dot blots) for the forward allele-specific oligonucleotide (ASO) assay, whereas the PCR products are labeled with the RDB hybridization assay.

35. **F**. According to the CAP ACMG Standards and Guidelines for Clinical Genetics Laboratories, 2008 Edition, G8.2, "An alternative approach to forward allele-specific oligonucleotide (ASO) is reverse dot-blot (RDB) hybridization. In this method, the roles of the oligonucleotide probe and the target amplified DNA are reversed. Probe pairs, complementary to mutant and normal DNA sequences, are bound to nylon membranes in the form of dots or slots. DNA that has been amplified in multiplex reaction(s) and labeled using end-labeled primers or internal incorporation of biotinylated dUTP, is hybridized to the membrane."

"RDB strips can be produced manually. *Alternatively, this process is amenable to the robotic production of large strip lots that can then be stored at room temperature until use.* Each lot of strips should be compared to a previous lot to verify consistency with respect to each allele detected in the assay as well as a negative (no DNA) control. For in-house developed strip production, it is often necessary to adjust the amount of new lots of probe that is applied to the strips in order to optimize hybridization signal."

Therefore, the probe spotted membranes may be stored at room temperature (choice F).

36. **A**. According to the CAP ACMG Standards and Guidelines for Clinical Genetics Laboratories, 2008 Edition, G8.1, G8.2, G8.4, and G8.5, "The *Forward allele-specific oligonucleotide (ASO)* method is based upon hybridization of a labeled *oligonucleotide probe containing either wild-type sequence or known mutant sequence* to the target, patient DNA. Generally, PCR products from multiplex PCR reactions of patient DNAs are manually or robotically spotted onto replicate filters (dot blots) and then hybridized to label ASOs under specific conditions. Design of the multiplex PCR conditions, ASOs, hybridization and wash conditions, and detection is complex. An advantage of this method is that pathogenic variants can be readily added to an already existing panel. There are a number of issues that must be considered in the development of this test platform."

"Reverse Dot Blot Hybridization (RDB): An alternative approach to ASO is reverse dot-blot (RDB) hybridization. In this method, the roles of the oligonucleotide probe and the target amplified DNA are reversed. *Probe pairs, complementary to mutant and normal DNA sequences,* are bound to nylon membranes in the form of dots or slots. DNA that has been amplified in multiplex reaction (s) and labeled using end-labeled primers or internal incorporation of biotinylated dUTP, is hybridized to the membrane. This procedure is very amenable to high throughput analysis of high mutation spectrum genes. Although probe design and production of the spotted membranes may be complex, mutation detection using this method is nonradioactive, convenient, rapid, robust and requires no specialized interpretation skills. This technology, while robust, is relatively inflexible and not easily expanded to include additional pathogenic variants."

"Oligonucleotide Ligation Assay (OLA): The oligonucleotide ligation assay (OLA) is a novel approach to detect point pathogenic variants, small deletions and small insertions. This method consists of PCR amplification of the target sequence followed by hybridization and ligation. *Hybridization involves 3 probes, one specific for the normal allele, a competing probe specific for the mutant allele, and a common probe that binds to both alleles.* The 5′ probe is an allele-specific oligonucleotide (ASO) designed with either the normal or the mutant nucleotide(s) at the ultimate 3′ end. The 3′ probe is a ligation-specific oligonucleotide (LSO) which binds immediately adjacent to the site to be interrogated. This common probe is phosphorylated at the 5′ end to enable the ligation reaction. A thermostable DNA ligase is used to ligate either the normal or mutant ASO to the LSO. Ligation only occurs in the presence of a perfect match between the ASO, LSO and amplicon."

"Fluorescence Resonance Energy Transfer (FRET): The fluorescence resonance energy transfer (FRET) assay involves two concurrent reactions in a single well on a 96-well plate. *The primary reaction utilizes two different oligonucleotide probes, one specific for the normal sequence and the other specific for the mutant sequence.* Both probes hybridize to the target genomic DNA, forming an overlapping structure. This structure is recognized by a proprietary enzyme, resulting in the release of a DNA fragment, which forms the substrate for the secondary reaction. The secondary reaction involves the binding of the released DNA fragment to a FRET cassette containing a fluorescent reporter and quencher molecule. The overlapping structure created by the binding of the released DNA fragment to the cassette is recognized by the same enzyme as the primary reaction. The second structure is cleaved, separating the fluorophore and quencher, generating a detectable fluorescence signal. Mismatch between the mutant probe and wild-type target DNA or wild-type probe and mutant target DNA in the primary reaction prevents the formation of the overlapping structure and the generation of the subsequent fluorescent signal. By utilizing two different allele-specific (normal and mutant) probes in the primary reaction, with each binding to a different FRET cassette with a unique spectral fluorophore, 2 sequence variants (normal and mutant) at a single site can be detected in the same well."

Therefore, the similarity of these techniques is probes are for different alleles.

37. **D.** According to the CAP ACMG Standards and Guidelines for Clinical Genetics Laboratories, 2008 Edition, G8.1, G8.2, G8.3, and G8.4, and G8.5, "The oligonucleotide ligation assay (OLA) consists of PCR amplification of the target sequence followed by hybridization and ligation. *Hybridization involves 3 probes, one specific for the normal allele, a competing probe specific for the mutant allele, and a common probe that binds to both alleles.* The 5′ probe is an allele-specific oligonucleotide (ASO) designed with either the normal or the mutant nucleotide(s) at the ultimate 3′ end. The 3′ probe is a ligation-specific oligonucleotide (LSO) which binds immediately adjacent to the site to be interrogated. This common probe is phosphorylated at the 5′ end to enable the ligation reaction. A thermostable DNA ligase is used to ligate either the normal or mutant ASO to the LSO. Ligation only occurs in the presence of a perfect match between the ASO, LSO and amplicon." The forward allele-specific oligonucleotide (ASO) method, Reverse Dot Blot Hybridization (RDB), and amplification Refractory Mutation System (ARMS) are relatively old assays, which have been replaced by newer techniques for low throughput.

Therefore, oligonucleotide ligation assay (OLA) is relatively higher throughput and more accurate in the detection of pathogenic variants in the *CFTR* gene than ASO, RDB, and ARMS, according to the ACMG Standards and Guidelines for Clinical Genetics Laboratories.

38. **C.** According to the CAP ACMG Standards and Guidelines for Clinical Genetics Laboratories, 2008 Edition, G8.4, "The oligonucleotide ligation assay (OLA) is a novel approach to detect point pathogenic variants, small deletions and small

insertions. This method consists of PCR amplification of the target sequence followed by hybridization and ligation. *Hybridization involves 3 probes, one specific for the normal allele, a competing probe specific for the mutant allele, and a common probe that binds to both alleles.* The 5′ probe is an allele-specific oligonucleotide (ASO) designed with either the normal or the mutant nucleotide(s) at the ultimate 3′ end. The 3′ probe is a ligation-specific oligonucleotide (LSO) which binds immediately adjacent to the site to be interrogated. This common probe is phosphorylated at the 5′ end to enable the ligation reaction. A thermostable DNA ligase is used to ligate either the normal or mutant ASO to the LSO. Ligation only occurs in the presence of a perfect match between the ASO, LSO and amplicon."

Therefore, Dr. Z will use three probes for each pathogenic variant in the *CFTR* gene, according to the ACMG Standards and Guidelines for Clinical Genetics Laboratories.

39. **A.** According to the CAP ACMG Standards and Guidelines for Clinical Genetics Laboratories, 2008 Edition, G8.4, "*The oligonucleotide ligation assay (OLA) has reagents for both mutant allele and the wild type allele together in one reaction, then separate them by either different fluorescent dye or different size of the alleles.* One method of allele detection involves the addition of a mobility modifying tail at the 5′ end of each ASO, with the tail length differing between the mutant and normal alleles. This allows for electrophoretic size separation and therefore differentiation between the normal and mutant alleles. In this case, the LSO probe contains a fluorescent dye marker at the 3′ end to allow detection upon separation. A second method of allele detection involves labeling the 5′ end of the normal and mutant ASO with two different fluorescent dye markers. In this case, the OLA products are the same size but are differentiated by the fluorescence signal detected."

Therefore, one tube of reaction may be used to detect both alleles with oligonucleotide ligation assays (OLA), according to the ACMG Standards and Guidelines for Clinical Genetics Laboratories.

40. **B.** According to the CAP ACMG Standards and Guidelines for Clinical Genetics Laboratories, 2008 Edition, G8.8, "The fluorescence resonance energy transfer (FRET) assay involves two concurrent reactions in a single well on a 96-well plate. *The primary reaction utilizes two different oligonucleotide probes, one specific for the normal sequence and the other specific for the mutant sequence.* Both probes hybridize to the target genomic DNA, forming an overlapping structure. This structure is recognized

by a proprietary enzyme, resulting in the release of a DNA fragment, which forms the substrate for the secondary reaction. The secondary reaction involves the binding of the released DNA fragment to a FRET cassette containing a fluorescent reporter and quencher molecule. The overlapping structure created by the binding of the released DNA fragment to the cassette is recognized by the same enzyme as the primary reaction. The second structure is cleaved, separating the fluorophore and quencher, generating a detectable fluorescence signal. Mismatch between the mutant probe and wild-type target DNA or wild-type probe and mutant target DNA in the primary reaction prevents the formation of the overlapping structure and the generation of the subsequent fluorescent signal. By utilizing two different allele-specific (normal and mutant) probes in the primary reaction, with each binding to a different FRET cassette with a unique spectral fluorophore, 2 sequence variants (normal and mutant) at a single site can be detected in the same well."

Therefore, Dr. Z will use two probes for each pathogenic variant in the *CFTR* gene, according to the ACMG Standards and Guidelines for Clinical Genetics Laboratories.

41. **B.** According to the CAP ACMG Standards and Guidelines for Clinical Genetics Laboratories, 2008 Edition, G8.5 "Some systems (Taqman(r)) use only single labeled probes. This system uses a single internal oligonucleotide probe bearing a 5′ reporter fluorophore (e.g., 6-carboxy-fluorescein) and a 3′ quencher fluorophore (e.g., 6-carboxy-tetra-methyl-rhodamine). During the extension phase the TaqMan(r) probe is hydrolyzed by the nuclease activity of the Taq polymerase, resulting in separation of the reporter and quencher fluorochromes and consequently in an increase in fluorescence. In this technology, the number of PCR cycles necessary to detect a signal above the threshold is called the cycle threshold (Ct) and is directly proportional to the amount of target present at the beginning of the assay. The change in the amount of signal corresponds to the increase in fluorescence intensity when the plateau phase is reached. Using standards or calibrators with a known number of molecules, one can establish a standard curve and determine the precise amount of target present in the test sample."

Therefore, the TaqMan assay has one probe for the *JAK2* V617F variant and another probe for the wild type.

42. **B.** According to the CAP ACMG Standards and Guidelines for Clinical Genetics Laboratories,

2008 Edition, G8.9.1, "Denaturing high performance liquid chromatography (dHPLC) can be used for rapid, automated, and high-throughput mutation detection based on principles similar to those for heteroduplex analysis. . . . This technology is particularly suited for detection of point pathogenic variants, small deletions and insertions. It has also been applied for analysis of fragment size differences and for sensitive detection of sequence differences in minor cell populations such as tumors. The basic principle is that DNA is negatively charged, the column cartridge is neutral, and a positively charged binding ion--triethylammonium acetate (TEAA)--links the two. Heterozygous pathogenic variants are detected through differential binding of homo- and heteroduplexes to the column. Analysis is performed at a temperature sufficient to partially denature heteroduplexes. The melted heteroduplexes are resolved from the corresponding homoduplex by HPLC. Denaturation leads to a reduced double-stranded PCR fragment. *Single-stranded fragments elute earlier than double-stranded fragments due to the reduced negative charge.*"

According to the CAP ACMG Standards and Guidelines for Clinical Genetics Laboratories, 2008 Edition, G8.9.6, "The observation of heteroduplex peaks in a chromatogram indicates the presence of a sequence variant, while samples without base mismatches resolve as homoduplex. *Heteroduplex peaks elute earlier than homoduplex, and can be observed as separate peaks or as shoulders on the leading edge of homoduplex peaks.* The manner in which a heteroduplex peak resolves is influenced by the specific nucleotide mismatch present and the melting characteristics of the surrounding bases. Elution profiles that differ from the wild-type or reference DNA indicate the presence of sequence alterations in the form of base substitutions, deletions, or insertions. One cannot predict the type of mutation (i.e., deletion, insertion, nonsense, etc.) from the heteroduplex pattern."

Therefore, single-stranded fragments are eluted first by the column, followed by heteroduplex, then homoduplex.

43. **D**. Denaturing high-performance liquid chromatography (dHPLC) is designed to detect heteroduplex, and heteroduplexes elute prior to homoduplexes. And "For individuals who are heterozygous for a sequence alteration, heating to 95°C and slowly cooling produces a mixture of heteroduplexes and homoduplexes. However, *for detection of homozygotes, the PCR product from the*

patient is mixed with a comparable amount of wild-type PCR product in order to obtain heteroduplexes."

According to the CAP ACMG Standards and Guidelines for Clinical Genetics Laboratories, 2008 Edition, G8.9.2, "PCR fragment design is critical to the success of dHPLC analysis. dHPLC can be used for fragments up to 600 bp; however, generally optimum separation is achieved with fragments of 200 to 400 bp. For PCR fragment design of regions of large size, it is recommended that overlapping sets of primers be used. It is suggested that the overlap region be a minimum of 50 bp."

Sanger sequencing is the gold standard for the detection of pathogenic variants. In G8.9.1, it states, "Sensitivity depends upon the size and sequence of the PCR fragment, in particular the melting profile, as well as the conditions of analysis, including temperature and buffer concentration. At present, there is no reliable way to predict the sensitivity of detection for novel pathogenic variants, which have been reported in various genes to exceed well over 90%."

dHPLC is a screening tool for pathogenic variants. In G8.9.7 it states "All samples identified as heteroduplexes by dHPLC analysis must be sequenced in both directions to confirm and determine the nature of the sequence change. Each sequence change within a DNA fragment is predicted to have a unique heteroduplex pattern. It is recommended that a pattern file be established for quick identification of specific sequence changes. However, pattern recognition alone is not considered sufficient for diagnostic purposes, particularly when scanning genes for unknown pathogenic variants. In the case of a recurring mutation within a well characterized DNA fragment such as a targeted mutation test, pattern recognition alone may be sufficient for mutation identification. However, sufficient validation is required by the laboratory prior to introduction of such tests."

Therefore, dHPLC is more sensitive for the detection of heterozygotes than homozygotes.

44. **A**. According to the CAP ACMG Standards and Guidelines for Clinical Genetics Laboratories, 2008 Edition, G9.5, "*Stutter artifact tends to be more noticeable with the smaller STR repeat types (mono- and dinucleotide repeats) than with larger repeat units (tetranucleotide repeats).*" There is high error rate during polymerase chain reactions (PCRs) at mononucleotide and dinucleotide repeat sequence motifs. And repeats generally contract during PCR because of the loss of repeat units.

Therefore, mononucleotide repeats tend to be more noticeable for stutter artifact than trinucleotide repeats and pentanucleotide repeats.

45. D. According to the CAP ACMG Standards and Guidelines for Clinical Genetics Laboratories, 2008 Edition, G11.1, "There are several screening methods for the detection of point pathogenic variants, such as single-stranded conformation polymorphism, heteroduplex analysis, denaturing gradient gel electrophoresis, and chemical cleavage. These are powerful tools for the identification of small sequence changes, but fail to detect heterozygous deletions or duplications of exons, genes or chromosomes." *Multiplex ligation-dependent probe amplification (MLPA) is one of standard technologies in the molecular genetics laboratory to detect copy-number changes in targeted genes.*

Therefore, multiplex ligation-dependent probe amplification (MLPA) may be used to detect heterozygous deletions or duplications of exons, genes, or chromosomes.

46. E. *Xeroderma pigmentosum is a defect of nucleotide excision repair causing by pathogenic variants affecting the global genome repair subpathway of nucleotide excision repair or by pathogenic variants affecting postreplication repair.* It is inherited in autosomal recessive matter causing by pathogenic variants in at least eight genes (https://www.ncbi.nlm.nih.gov/books/NBK1397/). Usually missence variants in the genes cause xeroderma pigmentosum. There are a list of disorders primarily caused by defect either due to allelic deletions or duplications, such as Duchenne muscular dystrophy, spinal muscular atrophy, alpha thalassemia, Charcot Marie Tooth type 1, growth hormone deficiency, familial hypercholesterolemia, etc.

Therefore, xeroderma pigmentosum is NOT commonly caused by heterozygous deletions or duplications of exons, genes, or chromosomes.

47. C. According to the CAP ACMG Standards and Guidelines for Clinical Genetics Laboratories, 2008 Edition, G13.1, "When working with RNA, care should be taken to avoid contamination of reagents, lab equipment and disposables with RNases. Methods for RNA isolation may use strong denaturants such as guanidinium hydrochloride or guanidinium thiocyanate to denature endogenous RNases. Gloved hands, new plasticware, barrier tips, and DEPC-treated glassware should be used to minimize contamination with RNases. Specimen temperature is an important consideration. Storage and shipping condition of samples can influence the stability of RNA. *Bone marrow and blood should not be frozen. They should be transported to the lab on wet ice. Solid tissues should be snap frozen and transported on dry ice. RNA stabilizers can be used prior to RNA isolation."*

A quantitative real time RT-PCR assay for the *BCR-ABL1* fusion gene is a RNA-based test. Therefore, bone marrow and peripheral blood specimens should be transported to the lab on wet ice, whereas solid tissues should be transported on dry ice.

48. B. Primers are critical component of the PCR because they determine the specificity of the PCR. Primers are designed to contain sequences complementary to sites flanking the region to be analyzed. *Primers are single-stranded DNA fragments, usually approximately 25 bp in length.* The forward primer hybridizes to the target DNA sequence on the opposite strand just 5-prime (5′) to the sequences to be amplified. The reverse primer hybridizes just 3-prime (3′) to the sequence to be amplified.

Therefore, the primers for both the specificity and efficiency are usually approximately 25 bp.

49. C. Polymerase chain reaction (PCR) is a revolutionary method that was developed by Kary Mullis in the 1980s. *Each cycle of PCR includes three steps: template denaturation, primer annealing, and primer extension.* The initial step denatures the target DNA by heating it to 94°C or higher for 15 s to 2 min. In the denaturation process, the two intertwined strands of DNA separate from one another, producing the necessary single-stranded DNA template for replication by the thermostable DNA polymerase. In the next step of a cycle, the temperature is reduced to approximately 40°C−60°C. At this temperature, the oligonucleotide primers can form stable associations (anneal) with the denatured target DNA and serve as primers for the DNA polymerase. This step lasts approximately 15−60 s. Finally, the synthesis of new DNA begins as the reaction temperature is raised to the optimum for the DNA polymerase. For most thermostable DNA polymerases, this temperature is in the range of 70°C−74°C. The extension step lasts approximately 1−2 min. The next cycle begins with a return to 94°C for denaturation.

Therefore, the correct order for each cycle of PCR reaction is denaturation → annealing → extension.

50. A. *Primer dimmers occur when the forward and reverse primers hybridize to each other owing to the complementary sequence in the primers.* High concentration of primers may inhibit PCR reaction by decreasing the activity of Taq polymerase, but may not cause primer dimer. Low annealing temperature increases random annealing of the primer with nonspecific templates, which increases nonspecific PCR products. High GC content in the primer sequence significantly increases the required annealing temperature, which may interrupt the extension and cause low productivity.

Therefore, complementarity in the primer sequences most likely is the reason for the primer dimer band in this amplicon. Redesigning primers may solve the problem.

51. **D.** *Nonspecific products occur when primers bind to regions other than the intended target, which could be caused by low annealing temperature, high concentration of primers, and pseudogenes.*

Therefore, low annealing temperature, high concentration of primers, and pseudogenes may all result in nonspecific PCR products.

52. **D.** Nonspecific products occur when primers bind to regions other than the intended target, which could be caused by low annealing temperature, high concentration of primers, and pseudogenes.

Therefore, decreasing the concentration of the primers, increasing annealing temperature, and redesigning primers to avoid pseudogenes may all be used to decrease nonspecific PCR products.

53. **E.** One of the biggest strengths of PCR for DNA typing is the degree to which DNA can be amplified. But it can cause problems if great care is not taken to avoid contaminating the reaction with exogenous DNA. In a DNA-typing laboratory, every precaution must be taken to ensure that results are accurate and that unexpected peaks or bands do not cast doubt on the data. *One of the most efficient safeguards to prevent contamination is the separation of preamplification and postamplification areas and equipment.* Use a dedicated set of pipettes, preferably with aerosol-resistant (barrier) tips, in the preamplification area. Do not enter the preamplification area after handling amplified samples or allelic ladders. The use of gloves is essential; be sure to change gloves whenever you move from the preamplification area to the postamplification areas. As much as possible, avoid touching any surfaces or objects with your gloved hands. *For every set of reactions, assemble a negative control reaction and scrutinize the reactions for the presence of unexpected peaks.* After setting up reactions, wash all surfaces with a dilute bleach solution. *PCR contamination can also be limited by using fewer PCR cycles.*

Therefore, a nontemplate control, a reagent blank control, a separate area for PCR setup, and fewer PCR cycle may all be parts of quality control for PCR contamination.

54. **D.** The number of copies of DNA obtained after n cycles $= 2^{(n+1)}$.

55. **D.** 2% agarose gel is best to separate the DNA fragments between 100 bp and 500 bp.

Recommended % agarose	Optimal resolution for linear DNA (bp)
0.5	1000–30,000
0.7	800–12,000
1	500–10,000
1.2	400–7000
1.5	200–3000
2	50–2000

Therefore, 2% agarose gel will be used to resolve the fragments.

56. **B.** 0.5% agarose gel is best to separate the DNA fragments between 2000 and 8000 bp.

Recommended % agarose	Optimal resolution for linear DNA (bp)
0.5	1000–30,000
0.7	800–12,000
1	500–10,000
1.2	400–7000
1.5	200–3000
2	50–2000

Therefore, 0.5% agarose gels will be use to resolve the fragments.

57. **F.** DNA fragments are negatively charged in the buffer and migrate from cathode (−) toward anode (+) in an electric field. *The biggest fragment migrates slower than others.* The smallest fragment migrates faster than others.

Therefore, the biggest PCR product is sample F in this agarose gel.

58. **B.** DNA fragments are negatively charged in the buffer and migrate from cathode (−) toward anode (+) in an electric field. The biggest fragment migrates more slowly than the others. *The smallest fragment migrates faster than others.*

Therefore, the smallest PCR product is sample B in this agarose gel.

59. **F.** Hereditary hemochromatosis (HH) is an autosomal recessive disorder characterized by enhanced intestinal absorption of dietary iron. *The major mutation associated with HH is the p. Cys282Tyr (c.845G > A) in the HFE gene that occurs in approximately 80% of HH cases.* In addition, a high proportion of the remaining patients are compound heterozygous for the p.Cys282Tyr and the common p.His63Asp (c.187C > G) alteration.

A third mutation may also be assessed, which is the substitution of cysteine for serine at amino acid position 65 (p.Ser65Cys, c.193A > T). p. Cys282Tyr may be detected with Rsa 1, and p. His63Asp is detected with Mbo I. Sample A has exactly the same digested fragment pattern as C.

Therefore, the sample A genotype is homozygous for p.C282Y/p.C282Y.

60. **A**. Hereditary hemochromatosis (HH) is an autosomal recessive disorder characterized by enhanced intestinal absorption of dietary iron. The major mutation associated with HH is the p. Cys282Tyr (c.845G > A) in the *HFE* gene that occurs in approximately 80% of HH cases. In addition, a high proportion of the remaining patients are compound heterozygous for the p. Cys282Tyr and the common p.His63Asp (c.187C > G) alteration. A third mutation may also be assessed, which is the substitution of cysteine for serine at amino acid position 65 (p.Ser65Cys, c.193A > T). p.Cys282Tyr may be detected with Rsa 1, and p.His63Asp is detected with Mbo I. *Sample B shows no p.C282Y digestion on the top part of the gel, and no p.H63D digestion on the bottom part of the gel as compared with the homozygous p.C282Y/ p.C282Y control ("C"), and the compound heterozygous p.C282Y/p.H63D control ("D").*

Therefore, sample B is homozygous for wild type/wild type.

61. **C**. All the chemistries in the question can be used to detect DNA. *Radioactive P^{32} remains the most sensitive one, followed by fluorescence and luciferase.* Silver stain and ethidium bromide are less sensitive than the others.

Therefore, isotopic P^{32} is the most sensitive for DNA detection.

62. **A**. According to the ACMG Standards and Guidelines for Fragile X test, 2013, fragile X syndrome is caused by the deficiency or absence of FMR1 protein. Theoretically, this can occur through any type of deletion or inactivation mutation, but in more than 99% of cases, there is an expansion of a segment of CGG repeats in the 5′ untranslated region of *FMR1*. Large CGG expansions in this region are associated with hypermethylation and inhibition of transcription.

Laboratories will likely need to use more than one method, because no single method can characterize all aspects of the *FMR1* full mutation, and precision in determining allele size varies between PCR and Southern blot analysis. For mosaic samples spanning the premutation and full mutation ranges, traditional PCR may amplify the premutation population but not the subpopulation with the full mutation. The expected phenotype for an individual with a premutation versus mosaicism for a premutation and full mutation is very different. Therefore, not detecting the full mutation would result in a different risk assessment for fragile X, FXTAS and FXPOI. For this reason, the ACMG policy statement recommends that Southern blot analysis always be performed along with traditional PCR, even if a premutation allele is identified by traditional PCR.

Amplification of CG-rich regions is difficult, and special conditions are required. The difficulty increases with increasing numbers of CGG repeats. Therefore, *many PCR strategies do not attempt to detect large alleles.* When a PCR strategy is capable of detecting large alleles, amplification nevertheless may favor the smaller allele in any specimen with multiple alleles (i.e., females and mosaics). Basic PCR amplification is not affected by methylation. Although PCR tests specifically modified to detect methylation status have been described, the original PCR strategies that have been in use for many years are completely independent of methylation.

When Southern blot analysis uses the StB12.3 probe and genomic DNA digested with EagI/ EcoRI, it may take 3–4 days. The size of the digestion products is between 2000 and 8000 bp. It may detect full mutation and review methylation status of the alleles. It helps to discriminate between prepathogenic variants and full pathogenic variants for the alleles that fall near the boundary (i.e., around 200 repeats) and in the detection of individuals who are methylation mosaics.

Therefore, the analyzable DNA fragments for PCR are usually smaller than the ones for Southern blot.

63. **C**. Conditions for Southern blot hybridization must be empirically optimized for each nucleic acid target. If the stringency is too high, faint or no bands will be present on the autoradiogram. Several factors affect stringency. These include temperature of hybridization, salt concentration of the hybridization buffer, and concentration of denaturant such as formamide in the buffer (high temperature, high formamide, and low salt is more stringent). *Decreasing the hybridization temperature makes the hybridization less stringent, which increases the chance that probe will anneal with the target genomic DNA in the sample.* The length and nature of the probe sequence can also influence the level of stringency. A long probe or one with a higher percentage of G and C bases will bind under more stringent conditions than a

short probe or one with greater numbers of A and T bases. Formamide in the hybridization buffer effectively lowers the optimal hybridization temperature. Switching to another company is never a good option.

Therefore, in this case, the hybridization temperature may be decreased to increase hybridization.

64. **B**. Conditions for Southern blot hybridization must be empirically optimized for each nucleic acid target. If the stringency is too high, faint or no bands will be present on the autoradiogram. Several factors affect stringency. These include temperature of hybridization, salt concentration of the hybridization buffer, and concentration of denaturant such as formamide in the buffer (high temperature, high formamide, and low salt is more stringent). *Increasing the NaCl concentration makes the hybridization less stringent, which increases the chance that probe will anneal with the target genomic DNA in the sample.* The length and nature of the probe sequence can also influence the level of stringency. A long probe or one with a higher percentage of G and C bases will bind under more stringent conditions than a short probe or one with greater numbers of A and T bases. Formamide in the hybridization buffer effectively lowers the optimal hybridization temperature. Switching to another company is never a good option.

Therefore, in this case, the concentration of NaCl in the hybridization buffer may be increased to increase hybridization.

65. **A**. Southern blot hybridization condition must be empirically optimized for each nucleic acid target. If the stringency is too high, faint or no bands will be present on the autoradiogram. Several factors affect stringency. These include temperature of hybridization, salt concentration of the hybridization buffer, and the concentration of denaturant such as formamide in the buffer (high temperature, high formamide, and low salt is more stringent). *Decreasing the formamide concentration makes the hybridization less stringent, which increases the chance that probe anneals with the target genomic DNA in the sample.* The length and nature of the probe sequence can also influence the level of stringency. A long probe or one with a higher percentage of G and C bases will bind under more stringent conditions than a short probe or one with greater number s of A and T bases will bind. Formamide in the hybridization buffer effectively lowers the optimal hybridization temperature. Switch to another company is never a good option.

Therefore, in this case, the formamide in the hybridization buffer may be decreased to increase hybridization.

66. **A**. The ideal hybridization conditions are estimated from calculation of the melting temperature, or T_m, of the probe sequence. The T_m is a way to express the amount of energy required to separate the hybridized strands of a given sequence. At the T_m, half of the sequence is double-stranded and half is single-stranded. The T_m for short probes (14–20 bases) can be calculated by a simplified formula:

$$T_m = 4°C \times \text{number of GC pairs} + 2°C \times \text{number of AT pairs}$$

The hybridization temperature of oligonucleotide probes is about 5°C below the melting temperature.[4] The sequence in choice A has a high GC content. Therefore, the prime in choice A has the highest T_m value.

67. **C**. DNA fragments are negatively charged in the buffer and migrate from cathode (−) toward anode (+) in an electric field. This is an autoradiogram of a dideoxy sequencing gel. The letters over the lanes in the figure indicate which dideoxynucleotide was used in the sample being represented by that lane. *When you read from the bottom up, you are reading the DNA sequence.*

Therefore, the correct DNA sequence is GACCGTTATACGGGTACTTGCA (choice C).

68. **D**. Automated DNA sequencers generate a four-color chromatogram showing the results of the sequencing run. A single peak position within a trace may have two peaks of different colors instead of just one. This is common when sequencing a PCR product derived from diploid genomic DNA, where polymorphic positions will show both nucleotides simultaneously. Note that the software may list that base position as an "N" or it may simply call it the larger of the two peaks. The figure in the question is an example of a chromatogram of a DNA sequence with a heterozygous single-nucleotide polymorphism (SNP).

In this case, one allele carries a "C," while the other one has a "T." Both peaks are present, but at roughly half the height they would show if they were homozygous. Therefore, it is a C/T heterozygote (choice D).

69. **D**. Automated DNA sequencers generate a four-color chromatogram showing the results of the sequencing run. A single peak position within a trace may have two peaks of different colors instead of just one. This is common when sequencing a PCR product derived from diploid genomic DNA, where polymorphic positions will

show both nucleotides simultaneously. Note that the software may list that base position as an "N," or it may simply call it the larger of the two peaks. The figure in the question is an example of chromatogram of a DNA sequence with a heterozygous single-nucleotide polymorphism (SNP). In this case, one allele carries a C, while the other has a T. Both peaks are present, but at roughly half the height they would show if they were homozygous.

SNPs may cause silent, missense, nonsense, and splicing site pathogenic variants, but not frameshift mutation. Therefore, the patient does NOT have a frameshift mutation according to this chromatograph.

70. **D**. The sequencing peaks are not "clean." It looks like multiple peaks with the same height or different heights overlapping one another.

Therefore, all three reasons listed in the question are possible.

71. **B**. *Locus heterogeneity means that variations in completely unrelated genes cause one disorder*. For example, long-QT syndrome may be caused by pathogenic variants from more than 15 genes with the autosomal dominant, autosomal recessive, or X-linked inherited mode.

In contrast, pleiotropy means that one gene may cause multiple phenotypic expressions or disorders. For example, phenylketonuria affects multiple organ systems but is caused by one gene defect, *PAH*. Allelic heterogeneity means that different pathogenic variants within one gene cause the same phenotypic expression. For example, there are over 1000 known mutant alleles of the *CFTR* gene that cause CF. Epistasis is a phenomenon that consists of the effect of one gene being dependent on the presence of one or more modifier genes (genetic background). A haplotype is a set of DNA variations, or polymorphisms, that tend to be inherited together (http://ghr.nlm.nih.gov).

Therefore, this is an example of locus heterogeneity.

72. **C**. *Restriction sites are the recognition site of restriction enzymes, which are usually palindromic sequences*. A particular restriction enzyme may cut the sequence between two nucleotides within its recognition site or somewhere nearby. For example, HindIII, a common restriction enzyme, recognizes the palindromic sequence AAGCTT and cuts between the two As, leaving an 5' overhang on each end. *The GAATTC is the EcoRI recognition site. The cutting site is between G and A, also leaving a 5' overhang.*

Therefore, GAATTC is most likely to be a recognition site of a restriction enzyme.

73. **C**. *A potential single nucleotide polymorphism (SNP) at the 5' end of a primer, but not 3' SNP in the primer, is tolerable for PCR reaction.* A 3' end SNP may cause and allelic drop during PCR, which may cause a heterozygous mutation in the amplicon to be missed or to be misinterpreted as a homozygous mutation.

Therefore, 5' GCCACCACGCTCTTCTGTCt/c most likely won't work.

74. **A**. One of the most important factors in successful automated DNA sequencing is proper primer design. Here are a few things to remember about how to examine a DNA sequence to choose an appropriate primer sequence (https://seqcore. brcf.med.umich.edu/sites/default/files/html/ primers.html):
- Length should be between 18 and 30 nt, with optimal being 20–25 nt.
- GC content of 40%–60% is desirable.
- The T_m should be between 55°C and 75°C.
- Discard candidate primers that show undesirable self-hybridization (option C).
- More than seven consecutive homologous nucleotides at the 3' end (option B).

5' Gc/tCACCACGCTCTTCTGTCT has a SNP at the 5' end of the primer, which is tolerable for PCR reaction. 5' GACGGCACACCACACCTCt/c has a SNP at the 3' end of the primer. 5' AAGGGGGACAGC ATCCCCCC has poly G and poly C, which may self-hybridize. 5' CCTCGGACGCCCACCCACCGG has high GC content. Therefore, the correct answer is choice A.

75. **C**. Primers are used to determine the DNA fragment to be amplified by the PCR process and are always written from 5' to 3'. One of the two primers will anneal to one strand, and another primer will anneal to the opposite strand. Pairs of primers should have similar melting temperatures, since annealing in a PCR occurs for both simultaneously. Primer sequences need to be chosen to uniquely select for a region of DNA, avoiding the possibility of mishybridization to a similar sequence nearby. Mononucleotide and dinucleotide repeats should be avoided, as loop formation can occur and contribute to mishybridization.

Therefore, the correct answer that 5' GTACCACGCTCTTCTGTCT and GGCGACTGTACGCTTCGGTTC are the pair of primer for exon 3 of the oncogene.

76. **A**. "Reverse complement" is also called "antiparallel." One example is the sequence ATGC converted to GCAT.

Therefore, GUUCA and UGAAC in choice A are reverse complementary sequences.

77. **A**. According to ACMG guidelines, there are five interpretive categories of sequence variations:

- Pathogenic: sequence variation is previously reported to cause the disorder.
- Likely pathogenic: sequence variation is previously unreported and is expected cause the disorder.
- Unknown clinical significance: sequence variation is previously unreported and is of the type which may or may not be causative of the disorder.
- Likely benign: sequence variation is previously unreported and is probably not causative of the disorder.
- *Benign: sequence variation is previously reported and is a recognized neutral variant.*

A variant seen in 10% of any normal population is a benign (neutral) variant regardless of the population it presents. Therefore, this $G > T$ variant is benign.

78. **D**. The 2-bp deletion is a de novo variant and has not been identified in normal populations. It is in the middle of an exon of an OMIM disease gene for an autosomal dominant disease, which causes frameshift. So it has the potential to alter the function of the protein. However, since it has not been identified in any patients, it should be called "likely pathogenic," according to ACMG guidelines.

Therefore, this variant is considered to be likely pathogenic.

79. **E**. *TAA, TAG, and TGA are stop codons. TGG codes for tryptophan (Trp/W).* A terminal codon changes to a tryptophan in this case, which cause a nonstop change in the amino acid sequence.

Therefore, this variant is a nonstop variant.

80. **D**. The mutation is a de novo mutation, and has not been identified in normal populations. It is a nonstop mutation, which changes the terminal codon to tryptophan, so it has the potential to alter the function of the protein. However, since it has not been identified in any patients, it should be called "likely pathogenic," according to ACMG guidelines.

Therefore, this variant is considered to be likely pathogenic.

81. **C**. *EDTA in the buffer reduces DNase activity.* EDTA is a chelating agent, which chelates the magnesium ions in solution. Magnesium ions are cofactors for nuclease (DNase and RNase). In the presence of EDTA, magnesium ions will not be available for DNase. DNase-free reagents also may be used to prevent a DNA sample from

degrading. However, it is very costly and labor-intensive to run DNase-free gels.

Therefore, EDTA would be most appropriate for him to use to prevent nucleic acid samples from degrading during gel electrophoresis.

82. **D**. *TGG is the codon for tryptophan.* TAA, TAG, and TGA are all stop codons.

TGG is NOT a stop codon.

83. **B**. TAA, TAG, and TGA are all stop codons. *TAT and TAC code for tyrosine (Tyr/Y).*

Therefore, TAT is NOT a stop codon.

84. **A**. *TAA, TAG, and TGA are stop codons.* TAT and TAC code for tyrosine (Tyr/Y). TTA and TTG code for leucine (Leu/L). TGT and TGC code for cysteine (Cys/C).

Therefore, TAG is a stop codon.

85. **C**. *TAA, TAG, and TGA are stop codons.* TAT and TAC code for tyrosine (Tyr/Y). *TGT and TGC code for cysteine (Cys/C).*

Therefore, TGA is a stop codon.

86. **B**. *ATG codes for methionine and also serves as the transcript initiation site.* ATT, ATC, and ATA code for isoleucine (Ile/I). *TAA, TAG, and TGA are stop codons.*

Therefore, ATG is the start codon.

87. **D**. Nearly all splice sites conform to consensus sequences. *These consensus sequences include nearly invariant dinucleotides at each end of the intron, GT at the 5′ end of the intron and AG at the 3′ end.* When a splice-site mutation occurs, the mRNA transcript possesses information from these introns that normally should not be included.

Therefore, the variant in the question may be a splice-site mutation.

88. **B**. Alport syndrome (AS) is a heterogeneous disorder, characterized by renal, cochlear, and ocular dysfunction. It is caused by pathogenic variants in the type IV collagen genes, *COL4A3, COL4A4,* and *COL4A5. Variants in the* COL4A5 *gene cause X-linked AS.*

The high-resolution melting analysis (HRMA) assay is sensitive for the detection of heterozygosity, or a homozygosity/hemizygosity variant mixed with a wild- type control. The amplicons are melted slowly by increasing the temperature to 95°C−96°C at a rate of 0.1°C/s. This forces the heteroduplex of the mutant allele and the wild-type allele in the heterozygous carrier, or the mixture of a hemizygosity and a wild-type control, melting more easily than homoduplexes of homozygous mutant or normal alleles.

Therefore, a peripheral-blood specimen from this patient mixed with a wild-type control in a 1:1 ratio will most likely show a positive result with the HRMA assay if the patient has a *COL4A5* hemizygous variant.

89. **E.** The disease in the pedigree is X-linked, which affects only males and skips generations. The mother of the proband carries one normal copy and one abnormal copy of the gene for the disease. *X inactivation is the mechanism by which one of the two chromosome Xs is randomly silenced in each cell of females.* Female carriers of an X-linked recessive disease are usually NOT affected or are only mildly affected except in cases of extremely skewed X activation.

When a mutation happens during mitosis and passes on to the next generation, it is a de novo mutation, rather than an inherited one. Penetrance refers to the proportion of people with a particular genetic change who exhibit signs and symptoms of a genetic disorder. If some people with the mutation do not develop features of the disorder, the condition is said to have reduced or incomplete penetrance. For example, many people with a mutation in the *BRCA1* or *BRCA2* gene will develop cancer during their lifetime, but some people will not. Physicians cannot predict which individual with these pathogenic variants will develop cancer or when the tumors will develop (http://ghr.nlm.nih.gov). *Variable expression* refers to the range of signs and symptoms that can occur in different people with the same genetic condition. For example, the features of Marfan syndrome vary widely—some people have only mild symptoms (such as being tall and thin with long, slender fingers), while others also experience life-threatening complications involving the heart and blood vessels. Although the features are highly variable, most people with this disorder have a mutation in *FBN1*. There is no clear definition for clinical heterogeneity.

Therefore, the mother of the proband in this question does NOT have symptoms owing to X inactivation.

90. **C.** *The disease in the pedigree looks like an autosomal dominant disease with reduced penetrance.* Penetrance refers to the proportion of people with a particular genetic change who exhibit signs and symptoms of a genetic disorder. If some people with the mutation do not develop features of the disorder, the condition is said to have reduced or incomplete penetrance. For example, many people with a mutation in the *BRCA1* or *BRCA2* gene will develop cancer during their lifetime, but some people will not. Physicians cannot predict which individual with these pathogenic variants will develop cancer or when the tumors will develop (http://ghr.nlm.nih.gov).

When a mutation happens during mitosis and passes on to the next generation, it is a de novo mutation, rather than an inherited one. Variable expressivity refers to the range of signs and symptoms that can occur in different people with the same genetic condition. For example, the features of Marfan syndrome vary widely—some people have only mild symptoms (such as being tall and thin with long, slender fingers), while others also experience life-threatening complications involving the heart and blood vessels. Although the features are highly variable, most people with this disorder have a mutation in *FBN1*. X inactivation is the mechanism by which one of the two chromosome Xs is randomly silenced in each cell of females. Therefore, female carriers of an X-linked recessive disease are usually NOT affected or are only mildly affected except in cases of extremely skewed X activation. There is no clear definition for clinical heterogeneity.

Therefore, reduced penetrance most likely explains the reason why the proband's mother does NOT have symptoms of this disorder.

91. **C.** The Philadelphia chromosome (Ph), a reciprocal translocation of the long arms of chromosomes 9 and 22, is found in >90% patients with chronic myeloid leukemia (CML) and 15%–25% of patients with acute lymphoblastic leukemia (ALL). This translocation transposes the *ABL1* oncogene from chromosome 9q34 to the *BCR* gene on chromosome 22q11. The fused *BCR-ABL1* gene and its gene products provide specific markers for diagnosis and disease monitoring. Since there are lots of breakpoints on *BCR* and *ABL1* genes, it is technically hard to amplify the fusion gene by genomic DNA (gDNA) analysis. *Also for better monitoring of disease progress, and efficacy of therapy, mRNA from specimens is used to test BCR-ABL.* Messenger RNA (mRNA) conveys genetic codes from DNA to RNA, then the codes in the mRNA translated into amino acid sequence. Reverse transcriptase is used first to convert mRNA into cDNA before quantitative PCR.

A transfer RNA (tRNA) serves as the physical link between the mRNA and the amino acid sequence of proteins. It does this by carrying an amino acid to ribosomes as directed by a codon in an mRNA sequence. The specific nucleotide sequence of an mRNA specifies which amino acid is incorporated into the protein product of the gene from which the mRNA is transcribed, and the role of tRNA is to specify which sequence from the genetic code corresponds to which amino acid. Complementary DNA (cDNA) is single-stranded DNA synthesized from mRNA templates by reverse transcriptase.

Therefore, mRNA would be extracted from the specimen for the test.

92. **A**. *As the concentration of the fusion gene increases, the growth curves shift to earlier cycles.* Therefore, the curve would be shifted to the left if the concentration of the target increased (was not diluted).

93. **A**. *For quantitative PCR, as the concentration of the fusion gene increases, the growth curves shift to earlier cycles.* Therefore, the leftmost growth curve (A) corresponds to the highest concentration of fusion gene, whereas, the rightmost growth curve (D) corresponds to the lowest concentration of fusion gene.

94. **A**. The slope of a standard curve is commonly used to estimate the PCR amplification efficiency of a real-time PCR reaction. The standard curve plots the log of starting template versus the PCR cycle number (copy numbers of PCR products). A linear fit with a slope between approximately -3.1 and -3.6, equivalent to a calculated 90%–110% reaction efficiency, is typically acceptable for most applications requiring accurate quantification. If the amplification reaction is not efficient at the point being used to extrapolate back to the amount of starting material (usually the C_t is used for this purpose), then the calculated quantities may not be accurate. Since the PCR reaction is based on exponential amplification, if the efficiency of PCR amplification is 100%, the amount of the total template is expected to double with each cycle. This assumption allows the reliable calculation of quantity from Ct, and thus $\sim$100% qPCR efficiency needs to be assessed and verified prior to running valuable samples. Slopes more negative than -3.32 (e.g., -4.2) indicate reactions that are less than 100% efficient, and it takes longer to reach the C_t value. Panel A is expressed as $Y = b - aX$ (e.g., $Y = 20 - 3.32X$). Panel B is expressed as $Y = b + aX$ (e.g., $Y = 20 + 3.32X$). Panel C is $Y = -b + aX$ (e.g., $Y = -20 + 3.32X$). Panel D is $Y = -b - aX$ (e.g., $Y = -20 - 3.32X$). "a" and "b" are any numbers from 1 to 9. "$-a$" represents the slope. "i" represents the value on the Y axis when the $X = 0$.

Therefore, Panel A is the correct one.

95. **D**. PCR amplification efficiency is the rate at which a PCR amplicon is generated commonly expressed as a percentage value. If a particular PCR amplicon doubles in quantity during the geometric phase of its PCR amplification, then the PCR assay has 100% efficiency. The slope of a standard curve is commonly used to estimate the PCR amplification efficiency of a real-time PCR reaction. A real-time PCR standard curve is graphically represented as a semilog regression line plot of C_t value versus the log of input nucleic acid. *A standard curve slope of -3.32 indicates a PCR reaction with 100% efficiency.* Slopes more negative than -3.32 (e.g., -3.9) indicate reactions that are less than 100% efficient. Slopes more positive than -3.32 (e.g., -2.5) may indicate sample quality or pipetting problems. A 100% efficient reaction will yield a 10-fold increase in PCR amplicon every 3.32 cycles during the exponential phase of amplification. If we use the equation $Y = -aX + b$, then "$-a$" represents the slope and "b" represents the value on the Y-axis when the $X = 0$.

Therefore, choice D is the correct one.

96. **D**. The slope of a standard curve is commonly used to estimate the PCR amplification efficiency of a real-time PCR reaction. The standard curve plots the log of the starting template versus the PCR cycle number (copy numbers of PCR products). A linear fit with a slope between approximately -3.1 and -3.6, equivalent to a calculated 90%–110% reaction efficiency, is typically acceptable for most applications requiring accurate quantification. If the amplification reaction is not efficient at the point being used to extrapolate back to the amount of starting material (usually the C_t is used for this purpose), then the calculated quantities may not be accurate. Since the PCR reaction is based on exponential amplification, if the efficiency of PCR amplification is 100%, the amount of the total template is expected to double with each cycle. This assumption allows the reliable calculation of quantity from Ct, and thus $\sim$100% qPCR efficiency needs to be assessed and verified prior to running valuable samples. *Slopes more negative than -3.32 (e.g., in choices A, B, and C) indicate reactions that are less than 100% efficient, and it takes longer to reach Ct value.*

Therefore, choice D is the most efficient one.

97. **A**. The TaqMan assay was named after *Taq* DNA polymerase, which was one of the earliest methods introduced for real-time PCR reaction monitoring and has been widely adopted for both the quantification of mRNAs and for detecting variation. *The method exploits the 5' endonuclease activity of Taq DNA polymerase to cleave an*

oligonucleotide probe during PCR, thereby release the fluorescence from the quencher to generate a detectable signal. TaqMan probes consist of a fluorophore covalently attached to the 5′ end of the oligonucleotide probe and a quencher at the 3′ end. Specificity is conferred at three levels: via two PCR primers and the probe. Applied Biosystems (ABI) probes also include a minor groove binder for added specificity.

Therefore, probes are fluorescence-labeled for signal detection in TaqMan assays.

98. **E.** The TaqMan method was first reported in 1991 by researchers at Cetus Corporation. TaqMan probes consist of a fluorophore covalently attached to the 5′ end of the oligonucleotide probe and a quencher at the 3′ end. The quencher molecule quenches the fluorescence emitted by the fluorophore when excited by the cycler's light source via FRET (Fluorescence Resonance Energy Transfer). *The TaqMan principle relies on the 5′−3′ exonuclease activity of Taq polymerase to cleave a dual-labeled probe (fluorescence and quencher) during hybridization to the complementary target sequence and fluorophore-based detection.* As the Taq polymerase extends the primer and synthesizes the reverse complement strand, the 5′−3′ exonuclease activity of the Taq polymerase degrades the probe that has annealed to the template. Degradation of the probe releases the fluorophore from it and breaks the close proximity to the quencher, relieving the quenching effect and allowing fluorescence of the fluorophore. Hence, fluorescence detected in the quantitative PCR thermal cycler is directly proportional to the fluorophore released and the amount of DNA template present in the PCR.

Therefore, TaqMan assay uses Taq polymerase's 5′−3′ exonuclease activity to release fluorescence signal from quencher.

99. **A.** V600E (c.1799T > A) is the most common mutation in the *BRAF* gene associated with melanomas, nonsmall-cell lung cancers, colorectal cancer, papillary thyroid carcinoma, and Langerhans-cell histiocytosis patients. V600K (c.1798_1799GT > AA) is one of less common mutations in *BRAF*. Inhibition of *BRAF* with vemurafenib improves survival in patients with V600E mutation and in patients with the less common V600K mutation. TaqMan method exploits the 5′ endonuclease activity of *Taq* DNA polymerase to cleave an oligonucleotide probe during PCR, thereby releasing the fluorescence from the quencher to generate a detectable signal.

For SNP genotyping, TaqMan assays two probes for two alleles that are fluorescently labeled at their 5′ end with FAM or VIC, respectively. The 3′ end of the probes is the quencher. The TaqMan for V600E in *BRAF* only has probes for T or A at location 1799. *Since the TaqMan probes are allelic-specific, the assay for V600E cannot detect the V600K (c.1798_1799GT > AA) allele.*

Therefore, a heterozygous V600K mutation will be recognized as homozygous wild type, since there will be a signal for wild type, but no signal from the V600E mutant allele.

100. **B.** *The pedigree and the genotyping results indicate that the maternal grandfather, the mother, and BJ share a null allele in the gene associated with this late-onset autosomal dominant disease, which is not in other family members.* The null allele may be caused by a gross deletion beyond the PCR region for this marker. It is also possible that there is a mutation in the primer region, which cosegregates with the disease in this family. Re-PCR and Sanger sequencing with another pair of primers outside of the current primers will clarify the possibility of a mutation in the primer region.

Therefore, there is a good chance BJ will have this disease, since the null allele segregates with the disease in the family.

101. **B.** *The pedigree and the genotyping results indicate that the maternal grandfather, the mother, and BJ share a null allele in the gene associated with this late-onset autosomal dominant disease, which is not in other family members.* The null allele segregates with the disease in the family. The null allele may be caused by a gross deletion beyond the PCR region for this marker. It is also possible that there is a mutation in the primer region, which cosegregates with the disease in this family. Re-PCR and Sanger sequencing with another pair of primers outside of the current primers will clarify the possibility of a mutation in the primer region.

Therefore, most likely BJ is heterozygous for a deletion (genotype: 1/deletion).

102. **B.** The most common way to detect microsatellites (short tandem repeats, STR) is to use PCR primers that are unique and are on either side of the repeated portion. The PCR products are then separated by either gel electrophoresis or fluorescence capillary electrophoresis. The size of the PCR product can be determined. Thus, copies of the repeats for each allele can be determined. *PCR with capillary electrophoresis is more commonly used than gel electrophoresis, since it less labor-intensive and*

potentially has higher throughput than gel electrophoresis. Applied Biosystems (ABI) and Promega have premade kits for sets of STR markers for forensic genetic analysis.

Allelic-specific PCR, PCR-RFLP, and TaqMan genotyping assay are methods for single-nucleotide polymorphism (SNP) analysis instead of STR.

Therefore, PCR and fluorescence capillary electrophoresis would be most commonly used for microsatellite analysis in clinical laboratories nowadays.

103. **B**. A genome-wide association study (GWAS) is an approach that involves rapidly scanning markers across the complete sets of human genomes of many people to find genetic variations associated with common diseases, such as coronary artery disease. Once new genetic associations are identified, researchers can use the information to develop better strategies to detect, treat, and prevent the disease. Such studies are particularly useful in finding genetic variations that contribute to common, complex diseases, such as asthma, cancer, diabetes, heart disease, and mental illnesses. There are roughly 1 million "effectively independent" common single nucleotide polymorphisms (SNPs) in the human genome, which makes it is the most abundant type of polymorphism. *GWASs were made possible by the availability of chip-based microarray technology for assaying 1 million or more SNPs, since SNPs typically have two alleles.*

The number of RFLP markers in the human genome is limited by the restriction enzyme recognition sites. STR (microsatellites, short tandem repeats, STR) markers are highly polymorphic; however, it is hard to develop high-throughput methods for STR analysis. Besides, STR markers are not as abundant as SNP markers in human genome. VNTRs are relatively large genetic markers, which are difficult to detect with STRs and SNPs.

Therefore, SNPs would be more appropriate markers for this study than the other choices listed.

104. **B**. *A genome-wide association study (GWAS) is an approach that involves rapidly scanning markers across the complete sets of human genomes of many people to find genetic variations associated with common diseases, such as Crohn disease, hypertension, diabetes, and bipolar disorder.* The remaining diseases in the question are not common. Smith–Magenis is an autosomal dominant microdeletion syndrome. Genetic forms of

hearing loss could be autosomal dominant, autosomal recessive, or X-linked recessive. Autosomal recessive hearing loss may be studied with exome sequencing, but not GWAS. And Myoclonic Epilepsy with Ragged Red Fibers (MERRF) is a mitochondrial inherited disease.

Therefore, Crohn disease would be more appropriate for GWAS studies than the other choices listed.

105. **C**. The four affected children in the family have a same genotype for this tetranucleotide repeat. *The first of the four affected children sets the phase. For each subsequent affected child, the chance of receiving the same genotype is 1/4.* Therefore, the probability that all of the subsequent affected children would inherited the same tetranucleotide genotype is $1/4 \times 1/4 \times 1/4 = 1/64$.

Therefore, the odds of obtaining a result linkage by chance would be 1 in 64.

106. **A**. The three affected children in the family have the same genotype for this tetranucleotide repeat. *The first of the three affected children in this family sets the phase. For each subsequent affected child, the chance of receiving the same genotype is 1/4.* Therefore, the probability that all of the subsequent affected children would inherited the same tetranucleotide genotype is $1/4 \times 1/4 = 1/16$.

Therefore, the odds of obtaining a result linkage by chance would be 1 in 16.

107. **B**. *Genetic heterogeneity is used to describe disorders or traits caused by genetic and nongenetic factors. Another example of genetic heterogeneity is diabetes, which has both genetic and environmental components.*

Penetrance refers to the proportion of people with a particular mutation in a specific gene who exhibit signs and symptoms of a genetic disorder. If some people with the mutation do not develop features of the disorder, the condition is said to have reduced (or incomplete) penetrance. One example of reduced penetrance is familial cancer syndromes, such as *BRCA1*- and *BRCA2*-related hereditary breast cancer. Not everyone with mutation(s) in *BRCA1* or *BRCA2* has breast cancer (http://ghr.nlm.nih.gov). Variable expressivity refers to the range of signs and symptoms that can occur in different people with the same genetic condition. One example of variable expression is Marfan syndrome. Marfan syndrome may have variable severity of symptoms even in the same family (http://ghr.nlm.nih.gov). Dominant-negative is used to describe a mutation whose gene product adversely affects the normal, wild-type gene product within the same cell, usually by dimerizing (combining) with it. In cases of polymeric molecules, such as collagen, dominant-negative pathogenic variants are often more deleterious than pathogenic variants causing the production of no gene product (null pathogenic variants or null alleles). One example of a dominant-negative mutation is osteogenesis imperfecta (OI) caused by pathogenic variants in *COL1A1* and *COL1A2* (http://ghr.nlm.nih.gov). Pleiotropy is used to describe multiple, often seemingly unrelated, physical effects caused by a single altered gene or pair of altered genes. One example of it is pathogenic variants in *KCNQ1*, which may cause autosomal dominant Romano–Ward syndrome or autosomal recessive Jervell and Lange–Nielsen syndrome.

Therefore, genetic heterogeneity may be used to describe the complex inheritance mode of age-related macular degeneration (AMD).

108. **C.** An odds ratio (OR) is a measure of association between an exposure and an outcome. The OR represents the odds that an outcome will occur given a particular exposure, compared to the odds of the outcome occurring in the absence of that exposure. Odds ratios are most commonly used in case–control studies; however, they can also be used in cross-sectional and cohort study designs as well (with some modifications and/or assumptions).

		Outcome status	
		+	–
Exposure status	+	*a*	*B*
	–	*c*	*D*

$$OR = \frac{a/b}{c/d} = \frac{30/70}{10/90} = \frac{2700}{700} = 3.86$$

Therefore, 3.86 is the most likely odds that AMD is associated with smoking status.

109. **B.** Relative risk or risk ratio (RR) is the ratio of the probability of an event occurring (e.g., developing a disease) in an exposed group to the probability of the event occurring in a comparison, nonexposed group.

		Outcome status	
		+	–
Exposure status	+	*a*	*B*
	–	*c*	*D*

$$RR = \frac{a/(a+b)}{c/(c+d)} = \frac{30/100}{10/100} = 3$$

Therefore, 3 most likely is the relative risk for AMD with smoking status.

110. **A.** *Dominant-negative mutation is used to describe a mutation whose gene product adversely affects the normal, wild-type gene product within the same cell, usually by dimerizing (combining) with it.* In cases of polymeric molecules, such as collagen, dominant-negative pathogenic variants are often more deleterious than pathogenic variants, causing the production of no gene product (null pathogenic variants or null alleles). Osteogenesis imperfecta (OI) is a good example of a dominant-negative mutation, which is caused by pathogenic variants in *COL1A1* and *COL1A2* (http://ghr.nlm.nih.gov).

Genetic heterogeneity is used to describe disorders or traits caused by genetic and nongenetic factors. One example of genetic heterogeneity is Crohn disease, which has both genetic and environmental components (http://ghr.nlm.nih.gov). Penetrance refers to the proportion of people with a mutation in a specific gene who exhibit signs and symptoms of a genetic disorder. If some people with the mutation do not develop features of the disorder, the condition is said to have reduced (or incomplete) penetrance. One example of reduced penetrance is familial cancer syndromes, such as *BRCA1*- and *BRCA2*-related hereditary breast cancer. Not everyone with mutation(s) in *BRCA1* or *BRCA2* has breast cancer (http://ghr.nlm.nih.gov). Variable expressivity refers to the range of signs and symptoms that can occur in different people with the same genetic condition. One example of variable expression is ataxia–telangiectasia (AT), which is caused by pathogenic variants in the *ATM* gene. AT may have variable severity of symptoms even in the same family. Pleiotropy is used to describe multiple, often seemingly unrelated, physical effects caused by a single altered gene or pair of altered genes. One example of it—pathogenic variants in *KCNQ1*—may cause both autosomal dominant Romano–Ward syndrome, or autosomal recessive Jervell and Lange–Nielsen syndrome (http://ghr.nlm.nih.gov).

Therefore, dominant-negative explains the more deleterious effect of pathogenic variants in either the *COL1A1* or *COL1A2* gene than pathogenic variants causing the production of no gene product.

111. B. *Genetic heterogeneity is used to describe disorders or traits caused by genetic factors and nongenetic factors. Another example of genetic heterogeneity is obesity, which has both genetic and environmental components* (http://ghr.nlm.nih.gov).

Penetrance refers to the proportion of people with a particular mutation in a specific gene who exhibit signs and symptoms of a genetic disorder. If some people with the mutation do not develop features of the disorder, the condition is said to have reduced (or incomplete) penetrance. One example of reduced penetrance is familial cancer syndromes, such as *BRCA1*- and *BRCA2*-related hereditary breast cancer. Not everyone with mutation(s) in *BRCA1* or *BRCA2* has breast cancer (http://ghr.nlm.nih.gov). Variable expressivity refers to the range of signs and symptoms that can occur in different people with the same genetic condition. One example of variable expression is Marfan syndrome. Marfan syndrome may have variable severity of symptoms even in the same family (http://ghr.nlm.nih.gov). Dominant-negative mutation is used to describe a mutation whose gene product adversely affects the normal, wild-type gene product within the same cell, usually by dimerizing (combining) with it. In cases of polymeric molecules, such as collagen, dominant-negative pathogenic variants are often more deleterious than pathogenic variants causing the production of no gene product (null pathogenic variants or null alleles). One example of dominant-negative mutation is Osteogenesis imperfecta (OI) caused by pathogenic variants in *COL1A1* and *COL1A2* (http://ghr.nlm.nih.gov). Pleiotropy is used to describe multiple, often seemingly unrelated, physical effects caused by a single altered gene or pair of altered genes. One example of it is pathogenic variants in *KCNQ1* that may cause autosomal dominant Romano–Ward syndrome or autosomal recessive Jervell and Lange–Nielsen syndrome (http://ghr.nlm.nih.gov).

Therefore, genetic heterogeneity may be used to describe one disorder caused by multiple genes, such as Charcot–Marie–Tooth (CMT) disease.

112. D. *Pleiotropy is used to describe multiple, often seemingly unrelated, physical effects caused by a single altered gene or pair of altered genes.* Another example of it is pathogenic variants in *KCNQ1*, which may cause autosomal dominant Romano–Ward syndrome or autosomal recessive Jervell and Lange–Nielsen syndrome.

Genetic heterogeneity is used to describe disorders or traits caused by genetic and nongenetic factors. One example of genetic heterogeneity is learning disability, which has both genetic and environmental components (http://ghr.nlm.nih.gov). Penetrance refers to the proportion of people with a particular mutation in a specific gene who exhibit signs and symptoms of a genetic disorder. If some people with the mutation do not develop features of the disorder, the condition is said to have reduced (or incomplete) penetrance. One example of reduced penetrance is familial cancer syndromes, such as *BRCA1*- and *BRCA2*-related hereditary breast cancer. Not everyone with mutation(s) in *BRCA1* or *BRCA2* has breast cancer (http://ghr.nlm.nih.gov). Variable expressivity refers to the range of signs and symptoms that can occur in different people with the same genetic condition. One example of variable expression is Fabry disease, which is caused by pathogenic variants in the *GLA* gene on the X chromosome. Fabry disease may have variable severity of symptoms even in the same family (http://ghr.nlm.nih.gov). Dominant-negative mutation is used to describe a mutation whose gene product adversely affects the normal, wild-type gene product within the same cell, usually by dimerizing (combining) with it. In cases of polymeric molecules, such as collagen, dominant-negative pathogenic variants are often more deleterious than pathogenic variants causing the production of no gene product (null pathogenic variants or null alleles). One example of dominant-negative mutation is osteogenesis imperfecta (OI) caused by pathogenic variants in *COL1A1* and *COL1A2* (http://ghr.nlm.nih.gov).

Therefore, pleiotropy, used to describe pathogenic variant(s) in one gene, *CHD7*, leads all the symptoms in different organs and systems for CHARGE.

113. B. Sanger sequencing was developed by Frederick Sanger and colleagues in 1977. It has been the most widely used classical chain-termination sequencing method for approximately 25 years. The Human Genome Project was done by Sanger sequencing. *A nonsense mutation is a point mutation in a sequence of DNA that results in a premature stop codon, which can be detected by Sanger sequencing.*

The Sanger method is still considered by the research community as the gold standard for sequencing; however, it has several limitations. Common challenges include poor quality in the first 15–40 bases of the sequence due to primer binding and deteriorating quality of sequencing traces after 700–900 bases. And Sanger sequencing has very restricted ability to handle and analyze allele frequencies. Often, even finding a heterozygous SNP in a PCR product is cumbersome, let alone any bases that are not represented at 1:1 ratios. So it is challenging to detect mosaic pathogenic variants in tissues. If there is a single-nucleotide polymorphism (SNP) in the primer region, it may cause allelic drop during PCR, which may lead to false positive or false negative sequencing results. Lastly, if a deletion or duplication is larger than the amplicon for the sequencing reaction, the sequencing will recognize it as homozygous for wild type, which lead to false negative results. One example of it is Duchenne muscular dystrophy (DMD) and Becker muscular dystrophy (BMD) caused by pathogenic variants in the *DMD* gene on the X chromosome. Deletions of one or more exons of DMD account for approximately 60%–70% of pathogenic variants in individuals with DMA or BMD. This type of deletion/duplication is not suitable with Sanger sequencing. It is also well known that qualtiy of sequencing data becomes poor after a stretch of seven or more nucleotides of the same base.

Therefore, nonsense mutation is NOT one of the limitations of Sanger sequencing.

114. **D**. *Locus heterogeneity is a disorder or trait caused by pathogenic variants in genes at different chromosomal loci* (http://ghr.nlm.nih.gov). In addition to HCM, another example is Fanconi anemia (FA). There are at least 15 genes responsible for FA.

Allelic heterogeneity is the phenomenon in which different pathogenic variants at the same gene cause a similar phenotype (http://ghr.nlm.nih.gov). Genetic heterogeneity is a phenomenon in which a single phenotype or genetic disorder may be caused by any one of multiple alleles or nonallele (locus) pathogenic variants and nongenetic factors. An example of genetic heterogeneity is Hirschsprung disease, which could be caused by chromosome abnormalities, single-gene pathogenic variants, and unknown environmental factors (http://ghr.nlm.nih.gov). Penetrance refers to the proportion of people with a particular mutation in a specific gene who exhibit signs and symptoms of a genetic disorder. If some people with the mutation do not develop features of the disorder, the condition is said to have reduced (or incomplete) penetrance. One example of reduced penetrance is familial cancer

syndromes, such as *BRCA1*- and *BRCA2*-related hereditary breast cancer. Not everyone with mutation(s) in *BRCA1* or *BRCA2* has breast cancer (http://ghr.nlm.nih.gov). Variable expressivity refers to the range of signs and symptoms that can occur in different people with the same genetic condition. One example of variable expression is Marfan syndrome. Marfan syndrome may have variable severity of symptoms even in the same family. Pleiotropy is used to describe multiple, often seemingly unrelated, physical effects caused by a single altered gene or pair of altered genes. One example is pathogenic variants in *KCNQ1,* which may cause both autosomal dominant Romano–Ward syndrome or autosomal recessive Jervell and Lange–Nielsen syndrome (http://ghr. nlm.nih.gov). Dominant-negative mutation is used to describe a mutation whose gene product adversely affects the normal, wild-type gene product within the same cell, usually by dimerizing (combining) with it. In cases of polymeric molecules, such as collagen, dominant-negative pathogenic variants are often more deleterious than pathogenic variants causing the production of no gene product (null pathogenic variants or null alleles). One example of a dominant-negative mutation is osteogenesis imperfecta (OI) caused by pathogenic variants in *COL1A1* and *COL1A2*. (http://ghr.nlm.nih.gov).

Therefore, locus heterogeneity is a more accurate genetic term than genetic heterogeneity to describe multiple genes that contribute to the pathogenesis of hypertrophic cardiomyopathy (HCM).

115. **A**. In an autosomal dominant condition, a mutation in one copy of the gene is sufficient to impair cell function, leading to disease. Each affected person usually has one affected parent. *Autosomal dominant disorders tend to occur in every generation of an affected family, with male-to-male transmission.* One example of autosomal dominant syndromic hearing loss is branchio-oto-renal syndrome.

Therefore, BJ may have an autosomal dominant disorder.

116. **B**. In an autosomal recessive condition, two mutated copies of the gene are present in each cell leading to dysfunction and disorder. *An affected person usually has unaffected parents who each carry a single copy of the mutated gene. Autosomal recessive disorders are typically not seen in every generation of an affected family.* One example

of autosomal recessive syndromic hearing loss is Jervell and Lange–Nielsen syndrome.

Therefore, BJ may have an autosomal recessive disorder, based on the pedigree.

117. E. *Mitochondrial diseases, also known as "maternal inheritance," are caused by genes in mitochondrial DNA.* Mitochondria are structures in each cell that convert molecules into energy, and each contains a small amount of DNA. Because only egg cells contribute mitochondria to the developing embryo, only females can pass on mitochondrial pathogenic variants to their children. Disorders resulting from pathogenic variants in mitochondrial DNA can appear in every generation of a family and can affect both males and females, but fathers do not pass these disorders to their children.[13] Hearing loss is common in mitochondrial disorders including MELAS (mitochondrial encephalomyopathy, lactic acidosis, and stroke-like episodes), Kearns–Sayre syndrome and MERRF (myoclonic epilepsy with ragged red fibers).

Therefore, BJ may have a mitochondrial disorder because of the maternally inherited pattern shown in the pedigree.

118. D. X-linked recessive disorders are caused by pathogenic variants in genes on the X chromosome. Families with an X-linked recessive disorders often have affected males but rarely have affected females, owing to random X inactivation in each generation. A characteristic of X-linked inheritance is that fathers cannot pass X-linked traits to their sons (no male-to-male transmission). One example of X-linked recessive conditions is hemophilia A/B.

Therefore, BJ may have an X-linked recessive disorder because the disease affects only the males in the family and does not support male-to-male transmission.

119. C. X-linked dominant disorders are caused by pathogenic variants in genes on the X chromosome. Families with an X-linked dominant disorder may have both affected males and affected females in each generation. However, some X-linked dominant disorders may be lethal to males. A characteristic of X-linked inheritance is that fathers cannot pass X-linked traits to their sons (no male-to-male transmission). One example of the X-linked dominant conditions is Rett syndrome. X-linked dominant Charcot–Marie–Tooth (CMT) may cause hearing loss.

Therefore, BJ may have an X-linked dominant disorder, based on the pedigree.

120. E. *A disease expressed in both sexes but with no evidence of paternal transmission is strongly suggestive of a mitochondrial disease.* Mitochondrial heteroplasmy is the presence of more than one type of mtDNA within a cell or individual. It is an important factor in considering the severity of mitochondrial diseases. mtDNA can be passed only from the mother (maternal inheritance). A mother with a mtDNA gene mutation will pass this abnormal gene to all of her children. The children will all be affected, with different degrees of severity. The threshold for expression depends on the proportion of mutant mtDNA in a heteroplasmic mtDNA pool. One example of mitochondrial diseases with heteroplasmy is myoclonic epilepsy with ragged-red fibers (MERRF).

Therefore, BJ may have a mitochondrial inherited disorder, since there is no evidence of paternal transmission.

121. C. This question asks which disease in the list is an autosomal recessive condition since BJs parents are second cousins. *Inbreeding causes offspring to be subject to autosomal recessive diseases.* All six diseases in the question may cause severe hypotonia in newborns. *The only autosomal recessive disease in the question is Krabbe disease.*

Achondroplasia is an autosomal dominant condition caused by de novo pathogenic variants in most patients. Prader–Willi is an autosomal dominant disorder caused by deletion of the paternal copy of 15q11.2, uniparental disomy of 15q11.2, or pathogenic variants in the *SNRPN* gene. Fragile X syndrome is an X-linked condition that affects males more often than females and it is a trinucleotide repeat expansion disorder with anticipation. X-linked adrenoleukodystrophy is an X-linked recessive disease with higher prevalence in males than in females. Mitochondrial Encephalomyopathy Lactic Acidosis and Stroke like Episodes (MELAS) is a mitochondrial disease, which is inherited from the mother.

Therefore, BJ most likely has Krabbe disease because of consanguinity.

122. D. *This question asks which disease in the list is a mitochondrial disease, since the disease is maternally inherited in this family.* Mitochondria are structures in each cell that convert molecules into energy, and each contains a small amount of DNA. Because only egg cells contribute mitochondria to the developing embryo, only females can pass on mitochondrial pathogenic variants to their children. Disorders resulting from pathogenic variants in mitochondrial DNA can appear in

every generation of a family and can affect both males and females, but fathers do not pass these disorders to their children. All six diseases in the question may cause severe hypotonia in newborns. The only mitochondrial disease in the question is mitochondrial encephalomyopathy lactic acidosis and stroke-like episodes (MELAS).

Krabbe disease is an autosomal recessive lysosomal disease. Achondroplasia is an autosomal dominant condition caused by de novo pathogenic variants in most patients, and severe hypotonia is not one of its symptoms. Prader–Willi is an autosomal dominant disorder caused by deletion of the paternal copy of 15q11.2, uniparental disomy of 15q11.2, or pathogenic variants in the *SNRPN* gene. Fragile X syndrome is an X-linked condition that affects males more often than females, and it is a trinucleotide repeat expansion disorder with anticipation. X-linked adrenoleukodystrophy is a X-linked recessive disease with higher prevalence in males than females.

Therefore, BJ most likely have mitochondrial encephalomyopathy lactic acidosis and stroke-like episodes (MELAS) because of the maternally inherited pattern shown in the pedigree.

123. **F.** *This question asks which disease in the list is an X-linked recessive disease.* Families with an X-linked recessive disorders often have affected males, but rarely affected females due to random X inactivation, in each generation. A characteristic of X-linked inheritance is that fathers cannot pass X-linked traits to their sons (no male-to-male transmission). All six diseases in the question may cause severe hypotonia in newborns. The only X-linked recessive disease is X-linked adrenoleukodystrophy.

Krabbe disease is an autosomal recessive lysosomal disease. Achondroplasia is an autosomal dominant condition caused by de novo pathogenic variants in most patients, and severe hypotonia is not one of its symptoms. Prader–Willi is an autosomal dominant disorder caused by deletion of the paternal copy of 15q11.2, uniparental disomy of 15q11.2, or pathogenic variants in the *SNRPN* gene. Fragile X syndrome is an X-linked condition that affects males more often than females and is a trinucleotide repeat expansion disorder with anticipation. Mitochondrial encephalomyopathy lactic acidosis and stroke (MELAS)-like episodes is a mitochondrial disease, which is maternal inherited.

Therefore, BJ most likely has X-linked adrenoleukodystrophy because the disorder appears only in males in this family and it does not transmit from a male to males.

124. **C.** The proband had myoclonic epilepsy with ragged-red fibers (MERRF), which is a mitochondrial disease. *Patients with MERRF are nearly always heteroplasmic for the mutant mitochondria.* Heteroplasmy describes a situation in which, within a single cell, there is a mixture of mitochondria, some containing mutant DNA and some containing normal DNA. The threshold for expression depends on the proportion of mutant mtDNA in a heteroplasmic mtDNA pool.

The mitochondrial genome has a mutation rate 10 times that of nuclear DNA, is not protected by histones, and consists only of exons. Each cell has about 100 mitochondria, and each mitochondrion has about 5 mitochondrial genomes. Mitochondrial genomes encode part of the electron transport chain, while nuclear genomes encode others.

Therefore, heteroplasmy may explains why the maternal aunt does not have symptoms of MERRF.

125. **E.** *A lot of disorders caused by pathogenic variants in mtDNAs are heteroplasmic, and the risk to children of affected or unaffected females cannot be estimated accurately.* The risk to children of affected males is zero because children do not inherit paternal DNA.

The mitochondrial genome has a mutation rate 10 times that of the nuclear DNA (gDNA), is not protected by histones, and consists only of exons. Each cell has about 100 mitochondria, and each mitochondrion has about 5 mitochondrial genomes. Mitochondrial genomes encode part of the electron transport chain, while nuclear genomes encode others.

Therefore, the risk to children of affected females is NOT necessarily 100%, 50%, or 0%.

126. **E.** *The mitochondrial genome consists of only exons.* mtDNA has a mutation rate 10 times that of the nuclear DNA and is not protected by histones. Each cell has about 100 mitochondria, and each mitochondrion has about 5 mitochondrial genomes. Mitochondrial genomes encode part of the electron transport chain, while nuclear genomes encode others.

Therefore, there are no introns in the mitochondria genome.

127. **B.** LOD stands for "logarithm of the odds." In genetics, the LOD score is a statistical estimate of whether two genes, or a gene and a disease gene,

are likely to be located near each other on a chromosome and are therefore likely to be inherited. A LOD score of 3 or higher is generally understood to mean that two genes are located close to each other on the chromosome. In terms of significance, a LOD score of 3 means that the odds are a thousand to one that the two genes are linked and, therefore, inherited together. LOD = Z = log10 (likelihood if linked/likelihood if the loci are unlinked). *LOD in all five families is the summary of the LOD score in each family.*

Therefore, the LOD score of the five families together is: $1.41 + 0.51 + (-0.69) + 1.12 + (-0.21) = 2.14$.

128. **A**. In genetics, the LOD score is a statistical estimate of whether two genes, or a gene and a disease gene, are likely to be located near each other on a chromosome and are therefore likely to be inherited. A LOD score of 3 or higher is generally understood to mean that two genes are located close to each other on the chromosome. In terms of significance, a LOD score of 3 means that the odds are a thousand to one that the two genes are linked and, therefore, inherited together. LOD = Z = log10 (likelihood if linked/likelihood if the loci are unlinked). The bigger the LOD score, the greater the possibility that the locus and the disease gene are in linkage. θ is used to measure recombination frequency (genetic distance). $\theta = 0.05$ means the genetic distance of the locus and the disease gene is 5 cM.

Therefore, the peak LOD score, 6, occurs at 5 cM.

129. **C**. In genetics, the LOD score is a statistical estimate of whether two genes, or a gene and a disease gene, are likely to be located near each other on a chromosome and are therefore likely to be inherited. A LOD score of 3 or higher is generally understood to mean that two genes are located close to each other on the chromosome. In terms of significance, a LOD score of 3 means that the odds are a thousand to one that the two genes are linked and, therefore, inherited together. LOD = Z = log10 (likelihood if linked/likelihood if the loci are unlinked). The bigger the LOD score, the greater the possibility that the locus and the disease gene are in linkage.

Therefore, the LOD score is 4 for this SNP marker.

130. **F**. Heteroplasmy describes the presences of a mixture of mutant and normal mtDNA molecules within one cell. Therefore, the symptoms associated with a mtDNA mutation will depend on the relative proportion of normal and mutant mtDNA in the cells of a particular tissue.

Each cell has about 100 mitochondria, and each mitochondrion has about 5 mitochondrial genomes. Mitochondrial genomes encode part of the electron transport chain, while nuclear genomes encode others. The mitochondrial genome has a mutation rate 10 times that of the nuclear DNA and is not protected by histones, and it consists of only exons.

Therefore, mtDNA has all the characteristics listed in the question.

131. **A**. Positive predictive value is the probability that subjects with a positive screening test truly have the disease. Therefore, the positive predictive value in this case is $A/(A + B) = 9/(9 + 180) < 5\%$.

	Disease	No disease
Positive	A (9)	B (180)
Negative	C (1)	D (720)

132. **D**. Negative predictive value is the probability that subjects with a negative screening test truly do not have the disease. Therefore, the negative predict value in this case is $D/(C + D) = 630/(2 + 630) > 99\%$.

	Disease	No disease
Positive	A (8)	B (270)
Negative	C (2)	D (630)

133. **B**. Epigenetics is one of the fastest-growing areas of science. Based on current understanding, epigenetic mechanisms include histone modifications, DNA methylation, small and noncoding RNAs (e.g., microRNA), and chromatin architecture. These mechanisms, in addition to other transcriptional regulatory events, ultimately regulate gene activity and expression during development and differentiation or in response to environmental stimuli. Methylation of DNA is the main mechanism of genomic imprinting, the gamete-specific silencing of genes.

Prader—Willi syndrome (PWS) and Angelman syndrome (AS) are clinically distinct neurodevelopmental genetic disorders that map to 15q11-q13. The primary phenotypes are attributable to loss of expression of imprinted genes within this region, which can arise by means of a number of mechanisms. *The most sensitive single approach to diagnosing both PWS and*

AS is to study methylation patterns within 15q11–q13 irrespective of the molecular class.

Therefore, methylation status is altered in patients with PWS/AS.

134. **A.** DNA methylation is a process by which methyl groups are added to DNA; this occurs primarily at C5 of the cytosine ring within cytosine–guanine (CpG) dinucleotides. *It is frequently found clustered at gene regulatory sites such as promoter regions.* 5-Methylcytosine (5-mC)-based DNA methylation occurs by the covalent addition of a methyl (CH3) group at the 5-carbon of the cytosine ring resulting in 5-methylcytosine (5-mC). These methyl groups project into the major groove of DNA and inhibit transcription. Methylated C residues spontaneously deaminate to form T residues over time.

DNA methylation is essential for normal development and is associated with a number of key processes, including genomic imprinting, X-chromosome inactivation, suppression of repetitive elements, and carcinogenesis. The pattern of X-chromosome inactivation in females is currently evaluated by assays of differential methylation in the genes between the active and the inactive X chromosomes, with methylation-sensitive enzymes.

Therefore, the promoter region is usually the target for methylation study.

135. **C.** Prader–Willi syndrome (PWS) and Angelman syndrome (AS) are clinically distinct neurodevelopmental genetic disorders that map to 15q11–q13. The primary phenotypes are attributable to loss of expression of imprinted genes within this region, which can arise by means of a number of mechanisms. The most sensitive single approach to diagnosing both PWS and AS is to study methylation patterns within 15q11–q13 irrespective of the molecular class. The imprinting center for the PWS/AS critical region is located at the promoter region of *SNRPN*, which is methylated on the maternal chromosome, leading to silencing the maternal allele. Therefore, *the promoter region of the SNRPN gene usually has been tested for the methylation patterns within 15q11–q13. SNRPN* DNA methylation analysis results in detection in greater than 99% of PWS cases and approximately 80% AS cases. However, this molecular assay cannot be used to tell whether the PWS/AS is cause by deletion, uniparental disomy (UPD), imprinting defect, or mutation *UBE3A. NIPA1* and *NIPA2* are located at the nonimprinted region of 15q11.2, proximate to the *SNRPN* gene.

Therefore, the promoter region of *SNRPN* should be the target of the methylation study.

136. **E.** DNA methylation is a process by which methyl groups are added to DNA, which primarily occurs at C5 of the cytosine ring within cytosine–guanine (CpG) dinucleotides. It is frequently found clustered at gene regulatory sites such as promoter regions. 5-Methylcytosine-based DNA methylation occurs by the covalent addition of a methyl (CH3) group at the 5-carbon of the cytosine ring, resulting in 5-methylcytosine (5-mC). These methyl groups project into the major groove of DNA and inhibit transcription. Methylated C residues spontaneously deaminate to form T residues over time.

DNA methylation is essential for normal development and is associated with a number of key processes, including genomic imprinting, X-chromosome inactivation, suppression of repetitive elements, and carcinogenesis. The pattern of X-chromosome inactivation in females is currently evaluated by assays of differential methylation in the genes between the active and the inactive X chromosomes, with methylation-sensitive enzymes.

Treatment of DNA with sodium bisulfite converts cytosine residues to uracil but leaves 5-methylcytosine residues unaffected. If conversion is incomplete, the subsequent analysis will incorrectly interpret the unconverted unmethylated cytosines as methylated cytosines, resulting in false positive results for methylation.

Therefore, treatment of DNA with sodium bisulfite converts cytosine residues to uracil instead of methylcytosine.

137. **B.** Epigenetics is one of the fastest-growing areas of science. Based on current understanding, epigenetic mechanisms include histone modifications, DNA methylation, small and noncoding RNAs, and chromatin architecture. These mechanisms, in addition to other transcriptional regulatory events, ultimately regulate gene activity and expression during development and differentiation or in response to environmental stimuli. DNA methylation and small and noncoding RNAs (siRNA and miRNA) decrease gene expression, while *histone modifications (histone acetylation) increase gene expression.* miRNAs are small RNAs that regulate gene expression posttranscription by binding to the 3' end of mRNA and preventing its translation into protein. siRNA is a class of double-stranded RNA molecules; it functions by causing mRNA to be broken down after transcription, resulting in no translation.

Therefore, histone acetylation increases gene expression, but not methylation, miRNAs, or siRNA.

138. **D**. *Bisulfite conversion, also known as bisulfite treatment, is used to deaminate unmethylated cytosine to produce uracil in DNA.* Methylated cytosines are protected from the conversion to uracil, allowing the use of direct sequencing to determine the locations of unmethylated cytosines and 5-methylcytosines at single-nucleotide resolution.

Therefore, methylation study with sodium bisulfite converts C to U.

139. **C**. DNA methylation is a process by which methyl groups are added to DNA. 5-Methylcytosine-based DNA methylation occurs by the covalent addition of a methyl (CH3) group at the 5-carbon of the cytosine ring, resulting in 5-methylcytosine (5-mC). *Treatment of DNA with bisulfite converts cytosine residues to uracil, but leaves 5-methylcytosine residues unaffected.*

Therefore, bisulfite converts an unmethylated cytosine to uracil in DNA.

140. **E**. Bisulfite conversion is the most widely used technique for studying DNA methylation; however, complications have arisen. First, it cannot distinguish 5-methylcytosine (5-mC) from 5-hydroxymethylcytosine (hmC). 5-hmC is the first oxidative product in the active demethylation of 5-mC, which is further oxidized to 5-formylcytosine and 5-carboxycytosine, eventually removing the methyl group from 5-mC. Bisulfite sequencing relies on the conversion of every single unmethylated cytosine residue to uracil. If conversion is incomplete, the subsequent analysis will incorrectly interpret the unconverted unmethylated cytosines as methylated cytosines, resulting in false positive results for methylation.

Another challenge in bisulfite sequencing is the degradation of DNA that takes place concurrently with the conversion. The conditions necessary for complete conversion, such as long incubation times, elevated temperature, and high bisulfite concentration, can lead to the degradation of about 90% of the incubated DNA. Given that the starting amount of DNA is often limited, such extensive degradation can be problematic. The degradation occurs as depurinations, resulting in random strand breaks.

Therefore, all the points listed in the question are the technical difficulties of sodium bisulfite—mediated methylation study.

141. **B**. *All the methods list can be used to detect single nucleotide polymorphisms (SNPs), including methylated nucleotide, but not chromosome microarray (CMA).* CMA is a genomewide approach to

detecting copy-number variants (CNVs) instead of single-nucleotide pathogenic variants.

Therefore, chromosome microarray analysis cannot be used as a downstream method for sodium bisulfite—mediated methylation study.

142. **D**. Methylation of the MGMT promoter is found in 35%−45% of malignant gliomas (WHO grades III and IV) and in about 80% of WHO grade II gliomas. The methylation status of the MGMT promoter has been identified as a strong and independent predictive factor of favorable survival in glioblastoma patients undergoing chemotherapy with alkylating agents. The median survival for patients with a methylated MGMT promoter was 21.7 months, compared with 12.7 months for patients without this promoter. *The sequence for the methylated strand was determined by converting all cytosines to thymines, with the exception of those in the CpG dinucleotide after sodium bisulfite treatment.*

Therefore, in the example the methylated strand was converted to 5′ TTT CGA CGT TCG TAG GTT TTC GCG TAT TTT TTC GAA AAT GAA ACG (choice D) by sodium bisulfite.

143. **C**. Methylation of the *MGMT* promoter is found in 35%−45% of malignant gliomas (WHO grades III and IV) and in about 80% of WHO grade II gliomas. The methylation status of the *MGMT* promoter has been identified as a strong and independent predictive factor of favorable survival in glioblastoma patients undergoing chemotherapy with alkylating agents. The median survival for patients with a methylated *MGMT* promoter was 21.7 months, compared with 12.7 months for patients without this promoter. *The sequence for the unmethylated strand was determined by converting all cytosines to thymines, including of those in the CpG dinucleotide after sodium bisulfite treatment.*

Therefore, in the example the unmethylated strand was converted to 5′ TTT TGA TGT TTG TAG GTT TTT GTG TAT TTT TTT GAA AAT GAA ATG (choice C) by sodium bisulfite.

144. **B**. Prader−Willi syndrome (PWS) and Angelman syndrome (AS) are clinically distinct neurodevelopmental genetic disorders that map to 15q11-q13. The primary phenotypes are attributable to loss of expression of imprinted genes within this region, which can arise by means of a number of mechanisms. The most sensitive single approach to diagnosing both PWS and AS is to study methylation patterns within 15q11-q13. So far, several genes preferentially or exclusively expressed from the paternal chromosome have been described. They are

MKRN3, MAGEL2, NDN, PWRN1, C15orf2, SNURF-SNRPN, and several C/D box small nucleolar RNA (snoRNA) genes. At least two of these genes, *SNRPN* and *NDN*, have differentially methylated CpG islands in their promoter regions that are methylated on the maternal chromosome, leading to silencing of the maternal allele. *Treatment of DNA with bisulfite converts cytosine residues to uracil, but leaves 5-methylcytosine residues at the CpG islands unaffected if the strands were methylated.* Uracil will be replaced by thymidine during PCR reaction.

In the example the methylated strand was converted to 5′ tgcgcggtcgtagaggtaggttggcgcg (choice C) by sodium bisulfite. Therefore, the methylation-specific primer is 5′ cgcgccaacctacctctacgaccgcgca (choice B).

145. **A**. Prader—Willi syndrome (PWS) and Angelman syndrome (AS) are clinically distinct neurodevelopmental genetic disorders that map to 15q11-q13. The primary phenotypes are attributable to loss of expression of imprinted genes within this region, which can arise by means of a number of mechanisms. The most sensitive single approach to diagnosing both PWS and AS is to study methylation patterns within 15q11-q13. So far, several genes preferentially or exclusively expressed from the paternal chromosome have been described. They are *MKRN3, MAGEL2, NDN, PWRN1, C15orf2, SNURF-SNRPN*, and several C/D box small nucleolar RNA (snoRNA) genes. At least two of these genes, *SNRPN* and *NDN*, have differentially methylated CpG islands in their promoter regions that are methylated on the maternal chromosome, leading to silencing of the maternal allele. *Treatment of DNA with bisulfite converts cytosine residues to uracil, including those cytosines at the CpG islands if the strands were unmethylated.* Uracil will be replaced by thymidine during PCR reaction.

In the example the unmethylated strand was converted to 5′ tgtgtggttgtagaggtaggttggtgtg (choice D). Therefore, the unmethylation-specific primer is 5′ cacaccaacctacctctacaaccacaca (choice A).

146. **E**. Pyrosequencing is a sequencing-by-synthesis—based method of DNA sequencing. A sequencing primer is hybridized to a single-stranded amplified DNA template with the presence of DNA polymerase, ATP sulfurylase, luciferase and apyrase, adenosine 5′ phosphosulfate (APS), and luciferin. Then the first of four dNTPs is added to the reaction.

DNA polymerase catalyzes the incorporation of the deoxyribonucleotide triphosphate into the DNA strand, if it is complementary to the base in the template strand. *Each incorporation event is accompanied by release of pyrophosphate (PPi) in a quantity equimolar to the amount of incorporated nucleotide. ATP sulfurylase quantitatively converts PPi to ATP in the presence of APS. This ATP drives the luciferase-mediated conversion of luciferin to oxyluciferin, which generates visible light in amounts that are proportional to the amount of ATP.* The light produced in the luciferase-catalyzed reaction is detected by a charge-coupled device (CCD) camera and seen as a peak in a pyrogram. The height of each peak (light signal) is proportional to the number of nucleotides incorporated.

Therefore, none of the reagents for pyrosequencing is fluorescently labeled.

147. **D**. *Sanger sequencing is a classical chain-termination method based on the selective incorporation of chain-terminating dideoxynucleotides by DNA polymerase during in vitro DNA replication.* It requires a single-stranded DNA template, a DNA primer, a DNA polymerase, normal deoxynucleosidetriphosphates (dNTPs), and modified dideoxynucleotide triphosphates (ddNTPs), the latter of which terminate DNA strand elongation. These chain-terminating nucleotides lack a 3′-OH group required for the formation of a phosphodiester bond between two nucleotides, causing DNA polymerase to cease extension of DNA when a modified ddNTP is incorporated. The ddNTPs may be radioactively or fluorescently labeled for detection in automated sequencing machines.

Pyrosequencing is a method of DNA sequencing based on the sequencing by synthesis. The DNA sequence is able to be determined by light emitted upon incorporation of the next complementary nucleotide. Since only one dNTPs is added at a time, only one nucleotide can be incorporated on the single-stranded template. The intensity of the light determines whether there is more than one of this nucleotide in a row. The previous dNTP is degraded before the next nucleotide is added for synthesis. This process is repeated with each of the four letters until the DNA sequence of the single-stranded template is determined. Roche 454 sequencing is one of the next generation sequencing (NGS) methods, which adopts the pyrosequencing chemistry. Illumina genomic DNA sequencing is also an NGS method. Although it is different from Roche

454, it also uses the sequencing by synthesis principle.

Therefore, Sanger sequencing is the only one in the list that is not based on the sequencing by synthesis.

148. **B.** Pyrosequencing is a method of DNA sequencing based on sequencing by synthesis. The DNA sequence is able to be determined by light emitted upon incorporation of the next complementary nucleotide. Since only one dNTPs is added at a time, only one nucleotide can be incorporated on the single-stranded template. The intensity of the light determines whether there is more than one of this nucleotide in a row. The previous dNTP is degraded before the next nucleotide is added for synthesis. This process is repeated with each of the four letters until the DNA sequence of the single-stranded template is determined.

Therefore, the correct sequence is GCAGGCCT.

149. **C.** The Southern blot method is used to detect specific DNA sequences. It combines transfer of electrophoresis-separated DNA fragments to a filter membrane and subsequent fragment detection by probe hybridization. First, DNA samples are digested with a restriction enzyme and separated by gel electrophoresis. Second, the DNA is denatured into single strands by incubation with NaOH. Third, the DNA is transferred to a membrane. On the membranes, the DNA fragments retain the same pattern of separation as they had on the gel. Fourth, the blot is incubated with probes. The probe will form base pairs with its complementary DNA sequence on the membrane and bind to form a double-stranded DNA molecule. Lastly, the location of the probe is revealed by incubating it with a colorless substrate that the attached enzyme converts to a colored product that can be seen or gives off light, which will expose X-ray film. If the probe was labeled with radioactivity, it can expose X-ray film directly.

Therefore, 3, 4, 1, 6, 5, 2 is the correct order for Southern blotting.

150. **D.** The Southern blot method is used to separate DNA strands by length. Southern blotting combines transfer of electrophoresis-separated DNA fragments to a filter membrane and subsequent fragment detection by probe hybridization. The method is named after its inventor, the British biologist Edwin Southern. Comparing with PCR-based methods for DNA detection, Southern blotting can detect a large DNA fragment and well tolerate the high CG sequence in the region. *However, it usually takes about 3–4 days to run a Southern blot once.*

The polymerase chain reaction (PCR) provides an extremely sensitive means of amplifying small quantities of DNA. The development of this technique resulted in an explosion of new techniques in molecular biology. Therefore, Kary Mullins won a Nobel Prize in 1993 for inventing it. Since this technique involves amplification of DNA, the most obvious application of the method is in the detection of minuscule amounts of specific DNAs. This is important in the detection of low-level bacterial infections or rapid changes in transcription at the single cell level, as well as the detection of fragmented DNA (low quality) in forensic science (like in the O.J. trial). It can also be used in DNA sequencing, screening for genetic disorders, site-specific mutation of DNA, or cloning or subcloning of cDNAs. PCR is a relatively simple technique, which takes about 2 h. And it is considered a fast technique compared with other molecular DNA-detection methods. Multiplex PCR is an adaptation of PCR that allows simultaneous amplification of many sequences. However, it is harder to amplify large DNA fragments than the smaller ones (the optimal size is less than 1000 bp). One example is the molecular test for fragile X syndrome. It is technically changing to amplify CGG repeats in *FMR1*, especially when CGG expansion is in the full mutation range (greater than 200 copies). With increasing CGG repeats, the DNA melting temperature also increases, thus limiting the efficiency of the PCR due to impaired DNA strand separation. Southern blot analysis can overcome this limitation but has limited resolution of accurate DNA fragment size.

Therefore, Southern blot is much more labor-intensive and costly than PCR.

151. **B.** *A heterozygote advantage describes the case in which the heterozygote genotype has a higher relative fitness than either the homozygote dominant or homozygote recessive genotype.* Sickle cell anemia is a well-established case of heterozygote advantage (http://ghr.nlm.nih.gov).

Genetic drift is the change in the allele frequency of a gene in a population due to random chance. Natural selection is the differential survival and reproduction of individuals due to differences in phenotype; it is a key mechanism of evolution. In natural selection, negative selection is the selective removal of alleles that are deleterious. This can result in stabilizing selection through the purging of deleterious variations that arise, such as that carriers of the harmful point mutation may have fewer offspring each generation. Eventually, it reduces the frequency of the mutation in the gene pool. Positive selection, also known as Darwinian selection, is the process by which new advantageous genetic variants sweep a population. Heterozygote advantage is an example of positive selection, where the presence of one copy of the sickle cell mutation increases the fitness of the individual. A phenocopy describes a variation of phenotype that is caused by environmental conditions, and this phenotype matches a phenotype that is determined by genetic factors (http://ghr.nlm.nih.gov).

Therefore, heterozygote advantage may be used to describe carriers of sickle cell anemia with greater resistance to *P. falciparum* malaria than normal individuals.

152. **E.** *Restriction enzymes usually recognize inverted repeat palindrome DNA sequences and produce a double-stranded cut in the DNA.* The length of restriction recognition sites usually varies from 4 bp to 8 bp. A few restriction enzymes will cleave single stranded DNA, although usually at low efficiency. The restriction enzymes most used in molecular biology labs cut within their recognition sites and generate one of three different types of ends—5′ overhangs (*EcoR* I), 3′ overhangs (*Kpn* I), and blunts ends (*Sma* I)—but there are exceptions. For example, *EcoR* I recognizes and cuts at 5′ G↓AATTC3′/ 3′CTTAA↑G 5′, and generates 3′ overhangs. *Kpn* I recognizes and cuts at 5′ GGTAC↓C3′/ 3′C↑CATGG 5′, and generates 5′ overhangs. *Sma* I recognizes and cuts at 5′ CCC↓GGG3′/ 3′GGGG↑CCC 5′, and generates blunts ends.

Therefore, restriction enzymes usually cut an inverted repeat palindromic double-stranded DNA sequence.

153. **D.** *5′ GAT↓ATC is the EcoRV recognition site.* Restriction enzymes usually recognize inverted repeat palindrome DNA sequences and produce a double-stranded cut in the DNA. The length of restriction recognition sites usually varies from 4 bp to 8 bp. A few restriction enzymes will cleave single-stranded DNA, although usually at low efficiency. The restriction enzymes most used in molecular biology labs cut within their recognition sites and generate one of three different types of ends—5′ overhangs (*EcoR* I), 3′ overhangs (*Kpn* I), and blunts ends (*Sma* I)—but there are exceptions. For example, *EcoR* I recognizes and cuts at 5′ G↓AATTC3′/ 3′CTTAA↑G 5′, and generates 3′ overhangs. *Kpn* I

recognizes and cuts at 5′ GGTAC↓C3′/ 3′C↑CATGG 5′, and generates 5′ overhangs. *Sma* I recognizes and cuts at 5′ CCC↓GGG3′/ 3′GGGG↑CCC 5′, and generates blunts ends. *EcoRV* recognizes and cuts 5′ GAT↓ATC3′/ 3′CTA↑TAG 5′, and generates blunts ends.

Therefore, GATATC most likely is a restriction-enzyme recognition site (from 5′–3′).

154. **A.** *A founder effect can result either from a true founder event (e.g., the establishment of a new population from individuals derived from a much larger population) or from an extreme reduction in population size (e.g., a bottleneck in size).* In either case, alleles present in one copy immediately after the founder event or bottlenecks may be found at a much higher frequency than they were previously and can reach even higher frequencies because of strong genetic drift occurring while the population is still small (http://ghr.nlm.nih.gov). The founder effect has been invoked to account for several disease-associated alleles in the Ashkenazi Jewish population.

A heterozygote advantage describes the case in which the heterozygote genotype has a higher relative fitness than either the homozygote dominant or homozygote recessive genotype. Sickle cell anemia is a well-established case of heterozygote advantage. Natural selection is the differential survival and reproduction of individuals due to differences in phenotype. It is a key mechanism of evolution. In natural selection, negative selection is the selective removal of alleles that are deleterious. This can result in stabilizing selection through the purging of deleterious variations that arise, such as that carriers of the harmful point mutation may have fewer offspring each generation. Eventually, it reduces the frequency of the mutation in the gene pool. Positive selection, also known as Darwinian selection, is the process by which new advantageous genetic variants sweep a population. Heterozygote advantage is an example of positive selection, where the presence of one copy of the sickle cell mutation increases the fitness of the individual. A phenocopy is a variation of phenotype which is caused by environmental conditions, and this phenotype matches a phenotype which is determined by genetic factors (http://ghr.nlm.nih.gov).

Therefore, founder effect may be used to explain why certain genetic disorders are enriched in the Ashkenazi Jewish population.

155. **D.** *The term phenocopy is used to describe the situation where an environmental exposure could produce the same outcome as was produced by a*

genetic mutation. In human genetics, the term phenocopy refers to an environmentally produced disease state that is similar to a clear genetic syndrome. For example, the niacin deficiency disease, pellagra, is clinically similar to the autosomal recessive condition Hartnup disease. Therefore, pellagra has been referred to as a phenocopy of the genetic disorder. Hartnup disease is due to reduced neutral amino acid absorption from the intestine and reabsorption from the kidney, leading to low levels of blood tryptophan, which in turn leads to a biochemical anomaly that is similar to that seen when the diet is deficient in niacin (http://ghr.nlm.nih.gov).

Founder effect is used to describe a minor allele that may be found at a much higher frequency than they were previously after the establishment of a new population of individuals derived from a much larger population or after a bottleneck in size from an extreme reduction of strong genetic drift. The founder effect has been invoked to account for several disease-associated alleles in the Ashkenazi Jewish population. A heterozygote advantage describes the case in which the heterozygote genotype has a higher relative fitness than either the homozygote dominant or homozygote recessive genotype. Sickle cell anemia is a well-established case of heterozygote advantage. Natural selection is the differential survival and reproduction of individuals due to differences in phenotype. It is a key mechanism of evolution. In natural selection, negative selection is the selective removal of alleles that are deleterious. This can result in stabilizing selection through the purging of deleterious variations that arise, such as that carriers of the harmful point mutation may have fewer offspring each generation. Eventually, it reduces the frequency of the mutation in the gene pool. Positive selection, also known as Darwinian selection, is the process by which new advantageous genetic variants sweep a population. Heterozygote advantage is an example of positive selection, where the presence of one copy of the sickle cell mutation increases the fitness of the individual (http://ghr.nlm.nih.gov).

Therefore, phenocopy may be used to describe the similar clinical presentation between Hartnup disease and niacin deficiency.

156. **B**. Mitochondrial DNA (mtDNA) is not transmitted through nuclear DNA. In humans, mtDNA is inherited only from the mother's ovum. So it is non-Mendelian. *Eighty percent of mtDNA codes proteins are involved in the electron transport chain, therefore most mtDNA pathogenic variants lead to functional problems, which may be manifested as myopathies.* Each human mitochondrion contains, on average, approximately five such mtDNA molecules, with the quantity ranging between 1 and 15. Each human cell contains approximately 100 mitochondria, giving a total number of mtDNA molecules per human cell of approximately 500. It was originally believed that the mitochondrial genome contained 13 protein-coding genes, all of them encoding proteins of the electron transport chain. However, in 2001, a 14th biologically active protein, called "humanin," was discovered and was found to be encoded by the mitochondrial gene MT-RNR2.

Therefore, the most common symptom caused by pathogenic variants in mtDNA is myopathy.

157. **B**. The cell cycle or cell-division cycle is the series of events that take place in a cell leading to its division and duplication of its DNA (DNA replication) to produce two daughter cells. *The stages are G0-G1-S-G2-M.* The G0 stage is a resting phase, where the cell has left the cycle and has stopped dividing. G1 stands for "GAP 1," also called the "growth phase"; in this phase, the cell increases its supply of proteins, increases the number of organelles (such as mitochondria and ribosomes), and grows in size. The S stage stands for "synthesis." During this phase, the amount of DNA in the cell has effectively doubled, though the ploidy of the cell remains the same. G2 stands for "GAP 2." In this phase, the cell will continue to grow. Mitosis is when nuclear (chromosomes separate) and cytoplasmic (cytokinesis) division occur. Mitosis is further divided into five phases—prophase, metaphase, anaphase, telophase, and cytokinesis.

Therefore, the correct order of cell cycle is: G0→G1→S→G2→mitosis.

158. **C**. Degeneracy of codons is the redundancy of the genetic code, exhibited as the multiplicity of three-codon combinations specifying an amino acid. The degeneracy of the genetic code is what accounts for the existence of synonymous pathogenic variants. The codons encoding one amino acid may differ in any of their three positions; however, more often than not, this difference is in the second or third position. For instance, the amino acid glutamic acid is specified by GAA and GAG codons (difference in the third position). ATG is the only codon for methionine, which is also the start the codon for an amino acid sequence. If the start codon has an error, it may lead to no transcripts or an alternative start point of mRNA synthesis. Therefore, a change

from GCG to GCA is most likely to be benign as compared with the others, since the third position of the codon is changed in this choice.

Therefore, it is more likely to be synonymous (benign) if the third base pair in a codon is altered, as from ATG GCG CAT to ATG GCA CAT in this question.

159. **D**. Sanger sequencing may be used to detect small deletions and duplications, such as 10 bp. *However, large deletions/duplications are not readily detectable by Sanger sequence analysis of the coding and flanking intronic regions of genomic DNA, since each PCR product is usually less than 1,000 bp.* Quantitative PCR, long-range PCR, multiplex ligation-dependent probe amplification (MLPA), and chromosomal microarray (CMA) may be used to detect large deletions/duplications on the other side.

The dystrophinopathies include a spectrum of muscle disease caused by pathogenic variants in *DMD*, which encodes the protein dystrophin. The severe end of the spectrum includes progressive muscle diseases that are classified as Duchenne/Becker muscular dystrophy (DMD/BMD) when skeletal muscle is primarily affected and as *DMD*-associated dilated cardiomyopathy (DCM) when the heart is primarily affected. Deletions of one or more exons account for approximately 60%–70% of pathogenic variants in individuals with DMD and BMD. Duplications may lead to in-frame or out-of-frame transcripts and account for the pathogenic variants in approximately 5%–10% of males with DMD and BMD (https://www.ncbi.nlm.nih.gov/books/NBK1119/).

Therefore, Sanger sequencing is not an appropriate test to detect deletions/duplications in the *DMD* gene for Duchenne/Becker muscular dystrophy (DMD/BMD).

160. **D**. The hemolytic disease of the fetus and newborn (HDFN) is caused by alloimmunization of the mother by exposure to fetal red blood cells, which display a paternally inherited form of an antigen that is different from those in the mother. *Anti-D accounts for the majority of HDFN, followed by anti-K, anti-c, and anti-E. It can also occur in women with blood type O.* The frequency of Rh-negative individuals is more common in Caucasian than in other ethnic groups. The most common *RhD*-negative allele results from the deletion of *RHD*. The *RHD* pseudogene (RHDΨ) is a common *RhD* negative allele, which is not expressed (https://www.ncbi.nlm.nih.gov/books/NBK2269/).

Two Rh genes, *RHD* and *RHCE*, are tandemly located on 1p. They are more than 95% homologous. The D antigen is expressed from RHD. And the C and E antigens are expressed from RHCE. The alleles are inherited as haplotypes in eight possible combinations, DCe, dce, DcE, Dce, dCe, dcE, DCE, and dCE. Variable alleles have been identified because of gene conversions between RHD and RHCE or single-base-pair pathogenic variants. Hybrid RHD-CE-D alleles may result in either RhD-positive or RhD-negative haplotypes. Most variable *RhD* positive alleles encode proteins that do not express all the RhD epitopes. It is possible for an RhD-negative mother to be alloimmunized by a partial D antigen. In addition, a mother with a partial D can be alloimmunized by a normal RhD antigen.

Therefore, anti-RhD is the most common type of the HDFN.

161. **A**. The Hardy–Weinberg equilibrium is a principle stating that the genetic variation in a population will remain constant from one generation to the next in the absence of disturbing factors. When mating is random in a large population with no disruptive circumstances, the law predicts that both genotype and allele frequencies will remain constant because they are in equilibrium. Given a set of assumptions, this theory states that if the allele frequencies in a population with two alleles at a locus are p and q, then the expected genotype frequencies are p^2, $2pq$, and q^2. For example, if the frequency of allele A in the population is p and the frequency of allele a in the population is q, then the frequency of genotype AA is p^2, the frequency of genotype Aa is $2pq$, and the frequency of genotype aa is q^2. If there are only two alleles at a locus, then $p + q$, by mathematical necessity, equals 1. The Hardy–Weinberg genotype frequencies, $p^2 + 2pq + q^2$, represent the binomial expansion of $(p + q)^2$, and also sum to 1 (http://www.nature.com/scitable).

The answer may be calculated with the Hardy–Weinberg equation ($p^2 + 2pq + q^2$). The 9% (1%–91%) of the population is RhD-negative ($q^2 = 0.09$). So $q = 0.3$, and $p = 0.7$. Therefore, DD is 49% (p^2), while Dd is 42% ($2pq$).

162. **B**. One of the most important ideas in cancer research is the two-hit hypothesis, also called Knudson hypothesis or multiple-hit hypothesis, which is the hypothesis that cancer is the result of accumulated pathogenic variants to a cell's DNA. *This hypothesis applies to both hereditary and acquired cancers.*

One example of the Knudson hypothesis is inherited retinoblastoma. It occurs at a younger age than the sporadic disease. In addition, children with inherited retinoblastoma often developed the tumor in both eyes, suggesting an underlying predisposition. The Knudson hypothesis suggested that multiple "hits" to DNA were necessary to cause cancer. In the children with inherited retinoblastoma, the first insult was inherited in the DNA, and any second insult would rapidly lead to cancer. In noninherited retinoblastoma, two "hits" had to take place before a tumor could develop, explaining the age difference. However, it is worth pointing out that the Knudson hypothesis refers specifically to the heterozygosity of tumor suppressor genes, but not proto-oncogenes. Pathogenic variants in both alleles of a tumor suppressor gene are required for tumor genesis. Mutation in one allele of a proto-oncogene is sufficient for tumor genesis.

Chromothripsis similarly involves multiple pathogenic variants, but it asserts that they may all appear at once. This idea involves the catastrophic shattering of a chromosome into tens or hundreds of pieces and then being patched back together incorrectly. This shattering, it is presumed, takes place when the chromosomes are compacted during normal cell division, but the trigger for the shattering is unknown. In this model, cancer arises as the result of a single, isolated event, rather than as the slow accumulation of multiple pathogenic variants.

Therefore, the Knudson hypothesis applies to both hereditary and acquired cancers.

163. **C.** One of the most important ideas in cancer research is the two-hit hypothesis, also called Knudson hypothesis, or multiple-hit hypothesis, which is the hypothesis that cancer is the result of accumulated pathogenic variants to a cell's DNA. This hypothesis applies to both hereditary and acquired cancers.

One example is inherited retinoblastoma. It occurs at a younger age than the sporadic disease. In addition, children with inherited retinoblastoma often developed the tumor in both eyes, suggesting an underlying predisposition. The Knudson hypothesis suggested that multiple "hits" to DNA were necessary to cause cancer. In the children with inherited retinoblastoma, the first insult was inherited in the DNA, and any second insult would rapidly lead to cancer. In noninherited retinoblastoma, two "hits" had to take place before a tumor could develop, explaining the age difference. However, it is worth pointing out that *the Knudson hypothesis refers specifically to the heterozygosity of tumor suppressor genes, but not proto-oncogenes.* Pathogenic variants in both alleles of a tumor suppressor gene are required for tumor genesis.

Mutation in one allele of a proto-oncogene is sufficient for tumor genesis.

Pathogenic variants in the *RB1* gene cause retinoblastoma. Pathogenic variants in the *WT1* gene cause Wilms tumor. Pathogenic variants in the *TP53* gene cause Li–Fraumeni syndrome. Pathogenic variants in the *APC* gene cause colon cancer. Pathogenic variants in the RET gene cause multiple endocrine neoplasia type 2 (MEN2). *RB1, WT1, TP53, and APC are all tumor suppressor genes, but RET is a proto-oncogene.*

Therefore, MEN2 does not fit the Knudson hypothesis.

164. **C.** One of the most important ideas in cancer research is the two-hit hypothesis, also called Knudson hypothesis or multiple-hit hypothesis, which is the hypothesis that cancer is the result of accumulated pathogenic variants to a cell's DNA. This hypothesis applies to both hereditary and acquired cancers.

One example is inherited retinoblastoma. It occurs at a younger age than the sporadic disease. In addition, children with inherited retinoblastoma often developed the tumor in both eyes, suggesting an underlying predisposition. The Knudson hypothesis suggested that multiple "hits" to DNA were necessary to cause cancer. In the children with inherited retinoblastoma, the first insult was inherited in the DNA, and any second insult would rapidly lead to cancer. In noninherited retinoblastoma, two "hits" had to take place before a tumor could develop, explaining the age difference. However, it is worth pointing out that *the Knudson hypothesis refers specifically to the heterozygosity of tumor suppressor genes, but not proto-oncogenes.* Pathogenic variants in both alleles of a tumor suppressor gene are required for tumor genesis. Mutation in one allele of a proto-oncogene is sufficient for tumor genesis.

BRCA1 and *BRCA2* (breast/ovarian cancer), *RB1* (retinoblastoma), and *VHL* (von Hippel–Lindau syndrome) are tumor suppressor genes. *MLH1, MSH2, MSH6,* and *PMS2* for Lynch syndrome are involved in DNA mismatch repair. *Noonan syndrome is caused by pathogenic variants in PTPN11, RAF1, BRAF, and MAP2K1, which are proto-oncogenes.*

Therefore, Noonan syndrome does not fit the Knudson hypothesis.

165. **D.** The human genome contains approximately 3 billion base pairs and an estimated 30,000 genes. In genetics, a centimorgan (cM) is a unit for measuring genetic linkage, which is defined as the distance between genetic markers for which

the expected average number of intervening chromosomal crossovers (recombination) in a single generation is 0.01. *On average, 1 cM corresponds to approximately 1 million base pairs in humans.* The sex-average genetic map is about 3614.7 cM. The female map (4460 cM) is greater than the male map (2590.5 cM). The data are calculated from 1257 meiotic events from 146 Icelandic families using 5146 microsatellite markers.

Therefore, on average, 1 cM corresponds to approximately 1 Mb (1,000,000 bp) in the human genome.

166. **C.** The human genome contains approximately 3 billion base pairs and an estimated 30,000 genes. The sex-average genetic map is about 3614.7 cM. *The female map (4460 cM) is greater than the male map (2590.5 cM).* The data are calculated from 1257 meiotic events from 146 Icelandic families using 5146 microsatellite markers.

Therefore, the genetic length of the human genome is approximately 4400 cM for females.

167. **E.** The human genome contains approximately 3 billion base pairs and an estimated 30,000 genes. The sex-average genetic map is about 3614.7 cM. *The female map (4460 cM) is greater than the male map (2590.5 cM).* The data are calculated from 1257 meiotic events from 146 Icelandic families using 5146 microsatellite markers.

Therefore, the genetic length of human genome is approximately 2700 cM for males.

168. **D.** The human genome contains approximately 3 billion base pairs, and estimated 30,000 genes. *The sex-average genetic map is about 3614.7 cM.* The female map (4460 cM) is greater than the male map (2590.5 cM). The data are calculated from 1257 meiotic events from 146 Icelandic families using 5146 microsatellite markers.

Therefore, the sex-average genetic length of human genome is approximately 3700 cM.

169. **C.** *There are 180,000 exons in human genome, which constitute about 1% of the human genome, or approximately 30 million base pairs.* Pathogenic variants in these sequences are much more likely to have severe consequences than in the remaining 99%.

Therefore, exome sequencing usually covers 30 Mb.

170. **B.** *There are 180,000 exons in the human genome, which constitute about 1% of the human genome, or approximately 30 million base pairs.* Pathogenic variants in these sequences are much more likely to have severe consequences than in the remaining 99%.

Therefore, exome sequencing usually covers 1% of the human genome.

171. **E.** The Human Genome Project was started in 1990, and completed in 2001.[1] It remains the world's largest collaborative biological project performed in 20 universities and research centers in the United States, the United Kingdom, Japan, France, Germany, and China. *The decision was made to use a composite template from multiple individuals rather a single genome from one donor, which was done by mass shotgun Sanger sequencing.* Sanger sequencing is a method of DNA sequencing based on the selective incorporation of chain-terminating dideoxynucleotides by DNA polymerase during in vitro DNA replication, which is good for DNA fragments between 500 bp and 1000 bp.

Pyrosequencing is a method of DNA sequencing based on the sequencing by synthesis. It sequences about 25 bp a time. This technology is relatively good at quantitative analysis as compared with Sanger sequencing. So it has been widely used in methylation studies for tumors. Roche 454 sequencing, SOLiD DNA sequencing, Illumina DNA sequencing, and Iron Torrent sequencing are all so-called next generation sequencing, which may finish sequencing one human genome in days instead of years.

Therefore, Sanger sequencing was used for the Human Genome Project.

172. **C.** Sanger sequencing is a method of DNA sequencing based on the selective incorporation of chain-terminating dideoxynucleotides (ddNTPs) by DNA polymerase during in vitro DNA replication. Developed by Frederick Sanger and colleagues in 1977, it was the most widely used sequencing method for approximately 25 years. Nowadays scientists prefer to directly sequence a PCR product without first cloning the fragment into bacteria, which significantly increased the efficiency.

After DNA extraction from the samples, PCR amplification is performed to increase the concentration of the targeted genomic region. Then gel electrophoresis is used to make sure the fragment amplification is as expected. Then the amplicons from the PCR reaction have to be purified to get rid of PCR primers and dNTPs. Finally, sequencing reaction may be done with the sequencing primer, dNTPs, and ddNTPs, which is followed by capillary electrophoresis to separate and examining the fluorescent signals.

Therefore, the correct order for Sanger sequencing is DNA extraction → PCR amplification→gel electrophoresis→DNA purification→sequencing reaction→capillary electrophoresis. Nowadays, DNA purification is simplified with ExoSAP (Exonuclease I-Shrimp Alkaline Phosphatase), which replaces "gel electrophoresis→DNA purification" for Sanger sequencing in most laboratories.

173. **B**. Pyrosequencing is called "sequencing by synthesis" and involves taking a single strand of the DNA to be sequenced and then synthesizing its complementary strand enzymatically. The pyrosequencing method is based on detecting the activity of DNA polymerase with luciferase. Essentially, the method allows sequencing of a single strand of DNA by synthesizing the complementary strand along it, one base pair at a time, and detecting which base was actually added at each step. The template DNA is immobile, and solutions of A, C, G, and T nucleotides are sequentially added and removed from the reaction. Light is produced only when the nucleotide solution complements the first unpaired base of the template. The sequence of solutions that produce chemiluminescent signals allows the determination of the sequence of the template.

After DNA is extracted from the samples, PCR amplification is performed to increase the concentration of the targeted genomic region with a biotinylated primer. Then magnet beads are used to capture the biotin-labeled single-stranded DNA. This single-stranded DNA as the pyrosequencing template is incubated together with DNA polymerase and A, C, G, or T nucleotides one at a time.

Therefore, the correct order for pyrosequencing is DNA extraction→PCR amplification→DNA purification/template preparation→pyrosequencing reaction.

174. **D**. Bone-marrow transplantation is used to treat malignant and nonmalignant blood disorders, as well as some solid tumors. Once successful engraftment of donor cells is established, the recipient is a genetic chimera. DNA typing has become the method of choice for engraftment monitoring because all individuals, except identical twins, have unique DNA polymorphisms. Donor cells are monitored by following donor-specific alleles of polymorphic markers in the recipient blood and bone marrow.

STR markers are highly polymorphic. They can easily be detected by PCR amplification with fluorescence-labeled primers and can be multiplied in one reaction. *For these reasons, STRs have been widely used in forensic identification, paternity testing, engraftment, and maternal-cell contamination tests, especially after automatic forensic multiple STRs kits with capillary electrophoresis became available.* In a laboratory, there are two parts to engraftment/chimerism DNA testing. Before the transplantation, several STRs in the donor and recipient cells must be screened to find at least one informative marker. The second part of the testing process is the engraftment analysis, which is performed at specified intervals after the transplantation.

Copy number and epigenetic markers are usually labor-intensive and have limited alleles if they are not done on a genomewide scale. SNP markers usually have only two alleles, which may have a lot of noninformative loci for engraftment analysis. Mitochondrial DNA is maternally inherited and can be used to test whether a member belongs to a family on the maternal side. Variable-number tandem repeats (VNTRs) are bigger genetic markers than STRs, which usually cannot easily be amplified by PCR. This has limited the utility of VNTRs in personal identification, including engraftment and maternal-cell analyses.

Therefore, currently STRs are widely used for engraftment monitoring. In the future, a more cost-effective method may change the dynamics, making SNPs or CNVs more suitable for engraftment monitoring.

175. **D**. The potential presence of maternal-cell contamination (MCC) in chorionic villi, amniotic fluid, and product-of-conception (POC) samples can mask the results of any genetic testing performed on the fetal cells. STR markers are highly polymorphic. They can easily be detected by PCR amplification with fluorescence-labeled primers and can be multiplied in one reaction. *For these reasons, STRs have been widely used in forensic identification, paternity testing, engraftment, and maternal cell contamination testing, especially after automatic forensic multiple STRs kits with capillary electrophoresis became available.* To rule out the presence of MCC, a maternal blood specimen is necessary for comparison of maternal and fetal genetic markers. MCC is confirmed when both alleles in the fetus are maternal.

Copy number and epigenetic markers are usually labor-intensive and have limited alleles if they are not done on a genomewide scale. SNP markers usually have only two alleles, which may have a lot of noninformative loci for engraftment analysis. Mitochondrial DNA is maternally inherited and can be used to test whether a member belongs to a family on the maternal side. Variable-number tandem repeats (VNTRs) are bigger genetic markers than STRs, which usually cannot easily be amplified by PCR. This limits the utility of VNTRs in personal identification, including engraftment and maternal-cell analyses.

Therefore, currently STRs are widely used for MCC. In the future, a more cost-effective method may change the dynamics, making SNPs or CNVs more suitable for MCC.

176. **F.** Mitochondrial DNAs (mtDNA) are maternal inherited, which can be used to track family trees from maternal side. With the living family member, Prince Philip, the great nephew of the last queen, the scientist may be able to tell whether the bones belong to the Russian royal family. Prince Philip, Duke of Edinburgh, is the husband of Queen Elizabeth II in the British royal family.

Copy-number variants and epigenetic markers are usually labor-intensive and have limited alleles if they are not done on a genomewide scale. SNP markers usually have only two alleles, which may have a lot of noninformative loci for engraftment analysis. Mitochondrial DNA is maternally inherited and can be used to test whether a member belongs to a family on the maternal side. Variable-number tandem repeats (VNTRs) are bigger genetic markers than STRs, which usually cannot easily be amplified by PCR. This limits the utility of VNTRs in the engraftment analysis. STRs are highly polymorphic; they can easily be detected by PCR amplification with fluorescence-labeled primers and can be multiplied in one reaction. Therefore, STRs have been widely used in forensic identification, paternity testing, engraftment, and maternal-cell contamination tests, especially after automatic forensic multiple STRs kits with capillary electrophoresis became available. Nowadays, the forensic STR kits may detect fragmented DNA to as small as 100−200 bp. With 10−20 of this kind of STR makers, scientists may be able to tell whether these bones belong to one family. However, STRs cannot be used to tell whether the bones belong to the Russian royal family.

Therefore, mtDNA was used to confirm whether the bones belong to the Russian family, using a specimen from Prince Philip.

177. **C.** Canavan disease (CD) is an autosomal recessive disease, caused by pathogenic variants in the ASPA gene. Only if both of a couple are carriers of CD would their offspring be at risk for CD. *If the assay is performed for the four common pathogenic variants representing 99% of the pathogenic variants, 99% × 99% = 98% of carrier couples could be detected.* If the assay is performed for the two most common pathogenic variants representing 97.4% of the pathogenic variants, 97.4% × 97.4% = 94.9% of carrier couples could be detected.

Therefore, the clinical sensitivity is approximately 98% for predicting whether offspring may have CD when a Ashkenazi Jewish couple is tested for all four pathogenic variants.

178. **E.** Analytical sensitivity is the ability of a test to detect a target analyte (e.g., a mutation in a gene). In practice, the way in which analytic sensitivity is calculated varies according to the laboratory, with differing replicates and matrices. *In clinical molecular practice, analytical sensitivity is usually calculated as number of true positive samples with positive test results/number of true positive sample = 90/(10 + 90) = 90%.*

		Disease	
		+	−
Test	+	90	20
	−	10	80

Therefore, the analytical sensitivity of this assay for CF is 90%.

179. **C.** Analytical specificity refers to freedom from interference by any element or compound other than the analyte. *In clinical molecular practice, analytical specificity calculated as number of true negatives with negative test results/number of true negative samples = 80/(20 + 80) = 80%.*

		Disease	
		+	−
Test	+	90	20
	−	10	80

Therefore, the analytical specificity of this assay for Tay−Sachs disease is 80%.

180. **D.** Accuracy refers to the extent to which all measurements agree with the true value of what is being measured. Put another way, accuracy refers to how close a value is to the true value. *In clinical molecular practice, analytical accuracy is calculated as (number of true positives with positive test results + number of true negatives with negative test results)/(number of true positive + number of true negative) = (90 + 80)/(100 + 100) = 85%.*

		Disease	
		+	–
Test	+	90	20
	–	10	80

Therefore, the analytical accuracy of this assay for CD is 85%.

181. **B**. *Positive predictive value (PPV) is defined as number of true positives with positive test results/ (number of true positives with positive test results + number of true negatives with positive test results) = 90/(90 + 20) = 82%.*

		Disease	
		+	–
Test	+	90	20
	–	10	80

Therefore, the positive predict value of this assay for NPD is 82% if the prevalence of NPD is not taken into the consideration.

182. **D**. *Negative predictive value (NPV) is defined as number of true negatives with negative test results/ (number of true negatives with negative test results + number of true positives with negative test results) = 80/(80 + 10) = 88%.*

		Disease	
		+	–
Test	+	90	20
	–	10	80

Therefore, the negative predict value of this assay for NPD is 88% if the prevalence of NPD is not taken into the consideration.

183. **B**. Clinical negative predictive value is defined as the probability that a negative test result is correct. Assuming analytic sensitivity and a specificity of 100%, a false negative result will occur because the mutation present is not being tested by the laboratory. In this case, the detection rate of the two pathogenic variants in *MCOLN1* for MLIV is 95%. About 5% of pathogenic variants will not be identified by the assay testing the two pathogenic variants. Since the carrier risk frequency is 1 in 127, there are approximately 20 carriers in 2540 Ashkenazi Jews. An assay for the two pathogenic alleles may detect 19 of 20 carriers.

Therefore, the clinical negative predictive value is 2520/2521.

		Disease	
		+	–
Test	+	19	0
	–	1	2520

184. **A**. *Next-generation sequencing (NGS) is often referred to as massively parallel sequencing, which means that millions of small fragments of DNA can be sequenced at the same time, creating a massive pool of data. This pool of data can reach gigabytes in size, which is the equivalent of 1 billion (1,000,000,000) base pairs of DNA. In comparison, previous methods could sequence 1 DNA fragment at a time, perhaps generating 500–1000 base pairs of DNA in a single reaction. A lot of overlapped short sequence reads will be assembled together on the basis of their overlapping areas as shown in the figure.*

The mean mapped read depth (or mean read depth) is the sum of the mapped read depths at each reference base position divided by the number of known bases in the reference. The mean read depth metric indicates how many reads, on average, are likely to be aligned at a given reference base position. Deep sequencing refers to sequencing a genomic region multiple times, sometimes hundreds or even thousands of times.

Sequencing coverage describes the average number of reads that align to, or "cover," known reference bases. The NGS (next-generation sequencing) coverage level often determines whether variant discovery can be made with a certain degree of confidence at particular base positions. Sequencing coverage requirements vary by application, as noted below. At higher levels of coverage, each base is covered by a greater number of aligned sequence reads, so base calls can be made with a higher degree of confidence.

In the methods listed in the question only Illumina DNA sequencing by synthesis is NGS sequencing. Therefore, B is the answer of choice.

185. **D**. *In the pop-out TXT window covering part of the aligned reads, it showed total count: 341. For the variant, 62 reads were with C and 279 with G. No reads were with A or T.*

Therefore, the reading depth at this point was 341.

186. E. *Sequencing coverage describes the average number of reads that align to, or "cover," known reference bases.* The NGS (next-generation sequencing) coverage level often determines whether variant discovery can be made with a certain degree of confidence at particular base positions. Sequencing coverage requirements vary by application, as noted below. At higher levels of coverage, each base is covered by a greater number of aligned sequence reads, so base calls can be made with a higher degree of confidence.

In the pop-out TXT window covering part of the aligned reads, it showed total count: 341. For the variant, 62 reads were with C and 279 with G. No reads were with A or T.

In this case, the sequencing coverage is not shown in the figure. Therefore, the coverage of this region is unclear according to the figure in the question.

187. B. In the pop-out TXT window covering part of the aligned reads, it showed total count: 341. For the variant, 62 reads were with and 279 with G. No reads were with A or T. The left side of the figure it showed the reads were aligned to the build 37 human reference sequences. On the top of the figure we may find that the location of the sequence was on 11p13, and the bottom of the figure pointed out that the region was in the *WT1* gene. *It is possible that the mutation is mosaic constitutional, but based on the patient's age, indication, and the ratio of reverse to forward reads (C: G = 62:279), most likely the mutation was acquired instead of constitutional.*

Therefore, the result indicated that the patient had an acquired deleterious variant in the *WT1* gene instead of a constitutional one.

188. A. *Based on the patient's age, morphological pathology diagnosis, and the nature of the mutation in the* FLT3 *gene, most likely the mutation was acquired* instead of constitutional. The internal tandem duplication of the *FLT3* gene is one of the recurrent abnormalities in acute myeloid leukemia (AML).

Therefore, it is most like to be an acquired mutation.

189. C. *Roche 454 sequencing is the only next-generation sequencing (NGS) technique using a large-scale parallel pyrosequencing system, which is capable of sequencing roughly 400–600 megabases of DNA per 10-h run on the Genome Sequencer FLX with GS FLX Titanium series reagents.* It is based on the sequencing-by-synthesis method. During the nucleotide flow, millions of copies of DNA bound to each of the beads are sequenced in parallel. When a nucleotide complementary to the template strand is added to a well, the polymerase extends the existing DNA strand by adding nucleotide(s).

Addition of one (or more) nucleotide(s) generates a light signal that is recorded by the CCD camera in the instrument. The height of each peak (light signal) is proportional to the number of nucleotides incorporated.

Therefore, Roche 454 sequencing is technologically similar to pyrosequencing.

190. D. *SOLiD (sequencing by oligonucleotide ligation and detection) is a next-generation DNA sequencing technology developed by Life Technologies, and by definition it is based on the sequencing-by-ligation method.* The rest of the next-generation sequencing (NGS) techniques are based on the sequencing-by-synthesis method.

Therefore, SOLiD is NOT based on sequencing-by-synthesis method.

191. A. Illumina genome sequencing and Roche 454 sequencing are next-generation sequencing (NGS), but not Pyrosequencing or Sanger sequencing. Roche 454 sequencing can produce read lengths approximately 400–700 bp, while Illumina genome sequencing can generate read length of only around 90 bp.

Therefore, Illumina genome sequencing produces the shortest reading length.

192. A. Iron Torrent DNA sequencing and Roche 454 sequencing are next-generation sequencing (NGS), but not Pyrosequencing or Sanger sequencing. Roche 454 sequencing can produce read lengths of approximately 400–700 bp, while Iron Torrent DNA sequencing can generate read lengths of only around 90 bp.

Therefore, Iron Torrent DNA sequencing produces the shortest reading length.

193. D. Illumina genome sequencing, Iron Torrent DNA sequencing, Roche 454 sequencing, and SOLiD (Sequencing by Oligonucleotide Ligation and Detection) are next-generation sequencing (NGS), but not Sanger sequencing. NGS has a higher false positive base pair reading than Sanger sequencing. Therefore, a lot of clinical laboratories still use Sanger sequencing to confirm the findings by NGS or use one NGS chemical to confirm the findings from another NGS chemical.

Therefore, Sanger sequencing has the highest accuracy and remains the gold standard for sequencing.

194. C. *Next-generation sequencing (NGS) usually starts with library preparation.* This step includes the targeted genomic region enrichment (library preparation) if a panel or exome sequencing is the goal. Adapters with nonhuman sequencing will be added to each fragment for the follow-up PCR reaction to increase the number of targeted sequences. Then NGS reactions will produce massively parallel sequences of the targeted regions. Bioinformatics will be followed for data analysis.

Therefore, the first step for next-generation sequencing (NGS) assays is library preparation.

195. D. For next-generation sequencing (NGS), translating the raw sequencing data into the final SNP and genotype calls requires two essential steps: read mapping and SNP/genotype inference. First, reads are aligned onto an available reference genome, then variable sites are identified and genotypes at those sites are determined. SNP and genotype calling suffers from high error rates that are due to the following factors. Poor quality or low-quality tails prevent reads from being properly mapped. Each read is aligned independently, causing many reads that span in/dels to be misaligned. The raw base-calling quality scores often co-vary with features like sequence technology, machine cycle and sequence context and, thus, cannot reflect the true base-calling error rates. These alignment and base-calling errors propagate into SNP and genotype inference and lead to false variant detection. Moreover, low-coverage sequencing (reading deeps) always introduces considerable uncertainty into the results and makes accurate SNP and genotype calling difficult. Furthermore, poor-quality tails of reads (location of the variant in the fragments) were evidenced with most NGS techniques. The ratio of the number of transitions to the number of transversions and ratio of the forward to reverse reading are helpful for assessing the quality of SNP calls.

Since NGS has higher false positive base pair reading than Sanger sequencing, a lot of clinical laboratories still use Sanger sequencing to confirm the findings by NGS, or use one NGS chemical to confirm the findings from another NGS chemical.

Therefore, reading deeps, location of variants in the fragments, and ratio of the forward to reverse reading usually are all monitored to assess the accuracy of the detections to decrease the false positive findings.

References

1. Mullis K, Faloona F, Scharf S, Saiki R, Horn G, Erlich H. Specific enzymatic amplification of DNA in vitro: the polymerase chain reaction. *Cold Spring Harb Symp Quant Biol* 1986;**51**(Pt 1):263–73 PubMed PMID: 3472723.
2. Gemeinholzer B, et al. The DNA bank network: the start from a german initiative. *Biopreserv Biobank* 2011;**9**(1):51–5.
3. Gallagher SR. Quantitation of DNA and RNA with absorption and fluorescence spectroscopy. *Curr Protoc Immunol* 2001. Appendix 3: p. Appendix3L.
4. Buckingham L. *Molecular diagnostics: fundamentals, methods, and clinical applications.* 2nd ed Philadelphia: F.A. Davis Co; 2012. xvi, 558 p.
5. Committee Opinion No. 640: Cell-Free DNA Screening For Fetal Aneuploidy. *Obstet Gynecol* 2015;**126**(3):e31–7.
6. Ashoor G, et al. Fetal fraction in maternal plasma cell-free DNA at 11-13 weeks' gestation: relation to maternal and fetal characteristics. *Ultrasound Obstet Gynecol* 2013;**41**(1):26–32.
7. Brar H, et al. The fetal fraction of cell-free DNA in maternal plasma is not affected by a priori risk of fetal trisomy. *J Matern Fetal Neonatal Med* 2013;**26**(2):143–5.
8. Suzumori N, et al. Fetal cell-free DNA fraction in maternal plasma is affected by fetal trisomy. *J Hum Genet* 2016;**61**(7):647–52.
9. *ACMG standards and guidelines for clinical, CF and Section G.* 2008 (http://www.acmg.net/PDFLibrary/Standards-Guidelines-Clinical-Molecular-Genetics.pdf).
10. Monaghan KG, et al. ACMG Standards and Guidelines for fragile X testing: a revision to the disease-specific supplements to the Standards and Guidelines for Clinical Genetics Laboratories of the American College of Medical Genetics and Genomics. *Genet Med* 2013;**15**(7):575–86.
11. Richards CS, et al. ACMG recommendations for standards for interpretation and reporting of sequence variations: Revisions 2007. *Genet Med* 2008;**10**(4):294–300.
12. Richards S, et al. Standards and guidelines for the interpretation of sequence variants: a joint consensus recommendation of the American College of Medical Genetics and Genomics and the Association for Molecular Pathology. *Genet Med* 2015;**17**(5):405–24.
13. Nussbaum RL, McInnes RR, Willard HF. *Thompson & Thompsongenetics in medicine.* 8th ed. Philadelphia: Elsevier; 2016. xi, 546 pages.
14. Bush WS, Moore JH. Chapter 11: Genome-wide association studies. *PLoS Comput Biol* 2012;**8**(12):e1002822.
15. Szumilas M. Explaining odds ratios. *J Can Acad Child Adolesc Psychiatry* 2010;**19**(3):227–9.
16. Thron CD. Calculation of relative risk. *N Engl J Med* 1972;**287**(18):937.
17. Garibyan L, Avashia N. Polymerase chain reaction. *J Invest Dermatol* 2013;**133**(3):e6.
18. Knudson A. Alfred Knudson and his two-hit hypothesis. (Interview by Ezzie Hutchinson). *Lancet Oncol* 2001;**2**(10):642–5.
19. Pannett AA, Thakker RV. Somatic mutations in MEN type 1 tumors, consistent with the Knudson "two-hit" hypothesis. *J Clin Endocrinol Metab* 2001;**86**(9):4371–4.
20. Rode A, et al. Chromothripsis in cancer cells: An update. *Int J Cancer* 2015.
21. Mohrenweiser HW, et al. Regions of sex-specific hypo- and hyper-recombination identified through integration of 180 genetic markers into the metric physical map of human chromosome 19. *Genomics* 1998;**47**(2):153–62.
22. Sachidanandam R, et al. A map of human genome sequence variation containing 1.42 million single nucleotide polymorphisms. *Nature* 2001;**409**(6822):928–33.
23. van Dijk EL, et al. Ten years of next-generation sequencing technology. *Trends Genet* 2014;**30**(9):418–26.

Further Reading

- Human Genome Project: https://www.genome.gov/12011238/an-overview-of-the-human-genome-project/
- 1000 Human Genome Project: http://www.internationalgenome.org/about/
- Exome Aggregation Consortium (ExAC): http://exac.broadinstitute.org/

2

Regulations From Oversight Agencies

Clinical genetics laboratories have many regulatory agencies with which they must contend. The responsibility of genetic test quality regulation is often divided among several regulatory agencies, which safeguard different elements of the testing process. This introduction is an overview of the regulatory agencies for clinical genetics laboratories.

LABORATORY ACCREDITATION BODIES

Laboratory procedures, setup, and general quality assurance mechanisms are held to standards that are mandated and enforced by laboratory accreditation organizations.

CLIA'88 (Clinical Laboratory Improvement Amendments of 1988): These federal regulatory standards apply to all clinical laboratory testing performed on patient specimens, except clinical trials and basic research, in order to ensure accurate and reliable test results. Three federal agencies are responsible for CLIA: the Food and Drug Administration (FDA), the Center for Medicare and Medicaid Services (CMS), and the Centers for Disease Control and Prevention (CDC). The CMS has primary responsibility for the operation of the CLIA Program.

CAP (College of American Pathologists). CAP inspects and accredits medical laboratories under the authority of the CMS. The CAP Laboratory Accreditation Program advances the quality of pathology and laboratory services, including molecular diagnosis through education and standard setting and ensuring that laboratories meet or exceed regulatory requirements. With more than 600 surveys, the CAP Proficiency Testing/External Quality Assurance (PT/ EQA) is the largest laboratory peer-comparison program in the world. Through these programs, the CAP provides individual laboratories with unknown specimens for testing. The participants analyze the specimens and return the results to the CAP for evaluation. Then, each participating laboratory receives a report of

its performance as well as a report summarizing the results of all participating laboratories.

CONSUMER PROTECTION AGENCIES

Genetic tests are subject to regulations mandated by consumer protection agencies. Regulation must ensure that tests that are offered are of an acceptable efficacy.

FDA (US Food and Drug Administration). The FDA is an agency within the US Department of Health and Human Services that classifies tests as waived, moderately complex, or highly complex on the basis of complexity. None of molecular genetic tests are classified as waived. The FDA categorizes medical devices into three separate classes, ranging from class I, for relatively low risk products, to class III, where tests are subject to the greatest level of scrutiny. Tests that are marketed and distributed by private genetic test developers to laboratories in self-contained kits are regulated by the FDA for their accuracy and reliability. However, more commonly, a test comes to market as a laboratory-developed test (LDT)—a test that is developed and performed by a single laboratory as an "in-house" test and for which specimen samples are sent to that laboratory to be tested. The FDA has practiced "enforcement discretion" for LDTs, and we will find out where it leads to. The FDA also oversees marketed drugs to ensure that manufacturers provide information on drug labels about genetic markers that are relevant for drug safety and effectiveness.

PROFESSIONAL LICENSING ORGANIZATIONS

Professional licensing organizations uphold the qualification of clinical molecular geneticists by licensing only professionals who have been trained to perform required tasks. Professional certification also requires that clinical molecular geneticists participate in continuing education to maintain and develop professional knowledge. Certificates may be revoked in cases of inadequate performance.

ABMGG (American Board of Medical Genetics and Genomics). This member of the American Board of Medical Specialties (ABMS) accredits medical genetics and genomics laboratory training programs, credentials and certifies practitioners of medical genetics and genomics, and fosters lifelong learning through maintenance of certification.

ACMG (American College of Medical Genetics and Genomics). This professional organization has more than 1600 board-certified clinical and laboratory genetics professionals. The ACMG publishes serial standards "as an educational resource to assist medical geneticists in providing accurate and reliable diagnostic genetics laboratory testing consistent with currently available technology and procedures in the areas of clinical cytogenetics, biochemical genetics and molecular diagnostics." These standards establish minimum criteria for clinical genetics laboratories (http://www.acmg.net/ ACMG/Medical-Genetics-Practice-Resources/ACMG/ Medical-Genetics-Practice-Resources/Medical-Genetics-Practice-Resources.aspx?hkey = 9b68bf77-2376-489d-a567-c0130b2473e9.

OTHER REGULATORY BODIES

OSHA (Occupational Safety and Health Administration). OSHA is an agency of the US Department of Labor. Its mission is to prevent work-related injuries, illnesses, and deaths by issuing and enforcing rules for workplace safety and health.

HIPAA (Health Insurance Portability and Accountability Act). The HIPAA law was created in 1996 to protect millions of working Americans and their family members with medical problems. These people often had trouble getting health insurance because of a medical problem they had before they tried to buy health insurance (called a "preexisting condition"). In fact, before the important protections of the health care law known as the Affordable Care Act took effect, many people with serious health problems couldn't get health insurance.

FTC (Federal Trade Commission). The FTC has the authority to protect consumers from unfair and deceptive trade practices (including false and misleading advertising claims) under Section 5(a) of the FTC Act, 15 U.S.C. 45(a)(1). The FTC also enforces posted corporate privacy policies. In July 2006, the FTC issued a consumer alert warning consumers to be skeptical of claims made by direct-to-consumer (DTC) test providers and to discuss test results with a health care provider.

GINA (Genetic Information Nondiscrimination Act). This 2008 federal law protects individuals from genetic discrimination in health insurance and employment. GINA, together with already existing nondiscrimination provisions of the HIPAA, generally prohibits health insurers or health plan administrators from requesting or requiring genetic information from an individual or the individual's family members or using it for decisions regarding coverage, rates, or preexisting conditions. The law also prohibits most employers from using genetic information for hiring, firing, or promotion decisions and for any decisions regarding terms of employment.

NPI (National Provider Identifier Standard). The NPI is a HIPAA Administrative Simplification Standard. The NPI is a unique identification number for covered health care providers. Covered health care providers and all health plans and health care clearinghouses must use the NPIs in the administrative and financial transactions adopted under HIPAA. The NPI is a 10-position, intelligence-free numeric identifier (10-digit number). This means that the numbers do not carry other information about health care providers, such as the state in which they live or their medical specialty.

In this chapter, we will mainly review the CAP Accreditation Checklists dated July 28, 2015, including All Common, Laboratory General, Molecular Pathology, and Team Leader Assessment of Director and Quality. Those checklists contain the CAP accreditation program requirements.

QUESTIONS

1. According to CLIA and CAP regulations, which one of the following individuals is considered to be a director of a clinical molecular laboratory?[1]
   A. Dr. A, a member of the corresponding academic society
   B. Dr. B, appointed by the institute as the director laboratory
   C. Dr. C, board certified in the corresponding specialty
   D. Dr. D, listed on the laboratory's CAP and CLIA certificate as the lab director
   E. All of the above
   F. None of the above
2. A scientist plans to develop a Sanger sequencing—based test for the *FAS* (*TNFRSF6*) gene to assist diagnosis of autoimmune lymphoproliferative syndrome in a clinical molecular laboratory. There are no commercially available FDA-cleared/approved assays for it. According to the Clinical Laboratory Improvement Amendments (CLIA) regulations,

which one of the following descriptions most appropriately describes this test?

A. Waived test

B. Nonwaived test

C. Moderate-complexity test

D. High-complexity test

E. None of the above

3. A scientist plans to develop a quantitative PCR−based test for pathogenic variants in the *NPM1* gene to assist in the diagnosis of acute myeloid leukemia (AML) in a clinical molecular laboratory. There are no commercially available FDA-cleared/approved assays for it. According to the Clinical Laboratory Improvement Amendments (CLIA) program, which one of the following descriptions most appropriately describes this test?

A. Waived test

B. Nonwaived test

C. Moderate-complexity test

D. High-complexity test

E. None of the above

4. A scientist plans to validate a quantitative HIV-1 RNA assay for viral load assessment with the Bayer VERSANT HIV-1 RNA 3.0 Assay (bDNA), a FDA-approved commercially available assay, in a clinical molecular laboratory. According to the Clinical Laboratory Improvement Amendments (CLIA) program, which one of the following descriptions most appropriately describes this test?

A. Waived test

B. Nonwaived test

C. Moderate-complexity test

D. High-complexity test

E. None of the above

5. A scientist developed a quantitative PCR-based test for pathogenic variants in the *NPM1* gene to assist in the diagnosis of acute myeloid leukemia (AML) in a clinical molecular laboratory. He used the data published in a peer-reviewed article, since there were no commercially available FDA-cleared/approved assays for it. The validation was done as planned, and the summary was written. Who has the authority to review and approve the validation, according to the College of American Pathologist (CAP)'s regulations, if applicable?[1]

A. Clinical Laboratory Improvement Amendments (CLIA)

B. College of American Pathologist (CAP)

C. The chair of the department

D. The laboratory director

E. The supervisor of the laboratory

F. All of the above

G. None of the above

6. A scientist planned to validate the bioMérieux THxID *BRAF* assay, an FDA-approved commercially available assay, to detect somatic mutations in order to guide the therapy of metastatic melanoma in a clinical molecular laboratory. The protocol received from bioMérieux was for 20-μL total volume for each reaction. To save money, the scientist decided to use 10 μL for each reaction. Which validation stringency should he follow for the validation, according to the College of American Pathologist (CAP)'s regulations, if applicable?[1,2]

A. Follow the validation procedure for FDA-approved assay.

B. Follow the validation procedure for FDA-approved assay, and add analytical sensitivity and specificity.

C. Follow the validation procedure for FDA-approved assay with both 20-μL and 10-μL reactions.

D. Follow the validation procedure for a laboratory-developed assay.

E. None of the above.

7. A scientist reviewed last month's data in a clinical molecular laboratory and found that the failure rate of the *KRAS* test was 10% higher than that for the previous 6 months and for the same month last year. Which one of the following is the most appropriate term used to define the nature of this monthly review of failure rate, according to the College of American Pathologist (CAP)'s regulations, if applicable?[1,2]

A. Quality assurance

B. Quality control

C. Quality improvement

D. Quality planning

E. All of the above

F. None of the above

8. A scientist reviewed last month's quality control data in a clinical molecular laboratory and found that the failure rate of the *KRAS* test was 10% higher than that for the previous 6 months and for the same month last year. Which one of following actions should he take to resolve the problem, according to the College of American Pathologist (CAP)'s regulations, if applicable?[1,2]

A. Quality assurance

B. Quality control

C. Quality improvement

D. Quality planning

E. All of the above

F. None of the above

9. A clinical molecular genetic scientist has been working in a start-up company for 2 months. He has been purchasing reagents and writing policies and procedures for this new laboratory. Which one of the following should be included in his quality management plan for the clinical laboratory, according to the College of American Pathologist (CAP)'s regulations, if applicable?[1,2]
   A. Calibrating the pipette at least once a year
   B. Checking the quality of new lots and new shipments of reagents against old ones
   C. Having a written quality management plan
   D. Maintaining discontinued procedures for at least 2 years
   E. Participating in the CAP Proficiency Test (PT)
   F. All of the above
   G. None of the above

10. A courier picked up a peripheral-blood sample (lavender) from an outreach draw station for BCR-ABL1 quantitative testing at the main hospital. He checked the identifiers of the sample on the requisition form and the tube to make sure the identity of the sample matched. At a minimum, how many identifiers have to be on the tube for a collected peripheral-blood sample, according to the College of American Pathologist (CAP)'s regulations, if applicable?[2]
   A. At least one
   B. At least two
   C. At least three
   D. At least four
   E. None of above

11. A courier picked up a peripheral-blood sample (lavender) from a local obstetrician/gynecologist (Ob/Gyn) practice for cystic fibrosis testing in the main hospital. He noticed the patient's name was donor BJ. And the only usable identifier on the requisition form and the tube was patient's medical record number. Which type of deficiency would an on-site College of American Pathologist (CAP) inspector find it to be, according to the College of American Pathologist (CAP)'s regulations, if applicable?[1]
   A. Phase 0
   B. Phase I
   C. Phase II
   D. Phase III
   E. None of above

12. A scientist just finished validation of a HER2 FISH assay with archived formalin-fixed, paraffin-embedded (FFPE) tissue samples in a clinical molecular laboratory at a hospital. According to procedure, he sends samples to the cytology laboratory in the same hospital for hybridization, then takes the slides back for analysis. How should the clinical molecular laboratory perform proficiency test on this HER2 FISH assay, according to the College of American Pathologist (CAP)'s regulations, if applicable?[1]
   A. Enroll in the College of American Pathologist (CAP) HER2 immunohistochemistry (IHC) proficiency test.
   B. Enroll in the College of American Pathologist (CAP) HER2 FISH proficiency test.
   C. Perform an alternative HER2 FISH proficiency test.
   D. All of the above.
   E. None of the above.

13. A scientist in a clinical molecular laboratory of a hospital just finished validation of a HER2 FISH assay with archived formalin-fixed, paraffin-embedded (FFPE) tissue samples. According to procedure, she sends samples to the cytology laboratory in the same hospital for hybridization, then takes the slides back for analysis. Therefore, the clinical molecular laboratory must perform an alternative assessment of the HER2 FISH assay instead of the CAP formal proficiency test. At a minimum, how frequently should the laboratory perform the alternative assessment of the HER2 FISH assay, according to the College of American Pathologist (CAP)'s regulations, if applicable?[1]
   A. Every quarter
   B. Semiannually
   C. Annually
   D. Biennially
   E. None of the above

14. A clinical molecular laboratory in a hospital received specimens for proficiency test of a BRAF assay from the College of American Pathologist (CAP) last week. The specimens were treated as regular clinical samples, and were signed out in the electronic reporting system in the laboratory. Who should sign the Proficiency Test (PT) Attestation Statement according to the College of American Pathologist (CAP)'s regulations, if applicable?[1]
   a. The laboratory director or designee
   b. All individuals involved in the testing process
   c. All staff in this laboratory
   d. The quality control office of the hospital
   A. a, b, and d
   B. a, c, and d
   C. a and b
   D. a and c
   E. a, b, c, and d

15. A clinical molecular laboratory in a hospital received specimens for a proficiency test of a BRAF assay from the College of American Pathologist (CAP) last week, which was 3 months

after test was launched. The specimens were treated as regular clinical samples and were signed out in the electronic reporting system in the laboratory. At a minimum, how frequently should proficiency tests (PT) of this assay be done according to the Clinical Laboratory Improvement Amendments (CLIAs) 1988?[1]

A. Annually
B. Biennially
C. Twice a year
D. Three times a year
E. None of above

16. A director of a CAP/CLIA-certified clinical molecular laboratory received specimens for a proficiency test (PT) of a *BRAF* assay from the College of American Pathologist (CAP). One of the samples showed unacceptable results. Which type of deficiency would this discrepancy be, according to the College of American Pathologist (CAP)'s regulations, if applicable?

A. Phase 0
B. Phase I
C. Phase II
D. Phase III
E. None of above

17. A CAP inspection team comes to the molecular pathology laboratory in the department of pathology of a hospital for an on-site inspection. The team member for the molecular laboratory finds that the *CYP2C19* test is on the test menu of the laboratory, but not on the current College of American Pathologist (CAP) activity menu. The director explains that the test was developed 6 months ago, and he has not had a chance to add it to the CAP activity menu. Which type of deficiency would this discrepancy be, according to the College of American Pathologist (CAP)'s regulations, if applicable?[1]

A. Phase 0
B. Phase I
C. Phase II
D. Phase III
E. None of above

18. A clinical molecular scientist reviewed last month's quality control data in the laboratory, and found that the detection rate of the *KRAS* test was 50% lower than it had been in the previous 6 months and in the same month last year. He started to investigate the reason while sending the samples to a reference laboratory. During investigation, the laboratory received CAP proficiency test (PT) specimens for this test. One of the ideas was to send the specimens to the reference laboratory as clinical samples. Which type of deficiency would it be if the laboratory

sent the CAP specimens to a reference laboratory, according to the College of American Pathologist (CAP)'s regulations, if applicable?[1]

A. Phase 0
B. Phase I
C. Phase II
D. Phase III
E. None of above

19. A clinical molecular laboratory in a hospital received specimens for proficiency test (PT) of a *BRAF* assay from the College of American Pathologist (CAP) last week, which was 3 months after test was launched. The specimens were treated as regular clinical samples and were signed out in the electronic reporting system in the laboratory. How long should the primary records of the proficiency test (PT) be retained, according to the Clinical Laboratory Improvement Amendments (CLIA) 1988?[1]

A. At least 1 year
B. At least 2 years
C. At least 3 years
D. At least 4 years
E. At least 5 years
F. At least 10 years

20. A start-up clinical molecular genetics laboratory in the state of Arizona welcomed its first on-site inspector on a Monday morning. There were only two tests in this laboratory—factor V Leiden and factor II. The director shared with the inspector that he used an alternative approach for the proficiency test (PT) in order to save money. Which type of deficiency would it be, according to the College of American Pathologist (CAP)'s regulations, if applicable?[1]

A. Phase 0
B. Phase I
C. Phase II
D. Phase III
E. None of above

21. A start-up clinical molecular genetics laboratory in the state of Arizona welcomed its first on-site inspector on a Monday morning. There were only two tests in this laboratory—*BRAF* and *EGFR*. The director shared with the inspector that he used an alternative approach for the proficiency test (PT) in order to save money. Which type of deficiency would it be, according to the College of American Pathologist (CAP)'s regulations, if applicable?[1]

A. Phase 0
B. Phase I
C. Phase II
D. Phase III
E. None of above

22. According to the Centers for Disease Control and Prevention (CDC) classification of biohazardous waste, the risk group 1 agents are:[3]
   A. Agents that are not associated with disease in healthy adult humans.
   B. Agents that are associated with serious or lethal human disease for which preventive or therapeutic interventions may be available (high individual risk but low community risk).
   C. Agents that are associated with human disease that is rarely serious and for which preventive or therapeutic interventions are often available.
   D. Agents that are likely to cause serious or lethal human disease for which preventive or therapeutic interventions are not usually available (high individual risk and high community risk).

23. According to the Centers for Disease Control and Prevention (CDC) classification of biohazardous waste, the Risk Group 4 agents are:
   A. Agents that are not associated with disease in healthy adult humans.
   B. Agents that are associated with serious or lethal human disease for which preventive or therapeutic interventions may be available (high individual risk but low community risk).
   C. Agents that are associated with human disease that is rarely serious and for which preventive or therapeutic interventions are often available.
   D. Agents that are likely to cause serious or lethal human disease for which preventive or therapeutic interventions are not usually available (high individual risk and high community risk).

24. According to the Centers for Disease Control and Prevention (CDC) classification of biohazardous waste, the Risk Group 2 agents are:
   A. Agents that are not associated with disease in healthy adult humans.
   B. Agents that are associated with serious or lethal human disease for which preventive or therapeutic interventions may be available (high individual risk but low community risk).
   C. Agents that are associated with human disease that is rarely serious and for which preventive or therapeutic interventions are often available
   D. Agents that are likely to cause serious or lethal human disease for which preventive or therapeutic interventions are not usually available (high individual risk and high community risk).

25. According to the Disease Control and Prevention (CDC) classification of biohazardous waste, the risk group 3 agents are:

   A. Agents that are not associated with disease in healthy adult humans.
   B. Agents that are associated with serious or lethal human disease for which preventive or therapeutic interventions may be available (high individual risk but low community risk).
   C. Agents that are associated with human disease that is rarely serious and for which preventive or therapeutic interventions are often available.
   D. Agents that are likely to cause serious or lethal human disease for which preventive or therapeutic interventions are not usually available (high individual risk and high community risk).

26. Human immunodeficiency virus (HIV) spreads through certain body fluids and attacks a person's immune system by destroying CD4-positive T cells. This makes it harder and harder for the body to fight infections and other diseases. Currently, no effective cure exists for HIV. But with proper medical care, HIV can be controlled. According to the Centers for Disease Control and Prevention (CDC) classification of biohazardous waste, to which risk group does the HIV-1 virus belong?
   A. Risk Group 1
   B. Risk Group 2
   C. Risk Group 3
   D. Risk Group 4
   E. Risk Group 5

27. The Ebola virus causes an acute and serious illness that is often fatal if left untreated. Ebola virus disease (EVD) first appeared in 1976 in two simultaneous outbreaks, one in what is now, Nzara, South Sudan, and the other in Yambuku, Democratic Republic of Congo. The latter occurred in a village near the Ebola River, from which the disease takes its name. According to the Centers for Disease Control and Prevention (CDC) classification of biohazardous waste, to which risk group does the Ebola virus belong?
   A. Risk Group 1
   B. Risk Group 2
   C. Risk Group 3
   D. Risk Group 4
   E. Risk Group 5

28. According to the Centers for Disease Control and Prevention (CDC) classification of biohazardous waste, to which risk group do hepatitis B, cytomegalovirus (CMV), Epstein–Barr virus (EBV), and herpes simplex types 1 and 2 viruses belong?
   A. Risk Group 1
   B. Risk Group 2
   C. Risk Group 3
   D. Risk Group 4
   E. Risk Group 5

29. Rabies virus has a nonsegmented and negative-stranded RNA genome. Rabies disease is most often transmitted through the bite of a rabid animal such as raccoons, skunks, bats, and foxes. According to the Centers for Disease Control and Prevention (CDC) classification of biohazardous waste, to which risk group does rabies virus belong?
   A. Risk Group 1
   B. Risk Group 2
   C. Risk Group 3
   D. Risk Group 4
   E. Risk Group 5

30. An ACMG board-certified molecular geneticist started a job as a director in a commercial laboratory. He planned to review all the procedures and policies in the laboratory in the first 2 months. He found that one of the procedures stated that a designee of the director would review and assess instrument and equipment maintenance and function-check records semiannually. He felt it was wrong. How frequently should he or his designee review and assess instrument and equipment maintenance and function check records, according to the College of American Pathologist (CAP)'s regulations, if applicable?[1]
   A. At least monthly
   B. At least quarterly
   C. At least twice a year
   D. At least annually
   E. At least biennially

31. An ACMG board-certified molecular geneticist started a job as a director in a commercial laboratory. He planned to review all the procedures and policies in the laboratory in 2 months. He found that one of the procedures stated that a designee of the director would check the 20 thermal cyclers against each other once a year. He noticed that 10 of the thermal cyclers were from Applied Biosystems (ABI), 5 were from Eppendorf, and the remaining 5 were from Thermo Fisher Scientific. Which one of the following statements is correct, according to the College of American Pathologist (CAP)'s regulations, if applicable?[1]
   A. He should check the thermal cyclers from the same manufacturer against each other at least once a year.
   B. He should check all 20 thermal cyclers against each other at least once a year.
   C. He should check the thermal cyclers from the same manufacturer against each other at least twice a year.
   D. He should check all 20 thermal cyclers against each other at least twice a year.
   E. None of the above.

32. An ACMG board-certified molecular geneticist started a job as a director in a commercial laboratory. He planned to review all the procedures and policies in the laboratory in the first month. He found that one of the procedures stated that a designee of the director would check the 20 thermal cyclers against each other once a year. He noticed that 10 of the thermal cyclers were from Applied Biosystems (ABI) and the rest were from Eppendorf or Thermo Fisher Scientific. How frequently should he or a designee check the thermal cyclers against each other for comparability of results in the laboratory, according to the College of American Pathologist (CAP)'s regulations, if applicable?[1]
   A. At least monthly
   B. At least quarterly
   C. At least twice a year
   D. At least annually
   E. At least biennially

33. A newly ACMG board-certified molecular geneticist started a job as a director in a commercial laboratory 2 months ago. While he reviewed the procedures and policies, he found that the laboratory used a triplet primer PCR assay without methylation-sensitive confirmation for the fragile X test. Before taking any action on it, the laboratory received specimens from the College of American Pathologist (CAP) for proficiency testing on fragile X. One of the specimens was homozygous for allele 30. Since the gender of the specimen was unknown, the director was concerned about whether there was a gross deletion or a mutation in the primer region leading to allelic drop. He called a director at another institute to discuss the result before finalizing it. Which type of deficiency would it be if they discussed the results, according to the College of American Pathologist (CAP)'s regulations, if applicable?[1]
   A. Phase 0
   B. Phase I
   C. Phase II
   D. Phase III
   E. None of above

34. Dr. A, a newly board-certified molecular geneticist, started to work for a hospital 10 days ago. He planned to review all the procedures and policies in the laboratory in the first 2 months. He found that some of the procedures had not been reviewed for more than 5 years. How frequently should the technical policies and procedures be reviewed by the current

laboratory director or designee in a clinical molecular genetics laboratory, according to the College of American Pathology (CAP) regulations, if applicable?[1]

A. At least monthly
B. At least quarterly
C. At least twice a year
D. At least annually
E. At least biennially
F. At least once in 5 years

35. Dr. A, a newly board-certified molecular geneticist, started to work for a hospital 10 days ago. He planned to review all the procedures and policies in the laboratory in the first 2 months. He found that some of the procedures had not been reviewed for more than 5 years. Which type of deficiency would it be, according to the College of American Pathologist (CAP)'s regulations, if applicable?[1]

A. Phase 0
B. Phase I
C. Phase II
D. Phase III
E. None of above

36. Dr. B, a director of a clinical molecular genetics laboratory in an academic center, validated a clinical next-generation sequencing (NGS) panel for somatic mutations in solid tumors. When should the procedure for this new test be reviewed and approved, according to the College of American Pathologist (CAP)'s regulations, if applicable?[1]

A. It should be reviewed and approved 30 days before implementation.
B. It should be reviewed and approved 15 days before implementation.
C. It should be reviewed and approved before implementation.
D. It should be reviewed and approved within 1 month after implementation.
E. None of above.

37. Dr. B, the only director of a clinical molecular genetics laboratory in an academic center, validated a clinical next-generation sequencing (NGS) panel for somatic pathogenic variants in solid tumors. By whom should this procedure for the new test be reviewed and approved, according to the College of American Pathologist (CAP)'s regulations, if applicable?[1]

A. BJ, the supervisor of the laboratory
B. Dr. B
C. Dr. C, the chair of the department
D. Dr. D, the chief medical officer of the hospital
E. College of American Pathologist (CAP)

F. All of the above
G. None of above

38. JJ, a technologist in a clinical molecular genetics laboratory, came to Dr. E, the director, to complain about the speed of the computer. The laboratory support team assessed the situation and suggested the purchase of a new remote drive or the deletion some files in the current hard drive to free some space. Dr. E decided to delete some of the discontinued procedures. How long should the discontinued procedures be maintained in a clinical molecular genetics laboratory, according to the College of American Pathologist (CAP)'s regulations, if applicable?[1]

A. At least 1 year
B. At least 2 years
C. At least 5 years
D. At least 7 years
E. At least 16 years
F. At least 23 years
G. Forever

39. Dr. J, a clinical molecular geneticist, called Dr. G, an oncologist in the same hospital, about a patient's abnormal *PML/RARA* quantitative results. What information should be recorded in the patient's record for this communication, according to the College of American Pathologist (CAP)'s regulations, if applicable?[1]

a. Patient ID
b. Date of the phone call
c. Time of the phone call
d. Laboratory individual responsible for the phone call
e. Person notified in the physician office (first and last name)
f. Test results
g. Recommendations
h. "Read-back" of the results

A. a, b, d, e, and h
B. a, b, d, e, f, and h
C. a, b, c, d, e, f, and h
D. a, b, d, e, f, and h
E. a, b, c, d, e, f, g, and h
F. None of above

40. Dr. D, a director of a clinical laboratory in Wisconsin, found that a lot of restriction enzymes in the laboratory had passed the expiration date. It would be a huge waste to throw them away, so he tested the enzymes with positive controls, negative controls, and 10 previous patient samples. All the results were correct, so he decided to keep using those enzymes clinically. Which type of deficiency would this decision be, according to the College

of American Pathologist (CAP)'s regulations, if applicable?[1]

- **A.** Phase 0
- **B.** Phase I
- **C.** Phase II
- **D.** Phase III
- **E.** None of above

41. Dr. A, an ACMG board-certified molecular geneticist, started a job as a senior director in a commercial laboratory 2 months ago. When reviewing the procedures and policies in the laboratory, he found that the laboratory only checked new reagent lots against old reagent lots, but not against new reagent shipments in the same lot. The manager explained that it was done that way in order to save money. Dr. A changed the procedure to check new reagent lots and new shipments against old reagent lots and old shipments. Why did Dr. A make the change, according to the College of American Pathologist (CAP)'s regulations, if applicable?[1]

- **A.** Because it is a Phase 0 deficiency if the laboratory doesn't check new shipments in the same lot.
- **B.** Because it is a Phase I deficiency if the laboratory doesn't check new shipments in the same lot.
- **C.** Because it is a Phase II deficiency if the laboratory doesn't check new shipments in the same lot.
- **D.** Because it is a Phase III deficiency if the laboratory doesn't check new shipments in the same lot.
- **E.** Because it makes Dr. A feel more comfortable to have both new lots and new shipments checked.
- **F.** None of above.

42. Dr. A, an ACMG board-certified molecular geneticist, started a job as a senior director in a commercial laboratory 2 months ago. He observed the staff performing each test. When he was observing JJ, a technologist, setting up a quantitative PCR reaction for *BCR-ABL1*, JJ found that the reagents in the kit were not enough for this run. JJ took out another kit with a different lot number from the freezer. The new lot was checked and verified. JJ pipetted the remaining reagents from the old kit to the new kit and explained to Dr. A that this was a new policy in the laboratory to save money. Dr. A stopped JJ and changed the procedure immediately. Why did Dr. A stop JJ and make the change to the procedure, according to the College of American Pathologist (CAP)'s regulations, if applicable?[1]

- **A.** Because it is a Phase 0 deficiency to mix kit components from different lots.
- **B.** Because it is a Phase I deficiency to mix kit components from different lots.
- **C.** Because it is a Phase II deficiency to mix kit components from different lots.
- **D.** Because it is a Phase III deficiency to mix kit components from different lots.
- **E.** Because Dr. G did not feel that it was right to mix kit components from different lots.
- **F.** None of above.

43. Dr. G, an ACMG board-certified molecular geneticist, started a job as a senior director of a clinical molecular pathology laboratory in a hospital 2 months ago. He started to observe the staff to performing each test. When he was observing BJ, a technologist, as he set up a quantitative PCR reaction for *BCR-ABL1*, a man put an Eppendorf thermal cycler on the bench, and told BJ it was fixed. BJ explained to Dr. G that the Eppendorf thermal cycler had had a problem and that a clinical engineer took it a few days ago. While they were talking, Emily, another technologist, walked in with her PCR plate. Emily started to set up her PCR in the newly fixed thermal cycler. Dr. G suggested that Emily use other thermal cyclers in the laboratory. Why did Dr. G suggest the use of other thermal cyclers in the laboratory, according to the College of American Pathologist (CAP)'s regulations, if applicable?[1]

- **A.** It is a Phase 0 deficiency to use newly fixed instruments/equipment before performance verification.
- **B.** It is a Phase I deficiency to use newly fixed instruments/equipment before performance verification.
- **C.** It is a Phase II deficiency to use newly fixed instruments/equipment before performance verification.
- **D.** It is a Phase III deficiency to use newly fixed instruments/equipment before performance verification.
- **E.** Dr. G felt that using newly fixed instruments/equipment before performance verification did not feel right.
- **F.** None of above.

44. A start-up CAP/CLIA-certified clinical molecular genetics laboratory has only two technologists, one part-time on-site supervisor, and one part-time off-site director. The technologists validated a *BRAF* assay with formalin-fixed and paraffin-embedded (FFPE) tissue samples. The supervisor approved the validation summary and sent it to the director.

Before the director replied, the husband of the supervisor, a physician in the same hospital, sent a FFPE sample for the *BRAF* test. How should the laboratory treat this sample, according to the College of American Pathologist (CAP)'s regulations, if applicable?[1]

A. Set up the sample for the *BRAF* test while waiting for the director to approve the validation for the final report.

B. Set up the sample for the *BRAF* test, giving the preliminary results to the ordering physician while waiting for the director to approve the validation for the final report.

C. Set up the sample for the *BRAF* test, reporting it out before the director approves the validation.

D. Hold the sample while waiting for the director to approve the validation.

E. Explain to the ordering physician that the method for the *BRAF* test has not been validated in this laboratory.

F. None of above.

45. Dr. Z has been validating the FDA-cleared/approved quantitative COBAS AmpliPrep/COBAS TaqMan CMV test from Roche Molecular Systems for cytomegalovirus (CMV) in a clinical molecular pathology laboratory in Florida. He gathered all the data to write the validation summary. What components should he include in the validation summary, according to the College of American Pathologist (CAP)'s regulations, if applicable?[1]

a. Analytical accuracy
b. Analytical precision
c. Analytical sensitivity
d. Analytical specificity
e. Cross-contamination
f. Interferences
g. Reportable range
A. a, b, c, and d
B. a, b, and g
C. a, b, f, and g
D. c, d, f, and g
E. a, b, c, d, e, f, and g
F. None of the above

46. Dr. Y has been validating the FDA-cleared/approved quantitative COBAS AmpliPrep/COBAS TaqMan CMV test from Roche Molecular Systems for cytomegalovirus (CMV) in a clinical molecular pathology laboratory in Florida. And he planned to use the assay on cerebrospinal fluid (CSF) specimens, too, which was not been approved or cleared by the FDA. He gathered all the data to write the validation summary. What

components should he include in the validation summary according to the College of American Pathologist (CAP) regulations, if applicable?[1]

a. Analytical accuracy
b. Analytical precision
c. Analytical sensitivity
d. Analytical specificity
e. Cross-contamination
f. Interferences
g. Reportable range
A. a, b, c, and d
B. a, b, and g
C. a, b, f, and g
D. c, d, e, f, and g
E. a, b, c, d, e, f, and g
F. None of the above

47. A clinical molecular pathology laboratory decides to discontinue its *CYP2C19* test used to predict therapeutic response to clopidogrel (commonly known as Plavix) as an antiplatelet agent for cardiovascular disorders, because it is an extremely low volume test. How long should the laboratory keep the procedure for the *CYP2C19* test after discontinuation, according to the College of American Pathologist (CAP)'s regulations, if applicable?[1]

A. At least 1 year
B. At least 2 years
C. At least 5 years
D. At least 7 years
E. At least 16 years
F. At least 23 years
G. Forever

48. A clinical molecular pathology laboratory in Florida has been offering a quantitative cytomegalovirus (CMV) test with the FDA-cleared/approved COBAS AmpliPrep/COBAS TaqMan CMV assay from Roche Molecular Systems for more than 2 years. Last month the laboratory moved from the main hospital to a remote facility with the rest of the department of pathology. Which of the following parameters should be included in the verification after the move, according to the College of American Pathologist (CAP)'s regulations, if applicable?[1]

a. Analytical accuracy
b. Analytical precision
c. Analytical sensitivity
d. Analytical specificity
e. Cross-contamination
f. Interferences
g. Reportable range
A. a, b, c, and d
B. a, b, and g

C. a, b, f, and g

D. c, d, e, f, and g

E. a, b, c, d, e, f, and g

F. None of the above

49. A clinical molecular pathology laboratory used a *CYP2C19* assay to predict therapeutic response to clopidogrel (commonly known as Plavix) as an antiplatelet agent for cardiovascular disorders. Two years ago, the laboratory discontinued the test because of low volume. Recently, the data from the send-outs indicated the increase of volume for *CYP2C19*. The laboratory is considering bringing the assay back. Which one of the following requirements must be met in order to put the test back into production, according to the College of American Pathologist (CAP)'s regulations, if applicable?[1]

A. PT or alternative assessment performed within 30 days prior to restarting patient testing

B. Method of performance specifications verified, as applicable, within 30 days prior to restarting patient testing

C. Competency assessed for analysts within 12 months prior to restarting patient testing

D. All of the above

E. None of the above

50. A clinical molecular pathology laboratory has been offering an FDA-approved quantitative HIV-1 RNA test for 1 year. However, the test has been suspended for a month, and the laboratory cannot participate in the most recent CAP proficiency test (PT) because of an instrument breakdown. Which one of the following requirements must be met in order to put the test back into production, according to the College of American Pathologist (CAP)'s regulations, if applicable?[1]

A. PT or alternative assessment performed within 30 days prior to restarting patient testing

B. Method of performance specifications verified, as applicable, within 30 days prior to restarting patient testing

C. Competency assessed for analysts within 12 months prior to restarting patient testing

D. Perform alternative proficiency test (PT) assessment

E. All of the above

F. None of the above

51. Dr. Z, a director of a clinical molecular pathology laboratory, wants to validate the FDA-cleared/approved Cystic Fibrosis 139-Variant Assay. However, the laboratory has Illumina MiSeq instead of Illumina MiSeqDx. Dr. Z decides to validate the assay with Illumina MiSeq (MiSeqDX

is the instrument for the FDA-cleared/approved Cystic Fibrosis 139-Variant Assay). Which of the following parameters should Dr. Z include in the verification, according to the College of American Pathologist (CAP)'s regulations, if applicable?[1]

a. Analytical accuracy

b. Analytical precision

c. Analytical sensitivity

d. Analytical specificity

e. Cross-contamination

f. Interferences

g. Reportable range

A. a, b, c, and d

B. a, b, and g

C. a, b, f, and g

D. c, d, e, f, and g

E. a, b, c, d, e, f, and g

F. None of the above

52. Which one of the following efforts is used to verify or establish analytical accuracy, according to the College of American Pathologist (CAP)'s regulations?[1]

A. Using reference materials or other materials with known concentrations or activities

B. Comparing results to an established comparative method

C. Repeating measurement of samples at varying concentrations or activities within-run and between-run over a period of time

D. Testing the lower detection limit of an assay

E. A and B

F. A, B, and C

G. C and D

H. None of the above

53. Dr. Y, a director of a clinical molecular pathology laboratory in Florida, decided to validate a quantitative cytomegalovirus (CMV) assay with the FDA-cleared/approved COBAS AmpliPrep/ COBAS TaqMan CMV test from Roche Molecular Systems. He planned to use the assay on cerebrospinal fluid (CSF) specimens, too, which was not been approved or cleared by the FDA. How many samples should Dr. Y include in this validation according to the College of American Pathologist (CAP)'s regulations, if applicable?[1]

A. At least 5 samples

B. At least 10 samples

C. At least 20 samples

D. At least 40 samples

E. At least 60 samples

F. None of the above

54. Dr. Y, a director of clinical molecular pathology laboratory in Florida, decides to validate an assay

for hereditary hemochromatosis (HH). There is no-FDA-cleared/approved assay available for HH. How many samples should Dr. Y include in this validation, according to the College of American Pathologist (CAP)'s regulations, if applicable?[1]

A. At least 5 samples

B. At least 10 samples

C. At least 20 samples

D. At least 40 samples

E. At least 60 samples

F. None of the above

55. The most recent College of American Pathologist (CAP) All Common Checklist, dated July 28, 2015, states that a laboratory must make the summary of the analytical performance specifications for each method available to clients and the inspection team upon request. Which one of the following is a client, according to this statement?[1]

A. Health care entities

B. Licensed independent practitioners

C. Patients

D. Patient's family members

E. A and B

F. A, B, and C

G. A, B, C, and D

H. None of the above

56. In the most recent College of American Pathologist (CAP) All Common Checklist, dated July 28, 2015, a new chapter named "Individualized Quality Control Plan (IQCP)" was added. Which one of the following statements regarding this plan is correct?[1]

A. This IQCP is a quality control plan lower than the standard defined in the CLIA regulation.

B. This IQCP is a quality control plan lower than the standard defined in the CAP checklist.

C. This IQCP is a quality control plan higher than the standard defined in the CLIA regulation.

D. This IQCP is a quality control plan higher than the standard defined in the CAP checklist.

E. A and B.

F. C and D.

G. A and D.

H. B and C.

I. None of the above.

57. In the most recent College of American Pathologist (CAP) All Common Checklist, dated July 28, 2015, a new chapter named "Individualized Quality Control Plan (IQCP)"

was added. Which one of the following statements regarding this plan is correct?[1]

A. This IQCP allows a laboratory to perform quality control less frequently than indicated in the manufacturer's instructions.

B. This IQCP allows a laboratory to perform quality control less frequently than CAP accreditation requirements.

C. FISH testing is not eligible for use of an IQCP.

D. IQCP can be used in any US state.

E. IQCP does not apply to waived tests.

F. All of the above.

G. None of the above.

58. In the most recent College of American Pathologist (CAP) All Common Checklist, dated July 28, 2015, a new chapter named "Individualized Quality Control Plan (IQCP)" was added. If an IQCP plan is in use in a laboratory, which one of the following should the laboratory do, according to this CAP regulation?[1]

A. Identify all tests using an IQCP in the laboratory.

B. Check the eligibility of those tests using this CAP checklist.

C. Complete the CAP form for all tests using an IQCP.

D. Assess the risks for each IQCP test/device/instrument.

E. Write a quality control plan for IQCP with approval from the laboratory director.

F. Reassess and reapprove the quality control annually.

G. All of the above.

H. None of the above.

59. In the most recent College of American Pathologist (CAP) All Common Checklist, dated July 28, 2015, a new chapter named "Individualized Quality Control Plan (IQCP)" was added. If an IQCP plan is in use in a laboratory, how frequently should the director reassess and reapprove the quality control plan for the IQCP?[1]

A. At least monthly

B. At lease semiannually

C. At least annually

D. At least biennially

E. At least every 5 years

F. None of the above

60. In the most recent College of American Pathologist (CAP) All Common Checklist, dated July 28, 2015, a new chapter named

"Individualized Quality Control Plan (IQCP)" was added. If an IQCP plan is in use in a laboratory, how frequently should the director review quality control and instrument/equipment maintenance and function for the IQCP?[1]

A. At least every week
B. At least every 2 weeks
C. At least monthly
D. At lease semiannually
E. At least annually
F. At least biennially
G. None of the above

61. In the most recent College of American Pathologist (CAP) All Common Checklist, dated July 28, 2015, a new chapter named "Individualized Quality Control Plan (IQCP)" was added. Dr. Z, a director in a clinical molecular genetics laboratory, identified one test for IQCP. There was no special indication in the manufacturer's instruction for using external control material samples. How frequently must the external control material samples be analyzed, according to the College of American Pathologist (CAP)'s regulations, if applicable?[1]

A. At least every 5 business days
B. At least every 14 days
C. At least every 31 days
D. At least every 3 months
E. At least every 6 months
F. None of the above

62. In the most recent College of American Pathologist (CAP) All Common Checklist, dated July 28, 2015, a new chapter named "Individualized Quality Control Plan (IQCP)" was added. Dr. Z, a director in a clinical molecular genetics laboratory, identified one test for IQCP. The manufacturer's instruction indicated that it was better to use external control material samples every week. How frequently must the external control material samples be analyzed, according to the College of American Pathologist (CAP)'s regulations, if applicable?[1]

A. At least every week
B. At least every 2 weeks
C. At least every 31 days
D. At least every 3 months
E. At least every 6 months
F. None of the above

63. How frequently should a director of a clinical molecular laboratory review the maintenance and function check records of centrifuges, according

to the College of American Pathologist (CAP)'s regulations, if applicable?[1]

A. Biennially
B. Annually
C. Semiannually
D. Quarterly
E. Monthly

64. How frequently should a director of a clinical molecular laboratory review the maintenance and function check records of thermal cyclers, according to the College of American Pathologist (CAP)'s regulations, if applicable?[1]

A. Once every 5 years
B. Biennially
C. Annually
D. Semiannually
E. Monthly

65. Which one of the following samples may be used to compare a new lot against an old lot for quantitative nonwaived tests, according to the College of American Pathologist (CAP)'s regulations, if applicable?[1]

A. Patient specimens
B. Reference materials provided by the manufacturer
C. Proficiency testing materials with peer group−established means
D. QC materials with peer group−established means
E. QC materials used to test the current lot
F. All of the above

66. Which one of the following tests is NOT considered to be a laboratory-developed test (LDT) according to the College of American Pathologist (CAP)'s regulations, if applicable?[1]

A. An unmodified FDA-cleared/approved test.
B. A modified FDA-cleared/approved test.
C. The test is performed by the clinical laboratory in which the test was developed.
D. The test was developed and launched by the clinical laboratory in 2005.
E. The test is performed by the clinical laboratory, while the test procedure was created by another laboratory.

67. According to the US Food and Drug Administration (FDA) regulations, a laboratory-developed Sanger sequencing assay for Gaucher disease is a(n):

A. High-complexity test
B. Moderate-complexity test
C. Low-complexity test
D. FDA-cleared test
E. Waived test

68. An ACMG board-certified molecular geneticist started a job as a director in a commercial laboratory. He planned to review all the procedures and policies in the laboratory in 2 months. He found that the quality management procedure stated that a designee of the director would review this procedure biennially. How frequently should a clinical molecular laboratory review its quality management procedure, according to the College of American Pathologist (CAP)'s regulations, if applicable?[2]
    A. At least monthly
    B. At least quarterly
    C. At least twice a year
    D. At least annually
    E. At least biennially

69. An ACMG board-certified molecular geneticist started a job as a director in a commercial laboratory. He planned to review all the procedures and policies in the laboratory in 2 months. He found that the quality management procedure stated that the competency assessment records should be kept for 1 year. How frequently should a clinical molecular laboratory retain the competency assessment records?[2]
    A. At least 1 year
    B. At least 2 years
    C. At least 5 years
    D. At least 10 years
    E. At least 20 years

70. An ACMG board-certified molecular geneticist started a job as a director in a commercial laboratory. He planned to review all the procedures and policies in the laboratory in 2 months. He found that the quality management procedure stated that the quality control records should be kept for 1 year. How frequently should a clinical molecular laboratory retain the quality control records?[2]
    A. At least 1 year
    B. At least 2 years
    C. At least 5 years
    D. At least 10 years
    E. At least 20 years

71. In which one of following circumstances must a clinical molecular laboratory notify CAP?[2]
    A. Investigation of the laboratory by a government entity or other oversight agency
    B. Discovery of actions by laboratory personnel that violate national, state, or local regulations
    C. Change in laboratory test menu
    D. Change in location, ownership, or directorship of the laboratory
    E. All of the above
    F. None of the above

72. Dr. G has been the only director of a genetics laboratory in a small hospital for more than 30 years. His name has been listed on the laboratory's CAP and CLIA certificate as the lab director. Yesterday he announced that he would retire in 4 month and that his last day would be June 30. Which one of following statements is appropriate, according to the College of American Pathologist (CAP)'s regulations, if applicable?[2]
    A. The laboratory should notify CAP immediately.
    B. The laboratory should notify CAP before May 30.
    C. The laboratory should notify CAP before June 15.
    D. The laboratory should notify CAP any time before Dr. G's last day.
    E. There is no need to notify the CAP about this change.
    F. None of the above.

73. Dr. G, a director of a clinical molecular genetics laboratory in an academic center, validated a clinical exome-sequencing test in the laboratory. Which one of following statements is appropriate, according to the College of American Pathologist (CAP)'s regulations, if applicable?[2]
    A. Dr. G should notify CAP immediately.
    B. Dr. G should notify CAP 30 days before launching the test.
    C. Dr. G should notify CAP 15 days before launching the test.
    D. Dr. G should notify CAP any time before launching the test.
    E. There is no need to notify the CAP about this change.
    F. None of the above.

74. How frequently should a director review the quality management (QM) plan in a clinical laboratory according to the College of American Pathologist (CAP)'s regulations, if applicable?[2]
    A. At least biannually
    B. At least annually
    C. At least biennially
    D. At least once every 5 years
    E. At least once every 10 years

75. Dr. A, a director of a clinical molecular genetics laboratory, received a phone call from Dr. G, an oncologist in the same institute. Dr. G asked Dr. A to add a *JAK2* test for a specimen that was sent 2 days ago for a *BCR-ABL1* quantitative test. Dr. A checked with laboratory staff and confirmed that no specimens were received for a *BCR-ABL1*

quantitative test in the past 2 days. After checking with laboratory support team, he found that the bone marrow specimen had been sent to a reference laboratory for TB test by mistake. What should Dr. A do at this point as part of the quality management program, according to College of American Pathologist (CAP)'s regulations, if applicable?[2]

A. Dr. A should perform root-cause analysis.
B. Dr. A should send a gift and a letter to Dr. G to apologize.
C. Dr. A should take 2 weeks off to avoid Dr. G.
D. Dr. A should ask Dr. G for another specimen and promise no charge.
E. Dr. A should get the specimen back from the reference laboratory for the ordered tests.
F. None of the above.

76. Dr. Z, a clinical molecular genetic scientist, has been working for a start-up company in the state of California for 2 months. He has been applying for CLIA and CAP certificates for the laboratory while registering with the Centers for Medicare and Medicaid Services (CMS). Which one of the following types of CLIA certificate must Dr. Z obtain for this laboratory?[2]

A. Certificate of Accreditation
B. Certificate of Compliance
C. Certificate of Registration
D. Certificate of Waiver
E. All of the above
F. None of the above

77. According to the American Pathologist (CAP)'s regulations, a US-regulated clinical molecular laboratory should have a procedure to report device-related adverse patient events to the FDA and to the device manufacturer if the event is death. How soon must the reports be submitted to the FDA?[2]

A. As soon as practical, but no later than 5 days from the time medical personnel become aware of the event
B. As soon as practical, but no later than 10 days from the time medical personnel become aware of the event
C. As soon as practical, but no later than 15 days from the time medical personnel become aware of the event
D. As soon as practical, but no later than 20 days from the time medical personnel become aware of the event
E. As soon as practical, but no later than 1 month from the time medical personnel become aware of the event

78. A US-regulated clinical molecular laboratory should have a procedure to report device-related adverse patient events to the FDA and to the device manufacturer if the event is death. If the FDA investigates a laboratory performance, which other regulatory or oversight agency must the laboratory notify?[2]

A. Centers for Medicare and Medicaid Services (CMS)
B. Clinical Laboratory Improvement Amendments (CLIA) of 1988
C. College of American Pathologist (CAP)
D. Occupational Safety and Health Administration (OSHA)
E. US Department of Health and Human Services
F. All of the above
G. None of the above

79. A US clinical molecular laboratory should have a procedure to report device-related adverse patient events to the FDA and to the device manufacturer if the event is death. If the FDA investigates a laboratory's performance, how soon must the laboratory notify the College of American Pathology (CAP)?[2]

A. No later than 8 hours
B. No later than 2 working days
C. No later than 5 working days
D. No later than 2 weeks
E. No later than 1 month
F. None of the above

80. According to the College of American Pathology (CAP) regulations, a clinical molecular laboratory should report device-related adverse patient events to the FDA and to the device manufacturer if the event is death. Also, the laboratory must submit an annual report of device-related deaths and serious injuries to the FDA if any such event was reported during the previous year. How long must the laboratory keep the records of the FDA MDR (medical-device reporting) reports if applicable?[2]

A. 1 year
B. 2 years
C. 3 years
D. 4 years
E. 10 years

81. ZZ, a technologist on probation, broke a tube of patient blood in a clinical molecular genetics laboratory. He quickly cleaned up the area with bleach without telling anyone. The next day BJ, a technologist, rotating in the wet lab worked in the same area with bare feet because her new high heel shoes hurt her so much. BJ cut her foot on a piece of glass and got stitches at the employee health center. One month later, BJ was diagnosed with HIV-1 infection when she tried to donate

blood. Then ZZ confessed to the accident and the director found that the broken tube of blood was from a patient with HIV-1 infection. Occupational Safety and Health Administration (OSHA) started to investigate the incident. Which one of following statements is appropriate, according to the College of American Pathologist (CAP)'s regulations, if applicable?[2]

A. The laboratory should notify CAP immediately after the adverse incident.

B. The laboratory should notify CAP within 30 days after OSHA started the investigation.

C. The laboratory should notify CAP within 15 days after OSHA started the investigation.

D. The laboratory should notify CAP within 2 days after OSHA started the investigation.

E. There is no need to notify the CAP about this investigation.

F. None of the above.

82. How often must a director of a clinical molecular laboratory review policies and procedures, according to College of American Pathologist (CAP)'s regulations, if applicable?[2]

A. At least once every 10 years

B. At least once every 5 years

C. At least once every 4 years

D. At least once every 2 years

E. At least annually

83. Dr. G, a director in a clinical molecular pathology laboratory in Massachusetts, validated the FDA-cleared/approved Cystic Fibrosis 139-Variant Assay with Illumina MiSeqDx a month ago. Previously the laboratory used xTAG Cystic Fibrosis 60 Kit v2 from Luminex Molecular Diagnostics. Dr. G reviewed and approved the new assay and discontinued the old one. How long should the laboratory keep the discontinued procedure for the cystic fibrosis test?[2]

A. A minimum of 23 years

B. A minimum of 12 years

C. A minimum of 5 years

D. A minimum of 2 years

E. A minimum of 1 year

84. Dr. G, a director of a clinical molecular pathology laboratory in Massachusetts, validated the FDA-cleared/approved Cystic Fibrosis 139-Variant Assay with Illumina MiSeqDx a month ago. Previously, the laboratory had used xTAG Cystic Fibrosis 60 Kit v2 from Luminex Molecular Diagnostics. Dr. G reviewed and approved the new assay and discontinued the old one. Which regulatory or oversight agency must Dr. G notify for the change?[2]

A. Centers for Medicare and Medicaid Services (CMS)

B. Clinical Laboratory Improvement Amendments (CLIA) of 1988

C. College of American Pathologist (CAP)

D. Occupational Safety and Health Administration (OSHA)

E. US Food and Drug Administration (FDA)

F. US Department of Health and Human Services

G. All of the above

H. None of the above

85. Dr. J, a director of a clinical molecular laboratory, reviewed last month's quality control (QC) data. He found that the failure rate of the KRAS assay was 10% higher than it had been for the previous 6 months and for the same month last year. He temporarily discontinued the KRAS assay in the laboratory and sent the samples to a reference laboratory while investigating the reason. Which regulatory or oversight agency must Dr. J notify for the change?[2]

A. Centers for Medicare and Medicaid Services (CMS)

B. Clinical Laboratory Improvement Amendments (CLIA) of 1988

C. College of American Pathologist (CAP)

D. Occupational Safety and Health Administration (OSHA)

E. US Food and Drug Administration (FDA)

F. US Department of Health and Human Services

G. All of the above

H. None of the above

86. A small clinical molecular laboratory in the state of Florida is sold to LabCorp after 1 year of negotiation. When must the College of American Pathologist (CAP) be notified about this change to comply with the CAP terms of accreditation?[2]

A. No later than 60 days prior to the final date

B. No later than 30 days prior to the final date

C. No later than 2 weeks prior to the final date

D. No later than 2 working days afterward

E. No later than 2 weeks afterward

87. A small clinical molecular laboratory in the state of Florida is sold to LabCorp after 1 year of negotiation. The College of American Pathologist (CAP) was notified about this change 1 month before the change. Which additional regulatory or oversight agency must be notified to comply with the CAP terms of accreditation?[2]

A. Centers for Medicare and Medicaid Services (CMS)

B. Clinical Laboratory Improvement Amendments (CLIA) of 1988

C. College of American Pathologist (CAP)

D. Occupational Safety and Health Administration (OSHA)

E. US Food and Drug Administration (FDA)

F. US Department of Health and Human Services

G. All of the above

H. None of the above

88. It is time for an interim self-inspection in a clinical molecular laboratory. Who in the following list may the director of a clinical molecular genetics laboratory choose for self-inspection, according to the College of American Pathologist (CAP)'s regulations, if applicable?

A. Residents

B. Technologists

C. Fellows

D. Supervisor of the cytogenetics laboratory next door

E. All of the above

F. None of the above

89. One of the directors in a CAP/CLIA-certified clinical molecular genetics laboratory in New York City received a phone call from a physician to order fragile X test on a patient. When should the laboratory solicit written or electronic authorization for this verbal order, according to the College of American Pathologist (CAP)'s regulations, if applicable?[2]

A. Within 10 days

B. Within 15 days

C. Within 30 days

D. Within 2 months

E. Within 3 months

90. Dr. A, a medical geneticist, saw a patient who potentially had one of immunodeficiency disorders. She ordered a next-generation sequencing (NGS) panel for immunodeficiency disorders from a reference laboratory. The peripheral-blood sample was sent to the clinical molecular genetics laboratory in the hospital to be sent out. TM, a technologist, was the only staff member trained to pack human specimens for send-out. She was trained at the state health department 6 years ago. How frequently would recurring training be required for TM to keep her active status, according to the College of American Pathologist (CAP)'s regulations, if applicable?[2]

A. At least annually

B. At least biennially

C. At least every 3 years

D. At least every 5 years

E. None of the above

91. How long should a clinical molecular laboratory keep specimen requisitions, according to the College of American Pathologist (CAP)'s regulations, if applicable?[2]

A. A minimum of 10 years

B. A minimum of 5 years

C. A minimum of 4 years

D. A minimum of 2 years

E. A minimum of 1 year

92. How frequently should the operating speeds of centrifuges be checked in clinical molecular genetics laboratories, according to the College of American Pathologist (CAP)'s regulations, if applicable?[2]

A. At least once every 5 years

B. At least biennially

C. At least annually

D. At least semiannually

E. At least monthly

93. How frequently should a clinical molecular laboratory monitor refrigerator/freezer temperature, according to the College of American Pathologist (CAP)'s regulations, if applicable?[2]

A. Every day, including weekends and holidays

B. Every work day

C. Twice a day, including weekends and holidays

D. Twice a day, but only on work days

E. Once a week

94. How frequently should a director of a clinical molecular laboratory review and approve the content and format of patient reports?[2]

A. At least once every 5 years

B. At least biennially

C. At least annually

D. At least semiannually

E. At least monthly

95. How long must a clinical molecular laboratory in a local hospital retain patient charts, according to the College of American Pathologist (CAP)'s regulations, if applicable?[2]

A. Permanently

B. At least 23 years

C. At least 10 years

D. At least 5 years

E. At least 2 years

F. None of the above

96. A clinical molecular laboratory went paperless 2 years ago. Patients' electronic charts have been stored in a cloud-based computing system. There is a written procedure to address patient confidentiality during transfer of data to external servers. How frequently must the laboratory

audit compliance with the procedures, according to the College of American Pathologist (CAP)'s regulations, if applicable?[2]

A. At least once every 5 years

B. At least biennially

C. At least annually

D. At least semiannually

E. At least monthly

97. Dr. F, a director in a clinical molecular laboratory, received a phone call from a patient who asked for a copy of test results that were reported 2 years ago. She said she did not live in the area anymore and could not find the ordering physician. How should Dr. F address the patient's request, according to the College of American Pathologist (CAP)'s regulations, if applicable?[2]

A. Provide final test results to the patient within 30 days after such a request.

B. Provide final test results to the patient within 15 days of such a request.

C. Provide final test results to the patient within 5 business days of such a request.

D. Apologize to the patient, then ask her to have her current physician contact the laboratory.

E. None of the above.

98. Dr. F, a director in a clinical molecular genetics laboratory at an academic center, received a phone call from a genetic counselor, BJ, from a private practice. BJ asked for a copy of a patient's test result, which was ordered by a physician in a nonaffiliated hospital. BJ faxed a copy of a medical record release form signed by the patient to release the result to Dr. F. Under the HIPAA Privacy Rule, which one of the following individuals may have access to a patient's test results?[2]

A. The patient

B. The patient's personal representative

C. Authorized persons responsible for using the test reports

D. The laboratory that initially requested the test

E. All of the above

F. None of the above

99. The Health Insurance Portability and Accountability Act (HIPAA) was passed by the US Congress in 1996. What does HIPAA protect?

A. Patient health information privacy

B. Patient right to be treated equally

C. Patient informed consent

D. Patient protection and affordable care

E. All of the above

F. None of the above

100. "ObamaCare" was signed by President Barack Obama in 2010. What does "ObamaCare" mean?

A. Patient health information privacy

B. Patient right to be treated equally

C. Patient informed consent

D. Patient protection and affordable care

E. All of the above

F. None of the above

101. In a clinical molecular genetics laboratory the turnaround time (TAT) in the written policy is 5 business days for a *BCR-ABL1* test. Last week the technologist who was responsible for this test repeated the test on five samples four times to obtain reportable results. The real TAT was 7 days for those five samples. If the College of American Pathologist (CAP)–required TAT on this test is 10 days, did these five samples meet the required TAT?[2]

A. Yes

B. No

C. Not sure

102. A clinical molecular laboratory became paperless 2 years ago. Patient's electronic charts have been stored in a cloud-based computing system. There is a written procedure to address patient confidentially during transfer of data to external servers. Electronic copies of reports from reference laboratories have been stored in the same place. The director of the laboratory received a warning message to inform him that the server is almost full. To save money, he decided to delete some of archived reports, and stop saving new reports from reference laboratories. Which type of deficiency would it be if it were one?[2]

A. Phase 0

B. Phase I

C. Phase II

D. Phase III

E. Not a deficiency

F. None of the above

103. How frequently should a clinical molecular genetics laboratory test its water quality to make sure it is as claimed to be in each of its testing procedures?[2]

A. At least once every 5 years

B. At least biennially

C. At least annually

D. At least semiannually

E. At least monthly

104. How frequently should the autoverification process of documentation be tested after initial validation, according to the College of American Pathologist (CAP)'s regulations, if applicable?[2]

A. Annually

B. Biennially

C. Every 3 years

D. Every 4 years

E. Every 5 years

105. Dr. G, a director of a clinical molecular laboratory, plans to transfer the reports for cystic fibrosis carrier tests from Cerner to SunQuest. How many examples of reports must Dr. G test for the interface before the implementation?[2]

A. At least 1

B. At least 2

C. At least 10

D. At least 20

E. At least 30

106. Dr. A, an ACMG board-certified molecular geneticist, started a job as a senior director in a commercial laboratory 2 months ago. When he reviewed the procedures and policies in the laboratory, he found that the laboratory verified two examples of reports every 4 years to ensure the interface result integrity. Dr. A changed the policy immediately. What did Dr. A change the policy to, according to the College of American Pathologist (CAP)'s regulations, if applicable?[2]

A. At least 4 examples of reports every 2 years

B. At least 4 examples of reports every 4 years

C. At least 2 examples of reports every 2 years

D. At least 10 examples of reports every 10 years

E. None of the above

107. How many years of experience with high-complexity testing must an individual have to be qualified as a general supervisor of a clinical molecular pathology laboratory if he or she has a bachelor's degree in a chemical, physical, biological, or clinical laboratory science or medical technology, according to the College of American Pathologist (CAP)'s regulations, if applicable?[2]

A. At least 1 year

B. At least 2 years

C. At least 4 years

D. At least 10 years

E. At least 15 years

108. According to the College of American Pathologist (CAP)'s regulations, a technical consultant in a clinical molecular laboratory must have at least a(n):[2]

A. Doctoral degree (MD or PhD)

B. Master's degree

C. Bachelor's degree

D. Associate's degree

E. High school diploma

109. According to the College of American Pathologist (CAP)'s regulations, a clinical consultant in a clinical molecular laboratory must have at least a(n):[2]

A. Doctoral degree (MD or PhD)

B. Master's degree

C. Bachelor's degree

D. Associate's degree

E. High school diploma

110. A technologist was hired into a clinical molecular laboratory 1 month ago and was trained to run the BRAF V600E qualitative assay. How frequently should this technologist be assessed for competency on this test after the initial training, according to the College of American Pathologist (CAP)'s regulations, if applicable?[2]

A. At least once every 5 years

B. At least biennially

C. At least annually

D. At least semiannually

E. At least monthly

111. Dr. B, an on-site College of American Pathologist (CAP) inspector, presented herself to the staff in a clinical molecular genetics laboratory that she was assigned to inspect. She asked the supervisor whether new personnel had been hired in the past 2 years. OB, a technologist, had been hired into the laboratory 2 years ago. OB's personnel file showed that his initial training for the BRAF V600E qualitative test was on January 1, 2012. Which one of the following personnel files indicated that OB was competent to perform the BRAF V600E assay and fulfilled the minimal requirement of the College of American Pathologist (CAP)'s regulations?[2]

A. OB's competency was first assessed on June 30, 2012, and then on December 30, 2013.

B. OB's competency was first assessed on December 30, 2012, and then on December 30, 2013.

C. OB's competency was first assessed on June 30, 2012, and then on June 30, 2013.

D. OB's competency was first assessed on December 30, 2012, and then on December 30, 2014.

E. All of the above.

F. None of the above.

112. Who must be assessed for competency in a clinical molecular pathology laboratory, according to the College of American Pathologist (CAP)'s regulations, if applicable?[2]

A. Technologists

B. General supervisors

C. Technical consultants

D. Section directors

E. All of the above

F. None of the above

113. A technologist was hired into a clinical molecular laboratory 2 years ago. He has been competent to perform the *BRAF* V600E qualitative assay for 1 year. How frequently must his competency for the *BRAF* V600E qualitative assay be evaluated from now on, according to the College of American Pathologist (CAP)'s regulations, if applicable?[2]
    A. At least once every 5 years
    B. At least biannually
    C. At least annually
    D. At least semiannually
    E. At least monthly

114. Which one of the following should be included in competency assessments, according to the College of American Pathologist (CAP)'s regulations, if applicable?[2]
    A. Directly observing routine patient test performance
    B. Monitoring the recording and reporting of test results
    C. Reviewing intermediate test results or worksheets, quality control records, proficiency testing results, and preventive maintenance records
    D. Directing observation of performance of instrument maintenance and function checks
    E. Assessing test performance through testing previously analyzed specimens, internal blind testing samples, or external proficiency testing samples
    F. Evaluating problem-solving skills
    G. All of the above
    H. None of the above

115. BJ, a technologist at a clinical molecular laboratory, has been competent to perform the *BRAF* V600E qualitative assay for 3 years. However, he did not pass the competency assessment for this assay this year. What should be the next step for BJ, according to the College of American Pathologist (CAP)'s regulations, if applicable?[2]
    A. Layoff
    B. Reassignment of duties
    C. Reeducation and training
    D. Supervisory review of work
    E. None of the above

116. Dr. B, an on-site College of American Pathologist (CAP) inspector, presented herself to the staff in a clinical molecular genetics laboratory that she was assigned to inspect. She asked JJ, the supervisor, how frequently the laboratory's safe work practices were reviewed. JJ said they were reviewed biennially.

Dr. B cited Phase II deficiency on it. How frequently should a clinical molecular laboratory review its safe work practices to reduce hazards, according to the College of American Pathologist (CAP)'s regulations, if applicable?[2]
    A. At least once every 5 years
    B. At least biennially
    C. At least annually
    D. At least semiannually
    E. At least monthly

117. For US laboratories subject to OSHA regulations, all workplace fatalities must be reported to the Occupational Safety and Health Administration (OSHA). How soon should a clinical molecular laboratory report the accident to OSHA?[2]
    A. Within 4 hours
    B. Within 8 hours
    C. Within 24 hours
    D. Within 2 days
    E. Within 1 week

118. For US laboratories subject to OSHA regulations, all work-related inpatient hospitalizations, amputations, or losses of an eye must be reported to the Occupational Safety and Health Administration (OSHA). How soon should a clinical molecular laboratory report the accident to OSHA?[2]
    A. Within 4 hours
    B. Within 8 hours
    C. Within 24 hours
    D. Within 2 days
    E. Within 1 week

119. According to the College of American Pathologist (CAP)'s regulations, how frequently must sterilizing devices be monitored in a clinical molecular pathology laboratory?[2]
    A. Daily
    B. Weekly
    C. Biweekly
    D. Monthly
    E. Quarterly

120. After new employees pass fire safety training, how frequently should a fire safety review be conducted, according to the College of American Pathologist (CAP)'s regulations, if applicable?[2]
    A. At least once every 5 years
    B. At least biannually
    C. At least annually
    D. At least semiannually
    E. At least monthly

121. According to the College of American Pathologist (CAP)'s regulations, for laboratories subject to US

regulations, chemicals that must be handled as potential carcinogens include those defined by OSHA as "select carcinogens." The list of OSHA-defined select carcinogens does NOT include:[2]

A. Group 1 carcinogen listed by the IARC
B. Group 2A carcinogen listed by the IARC
C. Group 2B carcinogen listed by the IARC
D. Group 3 carcinogen listed by the IARC
E. A "known to be carcinogen" classified by the NTP
F. A "reasonably anticipated to be carcinogen" classified by the NTP

122. According to the College of American Pathologist (CAP)'s regulations, which one of the following locations is appropriate to store strong acid and bases?[2]

A. Storage above eye level
B. Storage near the floor
C. Storage containers of acids and bases together
D. Storage under sinks
E. Any one of the above
F. None of the above

123. Which one of the following individuals is qualified to be a section director/technical supervisor of a clinical molecular pathology laboratory, according to the College of American Pathologist (CAP)'s regulations, if applicable?[4]

A. A pathologist
B. An MD with an ACMG certification in clinical molecular genetics
C. A PhD with an ACMG certification in clinical molecular genetics
D. A technologist with an ASCP certification and 10 years of experiences in a molecular pathology laboratory
E. A, B, and C
F. All of the above
G. None of the above

124. How many years of experience must an individual have to be qualified to serve as a bench testing supervisor of a clinical molecular pathology laboratory if he or she has bachelor's degree in a chemical, physical, biological, or clinical laboratory science or medical technology, according to the College of American Pathologist (CAP)'s regulations, if applicable?[4]

A. At least 1 year
B. At least 2 years
C. At least 4 years
D. At least 10 years
E. At least 15 years

125. According to the College of American Pathologist (CAP)'s regulations, a technologist in a clinical molecular laboratory must have at least a(n):[4]

A. Certification as a clinical molecular genetics technologist
B. Master's degree
C. Bachelor's degree
D. Associate's degree
E. High school diploma

126. For quantitative molecular tests, which one of the following controls should be included in each run, according to the College of American Pathologist (CAP)'s regulations, if applicable?[4]

a. A no-template control
b. A wild-type control
c. A low-positive control
d. A high-positive control
e. An internal control
A. a, b, c, and d
B. a, b, c, d, and e
C. a and b
D. a, b, and d
E. a, b, d, and e

127. Which of the following parameters should be verified for FDA-cleared/approved tests during assay validation in a clinical molecular genetics laboratory, according to the College of American Pathologist (CAP)'s regulations, if applicable?[1]

a. Analytical accuracy
b. Analytical precision
c. Analytical sensitivity
d. Analytical specificity
e. Reference range
f. Reportable range
g. Positive predictive value
h. Negative predictive value
A. a, b, c, and d
B. a, b, c, d, and e
C. a, b, c, d, and f
D. a, b, e, and f
E. a, b, c, d e, and f
F. a, b, c, d, e, f, g, and h

128. Which of the following parameters should be verified for modified FDA-cleared/approved assays during validation in a clinical molecular genetics laboratory, according to the College of American Pathologist (CAP)'s regulations, if applicable?[1]

a. Analytical accuracy
b. Analytical precision
c. Analytical sensitivity

     d. Analytical specificity
     e. Reference range
     f. Reportable range
     g. Positive predictive value
     h. Negative predictive value
     A. a, b, c, and d
     B. a, b, c, d, and e
     C. a and b
     D. a, b, and d
     E. a, b, c, d, e, and f
     F. a, b, c, d, e, f, g, and h

129. A director planned to validate a quantitative *BCR-ABL1* TaqMan-based assay in a clinical molecular genetics laboratory at a hospital. He sent six peripheral-blood samples to a commercial laboratory for this validation. For one positive sample, the result from the commercial laboratory was 86% translocation-positive. The technologists in the laboratory repeated the sample three times in one run and repeated the run three times. The results for this sample were 66% ± 0.1% translocation-positive with all nine repeats. Which one of the following statements regarding the results is correct, according to the College of American Pathologist (CAP)'s regulations, if applicable?[4]

     A. The accuracy of the assay in this lab was high.
     B. The precision of the assay in this lab was low.
     C. The reproducibility of the assay in this lab was high.
     D. The analytical sensitivity of the assay in this lab was low.
     E. The analytical specificity of the assay in this lab was high.

130. A director planned to validate a quantitative *BCR-ABL1* TaqMan-based assay in a clinical molecular genetics laboratory at a hospital. He sent six peripheral-blood samples to a commercial laboratory for this validation. For one positive sample, the result from the commercial laboratory was 86% translocation-positive. The technologists in the laboratory repeated the sample three times in one run and repeated the run three times. The results for this sample were 85% ± 20% translocation-positive with all nine repeats. Which one of the statements below regarding the results is correct, according to the College of American Pathologist (CAP)'s regulations, if applicable?[4]

     A. The accuracy of the assay in this lab is high.
     B. The precision of the assay in this lab is high.
     C. The reproducibility of the assay in this lab is high.

     D. The analytical sensitivity of the assay in this lab is low.
     E. The analytical specificity of the assay in this lab is high.

132. Dr. Z, a director in a clinical molecular genetics laboratory at a hospital, plans to validate a quantitative *BCR-ABL1* TaqMan-based assay. Which one of the following values should be used to monitor precision/reproducibility for this validation, according to the College of American Pathologist (CAP)'s regulations, if applicable?[4]

     A. Ratios of concordance
     B. Standard deviation
     C. Coefficient of variation
     D. Standard score (Z score)
     E. Confidence interval

133. Dr. Z, a director in a clinical molecular genetics laboratory at a hospital, plans to validate a cystic fibrosis carrier test. Which one of the following parameters should be used to monitor precision/reproducibility for this validation, according to the College of American Pathologist (CAP)'s regulations, if applicable?[4]

     A. Ratios of concordance
     B. Standard deviation
     C. Coefficient of variation
     D. Standard score (Z score)
     E. Confidence interval

134. Dr. Z, a director in a clinical molecular genetics laboratory at a hospital, plans to validate an HIV-1 RNA viral load test. He expects that a few samples may be out of reportable range of this assay (lower than the reportable range). Which one of the following resolutions would NOT be acceptable for out of range samples, according to the College of American Pathologist (CAP)'s regulations, if applicable?

     A. Reporting it out as negative
     B. Concentrating the sample for rerun
     C. Reporting it out as low positive
     D. Reporting it out as <5% (low limit of reportable range)
     E. None of the above

135. Dr. Z, a director in a clinical molecular genetics laboratory at a hospital, plans to validate an HIV-1 RNA viral load test. He expects that a few samples may be out of reportable range of a quantitative assay (higher than the reportable range). Which one of the following resolutions would NOT be acceptable for out of range samples, according to the College of

American Pathologist (CAP)'s regulations, if applicable?[4]

A. Reporting it out as positive

B. Diluting the sample for rerun

C. Reporting it out as high positive

D. Reporting it out as >10,000 copies/mL (high limit of reportable range)

E. None of the above

136. According to the College of American Pathologist (CAP)'s regulations, in which of the following situations should calibration for quantitative assays typically be done, aside from initial validation?[4]

a. At changes of reagent lots.

b. When the results of the high-positive and low-positive controls consistently have been outside the laboratory's acceptable limits in the past month and the reasons cannot be identified.

c. When the ABI7900HT was shipped back to the lab yesterday after major repair at the manufacturer.

d. When recommended by the manufacturer.

e. At least every 3 months.

f. At least every 6 months.

g. At least every year.

h. At least every 2 years.

A. a, b, c, d, and e

B. a, b, c, d, and f

C. a, b, c, d, and g

D. a, b, c, d, and h

E. None of the above

137. According to the College of American Pathologist (CAP)'s regulations, how frequently should quality control (QC) statistics be calculated and reviewed for quantitative assays to define analytic imprecision and to monitor trends over time in a molecular pathology laboratory?[4]

A. At least monthly

B. At least every 2 months

C. At least every 3 months

D. At least every 6 months

E. At least every 1 year

F. None of the above

138. A laboratory has fewer than five samples for a quantitative JAK2 V617F test each month. So the test is only run when there are 10 samples in total. How frequently must quality control (QC) statistics be calculated and reviewed for this test in this laboratory, according to the College of American Pathologist (CAP)'s regulations, if applicable?[4]

A. At least monthly

B. At least every 2 months

C. At least every 3 months

D. At least every 6 months

E. At least every 1 year

F. When the tests are performed

139. A laboratory has a qualitative JAK2 V617F assay, and the cutoff for positivity is 5%. How frequently must the cutoff value be verified after been established initially according to the College of American Pathologist (CAP)'s regulations, if applicable?[4]

a. At changes of reagent lots.

b. The ABI7900HT, used for this test, was shipped back to the lab yesterday after major repair at the manufacturer.

c. When recommended by the manufacturer.

d. At least every 3 months.

e. At least every 6 months.

f. At least every 1 years.

g. At least every 2 years.

A. a, b, c, and d

B. a, b, c, and e

C. a, b, c, and f

D. a, b, c, and g

E. None of the above

140. Which one of the following is the most appropriate order of specimens set up for an amplification reaction according to the College of American Pathologist (CAP)'s regulations, if applicable?[4]

A. Negative controls, positive controls, and patient samples

B. Positive controls, patient samples, and negative controls

C. Patient samples, negative controls, and positive controls

D. Patient samples, positive controls, and negative controls

E. Negative controls, patient samples, and positive controls

141. Dr. Z, a director in a clinical molecular genetics laboratory at a local hospital, plans to validate a Sanger sequencing–based assay for mutations in the BCR-ABL1 kinase domain in order to assess Gleevec resistance in patients with chronic myeloid leukemia (CML). Which one of the following steps may be taken to prevent errors caused by unequivocal sequence readout, according to the College of American Pathologist (CAP)'s regulations, if applicable?[4]

A. Perform sequencing with more PCR products

B. Perform sequencing with more labeled ddNTPs

C. Perform sequencing in both directions

D. Add more EXOSAP to purify the PCR products

E. Perform sequencing with more of everything

F. None of the above

142. Dr. Z, a director in a clinical molecular genetics laboratory at a local hospital, plans to validate a Sanger sequencing–based assay for mutations in the *BCR-ABL1* kinase domain in order to assess Gleevec resistance in patients with chronic myeloid leukemia (CML). Which one of the following steps may be taken to prevent errors caused by unequivocal sequence readout, according to the College of American Pathologist (CAP)'s regulations?[4]

A. Perform sequencing with more PCR products

B. Perform sequencing with more labeled ddNTPs

C. Perform unidirectional coverage by replicate independent reads

D. Add more EXOSAP to purify the PCR products

E. Perform sequencing with more of everything

F. None of the above

143. Wiskott–Aldrich syndrome is a rare X-linked recessive disease characterized by eczema, thrombocytopenia, immune deficiency, and bloody diarrhea secondary to the thrombocytopenia. Dr. Z, a director in a clinical molecular genetics laboratory at a local hospital, plans to validate a Sanger sequencing–based assay for mutations in *WAS* for Wiskott–Aldrich syndrome. Which one of following professional oversight organization's guidelines should Dr. Z follow to classify variants?[4]

A. American Board of Medical Genetics and Genomics

B. American College of Medical Genetics and Genomics

C. Association for Molecular Pathology

D. College of American Pathologist

E. Human Genome Variation Society

F. All of the above

G. None of the above

144. According to the College of American Pathologist (CAP)'s regulations, samples should be drawn only over a specific gestational age range for noninvasive prenatal tests (NIPTs). What would usually be the earliest gestational age for NIPT?[4]

A. 5 weeks gestational age

B. 10 weeks gestational age

C. 15 weeks gestational age

D. 20 weeks gestational age

E. 25 weeks gestational age

145. Which one of the following is not essential in the requisitions for next-generation sequencing of maternal plasma to identify fetal aneuploidy readout, according to the College of American Pathologist (CAP)'s regulations, if applicable?

A. Gestational age

B. Ethnicity of the parents

C. Maternal age

D. Maternal weight

E. Parentage information

F. Multiple gestation

G. Family history

H. Prior pregnancy risk

146. According to the College of American Pathologist (CAP)'s regulations, a clinical molecular laboratory with noninvasive prenatal tests (NIPTs) should monitor the percentage of women with positive results for each targeted disorder, such as Down syndrome, Turner syndrome, test failure rates, and "inconclusive" test results. What is the recommended frequency of this monitoring?[4]

A. At least monthly

B. At least every 2 months

C. At least every 3 months

D. At least every 6 months

E. At least every 1 year

147. Which one of following must be included in patient reports for noninvasive prenatal tests (NIPTs), according to the College of American Pathologist (CAP)'s regulations, if applicable?[4]

A. A statement that a positive test result is diagnostic for aneuploidies.

B. A statement that this test is also intended to identify pregnancies at risk for open neural-tube defects.

C. Recommendations regarding next steps for women with uninformative results and/or test failures.

D. All of the above.

E. None of the above.

148. How long should a clinical laboratory retain images of FISH assays for t(9;22) according to the College of American Pathologist (CAP)'s regulations, if applicable?[4]

A. At least 1 years

B. At least 7 years

C. At least 10 years

D. At least 20 years

E. At least 30 years

149. How long should a clinical laboratory retain images of FISH assays for 22q11.2 deletion syndrome, according to the College of American Pathologist (CAP)'s regulations, if applicable?[4]
   A. At least 1 years
   B. At least 7 years
   C. At least 10 years
   D. At least 20 years
   E. At least 30 years

150. How many FISH images should a clinical laboratory retain for normal t(9;22), according to the College of American Pathologist (CAP)'s regulations, if applicable?[4]
   A. At least 1 cell
   B. At least 2 cells
   C. At least 3 cells
   D. At least 5 cells
   E. At least 10 cells

151. How many FISH images should a clinical laboratory retain for abnormal t(9;22), according to the College of American Pathologist (CAP)'s regulations, if applicable?[4]
   A. At least 1 cell
   B. At least 2 cells
   C. At least 3 cells
   D. At least 5 cells
   E. At least 10 cells

152. How many FISH images should a clinical laboratory retain for normal 4p− syndrome according to the College of American Pathologist (CAP)'s regulations, if applicable?[4]
   A. At least 1 cell
   B. At least 2 cells
   C. At least 3 cells
   D. At least 5 cells
   E. At least 10 cells

153. How many FISH images should a clinical laboratory retain for abnormal 4p− syndrome, according to the College of American Pathologist (CAP)'s regulations, if applicable?[4]
   A. At least 1 cell
   B. At least 2 cells
   C. At least 3 cells
   D. At least 5 cells
   E. At least 10 cells

154. How long should a sample for an HER2 FISH assay be fixed in 10% neutral buffered formalin according to the College of American Pathologist (CAP)'s regulations, if applicable?[4]
   A. At least 6 hours and no longer than 48 hours
   B. At least 12 hours and no longer than 96 hours
   C. At least 6 hours and no longer than 72 hours
   D. At least 6 hours and no longer than 96 hours
   E. At least 12 hours and no longer than 48 hours

155. How many samples should a clinical molecular laboratory use to validate an FDA-cleared/approved HER2 FISH assay, according to the College of American Pathologist (CAP)'s regulations, if applicable?[4]
   A. At least 40 samples
   B. At least 50 samples
   C. At least 20 positive and 20 negative samples
   D. At least 25 positive and 25 negative samples
   E. At least 40 positive and 40 negative samples

156. How many samples should a clinical molecular laboratory use to validate a laboratory-developed test (LDTs) HER2 FISH assay according to the College of American Pathologist (CAP)'s regulations, if applicable?[4]
   A. At least 40 samples
   B. At least 50 samples
   C. At least 20 positive and 20 negative samples
   D. At least 25 positive and 25 negative samples
   E. At least 40 positive and 40 negative samples

157. How many copies of the HER2 genes in one nucleus is the criterion for positive HER2 amplification in a FISH assay regardless of ratio of HER2 to CEP17, according to the College of American Pathologist (CAP)'s regulations, if applicable?[4]
   A. At least three copies
   B. At least four copies
   C. At least five copies
   D. At least six copies
   E. At least seven copies

158. Spectrophotometers are commonly used to quantify DNA/RNA in molecular pathology laboratories. How frequently must the filter and wavelength calibration be checked for appropriate function, according to the College of American Pathologist (CAP)'s regulations, if applicable?[4]
   A. At least monthly
   B. At least every 6 months
   C. At least annually
   D. At least biennially
   E. At least every 5 years

159. How frequently must pipettes used for quantitative dispensing of material be checked for accuracy and reproducibility in a clinical molecular genetics laboratory besides checking before being placed in service according to the College of American Pathologist (CAP)'s regulations, if applicable?[4]
   A. At least monthly
   B. At least every 3 months
   C. At least every 6 months
   D. At least every year
   E. At least every 2 years

160. How frequently must the individual wells (or a representative sample) of thermal cyclers be checked for temperature accuracy in a clinical molecular genetics laboratory in addition to being checked before being placed into service, according to the College of American Pathologist (CAP)'s regulations, if applicable?[4]
    A. At least monthly
    B. At least every 3 months
    C. At least every 6 months
    D. At least every year
    E. At least every 2 years

161. Dr. Z, a scientist, planned to validate a quantitative PCR–based assay for the V617F mutation in the *JAK2* gene-related chronic myeloid leukemia (CMA) in a clinical molecular laboratory. There is no commercially available FDA-cleared or approved assay for it. Dr. Z bought TaqMan genotyping assay from Applied Biosystems (ABI) for the validation. Which class of reagents do the primers of this assay belong to according to the analyte-specific reagents (ASRs) rule?[5–11]
    A. Class I
    B. Class II
    C. Class III
    D. Class IV
    E. None of the above

162. A molecular laboratory scientist planned to validate a quantitative HIV-1 RNA assay for viral load assessment with Bayer VERSANT HIV-1 RNA 3.0 Assay (bDNA), an FDA-approved commercially available assay. Which class of reagents do the primers of this assay belong to, according to the analyte-specific reagents (ASRs) rule?[5–11]
    A. Class I
    B. Class II
    C. Class III
    D. Class IV
    E. None of the above

163. In a molecular laboratory there are CMV, HBV, HCV, HBP, and KB virus tests, which use automatic COBAS instruments. And the reports are generated by computer without interpretation. Which one of following statements is correct, according to the College of American Pathologist (CAP)'s regulations, if applicable?[4]
    A. The section director need not review the report.
    B. The section director need not approve the report.
    C. The section director need not sign the report.
    D. All of the above.
    E. None of the above.

164. A 24-year-old patient asked a genetic counselor if she might pay out of her own pocket for the genetic test for Huntington disease so that the results would not be put into her medical record because she was concerned that abnormal results in her medical record might affect her insurance premium. What would be your answer to this question if you were the physician, according to the College of American Pathologist (CAP)'s regulations, if applicable (no need to take state laws into consideration)?[4]
    A. Yes, it may be done.
    B. No, it may not be done.
    C. Not sure.

165. Without a patient's express consent, a patient's molecular test results for Huntington disease may NOT be provided to:[4]
    A. The referring physician
    B. The genetic counselor
    C. The medical record
    D. The patient's husband
    E. Not sure

166. Without a patient's express consent, a patient's molecular test results for Huntington disease may be provided to:[4]
    A. The patient's cousin
    B. The patient's genetic counselor
    C. The patient's employer
    D. The patient's insurer
    E. The patient's husband

167. How long must a clinical molecular laboratory retain final reports for its *JAK2* assay, according to the College of American Pathologist (CAP)'s regulations, if applicable?[4]
    A. At least 1 year
    B. At least 7 years
    C. At least 10 years
    D. At least 20 years
    E. At least 30 years

168. How long must a clinical molecular laboratory retain final reports for Huntington disease according to the College of American Pathologist (CAP)'s regulations, if applicable?[4]
    A. At least 1 years
    B. At least 7 years
    C. At least 10 years
    D. At least 20 years
    E. At least 30 years

169. Which one of the following parameters need NOT be verified for FDA-cleared/approved tests, according to the College of American Pathologist (CAP)'s regulations, if applicable?[4]
    A. Analytical accuracy
    B. Analytical precision

C. Analytical sensitivity
D. Reportable range
E. Reference range

170. Which one of the following parameters need NOT be verified for FDA-cleared/approved tests according to the College of American Pathologist (CAP)'s regulations, if applicable?[4]
    A. Analytical accuracy
    B. Analytical precision
    C. Cross-contamination
    D. Reportable range
    E. Reference range

171. A molecular laboratory scientist planned to validate a quantitative HIV-1 RNA assay for viral load assessment with the Bayer VERSANT HIV-1 RNA 3.0 Assay (bDNA), an FDA-approved commercially available assay. At a minimum, which one of the following samples must be used to verify the analytical measurement range (AMR) of the assay after the initial implementation, according to the College of American Pathologist (CAP)'s regulation, if applicable?[4]
    A. One negative and one positive sample
    B. One negative, one low positive, and one high positive sample
    C. One negative, one low positive, one midrange positive, and one high positive sample
    D. One low positive, one midrange positive, and one high positive sample
    E. One low positive and one high positive sample
    F. One positive sample

172. Which of the following meets the criteria to be positive for an *HER2* FISH assay when probe on the centromere of chromosome 17 (CEP17) was used as internal control according to the College of American Pathologist (CAP)'s regulations, if applicable?[4]
    a. Ratios of HER2 to CEP17 is <2.0, average HER2 copy number signals <4.0 per cell
    b. Ratios of HER2 to CEP17 is <2.0, average HER2 copy number signals >4.0 and <6.0 per cell
    c. Ratios of HER2 to CEP17 is >2.0, average HER2 copy number signals >4.0 and <6.0 per cell
    d. Ratios of HER2 to CEP17 is >2.0, average HER2 copy number signals >6.0 per cell
    e. Ratios of HER2 to CEP17 is <2.0, average HER2 copy number signals >6.0 per cell
    A. a, b, c, d, and e
    B. b, c, d, and e
    C. c, d, and e
    D. c and d
    E. d and e

173. To comply with the College of American Pathologist (CAP)'s regulations, you, as a clinical molecular laboratory director, write in the policy to test and certify the biological safety cabinet at least:[4]
    A. Daily
    B. Weekly
    C. Monthly
    D. Semiannually
    E. Annually

174. How frequently must a clinical molecular laboratory decontaminate workbenches and sinks for radiation safety if radioactive reagents are used in this laboratory, according to the College of American Pathologist (CAP)'s regulations, if applicable?[4]
    A. Daily
    B. Weekly
    C. Monthly
    D. Semiannually
    E. Annually

175. How frequently must a clinical molecular laboratory check workbenches and sinks for the effectiveness of decontamination for radiation safety if radioactive reagents are used in this laboratory, according to the College of American Pathologist (CAP)'s regulations, if applicable?[4]
    A. Daily
    B. Weekly
    C. Monthly
    D. Semiannually
    E. Annually

176. How many times should DNA test results for parentage testing be interpreted independently, according to the College of American Pathologist (CAP)'s regulations, if applicable?[4]
    A. One time
    B. Two times
    C. Three times
    D. Four times
    E. Five times

177. A clinical molecular genetics laboratory had an on-site inspection in May. When should be the next on-site inspection occur, according to the College of American Pathologist (CAP)'s regulations, if applicable?[12]
    A. In 6 months
    B. In 1 year
    C. In 2 years
    D. In 3 years
    E. None of the above

178. Which one of the following is a responsibility of the director in a clinical molecular genetics laboratory, according to the College of

American Pathologist (CAP)'s regulations, if applicable?[12]

a. Effective quality management program
b. Sufficient proficiency testing, alternative assessment, and QC procedures
c. New method validation/verification
d. Communication of laboratory data and appropriate patient result reporting
e. Intralaboratory consultations and clinical consultations
f. Appropriate educational programs, strategic planning, and research and development
g. Sufficient numbers of personnel with appropriate educational qualifications
h. Implementation of a safe laboratory environment
i. Interaction with government and other agencies
j. Selection of all laboratory equipment, supplies, and services
A. a, b, c, d, e, and f
B. a, b, c, d, e, f, and i
C. a, b, c, d, e, f, I, and j
D. All of the above
E. None of the above

179. According to the ACMG Standards and Guidelines for Clinical Genetics Laboratories, which one of the following may be used as patient identifiers on specimen containers for genetic tests?[13]

a. Date of birth
b. Hospital number
c. Hospital room number
d. Insurance ID number
e. Laboratory number
f. Patient name
g. Social security number
A. a, b, e, and f
B. a, b, e, f, and g
C. a, b, d, e, and f
D. a, b, d, e, f, and g
E. None of the above

180. How should extracted DNA be stored to ensure long-term stability, according to the ACMG Standards and Guidelines for Clinical Genetics Laboratories?[14]

A. Room temperature
B. 0°C−5°C
C. Frozen
D. All of the above
E. None of the above

181. Dr. Z, a director of a clinical pathology laboratory, planned to validate a Sanger sequencing−based assay for the USH1A gene to assist in the diagnosis of Usher syndrome. Which

one of the following specimens may be used as a positive control in the validation, according to the ACMG Standards and Guidelines for Clinical Genetics Laboratories?[14]

a. A commercially available cell line with a mutation in the exon 3 of USH1A
b. A cell line with a mutation in the exon 3 of USH1A detected and shared by a research laboratory
c. A sample with a mutation in the exon 3 of USH1A detected and shared by a research laboratory
d. A sample with a mutation in the exon 3 of USH1A detected by a CAP-certified laboratory
e. A sample with a mutation in the exon 3 of USH1A detected by exome sequencing done in a CAP-certified laboratory
A. d
B. d and e
C. a, d, and e
D. a, c, d, and e
E. All of the above
F. None of the above

182. Dr. Z, a director of a clinical pathology laboratory, planned to validate a PCR and Southern blot combined assay for fragile X syndrome. Which one of the following statements is appropriate regarding southern blot test according to the ACMG Standards and Guidelines for Clinical Genetics Laboratories?[14]

A. Southern blots need higher quantity of DNA than PCR, but not quality.
B. Degradation of specimen is the only reason for incomplete digestion.
C. Southern blot testing is very straightforward. There is no need for human DNA control.
D. The gel run for Southern analysis may be dried as a hard copy of documentation of the digestion.
E. None of the above.

183. A clinical pathology laboratory has two physically distinct areas for pre- and post-PCR. BJ, a technologist in this laboratory, set up a PCR reaction with a 96-well plate in the order of patient samples, positive control and negative control at the pre-PCR area. After spinning the reagents down, he puts the plate into a thermal cycler in the same area. After the amplification reaction, BJ takes the plate out of the thermal cycler to the post-PCR area for gel electrophoresis. Which one of the following descriptions is appropriate, according to the ACMG Standards and Guidelines for Clinical Genetics Laboratories?[4]

A. The order of the samples in the 96-well plate should be negative control, positive control, and patient samples.

B. The reagents for PCR should be put into a thermal cycler directly without spinning down.

C. The thermal cycler should be kept in the post-PCR area instead of pre-PCR area.

D. There is no need for gel electrophoresis before Sanger sequencing.

E. None of the above.

184. A clinical pathology laboratory has two physically distinct areas for pre- and post-PCR. BJ, a technologist in this laboratory, was ready to set up a PCR reaction with a 96-well plate manually at the pre-PCR area. He made the master mix with the primers in, then aliquot 18 μL of the mix to each individual wells of a 96-well plate. After spinning down the patient samples in tubes, he added 2 μL of patient DNA samples into the wells from A1 to A6. Then BJ added 2 μL of positive control DNA into well A7. Lastly, he put 2 μL of water into well A8. After sealing the plate, BJ used 2% bleach to clean the bench and then took the plate to the post-PCR area for the centrifuge and thermal cycler. Which one of the following descriptions is appropriate, according to the ACMG Standards and Guidelines for Clinical Genetics Laboratories?[4,14]

A. The order of the samples in the 96-well plate should be positive control, patient samples, and negative control.

B. It is better to put samples in each individual well before adding master mix.

C. BJ should use 10% bleach to clean the bench instead of 2%.

D. The thermal cycler should be kept in the pre-PCR instead of the post-PCR area.

E. None of the above.

185. A director of a clinical pathology laboratory, planned to validate an oligonucleotide ligation assay (OLA) to detect carriers of cystic fibrosis. At a minimum, how many positive controls should be included in each run, according to the ACMG Standards and Guidelines for Clinical Genetics Laboratories?

A. 1
B. 2
C. 3
D. 4
E. All of mutations detectable with this assay
F. Not sure
G. None of the above

186. A technologist in a clinical molecular laboratory received two samples on a Friday afternoon. She confirmed that the two identifiers on the tubes matched up with the ones on the requisition forms. When she logged in the two samples, she found E84.9 for diagnosis. Which kind of code is it?

A. CPD code
B. CPT code
C. ICD code
D. ICT code
E. None of the above

187. A senior technologist reviewed the report for a chromosome microarray case in a clinical molecular laboratory. For billing, she confirmed that the code, 81229, was there. Which kind of code is it?

A. CPD code
B. CPT code
C. ICD code
D. ICT code
E. None of the above

188. A reference sequence in the table below is mutated to ... cag GGA GCC AAT CTT GCT AGC CCT AGA TTT GGT TCT ttt... tag GAC in a Caucasian patient. The gene is an OMIM gene, which is related to an autosomal dominant disease. The variant has not been reported in any patients, and it is not found in the parents of the patient. It is not a common variant in any general population either. Both SIFT and PolyPhen predicted it to be a pathogenic mutations. Which one of the following results will most likely be reported?[15]

A. Benign
B. Likely benign
C. Unknown clinical significance
D. Likely pathogenic
E. Pathogenic

	Exon 3												Exon 4
	26	27	28	29	30	31	32	33	34	35	36		37
	Gly	Ala	Asn	Leu	Ala	Ser	Pro	Arg	Phe	Gly	Ser		Asp
... cag	GGA	GCC	AAT	CTT	GCT	AGC	CCT	AGA	TTT	GGT	TCT	gtt ... tag	GAC
	76	79	82	85	88	91	94	97	100	103	106		109

189. A reference sequence in the table below is mutated to ... cag GGA GCC AAT CTT GCT AGC CCT AGA TTT GGT TA**A** gtt ... in a Caucasian patient. The gene is an OMIM gene, which is related to an autosomal dominant disease. The variant has not been reported in any patients, and it is not found in the parents of the patient. It is not a common variant in any general population either. Which one of the following most accurately describes the effect of this variant?[15]

A. Benign
B. Likely benign
C. Unknown clinical significance
D. Likely pathogenic
E. Pathogenic

				Exon 11								
	111	112	113	114	115	116	117	118	119	120		
	Gly	Ala	Asn	Leu	Ala	Ser	Pro	Arg	Phe	Gly		
... cag	GGA	GCC	AAT	CTT	GCT	AGC	CCT	AGA	TTT	GGT	TA**G**	gtt ...
	333	336	339	342	345	348	351	354	357	360	363	

190. A reference sequence in the table below is mutated to ... cag GGA GCC AAT CTT GCT AGC CCT AGA TTT GGT TA**T** gtt ... in a Caucasian patient. The gene is an OMIM gene, which is related to an autosomal dominant disease. The variant has not been reported in any patients, and it is not found in the parents of the patient. It is not a common variant in any general population either. Which one of the following most accurately describe the effect of this variant?[15]

A. Benign
B. Likely benign
C. Unknown clinical significance
D. Likely pathogenic
E. Pathogenic

				Exon 11								
	111	112	113	114	115	116	117	118	119	120		
	Gly	Ala	Asn	Leu	Ala	Ser	Pro	Arg	Phe	Gly		
... cag	GGA	GCC	AAT	CTT	GCT	AGC	CCT	AGA	TTT	GGT	TA**G**	gtt ...
	333	336	339	342	345	348	351	354	357	360	363	

191. A reference sequence in the table below is mutated to ... cag GGA GCC AAT CTT GCT AGC CCT AGA TTT GGT T**GA** gtt ... in a Caucasian patient. The gene is an OMIM gene, which is related to an autosomal dominant disease. The variant has not been reported in any patients, and it is not found in the parents of the patient. It is not a common variant in any general population either. Which one of the following most accurately describes the effect of this variant?[15]

A. Benign
B. Likely benign
C. Unknown clinical significance
D. Likely pathogenic
E. Pathogenic

				Exon 11								
	111	112	113	114	115	116	117	118	119	120		
	Gly	Ala	Asn	Leu	Ala	Ser	Pro	Arg	Phe	Gly		
... cag	GGA	GCC	AAT	CTT	GCT	AGC	CCT	AGA	TTT	GGT	TA**G**	gtt ...
	333	336	339	342	345	348	351	354	357	360	363	

ANSWERS

1. **D**. According to the College of American Pathology (CAP) All Common Checklist dated July 28, 2015, the "Laboratory Director is the individual who is responsible for the overall operation and administration of the laboratory, including provision of timely, reliable and clinically relevant test results and compliance with applicable regulations and accreditation requirements. This individual is *listed on the laboratory's CAP and CLIA certificate* (as applicable)." Most molecular tests are high complexity, according to CLIA regulations. The qualification of a director in a laboratory performing high-complexity tests are as follows:
   * MD, DO with current medical license in state of lab's location AND certified in anatomic and/or clinical pathology by ABP, AOBP, or equivalent qualifications.
   * MD, DO, DPM with current medical license in state of lab's location AND 1 year of laboratory training during medical residency.
   * MD, DO, DPM with current medical license in state of lab's location AND 2 years experience in directing/supervising high-complexity testing.
   * PhD in chemical, physical, biological, or clinical laboratory science AND certification by the HHS–approved boards (effective February 24, 2003).
   * Hold an earned PhD in chemical, physical, biological, or clinical laboratory science from an accredited institution AND, until December 31, 2002, must have served or be serving as director of a laboratory performing high-complexity testing AND must have at least 2 years of laboratory training or experience or both AND 2 years of experience directing or supervising high-complexity testing. (Directors meeting this qualification will be "grandfathered" in by CMS.).
   * ON OR BEFORE February 28, 1992: Serving as a laboratory director and must have previously qualified or could have qualified as a laboratory director under laboratory regulations published March 14, 1990.
   * ON OR BEFORE February 28, 1992: Qualified as director by the state in which the laboratory is located.[1]

   Therefore, Dr. D listed on the laboratory's CAP and CLIA certificate as the lab director should be considered to be the director of a clinical molecular laboratory.

2. **D**. The laboratory-developed Sanger sequencing assay for the *FAS* gene is *a high-complexity test system*. Clinical laboratories or other testing sites

need to know whether a test system is waived or moderate or high complexity for each test on their menu, as this determines the applicable CLIA requirements. The category of tests a laboratory offers is also a factor in determining the appropriate CLIA certificate for the laboratory.

As defined by CLIA, waived tests are simple tests with a low risk for an incorrect result. They include certain tests listed in the CLIA regulations, tests cleared by the FDA for home use, and tests approved for waiver by the FDA using the CLIA criteria. Sites performing only waived testing must have a CLIA certificate and follow the manufacturer's instructions; other CLIA requirements do not apply to these sites.

Nonwaived testing refers collectively to moderate- and high-complexity testing. Laboratories or sites that perform these tests need to have a CLIA certificate, must be inspected, and must meet the CLIA quality standards, such as those for proficiency testing, quality control, and personnel requirements, described in 42 CFR Subparts H, J, K, and M. (https://wwwn.cdc.gov/clia).

Clinical laboratory test systems are assigned to a moderate- or high-complexity category on the basis of seven criteria given in the CLIA regulations. The standards for moderate- and high-complexity testing differ only in the personnel requirements. For commercially available FDA-cleared/approved tests, the test complexity is determined by the FDA during the premarketing approval process. The final score is used to determine whether the test system is classified as moderate or high complexity (see 42 CFR 493.17). *For tests developed by the laboratory or that have been modified from the approved manufacturer's instructions, the complexity category defaults to high per the CLIA regulations* (see 42 CFR 493.17) (https://www.govinfo.gov/content/pkg/CFR-1996-title42-vol3/xml/CFR-1996-title42-vol3-sec493-17.xml).

Therefore, both choices B and D are correct, and choice D is the most appropriate answer.

3. **D**. The laboratory-developed quantitative PCR assay for the *NPM1* gene is *a high-complexity test system*. Clinical laboratories or other testing sites need to know whether a test system is waived or moderate or high complexity for each test on their menu, as this determines the applicable CLIA requirements. The category of tests a laboratory offers is also a factor in determining the appropriate CLIA certificate for the laboratory.

As defined by CLIA, waived tests are simple tests with a low risk for an incorrect result. They include certain tests listed in the CLIA regulations, tests cleared by the FDA for home use, and tests approved for waiver by the FDA using the CLIA criteria. Sites performing only waived testing must have a CLIA certificate and follow the manufacturer's instructions; other CLIA requirements do not apply to these sites.

Nonwaived testing refers collectively to moderate- and high-complexity testing. Laboratories or sites that perform these tests need to have a CLIA certificate, must be inspected, and must meet the CLIA quality standards, such as those for proficiency testing, quality control, and personnel requirements, described in 42 CFR Subparts H, J, K, and M (https://wwwn.cdc.gov/clia).

Clinical laboratory test systems are assigned to a moderate- or high-complexity category on the basis of seven criteria given in the CLIA regulations. The standards for moderate- and high-complexity testing differ only in the personnel requirements. For commercially available FDA-cleared/approved tests, the test complexity is determined by the FDA during the premarketing approval process. The final score is used to determine whether the test system is classified as moderate or high complexity (see 42 CFR 493.17). *For tests developed by the laboratory or that have been modified from the approved manufacturer's instructions, the complexity category defaults to high complexity per the CLIA regulations* (see 42 CFR 493.17) (https://www.govinfo.gov/content/pkg/CFR-1996-title42-vol3/xml/CFR-1996-title42-vol3-sec493-17.xml).

Therefore, both choices B and D are correct, and choice D is the most appropriate answer.

4. **D**. HIV-1 RNA quantitative PCR assay is *a high-complexity test system*. Clinical laboratories or other testing sites need to know whether a test system is waived or moderate or high complexity for each test on their menu, as this determines the applicable CLIA requirements. The category of tests a laboratory offers is also a factor in determining the appropriate CLIA certificate for the laboratory.

As defined by CLIA, waived tests are simple tests with a low risk for an incorrect result. They include certain tests listed in the CLIA regulations, tests cleared by the FDA for home use, and tests approved for waiver by the FDA using the CLIA criteria. Sites performing only waived testing must have a CLIA certificate and follow the manufacturer's instructions; other CLIA requirements do not apply to these sites.

Nonwaived testing refers collectively to moderate- and high-complexity testing. Laboratories or sites that perform these tests need to have a CLIA certificate, must be inspected, and must meet the

CLIA quality standards, such as those for proficiency testing, quality control, and personnel requirements, described in 42 CFR Subparts H, J, K, and M (https://wwwn.cdc.gov/clia).

Clinical laboratory test systems are assigned a moderate- or high-complexity category on the basis of seven criteria given in the CLIA regulations. The standards for moderate- and high-complexity testing differ only in the personnel requirements. For commercially available FDA-cleared/approved tests, the test complexity is determined by the FDA during the premarketing approval process. The final score is used to determine whether the test system is classified as moderate or high complexity (see 42 CFR 493.17). The complexity designation may be printed in the manufacturer's package insert or other instructions. In addition, the FDA and CMS websites have several resources: https://www.accessdata.fda.gov/scripts/cdrh/cfdocs/cfclia/search.cfm. *For tests developed by the laboratory or that have been modified from the approved manufacturer's instructions, the complexity category defaults to high complexity per the CLIA regulations (see 42 CFR 493.17).*

HIV-1 RNA quantitative PCR assay is a FDA-approved test, and according to FDA and CMS, it is a high-complexity test system. Therefore, both choices B and D are correct, and choice D is the most appropriate answer.

5. **D**. According to the College of American Pathology (CAP) All Common Checklist dated July 28, 2015, COM.40000, "There is a summary statement, *signed by the laboratory director (or designee who meets CAP director qualifications)* prior to use in patient testing, that includes the evaluation of validation/verification studies and approval of each test for clinical use."

For laboratory-developed test only the laboratory direct need review and approve it before launching it. The FDA defines a laboratory-developed test (LDT) as an in vitro diagnostic test that is manufactured by and used within a single laboratory (i.e., a laboratory with a single CLIA certificate). LDTs are also sometimes called "in-house developed tests" or "home brew tests." Similar to other in vitro diagnostic tests, LDTs are considered "devices," as defined by the Federal Food, Drug, and Cosmetic Act (FFDCA), and are therefore subject to regulatory oversight by FDA.

The Clinical Laboratory Improvement Amendments (CLIA) program regulates laboratories that perform testing on patient specimens in order to ensure accurate and reliable test results. The FDA regulates manufacturers and devices under the FFDCA to ensure that devices, including those intended for use in the diagnosis of disease or other conditions, or in the cure, mitigation, treatment, or prevention of disease, are reasonably safe and effective.

When a laboratory develops a test system such as an LDT in-house without receiving FDA clearance or approval, CLIA prohibits the release of any test results prior to the laboratory establishing certain performance characteristics relating to analytical validity for the use of that test system in the laboratory's own environment. See 42 CFR 493.1253(b) (establishment of performance specifications). This analytical validation is limited, however, to the specific conditions, staff, equipment and patient population of the particular laboratory, so the findings of these laboratory-specific analytical validation are not meaningful outside the laboratory that did the analysis. Furthermore, the laboratory's analytical validation of LDTs is reviewed during its routine biennial survey—after the laboratory has already started testing.

Therefore, this Sanger sequencing based test for the *FAS* (*TNFRSF6*) gene is a high complexity test.

6. **D.** According to the College of American Pathology (CAP) All Common Checklist dated July 28, 2015, "For FDA-cleared/approved tests, the needs of the user (intended use and clinical utility) have been defined and the performance characteristics established by the manufacturer. Laboratory validation of FDA-cleared/approved tests therefore only requires verification of analytical performance parameters: accuracy, precision, reference range, and reportable range."

According to the CAP Molecular Pathology Checklist dated July 28, 2015, "*If an FDA-cleared/approved test is modified to meet the needs of the user or if the test is developed by the laboratory (LDT), both analytical and clinical performance parameters need to be established.* Analytical performance parameters include, precision, reference range, reportable range, as well as analytical sensitivity, analytical specificity, and any other parameter that is considered important to assure the analytical performance of a particular test (e.g. specimen stability, reagent stability, linearity, carryover, cross-contamination, etc., as appropriate and applicable). The clinical validity, which includes clinical performance characteristics, such as clinical sensitivity, clinical specificity, positive and negative predictive values in defined populations or likelihood ratios, and clinical utility should also be considered, although individual laboratories may

not be able to assess these parameters within their own patient population, especially for rare diseases. However, patients without disease can typically be tested to assess clinical specificity. If clinical validation cannot be established within a laboratory, it is appropriate to cite scientific literature that established clinical sensitivity and specificity. Clinical performance characteristics should be determined relative to clinical data (e.g. biopsy findings, radiographic and clinical findings, other laboratory results, etc.) whenever possible."

Therefore, the scientist should follow the validation procedure for a laboratory-developed assay, since he modified the FDA-cleared/approved test.

7. **A.** *Quality assurance (QA)* is a way of preventing mistakes or defects in the process of testing clinical samples and avoiding problems when delivering the results to customers, which is the part of quality management focused on providing confidence that quality requirements will be fulfilled. This defect prevention in QA differs subtly from defect detection and rejection in quality control and has been referred to as a shift left, as it focuses on quality earlier in the process. Monitoring preanalytical, analytical, and postanalytical processes ensures the quality of the results. Maintaining instruments regularly is part of the QA process, too.

Quality management (QM) ensures that an organization, product, or service is consistent. It has four main components: quality planning, quality control, quality assurance, and quality improvement. Quality management is focused not only on product and service quality, but also on the means to achieve it. It, therefore, uses quality assurance and control of processes as well as products to achieve more consistent quality. Quality control (QC) is a process by which entities review the quality of all factors involved in production, which is defined as "A part of quality management focused on fulfilling quality requirements." An example of QC is using negative and positive controls in each experiment. Quality improvement (QI) is a formal approach to the analysis of performance and systematic efforts to improve it. In the example in this question, an investigation was done and showed that the reaction volume at the end of procedure became very low (from 20 μL to 5 μL) after the scientist in the question identified the potential problem. So the laboratory worked on two plans to solve the problem. This troubleshooting process is called "quality improvement."

QA is focused on planning, documenting, and agreeing on a set of guidelines that are necessary to ensure quality. QA planning is undertaken at the beginning of a project and draws on industry or company standards. Quality control, on the other hand, includes all activities that are designed to determine the level of quality, including monitoring the failure rate of a test. QC is a reactive means by which quality is gauged and monitored and includes all operational techniques and activities used to fulfill requirements for quality.

Monitoring the failure rate is part of QA plan under the umbrella of QM. Therefore, QA is the most appropriate answer for this question.

8. **C.** *Quality improvement (QI)* is a formal approach to the analysis of performance and systematic efforts to improve it. This question is a good example. The initial finding was the high failure rate based on the data gathered through the quality assurance program. Further investigation found that the reaction volume at the end of procedure became very low (from 20 µL to 5 µL). So the laboratory worked on two plans to solve the problem. This troubleshooting process is called quality improvement (QI).

Quality management ensures that an organization, product, or service is consistent. It has four main components: quality planning, quality control, quality assurance and quality improvement. Quality management is focused not only on product and service quality, but also on the means to achieve it. It, therefore, uses quality assurance and control of processes as well as products to achieve more consistent quality. Quality assurance (QA) is a way of preventing mistakes or defects in the process of testing clinical samples and avoiding problems when delivering the results to customers, which is part of quality management focused on providing confidence that quality requirements will be fulfilled. This defect prevention in quality assurance differs subtly from defect detection and rejection in quality control and has been referred to as a shift left, as it focuses on quality earlier in the process. Monitoring preanalytical, analytical, and postanalytical processes ensures the quality of the results. Maintaining instruments regularly is part of QA process, too. Quality control (QC) is a process by which entities review the quality of all factors involved in production, which is defined as "A part of quality management focused on fulfilling quality requirements." An example of QC is using negative and positive controls in each experiment.[1,2]

Therefore, investigation and troubleshooting is part of QI plan.

9. **F.** Quality management is a very important part of laboratory medicine. There is a chapter in College of American Pathology (CAP) Laboratory General Checklist dated July 28, 2015, and a chapter in CAP All Common Checklist dated July 28, 2015, dedicated to quality management. GEN.13806 states, "The laboratory has a written quality management (QM) program." GEN.20316 states, "The QM program includes monitoring key indicators of quality in the preanalytic, analytic, and postanalytic phases." GEN.20375 states, "The laboratory has a document control system to manage policies, procedures, and forms that are subject to CAP accreditation." GEN.20425 states, "The laboratory has a policy to ensure that all records, slides, blocks, and tissues are retained and available for appropriate times should the laboratory cease operation." GEN.30000 states, "There is a written quality control program that clearly defines policies and procedures for monitoring analytic performance." GEN.30070 states, "If the laboratory performs test procedures for which neither calibration nor control materials are available, procedures are established to validate the reliability of patient test results."

Quality management (QM) is big part of clinical laboratory practice. And QM plan infiltrates all parts of CAP Team Leader Assessment of Director & Quality, All Common, Molecular Pathology, and Microbiology Checklist for molecular genetic based test.

Therefore, all the plans listed in this question should be included in the quality management policy in a clinical laboratory.

10. **B.** According to the College of American Pathology (CAP) Laboratory General Checklist dated July 28, 2015, GEN.4049, "All primary specimen containers are labeled with *at least two patient-specific identifiers*." And according to the CAP All Common Checklist dated July 28, 2015, COM.06100, "All primary specimen containers are labeled with *at least two patient-specific identifiers*."

Therefore, at least 2 identifiers have to be on the tube for a collected peripheral blood sample according to the College of American Pathologist (CAP)'s regulation.

11. **E.** This is *not a deficiency*. According to the College of American Pathologists (CAP) All Common Checklist dated July 28, 2015, COM.06100, "All primary specimen containers are labeled with at least two patient-specific identifiers." However, it also states "In limited situations, a single identifier may be used if it can uniquely identify the specimen. For example, in a trauma situation,

where a patient's identification is not known, a specimen may be submitted for testing labeled with a unique code that is traceable to the trauma patient. Other examples may include forensic specimens, coded or deidentified research specimens, *or donor specimens labeled with a unique code decryptable only by the submitting location.*"

Phase 0 deficiency does not require a formal response, though it should be corrected by the laboratory. Phase I deficiency does not seriously affect the quality of patient care or significantly endanger the welfare of laboratory workers. Correction and a written response to the CAP are required, but not supportive documents. Phase II deficiency may seriously affect the quality of patient care or the health and safety of hospital or laboratory personnel. Correction requires both an action plan and supportive documentation that the plan has been implemented. There is no Phase III deficiency.

Therefore, there would be NO deficiency if an on-site College of American Pathologist (CAP) inspector had found it according to the CAP's regulation.

12. **C**. According to the College of American Pathologists (CAP) All Common Checklist dated July 28, 2015, COM.01300, "Proficiency testing for *HER2* (*ERBB2*) is method specific. If the laboratory performs *HER2* (*ERBB2*) testing by multiple methods, the laboratory must participate in PT for each method... If the laboratory sends its FISH (or ISH) slides for hybridization to another facility, the laboratory must perform *an alternative assessment* of the test twice annually and may not participate in formal (external) PT."

Therefore, an alternative *HER2* FISH proficiency test should be performed in this laboratory according to the College of American Pathologist (CAP)'s regulation.

13. **B**. According to the College of American Pathologists (CAP) All Common Checklist dated July 28, 2015, COM.01300, "Proficiency testing for *HER2* (*ERBB2*) is method specific. If the laboratory performs *HER2* (*ERBB2*) testing by multiple methods, the laboratory must participate in PT for each method... If the laboratory sends its FISH (or ISH) slides for hybridization to another facility, the laboratory must perform an alternative assessment of the test *twice annually* and may not participate in formal (external) PT."

Therefore, the laboratory should perform the alternative assessment of the *HER2* FISH assay minimally semi-annually according to the College of American Pathologist (CAP)'s regulation.

14. **C**. According to the College of American Pathology (CAP) All Common Checklist dated July 28, 2015, COM.01400, "The proficiency testing attestation statement is signed by *the laboratory director or designee and all individuals involved in the testing process.* ... Physical signatures must appear on a paper version of the attestation form. A listing of typed names on the attestation statement does not meet the intent of the requirement. The signature of the laboratory director or designee need not be obtained prior to reporting results to the proficiency testing provider."

Therefore, the laboratory director or designee and all individuals involved in the testing process should sign the Proficiency Test (PT) Attestation Statement according to CAP's regulation.

15. **C**. According to the College of American Pathology (CAP) All Common Checklist dated July 28, 2015, COM.01500, "For test for which CAP does not require PT, the laboratory *at least semi-annually* exercises an alternative performance assessment system for determining the reliability of analytic testing."

The molecular targeted *BRAF* test is not PT program required by CAP. Therefore, the laboratory may exercises an alternative performance assessment system at least semiannually.

16. **E**. *This is not a deficiency* according to the College of American Pathologist (CAP)'s regulations. However, the laboratory must have written procedures for the proper handling, analysis, review, and reporting of proficiency testing materials. There must be written procedure(s) for investigation and correction of problems that are identified by unacceptable proficiency testing results. The laboratory should also have procedures for investigation of results that, although acceptable show bias or trends suggesting a problem (CAP All Common Checklist dated July 28, 2015, COM.01000, COM.01700). And if the laboratory does not have written procedures for proficiency testing sufficient for the extent and complexity of testing done in the laboratory, it would be a Phase II deficiency.

Phase 0 deficiency does not require a formal response, though it should be corrected by the laboratory. Phase I deficiency does not seriously affect the quality of patient care or significantly endanger the welfare of laboratory workers. Correction and a written response to the CAP are required, but not supportive documents. Phase II deficiency may seriously affect the quality of patient care or the health and safety of hospital or laboratory personnel. Correction requires both an action plan and supportive documentation that the plan has been implemented. There is no Phase III deficiency.

Therefore, this discrepancy would NOT be a deficiency according to CAP's regulation.

17. **B**. This is a *Phase I deficiency* according to the College of American Pathologist (CAP)'s regulations. In the College of American Pathology (CAP) All Common Checklist dated July 28, 2015, COM.01200, it states "The laboratory's current CAP Activity Menu accurately reflects the testing performed." If the laboratory failed to inform CAP the change of the test menu, it would be a phase I deficiency. In the situation described in the question, "the inspector should contact the CAP (800-323-4040) for instructions and record on the appropriate section page in the Inspector's Summation Report (ISR) whether those tests were inspected or not inspected."

Phase 0 deficiency does not require a formal response though should be corrected by the laboratory. Phase I deficiency does not seriously affect the quality of patient care or significantly endanger the welfare of a laboratory worker. Correction and a written response to the CAP are required, but not supportive documents. Phase II deficiency may seriously affect the quality of patient care or the health and safety of hospital or laboratory personnel. Correction requires both action plan and supportive documentation that the plan has been implemented. There is no Phase III deficiency.

Therefore, this discrepancy would be a Phase I deficiency according to CAP's regulation.

18. **C**. Under CLIA'88 regulations, there is a strict prohibition against referring proficiency testing (PT) specimens to another laboratory with a different CLIA number, even if the second laboratory is in the same health care system. If a laboratory refers College of American Pathology (CAP) PT specimens to another laboratory in any circumstances, it is a *Phase II deficiency*. According to the CAP All Common Checklist dated April 21, 2014, COM.01900, "There is a policy that prohibits referral of proficiency testing specimens to another laboratory or acceptance from another laboratory."

Therefore, it would be a Phase II deficiency if the laboratory sent the CAP specimens to a reference laboratory according to CAP's regulation. In the situation described in the question, the laboratory must submit a PT result indicating that the test was not performed since the test was not performed in the referring laboratory.

19. **B**. According to the College of American Pathology (CAP) All Common Checklist dated April 21, 2014, COM.01700, "Primary records related to PT and alternative assessment testing are retained for *two years* (unless a longer retention period is required elsewhere in this checklist for specific analytes or disciplines). These include all instrument tapes, work cards, computer printouts, evaluation reports, evidence of review, and documentation of follow-up/ corrective action."

Therefore, the primary records of the proficiency test (PT) should be retained for at least 2 years according to the Clinical Laboratory Improvement Amendments (CLIA) 1988.

20. **C**. This is a *Phase II deficiency* according to the College of American Pathologist (CAP)'s regulations. According to the CAP All Common Checklist dated July 28, 2015, COM.01300, "The laboratory participates in the appropriate required proficiency testing (PT)/external quality assessment (EQA) program accepted by CAP for the patient testing performed." It also states, "Information on analytes that require enrollment and participation in a CAP-accepted PT program is available on the CAP website (http://www.cap.org/) through e-LAB Solutions Suite under CAP Accreditation Resources, Master Activity Menu Reports. Also, the inspection packet includes a report with this information for each laboratory section/ department." And "For laboratories subject to US regulations, participation in proficiency testing may be through CAP PT Programs or another proficiency testing provider accepted by CAP. Laboratories will not be penalized if they are unable to participate in an oversubscribed program. If unable to participate, however, the laboratory must implement an alternative assessment procedure for the affected analytes. For regulated analytes, if the CAP and CAP-accepted PT programs are oversubscribed, CMS requires the laboratory to attempt to enroll in another CMS-approved PT program" (http://www.cap.org/).

Phase 0 deficiency does not require a formal response, though it should be corrected by the laboratory. Phase I deficiency does not seriously affect the quality of patient care or significantly endanger the welfare of laboratory workers. Correction and a written response to the CAP are required, but not supportive documents. Phase II deficiency may seriously affect the quality of patient care or the health and safety of hospital or laboratory personnel. Correction requires both an action plan and supportive documentation that the plan has been implemented. There is no Phase III deficiency.

Factor V Leiden and factor II tests are PT program required by CAP. Therefore, sending specimens to another laboratory is not an acceptable alternative in this situation.

21. E. This is *not a deficiency* according to the College of American Pathologist (CAP)'s regulations. According to the CAP All Common Checklist dated July 28, 2015, COM.01300, "The laboratory participates in the appropriate required proficiency testing (PT)/external quality assessment (EQA) program accepted by CAP for the patient testing performed." And in COM.01500, "For tests for which CAP does not require PT, the laboratory at least semi-annually exercises an alternative performance assessment system for determining the reliability of analytic testing."

BRAF and *EGFR* molecular assays fall into this category, which requires alternative assessment. According to COM.01500, "Appropriate alternative performance assessment procedures include participation in an external PT program not required by CAP; participation in an ungraded/educational PT program; split sample analysis with reference or other laboratories, split samples with an established in-house method, assayed materials, clinical validation by chart review, or other suitable and documented means. It is the responsibility of the laboratory director to define such alternative assessment procedures and the criteria for successful performance in accordance with good clinical and scientific laboratory practice." Therefore, sending samples to a reference laboratory as an alternative PT assessment is acceptable.

Phase 0 deficiency does not require a formal response, though it should be corrected by the laboratory. Phase I deficiency does not seriously affect the quality of patient care or significantly endanger the welfare of laboratory workers. Correction and a written response to the CAP are required, but not supportive documents. Phase II deficiency may seriously affect the quality of patient care or the health and safety of hospital or laboratory personnel. Correction requires both an action plan and supportive documentation that the plan has been implemented. There is no Phase III deficiency.

Therefore, it would NOT be a deficiency if it were one according to CAP's regulation.

22. A. In a research laboratory, this would include solid waste generated from any work with human or nonhuman primate blood, tissue, or cells and microbiological agents that may cause human illness. The Basis for the Classification of Biohazardous Agents by Risk Group (RG) is as follows:
- *Risk Group 1 (RG1): Agents that are not associated with disease in healthy adult humans.*
- Risk Group 2 (RG2): Agents that are associated with human disease that is rarely serious and for which preventive or therapeutic interventions are often available.
- Risk Group 3 (RG3): Agents that are associated with serious or lethal human disease for which preventive or therapeutic interventions may be available (high individual risk but low community risk).
- Risk Group 4 (RG4): Agents that are likely to cause serious or lethal human disease for which preventive or therapeutic interventions are not usually available (high individual risk and high community risk).

Risk Group 1 (RG1) Agents: RG1 agents are not associated with disease in healthy adult humans. Examples of RG1 agents include asporogenic *Bacillus subtilis* or *Bacillus licheniformis* (see Appendix C-IV-A, *B. subtilis* or *B. licheniformis* Host-Vector Systems, Exceptions), adeno-associated virus (AAV) types 1 through 4, and recombinant AAV constructs, in which the transgene does not encode either a potentially tumorigenic gene product or a toxin molecule and are produced in the absence of a helper virus. A strain of *Escherichia coli* is an RG1 agent if it: (1) does not possess a complete lipopolysaccharide (i.e., lacks the O antigen); and (2) does not carry any active virulence factor (e.g., toxins) or colonization factors and does not carry any genes encoding these factors. (Page 38 of NIH Guidelines for Research Involving Recombinant DNA Molecules [September 2009].)

Agents that fall within Risk Groups 2, 3, and 4 are considered biohazardous and should be treated as such. Agents that fall within Risk Group 1 are considered to be biowaste and do not fall under the biohazardous waste requirements, although certain precautions still need to be followed (https://www.safety.caltech.edu).

Therefore, the risk group 1 agents are agents that are not associated with disease in healthy adult humans according to the Disease Control and Prevention (CDC) classification of biohazardous waste.

23. **D**. In a research laboratory, this would include solid waste generated from any work with human or nonhuman primate blood, tissue, or cells and microbiological agents that may cause human illness. The Basis for the Classification of Biohazardous Agents by Risk Group (RG) is as follows:
    - Risk Group 1 (RG1): Agents that are not associated with disease in healthy adult humans.
    - Risk Group 2 (RG2): Agents that are associated with human disease that is rarely serious and for which preventive or therapeutic interventions are often available.
    - Risk Group 3 (RG3): Agents that are associated with serious or lethal human disease for which preventive or therapeutic interventions may be available (high individual risk but low community risk).
    - *Risk Group 4 (RG4): Agents that are likely to cause serious or lethal human disease for which preventive or therapeutic interventions are not usually available (high individual risk and high community risk).*

    Agents that fall within Risk Groups 2, 3, and 4 are considered biohazardous and should be treated as such. Agents that fall within Risk Group 1 are considered to be biowaste and do not fall under the biohazardous waste requirements, although certain precautions still need to be followed (https://www.safety.caltech.edu).

    Therefore, the risk group 4 agents are agents that are likely to cause serious or lethal human disease for which preventive or therapeutic interventions are not usually available (high individual risk and high community risk) according to CDC classification of biohazardous waste.

24. **B**. In a research laboratory, this would include solid waste generated from any work with human or nonhuman primate blood, tissue, or cells and microbiological agents that may cause human illness. The Basis for the Classification of Biohazardous Agents by Risk Group (RG) is as follows:
    - Risk Group 1 (RG1): Agents that are not associated with disease in healthy adult humans.
    - *Risk Group 2 (RG2): Agents that are associated with human disease that is rarely serious and for which preventive or therapeutic interventions are often available.*
    - Risk Group 3 (RG3): Agents that are associated with serious or lethal human disease for which preventive or therapeutic interventions may be

available (high individual risk but low community risk).
    - Risk Group 4 (RG4): Agents that are likely to cause serious or lethal human disease for which preventive or therapeutic interventions are not usually available (high individual risk and high community risk).

    Agents that fall within Risk Groups 2, 3, and 4 are considered biohazardous and should be treated as such. Agents that fall within Risk Group 1 are considered to be biowaste and do not fall under the biohazardous waste requirements, although certain precautions still need to be followed (https://www.safety.caltech.edu).

    Therefore, the risk group 2 agents are agents that are associated with serious or lethal human disease for which preventive or therapeutic interventions may be available (high individual risk but low community risk) according to CDC classification of biohazardous waste.

25. **C**. In a research laboratory, this would include solid waste generated from any work with human or nonhuman primate blood, tissue, or cells and microbiological agents that may cause human illness. The Basis for the Classification of Biohazardous Agents by Risk Group (RG) is as follows:
    - Risk Group 1 (RG1): Agents that are not associated with disease in healthy adult humans.
    - Risk Group 2 (RG2): Agents that are associated with human disease that is rarely serious and for which preventive or therapeutic interventions are often available.
    - *Risk Group 3 (RG3): Agents that are associated with serious or lethal human disease for which preventive or therapeutic interventions may be available (high individual risk but low community risk).*
    - Risk Group 4 (RG4): Agents that are likely to cause serious or lethal human disease for which preventive or therapeutic interventions are not usually available (high individual risk and high community risk).

    Agents that fall within Risk Groups 2, 3, and 4 are considered biohazardous and should be treated as such. Agents that fall within Risk Group 1 are considered to be biowaste and do not fall under the biohazardous waste requirements, although certain precautions still need to be followed (https://www.safety.caltech.edu).

    Therefore, the risk group 2 agents are agents that are associated with human disease which is rarely serious and for which preventive or therapeutic are often available according to CDC classification of biohazardous waste.

26. **C**. *HIV-1 and 2 viruses are in the risk group 3* according to the Centers for Disease Control and Prevention (CDC) classification of biohazardous waste. The four risk groups are as follows:
   - Risk Group 1 (RG1): Agents that are not associated with disease in healthy adult humans.
   - Risk Group 2 (RG2): Agents that are associated with human disease that is rarely serious and for which preventive or therapeutic interventions are often available.
   - *Risk Group 3 (RG3): Agents that are associated with serious or lethal human disease for which preventive or therapeutic interventions may be available (high individual risk but low community risk).*
   - Risk Group 4 (RG4): Agents that are likely to cause serious or lethal human disease for which preventive or therapeutic interventions are not usually available (high individual risk and high community risk).

   There is no Risk Group 5. Agents that fall within Risk Groups 2, 3, and 4 are considered biohazardous and should be treated as such. Agents that fall within Risk Group 1 are considered to be biowaste and do not fall under the biohazardous waste requirements, although certain precautions still need to be followed (https://www.safety.caltech.edu).

   Therefore, HIV-1 virus belongs to risk group 3 according to CDC classification of biohazardous waste.

27. **D**. *Ebola virus is in the Risk Group 4* according to the Centers for Disease Control and Prevention (CDC) classification of biohazardous waste. The four risk groups are as follows:
   - Risk Group 1 (RG1): Agents that are not associated with disease in healthy adult humans.
   - Risk Group 2 (RG2): Agents that are associated with human disease that is rarely serious and for which preventive or therapeutic interventions are often available.
   - Risk Group 3 (RG3): Agents that are associated with serious or lethal human disease for which preventive or therapeutic interventions may be available (high individual risk but low community risk).
   - *Risk Group 4 (RG4): Agents that are likely to cause serious or lethal human disease for which preventive or therapeutic interventions are not usually available (high individual risk and high community risk).*

   There is no Risk Group 5. Agents that fall within Risk Groups 2, 3, and 4 are considered biohazardous and should be treated as such.

Agents that fall within Risk Group 1 are considered to be biowaste and do not fall under the biohazardous waste requirements, although certain precautions still need to be followed (https://www.safety.caltech.edu).

   Therefore, Ebola virus belongs to risk group 4 according to CDC classification of biohazardous waste.

28. **B**. *Hepatitis B, cytomegalovirus [CMV, Epstein—Barr virus (EBV)], and herpes simplex types 1 and 2 viruses are in risk group 2* according to the Centers for Disease Control and Prevention (CDC) classification of biohazardous waste. The four risk groups are as follows:
   - Risk Group 1 (RG1): Agents that are not associated with disease in healthy adult humans.
   - *Risk Group 2 (RG2): Agents that are associated with human disease that is rarely serious and for which preventive or therapeutic interventions are often available.*
   - Risk Group 3 (RG3): Agents that are associated with serious or lethal human disease for which preventive or therapeutic interventions may be available (high individual risk but low community risk).
   - Risk Group 4 (RG4): Agents that are likely to cause serious or lethal human disease for which preventive or therapeutic interventions are not usually available (high individual risk and high community risk).

   There is no Risk Group 5. Agents that fall within Risk Groups 2, 3, and 4 are considered biohazardous and should be treated as such. Agents that fall within Risk Group 1 are considered to be biowaste and do not fall under the biohazardous waste requirements, although certain precautions still need to be followed (https://www.safety.caltech.edu).

   Therefore, Hepatitis B, cytomegalovirus [CMV, Epstein—Barr virus (EBV)], and herpes simplex types 1 and 2 viruses belong to risk group 2 according to CDC classification of biohazardous waste.

29. **B**. *Rabies virus is in risk group 2* according to the Centers for Disease Control and Prevention (CDC) classification of biohazardous waste. The four risk groups are as follows:
   - Risk Group 1 (RG1): Agents that are not associated with disease in healthy adult humans.
   - *Risk Group 2 (RG2): Agents that are associated with human disease that is rarely serious and for which preventive or therapeutic interventions are often available.*

- Risk Group 3 (RG3): Agents that are associated with serious or lethal human disease for which preventive or therapeutic interventions may be available (high individual risk but low community risk).
- Risk Group 4 (RG4): Agents that are likely to cause serious or lethal human disease for which preventive or therapeutic interventions are not usually available (high individual risk and high community risk).

There is no Risk Group 5. Agents that fall within Risk Groups 2, 3, and 4 are considered biohazardous and should be treated as such. Agents that fall within Risk Group 1 are considered to be biowaste and do not fall under the biohazardous waste requirements, although certain precautions still need to be followed (https://www.safety.caltech.edu).

Therefore, Rabies virus belongs to risk group 2 according to CDC classification of biohazardous waste.

30. **A**. According to the College of American Pathology (CAP) All Common Checklist dated July 28, 2015, COM.04200, "Instrument and equipment maintenance and function check records are reviewed and assessed *at least monthly* by the laboratory director or designee."

Therefore, he or his designee should review and assess instrument and equipment maintenance and function check records at least monthly according to CAP's regulation.

31. **D**. According to the College of American Pathology (CAP) All Common Checklist dated July 28, 2015, COM.04250, "If the laboratory uses more than one nonwaived instrument/method to test for a given analyte, the instruments/methods are checked against each other *at least twice a year* for comparability of results." It also states, "This requirement applies to tests performed *on the same or different instrument makes/models or by different methods*." Please also be aware that "This comparison is required only for nonwaived instruments/methods accredited under a single CAP number."

Therefore, he should check all the 20 thermal cyclers against each other at least twice a year.

32. **C**. According to the College of American Pathology (CAP) All Common Checklist dated July 28, 2015, COM.04250, "If the laboratory uses more than one nonwaived instrument/method to test for a given analyte, the instruments/methods are checked against each other *at least twice a year* for comparability of results."

Therefore, he or designee should check the thermal cyclers against each other for comparability of results in the laboratory at least twice a year according to CAP's regulation.

33. **C**. It would be a *Phase II deficiency*. According to the College of American Pathology (CAP) All Common Checklist dated July 28, 2015, COM.01800, "Results must be reported by personnel within the laboratory. There is a strict prohibition against interlaboratory communications about proficiency testing samples or results until after the deadline for submission of data to the proficiency testing provider."

Phase 0 deficiency does not require a formal response, though should be corrected by the laboratory. Phase I deficiency does not seriously affect the quality of patient care or significantly endanger the welfare of laboratory workers. Correction and a written response to the CAP are required, but not supportive documents. Phase II deficiency may seriously affect the quality of patient care or the health and safety of hospital or laboratory personnel. Correction requires both an action plan and supportive documentation that the plan has been implemented. There is no Phase III deficiency.

Therefore, it would be a Phase II deficiency if they discussed the results according to CAP's regulation.

34. **E**. According to the College of American Pathology (CAP) All Common Checklist dated July 28, 2015, COM.10100 "There is documentation of review of all technical policies and procedures by the current laboratory director or designee *at least every two years*."

Therefore, the technical policies and procedures should be reviewed by the current laboratory director or designee at least biennially according to CAP's regulation.

35. **C**. It would be a *Phase II deficiency*. According to the College of American Pathology (CAP) All Common Checklist dated July 28, 2015, COM.10100, "There is documentation of review of all technical policies and procedures by the current laboratory director or designee at least every two years." If it is not done, it is a Phase II deficiency.

Phase 0 deficiency does not require a formal response, though should be corrected by the laboratory. Phase I deficiency does not seriously affect the quality of patient care or significantly endanger the welfare of laboratory workers. Correction and a written response to the CAP are required, but not supportive documents. Phase II deficiency may seriously affect the quality of patient care or the health and safety of hospital or laboratory personnel. Correction requires both an action plan and supportive documentation that the plan has been implemented. There is no Phase III deficiency.

Therefore, it would be a Phase II deficiency according to CAP's regulation.

36. **C.** According to the College of American Pathology (CAP) All Common Checklist dated July 28, 2015, COM.10200, "The laboratory director reviews and approves all new technical policies and procedures, as well as substantial changes to existing documents, *before implementation*. This review may not be delegated to designees in laboratories subject to the CLIA regulations. Paper/electronic signature review is required. A secure electronic signature is desirable, but not required."

Therefore, the procedure for this new test should be reviewed and approved before implementation according to CAP's regulation.

37. **B.** According to the College of American Pathology (CAP) All Common Checklist dated July 28, 2015, COM.10200, *"The laboratory director* reviews and approves all new technical policies and procedures, as well as substantial changes to existing documents, before implementation. This review may not be delegated to designees in laboratories subject to the CLIA regulations. Paper/electronic signature review is required. A secure electronic signature is desirable, but not required." In COM.10250, "For laboratories not subject to US regulations, the laboratory director or designee reviews and approves all new technical policies and procedures, as well as substantial changes to existing documents before implementation."

Therefore, Dr. B should review and approve the new procedure.

38. **F.** According to the College of American Pathology (CAP) All Common Checklist dated July 28, 2015, COM.10500, "When a procedure is discontinued, a paper or electronic copy is maintained for at least 2 years, recording initial date of use, and retirement date. For genetic testing, in order to meet the requirements of some states relating to the testing of minors (under the age of 21), it is recommended that laboratories retain procedures (paper or electronic) for *at least 23 years* (to cover the interval from fetal period to age 21)."

Therefore, the discontinued procedures should be maintained for at least 23 years in a clinical molecular genetics laboratory according to CAP's regulation.

39. **C.** According to the College of American Pathology (CAP) All Common Checklist dated

July 28, 2015, COM.30000, "Records must be maintained showing prompt notification of the appropriate clinical individual after obtaining results in the critical range. These records must include: *date, time, responsible laboratory individual, person notified* (the person's first name alone is not adequate documentation), and *test results.*" It also states, "When critical results are communicated by phone, *'read-back'* of the results is requested and recorded" in COM.30100.

PML/RARA translocation is diagnostic for acute promyelocytic leukemia (APML, APL). Individuals with APL are especially susceptible to developing bruises, small red dots under the skin (petechiae), nosebleeds, bleeding from the gums, blood in the urine (hematuria), or excessive menstrual bleeding. APL is unique among leukemias owing to its sensitivity to all-*trans* retinoic acid (ATRA). Currently, it is one of the most treatable forms of leukemia, with a 12-year progression-free survival rate of approximately 70%. Early diagnosis and treatment of acute promyelocytic leukemia (APL), the M3 subtype of acute myeloid leukemia (AML), is important because patients with APL can develop serious blood-clotting or bleeding problems. Therefore, the *PML/RARA* test should be treated as STAT, preliminary results should be given to the ordering physician ASAP. However, *recommendation is not necessary for preliminary results.*

Therefore, patient's ID (a), date and time of the phone call (b and c), responsible laboratory individual for the phone call (d), person notified in the physician office (first and last name) (e), test results (f), and "read-back" of the results (h) should be recorded in the patient's record according to CAP's regulation.

40. **C.** This is a *Phase II deficiency*, according to the College of American Pathologist (CAP)'s regulations. According to the CAP All Common Checklist dated July 28, 2015, COM.30400, "All reagents, chemicals, and media are *used within their indicated expiration date.*"

Phase 0 deficiency does not require a formal response, though it should be corrected by the laboratory. Phase I deficiency does not seriously affect the quality of patient care or significantly endanger the welfare of laboratory workers. Correction and a written response to the CAP are required, but not supportive documents. Phase II deficiency may seriously affect the quality of patient care or the health and safety of hospital or laboratory personnel. Correction requires both an action plan and supportive documentation that the plan has been implemented. There is no Phase III deficiency.

Therefore, this decision would be a Phase II deficiency if it were one according to CAP's regulation.

41. C. It would be a *Phase II deficiency* if the laboratory does not check new shipments according to the College of American Pathologist (CAP)'s regulations. According to the CAP All Common Checklist dated July 28, 2015, COM.30450, "New reagent lots and shipments are checked against old reagent lots or with suitable reference material before or concurrently with being placed in service." And "Improper storage conditions during shipping of reagents may have a negative impact on their ability to perform or exhibit the same levels of reactivity as intended."

Phase 0 deficiency does not require a formal response, though it should be corrected by the laboratory. Phase I deficiency does not seriously affect the quality of patient care or significantly endanger the welfare of laboratory workers. Correction and a written response to the CAP are required, but not supportive documents. Phase II deficiency may seriously affect the quality of patient care or the health and safety of hospital or laboratory personnel. Correction requires both an action plan and supportive documentation that the plan has been implemented. There is no Phase III deficiency.

Therefore, it is a Phase II deficiency if the laboratory don't check new shipments in the same lot according to CAP's regulation.

42. C. It would be a *Phase II deficiency* if JJ used reagents from kits within different kit lots, according to the College of American Pathologist (CAP)'s regulations. According to the CAP All Common Checklist dated July 28, 2015, COM.30500, "If there are multiple components of a reagent kit, the laboratory uses components of reagent kits only within the kit lot unless otherwise specified by the manufacturer." And laboratories should have "Written policy defining allowable exceptions for mixing kit components from different lots."

Phase 0 deficiency does not require a formal response, though it should be corrected by the laboratory. Phase I deficiency does not seriously affect the quality of patient care or significantly endanger the welfare of laboratory workers. Correction and a written response to the CAP are required, but not supportive documents. Phase II deficiency may seriously affect the quality of patient care or the health and safety of hospital or

laboratory personnel. Correction requires both an action plan and supportive documentation that the plan has been implemented. There is no Phase III deficiency.

Therefore, it is a Phase II deficiency to mix kit components from different lots according to CAP's regulation.

43. C. It would be a *Phase II deficiency* if Emily uses the newly fixed thermal cycler before performance verification, according to the College of American Pathologist (CAP)'s regulations. According to the CAP All Common Checklist dated July 28, 2015, COM.30550, "The performance of all instruments and equipment is verified upon installation and after major maintenance or service to ensure that they run according to expectations." It also states, "Performance verification is necessary after repairs or replacement of critical components of an instrument or item of equipment."[1]

Phase 0 deficiency does not require a formal response, though it should be corrected by the laboratory. Phase I deficiency does not seriously affect the quality of patient care or significantly endanger the welfare of laboratory workers. Correction and a written response to the CAP are required, but not supportive documents. Phase II deficiency may seriously affect the quality of patient care or the health and safety of hospital or laboratory personnel. Correction requires both an action plan and supportive documentation that the plan has been implemented. There is no Phase III deficiency.

Therefore, it is a Phase II deficiency to use newly fixed instrument/equipment before performance verification according to CAP's regulation.

44. E. The lab staff should explain to the ordering physician that the method for the *BRAF* test has not been validated in this laboratory, and the lab could not accept clinical specimens for this test yet. According to the College of American Pathologist (CAP) All Common Checklist dated July 28, 2015, COM.40000, *"There is a summary statement, signed by the laboratory director (or designee who meets CAP director qualifications) prior to use in patient testing*, that includes the evaluation of validation/verification studies and approval of each test for clinical use. In this case, the supervisor did not meet CAP director qualifications. Therefore, the laboratory had to wait for the director to approve the validation summary before accepting clinical specimens for tests. Since the director may ask for more experiments, such as adding an experiment to show that method performance specifications have been separately verified for both thermal cycler in the laboratory, holding the sample may delay delivering critical results to the physician/patient. If a laboratory accepts and performs a clinical test before the validation summary is approved by the laboratory director (or designee who meets CAP director qualifications), it is *a Phase II deficiency* according to CAP regulations."

Therefore, the laboratory should explain to the ordering physician the method for the *BRAF* test has not been validated in this laboratory.

45. **C.** The College of American Pathologist (CAP) has clearly different validation requirements for FDA-cleared/approved and non-FDA-cleared/approved tests. Non-FDA-cleared/approved tests include laboratory-developed tests (LTDs) and modified FDA-cleared/approved tests. According to the CAP All Common Checklist dated July 28, 2015, COM.40000, "For an FDA-cleared/approved test, a summary of the verification data must address analytical performance specifications, including *analytical accuracy, precision, interferences, and reportable range, as applicable.*" It also states that the summary statement must include a written assessment of the validation/verification study, including the acceptability of the data. The summary must also include a statement approving the test for clinical use with an approval signature such as, "This validation study has been reviewed, and the performance of the method is considered acceptable for patient testing."

The COBAS AmpliPrep/COBAS TaqMan CMV Test is an in vitro nucleic acid amplification test for the quantitation of cytomegalovirus (CMV) DNA in human plasma using the COBAS AmpliPrep Instrument for automated specimen processing and the COBAS TaqMan Analyzer or COBAS TaqMan 48 Analyzer for automated amplification and detection. It is an FDA-cleared/approved assay.

Therefore, analytical accuracy, precision, interferences, and reportable range should be in the validation summary for this FDA-cleared/approved assay.

46. **E.** The College of American Pathologist (CAP) has clearly different validation requirements to FDA-cleared/approved and non-FDA-cleared/approved tests. No-FDA-cleared/approved tests include laboratory-developed tests (LTDs) and modified FDA-cleared/approved tests. According to the CAP All Common Checklist dated July 28, 2015, COM.40000, "for modified FDA-cleared/

approved tests or LDTs, the summary must address *analytical sensitivity, analytical specificity*, and any other parameter that is considered important, to assure that the analytical performance of a test (e.g., *specimen stability, reagent stability, linearity, carryover, and cross-contamination*, etc.), as appropriate and applicable." It also states that the summary statement must include a written assessment of the validation/verification study, including the acceptability of the data. The summary must also include a statement approving the test for clinical use with an approval signature such as, "This validation study has been reviewed, and the performance of the method is considered acceptable for patient testing."

In the "Method Performance Specifications" part of the CAP All Common Checklist, it clearly states again, "For tests that are not FDA-cleared or approved (including tests developed in-house, LTD), or for FDA-cleared/approved tests modified by the laboratory, the laboratory must establish *accuracy, precision, analytical sensitivity, interferences, analytical specificity, and reportable range*, as applicable; data on interferences may be obtained from manufacturers or published literature, as applicable."

The COBAS AmpliPrep/COBAS TaqMan CMV Test is an in vitro nucleic acid amplification test for the quantitation of cytomegalovirus (CMV) DNA in human plasma using the COBAS AmpliPrep Instrument for automated specimen processing and the COBAS TaqMan Analyzer or COBAS TaqMan 48 Analyzer for automated amplification and detection. This assay is FDA-cleared/approved to be used with plasma sample, but not cerebrospinal fluid.

Therefore, the laboratory must treat the assay as an LTD to validate all the parameters listed above because of the modification.

47. **F.** According to the College of American Pathology (CAP) All Common Checklist dated July 28, 2015, COM.10500, "When a procedure is discontinued, a paper or electronic copy is maintained for at least 2 years, recording initial date of use, and retirement date. For genetic testing, in order to meet the requirements of some states relating to the testing of minors (under the age of 21), it is recommended that laboratories retain procedures (paper or electronic) for *at least 23 years* (to cover the interval from fetal period to age 21)."

Therefore, the laboratory should keep the procedure for the *CYP2C19* test for at least 23 years after discontinuation.

48. **B**. In the College of American Pathologist (CAP) All Common Checklist dated July 28, 2015, there is chapter dedicated to "Method Performance Specifications," which clearly states, "The method performance specifications must be validated or verified in the location in which patient testing will be performed. If an instrument is moved, the laboratory must verify the method performance specifications (i.e., *accuracy, precision, reportable range*) after the move to ensure that the test system was not affected by the relocation process or any changes due to the new environment (e.g., temperature, humidity, reagent storage conditions, etc.). The laboratory must follow manufacturer's instructions for instrument set up, maintenance, and system verification."

The COBAS AmpliPrep/COBAS TaqMan CMV Test is an in vitro nucleic acid amplification test for the quantitation of cytomegalovirus DNA in human plasma using the COBAS AmpliPrep Instrument for automated specimen processing and the COBAS TaqMan Analyzer or COBAS TaqMan 48 Analyzer for automated amplification and detection. It is an FDA-cleared/approved assay.

Therefore, analytical accuracy (a), analytical precision (b), and reportable range (g) should be included in the verification after the move.

49. **D**. According to the College of American Pathologist (CAP) All Common Checklist dated July 28, 2015, COM.40100, "When a test is put back into production, the following requirements must be met:

- *PT or alternative assessment performed within 30 days prior to restarting patient testing.*
- *Method performance specifications verified, as applicable, within 30 days prior to restarting patient testing.*
- *Competency assessed for analysts within 12 months prior to restarting patient testing."*

Also, a "test is considered to be taken out of production when (1) patient testing is not offered AND (2) PT or alternative assessment, as applicable, is suspended. It does not apply to situations where a proficiency testing challenge is not performed due to a temporary, short-term situation, such as a reagent back order or an instrument breakdown. In those situations, the laboratory must perform alternative assessment for that testing event."

Therefore, all the choices listed in the question are the requirements, which must be met in order to put the test back into production.

50. **D**. According to the College of American Pathologist (CAP) All Common Checklist dated July 28, 2015, COM.40100, intermittent testing "does not apply to situations where a proficiency testing challenge is not performed due to a temporary, short-term situation, such as a reagent back order or an instrument breakdown. In those situations, the laboratory must *perform alternative assessment for that testing event.*" The quantitative HIV-1 RNA test is one of the PT required tests. The laboratory should perform alternative assessment for the test.

Therefore, alternative proficiency test (PT) assessment must be performed in order to put the test back into production.

51. **E**. The College of American Pathologist (CAP) has clearly different validation requirements for FDA-cleared/approved and non-FDA-cleared/approved tests. Non-FDA-cleared/approved tests include laboratory-developed tests (LTDs) and modified FDA-cleared/approved tests. According to the CAP All Common Checklist dated July 28, 2015, COM.40000, "for modified FDA-cleared/approved tests or LDTs, the summary must address analytical sensitivity, analytical specificity, and any other parameter that is considered important, to assure that the analytical performance of a test (e.g., *specimen stability, reagent stability, linearity, carryover, and cross-contamination*, etc.), as appropriate and applicable." It also states that the summary statement must include a written assessment of the validation/verification study, including the acceptability of the data. The summary must also include a statement approving the test for clinical use with an approval signature such as, "This validation study has been reviewed, and the performance of the method is considered acceptable for patient testing."

In the "Method Performance Specifications" part of the CAP All Common Checklist, it states again "For tests that are not FDA-cleared or approved (including tests developed in-house, LTD), or for FDA-cleared/approved tests modified by the laboratory, the laboratory must establish accuracy, precision, analytical sensitivity, interferences, analytical specificity, and reportable range, as applicable; data on interferences may be obtained from manufacturers or published literature, as applicable." According to COM.40250, the different validation requirements for FDA-cleared/approved and non-FDA-cleared/approved tests are repeated again.

Illumina MiSeqDx Cystic Fibrosis 139-Variant Assay is an FDA-cleared/approved assay to be used with Illumina MiSeqDx. Modification of the instrument model modifies manufacturer's instructions, so the test is no longer an FDA-cleared/approved test. Therefore, because of the modification, the laboratory must treat the assay as an LTD to validate all the parameters listed above.

52. **E.** According to the College of American Pathologist (CAP) All Common Checklist dated July 28, 2015, COM.40300, "Where current technology permits, accuracy is established by *comparing results to a definitive or reference method*, or may be verified by *comparing results to an established comparative method*. Use of reference materials or other materials with known concentrations or activities is suggested in establishing or verifying accuracy." And "Precision is established by repeat measurement of samples at varying concentrations or activities within-run and between-run over a period of time." A lower detection limit establishes the analytical sensitivity of a test.

    Therefore, accuracy may be established by comparing results to a definitive or reference method, or be verified by comparing results to an established comparative method.

53. **C.** According to the College of American Pathologist (CAP) All Common Checklist dated July 28, 2015, COM.40350, "For modified FDA-cleared/approved and laboratory-developed tests (LDTs), validation of analytical accuracy includes testing with an appropriate number of samples." An appropriate number of samples is defined as *"minimum of 20 samples* with analyte concentrations distributed across the analytical measurement range should be used" for quantitative tests. "Proportionate mixtures of samples may be used to supplement the study population." It also states, "If the laboratory uses fewer samples, the laboratory director must record the criteria used to determine the appropriateness of the sample size. In many cases, a validation study with more samples is desirable."

    However, in the CAP checklist dated July 28, 2015, it also states "For modified FDA-cleared/approved tests and LDTs in use prior to July 31, 2016, for which limited validation studies are recorded, ongoing data supporting acceptable test performance may be used to meet the above minimum sample requirement, unless the laboratory director has recorded the criteria used to determine the acceptability of a smaller sample size. Examples of such ongoing data include records of proficiency testing, alternative performance assessment, and quality control."

Therefore, Dr. Y should include at least 20 samples in this validation.

54. **C.** According to the College of American Pathologist (CAP) All Common Checklist dated July 28, 2015, COM.40350, "For modified FDA-cleared/approved and laboratory-developed tests (LDTs), validation of analytical accuracy includes testing with an appropriate number of samples." An appropriate number of samples is defined as *"a minimum of 20 samples,* including positive, negative, and low-positive samples with concentrations near the lower level of detection should be used; equivocal samples should not be used" for qualitative tests. "Proportionate mixtures of samples may be used to supplement the study population." It also states, "If the laboratory uses fewer samples, the laboratory director must record the criteria used to determine the appropriateness of the sample size. In many cases, a validation study with more samples is desirable."

    However, in the CAP checklist dated July 28, 2015, it also states, "For modified FDA-cleared/approved tests and LDTs in use prior to July 31, 2016, for which limited validation studies are recorded, ongoing data supporting acceptable test performance may be used to meet the above minimum sample requirement, unless the laboratory director has recorded the criteria used to determine the acceptability of a smaller sample size. Examples of such ongoing data include records of proficiency testing, alternative performance assessment, and quality control."

    Therefore, Dr. Y should include at least 20 samples in this validation.

55. **E.** According to the College of American Pathologist (CAP) All Common Checklist dated July 28, 2015, COM.40700, "Clients include *healthcare entities, other laboratories, and licensed independent practitioners.* This requirement does not apply to patients or their authorized representatives."

    Therefore, healthcare entities (A) and licensed independent practitioners (B) may be client(s), but not patients and patient's family members.

56. **E.** According to the College of American Pathologist (CAP) All Common Checklist dated July 28, 2015, an individualized quality control plan (IQCP) is "approved by the laboratory director for nonwaived testing to reduce external control analysis to a frequency *less than the limits defined in the CLIA regulations and CAP checklists.*"

    Therefore, IQCP is a quality control plan lower than the standard defined in the CLIA regulation and CAP checklists.

57. **E**. According to the College of American
Pathologist (CAP) All Common Checklist dated
July 28, 2015, an individualized quality control
plan (IQCP) is applied to nonwaived tests.

"If a laboratory is located in a state that does
not accept IQCP as an option for reducing the
frequency of external quality control, the
laboratory must follow the state regulations and
perform external daily quality control following
the frequency defined in the state regulations
and CAP checklists." And "A laboratory may
not implement an IQCP that allows for quality
control to be performed less frequently than
indicated in the manufacturer's instructions. The
components of the quality control plan must
meet regulatory and CAP accreditation
requirements and be in compliance with the
manufacturer instructions and
recommendations, at minimum." As one of the
nonwaived tests, FISH may be classified as
either a histopathology or a cytogenetics test,
which is eligible for IQCP.

Therefore, IQCP does not apply to waived
tests.

58. **G**. According to the College of American
Pathologist (CAP) All Common Checklist dated
July 28, 2015, an individualized quality control
plan (IQCP) may be used by a clinical laboratory
for eligible nonwaived tests. First, a laboratory
should *identify all tests using an IQCP*. Second,
check on the eligibility of IQCP, according to CAP
and state regulations. Third, *complete the CAP form
for IQCP*, which may be downloaded from the
CAP website (http://www.cap.org) through the
e-LAB Solution Suite (COM.50200). Fourth, *assess
the risk of IQCP for a test/device/instrument*
(COM.50300). Fifth, *write a quality control plan*,
with approval from the laboratory director prior
to implementation (COM.50400). Six, *monitor
ongoing quality data*, including quality control and
instrument/equipment maintenance and function,
etc., at least monthly (COM.50600). Finally,
*reassess and reapprove the quality control plan
annually* (COM.50600).

Therefore, all the choices listed in the questions
are required for IQCP.

59. **C**. According to the College of American
Pathologist (CAP) All Common Checklist dated
July 28, 2015, COM.50600, "Ongoing quality
assessment monitoring is performed by the
laboratory to ensure that the quality control plan
is effective in mitigating the identified risks for
the IQCP, and include ... reapproval of the
quality control plan by the laboratory director or
designee *at least annually*."

Therefore, the director should reassess and reapprove the quality control plan for the IQCP at
least annually in the laboratory.

60. **C**. According to the College of American
Pathologist (CAP) All Common Checklist dated
July 28, 2015, COM.50600, "Ongoing quality
assessment monitoring is performed by the
laboratory to ensure that the quality control plan
is effective in mitigating the identified risks for
the IQCP, and include ... Review of quality
control and instrument/equipment maintenance
and function check data *at least monthly*."

Therefore, the director should review of quality
control and instrument/equipment maintenance
and function for the IQCP at least monthly.

61. **C**. According to the College of American
Pathologist (CAP) All Common Checklist dated
July 28, 2015, COM.50500, "External control
material samples must be analyzed *at least every
31 days* and with new lots and shipments of
reagents or more frequently if indicated in the
manufacturer's instructions." Therefore, in this
case, the laboratory must follow CAP regulations
to analyze external control material samples at
least every 31 days unless new lots and
shipments of reagents come in.

Therefore, the external control material
samples must be analyzed at least every 31 days.

62. **A**. According to the College of American
Pathologist (CAP) All Common Checklist dated
July 28, 2015, COM.50500, "External control
material samples must be analyzed at least every
31 days and with new lots and shipments of
reagents or *more frequently if indicated in the
manufacturer's instructions*." Therefore, in this case,
the laboratory must follow the manufacturer's
instruction to analyze external control material
samples at least every 5 business days (a week).

Therefore, the external control material
samples must be analyzed at least every week.

63. **E**. According to the College of American
Pathology (CAP) All Common Checklist dated
July 28, 2015, COM.0420, "Instrument and
equipment maintenance and function check
records are reviewed and assessed *at least monthly*
by the laboratory director or designee." And "The
review of the records related to tests that have an
approved Individualized quality control plan
(IQCP) must include an assessment of whether
further evaluation of the risk assessment and
quality control plan is needed based on problems
identified (e.g., trending for repeat failures, etc.)."

Therefore, a director of a clinical molecular
laboratory should review the maintenance and
function check records of centrifuges monthly.

64. E. According to the College of American Pathology (CAP) All Common Checklist dated July 28, 2015, COM.04200 "Instrument and equipment maintenance and function check records are reviewed and *assessed at least monthly* by the laboratory director or designee." And "The review of the records related to tests that have an approved Individualized quality control plan (IQCP) must include an assessment of whether further evaluation of the risk assessment and quality control plan is needed based on problems identified (e.g., trending for repeat failures, etc.)."

Therefore, a director should review the maintenance and function check records of thermal cyclers monthly.

65. F. According to the College of American Pathology (CAP) Common Checklist dated July 28, 2015, COM.30450, "New reagent lots and/or shipments are checked against old reagents lots or with suitable reference material before or concurrently with being placed in service." It also states, "For quantitative nonwaived tests, patient specimens should be used to compare a new lot against the old lot, when possible. Manufactured materials, such as proficiency testing (PT) or QC materials may be affected by matrix interference between different reagent lots, even if results show no change following a reagent lot change. The use of patient samples confirms the absence of matrix interference. Other than patient samples, the following materials may also be used:

- *Reference materials or QC products* provided by the manufacturer with method-specific and reagent lot–specific target values.
- *Proficiency testing materials* with peer group–established means.
- *OC materials with peer group–established means* based on interlaboratory comparison that is method-specific and include data from at least 10 laboratories.
- *Third-party general purpose reference materials* if the material is documented in the package insert or by the method manufacturer to be commutable with patient specimens for the method. Commutability between reference materials and patient samples can be demonstrated using the protocol in CLSI EP14-A2.
- *QC material used to test the current lot* is adequate alone to check a new shipment of the same reagent lot, as there should be no change in potential matrix interactions between the QC material and different shipments of the same lot number of reagents."

Therefore, all the choices listed in the question may be used to compare a new lot against old lot for quantitative nonwaived tests, according to the College of American Pathologist (CAP)'s regulations.

66. A. According to the College of American Pathology (CAP) All Common Checklist dated July 28, 2015, "For the purposes of interpreting the checklist requirements, a laboratory-developed test (LDT) is defined as follows: A test used in patient management that has both of the following features:

- *The test is performed by the clinical laboratory in which the test was developed wholly or in part;* AND
- *The test is neither FDA-cleared nor FDA-approved.*"

If a laboratory has made a modification to manufacturer's instructions for an FDA-cleared/approved test, the test is developed in part in this laboratory. Therefore, *modified FDA-cleared/approved tests may be considered as LDT tests* by this definition.

67. A. CLIA regulates laboratory testing and requires that clinical laboratories obtain a certificate before accepting materials derived from the human body for the purpose of providing information for the diagnosis, prevention, or treatment of any disease or the impairment of, or assessment of the health of human beings. The type of CLIA certificate a laboratory obtains depends upon the complexity of the tests it performs. CLIA regulations describe the following three levels of test complexity: waived tests, moderate-complexity tests, and high-complexity tests.

Clinical laboratory test systems are assigned a moderate- or high-complexity category on the basis of seven criteria given in the CLIA regulations. For commercially available FDA-cleared/approved tests, the test complexity is determined by the FDA during the premarketing approval process. *For tests developed by the laboratory or that have been modified from the approved manufacturer's instructions, the complexity category defaults to high complexity per the CLIA regulations* (https://www.govinfo.gov/content/pkg/CFR-1996-title42-vol3/xml/CFR-1996-title42-vol3-sec493-17.xml).

As defined by CLIA, waived tests are simple tests with a low risk for an incorrect result. They include certain tests listed in the CLIA regulations, tests cleared by the FDA for home use, and tests approved for waiver by the FDA using the CLIA criteria. Sites performing only waived testing must have a CLIA certificate and follow the manufacturer's instructions; other CLIA requirements do not apply to these sites. The current list of tests waived under CLIA may be found at https://wwwn.cdc.gov/clia/resources/waivedtests/default.aspx.

Nonwaived testing refers collectively to moderate- and high-complexity testing. Laboratories or sites that perform these tests need to have a CLIA certificate, must be inspected, and must meet the CLIA quality standards described in 42 CFR Subparts H, J, K, and M.

"FDA-cleared" means that a test system has been reviewed by the FDA and has been determined to be substantially equivalent to a test system already legally marketed for the same use. This could apply to waived, moderate-, or high-complexity test systems (https://wwwn.cdc.gov).

Therefore, the laboratory-developed Sanger sequencing assay for Gaucher disease described in this question is a high-complexity test by default, according to the CLIA regulations.

68. **D**. According to the CAP Laboratory General Checklist dated July 28, 2015, GEN.16902, "For laboratories that have been CAP accredited for more than 12 months, the QM plan is implemented as designed and is reviewed *annually* for effectiveness."

69. **B**. According to the CAP Laboratory General Checklist dated July 28, 2015, GEN.20377, "Competency assessment records must be retained for *at least 2 years.*"

70. **B**. According to the CAP Laboratory General Checklist dated July 28, 2015, GEN.20377, "Competency assessment records must be retained for at least 2 years." The following records must be retained for *at least 2 years:* specimen requisitions (the patient chart or medical record is included only if it was used as the requisition), patient test results and reports (both original and corrected), instrument printouts, accession records, quality control records, instrument maintenance records, proficiency testing records, and quality management records.

Therefore, a clinical molecular laboratory should retain the quality control records for at least two years.

71. **E**. According to the CAP Laboratory General Checklist dated July 28, 2015, GEN.26791, "The CAP terms of accreditation are listed in the laboratory's official notification of accreditation. The policy must include notification of CAP regarding the following:
- *Investigation of the laboratory by a government entity or other oversight agency*, or adverse media

attention related to laboratory performance; notification must occur no later than 2 working days after the laboratory learns of an investigation or adverse media attention. For laboratories subject to US regulations, this notification must include any complaint investigations conducted or warning letters issued by any oversight agency (i.e. CMS, State Department of Health, The Joint Commission, FDA, OSHA). For non-US laboratories, this notification must include discovery of actions by laboratory personnel that violate national, state or local regulations.
- A facility must notify the CAP as soon as it finds itself to be the subject of a validation inspection.
- *Discovery of actions by laboratory personnel that violate national, state or local regulations.*
- *Change in laboratory test menu* (notification must occur prior to starting new patient testing).
- *Change in location, ownership or directorship of the laboratory*; notification must occur no later than 30 days prior to the change(s); or, in the case of unexpected changes, no later than 2 working days afterwards.
  In addition, the policy must address:
- Provision of an inspection team comparable in size and scope if requested by CAP
- Cooperation with CAP when the laboratory is subject to a CAP investigation or inspection
- Adherence to the Terms of Use for the CAP Certification Mark of accreditation"

Therefore, a clinical molecular laboratory must notify CAP in all the circumstances listed in the question.

72. **B**. According to the CAP Laboratory General Checklist dated July 28, 2015, GEN.26791, "The CAP terms of accreditation are listed in the laboratory's official notification of accreditation." And "The policy must include notification of CAP regarding change in location, ownership or directorship of the laboratory; notification must occur *no later than 30 days prior to the change(s);* or, in the case of unexpected changes, no later than 2 working days afterwards."

Therefore, the laboratory should notify CAP regarding change in the directorship of the laboratory before May 30.

73. **D**. According to the CAP Laboratory General Checklist dated July 28, 2015, GEN.26791, "The CAP terms of accreditation are listed in the laboratory's official notification of accreditation." And "The policy must include notification of CAP regarding change in

laboratory test menu (*notification must occur prior to starting new patient testing*)."

Therefore, Dr. G should notify CAP before launching the test.

74. **B**. According to the College of American Pathology (CAP) Laboratory General Checklist dated July 28, 2015, GEN.16902, "For Laboratories that have been CAP accredited for more than 12 months, the QM plan is implemented as designed and is reviewed *annually* for effectiveness." And "Appraisal of program effectiveness may be evidenced by an annual written report, revisions to laboratory policies and procedures, or revisions to the QM plan, as appropriate."

Therefore, a director should review the quality management (QM) at least annually.

75. **A**. According to the College of American Pathology (CAP) Laboratory General Checklist dated July 28, 2015, GEN.20208, "Any problem that could potentially interfere with patient care or safety must be addressed. Clinical, rather than business/management issues, should be emphasized. The laboratory must record investigation and resolution of these problems. Laboratories must perform *root-cause analysis* of any unexpected event involving death or serious physical or psychological injury, or risk thereof (including 'near misses' and sentinel events). Laboratories must be able to demonstrate appropriate risk-reduction activities based on such root-cause analyses." It is an appropriate response for Dr. A getting the specimen back from the reference laboratory for the ordered tests. It is good patient care, but not part of quality management plan.

Therefore, Dr. A should perform root cause analysis.

76. **A**. CLIA regulates laboratory testing and requires that clinical laboratories obtain a certificate before accepting materials derived from the human body for the purpose of providing information for the diagnosis, prevention, or treatment of any disease or the impairment of, or assessment of the health of human beings. The type of CLIA certificate a laboratory obtains depends upon the complexity of the tests it performs. CLIA regulations describe the following three levels of test complexity: waived tests, moderate-complexity tests, and high-complexity tests.

According to the CAP Laboratory General Checklist dated July 28, 2015, GEN.20361, "Laboratories must obtain the CLIA certificate type that corresponds to their highest level of complexity. The CLIA certificate types include the following:

- Certificate of Waiver—waived tests only
- Certificate of Provider Performed Microscopy (PPM) Procedures—testing performed by a physician, midlevel practitioner, or dentist for specific microscopy procedures (moderate complexity) during the course of a patient's visit
- Certificate of Registration—nonwaived testing (moderate or high complexity) prior to initial laboratory inspection
- Certificate of Compliance—nonwaived testing with inspection by the State Department of Health (CLIA inspection)
- Certificate of Accreditation—nonwaived testing with inspection by a CMS-approved accrediting organization, such as the CAP accreditation programs"

A molecular genetics laboratory with LDTs, modified FDA-cleared/approved and FDA-cleared-approved tests must have Certificate of Accreditation from CLIA.

Therefore, Dr. Z must obtain Certificate of Accreditation from CLIA for this laboratory.

77. **B**. According to the College of American Pathology (CAP) Laboratory General Checklist dated July 28, 2015, GEN.20351, "The laboratory has a procedure for reporting device-related adverse patient events, as required by FDA." And "When information reasonably suggests that any laboratory instrument, reagent or other device has or may have caused or contributed to a patient death or serious patient injury, the FDA requires hospitals and outpatient diagnostic facilities, including independent laboratories, to report the event. If the event is death, the report must be made both to FDA and the device manufacturer. If the event is serious patient injury, the report must be submitted to FDA. Reports must be submitted on FDA Form 3500A as soon as practical but *no later than 10 days* from the time medical personnel become aware of the event."

Therefore, a US regulated clinical molecular laboratory should submit the reports as soon as practical but no later than 10 days from the time medical personnel become aware of the event.

78. **C**. According to the College of American Pathology (CAP) Laboratory General Checklist dated July 28, 2015, GEN.26791, "The CAP terms of accreditation are listed in the laboratory's official notification of accreditation. The policy must include *notification of CAP* regarding … Investigation of the laboratory by a government entity or other oversight agency, or adverse media attention related to laboratory performance; notification must occur no later than 2 working days after the laboratory learns of an

investigation or adverse media attention. For laboratories subject to US regulations, this notification must include any complaint investigations conducted or warning letters issued by any oversight agency (i.e. CMS, State Department of Health, The Joint Commission, FDA, OSHA). For non-US laboratories, this notification must include discovery of actions by laboratory personnel that violate national, state or local regulations."

Therefore, the laboratory must also notify CAP.

79. **B**. According to the College of American Pathology (CAP) Laboratory General Checklist dated July 28, 2015, GEN.26791, "The CAP terms of accreditation are listed in the laboratory's official notification of accreditation. The policy must include notification of CAP regarding ... Investigation of the laboratory by a government entity or other oversight agency, or adverse media attention related to laboratory performance; notification must occur *no later than 2 working days* after the laboratory learns of an investigation or adverse media attention. For laboratories subject to US regulations, this notification must include any complaint investigations conducted or warning letters issued by any oversight agency (i.e. CMS, State Department of Health, The Joint Commission, FDA, OSHA). For non-US laboratories, this notification must include discovery of actions by laboratory personnel that violate national, state or local regulations."

Therefore, the laboratory must notify CAP no later than 2 working days.

80. **B**. According to the College of American Pathology (CAP) Laboratory General Checklist dated July 28, 2015, GEN.20351, "The laboratory (or parent institution, as appropriate) must submit *an annual report* of device-related deaths and serious injuries to FDA, if any such event was reported during the previous year. Annual reports must be submitted on Form 3419 (for hospital-based laboratories only, or an electronic equivalent) or Form 3500 (for non-hospital-based laboratories) by January 1 of each year. The laboratory or institution must keep records of MDR reports for *2 years*."

Therefore, the laboratory must keep the records of the FDA MDR reports for 2 years.

81. **D**. According to the College of American Pathology (CAP) Laboratory General Checklist dated July 28, 2015, GEN.26791, "The CAP terms of accreditation are listed in the laboratory's official notification of accreditation. The policy must include notification of CAP regarding ...

Investigation of the laboratory by a government entity or other oversight agency, or adverse media attention related to laboratory performance; notification must occur *no later than 2 working days* after the laboratory learns of an investigation or adverse media attention. For laboratories subject to US regulations, this notification must include any complaint investigations conducted or warning letters issued by any oversight agency (i.e. CMS, State Department of Health, The Joint Commission, FDA, OSHA). For non-US laboratories, this notification must include discovery of actions by laboratory personnel that violate national, state or local regulations."

Therefore, the laboratory should notify CAP in 2 days after OSHA started the investigation.

82. **D**. According to the CAP Laboratory General Checklist dated July 29, 2013, "Document control requirements apply to all policies, procedures and forms (including quality management documents) and activities that are subject to CAP accreditation. The document control system must ensure ... that policies and procedures are reviewed *at least biannually* by the laboratory director or designee."

Therefore, a director must review policies and procedures at least once in 2 years.

83. **A**. According to the College of American Pathology (CAP) All Common Checklist dated July 28, 2015, COM.10500, "When a procedure is discontinued, a paper or electronic copy is maintained for at least 2 years, recording initial date of use, and retirement date. For genetic testing, in order to meet the requirements of some states relating to the testing of minors (under the age of 21), it is recommended that laboratories retain procedures (paper or electronic) for *at least 23 years* (to cover the interval from fetal period to age 21)."

Therefore, the laboratory should keep the discontinued procedure for cystic fibrosis test minimum for 23 years.

84. **C**. According to the College of American Pathology (CAP) Laboratory General Checklist dated July 28, 2015, GEN.26791, "The CAP terms of accreditation are listed in the laboratory's official notification of accreditation. The policy must include *notification of CAP* regarding ... Change in laboratory test menu prior to beginning that testing or the laboratory permanently or temporarily discontinues some or all testing."

Therefore, Dr. G must notify for the change CAP.

85. **C**. According to the College of American Pathology (CAP) Laboratory General Checklist dated July 28, 2015, GEN.26791 "The CAP terms of accreditation are listed in the laboratory's official notification of accreditation. The policy must include *notification of CAP* regarding ... Change in laboratory test menu prior to beginning that testing or the laboratory permanently or temporarily discontinues some or all testing."

Therefore, Dr. J must notify for the change CAP.

86. **B**. According to the College of American Pathology (CAP) Laboratory General Checklist dated July 28, 2015, GEN.26791, "The CAP terms of accreditation are listed in the laboratory's official notification of accreditation. The policy must include notification of CAP regarding ... Change in laboratory directorship, location, ownership, name, insolvency, or bankruptcy; notification must occur *no later than 30 days prior to the change(s);* or, in the case of unexpected changes, no later than two working days afterwards. Laboratories subject to US regulations must also notify the US Department of Health and Human Services."

Therefore, CAP must be notified about this change no later than 30 days prior to the final date.

87. **F**. According to the College of American Pathology (CAP) Laboratory General Checklist dated July 28, 2015, GEN.26791, "The CAP terms of accreditation are listed in the laboratory's official notification of accreditation. The policy must include notification of CAP regarding ... Change in laboratory directorship, location, ownership, name, insolvency, or bankruptcy; notification must occur no later than 30 days prior to the change(s); or, in the case of unexpected changes, no later than two working days afterwards. Laboratories subject to US regulations must also notify *the US Department of Health and Human Services.*"

Therefore, US Department of Health and Human Services must also be notified to comply with the CAP terms of accreditation.

88. **E**. According to the College of American Pathology (CAP) Laboratory General Checklist dated July 28, 2015, GEN.23584, "The interim self-inspection is an important aspect of continuing education and laboratory improvement. The use of a variety of mechanisms for self-inspection (*residents, technologists or others trained to perform inspections*) is strongly endorsed. Self inspection by personnel familiar with, but not directly involved in, the routine operation of the laboratory section to be inspected is a best practice. Record of performance of the interim self-inspection with correction of deficiencies is a requirement for maintaining accreditation. The laboratory must have a record to demonstrate that personnel responsible for each laboratory section have reviewed the findings of the interim self-inspection."

Therefore, residents, technologists, fellows , supervisor in cytogenetics may all perform self-inspection.

89. **C**. According to the College of American Pathology (CAP) Laboratory General Checklist dated July 28, 2015, GEN.40932, "For laboratories subject to US regulations, the laboratory solicits written or electronic authorization for verbal orders *within 30 days*. The laboratory must retain the written authorization or documentation of efforts made to obtain a written authorization. In a managed office where the staff assistants are not employees of the physician/clinician, the staff should not sign a test requisition for the physician without some type of provider services agreement. This agreement must specify how the clinician has accepted responsibility for the tests ordered from the off-site laboratory. (This situation is different from the hospital environment, where the physician has personally signed the order sheet.)"

Therefore, the laboratory should solicit written or electronic authorization for this verbal order with 30 days.

90. **C**. According to the College of American Pathology (CAP) Laboratory General Checklist dated July 28, 2015, GEN.40515, "All personnel who package infectious specimens for shipment must satisfactorily complete training in these requirements. Federal and international regulations mandate the proper packaging and transportation of infectious substances, also termed 'etiologic agents.' It is the laboratory's responsibility to determine whether specimens that are to be shipped are subject to the regulations, or are exempt. For US laboratories, specific requirements are set forth by the US Public Health Service, the US Department of Transportation and the US Postal Service. These apply to domestic transportation by land, air or sea, and to international air transportation. Recurrent training is required *every 3 years*. The laboratory should check with its local department of transportation or state health department for any recent revisions to these requirements."

In CAP Laboratory General Checklist dated July 28, 2015, GEN.74000, "Universal or standard precautions must be used when handling all blood and body fluid specimens. The term 'universal precautions' refers to a concept of bloodborne disease control requiring all human blood and other potentially infectious materials to be treated as if infectious for HIV, HBV, HCV or other bloodborne pathogens, regardless of the perceived 'low risk' status of a patient or patient population." And individuals with immunodeficiency disorders are prone to have infections. It is a precaution to assume that the peripheral-blood sample in this scenario is "infectious" and that the shipment is subject to the regulations.

Therefore, recurrent training is required for TM at least every 3 years to keep her active status.

91. **D**. According to the College of American Pathology (CAP) Laboratory General Checklist dated July 28, 2015, GEN.20377, "The following records must be retained for *at least 2 years*: specimen requisitions (including the patient chart or medical record only if used as the requisition), patient test results and reports (both original and corrected), instrument printouts, accession records, quality control records, instrument maintenance records, proficiency testing records, and quality management records."

Therefore, a clinical molecular laboratory should keep specimen requisitions for at least 2 years.

92. **C**. According to the College of American Pathology (CAP) Laboratory General Checklist dated July 28, 2015, GEN. 41017 "The operating speeds of centrifuges are checked *at least annually* as needed for the intended use, and this is done in a safe manner. For centrifuges having a safety mechanism preventing the opening of the lid while in operation, the checks of rpm should be performed only by an authorized service representative of the manufacturer or an appropriately trained clinical engineer."

Therefore, the operating speeds of centrifuges should be checked at least annually.

93. **A**. According to the College of American Pathology (CAP) Laboratory General Checklist dated July 28, 2015, GEN.41042, "Refrigerator/ freezer temperatures are checked and recorded daily using a calibrated thermometer" And *"Daily* means every day (7 days per week, 52 weeks per year). The laboratory must define the acceptable temperature ranges for these units. If temperature(s) are found to be outside the acceptable range, the laboratory must record

appropriate corrective action, which may include evaluation of contents for adverse effects."

"The two acceptable ways of recording temperatures are: (1) recording the numerical temperature, or (2) placing a mark on a graph that corresponds to a numerical temperature (either manually, or using a graphical recording device). The identity of the individual recording the temperature(s) must be recorded (the initials of the individual are adequate)."

Therefore, a clinical molecular laboratory should monitor refrigerator/freezer temperature everyday including weekends and holidays.

94. **B**. According to the College of American Pathology (CAP) Laboratory General Checklist dated July 28, 2015, GEN.41067, "An individual meeting CAP laboratory director qualifications reviews and approves the content and format of paper and electronic patient reports *at least every two years*." And "The laboratory director (or a designee who meets CAP qualifications for laboratory director) must review and, at least every two years, approve the content and format of laboratory patient reports (whether paper or computer screen images) to ensure that they effectively communicate patient test results, and that they meet the needs of the medical staff."

Therefore, a director should review and approve the content and format of patient reports at least biennially.

95. **A**. According to the College of American Pathology (CAP) Laboratory General Checklist dated July 28, 2015, GEN.41300, "The length of time that reported data are retained in the laboratory may vary; however, the reported results must be retained for that period encompassing a high frequency of requests for the data. In all circumstances, a hospital laboratory must have access to the patient's chart where the information is *permanently retained*."

Therefore, a clinical molecular laboratory must retain patient-charts permanently.

96. **C**. According to the College of American Pathology (CAP) Laboratory General Checklist dated July 28, 2015, GEN.41303, "The laboratory ensures that internal and external storage and transfer of data maintains patient confidentiality and security." And "Written procedures must address patient confidentially during transfer of data to external reference laboratories or other service providers. This must include cloud-based computing (e.g., for storage of confidential data), as appropriate." "The laboratory must audit compliance with the procedures *at least annually*."

Therefore, the laboratory must audit compliance with the procedures at least annually.

97. **A**. According to the College of American Pathology (CAP) Laboratory General Checklist dated July 28, 2015, GEN.41304, "Laboratories subject to US regulations must provide final test results to the patient or the patient's personal representative upon request. For completed tests, these results must generally be provided *no later than 30 days* after such a request."

    Therefore, Dr. F should address the patient's request by providing final test results to the patient in 30 days after such a request.

98. **E**. According to the College of American Pathology (CAP) Laboratory General Checklist dated July 28, 2015, GEN.41304 "Under the HIPAA Privacy Rule, only *the patient* or *a personal representative*, defined as an individual who has authority under applicable law to make health care decisions for the patient, can be given access to a patient's personal health data. Laboratories must take reasonable steps to verify the identity of the patient and the authority of a personal representative to have access to an individual's protected health information. The Rule also allows for the release of test reports to *authorized persons responsible for using the test reports* and to the *laboratory that initially requested the test*, if applicable."

    Therefore, the patients (A), the patient's personal representative (B), authorized persons responsible for using the test reports (C), and the laboratory that initially requested the test (D) may all have access to a patient's test results.

99. **A**. HIPAA is the acronym for the Health Insurance Portability and Accountability Act that was passed by Congress in 1996. HIPAA provides the ability to transfer and continue health insurance coverage for millions of American workers and their families when they change or lose their jobs; reduces health care fraud and abuse; mandates industry-wide standards for health care information on electronic billing and other processes; and *requires the protection and confidential handling of protected health information* (http://www.hhs.gov/hipaa/index.html).

    Informed consent is a process for getting permission before conducting a health care intervention on a person. A health care provider may ask a patient to consent to receive therapy before providing it, or a clinical researcher may ask a research participant before enrolling that person in a clinical trial. The official name for "ObamaCare" is the Patient Protection and Affordable Care Act (PPACA), or Affordable Care

Act (ACA) for short (http://obamacarefacts.com). The ACA was signed into law by President Barack Obama on March 23, 2010, in order to reform the health care industry; it was upheld by the Supreme Court on June 28, 2012. ObamaCare's goal is to give more Americans access to affordable, quality health insurance and to reduce the growth in US health care spending. The Affordable Care Act expands the affordability, quality, and availability of private and public health insurance through consumer protections, regulations, subsidies, taxes, insurance exchanges, and other reforms.

    Therefore, HIPAA protects patient health information privacy.

100. **D**. The official name for "ObamaCare" is the Patient Protection and Affordable Care Act (PPACA), or Affordable Care Act (ACA) for short. The ACA was signed into law by President Barack Obama on March 23, 2010, in order to reform the health care industry; it was upheld by the Supreme Court on June 28, 2012. ObamaCare's goal is to give more Americans access to affordable, quality health insurance and to reduce the growth in US health care spending. The Affordable Care Act expands the affordability, quality, and availability of private and public health insurance through consumer protections, regulations, subsidies, taxes, insurance exchanges, and other reforms (http://obamacarefacts.com).

    HIPAA is the acronym for the HIPPA that was passed by Congress in 1996. HIPAA provides the ability to transfer and continue health insurance coverage for millions of American workers and their families when they change or lose their jobs; reduces health care fraud and abuse; mandates industry-wide standards for health care information on electronic billing and other processes; and requires the protection and confidential handling of protected health information. Informed consent is a process for getting permission before conducting a health care intervention on a person. A health care provider may ask a patient to consent to receive therapy before providing it, or a clinical researcher may ask a research participant before enrolling that person into a clinical trial (http://www.hhs.gov/hipaa/index.html).

    Therefore, "ObamaCare" means patient protection and affordable care.

101. **B**. A laboratory's written policy defines test reporting turnaround time (TAT) in this laboratory, which is subject to the College of American Pathology (CAP) regulations. *In this*

case, the TAT in the written policy of the laboratory is acceptable according to CAP regulation, and it is the official TAT in this laboratory. Those five samples did not meet the laboratory-established TAT.

According to the College of American Pathology (CAP) Laboratory General Checklist dated July 28, 2015, GEN.41345, "The laboratory has defined turnaround times (i.e. the interval between specimen receipt by laboratory personnel and results reporting) for each of its tests, and it has a policy for notifying the requester when testing is delayed."

Therefore, these 5 samples did NOT meet the required TAT since the TAT was 5 business days according to the lab policy.

102. **C.** According to the College of American Pathology (CAP) Laboratory General Checklist dated July 28, 2015, GEN.41430, "For samples referred to another laboratory, the original or an exact copy of the testing laboratory's report is retained by the referring laboratory." And "The report may be retained on paper or in electronic format. Exceptions to this requirement may be made under special circumstances or for special categories, such as drugs of abuse or employee drug testing. The laboratory director may make these exceptions." Therefore, it is a *Phase II deficiency*, if the laboratory fails to do so.

103. **C.** According to the College of American Pathology (CAP) Laboratory General Checklist dated July 28, 2015, GEN.41500, "The laboratory defines the specific type of water required for each of its testing procedures and water quality is tested *at least annually.*"

Therefore, a clinical molecular genetics laboratory should test its water quality at least annually.

104. **A.** According to the College of American Pathology (CAP) Molecular Pathology Checklist April 21, 2015, GEN.43875, "Autoverification is the process by which patient results are generated from interfaced instruments and sent to the LIS, where they are compared against laboratory-defined acceptance parameters. There is documentation that the autoverification process was validated initially, and is tested *at least annually* and whenever there is a change to the system that could affect the autoverification logic."

Therefore, autoverification process of documentation should be tested annually after initial validation.

105. **B.** According to the College of American Pathology (CAP) Laboratory General Checklist dated July 28, 2015, GEN.48500, "There is a procedure to verify that patient results are

accurately transmitted from the point of data entry (interfaced instruments and manual input) to patient reports (whether paper or electronic)." And "At implementation of a new interface, or change to an existing interface, validation of *at least 2 examples* of reports from each of the following disciplines, where applicable, satisfies the intent of this checklist requirement. Subsequently, at least 2 examples of reports from at least 4 of these disciplines should be validated every 2 years. Not all of these report types will be applicable to every laboratory:
- Surgical pathology reports
- Cytopathology reports
- Clinical laboratory textual reports (e.g. *molecular*, protein electrophoresis, coagulation panel interpretation)
- Quantitative results (e.g. chemistry, hematology, or coagulation)
- Qualitative or categorical results (e.g. serology)
- Microbiology reports (e.g. culture and antimicrobial sensitivity)
- Blood bank reports (e.g. type and screen)

Interface validation should include examples of individual results, test packages or batteries, abnormal flags, and results with comments/footnotes. Initial interface validation should include verification that corrected results for clinical laboratory and anatomic pathology results are handled accurately in the receiving system."

Therefore, Dr. G must test at least 2 examples for the interface before the implementation.

106. **C.** According to the College of American Pathology (CAP) Laboratory General Checklist dated July 28, 2015, GEN.48500, "There is a procedure to verify that patient results are accurately transmitted from the point of data entry (interfaced instruments and manual input) to patient reports (whether paper or electronic)." And "At implementation of a new interface, or change to an existing interface, validation of at least 2 examples of reports from each of the following disciplines, where applicable, satisfies the intent of this checklist requirement. Subsequently, *at least 2 examples* of reports from at least 4 of these disciplines should be validated *every 2 years*. Not all of these report types will be applicable to every laboratory:
- Surgical pathology reports
- Cytopathology reports
- Clinical laboratory textual reports (e.g. molecular, protein electrophoresis, coagulation panel interpretation)
- Quantitative results (e.g. chemistry, hematology, or coagulation)

- Qualitative or categorical results (e.g. serology)
- Microbiology reports (e.g. culture and antimicrobial sensitivity)
- Blood bank reports (e.g. type and screen)
Interface validation should include examples of individual results, test packages or batteries, abnormal flags, and results with comments/footnotes. Initial interface validation should include verification that corrected results for clinical laboratory and anatomic pathology results are handled accurately in the receiving system."

Therefore, Dr. A changed the policy to validate at least 4 examples of reports every 4 years to make sure the interface result integrity.

107. **A**. According to the College of American Pathology (CAP) Laboratory General Checklist dated July 28, 2015, GEN.53600, "supervisors/general supervisors who do not qualify as a laboratory director or section director/technical supervisor must qualify as testing personnel and possess a:
- Bachelor's degree in a chemical, physical, biological or clinical laboratory science or medical technology with *at least one year of experience* with high complexity testing, or
- Associate degree in a laboratory science or medical technology program with at least two years experience with high complexity testing, or
- Have previously qualified or could have qualified as a general supervisor prior to 2/28/1992"

Therefore, a general supervisor of a clinical molecular pathology laboratory must have at least 1 year experience with high complexity testing if he/she has bachelor's degree in a chemical, physical, biological or clinical laboratory science or medical technology.

108. **C**. According to the College of American Pathology (CAP) Laboratory General Checklist dated July 28, 2015, GEN.53625, "The technical consultant (including the laboratory director who serves as a technical consultant) must be qualified by education and experience by one of the following combinations:
- MD or DO, licensed to practice medicine in the jurisdiction where the laboratory is located (if required), with certification in anatomic and/or clinical pathology, or qualifications equivalent to those required for board certification
- MD, DO, or DPM, licensed to practice in the jurisdiction where the laboratory is located (if required), with at least 1 year of training and/or experience in nonwaived testing (The

technical consultant's training and experience must be in the designated specialty or subspecialty area of service for which the consultant is responsible.); or
- Doctoral or masters degree in a chemical, physical, biological or clinical laboratory science with at least 1 year of training and/or experience in nonwaived testing (The technical consultant's training and experience must be in the designated specialty or subspecialty area of service for which the consultant is responsible.); or
- *Bachelor's degree* in a chemical, physical, biological or clinical laboratory science or medical technology with at least 2 years of experience in nonwaived testing (The technical consultant's training and experience must be in the designated specialty or subspecialty area of service for which the consultant is responsible.)."

Therefore, a technical consultant in a clinical molecular laboratory must have at least bachelor degree.

109. **A**. According to the College of American Pathology (CAP) Laboratory General Checklist dated July 28, 2015, GEN.53650, "Clinical consultants must be *a physician* licensed to practice medicine in the jurisdiction where the laboratory is located (if required) or *doctoral scientist* certified by a CLIA-approved board."

Therefore, a clinical consultant in a clinical molecular laboratory must have at least doctor degree (MD or PhD).

110. **D**. According to the College of American Pathology (CAP) Laboratory General Checklist dated July 28, 2015, GEN.55500 "Prior to starting patient testing and prior to reporting patient results for new methods or instruments, each individual must have training and be evaluated for proper test performance as required in GEN.55450. Thereafter, during the first year of an individual's duties, competency must be assessed *at least semiannually* for nonwaived testing. After an individual has performed his/her duties for one year, competency must be assessed annually for all duties. Retaining and reassessment of employee competency must occur when problems are identified with employee performance."

Therefore, this technologist should be assessed at least semiannually for competency on this test after the initial training.

111. **C**. According to the College of American Pathology (CAP) Laboratory General Checklist dated July 28, 2015, GEN.55450, "There are records that all staff has satisfactorily completed

initial training on all instruments/methods applicable to their designated job. The records must show that training specifically applies to the testing performed by each individual." GEN.55500 states, "During the first year of an individual's duties, competency must be assessed at least semiannually. After an individual has performed his/her duties for one year, competency must be assessed *at least annually*."

Therefore, if OB's first competency was assessed on 06/30/2012 and the second was on 06/30/2013, he was competent.

112. **E**. According to the College of American Pathology (CAP) Laboratory General Checklist dated July 28, 2015, GEN.55450, "There are records that *all staff* has satisfactorily completed initial training on all instruments/methods applicable to their designated job. The records must show that training specifically applies to the testing performed by each individual." GEN.55525 states, "The performance of *section directors/technical supervisors, general supervisors, and technical consultants* is assessed and satisfactory."

Therefore, technologists (A), general supervisors (B), technical consultants (C), and (section directors) must all be assessed for competency.

113. **C**. According to the College of American Pathology (CAP) Laboratory General Checklist dated July 28, 2015, GEN.55450, "There are records that all staff has satisfactorily completed initial training on all instruments/methods applicable to their designated job. The records must show that training specifically applies to the testing performed by each individual." GEN.55500 states, "During the first year of an individual's duties, competency must be assessed at least semiannually. After an individual has performed his/her duties for one year, competency must be assessed *at least annually*."

Therefore, his competency assessment for the *BRAF* V600E qualitative assay must be evaluated at least annually from now on.

114. **G**. According to the College of American Pathology (CAP) Laboratory General Checklist dated July 28, 2015, GEN.55500, "Elements of competency assessment include but are not limited to:
- *Direct observations of routine patient test performance*, including, as applicable;
- Patient identification and preparation; and specimen collection, handling, processing and testing;
- *Monitoring the recording and reporting of test results*, including, as applicable, reporting critical results;

- *Review of intermediate test results or worksheets, quality control records, proficiency testing results, and preventive maintenance records;*
- *Direct observation of performance of instrument maintenance and function checks;*
- *Assessment of test performance through testing previously analyzed specimens, internal blind testing samples or external proficiency testing samples;* and
- *Evaluation of problem-solving skills."*

Therefore, direct observations of routine patient test performance (A); monitoring the recording and reporting of test results (B); review of intermediate test results or worksheets, quality control records, proficiency testing results, and preventive maintenance records (C); direct observation of performance of instrument maintenance and function checks (D); assessment of test performance through testing previously analyzed specimens, internal blind testing samples or external proficiency testing samples (E); evaluation of problem-solving skills (F) are all elements of a test system. And they all should be included in the competency assessment.

115. **C**. BJ must undergo reeducation and training. According to the College of American Pathology (CAP) Laboratory General Checklist dated July 28, 2015, GEN.57000, "If an employee fails to demonstrate satisfactory performance on the competency assessment, the laboratory has a plan of corrective action to *retrain and reassess the employee's competency*." And "If it is determined that there are gaps in the individual's knowledge, the employee should be re-educated and allowed to retake the portions of the assessment that fell below the laboratory's guidelines. If, after reeducation and training, the employee is unable to satisfactorily pass the assessment, then further action should be taken which may include, supervisory review of work, reassignment of duties, or other actions deemed appropriate by the laboratory director."

Therefore, BJ should be re-educated and re-trained to re-gain his competency for the assay.

116. **C**. According to the College of American Pathology (CAP) Laboratory General Checklist dated July 28, 2015, GEN.73400 "There is documented periodic review (*at least annually*) of safe work practices to reduce hazards." And "Review must include bloodborne hazard control and chemical hygiene. If the review identifies a problem, the laboratory must investigate the cause and consider if modifications are needed to the safety policies and procedures to prevent

reoccurrence of the problem or mitigate potential risk."

Therefore, a clinical molecular laboratory should review its safe work practices at least annually to reduce hazards.

117. **B**. According to the College of American Pathology (CAP) Laboratory General Checklist dated July 28, 2015, GEN.73600, "For US laboratories subject to OSHA regulations, all workplace fatalities must be reported to the Occupational Safety and Health Administration (OSHA) *within eight hours* and work-related in-patient hospitalizations, amputations, or losses of an eye within 24 hours."

Therefore, a clinical molecular laboratory should report all workplace fatalities to OSHA within 8 hours.

118. **C**. According to the College of American Pathology (CAP) Laboratory General Checklist dated July 28, 2015, GEN.73600 "For US laboratories subject to OSHA regulations, all workplace fatalities must be reported to the Occupational Safety and Health Administration (OSHA) within eight hours and work-related in-patient hospitalizations, amputations, or losses of an eye *within 24 hours*."

Therefore, a clinical molecular laboratory should report the accident (all work-related in-patient hospitalizations, amputations, or losses of an eye) to OSHA within 24 hours.

119. **B**. According to the College of American Pathology (CAP) Laboratory General Checklist dated July 28, 2015, GEN.75000, "Each sterilizing device must be monitored periodically with a biologic indicator to measure the effectiveness of sterility. Chemical indicators that reflect sporicidal conditions may be used. The test must be performed under conditions that simulate actual use. One recommended method is to wrap the Bacillus stearothermophilus spore indicator strip in packaging identical to that used for a production run, and to include the test package with an actual sterilization procedure. *Weekly monitoring* is recommended."

Therefore, sterilizing devices must be monitored weekly.

120. **C**. According to the College of American Pathology (CAP) Laboratory General Checklist dated July 28, 2015, GEN.75400, "Fire safety training is performed for new employees, with a fire safety review conducted at least annually. Fire safety training must be recorded for all employees to show that they have been instructed on use and response to fire alarms and to execute duties as outlined in the fire safety plan. While

fire exit drills are not required, physical evaluation of the escape routes must be performed *annually*, to ensure that fire exit corridors and stairwells are clear and that all fire exit doors open properly (i.e., not rusted shut, blocked or locked). Paper or computerized testing of an individual's fire safety knowledge on the fire safety plan is acceptable; all personnel must participate *at least once a year*."

Therefore, a fire safety review should be conducted at least annually.

121. **D**. Agents classified by the International Agency for Research on Cancer (IARC) are: Group 1 (*Carcinogenic to humans*); Group 2A (*Probably carcinogenic to humans*); Group 2B (*Possibly carcinogenic to humans*); Group 3 (*Not classifiable as to its carcinogenicity to humans*); Group 4 (*Probably not carcinogenic to humans*). (https://monographs.iarc.fr/agents-classified-by-the-iarc/) According to the College of American Pathology (CAP) Laboratory General Checklist dated July 28, 2015, GEN.76000, "For laboratories subject to US regulations, chemicals that must be handled as potential carcinogens include those defined by OSHA as 'select carcinogens.' OSHA defines select carcinogens as any substance that is:

- Regulated as a carcinogen by OSHA, has been classified as "known to be carcinogenic" by the National Toxicology Program (NTP), or listed as a group I carcinogen by IARC.
- Has been classified as 'reasonably anticipated to be carcinogenic' by the NTP or listed as a group 2A or 2B carcinogen by the IARC if it meets the toxicological criteria listed in the January 31, 1990 Fed Register, pages 3319–3320.

OSHA also requires special containment procedures for substances that are reproductive toxins or are acutely hazardous." Therefore, *group 3 and group 4 agents are NOT OSHA-defined select carcinogens*.

122. **B**. According to the College of American Pathology (CAP) Laboratory General Checklist dated July 28, 2015, GEN.76700, "Supplies of concentrated acids and bases are stored safely. (1) Storage must be below eye level. *Storage near the floor is recommended*. (2) Strong acids and bases must not be stored under sinks, where contamination by moisture may occur. (3) Storage containers of acids and bases should be adequately separated to prevent a chemical reaction in the event of an accident/spill/leak. (4) Bottle carriers are used to transport all glass containers larger than 500 mL that contain hazardous chemicals."

Therefore, strong acid and bases should be stored near the floor.

123. **E.** According to the College of American Pathology (CAP) Molecular Pathology checklist dated July 28, 2015, MOL.49650, "The section director/technical supervisor of the molecular pathology laboratory is *a pathologist, board-certified physician in a specialty other than pathology, or doctoral scientist in a chemical, physical, or biologic science, with specialized training and/or appropriate experience in molecular pathology*." An individual with qualifications described in choice D may be a "bench testing/section supervisor" (MOL.49655).

Therefore, a pathologist (A), a MD with an ACMG certification in clinical molecular genetics (B), and a PhD with an ACMG certification in clinical molecular genetics (C) are qualified to be a section director/technical supervisor of a clinical molecular pathology laboratory.

124. **C.** According to the College of American Pathology (CAP) Molecular Pathology checklist dated July 28, 2015, MOL.49655, "Bench testing supervision is the person in charge of bench testing/section supervisor of the molecular pathology laboratory, who is qualified as one of the following:

- Person who qualifies as a section director/technical supervisor
- Bachelor's degree in a chemical, physical, biological, or clinical laboratory science or medical technology with *at least 4 years* of experience (at least 1 of which is in molecular pathology methods) under a qualified section director."

Therefore, this person has to have at lest 4 years of experience in order to serve as a bench testing supervisor.

125. **D.** According to the College of American Pathology (CAP) Molecular Pathology checklist dated July 28, 2015, MOL.49660 "Personnel performing the technical work of molecular pathology have appropriate experience in molecular pathology methods and qualify as high complexity testing personnel with a minimum of the following:

- Bachelor's degree in a chemical, physical, biological or clinical laboratory science or medical technology; or
- *Associate degree* in a laboratory science or medical laboratory technology from an accredited institution, or equivalent laboratory training and experience meeting the requirements defined in the CLIA regulation 42CFR493.1489. The qualifications to perform

high complexity testing can be assessed using the following link: CAP Personnel Requirements by Testing Complexity."

Therefore, a technologist in a clinical molecular laboratory must have at least an associate degree.

126. **B.** According to the College of American Pathology (CAP) Molecular Pathology checklist dated July 28, 2015, MOL.30440, "Quantitative molecular tests require that the dynamic range of the assay be defined and assay performance tested with controls in each run including *a negative, low positive, and a high positive control*." Usually *a wild-type control* is also used as a negative control for cross-reaction between the mutant and wild type. *The internal control* is used to confirm the quantity and quality of the sample for the assay.

Therefore, a no-template control (a), a wild type control (b), a low positive control (c), a high positive control (d), and an internal control (e) should all be included in each run.

127. **D.** According to the College of American Pathology (CAP) Molecular Pathology Checklist dated July 28, 2015, "For unmodified FDA-cleared/approved tests, the laboratory need only verify *accuracy, precision, reportable range, and reference range*." This is also stated in CAP All Common Checklist dated July 28, 2015, COM.40000.

Therefore, analytical accuracy (a), analytical precision (b), reference range (e), and reportable range (f) should be verified for FDA-cleared/approved tests during assay validation.

128. **F.** According to the College of American Pathology (CAP) Molecular Pathology Checklist dated July 28, 2015, "If an FDA-cleared/approved test is modified to meet the needs of the user or if the test is developed by the laboratory (LDT), both analytical and clinical performance parameters need to be established. *Analytical performance parameters* include, *precision, reference range, reportable range*, as well as *analytical sensitivity, analytical specificity*, and any other parameter that is considered important to assure the analytical performance of a particular test (e.g. *specimen stability, reagent stability, linearity, carryover, cross-contamination*, etc., as appropriate and applicable). The *clinical validity*, which includes clinical performance characteristics, such as *clinical sensitivity, clinical specificity, positive and negative predictive values* in defined populations or *likelihood ratios*, and *clinical utility* should also be considered, although individual laboratories may not be able to assess these parameters within their

own patient population, especially for rare diseases. However, patients without disease can typically be tested to assess clinical specificity. If clinical validation cannot be established within a laboratory, it is appropriate to cite scientific literature that has established clinical sensitivity and specificity. Clinical performance characteristics should be determined relative to clinical data (e.g. biopsy findings, radiographic and clinical findings, other laboratory results, etc.) whenever possible." The same concept is stated in the CAP All Common Checklist dated July 28, 2015.

Therefore, analytical accuracy (a), analytical precision (b), analytical sensitivity (c), analytical specificity (d), reference range (e), reportable range (f), positive predictive value (g), and negative predictive value (h) all should be verified for modified FDA-cleared/approved assays during validation.

129. **C.** Intermediate precision expresses within-laboratories variations, such as different days, different analysts, different equipment, etc. *Repeatability* expresses the precision under the same operating conditions over a short interval of time. Repeatability is also termed intraassay precision. According to the College of American Pathology (CAP) Molecular Pathology Checklist dated July 28, 2015, MOL.31145, "The laboratory must show recorded evidence that a test will return the same result regardless of minor variations in testing conditions that can cause random error, such as different technologists, instruments, reagent lots, days, etc. This is usually determined by repeated measures of samples throughout the reportable range, and for a quantitative test, represented as the coefficient of variation, whereas for a qualitative test, represented as ratios of concordant results."

The accuracy of an analytical procedure expresses the closeness of agreement between the value which is accepted either as a conventional true value or an accepted reference value and the value found. According to the CAP Molecular Pathology Checklist dated July 28, 2015, MOL.31015, "For a quantitative test, accuracy refers to 'closeness to true' whereas for a qualitative test it refers to correlation to a comparative test or tests that are used to establish 'true.' Accuracy can be assessed using well-characterized reference material together with appropriate biological matrix or by comparison to another valid test method, such as through specimen exchange."

According to the CAP Molecular Pathology Checklist dated July 28, 2015, MOL.31360, "The analytical sensitivity corresponds to the lower limit of detection. It refers to the ability of a test to confidently or consistently detect a minor allele or variant in a background of appropriate biological matrix (e.g. pathogens, rare mutants, chimerism, mosaicism, etc.)." CAP Molecular Pathology Checklist dated July 28, 2015, MOL.31375, states, "The analytical specificity refers to the ability of a test or procedure to correctly identify or quantify an entity in the presence of interfering or cross-reactive substances that might be expected to be present."

Therefore, the accuracy of this assay was low in this lab, the precision was high, and the reproducibility was high.

130. **A.** The *accuracy* of an analytical procedure expresses the closeness of agreement between the value that is accepted either as a conventional true value or an accepted reference value and the value found. According to the CAP Molecular Pathology Checklist dated July 28, 2015, MOL.31015, "For a quantitative test, accuracy refers to 'closeness to true' whereas for a qualitative test it refers to correlation to a comparative test or tests that are used to establish 'true.' Accuracy can be assessed using well-characterized reference material together with appropriate biological matrix or by comparison to another valid test method, such as through specimen exchange."

Intermediate precision expresses within-laboratories variations, such as different days, different analysts, different equipment, etc. Repeatability expresses the precision under the same operating conditions over a short interval of time. Repeatability is also termed intraassay precision. According to the College of American Pathology (CAP) Molecular Pathology Checklist dated July 28, 2015, MOL.31145, "The laboratory must show recorded evidence that a test will return the same result regardless of minor variations in testing conditions that can cause random error, such as different technologists, instruments, reagent lots, days, etc. This is usually determined by repeated measures of samples throughout the reportable range, and for a quantitative test, represented as the coefficient of variation, whereas for a qualitative test, represented as ratios of concordant results."

According to the CAP Molecular Pathology Checklist dated July 28, 2015, MOL.31360, "The analytical sensitivity corresponds to the lower limit of detection. It refers to the ability of a test to confidently or consistently detect a minor allele or variant in a background of appropriate biological matrix (e.g. pathogens, rare mutants, chimerism, mosaicism, etc.)." CAP Molecular Pathology Checklist dated July 28, 2015, MOL.31375, states "The analytical specificity refers to the ability of a test or procedure to correctly identify or quantify an entity in the presence of interfering or cross-reactive substances that might be expected to be present."

Therefore, the accuracy of this assay was high in this lab, the precision was low, and the reproducibility was low.

131. **C**. According to the College of American Pathology (CAP) Molecular Pathology Checklist dated July 28, 2015, MOL.31145, "The laboratory must show documented evidence that a test will return the same result regardless of minor variations in testing conditions that can cause random error, such as different technologists, instruments, reagent lots, days, etc. This is usually determined by repeated measures of samples throughout the reportable range, and for a quantitative test, represented as the *coefficient of variation*, whereas for a qualitative test, represented as ratios of concordant results. Laboratories are encouraged to review the cited references for guidance and provide confidence intervals to estimated performance characteristics."

Therefore, coefficient of variation should be used to monitor precision/reproducibility for the validation of the quantitative *BCR-ABL1* assay.

132. **A**. According to the College of American Pathology (CAP) Molecular Pathology Checklist dated July 28, 2015, MOL.31145, "The laboratory must show documented evidence that a test will return the same result regardless of minor variations in testing conditions that can cause random error, such as different technologists, instruments, reagent lots, days, etc. This is usually determined by repeated measures of samples throughout the reportable range, and for a quantitative test, represented as the coefficient of variation, whereas for a qualitative test, represented as *ratios of concordant* results. Laboratories are encouraged to review the cited references for guidance and provide confidence intervals to estimated performance characteristics."

Therefore, ratios of concordant should be used to monitor precision/reproducibility for the validation of the cystic fibrosis carrier assay.

133. **A**. According to the College of American Pathology (CAP) Molecular Pathology Checklist

dated July 28, 2015, MOL.31245, "The reportable range encompasses the full range of reported values. For qualitative tests that would include all reportable outcomes (e.g. homozygous wild type, heterozygous or homozygous mutant). For quantitative tests, the laboratory must define the analytic measurement range (AMR) as described in the Quantitative Assays; Calibration and Standards section of the checklist. The laboratory must also determine how to handle positive patient results below or above the AMR, since numerical values outside the AMR may be inaccurate. For example, these may be *reported as* <*x* or >y, or they may be *reported as low positive* or high positive along with an explanation that values outside the linear range cannot be quantified, or the sample may be *concentrated or diluted and rerun* to calculate an accurate value within the reportable range."

Therefore, it is not encouraged to report it out as negative without further investigation, considering the risk of a false negative result.

134. **A**. According to the CAP Molecular Pathology Checklist dated July 28, 2015, MOL.31245, "The reportable range encompasses the full range of reported values. For qualitative tests that would include all reportable outcomes (e.g. homozygous wild type, heterozygous or homozygous mutant). For quantitative tests, the laboratory must define the analytic measurement range (AMR) as described in the Quantitative Assays; Calibration and Standards section of the checklist. The laboratory must also determine how to handle positive patient results below or above the AMR, since numerical values outside the AMR may be inaccurate. For example, these may be *reported as* <*x or* >*y*, or they may be *reported as low positive or high positive* along with an explanation that values outside the linear range cannot be quantified, or the sample may be *concentrated or diluted and rerun* to calculate an accurate value within the reportable range."

Therefore, it is NOT acceptable to report out of range samples as positive because of the risk of false positive.

135. **B**. According to the College of American Pathology (CAP) Molecular Pathology Checklist dated July 28, 2015, MOL.33860, "Criteria are established for frequency of calibration or calibration verification, and the acceptability of results. Criteria typically include the following:
1. *At changes of reagent lots*, unless the laboratory can demonstrate that the use of different lots does not affect the accuracy of patient/client

test results and the range used to report patient/client test data.

2. *If QC materials reflect an unusual trend or shift or are outside of the laboratory's acceptable limits*, and other means of assessing and correcting unacceptable control values fail to identify and correct the problem.

3. *Major maintenance or service.*

4. *When recommended by the manufacturer.*

5. *At least every six months.*"

Therefore, quantitative assays typically should be calibrated: at changes of reagent lots (a), when the results of the high positive and low positive controls consistently have been outside of the laboratory's acceptable limits in the past one month, and the reasons cannot be identified (b), the ABI7900HT was shipped back to the lab yesterday after major repair at the manufacturer (c), when recommended by the manufacturer (d), and at least every 6 months (f).

136. **A**. According to the College of American Pathology (CAP) Molecular Pathology Checklist dated July 28, 2015, MOL.34475, "For quantitative assays, quality control statistics are performed *at least monthly* to define analytic imprecision and to monitor trends over time." And "The laboratory must use statistical methods such as calculating SD and CV at specified intervals to evaluate variance in numeric QC data." MOL.34495 states, "The QC data for tests performed less frequently than once per month should be reviewed when the tests are performed."

Therefore, quality control (QC) statistics should be calculated and reviewed at least monthly.

137. **F**. According to the College of American Pathology (CAP) Molecular Pathology Checklist dated July 28, 2015, MOL.34475, "For quantitative assays, quality control statistics are performed at least monthly to define analytic imprecision and to monitor trends over time." And "The laboratory must use statistical methods such as calculating SD and CV at specified intervals to evaluate variance in numeric QC data." In MOL.34495 "The QC data for tests performed less frequently than once per month should be *reviewed when the tests are performed.*"

Therefore, quality control (QC) statistics should be calculated and reviewed when this test is performed in this laboratory.

138. **B**. According to the College of American Pathology (CAP) Molecular Pathology Checklist dated July 28, 2015, MOL.34516, "For qualitative tests that use a cutoff value to distinguish positive from negative, the cutoff value is established

initially, and verified with *every change in lot* or *at least every six months.*" And "The threshold value that distinguishes a positive from a negative result must be established or verified when the test is initially placed in service, and verified with every change in lot (e.g. new master mix), instrument maintenance, or at least every six months thereafter. Note that a low-positive control that is close to the threshold value can satisfy this checklist requirement, but must be external to the kit (e.g. weak-positive patient sample or reference material prepared in appropriate matrix)."

Therefore, the cutoff value must be verified at changes of reagent lots (a); when the ABI7900HT, used for this test, was shipped back to the lab yesterday after major repair at the manufacturer (b); when recommended by the manufacturer (c); and at least every 6 months (e) after been established initially.

139. **D**. According to the College of American Pathology (CAP) Molecular Pathology Checklist dated July 28, 2015, MOL.35350, "Nucleic acid amplification procedures (e.g. PCR) are designed to minimize carryover (false positive results) using appropriate physical containment and procedural controls. This item is primarily directed at ensuring adequate physical separation of pre- and post-amplification samples to avoid amplicon contamination. ... In a given run, specimens should be ordered in the flowing sequence: *patient samples, positive controls, negative controls* (including 'no template' controls in which DNA is omitted and therefore no products are expected)."

Therefore, the most appropriate order of specimens set up for an amplification reaction is patient samples, positive controls, and negative controls.

140. **C**. According to the College of American Pathology (CAP) Molecular Pathology Checklist dated July 28, 2015, MOL.35805, "Sequencing assays differ from most other molecular pathology assays in that many targets (individual nucleotides) are examined at once, rather than addressing a discrete nucleotide mutation site. Assay procedures must assure that each of these targets is visualized adequately to produce an unequivocal sequence readout, whether this is done by manual or automated methods. Single nucleotide variants with low allele proportions in particular may be overlooked if the signals are low or unequal. Approaches to prevent this problem include *performing bidirectional sequencing of both sense and antisense strands or unidirectional*

coverage by replicate independent reads." And "For mutation testing on mixed cellular populations, e.g. tumor/normal, it is extremely important to distinguish low level signals from analytical background noise. Therefore, special care must be taken to optimize the assay to minimize background noise, and to preserve adequate signal strength. In addition, because of formalin-induced DNA crosslinking, sequencing performed on DNA derived from FFPE tissue is prone to artifacts that could potentially lead to false positive results. *Bidirectional sequencing is necessary to consistently achieve required accuracy in somatic applications.*"

Therefore, sequencing in both directions may be used to prevent errors caused by unequivocal sequence readout from happening.

141. **C**. According to the College of American Pathology (CAP) Molecular Pathology Checklist dated July 28, 2015, MOL.35805, "Sequencing assays differ from most other molecular pathology assays in that many targets (individual nucleotides) are examined at once, rather than addressing a discrete nucleotide mutation site. Assay procedures must assure that each of these targets is visualized adequately to produce an unequivocal sequence readout, whether this is done by manual or automated methods. Single nucleotide variants with low allele proportions in particular may be overlooked if the signals are low or unequal. Approaches to prevent this problem include *performing bidirectional sequencing of both sense and antisense strands or unidirectional coverage by replicate independent reads.*" And "For mutation testing on mixed cellular populations, e.g. tumor/normal, it is extremely important to distinguish low level signals from analytical background noise. Therefore, special care must be taken to optimize the assay to minimize background noise, and to preserve adequate signal strength. In addition, because of formalin-induced DNA crosslinking, sequencing performed on DNA derived from FFPE tissue is prone to artifacts that could potentially lead to false positive results. Bidirectional sequencing is necessary to consistently achieve required accuracy in somatic applications."

Therefore, unidirectional coverage by replicate independent reads may be used to prevent errors caused by unequivocal sequence readout.

142. **B**. According to the College of American Pathology (CAP) Molecular Pathology Checklist dated July 28, 2015, MOL.35820, "The laboratory should have an algorithm for decision-making in interpretation of pathogenic variants, benign

variants and variants of unknown clinical significance. The *ACMG guidelines* for classification of variants should be used for interpretation of germline variants associated with inherited diseases. For clinical interpretation of somatic variants, such as in tumor samples, the laboratory should have a written protocol for variant interpretation that considers frequency in the affected tumor (e.g., as reported in the COSMIC database), gene specific functional data, availability of targeted therapy, and other patient-specific clinical/pathological factors."

Therefore, Dr. Z should follow American College of Medical Genetics and Genomics (ACMG)'s guideline to classify variants.

143. **B**. According to the College of American Pathology (CAP) Molecular Pathology Checklist dated July 28, 2015, MOL.36310, "Relevant clinical validation studies included samples drawn only over a specific gestational age range (*e.g. 10 to 20 completed weeks gestation*). Knowing the estimated gestational age allows for the exclusion of samples collected too early in gestation where the test has not been validated (or is not valid). Fetal fraction increases slightly between 10 and 22 weeks gestation, but this increase is not sufficiently large to require gestational age specific test interpretations. Although less data are available for late second trimester or third trimester pregnancies, they strongly suggest that these tests will be reliable later in gestation. Laboratories can modify risk estimates to be specific to the pregnancy's gestational age (e.g. trisomies are more common in the first trimester than in the second trimester or term)."

Therefore, the earliest gestational age for NIPT would be 10 weeks of gestation age.

144. **B**. According to the College of American Pathology (CAP) Molecular Pathology Checklist dated July 28, 2015, from MOL.36310 to MOL.36370, requisitions for next-generation sequencing of maternal plasma to identify fetal aneuploidy should include *gestational age, maternal age, maternal weight, parentage information, multiple gestation, family history, and prior pregnancy risk.* Therefore, ethnicity of the couple is not essential for noninvasive prenatal tests (NIPTs). Therefore, ethnicity of the parents is not essential information for NIPT test.

145. **C**. According to the College of American Pathology (CAP) Molecular Pathology Checklist dated July 28, 2015, MOL.36410, "The percentage of women with positive results for each targeted disorders (e.g. Down syndrome, Turner syndrome), test failure rates (e.g. low fetal

fraction), and 'inconclusive' (e.g. gray zone) test results are calculated and reviewed *at least quarterly*." And "Since this type of testing may be performed in a mixed risk population (e.g. high or low risk woman in the general population), the proportion of women with positive results will likely vary by laboratory. If possible, laboratories should stratify test results and rates by indication of testing (e.g. low risk, high risk). In many instances, the pregnancy is at high risk for only one or two of the aneuploidies, offering the opportunity to establish relatively robust general population positive rates (both initial positive and false positive) for at risk and not at risk for specific chromosome abnormalities. These rates may be compared to the expected positive rates based on prevalence and clinical sensitivity and specificity. Monitoring test failure and inconclusive rates may be chromosome-specific or combined."

Therefore, monitoring for NIPT testing should be done in at least every 3 months.

146. **C**. According to the College of American Pathology (CAP) Molecular Pathology Checklist dated July 28, 2015, MOL.36430, "The patient report includes the following information as appropriate: (1) a recommendation for follow-up diagnostic testing for all pregnancies with a positive test result; (2) a statement that this test is not intended to identify pregnancies at risk for open neural-tube defects; and (3) *recommendations regarding next steps for women with uninformative results and/or test failures*."

Therefore, a recommendations regarding next steps for women with uninformative results and/or test failures must be included in patient's reports for noninvasive prenatal tests (NIPT).

147. **C**. According to the College of American Pathology (CAP) Molecular Pathology Checklist dated July 28, 2015, MOL.39288, "Images of FISH assays for neoplastic disorders must be retained for *10 years*; images of FISH assays for constitutional disorders must be retained for 20 years. Brightfield ISH slides or images must be retained for the same time periods."

Therefore, images of FISH assays for t(9;22) should be retained for at least 10 years.

148. **D**. According to the College of American Pathology (CAP) Molecular Pathology Checklist dated July 28, 2015, MOL.39288 "Images of FISH assays for neoplastic disorders must be retained for 10 years; images of FISH assays for constitutional disorders must be retained for *20 years*. Brightfield ISH slides or images must be retained for the same time periods."

Therefore, images of FISH assays for 22q11.2 deletion syndrome should be retained for at least 20 years.

149. **A**. According to the College of American Pathology (CAP) Molecular Pathology Checklist dated July 28, 2015, MOL.39288, "Photographic or digitized images are retained for documentation of all FISH assays (*at least one cell* for assays with normal results and at least two cells for assays with abnormal results)."

Therefore, a clinical laboratory should retain at least 1 FISH image for normal t(9;22).

150. **B**. According to the College of American Pathology (CAP) Molecular Pathology Checklist dated July 28, 2015, MOL.39288, "Photographic or digitized images are retained for documentation of all FISH assays (at least one cell for assays with normal results and *at least two cells* for assays with abnormal results)."

Therefore, a clinical laboratory should retain at least 2 FISH images for abnormal t(9;22).

151. **A**. According to the College of American Pathology (CAP) Molecular Pathology Checklist dated July 28, 2015, MOL.39288, "Photographic or digitized images are retained for documentation of all FISH assays (*at least one cell* for assays with normal results and at least two cells for assays with abnormal results)."

Therefore, a clinical laboratory should retain at least 1 FISH image for normal 4p- syndrome.

152. **B**. According to the College of American Pathology (CAP) Molecular Pathology Checklist dated July 28, 2015, MOL.39288 "Photographic or digitized images are retained for documentation of all FISH assays (at least one cell for assays with normal results and *at least two cells* for assays with abnormal results)."

Therefore, a clinical laboratory should retain at least 2 FISH images for abnormal 4p- syndrome.

153. **C**. According to the College of American Pathology (CAP) Molecular Pathology Checklist dated July 28, 2015, MOL.39358, "Specimens subject to *HER2* testing should be fixed in 10% neutral buffered formalin for *at least 6 hours* and *no longer than 72 hours*. The volume of formalin should be at least 10 times the volume of the specimen. Decalcification solutions with strong acids should not be used. While fixation outside these time limits is not an absolute exclusion criterion for *HER2* testing, laboratories should qualify any negative results for specimens fixed for less than 6 or longer than 72 hours."

Therefore, a sample for an *HER2* FISH assay be fixed in 10% neutral buffered formalin for at least 6 hours and no longer than 72 hours.

154. **C**. According to the College of American Pathology (CAP) Molecular Pathology Checklist dated July 28, 2015, MOL.39323, "the laboratory tests for *HER2* gene amplification by in situ hybridization (e.g. FISH, CISH, SISH, etc.), the laboratory has documented appropriate validation for the assay(s). NOTE: This requirement applies to both new and existing assays. Initial test validation must be performed on a minimum of *20 positive and 20 negative* samples for FDA-cleared/approved assays; or 40 positive and 40 negative samples for laboratory-developed tests (LDTs). Equivocal samples need not be used for validation studies. If the initial validation of existing assays does not meet the current standard, it must be supplemented and brought into compliance. It is permissible to do this retroactively by review of performance on past proficiency testing challenges or by sending unstained slides from recent cases to a reference laboratory for correlation. If no documentation exists from the initial validation, the assay must be fully revalidated and documented."

Therefore, a clinical molecular laboratory should use at least 20 positive and 20 negative samples to validate a FDA clear/approved *HER2* FISH assay.

155. **E**. According to the College of American Pathology (CAP) Molecular Pathology Checklist dated July 28, 2015, MOL.39323, "the laboratory tests for *HER2* gene amplification by in situ hybridization (e.g. FISH, CISH*, SISH*, etc.), the laboratory has documented appropriate validation for the assay(s). NOTE: This requirement applies to both new and existing assays. Initial test validation must be performed on a minimum of 20 positive and 20 negative samples for FDA-cleared/approved assays; or *40 positive and 40 negative* samples for laboratory-developed tests (LDTs). Equivocal samples need not be used for validation studies. If the initial validation of existing assays does not meet the current standard, it must be supplemented and brought into compliance. It is permissible to do this retroactively by review of performance on past proficiency testing challenges or by sending unstained slides from recent cases to a reference laboratory for correlation. If no documentation exists from the initial validation, the assay must be fully revalidated and documented."

Therefore, a clinical molecular laboratory should use at least 40 positive and 40 negative samples to validate a laboratory-developed test (LDTs) *HER2* FISH assay.

156. **D**. According to the College of American Pathology (CAP) Molecular Pathology Checklist dated July 28, 2015, MOL.39393, "For *HER2* gene status determined by in-situ hybridization, positive (amplified) cases are those with ratios of *HER2* to CEP17 of >2.2. Negative cases are defined as those with ratios of <1.8. Equivocal cases are those with a ratio of 1.8-2.2. For test systems without an internal control probe, positive (amplified) cases are those with an average *HER2* gene copy number > *six signals/nucleus*, negative cases are those with < four to six signals/nucleus, and equivocal cases are those with an average *HER2* gene copy number of four to six signals/nucleus. Careful attention should be paid to the recommended exclusion criteria for performing or interpreting in situ hybridization for *HER2*."

Therefore, at least 6 copies of the *HER2* genes in one nucleus is the criterion for positive *HER2* amplification in a FISH assay regardless of ratio of *HER2* to CEP17.

157. **C**. According to the College of American Pathology (CAP) Molecular Pathology Checklist dated July 28, 2015, MOL.44394 and MOL.448603, "Filters (filter photometers) are checked at least annually to ensure they are in good condition (e.g. clean, free of scratches)." And "Spectrophotometer wavelength calibration is checked with appropriate solutions, filters or emission line source lamps, *at least annually* (or as often as specified by the manufacturer)."

Therefore, the filter and wavelength calibration must be checked at least annually for appropriate function.

158. **D**. According to the College of American Pathology (CAP) Molecular Pathology Checklist dated July 28, 2015, MOL.48588, "Pipettors that are used for quantitative dispensing of material are checked for accuracy and reproducibility before being placed in service and at defined intervals (*at least annually*), and records maintained." And "Pipette checks must be performed following manufacturer's instructions, at minimum, and as defined in laboratory procedure. Such checks are most simply done gravimetrically. This consists of transferring a number of measured samples of water from the pipette to a balance. Each weight is recorded, the weights are converted to volumes, then means (for accuracy), and SD/CV (for imprecision) are calculated. Alternative approaches include spectrophotometry or (less frequently) the use of radioactive isotopes, and commercial kits are available from a number of vendors. Computer

software is useful where there are many pipettes, and provides convenient records."

Therefore, pipettes must be checked at least once in every 1 year for accuracy and reproducibility.

159. **D.** According to the College of American Pathology (CAP) Molecular Pathology Checklist dated July 28, 2015, MOL.49520, "Individual wells (or a representative sample thereof) of thermal cyclers are checked for temperature accuracy before being placed in service and *at least annually* thereafter." And "A downstream measure of well-temperature accuracy (such as productivity of amplification) may be substituted to functionally meet this requirement. For closed systems this function should be performed as a component of the manufacturer-provided preventive maintenance."

Therefore, the individual wells (or a representative sample) of thermal cyclers must be checked once in at least every 1 year for temperature accuracy.

160. **A.** According to the US Food and Drug Administration (FDA), analyte-specific reagents (ASRs) are defined as "antibodies, both polyclonal and monoclonal, specific receptor proteins, ligands, nucleic acid sequences, and similar reagents which, through specific binding or chemical reactions with substances in a specimen, are intended for use in a diagnostic application for identification and quantification of an individual chemical substance or ligand in biological specimens. ASRs are medical devices that are regulated by FDA."

"The ASR rule was designed to accomplish several policy objectives. One of the primary goals of the rule was to ensure the quality of the primary, active reagents of finished IVDs or LDTs. Another focus of the rule is the requirement for appropriate labeling to be appended to test results when ASRs are used by clinical laboratories in LDTs, so that healthcare users can understand when tests are being developed and validated by the laboratory and have not undergone FDA clearance or approval."

"The rule classifies *most ASRs as Class I* devices subject to general controls under section 513(a)(1)(A) of the Act, but exempt from premarket notification. The general controls require ASR manufacturers to register and list their devices, 21 CFR 807.20(a), submit medical device reports (21 CFR Part 803), follow labeling requirements, 21 CFR 809.10(e), and follow cGMPs, 21 CFR 809.20 (b). The rule also restricts the sale, use, distribution, labeling, advertising and promotion

of ASRs. 21 CFR 809.30. One of these restrictions allows only physicians and other persons authorized by applicable State law to order LDTs that are developed using ASRs. 21 CFR 809.30(f). Another restriction requires the laboratory that develops an LDT using an ASR to add a statement disclosing that the laboratory developed the test and it has not been cleared or approved by FDA when reporting the test result to the practitioner. 21 CFR 809.30(e)."

"Although most ASRs are Class I, there are some ASRs that are Class II and Class III and that must be cleared or approved by FDA before they can be marketed in the United States. 21 CFR 864.4020. FDA classifies medical devices, including diagnostic devices such as ASRs, into Class I, II, or III according to the level of regulatory control that is necessary to provide a reasonable assurance of safety and effectiveness. These classifications include consideration of the level of risk associated with the device. 21 U.S.C. 360c. The classification of an ASR determines the appropriate premarket process."

"An ASR is a Class II device if the reagent is used as a component in a blood banking test of a type that has been classified as a Class II device (e.g., certain cytomegalovirus serological and treponema pallidum nontreponemal test reagents). 21 CFR 864.4020(b)(2)."

"An ASR is *a Class III device* if the reagent is intended as a component in tests intended either:
- to diagnose a contagious condition that is highly likely to result in a fatal outcome and prompt, accurate diagnosis offers the opportunity to mitigate the public health impact of the condition [e.g., human immunodeficiency virus (HIV/AIDS) or tuberculosis (TB)]; or
- for use in donor screening for conditions for which FDA has recommended or required testing in order to safeguard the blood supply or establish the safe use of blood and blood products (e.g., tests for hepatitis or for identifying blood groups). 21 CFR 864.4020(b)(3).

FDA considers ASRs intended to be used as a component in tests for diagnosis of HIV (including monitoring for viral load or HIV drug resistance mutations) to be Class III ASRs" (http://www.fda.gov/downloads/medicaldevices/deviceregulationandguidance/guidancedocuments/ucm071269.pdf).

There is no Class IV for ASRs.

Therefore, the primers of this assay belong to Class I reagents.

161. C. According to US Food and Drug Administration (FDA), analyte-specific reagents (ASRs) are defined as "antibodies, both polyclonal and monoclonal, specific receptor proteins, ligands, nucleic acid sequences, and similar reagents which, through specific binding or chemical reactions with substances in a specimen, are intended for use in a diagnostic application for identification and quantification of an individual chemical substance or ligand in biological specimens. ASRs are medical devices that are regulated by FDA."

"The ASR rule was designed to accomplish several policy objectives. One of the primary goals of the rule was to ensure the quality of the primary, active reagents of finished IVDs or LDTs. Another focus of the rule is the requirement for appropriate labeling to be appended to test results when ASRs are used by clinical laboratories in LDTs, so that healthcare users can understand when tests are being developed and validated by the laboratory and have not undergone FDA clearance or approval."

"The rule classifies most ASRs as Class I devices subject to general controls under section 513(a)(1)(A) of the Act, but exempt from premarket notification. The general controls require ASR manufacturers to register and list their devices, 21 CFR 807.20(a), submit medical device reports (21 CFR Part 803), follow labeling requirements, 21 CFR 809.10(e), and follow cGMPs, 21 CFR 809.20(b). The rule also restricts the sale, use, distribution, labeling, advertising and promotion of ASRs. 21 CFR 809.30. One of these restrictions allows only physicians and other persons authorized by applicable State law to order LDTs that are developed using ASRs. 21 CFR 809.30(f). Another restriction requires the laboratory that develops an LDT using an ASR to add a statement disclosing that the laboratory developed the test and it has not been cleared or approved by FDA when reporting the test result to the practitioner. 21 CFR 809.30(e)."

"Although most ASRs are Class I, there are some ASRs that are Class II and Class III and that must be cleared or approved by FDA before they can be marketed in the United States. 21 CFR 864.4020. FDA classifies medical devices, including diagnostic devices such as ASRs, into Class I, II, or III according to the level of regulatory control that is necessary to provide a reasonable assurance of safety and effectiveness. These classifications include consideration of the level of risk associated with the device. 21 U.S.C. 360c. The classification of an ASR determines the appropriate premarket process."

"An ASR is a Class II device if the reagent is used as a component in a blood banking test of a type that has been classified as a Class II device (e.g., certain cytomegalovirus serological and treponema pallidum nontreponemal test reagents). 21 CFR 864.4020(b)(2)."

"An ASR is a *Class III device* if the reagent is intended as a component in tests intended either:
- to diagnose a contagious condition that is highly likely to result in a fatal outcome and prompt, accurate diagnosis offers the opportunity to mitigate the public health impact of the condition (e.g., human immunodeficiency virus (HIV/AIDS) or tuberculosis (TB)); or
- for use in donor screening for conditions for which FDA has recommended or required testing in order to safeguard the blood supply or establish the safe use of blood and blood products (e.g., tests for hepatitis or for identifying blood groups). 21 CFR 864.4020(b)(3).
FDA considers ASRs intended to be used as a component in tests for diagnosis of HIV (including monitoring for viral load or HIV drug resistance mutations) to be Class III ASRs" (http://www.fda.gov/downloads/medicaldevices/deviceregulationandguidance/guidancedocuments/ucm071269.pdf).

There is no class IV for ASRs.

Therefore, the primers of this assay belong to Class III reagents.

162. C. According to the College of American Pathology (CAP) Molecular Pathology Checklist dated July 28, 2015, MOL.49585, "The final report is reviewed and signed by the section director (or designee who meets section director qualifications) if there is a subjective or an interpretive component to the test." However, "When diagnostic reports are generated by computer or telecommunications equipment, *the actual signature or initials of the section director need not appear on the report*. Nevertheless, the laboratory must have a procedure that ensures that *the report has been reviewed and approved before its release*, and that records exist of the review and approval."

Therefore, the section director needs not to sign the report.

163. A. According to the College of American Pathology (CAP) Molecular Pathology Checklist dated July 28, 2015, MOL.49590 "Some patients, aware of the insurability risks, will choose to pay for testing out-of-pocket and request that the results not be recorded in their medical record;

such requests should be honored by the laboratory to the extent allowable under applicable laws."

Therefore, this patient may pay out of her own pocket for for the genetic test for Huntington disease.

164. **D**. According to the College of American Pathology (CAP) Molecular Pathology Checklist dated July 28, 2015, MOL.49590, "Molecular genetic test reports are released and transmitted in a manner adequate to maintain patient confidentiality at a level appropriate for the particular test." And "In view of the recognized risks of genetic discrimination and stigmatization, confidentiality of molecular test results is an important consideration. Results should be communicated only to the referring physician, genetic counselor, the medical record, or (in some cases) the patient. Potentially non-confidential media (e.g. FAX) should be used with caution. Some patients, aware of the insurability risks, will choose to pay for testing out-of-pocket and request that the results not be recorded in their medical record; such requests should be honored by the laboratory to the extent allowable under applicable laws. *Under no circumstances should results be provided to outside parties such as employers, insurers or other family members, without the patient's express consent*, despite the fact that there will be cases in which such action would appear to be in the best interest of the patient, family, or society."

Therefore, a patient's molecular test results for Huntington disease may NOT be provided to her husband without her express consent.

165. **B**. According to the College of American Pathology (CAP) Molecular Pathology Checklist dated July 28, 2015, MOL.49590, "In view of the recognized risks of genetic discrimination and stigmatization, confidentiality of molecular test results is an important consideration. *Results should be communicated only to the referring physician, genetic counselor, the medical record, or (in some cases) the patient*. Potentially non-confidential media (e.g. FAX) should be used with caution. Some patients, aware of the insurability risks, will choose to pay for testing out-of-pocket and request that the results not be recorded in their medical record; such requests should be honored by the laboratory to the extent allowable under applicable laws. Under no circumstances should results be provided to outside parties such as employers, insurers or other family members, without the patient's express consent, despite the fact that there will be cases in which such action would appear to be in the best interest of the patient, family, or society."

Therefore, a patient's molecular test results for Huntington disease may be provided to her genetic counselor without her express consent.

166. **C**. According to the College of American Pathology (CAP) Molecular Pathology Checklist dated July 28, 2015, MOL.49640, "CAP requires that test reports for neoplastic conditions be retained for *10 years*, and that test reports for constitutional/genetic conditions be retained for 20 years. Electronic versions are acceptable." *JAK2* assay is for neoplastic conditions.

Therefore, the final reports must be retained for at least 10 years.

167. **D**. According to the College of American Pathology (CAP) Molecular Pathology Checklist dated July 28, 2015, MOL.49640, "CAP requires that test reports for neoplastic conditions be retained for 10 years, and that test reports for constitutional/genetic conditions be retained for *20 years*. Electronic versions are acceptable." Huntington disease is a constitutional condition.

Therefore, final reports must be retained for at least 20 years.

168. **C**. According to the College of American Pathology (CAP) Molecular Pathology Checklist dated July 28, 2015, MOL.30785 to MOL.31705, "For an FDA-cleared/approved test a summary of the validation data should address accuracy, precision, reportable range, and reference range." Therefore, *analytical sensitivity* need NOT be verified for an FDA-cleared/approved test.

169. **C**. According to the College of American Pathology (CAP) Molecular Pathology Checklist dated July 28, 2015, MOL.30785 to MOL.31705, "For an FDA-cleared/approved test a summary of the validation data should address accuracy, precision, reportable range, and reference range." Therefore, *cross-contamination* need NOT be verified for an FDA-cleared/approved test.

170. **C**. According to the College of American Pathology (CAP) Molecular Pathology Checklist dated July 28, 2015, MOL.31245, "The ANALYTICAL MEASUREMENT RANGE (AMR) is the range of analyte values that a method can directly measure on the specimen without any dilution, concentration, or other pretreatment not part of the usual assay process." And "An important concept in verifying the AMR is that a plot of measured values from test samples vs. their actual (or expected) concentration or relative concentrations must be linear within defined acceptance criteria over the AMR. Verifying linearity using such a plot verifies the AMR. Beyond the limits of the AMR, there may not be a linear relationship between measured and actual

analyte concentrations, and test results may therefore be unreliable. For patient samples, only measured values that fall within the AMR (or can be brought into the AMR by sample dilution or concentration) should be reported. Values that fall outside the AMR may be reported as 'less than' or 'greater than' the limits of the AMR (see the note below, Patent Samples with Unusually High Concentrations of Analyte)."

CALIBRATION VERIFICATION denotes the process of confirming that the current calibration settings for each analyte remain valid for a test system. "Minimum requirements can be met by using matrix appropriate materials, which include *the low, mid and high concentration* or activity range of the AMR and recovering appropriate target values, within defined acceptance criteria. Records of AMR verification must be available."

Therefore, one negative, one low positive, one mid range positive, and one high positive samples must be used to verify the analytical measurement range (AMR) of this assay.

171. **C**. According to the College of American Pathology (CAP) Molecular Pathology Checklist dated July 28, 2015, MOL.39393, "If the laboratory interprets *HER2* gene amplification by in situ hybridization (e.g. FISH, CISH, SISH), results are reported using either the American Society of Clinical Oncology (ASCO)/CAP scoring criteria or the manufacturer's instructions. The table below contains the ASCO/CAP scoring criteria used to determine *HER2* gene status by in-situ hybridization [Table 2.1]."

TABLE 2.1 *HER2* FISH Diagnostic Criteria

Method	Result	Ratios of HER2 to CEP17[a]	Average HER2 Copy Number (Signals/Cell)[a]
HER2 ISH test systems with internal control probe	Positive (amplified)	> 2.0	N/A
		< 2.0	≥ 6.0
	Negative	<2.0	<4.0
	Equivocal	<2.0	≥ 4.0 and <6.0
HER2 ISH test systems without an internal control	Positive (amplified)	N/A	≥ 6.0
	Negative N/A <4.0	N/A	<4.0
	Equivocal	N/A	≥ 4.0 and <6.0

[a]*Criteria in both columns must be met for tests with internal control probes. For example, for a result to be negative, the ratio must be <2.0 and the average copy number must be <4.0.*

© *201X College of American Pathologists. Reprinted with permission of the College of American Pathologists. OR College of American Pathologists: (201X). CAP Accreditation Checklists: Molecular Pathology Checklist. Northfield, IL.*

172. **E**. According to the College of American Pathology (CAP) Molecular Pathology Checklist dated July 28, 2015, MOL.54570, "A biological safety cabinet (or hood) is available, when appropriate, and is certified *at least annually* to ensure that filters function properly and that airflow rates meet specifications."

173. **A**. According to the College of American Pathology (CAP) Molecular Pathology Checklist dated July 28, 2015, MOL.61055, "Workbenches and sinks are decontaminated *each day of use,* and the effectiveness checked at least monthly."

174. **C**. According to the College of American Pathology (CAP) Molecular Pathology Checklist dated July 28, 2015, MOL.61055, "Workbenches and sinks are decontaminated each day of use, and the effectiveness checked *at least monthly*."

175. **B**. According to the College of American Pathology (CAP) Molecular Pathology Checklist dated July 28, 2015, MOL.38294, "For parentage testing, DNA results (RFLP, STR, SNP) are interpreted *twice*, independently."

176. **C**. According to the CAP Team Leader Assessment of Director & Quality Checklist dated July 28, 2015, "Inspection method: *two-year accreditation cycle;* use of active laboratorians as inspectors; educational value to inspector and inspected laboratory."

177. **D**. According to the CAP Team Leader Assessment of Director & Quality Checklist dated July 28, 2015, TCL.10440 to TCL.11475, all of the items in the list are the responsibilities of the director in a molecular genetic laboratory.

178. **B**. According to the CAP ACMG Standards and Guidelines for Clinical Genetics Laboratories, 2008 Edition, C2.1, "Specimen containers arriving in the lab must include two identifiers, which may be the *patient's name, date of birth, hospital number, lab number or other unique identifier.* The date of specimen collection and, when appropriate, the time of collection, should be included. *Patient's hospital room number and insurance card number are subject to change, which cannot be used as specimen identifiers*."

Therefore, Date of birth (a), Hospital number (b), Laboratory number (e), Patient's name (f), and Social security number (SSN) (g) may be used as patient's identifiers on specimen containers for genetic tests.

179. **C**. According to the CAP ACMG Standards and Guidelines for Clinical Genetics Laboratories, 2008 Edition, G3.3, "Excess sample material (isolated DNA) should be stored at a temperature

no higher than 0–5°C. To ensure long-term stability, the DNA should be *stored frozen.*"

180. **C.** According to the CAP ACMG Standards and Guidelines for Clinical Genetics Laboratories, 2008 Edition, G5.1, "Each laboratory must determine the analytic validity (sensitivity, specificity, reproducibility) of the technique chosen for analysis of each gene. Validation with well-characterized samples is critical. Where available, performance characteristics should be compared with an existing 'gold standard' assay. In the absence of 'gold standards' for comparison of results of new assays, the splitting of samples with another laboratory with an established clinical assay may be considered. Documentation of validation results must be available for review (see section C8 and section CF2.11.1 in the Technical Standards and Guidelines for CFTR Mutation Testing)." *Test results from research laboratories cannot be used as "gold standards"* before being confirmed in a CAP/CLIA-certified laboratory.

Therefore, "b" and "c" cannot be used as positive controls in a validation.

181. **E.** According to the CAP ACMG Standards and Guidelines for Clinical Genetics Laboratories, 2008 Edition, G3.2, "*Southern analysis calls for DNA of higher quantity and quality than that required for PCR.*" In G6 it is explained *a partial digestion and a degraded specimen can both lead to incomplete digestion.* "*Each test must include human DNA control(s)* with a documented genotype at the locus tested." "Each test must include human DNA control(s) with a documented genotype at the locus tested." And "Prior to transfer, the gel run for Southern analysis must be photographed to provide a hard copy documentation of the gel." Because DNA in the gel will be transferred to a membrane, *a dried gel cannot be used as a hard copy documentation of the gel.* Therefore, none of the statements in the answer choices is correct.

182. **C.** According to the CAP ACMG Standards and Guidelines for Clinical Genetics Laboratories, 2008 Edition, G7.1.1, "An ideal laboratory design would include three physically distinct areas for reagent preparation, sample preparation, amplification and PCR product detection. At a minimum a pre-PCR and post-PCR area is required. The pre-PCR area requires that strict guidelines be in place to prevent contamination of the workspace. When possible, the workflow should be designed to be unidirectional from pre to post-PCR areas and to minimize traffic from post-PCR to pre-PCR areas. PCR workstations are useful for preventing contamination from other areas in the lab. The workstation area can be UV-treated and cleaned more easily than an open lab area." After PCR reaction, the targeted region in human genome is amplified million times. Therefore, *thermal cyclers should be kept in post-PCR area to separate the PCR products from the pre-PCR area.*

According to the College of American Pathology (CAP) Molecular Pathology Checklist dated July 28, 2015, MOL.35350, "Nucleic acid amplification procedures (e.g. PCR) are designed to minimize carryover (false positive results) using appropriate physical containment and procedural controls. This item is primarily directed at ensuring adequate physical separation of pre- and post-amplification samples to avoid amplicon contamination. ... In a given run, specimens should be ordered in the flowing sequence: patient samples, positive controls, negative controls (including 'no template' controls in which DNA is omitted and therefore no products are expected)."

And gel electrophoresis is commonly done after PCR and before Sanger sequencing to identify the efficiency and specificity of PCR, so the technologist may use the appropriate amount of PCR products for Sanger sequencing or rerun the PCR. It is cost-effective approach. And the use of centrifuges before putting PCR tubes or plates to thermal cyclers helps to keep all the liquid together so that the concentration of each reagents would be as it is supposed to be.

Therefore, there is no need for gel electrophoresis before Sanger sequencing.

183. **C.** According to the CAP ACMG Standards and Guidelines for Clinical Genetics Laboratories, 2008 Edition, G7.1.2.5, "Preventive cleaning of the pre-PCR work area (e.g., bench tops, floors, racks, and pipettes) can be accomplished by periodically wiping nonmetallic surfaces with freshly prepared *10% bleach.* In addition, contaminating DNA can be inactivated with UV irradiation."

According to the CAP ACMG Standards and Guidelines for Clinical Genetics Laboratories, 2008 Edition, G7.1.1, "An ideal laboratory design would include three physically distinct areas for reagent preparation, sample preparation, amplification and PCR product detection. At a minimum a pre-PCR and post-PCR area is required. The pre-PCR area requires that strict guidelines be in place to prevent contamination of the workspace. When possible, the workflow should be designed to be unidirectional from pre to post-PCR areas and to minimize traffic from post-PCR to pre-PCR areas. PCR workstations are useful for preventing contamination from other areas in the lab. The workstation area can be UV-treated and cleaned more easily than an open lab area." After PCR reaction, the targeted region in human genome is amplified million times. Therefore, thermal cyclers should be kept in the post-PCR area to separate the PCR products from the pre-PCR area.

In G7.1.2.3, "To decrease the chance of contamination, reagents should be aliquoted into small volumes. This will minimize the manipulation of reagents by repeated opening of the tubes. In the event that an aliquot of reagent is contaminated, only that aliquot would need to be discarded, sparing the laboratory the expense of discarding the entire lot of reagent. The assembly of PCR reagents into master mixes also decreases the chance of contamination."

According to the College of American Pathology (CAP) Molecular Pathology Checklist dated July 28, 2015, MOL.35350, "Nucleic acid amplification procedures (e.g. PCR) are designed to minimize carryover (false positive results) using appropriate physical containment and procedural controls. This item is primarily directed at ensuring adequate physical separation of pre- and post-amplification samples to avoid amplicon contamination. . . . In a given run, specimens should be ordered in the flowing sequence: patient samples, positive controls, negative controls (including "no template" controls in which DNA is omitted and therefore no products are expected)."

Therefore, BJ should use 10% bleach to clean the bench instead of 2%.

184. **A**. According to the CAP ACMG Standards and Guidelines for Clinical Genetics Laboratories, 2008 Edition, G8.4, "If practical for the laboratory, it is desirable to include all positive controls in each assay. However, for tests with several mutations it may not be feasible to include numerous positive controls in each assay run. Minimally, a normal control, *a positive control*, and a negative or 'no DNA' control should be included in each run. Additional positive controls should be rotated among assay runs."

Therefore, minimally 1 positive controls should be included in each run for this assay.

185. **C**. *ICD-10-CM* (*International Classification of Diseases*, 10th edition, Clinical Modification) is a set of codes used by physicians, hospitals, and allied health workers to indicate diagnoses for all

patient encounters. The ICD-10-CM is the HIPAA transaction code set for diagnosis coding (https://www.cms.gov/medicare-coverage-database). E84.9 is the ICD-10-CM code for unspecified cystic fibrosis.

CPT codes are five-digit numeric codes that are used to describe medical, surgical, radiology, laboratory, anesthesiology, and evaluation/management services of physicians, hospitals, and other health care providers. CPT codes are used for medical billing (http://www.ama-assn.org). CPD and ICT are not codes.

Therefore, E84.9 for diagnosis is a ICD code.

186. **B**. *CPT codes* are five-digit numeric codes that are used to describe medical, surgical, radiology, laboratory, anesthesiology, and evaluation/management services of physicians, hospitals, and other health care providers. CPT codes are used for medical billing (http://www.ama-assn.org). 81229 is the CPT code for SNP chromosome microarray.

ICD-10-CM (*International Classification of Diseases*, 10th edition, Clinical Modification) is a set of codes used by physicians, hospitals, and allied health workers to indicate diagnosis for all patient encounters. The ICD-10-CM is the HIPAA transaction code set for diagnosis coding (https://www.cms.gov/medicare-coverage-database). CPD and ICT are not codes.

Therefore, 81229 is a CPT code.

187. **D**. According to ACMG Recommendations for Standards for Interpretation and Reporting of Sequence Variations: Revisions 2007, there are six interpretive categories of sequence variations[15]:
- Sequence variation is previously reported to cause the disorder.
- Sequence variation is previously unreported and is expected cause the disorder.
- Sequence variation is previously unreported and is of the type that may or may not be causative of the disorder.
- Sequence variation is previously unreported and is probably not the cause of the disorder.
- Sequence variation is previously reported and is a recognized neutral variant.
- Sequence variation is previously not known or expected to be causative of disease, but is found to be associated with a clinical presentation.

A de novo splicing mutation in this case may cause exon 4 be spliced out, which may be expected to be pathogenic. However, since it has not been reported in patients, it is appropriate to classify it as *likely pathogenic*.

188. **A**. *"TAG," "TAA,"* and *"TGA"* are all stop codons. Any changes between them most likely are benign. According to "ACMG recommendations for standards for interpretation and reporting of sequence variations: revisions 2007," there are six interpretive categories of sequence variations:
    - Sequence variation is previously reported to cause the disorder.
    - Sequence variation is previously unreported and is expected cause the disorder.
    - Sequence variation is previously unreported and is of the type that may or may not cause the disorder.
    - Sequence variation is previously unreported and is probably not causative of the disorder.
    - Sequence variation is previously reported and is a recognized neutral variant.
    - Sequence variation is previously not known or expected to be causative of disease, but is found to be associated with a clinical presentation.

    Therefore, this mutation may be predicted to *benign*.

189. **D**. *TAG* is a stop codon. *TAT* is a codon for tyrosine (Tyr/T). According to "ACMG recommendations for standards for interpretation and reporting of sequence variations: revisions 2007", there are six interpretive categories of sequence variations:
    - Sequence variation is previously reported to cause the disorder.
    - Sequence variation is previously unreported and is expected cause the disorder.
    - Sequence variation is previously unreported and is of the type that may or may not cause the disorder.
    - Sequence variation is previously unreported and is probably not causative of the disorder.
    - Sequence variation is previously reported and is a recognized neutral variant.
    - Sequence variation is previously not known or expected to be causative of disease, but is found to be associated with a clinical presentation.

    A nonstop change affecting the translation termination codon leads to extension of the amino acid sequence, which most likely causes the disease. Therefore, this mutation may be predicted to *likely pathogenic*.

190. **A**. *"TAG,",* "TAA," and *"TGA"* are all stop codons. Any changes between them most likely are benign. According to "ACMG recommendations for standards for interpretation and reporting of sequence variations: revisions 2007," there are six interpretive categories of sequence variations:
    - Sequence variation is previously reported to cause the disorder.
    - Sequence variation is previously unreported and is expected cause the disorder.
    - Sequence variation is previously unreported and is of the type which may or may not be causative of the disorder.
    - Sequence variation is previously unreported and is probably not causative of the disorder.
    - Sequence variation is previously reported and is a recognized neutral variant.
    - Sequence variation is previously not known or expected to be causative of disease, but is found to be associated with a clinical presentation.

    Therefore, this mutation may be predicted to *benign*.

References

1. CAP, *All common checklist*. 2015.
2. CAP, *Laboratory general checklist*. 2015.
3. https://www.safety.caltech.edu/documents/22-biohazardous_agent_classification.pdf.
4. CAP, *Molecular pathology checklist*. 2015.
5. *Medical devices; classification/reclassification; restricted devices; analyte specific reagents—FDA. Final rule*. Fed Regist, 1997;**62**(225): p. 62243-60.
6. Garrett CT, Ferreira-Gonzalez A. FDA regulation of analyte-specific reagents (ASRs). Implications for nucleic acid-based molecular testing. *Diagn Mol Pathol* 1996;**5**(3):151–3.
7. Garrett CT, Leonard DG. Regulation of analyte-specific reagents. *Mol Diagn* 1996;**1**(3):276–7.
8. Johnson RL. Analyte specific reagents: FDA final rule and implications for your clinical flow cytometry laboratory. *Cytometry* 1999;**38**(1):40–1.
9. Leonard DG. FDA proposal for classification of "analyte-specific reagents". *Mol Diagn* 1996;**1**(2):153–4.
10. Press RD. Analyte-specific reagents. *Mol Diagn* 1999;**4**(1):71.
11. Tubbs RR, Abbott D. Analyte-specific reagents and the clinical laboratory. *Arch Pathol Lab Med* 1998;**122**(7):585–6.
12. CAP, Team leader assessment of director & quality checklist; 2015.
13. ACMG, *ACMG standards and guidelines for clinical genetics laboratories, Section C*; 2006.
14. Genetics, A.C.o.M., *ACMG standards and guidelines for clinical, CF and Section G*; 2011.
15. Richards CS, et al. ACMG recommendations for standards for interpretation and reporting of sequence variations: revisions 2007. *Genet Med* 2008;**10**(4):294–300.

Further Reading

- American Board of Medical Genetics and Genomics (ABMGG) (http://www.abmgg.org/).
- American College of Medical Genetics and Genomics (ACMG) (https://www.acmg.net/).
- American Society of Clinical Oncology (https://www.asco.org/).

- Association for Molecular Pathology (AMP) (https://www.amp.org/).
- Centers for Medicare & Medicaid Services (CMS) (https://www.cms.gov/).
- Clinical Laboratory Improvement Amendments (CLIA) (https://wwwn.cdc.gov/clia/).
- College of American Pathologists (CAP) (https://www.cap.org/).
- Current Procedural Terminology (CPT®) (https://www.ama-assn.org/amaone/cpt-current-procedural-terminology.
- Federal Trade Commission (FDC) (https://www.ftc.gov/).
- GINA help (http://ginahelp.org/).
- Health Information Privacy (https://www.hhs.gov/hipaa/index.html).
- International Classification of Diseases, Tenth Revision, Clinical Modification (ICD-10-CM) (https://www.cdc.gov/nchs/icd/icd10cm.htm).
- Occupational Safety and Health Administration (OSHA) (https://www.osha.gov/).
- Regulatory Bodies from World Health Organization (WHO) (http://www.who.int/genomics/policy/regulatory_bodies/en/).
- U.S. Department of Health and Human Services (HHS) (https://www.hhs.gov/).
- U S Food and Drug Administration (FDA) (https://www.fda.gov/).

SELF-ASSESSMENT QUESTIONS FOR CLINICAL MOLECULAR GENETICS

3

Molecular Genetic Nomenclature

It is essential that consensus nomenclatures of genes and variations in human genome are communicated easily and unequivocally for accurate reporting among laboratories.

HGNC (HUGO Gene Nomenclature Committee), founded by the NIH and the Wellcome Trust, is responsible for approving unique symbols and names for human loci, including protein-coding genes, noncoding RNA genes, and pseudogenes, to allow unambiguous scientific communication[1,2] (http://www.genenames.org/). By the time of publishing this book, almost 33,000 symbols have been approved by the HGNC. The vast majority of these are protein-coding genes, but also included are symbols for pseudogenes, noncoding RNAs, phenotypes and genomic features. All approved symbols are stored in the HGNC database.

HGVS (Human Genome Variation Society): provides the recommendations for the description of sequence variants.[3,4] HGVS nomenclature is used to report and exchange information regarding variants found in DNA, RNA, and protein sequences and serves as an international standard in DNA diagnostics.[5,6] In addition to the HGVS, the HGVS nomenclature is authorized by the Human Genome Variation Society (HGVS), the Human Variome Project (HVP) and the Human Genome Organization (HUGO) (http://varnomen.hgvs.org/).

This chapter is focuses mainly on the nomenclature of sequence variants at the DNA level as recommended by the HGVS.

QUESTIONS

1. BJ, a technologist, comes to Dr. Z, the director of a clinical pathology laboratory, with a question about the nomenclature of genomic variants. This is the first time that BJ has worked on reviewing wet laboratory results and writing nomenclature. Dr. Z explains to BJ what "c.," "g.," "m.," "n.,"

"r.," and "p." stand for in nomenclature, with examples. One of examples is myoclonic epilepsy with ragged red fibers (MERRF). Which one of the following nomenclatures may be used to describe a functional, effective variant for MERRF?[6]
   A. c.8344A > G
   B. g.8344A > G
   C. m.8344A > G
   D. n.8344A > G
   E. r.8344A > G
   F. p.8344A > G
   G. None of the above

2. John was evaluated for the genetic etiology of his recurrent respiratory infection and cardiomyopathy when he was 18 months old. His developmental milestones were normal. Family history indicated an X-linked recessive trait. Barth syndrome was at the top of the list of differential diagnoses. Sanger sequencing of the *TAZ* gene on Xq28 for Barth syndrome was ordered. A C-to-G transversion in exon 5 was detected in John's peripheral-blood sample, which was a nonsense mutation. Which one of the following nomenclatures may be used to describe this functional, effective variant?[6]
   A. c.153C > G
   B. g.153C > G
   C. m.153C > G
   D. n.153C > G
   E. r.153C > G
   F. p.153C > G
   G. None of the above

3. Dr. Z, a director of a clinical pathology laboratory, reviewed a patient's Sanger sequencing results on *USH1A* for Usher syndrome. By sequencing only the exons and 20-bp introns on either side of the exons, one variant of unknown clinical significance (VUCS) was found, which changed an aspartic acid (Asp/D) into tyrosine (Tyr/Y). Which one of

Self-assessment Questions for Clinical Molecular Genetics.
DOI: https://doi.org/10.1016/B978-0-12-809967-4.00003-X

the nomenclatures may Dr. Z use to describe this variant at the DNA level?[6,7]

A. a.1268C > T

B. c.1268C > T

C. g.1268C > T

D. p.1268C > T

E. All of the above

F. None of the above

4. Dr. Z, a director of a clinical pathology laboratory, reviewed a patient's Sanger sequencing results on *USH1A* for Usher syndrome. By sequencing only the exons and 20-bp introns on either side of the exons, one variant of unknown clinical significance (VUCS) was found, which changed an aspartic acid (Asp/D) into tyrosine (Tyr/Y). Which one of the nomenclatures may Dr. Z use to describe this variant at the amino acid level?[6,7]

A. a.D401Y

B. c.D401Y

C. g.D401Y

D. p.D401Y

E. All of the above

F. None of the above

5. Which one of the following nomenclatures should be used to describe ACTTTGTGCC to ACTTTGTGGCC?[6]

A. c.8dupG

B. c.8Gdup

C. c.8_9insG

D. c.8_9Gins

E. None of the above

6. Autosomal recessive nonsyndromic hearing loss and deafness (DFNB1) is characterized by congenital, nonprogressive, mild to profound sensorineural hearing impairment. The majority of individuals with DFNB1 have two identifiable variants in the *GJB2* gene, but some have compound heterozygous variants of the *GJB2* and *GJB6* genes. If an individual has a maternally inherited c.35delG in *GJB2* and a paternally inherited c.14C > T in *GJB6*, which one of the following nomenclatures would be appropriate to use in the molecular report?[6]

A. GJB2:c.35delG;GJB6:c.14C > T

B. GJB2:c.[35delG];GJB6:c.[14C > T]

C. GJB6:c.14C > T;GJB2:c.35delG

D. GJB6:c.[14C > T];GJB2:c.[35delG]

E. A and C

F. B and D

G. None of the above

7. Which one of the following nomenclatures is appropriate, according to published nomenclature for the description of sequence

variants by the Human Genome Variation Society in 2016?[6,8]

A. c.IVS2 + 2T > G

B. LRG_1:g.8463-2G > C

C. c.88 + 2U > G

D. c.*46T > A

E. All of the above

F. None of the above

8. Which one of the following nomenclatures may be used to describe a start codon, methionine (Met, M), is changed to valine (Val, V), which activates an upstream translation initiation site at position −12?[6]

A. p.-12Met

B. p.-12Met1

C. p.-12Met1Val

D. p.Met1Valext-12

E. None of the above

9. Which one of the following nomenclatures may be used to describe a variant in the stop codon at position 110 of an amino acid sequence, changing it to a codon for glutamine (Gln, Q) and adding a tail of 17 new amino acids (including Gln/Q) to the protein's C-terminus ending at a new stop codon?[6]

A. p.*110Glnext*17

B. p.Ter110Glnext*17

C. p.Ter110Gln

D. p.*110GlnextTer17

E. p.*110Gln

10. Which one of the following nomenclatures may be used to describe a chimeric organism in which a chromosome in some cells contains a normal sequence (arginine, Arg/R) at position 83, while other cells contain another chromosome with serine (Ser/S) at this position?[6]

A. p.[Arg83 = /Arg83Ser]

B. p.[Arg83 = //Arg83Ser]

C. p.[Arg83 =];[Arg83Ser]

D. p.[Arg83 = ;Arg83Ser]

E. p.[Arg83 = (;)Arg83Ser]

F. None of the above

11. Which one of the following nomenclatures may be used to describe a somatic mosaic case in which a chromosome in some cells contains a normal sequence (arginine, Arg/R) at position 83, while other cells contain a serine (Ser/S) at this position?[6]

A. p.[Arg83 = /Arg83Ser]

B. p.[Arg83 = //Arg83Ser]

C. p.[Arg83 =];[Arg83Ser]

D. p.[Arg83 = ;Arg83Ser]

E. p.[Arg83 = (;)Arg83Ser]

F. None of the above

12. Which one of the following nomenclatures may be used to describe two changes (amino acid alanine changes threonine at the position 25 and proline to leucine at the position 323, RNA or protein analyzed) were identified in one individual, but it is not known whether these changes are on the same chromosome (in cis) or on different chromosomes (in trans)?[6]
   A. p.[Arg83 = /Arg83Ser]
   B. p.[Arg83 = //Arg83Ser]
   C. p.[Arg83 =];[Arg83Ser]
   D. p.[Arg83 = ;Arg83Ser]
   E. p.[Arg83 = (;)Arg83Ser]
   F. None of the above

13. Which one of the following nomenclatures may be used to describe a homozygous A-to-C change at the nucleotide position 76 of a cDNA?[6]
   A. c.[76A > C];[76A > C]
   B. c.[76A > C];[(76A > C)]
   C. c.[76A > C];[=]
   D. c.[76A > C];[0]
   E. None of the above

14. Which one of the following nomenclatures may be used to describe a heterozygous A-to-C change at the nucleotide position 76 of a cDNA?[6]
   A. c.[76A > C];[76A > C]
   B. c.[76A > C];[(76A > C)]
   C. c.[76A > C];[=]
   D. c.[76A > C];[0]
   E. None of the above

15. Which one of the following nomenclatures may be used to describe a chimeric case in which at position 83, in addition to the normal sequence (a G), some cells are found containing another chromosome containing a C at this position?[6]
   A. c.[83G = /83G > C]
   B. c.[= /83G > C]
   C. c.[83G = //83G > C]
   D. c.[= //83G > C]
   E. None of the above

16. Which one of the following nomenclatures may be used to describe a mosaic case in which at position 83, in addition to the normal sequence (a G), chromosomes are also found containing a C?[6]
   A. c.[83G = /83G > C]
   B. c.[= /83G > C]
   C. c.[83G = //83G > C]
   D. c.[= //83G > C]
   E. None of the above

17. Which one of the following nomenclatures is appropriate according to recommendations for the description of sequence variants published by the Human Genome Variation Society in 2016?[6]
   A. m.[76u > c]
   B. m.[= ,73_88del]
   C. r.[76t > c]
   D. r.[= ,73_88del]
   E. None of the above

18. Which one of the following nomenclatures is appropriate, according to recommendations for the description of RNA sequence variants published by the Human Genome Variation Society in 2016?[6]
   A. r.[88G > A]
   B. r.[= ,73_88del]
   C. r.[76T > C]
   D. r.[76t > c,73_88del]
   E. None of the above

19. A reference sequence in the table below is mutated to ... cag ATG TCC AAT CTT GCT AGC CCT AGA TTT GGT TCT ... in a sample. Which one of the following nomenclatures is the most appropriate one to describe this change?[6]
   A. c.4C > T(p.2Ala > Ser)
   B. c.4C > T(p.Ala2Ser)
   C. c.C4T(p.Ala2Ser)
   D. c.4C > T(a.2Ala > Ser)
   E. None of the above

	Exon 1										
	1	2	3	4	5	6	7	8	9	10	11
	Met	Ala	Asn	Leu	Ala	Ser	Pro	Arg	Phe	Gly	Ser
... cag	ATG	GCC	AAT	CTT	GCT	AGC	CCT	AGA	TTT	GGT	TCT	...
	1	4	7	10	13	16	19	22	25	28	31

20. A reference sequence in the table below is mutated to ... cag ATG <u>T</u>CC AAT CTT GCT AGC CCT AGA TTT GGT TC<u>T</u> ... in a sample. Which one of the following nomenclatures is the most appropriate one to describe this change?[6]

- **A.** p.Ala2Ser
- **B.** p.(Ala2Ser)
- **C.** c.4C > T(p.Ala2Ser)
- **D.** c.C4T(p.Ala^{2}Ser)
- **E.** c.4C > T(p.ala2ser)
- **F.** None of the above

Exon 1										
1	2	3	4	5	6	7	8	9	10	11
Met	Ala	Asn	Leu	Ala	Ser	Pro	Arg	Phe	Gly	Ser
... cag ATG	<u>G</u>CC	AAT	CTT	GCT	AGC	CCT	AGA	TTT	GGT	TCT ...
1	4	7	10	13	16	19	22	25	28	31

21. A reference sequence in the table below is mutated to ... cag ATG <u>TG</u>C AAT CTT GCT AGC CCT AGA TTT GGT TCT ... in a sample. Which one of the following nomenclatures is the most appropriate one to describe this change?[6]

- **A.** c.4CG > TG(p.2Ala > Cys)
- **B.** c.4_5CG > TG(p.2delAlainsCys)
- **C.** c.4_5delGCinsTG(p.Ala2Cys)
- **D.** c.4_5delinsTG(p.2Cys)
- **E.** c.[4G > T(;)5C > G](a.Ala2Cys)
- **F.** None of the above

Exon 1										
1	2	3	4	5	6	7	8	9	10	11
Met	Ala	Asn	Leu	Ala	Ser	Pro	Arg	Phe	Gly	Ser
... cag ATG	<u>GC</u>C	AAT	CTT	GCT	AGC	CCT	AGA	TTT	GGT	TCT ...
1	4	7	10	13	16	19	22	25	28	31

22. A reference sequence in the table below is mutated to ... **tt**g ATG GCC AAT CTT GCT AGC CCT AGA TTT GGT TCT ... in a sample. Which one of the following nomenclatures is the most appropriate one to describe this change?[6]

- **A.** c.1-3_-2CA > TT
- **B.** c.-3CA > TT
- **C.** c.-3delCAinsTT
- **D.** c.-3_-2CA > TT
- **E.** c.-3_-2delCAinsTT
- **F.** None of the above

Exon 1										
1	2	3	4	5	6	7	8	9	10	11
Met	Ala	Asn	Leu	Ala	Ser	Pro	Arg	Phe	Gly	Ser
...<u>ca</u>g ATG	GCC	AAT	CTT	GCT	AGC	CCT	AGA	TTT	GGT	TCT ...
1	4	7	10	13	16	19	22	25	28	31

23. A reference sequence in the table below is mutated to ... cag ATG GCC AAT CTT GCT AGC CCT AGA TTT GGT TCT c<u>tt</u> ... in a sample. Which one of the following nomenclatures is the most appropriate one to describe this change?[6,8]
    c.33 + 2_ + 3CA > TT

A. c.33 + 2CA > TT
B. c. + 2CA > TT
C. c.33 + 2_ + 3delinsTT
D. c. + 2_ + 3delCAinsTT
E. c.IVS1 + 2_ + 3delinsTT
F. None of the above

				Exon 1							
	1	2	3	4	5	6	7	8	9	10	11
	Met	Ala	Asn	Leu	Ala	Ser	Pro	Arg	Phe	Gly	Ser
... cag	ATG	GCC	AAT	CTT	GCT	AGC	CCT	AGA	TTT	GGT	TCT	c**ca**...
	1	4	7	10	13	16	19	22	25	28	31	

24. A reference sequence in the table below is mutated to ... cag ATG GCC AAT CTT GCT AGC CCT AGA TTT GGT TCT c<u>tt</u> ... in a sample. Which one of the following nomenclatures is the most appropriate one to describe this change?[6,8]
    c.IVS1 + 2_ + 3CA > TT

A. IVS1 + 2_ + 3CA > TT
B. * + 2CA > TT
C. *2delCAinsTT
D. c.[33 + 2C > T;33 + 3A > T]
E. c.33[+ 2C > T; + 3A > T]
F. None of the above

				Exon 1							
	1	2	3	4	5	6	7	8	9	10	11
	Met	Ala	Asn	Leu	Ala	Ser	Pro	Arg	Phe	Gly	Ser
... cag	ATG	GCC	AAT	CTT	GCT	AGC	CCT	AGA	TTT	GGT	TCT	c**ca**...
	1	4	7	10	13	16	19	22	25	28	31	

25. A reference sequence the table below is mutated to ... **a**ag GGA GCC AAT CTT GCT AGC CCT CAT A̅GA TTT GGT TCT cat... in a sample. Which one of the following nomenclatures is the most appropriate one to describe this change?[6]

A. c.-3G > A
B. c.76-3G > A
C. *3G > A
D. c.73G > A
E. IVS3-3G > A
F. None of the above

				Exon 3							
	26	27	28	29	30	31	32	33	34	35	36
	Gly	Ala	Asn	Leu	Ala	Ser	Pro	Arg	Phe	Gly	Ser
...<u>c</u>ag	GGA	GCC	AAT	CTT	GCT	AGC	CCT	AGA	TTT	GGT	TCT	cat...
	76	79	82	85	88	91	94	97	100	103	106	

26. A reference sequence in the table below is mutated to . . . ca**a** GGA GCC AAT CTT GCT AGC CCT AGA TTT GGT TCT. Which one of the following nomenclatures is the most appropriate one to describe this change?[6]

A. c.76-1G > A
B. c.75G > A(p.Gly26fs)
C. c.76-1G > A(p.26Glyfs)
D. c.76-1G > A(p.Gly26*)
E. c.75G > A(p.Gly26Ter)
F. None of the above

		Exon 3										
	26	27	28	29	30	31	32	33	34	35	36	
	Gly	Ala	Asn	Leu	Ala	Ser	Pro	Arg	Phe	Gly	Ser	
. . . ca**g**	GGA	GCC	AAT	CTT	GCT	AGC	CCT	AGA	TTT	GGT	TCT	. . .
	76	79	82	85	88	91	94	97	100	103	106	

27. A reference sequence in the table below is mutated to . . . cag GGA GCC AAT CTT GCT AGC CCT AGA TTT GGT TCT g**c**t . . . tag GAC in a sample. Which one of the following nomenclatures is the most appropriate one to describe this change?

A. C.108 + 2T > C
B. c.108 + 2T > C(p.Asp37fs)
C. c.108 + 2T > C(p.37Asp > fs)
D. c.108 + 2T > C(p.Asp37*)
E. c.108 + 2T > C(p.Asp37Ter)
F. None of the above

		Exon 3												Exon 4
	26	27	28	29	30	31	32	33	34	35	36			37
	Gly	Ala	Asn	Leu	Ala	Ser	Pro	Arg	Phe	Gly	Ser			Asp
. . . cag	GGA	GCC	AAT	CTT	GCT	AGC	CCT	AGA	TTT	GGT	TCT	g**t**t . . . tag		GAC
	76	79	82	85	88	91	94	97	100	103	106			109

28. A reference sequence in the table below is mutated to . . . cag **T**GA GCC AAT CTT GCT AGC CCT AGA TTT GGT TCT gtt . . . tag GAC in a sample. Which one of the following nomenclatures is the most appropriate one to describe this change?[6]

A. p.Gly26Ter
B. c.76G > T(p.G26*)
C. c.76G > T(a.Gly26Ter)
D. c.76G > T(p.Gly26 =)
E. p.Gly26Tyr
F. None of the above

		Exon 3												Exon 4
	26	27	28	29	30	31	32	33	34	35	36			37
	Gly	Ala	Asn	Leu	Ala	Ser	Pro	Arg	Phe	Gly	Ser			Asp
. . . cag	**G**GA	GCC	AAT	CTT	GCT	AGC	CCT	AGA	TTT	GGT	TCT	gtt . . . tag		GAC
	76	79	82	85	88	91	94	97	100	103	106			109

29. A reference sequence in the table below is mutated to ... cag **T**GA GCC AAT CTT GCT AGC CCT AGA TTT GGT TCT gtt ... tag GAC in a sample. Which one of the following nomenclatures is the most appropriate one to describe this change?[6]

- **A.** c.76G > T(p.Gly26Ter)
- **B.** c.76G > T(p.Gly26*)
- **C.** c.76G > T(p.Gly26Phe)
- **D.** c.76G > T(p.Gly26Ser)
- **E.** A and B
- **F.** C and D
- **G.** None of the above

					Exon 3								Exon 4
	26	27	28	29	30	31	32	33	34	35	36		37
	Gly	Ala	Asn	Leu	Ala	Ser	Pro	Arg	Phe	Gly	Ser		Asp
... cag	**G**GA	GCC	AAT	CTT	GCT	AGC	CCT	AGA	TTT	GGT	TCT	gtt ... tag	GAC
	76	79	82	85	88	91	94	97	100	103	106		109

30. A reference sequence in the table below is mutated to ... cag GGA GCC AAT CTT GCT AGC CCT AGA TTT GGT TAG **t**tt ... in a sample. Which one of the following nomenclatures is the most appropriate one to describe this change?[6]

- **A.** c.365 + 1G > T
- **B.** c. + 1G > T
- **C.** c.G + 1T
- **D.** c.*1G > T
- **E.** c.IVS11 + 1G > T
- **F.** None of the above

					Exon 11						
	111	112	113	114	115	116	117	118	119	120	
	Gly	Ala	Asn	Leu	Ala	Ser	Pro	Arg	Phe	Gly	
...cag	GGA	GCC	AAT	CTT	GCT	AGC	CCT	AGA	TTT	GGT	TAG	**g**tt ...
	333	336	339	342	345	348	351	354	357	360	363	

31. A reference sequence in the table below is mutated to ... cag GGA GCC AAT CTT GCT AGC CCT AGA TTT GGT TA**T** gtt ... in a sample. Which one of the following nomenclatures is the most appropriate one to describe this change?[6]

- **A.** c.365G > T(p.Ter121TyrextTer22)
- **B.** c.365G > T(p.*121 =)
- **C.** c.365G > T(p.Ter121 =)
- **D.** c.365G > T(p.Ter121Tyrext*22)
- **E.** c.IVS11 + 3G > T(p.*121Tyrext*22)
- **F.** None of the above

					Exon 11						
	111	112	113	114	115	116	117	118	119	120	
	Gly	Ala	Asn	Leu	Ala	Ser	Pro	Arg	Phe	Gly	
...cag	GGA	GCC	AAT	CTT	GCT	AGC	CCT	AGA	TTT	GGT	TA**G**	gtt ...
	333	336	339	342	345	348	351	354	357	360	363	

32. A reference sequence in the table below is mutated to ... cag GGA GCC AAT CTT GCT AGC CCT AGA TTT GGT TA<u>T</u> gtt ... in a sample. Which one of the following nomenclatures is the most appropriate one to describe this change?[6]

    A. c.365G > T(p.Ter121 =)
    B. c.365g > t(p.*121*)
    C. c.365G > T(p.Ter121TyrextTer22)
    D. c.365G > T(p.ter121tyrextter22)
    E. None of the above

	Exon 11											
	111	112	113	114	115	116	117	118	119	120		
	Gly	Ala	Asn	Leu	Ala	Ser	Pro	Arg	Phe	Gly		
...cag	GGA	GCC	AAT	CTT	GCT	AGC	CCT	AGA	TTT	GGT	TA<u>G</u>	gtt ...
	333	336	339	342	345	348	351	354	357	360	363	

33. A reference sequence the table below is mutated to ... cag GGA GCC AAT CTT GCT AGC CCT AGA TTT GGT TA<u>A</u> gtt ... in a sample. Which one of the following nomenclatures is the most appropriate one to describe this change?[6]

    A. c. + 3G > T(p.Ter121*)
    B. c.365G > T(p.Ter121TyrextTer22)
    C. c.365G > T(p.Ter121 =)
    D. c.IVS11 + 3G > T(p.*121*)
    E. c.IVS11 + 3G > T(p.Ter121*)
    F. None of the above

	Exon 11											
	111	112	113	114	115	116	117	118	119	120		
	Gly	Ala	Asn	Leu	Ala	Ser	Pro	Arg	Phe	Gly		
...cag	GGA	GCC	AAT	CTT	GCT	AGC	CCT	AGA	TTT	GGT	TA<u>G</u>	gtt ...
	333	336	339	342	345	348	351	354	357	360	363	

34. A reference sequence in the table below is mutated to ... cag GGA GCC AAT CTT GCT AGC CCT AGA TTT GGT T<u>GA</u> gtt ... in a sample. Which one of the following nomenclatures is the most appropriate one to describe this change?[6]

    A. p.*121 =
    B. c.365G > T(p.121Tyrext*22)
    C. c.365G > T(p.ter121ter)
    D. c.365G > T(p.*121Tyrext*22)
    E. c.365G > T(p.*121 =)
    F. c.365G > T(p.Ter121TyrextTer22)
    G. None of the above

	Exon 11											
	111	112	113	114	115	116	117	118	119	120		
	Gly	Ala	Asn	Leu	Ala	Ser	Pro	Arg	Phe	Gly		
...cag	GGA	GCC	AAT	CTT	GCT	AGC	CCT	AGA	TTT	GGT	TA<u>G</u>	gtt ...
	333	336	339	342	345	348	351	354	357	360	363	

35. A reference sequence in the table below is mutated to … cag <u>T</u>TG GCC AAT CTT GCT AGC CCT AGA TTT GGT TCT … in a sample. Which one of the following nomenclatures is appropriate to describe this change?[6]

A. c.1A > T(p.Met1ext-5)
B. p.M1ext-5)
C. c.1A > T(p.met1ext-5)
D. c.1A > T(p.M^{1}ext-5)
E. p.Met1Leuext-5)
F. None of the above

	Exon 1										
	1	2	3	4	5	6	7	8	9	10	11
	Met	Ala	Asn	Leu	Ala	Ser	Pro	Arg	Phe	Gly	Ser
… cag	<u>A</u>TG	GCC	AAT	CTT	GCT	AGC	CCT	AGA	TTT	GGT	TCT	…
	1	4	7	10	13	16	19	22	25	28	31

36. A reference sequence in the table below is mutated to … cag <u>T</u>TG GCC AAT CTT GCT AGC CCT AGA TTT GGT TCT … in a sample. Which one of the following nomenclatures is appropriate to describe this change?[6]

A. p.Met1ext-5
B. c.1A > T(p.Met1LeuextMet-5)
C. c.1A > T(p.met1ext + 5)
D. c.1A > T(p.M^{1}ext-5)
E. c.1A > T(p.M1Lext + 5)
F. None of the above

	Exon 1										
	1	2	3	4	5	6	7	8	9	10	11
	Met	Ala	Asn	Leu	Ala	Ser	Pro	Arg	Phe	Gly	Ser
… cag	<u>A</u>TG	GCC	AAT	CTT	GCT	AGC	CCT	AGA	TTT	GGT	TCT	…
	1	4	7	10	13	16	19	22	25	28	31

37. A reference sequence in the table below is mutated to … cag GGA GCC AAT CTT G<u>C</u> <u>A</u>GC CCT AGA TTT GGT TCG gtt … tag GAC in a sample. Which one of the following nomenclatures is the most appropriate one to describe this change?[6]

A. c.90delT(p.Ala30 =)
B. c.90del(p.A30fs)
C. p.Ala30AlafsTer26
D. p.A30Afs*26
E. c.90delT(p.Ala30fs*26)
F. None of the above

	Exon 3												**Exon 4**
	26	27	28	29	30	31	32	33	34	35	36		37
	Gly	Ala	Asn	Leu	Ala	Ser	Pro	Arg	Phe	Gly	Ser		Asp
… cag	GGA	GCC	AAT	CTT	<u>GCT</u>	<u>A</u>GC	CCT	AGA	TTT	GGT	TCG	gtt … tag	GAC
	76	79	82	85	88	91	94	97	100	103	106		109

38. A reference sequence in the table below is mutated to … cag GGA GCC AAT CTT **G A**GC CCT AGA TTT GGT TCG gtt … tag GAC in a sample. Which one of the following nomenclatures is the most appropriate one to describe this change?[6]

A. c.89_90delCT(p.Ala30 =)
B. c.89_90del(p.Ala30Glu)
C. c.89_90delCT(p.Ala30GlufsTer3)
D. c.89_90del(p.A30Efs)
E. c.89_90delCT(p.Ala30fs*3)
F. None of the above

	Exon 3												Exon 4
	26	27	28	29	30	31	32	33	34	35	36		37
	Gly	Ala	Asn	Leu	Ala	Ser	Pro	Arg	Phe	Gly	Ser		Asp
… cag	GGA	GCC	AAT	CTT	G**CT**	**A**GC	CCT	AGA	TTT	GGT	TCG	gtt … tag	GAC
	76	79	82	85	88	91	94	97	100	103	106		109

39. A reference sequence in the table below is mutated to … cag GGA GCC AAT CTT **G G**C CCT AGA TTT GGT TCG gtt … tag GAC in a sample. Which one of the following nomenclatures is the most appropriate one to describe this change?[6]

A. c.89_91delCTA(p.Ala30 =)
B. c.89_91del(p.Ala30Gly)
C. c.89_91del(p.A30fs)
D. c.89_91delCTA(p.Ala30_Ser31delinsGly)
E. c.89_91delCTA(p.Ala30_Ser31insdelGly)
F. None of the above

	Exon 3												Exon 4
	26	27	28	29	30	31	32	33	34	35	36		37
	Gly	Ala	Asn	Leu	Ala	Ser	Pro	Arg	Phe	Gly	Ser		Asp
… cag	GGA	GCC	AAT	CTT	**GCT**	**A**GC	CCT	AGA	TTT	GGT	TCG	gtt … tag	GAC
	76	79	82	85	88	91	94	97	100	103	106		109

40. A reference sequence in the table below is mutated to … cag GGA GCC AAT CTT GCT AGC CCT AGA TTT GGT TC gtt … tag GAC in a sample. RNA analysis shows no effect on splicing. Which one of the following nomenclatures is the most appropriate one to describe this change?[6]

A. c.108delG(p.Ser36SerfsTer26)
B. c.108 + 1delG
C. c.108delG(p.Ser36Serfs)
D. c.108 + 1del(p.Ser36 =)
E. c.108del(p.Ser36fs*26)
F. None of the above

	Exon 3												Exon 4
	26	27	28	29	30	31	32	33	34	35	36		37
	Gly	Ala	Asn	Leu	Ala	Ser	Pro	Arg	Phe	Gly	Ser		Asp
… cag	GGA	GCC	AAT	CTT	GCT	AGC	CCT	AGA	TTT	GGT	TC**G**	**g**tt … tag	GAC
	76	79	82	85	88	91	94	97	100	103	106		109

41. A reference sequence in the table below is
mutated to … cag GGA GCC AAT CTT GCT
AGC CCT AGA TTT GGT T**C** g**t**t … tag GAC in a
sample. RNA analysis shows effect on
splicing. Which one of the following
nomenclatures is the most appropriate one to
describe this change?[6]

   A. c.108delG(p.Ser36SerfsTer26)
   B. c.108 + 1delG
   C. c.108delG(p.Ser36Serfs)
   D. c.108 + 1del(p.Ser36 =)
   E. c.108del(p.Ser36fs*26)
   F. None of the above

	Exon 3												Exon 4
	26	27	28	29	30	31	32	33	34	35	36		37
	Gly	Ala	Asn	Leu	Ala	Ser	Pro	Arg	Phe	Gly	Ser		Asp
… cag	GGA	GCC	AAT	CTT	GCT	AGC	CCT	AGA	TTT	GGT	T**CG**	**g**tt … tag	GAC
	76	79	82	85	88	91	94	97	100	103	106		109

42. A reference sequence in the table below is mutated
to … cag GGA GCC AAT CTT GC**T GGA A**GC
CCT AGA TTT GGT TCG gtt … tag GAC in a
sample. Which one of the following nomenclatures
is the most appropriate one to describe this
change?[6]

   A. c.90_91insGGA(p.Ala30AlaGly)
   B. c.90_91insGGA(p.Ala30_Ser31insGly)
   C. c.90_91insdelGGA(p.A30_Ser31insdelGly)
   D. c.90_91insGGA(p.Ala30_Ser31delinsGly)
   E. c.90_91delinsGGA(p.Ala30_Ser31delinsGly)
   F. None of the above

	Exon 3												Exon 4
	26	27	28	29	30	31	32	33	34	35	36		37
	Gly	Ala	Asn	Leu	Ala	Ser	Pro	Arg	Phe	Gly	Ser		Asp
… cag	GGA	GCC	AAT	CTT	GC**T**	**A**GC	CCT	AGA	TTT	GGT	TCG	gtt … tag	GAC
	76	79	82	85	88	91	94	97	100	103	106		109

43. A reference sequence in the table below is mutated
to … cag GGA GCC AAT CTT G**CGGAT** AGC
CCT AGA TTT GGT TCG gtt … tag GAC in a
sample. Which one of the following nomenclatures
is the most appropriate one to describe this
change?[6]

   A. c.89_90ins(p.Ala30AlaAsp)
   B. c.89_90ins(p.Ala30_Ser31insAsp)
   C. c.89_90insGGA(p.Ala30delinsAlaAsp)
   D. c.89_90insGGA(p.Ala30insAsp)
   E. c.89_90delinsGGA(p.AladelinsAsp)
   F. None of the above

	Exon 3												Exon 4
	26	27	28	29	30	31	32	33	34	35	36		37
	Gly	Ala	Asn	Leu	Ala	Ser	Pro	Arg	Phe	Gly	Ser		Asp
… cag	GGA	GCC	AAT	CTT	G**CT**	AGC	CCT	AGA	TTT	GGT	TCG	gtt … tag	GAC
	76	79	82	85	88	91	94	97	100	103	106		109

44. A reference sequence in the table below is mutated to … cag GGA GCC AAT CTT **GGA GCC** CCT AGA TTT GGT TCG gtt … tag GAC in a sample. Which one of the following nomenclatures is the most appropriate one to describe this change?[6]

A. c.88_93delinsGGAGCC
   (p.Ala30_Ser31delinsGlyAla)
B. c.88_93insdelGGAGCC
   (p.Ala30_Ser31insdelGlyAla)
C. c.88_93delGCTAGCinsGGAGCC
   (p.30_31delAlaSerinsGlyAla)
D. c.88_93insGGAGCCdelGCTAGC
   (p.Gly30_Ala31insdelAlaSer)
E. c.88_93insGGAGCCdelGCTAGC
   (p.30_31insGlyAladelAlaSer)
F. None of the above

	Exon 3												Exon 4
	26	27	28	29	30	31	32	33	34	35	36		37
	Gly	Ala	Asn	Leu	Ala	Ser	Pro	Arg	Phe	Gly	Ser		Asp
… cag	GGA	GCC	AAT	CTT	**GCT**	**AGC**	CCT	AGA	TTT	GGT	TCG	gtt … tag	GAC
	76	79	82	85	88	91	94	97	100	103	106		109

45. A reference sequence in the table below is mutated to … cag GGA GCC AAT CTT GC**AGCC** AGC CCT AGA TTT GGT TCG gtt … tag GAC in a sample. Which one of the following nomenclatures is the most appropriate one to describe this change?[6]

A. c.90T > AGCC(p.Ala30delinsAlaAla)
B. c.90insdelAGCC(p.Ala30insdelAlaALa)
C. c.90delinsAGCC(p.Ala30delinsAlaAla)
D. c.90insAGCCdelT(p.[Ala30 = ;
   Ala30_Ser31insAla)
E. None of the above

	Exon 3												Exon 4
	26	27	28	29	30	31	32	33	34	35	36		37
	Gly	Ala	Asn	Leu	Ala	Ser	Pro	Arg	Phe	Gly	Ser		Asp
… cag	GGA	GCC	AAT	CTT	GC**T**	AGC	CCT	AGA	TTT	GGT	TCG	gtt … tag	GAC
	76	79	82	85	88	91	94	97	100	103	106		109

46. A reference sequence in the table below is mutated to … cag ATG GCC AAT CTT GCT **AGC AGC** TTT GGT TCT … in a sample. ACG in exon 1 of this gene is not a common polymorphism in the general population. Which one of the following nomenclatures is right to describe this change?[6]

A. c.16_18del(p.Ser6del)
B. c.19_21del(p.Ser7del)
C. c.22_24del(p.Ser8del)
D. A and B
E. All of the above
F. None of the above

	Exon 1											
	1	2	3	4	5	6	7	8	9	10	11	
	Met	Ala	Asn	Leu	Ala	Ser	Ser	Ser	Phe	Gly	Ser	
… cag	ATG	GCC	AAT	CTT	GCT	**AGC**	**AGC**	**AGC**	TTT	GGT	TCT	…
	1	4	7	10	13	16	19	22	25	28	31	

47. A reference sequence in the table below is mutated to ... cag ATG GCC AAT CTT GCT **AGC AGC AGC** CGA TTT GGT TCT... in a sample. The variant is not a common polymorphism in the general population. Which one of the following nomenclatures is right to describe this change?[6]

A. c.16_18dupAGC(p.Ser6dup)
B. c.18_19insAGC(p.Ser6_Ser7insSer)
C. c.19_21dupAGC(p.Ser7dup)
D. c.21_22insAGC(p.Ser7_Arg8insSer)
E. All of the above
F. None of the above

Exon 1										
1	2	3	4	5	6	7	8	9	10	11
Met	Ala	Asn	Leu	Ala	Ser	Ser	Arg	Phe	Gly	Ser
ATG	GCC	AAT	CTT	GCT	**AGC**	**AGC**	CGA	TTT	GGT	TCT
1	4	7	10	13	16	19	22	25	28	31

... cag (before ATG) ... (after TCT)

48. A reference sequence in the table below is mutated to ... cag GGA GCC AAT CTT GCT AGC CCT AGA TTT GGT TCG g**ttt g**ac ... in a sample. The variant is not a common polymorphism in the general population. Which one of the following nomenclatures is the most appropriate one to describe this change?[6]

A. c.108 + 2dupT
B. c.108 + 3dupT
C. c.108 + 1_108 + 2insT
D. c.108 + 2_108 + 3insT
E. c.108 + 3_108 + 4insT
F. None of the above

Exon 3										
26	27	28	29	30	31	32	33	34	35	36
Gly	Ala	Asn	Leu	Ala	Ser	Pro	Arg	Phe	Gly	Ser
GGA	GCC	AAT	CTT	GCT	AGC	CCT	AGA	TTT	GGT	TCG
76	79	82	85	88	91	94	97	100	103	106

... cag (before GGA) ... g**tt** g**ac** (after TCG)

49. A reference sequence in the table below is mutated to ... cag ATG **TAA CCG** CTT GCT AGC CCT AGA TTT GGT TCT... in a sample. Which one of the following nomenclatures is correct to describe this change?[6]

A. c.4_9inv6(p.Ala2_Asn3*)
B. c.4_9inv(p.Ala2_Asn3delinsTer)
C. c.4_9inv(p.Ala2_Asn3invTer)
D. p.Ala2Ter
E. None of the above

Exon 1										
1	2	3	4	5	6	7	8	9	10	11
Met	Ala	Asn	Leu	Ala	Ser	Pro	Arg	Phe	Gly	Ser
ATG	**GCC**	**AAT**	CTT	GCT	AGC	CCT	AGA	TTT	GGT	TCT
1	4	7	10	13	16	19	22	25	28	31

... cag (before ATG) ... (after TCT)

50. A reference sequence in the table below is mutated to ... cag ATG **GCC GCC** AAT CTT GCT AGC CCT AGA TTT GGT TCT ... in a sample. Which one of the following nomenclatures is correct to describe this change?[6]

    A. c.4_6GCCdupGCCGCC(p.2Aladup)
    B. c.4_6dupGCC(p.Ala2dup)
    C. g.6_7insGCC(p.2dupAlaAla)
    D. m.4_6dupGCC(p.Ala2AlaAla)
    E. r.4_6GCC > GCCGCC(p.2Ala > AlaAla)

	Exon 1										
	1	2	3	4	5	6	7	8	9	10	11
	Met	Ala	Asn	Leu	Ala	Ser	Pro	Arg	Phe	Gly	Ser
... cag	ATG	**GCC**	AAT	CTT	GCT	AGC	CCT	AGA	TTT	GGT	TCT	...
	1	4	7	10	13	16	19	22	25	28	31

51. A reference sequence in the table below is mutated to ... cag **ATG AAT** CTT GCT AGC CCT AGA TTT GGT TCT ... in a sample. Which one of the following nomenclatures is correct to describe this change?[6]

    A. c.4_6del(p.Ala2del)
    B. c.4_6delGCC(p.Ala2 =)
    C. c.4_6del(p.Ala2_Asn3delinsAsn)
    D. c.4_6delGCC(p.Ala2ext)
    E. None of the above

	Exon 1										
	1	2	3	4	5	6	7	8	9	10	11
	Met	Ala	Asn	Leu	Ala	Ser	Pro	Arg	Phe	Gly	Ser
...cag	**ATG**	**GCC**	**AAT**	CTT	GCT	AGC	CCT	AGA	TTT	GGT	TCT	...
	1	4	7	10	13	16	19	22	25	28	31

52. A reference sequence in the table below is mutated to ... cag ATG GCC **AT C**TT GCT AGC CCT AGA TTT GGT TCT ... in a sample. Which one of the following nomenclatures is right to describe this change?[6]

    A. c.7delA(p.Asn3Ilefs)
    B. c.8delA(p.Asn3Ilefs)
    C. c.7del(p.Asn3fs)
    D. c.8del(p.Asn3fs)
    E. None of the above

	Exon 1										
	1	2	3	4	5	6	7	8	9	10	11
	Met	Ala	Asn	Leu	Ala	Ser	Pro	Arg	Phe	Gly	Ser
... cag	ATG	GCC	**AAT**	**C**TT	GCT	AGC	CCT	AGA	TTT	GGT	TCT	...
	1	4	7	10	13	16	19	22	25	28	31

53. A reference sequence in the table below is mutated to ... cag GGA GCC AAT CTT GCT AGC CCT AGA TTT GGT TCT g<u>tt t</u>a... in a sample. The variant is not a common polymorphism in the general population. Which one of the following nomenclatures is the most appropriate one to describe this change?[6]

A. c.365 + 2del
B. c.365 + 3del
C. c.365 + 4del
D. c.365 + 5del
E. None of the above

Exon 11										
111	112	113	114	115	116	117	118	119	120	121
Gly	Ala	Asn	Leu	Ala	Ser	Pro	Arg	Phe	Gly	Ser
GGA	GCC	AAT	CTT	GCT	AGC	CCT	AGA	TTT	GGT	TCT
333	336	339	342	345	348	351	354	357	360	363

... cag [before table]   g<u>tt tt</u>a... [after table]

54. A reference sequence in the table below is mutated to ... cag GGA GCC AAT CTT GCT AGC CCT AGA TTT GGT TCT gtg <u>tc</u> cat ... in a sample. Which one of the following nomenclatures is NOT appropriate to describe this change?[6]

A. c.365 + 5_365 + 6delGAinsC
B. c.[365 + 5delG;365 + 6A > C]
C. c.[365 + 5G > C;365 + 6delA]
D. c.365 + 5_365 + 6delinsC
E. None of the above

Exon 11										
111	112	113	114	115	116	117	118	119	120	121
Gly	Ala	Asn	Leu	Ala	Ser	Pro	Arg	Phe	Gly	Ser
GGA	GCC	AAT	CTT	GCT	AGC	CCT	AGA	TTT	GGT	TCT
333	336	339	342	345	348	351	354	357	360	363

...cag [before table]   gtg t**ga** cat... [after table]

55. A reference sequence in the table below is mutated to ... cag GGA GCC AAT CTT GCT AGC CCT AGA TTT GGT TCT g<u>tc tct ctc</u> aca t ... in a sample. The TG repeat in intron 11 of this gene is polymorphic in the general population. Which one of the following nomenclatures is appropriate to describe this change?[6]

A. c.365 + 2_365 + 3[4]
B. c.365 + 4_365 + 5[4]
C. c.365 + 2TC[4]
D. c.365 + 2_365 + 5dup
E. A and C
F. A, B, and C
G. All of the above

Exon 11										
111	112	113	114	115	116	117	118	119	120	121
Gly	Ala	Asn	Leu	Ala	Ser	Pro	Arg	Phe	Gly	Ser
GGA	GCC	AAT	CTT	GCT	AGC	CCT	AGA	TTT	GGT	TCT
333	336	339	342	345	348	351	354	357	360	363

... cag [before table]   g<u>tc t</u>ca cat ... [after table]

56. A reference sequence in the table below is mutated to … cag GGA GCC AAT CTT GCT AGC CCT AGA TTT GGT TCT gtc tct ctc aca t … in a sample. The TG repeat in intron 11 of this gene is polymorphic in the general population. Which one of the following nomenclatures is the most appropriate one to describe this change?[6]

  A. c.365 + 2TC[4]
  B. c.365 + 4TC[4]
  C. c.365 + 2_365 + 3TC[4]
  D. c.365 + 4_365 + 5TC[4]
  E. c.365 + 1_365 + 2insTCTC
  F. c.365 + 4_365 + 5ins(TC)2
  G. c.365 + 5_365 + 6insTCTC

	Exon 11											
	111	112	113	114	115	116	117	118	119	120	121	
	Gly	Ala	Asn	Leu	Ala	Ser	Pro	Arg	Phe	Gly	Ser	
… cag	GGA	GCC	AAT	CTT	GCT	AGC	CCT	AGA	TTT	GGT	TCT	gtc tca cat …
	333	336	339	342	345	348	351	354	357	360	363	

57. A reference sequence in the table below is mutated to … cag GGA GCC AAT CTT GCT AGC CCT AGA TTT GGT TCT gtc tct ctc aca t … in a sample. The TG repeat in intron 11 of this gene is polymorphic in the general population. Which one of the following nomenclatures is the most appropriate one to describe this change?[6]

  A. c.365 + 2[4]
  B. c.365 + 4[4]
  C. c.365 + 2_365 + 3[4]
  D. c.365 + 1_365 + 2insTCTC
  E. c.365 + 4_365 + 5ins(TC)2
  F. c.365 + 5_365 + 6insTCTC

	Exon 11											
	111	112	113	114	115	116	117	118	119	120	121	
	Gly	Ala	Asn	Leu	Ala	Ser	Pro	Arg	Phe	Gly	Ser	
… cag	GGA	GCC	AAT	CTT	GCT	AGC	CCT	AGA	TTT	GGT	TCT	gtc tca cat …
	333	336	339	342	345	348	351	354	357	360	363	

58. A reference sequence in the table below is mutated to … cag GGA GCC AAT CTT GCT AGC CCT AGA TTT GGT TCT gtc tct ctc aca t … in a sample. The TG repeat in intron 11 of this gene is polymorphic in the general population. Which one of the following nomenclatures is the most appropriate one to describe this change?[6]

  A. c.365 + 2[4]
  B. c.365 + 4[4]
  C. c.365 + 4_365 + 5[4]
  D. c.365 + 1_365 + 2insTCTC
  E. c.365 + 4_365 + 5ins(TC)2
  F. c.365 + 5_365 + 6insTCTC

	Exon 11											
	111	112	113	114	115	116	117	118	119	120	121	
	Gly	Ala	Asn	Leu	Ala	Ser	Pro	Arg	Phe	Gly	Ser	
… cag	GGA	GCC	AAT	CTT	GCT	AGC	CCT	AGA	TTT	GGT	TCT	gtc tca cat …
	333	336	339	342	345	348	351	354	357	360	363	

59. A technologist analyzed a peripheral-blood sample with an assay for hereditary hemochromatosis in a clinical molecular genetic laboratory. The patient had a C282Y and a H63D mutation in the *HFE* gene. Parental tests confirmed that the C282Y was from the mother, while H63D was from the father. Which one of the following nomenclatures is the most appropriate one for this patient?[6]
   A. p.H63D/C282Y
   B. p.[H63D;C282Y]
   C. p.[H63D];[C282Y]
   D. p.[H63D(;)C282Y]
   E. p.[H63D pat] + [C282Y mat]

60. A technologist analyzed a peripheral-blood sample with an assay for hereditary hemochromatosis in a clinical molecular genetic laboratory. The patient had a C282Y and a H63D mutation in the *HFE* gene. Parental tests have not been done. Which one of the following nomenclatures is the most appropriate one for this patient?[6]
   A. p.H63D/C282Y
   B. p.[H63D;C282Y]
   C. p.[H63D];[C282Y]
   D. p.[H63D(;)C282Y]
   E. p.[H63D pat] + [C282Y mat]

61. A technologist analyzed a peripheral-blood sample with an assay for hereditary hemochromatosis in a clinical molecular genetic laboratory. The patient had a C282Y and a H63D mutation in the *HFE* gene. Parental tests confirmed that both C282Y and H63D were maternal in origin. Which one of the following nomenclatures is the most appropriate one for this patient?[6]
   A. p.H63D/C282Y
   B. p.[H63D;C282Y]
   C. p.[H63D];[C282Y]
   D. p.[H63D(;)C282Y]
   E. p.[H63D pat] + [C282Y mat]

62. Fragile X molecular testing was ordered for a 4-year-old boy with mental retardation. PCR and Southern blot methods were used for the analysis, and they detected one methylated allele with approximately 1000 CGG repeats. Which one of the following nomenclatures is the most appropriate to describe this change?[9–11]
   A. c.-129CGG[1000]
   B. c.-129CGG(1000)
   C. c.-129CGG[1000];[0]
   D. c.-129CGG(1000);[0]
   E. c.-129CGG(1000);(1000)

63. A cystic fibrosis (CF) mutation panel was performed on a pregnant woman. The results showed an R117H mutation with a 5T allele. The parental tests confirmed that both of the variants were maternal in origin. Which one of the

following nomenclatures is the most appropriate one to describe these changes?[6]
   A. c.[350G > A(;)1210-12T[5]]
   B. c.[350G > A;1210-12T[5]]
   C. c.[350G > A];[1210-12T[5]]
   D. c.[350G > A];[(1210-12T[5])]
   E. c.[350G > A(;)1210-12[5]]
   F. c.[350G > A(;)1210-7_1210-6delTT]

64. A cystic fibrosis (CF) mutation panel was performed on a pregnant woman. The results showed an R117H mutation with a 5T allele. The parental tests confirmed that R117H was maternal in origin while 5T was paternal in origin. Which one of the following nomenclatures is the most appropriate one to describe these changes?[6]
   A. c.[350G > A(;)1210-12T[5]]
   B. c.[350G > A;1210-12T[5]]
   C. c.[350G > A];[1210-12T[5]]
   D. c.[350G > A(;)1210-12[5]]
   E. c.[350G > A(;)1210-12[5]]
   F. c.[350G > A;1210-12[5]]

65. A cystic fibrosis (CF) mutation panel was performed on a pregnant woman. The results showed an R117H mutation with a 5T allele. The parental tests have not been done. Which one of the following nomenclatures is the most appropriate one to describe these changes?[6]
   A. c.[350G > A(;)1210-12T[5]]
   B. c.[350G > A;1210-12T[5]]
   C. c.[350G > A];[1210-12T[5]]
   D. c.[350G > A(;)1210-12[5]]
   E. c.[350G > A(;)1210-12[5]]
   F. c.[350G > A;1210-12[5]]

66. A cystic fibrosis (CF) mutation panel was performed on a pregnant woman. The results showed a homozygous deltaF508 mutation. The parental tests have not been done. Which one of the following nomenclatures is the most appropriate one to describe this change?[6]
   A. c.[1521_1523delCTT];[1521_1523delCTT]
   B. c.[1521_1523delCTT];[(1521_1523delCTT)]
   C. c.[(1521_1523delCTT)];[(1521_1523delCTT)]
   D. c.[1521_1523delCTT];[=]
   E. c.[1521_1523delCTT];[0]
   F. None of the above

67. A cystic fibrosis (CF) mutation panel was performed on a pregnant woman. The results showed a heterozygous deltaF508 mutation. Which one of the following nomenclatures is the most appropriate one to describe this change?[6]
   A. c.[1521_1523delCTT];[1521_1523delCTT]
   B. c.[1521_1523delCTT];[(1521_1523delCTT)]
   C. c.[(1521_1523delCTT)];[(1521_1523delCTT)]
   D. c.[1521_1523delCTT];[=]
   E. c.[1521_1523delCTT];[0]
   F. None of the above

68. A reference sequence in the table below is mutated to … cag GGA GCC AAT CTT GCT AGC CCT AGA TTT GGT TCG gtt tga gca … in a sample. Which one of the following nomenclatures is the most appropriate one to describe this change?[6]

A. c.364A > C(p.*121Ser)
B. c.364A > C(p.Ter121Serext2)
C. c.364A > C(p.*121Serext*3)
D. c.362 + 2A > C(p.Ter121Ser)
E. c.364 + 2A > C(p.*121Serext)

	Exon 11											
	111	112	113	114	115	116	117	118	119	120		
	Gly	Ala	Asn	Leu	Ala	Ser	Pro	Arg	Phe	Gly		
… cag	GGA	GCC	AAT	CTT	GCT	AGC	CCT	AGA	TTT	GGT	TAG	gtt tga gca …
	333	336	339	342	345	348	351	354	357	360	363	

69. A reference sequence in the table below is mutated to … cag **ATG CTT** GCT AGC CCT AGA CCT AGA TTT GGT TCT … in a sample. Which one of the following nomenclatures is the most appropriate one to describe this change?[6]

A. c.4_9delGCCAAT(p.2_3del)
B. c.4_9del(p.2_3del)
C. c.4_9GCCAATdel(p.AlaAsn23del)
D. c.4_9del(p.Ala2_Asn3del)
E. g.4_9delGCCAAT(p.Ala2Asn3*)

	Exon 1										
	1	2	3	4	5	6	7	8	9	10	11
	Met	Ala	Asn	Leu	Ala	Ser	Pro	Arg	Phe	Gly	Ser
… cag	**ATG**	**GCC**	**AAT**	**CTT**	GCT	AGC	CCT	AGA	TTT	GGT	TCT	…
	1	4	7	10	13	16	19	22	25	28	31

70. A reference sequence in the table below is mutated to … cag ATG **GCC AAT GCC AAT** CTT GCT AGC CCT AGA TTT GGT TCT … in a sample. Which one of the following nomenclatures is the most appropriate one to describe this change?[6]

A. c.4_9dupGCCAAT(p.2_3dup)
B. c.4_9dup(p.2_3dup)
C. c.4_9dup(p.Ala2_Asn3dup)
D. c.9_10insGCCAAT(p.Ala2_Asn3dup)
E. g.9_10insGCCAAT(p.Asn3_Leu4insAlaAsn)

	Exon 1										
	1	2	3	4	5	6	7	8	9	10	11
	Met	Ala	Asn	Leu	Ala	Ser	Pro	Arg	Phe	Gly	Ser
… cag	ATG	**GCC**	**AAT**	CTT	GCT	AGC	CCT	AGA	TTT	GGT	TCT	…
	1	4	7	10	13	16	19	22	25	28	31

71. A reference sequence in the table below is mutated to ... cag ATG **GCC AGT GGG AAT** CTT GCT AGC CCT AGA TTT GGT TCT ... in a sample. Which one of the following nomenclatures is the most appropriate one to describe this change?[6]

A. c.6_7insAGTGGG(p.Ala2_Asn3insSerGly)

B. c.6_7ins(p.2_3ins)

C. c.6_7AGTGGGins(p.2_3insSerGly)

D. c.6_7ins(p.Ala2_Asn3ins)

E. g.6_7insAGTGGG(p.AlaAsn23insSerGly)

	Exon 1										
	1	2	3	4	5	6	7	8	9	10	11
	Met	Ala	Asn	Leu	Ala	Ser	Pro	Arg	Phe	Gly	Ser
... cag	ATG	**GCC**	**AAT**	CTT	GCT	AGC	CCT	AGA	TTT	GGT	TCT	...
	1	4	7	10	13	16	19	22	25	28	31

72. A reference sequence in the table below is mutated to ... cag ATG **CGA** CTT GCT AGC CCT AGA TTT GGT TCT ... in a sample. Which one of the following nomenclatures is the most appropriate one to describe this change?[6]

A. c.4_9delGCCAATinsCGA(p.Ala2_Asn3insArg)

B. c.4_9delinsCGA(p.2_3delinsArg)

C. c.4_9delGCCAATinsCGA(p. Ala2_Asn3delinsArg)

D. c.4_9delinsCGA(p.Ala2_Asn3insArg)

E. g.4_9insCGA(p.AlaAsn23insArg)

	Exon 1										
	1	2	3	4	5	6	7	8	9	10	11
	Met	Ala	Asn	Leu	Ala	Ser	Pro	Arg	Phe	Gly	Ser
... cag	ATG	**GCC**	**AAT**	CTT	GCT	AGC	CCT	AGA	TTT	GGT	TCT	...
	1	4	7	10	13	16	19	22	25	28	31

73. The chromatograph below shows sequence results of both directions with a peripheral-blood sample from a 6-year-old girl. A C in the reference sequence of a cDNA is mutated to a T at position 268 in a sample from the patient. Which one of the following nomenclatures is the most appropriate one?[6]

A. c.268C > T

B. c.[268C > T];[0]

C. c.[268C > T];[=]

D. c.[268C > T];[?]

E. c.[268C > T];[268C > T]

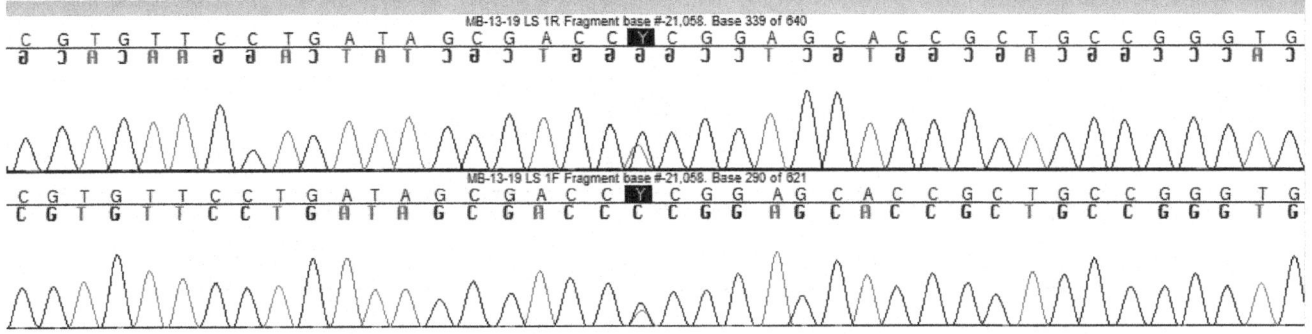

74. The chromatographs below shows sequence results of exon 6 and exon 8 of a gene from both directions with a peripheral-blood sample from a 6-year-old girl. A C in the reference sequence of a cDNA is mutated to a T at position 268 in exon 6, and a C to a T at position 343 in exon 12. The targeted parental tests on these two mutations were pending. Which one of the following nomenclatures is the most appropriate one for this patient?[6]

A. c.[268C > T;343C > T]
B. c.[268C > T];[343C > T]
C. c.[268C > T;343C > T/ =]
D. c.[268C > T(;)343C > T]
E. c.[268C > T/ = ; = /343C > T]

Exon 6

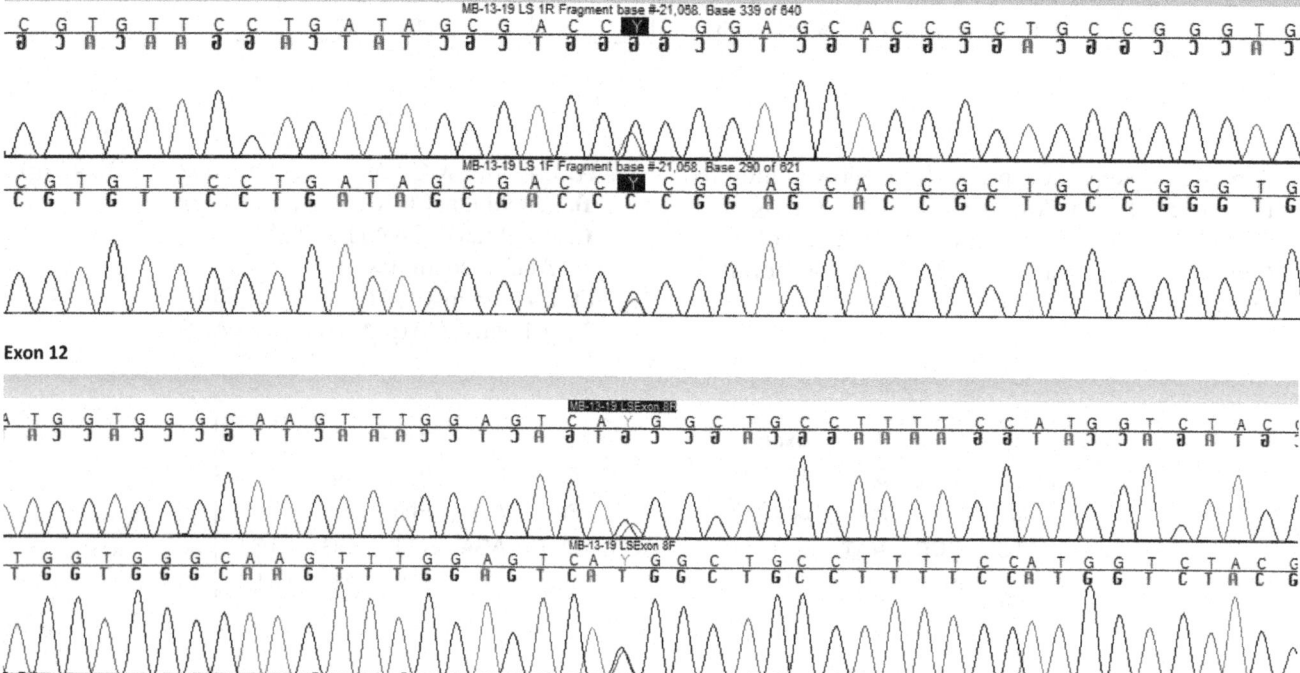

Exon 12

75. The chromatograph below shows sequence results of both directions with a peripheral-blood sample from a 6-year-old girl. A C in the reference sequence of a cDNA is mutated to a T at position 268 in a sample from the patient. The targeted parental tests on this mutation were pending. Which one of the following nomenclatures is the most appropriate one?[6]

A. c.[268C > T;268C > T]
B. c.[268C > T];[(268C > T)]
C. c.[268C > T];[=]
D. c.[268C > T];[268C > T]
E. c.[268C > T];[0]

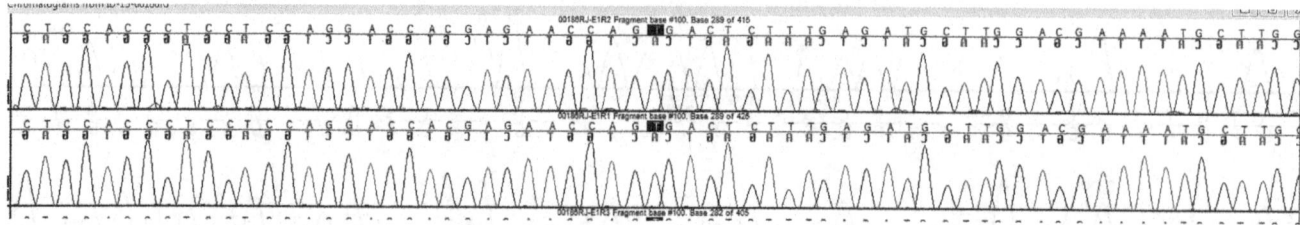

76. A 6-year-old boy was brought to a genetics clinic for developmental delay, intellectual disability, and hypotonia. His karyotype and chromosome microarray results are normal. A gene on chromosome X is suspected to be associated with his symptoms. The chromatograph below shows sequence results of exon 12 in both directions with a peripheral-blood sample from this patient. A C in the reference sequence of a cDNA is mutated to a T at position 268 in a sample from the patient. The targeted parental tests on this mutation were pending. Which one of the following nomenclatures is the most appropriate one?[6]

A. c.[268C > T;268C > T]
B. c.[268C > T];[(268C > T)]
C. c.[268C > T];[=]
D. c.[268C > T];[268C > T]
E. c.[268C > T];[0]

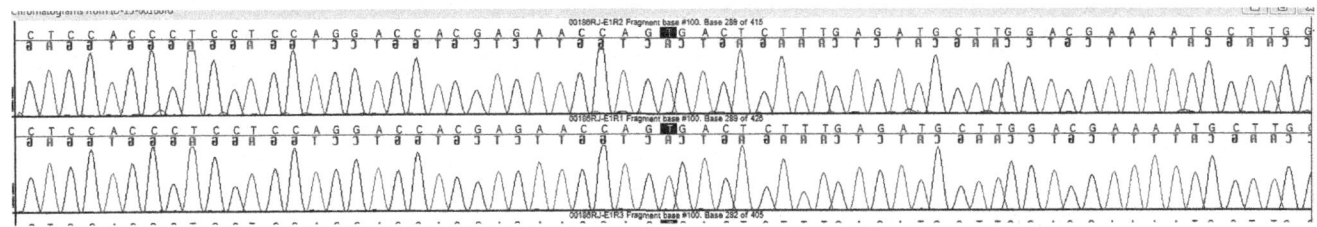

77. A reference sequence in the table below is mutated to ... cag GGA GCC GCA **GCT** AGC CCT AGA TTT GGT TCT gtt tta ... in a sample. Which one of the following nomenclatures is the most appropriate one to describe this change?[6]

A. c.342_344del(p.Ala114del)
B. c.343_345del(p.Ala114_Ala115delinsAla)
C. c.343_345del(p.[Ala114 = ;Ala115del])
D. c.344_346del (p.Ala114_Ala115delinsAla)
E. c.344_346del(p.[Ala114 = ;Ala115del])
F. c.345_347del(p.Ala115del)

			Exon 11							
111	112	113	114	115	116	117	118	119	120	121
Gly	Ala	Ala	Ala	Ala	Ser	Pro	Arg	Phe	Gly	Ser
... cag GGA	GCC	GCA	**GCT**	**GCT**	AGC	CCT	AGA	TTT	GGT	TCT	... gtt tta ...
333	336	339	342	345	348	351	354	357	360	363

78. A reference sequence in the table below is mutated to ... cag GGA GCC GCA GCG **GCT GCT** AGC CCT AGA TTT GGT TCT gtt tta ... in a sample. Which one of the following nomenclatures is the most appropriate one to describe this change?[6]

A. c.344_345insGCT(p.Ala114_Ala115insAla)
B. c.347_348insGCT(p.Ala115_Ser116insAla)
C. c.345dupGCT(p.Ala115dup)
D. c.345_347dupGCT(p.Ala115dupAla)
E. None of the above

			Exon 11							
111	112	113	114	115	116	117	118	119	120	121
Gly	Ala	Ala	Ala	Ala	Ser	Pro	Arg	Phe	Gly	Ser
... cag GGA	GCC	GCA	GCG	**GCT**	AGC	CCT	AGA	TTT	GGT	TCT	... gtt tta ...
333	336	339	342	345	348	351	354	357	360	363

79. A reference sequence in the table below is mutated to … ca**a** ATG GCC AAT CTT GCT AGC CCT AGA T̲T̲T̲ GGT TCT … in a sample. Which one of the following nomenclatures is the most appropriate one to describe this change?[6]

A. c.-1G > A(p.Met1ext)
B. c.1-1G > A(p.-1fs)
C. c.-1G > A(p.-1fs)
D. c.-1G > A
E. None of the above

	Exon 1											
	1	2	3	4	5	6	7	8	9	10	11	
	Met	Ala	Asn	Leu	Ala	Ser	Pro	Arg	Phe	Gly	Ser	
… ca**g**	ATG	GCC	AAT	CTT	GCT	AGC	CCT	AGA	TTT	GGT	TCT	…
	1	4	7	10	13	16	19	22	25	28	31	

80. A reference sequence in the table below is the last exon of a gene, which is mutated to … cag GGA GCC AAT CTT GCT AGC CCT AGA TTT GGT TAG a̲tt tga gca… in a sample. Which one of the following nomenclatures is the most appropriate one to describe this change?

A. c.* + 1G > A
B. c.362 + 4G > A(p.Ter121ext)
C. c.*1G > A
D. c.365 + 1G > A
E. c. + 1G > A(p.*121ext*?)

	Exon 11											
	111	112	113	114	115	116	117	118	119	120		
	Gly	Ala	Asn	Leu	Ala	Ser	Pro	Arg	Phe	Gly		
… cag	GGA	GCC	AAT	CTT	GCT	AGC	CCT	AGA	TTT	GGT	TAG	g̲tt tga gca …
	333	336	339	342	345	348	351	354	357	360	363	

ANSWERS

1. C. Myoclonic Epilepsy with Ragged Red Fibers syndrome is a mitochondrial disease. In over 80% of cases, it is caused by a maternally-inherited mutation at position 8344 in the mitochondrial genome.

According to updated nomenclature for the description of sequence variants by the Human Genome Variation Society in 2016 (http://varnomen.hgvs.org/), to avoid confusion in the description of a variant it should be preceded by a letter indicating the type of reference sequence used. The reference sequence used must contain the residue(s) described to be changed. Possible reference sequence types are the following:

- "c." for a coding DNA sequence (like c.76A > T)
- "g." for a genomic sequence (like g.476A > T)
- *"m." for a mitochondrial sequence (like m.8993T > C)*
- "n" for a noncoding RNA reference sequence (gene producing an RNA transcript but not a protein, see Community consultation 002)
- "r." for an RNA sequence (like r.76a > u)
- "p." for a protein sequence (like p.Lys76Asn)

Therefore, *m.8344A > G* is most likely to be a variant for MERRF.

2. A. Barth syndrome, also known as 3-methylglutaconic aciduria type II, is an X-linked recessive disorder. It is found almost exclusively in males, and is characterized by dilated cardiomyopathy, skeletal myopathy, recurrent infections due to neutropenia, and short stature. Mutations in the *TAZ* gene cause Barth syndrome.

According to updated nomenclature for the description of sequence variants by the Human Genome Variation Society in 2016 (http://varnomen.hgvs.org/), to avoid confusion in the description of a variant it should be preceded by a letter indicating the type of reference sequence used. The reference sequence used must contain the residue(s) described to be changed. Possible reference sequence types are the following:

- *"c." for a coding DNA sequence (like c.76A > T)*
- *"g." for a genomic sequence (like g.476A > T)*
- *"m." for a mitochondrial sequence (like m.8993T > C)*
- *"n." for a noncoding RNA reference sequence (gene producing an RNA transcript but not a protein, see Community consultation 002)*
- *"r." for an RNA sequence (like r.76a > u)*
- *"p." for a protein sequence (like p.Lys76Asn)*

Therefore, *c.153C > G (p.Tyr51Ter)* is most likely to be a functional, effective variant for Barth syndrome.

3. **B.** According to the CAP ACMG Standards and Guidelines for Clinical Genetics Laboratories, 2008 Edition, G1.5, "Clinical reports should describe the level at which the mutation is being described e.g. 'g.' for genomic sequence, 'c.' for cDNA sequence, 'p.' for protein, etc." (http://varnomen.hgvs.org/). In this case, Dr. Z only sequenced the exons of gene and splicing regions, therefore, the nomenclature is referred to cDNA sequence.

Therefore, it should be *c.1268C > T.*

4. **D.** According to the CAP ACMG Standards and Guidelines for Clinical Genetics Laboratories, 2008 Edition, G1.5 "Clinical reports should describe the level at which the mutation is being described e.g. 'g.' for genomic sequence, 'c.' for cDNA sequence, 'p.' for protein, etc." (http://varnomen.hgvs.org/). In this case, Dr. Z sequenced only the exons of gene and splicing regions, so the nomenclature is referred to the cDNA sequence.

Therefore, it should be *p.D401Y.*

5. **A.** There is a tandem duplication of G in the question. According to published nomenclature for the description of sequence variants by the Human Genome Variation Society in 2016 (http://varnomen.hgvs.org/), duplicating insertions are described as duplications, not as insertions; ACTTTGTGCC to ACTTTGT**GG**CC is described as *c.8dupG* (not as c.8_9insG).

Therefore, the correct nomenclature in this question is *c.8dupG.*

6. **F.** The patient in the question has compound heterozygous variants of the *GJB2* and *GJB6* genes. According to published nomenclature for the description of sequence variants by the

Human Genome Variation Society in 2016 (http://varnomen.hgvs.org/), descriptions of sequence changes in different genes (e.g., for recessive diseases) are listed between square brackets, separated by a semicolon and include a reference to the sequence (gene) changed; *DMD:c.[76A > C];GJB:c.[87delG].* There is no requirement with regard to the order of the two genes.

Therefore, both *GJB2:c.[35delG];GJB6:c.[14C > T]* and *GJB6:c.[14C > T];GJB2:c.[35delG]* are correct.

7. **D.** According to published nomenclature for the description of sequence variants by the Human Genome Variation Society in 2016 (http://varnomen.hgvs.org/), "c." is for a coding DNA sequence, such as A (adenine), C (cytosine), G (guanine), or T (thymidine). Uracil (U) presents only in RNA to replace T (thymidine) in DNA. "g." is for a genomic sequence including all nucleotides covering the sequence (gene) of interest. No + , −, or other signs should be used for a genomic sequence (g.). Initial recommendations suggested two alternative descriptions for variants in intron sequences based on a coding DNA reference sequence; the formats c.88 + 2T > G/c.89-1G > T and c.IVS2 + 2T > G/c.IVS2-1G > T. The current recommendation is that the format c.IVS2 + 2T > G/c.IVS2-1G > T should no longer be used. c.*46T > A denotes a T-to-A substitution 46 nucleotides 3′ of the translation termination codon.

Therefore, only *c.*46T > A* is a correct nomenclature in the question.

8. **D.** According to published nomenclature for the description of sequence variants by the Human Genome Variation Society in 2016 (http://varnomen.hgvs.org/), a change affecting the translation initiation codon (Met-1) introducing a new upstream initiation codon extending the N-terminus of the encoded protein described using "ext-#," where "-#" is the position of the new initiation codon (Met-#). For example, *p.Met1ext-5* describes a variant in the 5′ UTR activates a new upstream translation initiation site starting with amino acid Met-5 (methionine-5). Another example is *p.Met1Valext-12*, which is used to describe an amino acid Met1 is changed to Val activating an upstream translation initiation site at position −12 (methionine-12).

Therefore, in this question the appropriate nomenclature is *p.Met1ext-12, or p.Met1Valext-12.*

9. **A.** According to published nomenclature for the description of sequence variants by the Human Genome Variation Society in 2016 (http://varnomen.hgvs.org/), a change affecting the translation termination codon (Ter/*) introducing

a new downstream termination codon extending the C-terminus of the encoded protein described using "extTer#" (alternatively "ext*#"), where "#" is the position of the new stop codon (Ter#/*#). For example, *p.*110Glnext*17* (alternatively *p.Ter110GlnextTer17* or *p.*110Qext*17*) describes a variant in the stop codon (Ter/*) at position 110, changing it to a codon for glutamine (Gln, Q) and adding a tail of new amino acids to the protein's C-terminus ending at a new stop codon (Ter17/*17). Another example is *p.*327Argext*?* (alternatively, *p.Ter327ArgextTer?* or *p.*327Rext*?*), which describes a variant in the stop codon (Ter/*) at position 327, changing it to a codon for arginine (Arg, R) and adding a tail of new amino acids of unknown length since the shifted frame does not contain a new stop codon.

Therefore, in this question the appropriate nomenclature is *p.*110Glnext*17*, or *p.Ter110GlnextTer17*, or *p.*110Qext*17*.

10. **B.** According to published nomenclature for the description of sequence variants by the Human Genome Variation Society in 2016 (http://varnomen.hgvs.org/), chimerism is described using "//." For example, *p.[Arg83 = //Arg83Ser]* describes a chimeric organism in which a chromosome in some cells contains a normal sequence (Arg83 =), while other cells contain another chromosome with Ser at this position (p.Arg83Ser).

Mosaicism is described using "/." For example, p.[Arg83 = /Arg83Ser] describes a somatic case where a chromosome in some cells contains a normal sequence (p.Arg83 =), while other cells contain a Ser at this position (p.Arg83Ser). p.[Ala25Thr];[Gly28Val] describes two changes derived from a gene on each chromosome (one paternal, one maternal); the predicted change is amino acid alanine-25 to threonine on one chromosome and glycine-28 to valine on the other chromosome (RNA or protein analyzed). If two independent changes in one individual are derived from one chromosome, they are described as "[first change;second change]." For example, p.[(Ala25Thr; Gly28Val)] indicates two predicted changes derived from one chromosome (RNA or protein not analyzed); amino acid alanine-25 to threonine and glycine-28 to valine. Two sequence changes in one gene with chromosomes unknown are described as "[change 1(;)change 2]." For example, p.[Ala25Thr(;)Pro323Leu] describes that two changes were identified in one individual (amino acid alanine-25 to threonine and proline-323 to leucine, RNA or protein analyzed), but it is not known whether these changes are on the same

chromosome (in cis) or on different chromosomes (in trans).

Therefore, in this question the appropriate nomenclature is *p.[Arg83 = //Arg83Ser]*.

11. **A.** According to published nomenclature for the description of sequence variants by the Human Genome Variation Society in 2016 (http://varnomen.hgvs.org/), mosaicism is described using "/." For example, *p.[Arg83 = /Arg83Ser]* describes a somatic case in which a chromosome in some cells contains a normal sequence (p.Arg83 =), while other cells contain a Ser at this position (p.Arg83Ser).

Chimerism is described using "//." For example, p.[Arg83 = //Arg83Ser] describes a chimeric organism in which a chromosome in some cells contains a normal sequence (Arg83 =), while other cells contain another chromosome with Ser at this position (p.Arg83Ser). p.[Ala25Thr];[Gly28Val] describes two changes derived from a gene on each chromosome (one paternal, one maternal); the predicted change is amino acid alanine25 to threonine on one chromosome and glycine-28 to valine on the other chromosome (RNA or protein analyzed). If two independent changes in one individual are derived from one chromosome, they are described as "[first change; second change]." For example, p.[(Ala25Thr; Gly28Val)] indicates two predicted changes derived from one chromosome (RNA or protein not analyzed); amino acid alanine-25 to threonine and glycine-28 to valine. Two sequence changes in one gene with chromosomes unknown are described as "[change 1(;)change 2]." For example, p.[Ala25Thr(;)Pro323Leu] describes that two changes were identified in one individual (amino acid alanine-25 to threonine and proline-323 to leucine, RNA or protein analyzed), but it is not known whether these changes are on the same chromosome (in cis) or on different chromosomes (in trans).

Therefore, in this question the appropriate nomenclature is *p.[Arg83 = /Arg83Ser]*.

12. **E.** According to published nomenclature for the description of sequence variants by the Human Genome Variation Society in 2016 (http://varnomen.hgvs.org/), two sequence changes in one gene with chromosomes unknown are described as "[change 1(;)change 2]." For example, *p.[Ala25Thr(;)Pro323Leu]* describes that two changes were identified in one individual (amino acid alanine-25 to threonine and proline-323 to leucine, RNA or protein analyzed), but it is not known whether these changes are on the

same chromosome (in cis) or on different chromosomes (in trans).

Mosaicism is described using "/." For example, p.[Arg83 = /Arg83Ser] describes a somatic case in which a chromosome in some cells contains a normal sequence (p.Arg83 =), while other cells contain a Ser at this position (p.Arg83Ser). Chimerism is described using "//." For example, p.[Arg83 = //Arg83Ser] describes a chimeric organism in which a chromosome in some cells contain a normal sequence (Arg83 =), while other cells contain another chromosome with Ser at this position (p.Arg83Ser). p.[Ala25Thr];[Gly28Val] describes two changes derived from a gene on each chromosome (one paternal, one maternal); the predicted is change amino acid alanine-25 to threonine on one chromosome and glycine-28 to valine on the other chromosome (RNA or protein analyzed). If two independent changes in one individual are derived from one chromosome, they are described as "[first change;second change]." For example, p.[(Ala25Thr; Gly28Val)] indicates two predicted changes derived from one chromosome (RNA or protein not analyzed); amino acid alanine-25 to threonine and glycine-28 to valine.

Therefore, in this question the appropriate nomenclature is *p.[Ala25Thr(;)Pro323Leu]*.

13. **A.** According to published nomenclature for the description of sequence variants by the Human Genome Variation Society in 2016 (http://varnomen.hgvs.org/), *c.[76A > C];[76A > C]* denotes a homozygous A-to-C change at nucleotide 76.

c.[76A > C];[(76A > C)] denotes a homozygous A-to-C change at nucleotide 76, not confirmed by analysis of both parents, leaving the possibility of nonamplification of the sequences analyzed on the other chromosome (e.g., due to a primer mismatch or a deletion). c.[76A > C];[?] denotes an A-to-C change at nucleotide 76 in a gene on one chromosome and an expected not yet detected change on the other chromosome. c.[76A > C];[0] denotes an A-to-C change at nucleotide 76 in a gene on one chromosome and the absence of the entire coding DNA reference sequence on the other.

Therefore, in this question the appropriate nomenclature is *c.[76A > C];[76A > C]*.

14. **D.** According to published nomenclature for the description of sequence variants by the Human Genome Variation Society in 2016 (http://varnomen.hgvs.org/), *c.[76A > C];[0]* denotes a A-to-C change at nucleotide 76 in a gene on one chromosome and the absence of the entire coding

DNA Reference Sequence on the other chromosome.

c.[76A > C];[76A > C] denotes a homozygous A-to-C change at nucleotide 76. c.[76A > C];[(76A > C)] denotes a homozygous A-to-C change at nucleotide 76, not confirmed by analysis of both parents, leaving the possibility of nonamplification of the sequences analyzed on the other chromosome (e.g., due to a primer mismatch or a deletion). c.[76A > C];[?] denotes an A-to-C change at nucleotide 76 in a gene on one chromosome and an expected not yet detected change on the other chromosome.

Therefore, in this question the appropriate nomenclature is *c.[76A > C];[0]*.

15. **D.** According to published nomenclature for the description of sequence variants by the Human Genome Variation Society in 2016 (http://varnomen.hgvs.org/), chimeric is used to describe the occurrence in one individual of two or more cell populations, derived from different zygotes, with different sequences. Chimeric is expressed as "[= //nucleotide 2]." For example, *c.[= //83G > C]* describes a chimeric case in which at position 83, in addition the normal sequence (a G, described as " = "), cells are also found containing another chromosome containing a C at this position (c.83G > C).

Mosaicism—two different nucleotides in one position caused by somatic mosaicisms—are described as "[= /nucleotide 2]." For example, c.[83G = /83G > C] describes a mosaic case in which at position 83, in addition to the normal sequence (a G, described as " = "), chromosomes are also found containing a C (c.83G > C).

Therefore, in this question the appropriate nomenclature is *c.[= //83G > C]*.

16. **A.** According to published nomenclature for the description of sequence variants by the Human Genome Variation Society in 2016 (http://varnomen.hgvs.org/), mosaicism is used to describe the occurrence in one individual of two or more cell populations, derived from a single zygote, with different sequences. Mosaicisms are described as "[= /nucleotide 2]." For example, *c.[83G = /83G > C]* describes a mosaic case in which at position 83, in addition to the normal sequence (a G, described as " = ") chromosomes are also found containing a C (c.83G > C).

Chimerism is used to describe the occurrence in one individual of two or more cell populations, derived from different zygotes, with different sequences. Chimeric is expressed as "[= //nucleotide 2]." For example, c. [= //83G > C] describes a chimeric case in which at position 83, in addition to the normal sequence (a G, described as " = "), cells are also found containing another chromosome containing a C at this position (c.83G > C).

Therefore, in this question the appropriate nomenclature is *c.[83G = /83G > C]*.

17. **C.** According to published nomenclature for the description of sequence variants by the Human Genome Variation Society in 2016 (http://varnomen.hgvs.org/), an "r." is used to indicate that a change is described at the RNA level and nucleotides are designated by the bases (in lower case). T (tyrosine) is one of the bases for DNA, which is replaced by u (uracil) at RNA level. r.[76t > c] is not correct. And *r.78u > a* denotes that at nucleotide 78 a U is changed to an A. *r.[= ,73_88del]* denotes the nucleotide change c.76A > C causing the appearance of two RNA molecules, one normal transcript (r. =) and one containing a deletion of nucleotides 73−88 (shift of the splice donor site to within the exon).

"m." is for a mitochondrial sequence (like m.8993T > C). "U" is not a nucleotide in mitochondrial sequence. Mitochondrial DNAs are circulating DNAs in mitochondria, which are not diploid. So m.[= ,73_88del] and m.[76u > c] are not correct.

Therefore, in this question, *r.[= ,73_88del]* is the appropriate nomenclature.

18. **B.** According to published nomenclature for the description of sequence variants by the Human Genome Variation Society in 2016 (http://varnomen.hgvs.org/), an "r." is used to indicate that a change is described at the RNA level, and nucleotides are designated by the bases (in lower case). T (tyrosine) is one of the bases for DNA, which is replaced by u (uracil) at the RNA level. So r.[88G > A], r.[76T > C], and r.[76t > c,73_88del] are not appropriate nomenclatures.

r.[= , 73_88del] denotes the nucleotide change c.76A > C, causing the appearance of two RNA molecules, one normal transcript (r. =) and one containing a deletion of nucleotides 73−88 (shift of the splice donor site to within the exon). It is the only appropriate nomenclature in this question.

19. **B.** GCT, *GCC*, GCA, and GCG code for alanine (Ala/A). TCA, TCT, *TCC*, TCG, AGT, and AGC code for serine (Ser/S). There is a single base-pair substitution in the exon 1 of the gene, which causes a missense variant at the amino acid sequence. The alanine at position 2 is replaced by serine. This is an in-frame change.

According to published nomenclature for the description of sequence variants by the Human Genome Variation Society in 2016 (http://

varnomen.hgvs.org/), "c." is for a coding DNA sequence. *c.76A > C* denotes that at nucleotide 76 an A is changed to a C. A "p." preceding the change is used to indicate a description at the protein level. An example of missense variant is *p.Trp26Cys*, which denotes that amino acid tryptophan-26 (Trp, W) is changed to a cysteine (Cys).

In this case the second amino acid, alanine, is changed to serine. Therefore, in this question the appropriate nomenclature is *c.4C > T(p.A2S)*, or *c.4C > T(p.Ala2Ser)*.

20. **C.** GCT, *GCC*, GCA, and GCG code for alanine (Ala/A). TCA, TCT, *TCC*, TCG, AGT, and AGC code for serine (Ser/S). There is a single base-pair substitution in the exon 1 of the gene, which causes a missense variant at the amino acid sequence. The alanine at position 2 is replaced by serine. This is an in-frame change.

According to published nomenclature for the description of sequence variants by the Human Genome Variation Society in 2016 (http://varnomen.hgvs.org/), "c." is for a coding DNA sequence. *c.76A > C* denotes that at nucleotide 76 an A is changed to a C. *Descriptions at the protein level may only be given in addition to a description at DNA (and RNA) level. Amino acids are described as "Trp26" or "W26," that is, with capital first letter, not as "trp26" or "w26"), and the 3-letter amino acid code is preferred to describe the amino acid residues.* For example, *p. Trp26Cys* denotes that amino acid tryptophan-26 (Trp, W) is changed to a cysteine (Cys).

In this case the second amino acid, alanine, is changed to serine. Therefore, in this question the appropriate nomenclature is *c.4C > T(p.A2S)*, or *c.4C > T(p.Ala2Ser)*.

21. **C.** GCT, *GCC*, GCA, and GCG code for alanine (Ala/A). TGT and *TGC* code for cysteine (Cys/C). There is a 2-bp deletion in the exon 1 of the gene, which is accompanied by 2-bp insertion at the same location. This change causes a missense variant at the amino acid sequence. The alanine at position 2 is replaced by cysteine. This is an in-frame change.

According to published nomenclature for the description of sequence variants by the Human Genome Variation Society in 2016 (http://varnomen.hgvs.org/), "c." is for a coding DNA sequence (like c.76A > T). Deletion/insertions of two or more consecutive nucleotides (indels) are described as a deletion followed by an insertion. The description *c.76_77delinsTT* is preferred over c.[76G > T; 77G > T]. Based on the definition of a substitution this change cannot be described as a substitution (like c.76_77AG > TT or c.76AG > TT).

Two variations in one allele, separated by at least one nucleotide, are described as "[first change; second change]." For example, c.[76A > C; 83G > C] denotes two changes in one allele: an A-to-C change at nucleotide 76 and a G-to-C change at nucleotide 83.

"p." for a protein sequence (like p.Lys76Asn). "Amino acid substitutions (missense changes) replace one amino acid by one other amino acid and are described using the format p.Trp26Cys. The description does not use the ">" character used on DNA and RNA levels (indicating "changes to")."

Therefore, in this question the appropriate nomenclature is *c.4_5delinsTG(p.A2C)*, or *c.4_5delinsTG(p.Ala2Cys)*, or *c.4_5delGCinsTG(p.Ala2Cys)*. And c.[4G > T;5C > G](p.Ala2Cys) is correct, but not preferred.

22. **E.** There is a 2-bp deletion in the 5′ upstream region of the gene, which is accompanied by a 2-bp insertion at the same location. This change is not associated with amino acid change, but may cause a splicing change.

According to published nomenclature for the description of sequence variants by the Human Genome Variation Society in 2016 (http://varnomen.hgvs.org/), deletion/insertions of two or more consecutive nucleotides (indels) are described as a deletion followed by an insertion. The description *c.76_77delinsTT* is preferred over *c.[76G > T; 77G > T]*. Based on the definition of a substitution this change cannot be described as a substitution (like c.76_77AG > TT or c.76AG > TT). c.-14G > C denotes a G-to-C substitution 14 nucleotides 5′ of the ATG translation initiation codon.

Therefore, in this question the appropriate nomenclature is *c.-3_-2delCAinsTT*, or *c.-3_-2delinsTT*. And *c.[-3C > T;-2A > T]* is correct but is not preferred.

23. **D.** There is a 2-bp deletion in the intron 1 of the gene, which is accompanied by 2-bp insertion at the same location. This change is not associated with an amino acid change, but may cause a splicing change.

According to published nomenclature for the description of sequence variants by the Human Genome Variation Society in 2016 (http://varnomen.hgvs.org/), deletion/insertions of two or more consecutive nucleotides (indels) are described as a deletion followed by an insertion. The description *c.76_77delinsTT* is preferred over *c.[76G > T; 77G > T]*. Based on the definition of a substitution this change cannot be described as a substitution (like c.76_77AG > TT or c.76AG > TT).

c.88 + 1G > T denotes the G-to-T substitution at nucleotide +1 of an intron (in the coding DNA positioned between nucleotides 88 and 89). Initial recommendations suggested two alternative descriptions for variants in intron sequences based on a coding DNA reference sequence; the formats c.88 + 2T > G/c.89-1G > T and c.IVS2 + 2T > G/c.IVS2-1G > T. The current recommendation is that the format c.IVS2 + 2T > G/c.IVS2-1G > T should no longer be used.

Therefore, in this question the appropriate nomenclature is *c.33 + 2_ + 3delinsTT*, or *c.33 + 2_ + 3delCAinsTT*. Also, *c.[33 + 2C > T;33 + 3A > T]* is correct but is not preferred.

24. **E.** There is a 2-bp deletion in the intron 1 of the gene, which is accompanied by 2-bp insertion at the same location. This change is not associated with amino acid change, but it may cause a splicing change.

According to published nomenclature for the description of sequence variants by the Human Genome Variation Society in 2016 (http://varnomen.hgvs.org/), deletion/insertions of two or more consecutive nucleotides (indels) are described as a deletion followed by an insertion. The description *c.76_77delinsTT* is preferred over *c.[76G > T; 77G > T]*. Based on the definition of a substitution this change cannot be described as a substitution (like c.76_77AG > TT or c.76AG > TT).

c.88 + 1G > T denotes the G-to-T substitution at nucleotide +1 of an intron (in the coding DNA positioned between nucleotides 88 and 89). c.*46T > A denotes a T-to-A substitution 46 nucleotides 3′ of the translation termination codon. Initial recommendations suggested two alternative descriptions for variants in intron sequences based on a coding DNA reference sequence; the formats c.88 + 2T > G/c.89-1G > T and c.IVS2 + 2T > G/c.IVS2-1G > T. The current recommendation is that the format c.IVS2 + 2T > G/c.IVS2-1G > T should no longer be used.

Therefore, in this question the appropriate nomenclature is *c.33 + 2_ + 3delinsTT*, or *c.33 + 2_ + 3delCAinsTT*. Also, *c.[33 + 2C > T;33 + 3A > T]* is correct, but it is not preferred.

25. **B.** There is a single base-pair substitution in intron 2 of the gene. This change is not associated with an amino acid change, but it may cause a splicing change.

According to published nomenclature for the description of sequence variants by the Human Genome Variation Society in 2016 (http://varnomen.hgvs.org/), *c.89-2A > C* denotes the

A-to-C substitution at nucleotide-2 of an intron (in the coding DNA positioned between nucleotides 88 and 89).

c.76A > C denotes that at nucleotide 76 an A is changed to a C. c.-14G > C denotes a G-to-C substitution 14 nucleotides 5′ of the ATG translation initiation codon. c.88 + 1G > T denotes the G-to-T substitution at nucleotide +1 of an intron (in the coding DNA positioned between nucleotides 88 and 89). c.*46T > A denotes a T-to-A substitution 46 nucleotides 3′ of the translation termination codon.

Therefore, in this question the appropriate nomenclature is *c.76-3G > A.*

26. **A.** There is a single base-pair substitution in intron 2 of the gene. This change is not associated with an amino acid change, but it may cause a splicing change.

According to published nomenclature for the description of sequence variants by the Human Genome Variation Society in 2016 (http:// varnomen.hgvs.org/), *c.89-2A > C* denotes the A-to-C substitution at nucleotide-2 of an intron (in the coding DNA positioned between nucleotides 88 and 89). This variant may affect the 3′ splicing recognition site, "Acceptor," in intron 2. It may cause the whole exon 3 to be spliced out, or it may activate another potential acceptor site downstream. The effect at the amino acid level is hard to predict. So it is better to leave out the nomenclature for the protein variant.

Therefore, in this case the splicing change may be described as *c.76-1G > A.*

27. **A.** There is a single base-pair substitution in the intron 3 of the gene. This change is not associated with an amino acid change, but it may cause a splicing change.

According to published nomenclature for the description of sequence variants by the Human Genome Variation Society in 2016 (http:// varnomen.hgvs.org/), *c.88 + 1G > T* denotes the G-to-T substitution at nucleotide +1 of an intron (in the coding DNA positioned between nucleotides 88 and 89). This variant may affect the 5′ splicing recognition site, "donor," in intron 3. It may cause the whole intron 3 to be spliced in, or it may activate another potential donor site downstream. The effect at the amino acid level is hard to predict. So it is better to leave out the nomenclature for the protein variant.

Therefore, in this case the splicing change may be described as *c.108 + 2T > C.*

28. **B.** TAG, TAA, and *TGA* are stop codons. This change causes a missense variant at the amino acid sequence. The glycine at position 26 is replaced by a stop codon. This is a nonsense change.

According to published nomenclature for the description of sequence variants by the Human Genome Variation Society in 2016 (http:// varnomen.hgvs.org/), *c.76A > C* denotes that at nucleotide 76 an A is changed to a C. *Descriptions at the protein level may be given only in addition to a description at the DNA (and RNA) level.* Amino acids are described as "Trp26" or "W26," that is, with a capital first letter (not as "trp26" or "Trp26")—and the 3-letter amino acid code is preferred to describe the amino acid residues. The protein coding sequence ends at a translation termination codon (stop codon), described at protein level as *"Ter"* or *"*"* ("*" in 1- and 3-letter amino acid code). At the amino acid level, the nonsense variant is a special type of amino acid deletion introducing an immediate translation stop codon and is described like an amino acid substitution (*p. Trp26Ter* or *p.Trp26**).

Therefore, in this question the appropriate nomenclature is *c.76G > T(p.Gly26Ter)*, or *c.76G > T (p.Gly26*)*, or *c.76G > T(p.G26*)*.

29. **E.** TAG, TAA, and *TGA* are stop codons. This change causes a missense variant at the amino acid sequence. The glycine at position 26 is replaced by a stop codon. This is a nonsense change.

According to published nomenclature for the description of sequence variants by the Human Genome Variation Society in 2016 (http:// varnomen.hgvs.org/), *c.76A > C* denotes that at nucleotide 76 an A is changed to a C. The protein coding sequence ends at a translation termination codon (stop codon), described at the protein level as *"Ter"* or *"*"* ("*" in 1- and 3-letter amino acid code). And at the amino acid level, a nonsense variant is a special type of amino acid deletion introducing an immediate translation stop codon and is described like an amino acid substitution (*p. Trp26Ter* or *p.Trp26**).

Therefore, in this question the appropriate nomenclature is *c.76G > T(p.Gly26Ter)*, or *c.76G > T (p.Gly26*)*, or *c.76G > T(p.G26*)*.

30. **D.** *TAG*, TAA, and TGA are stop codons. There is a single base-pair substitution in the 3′ downstream region of the gene. This variant is not associated with amino acid change, but it may cause a nonstop change.

According to published nomenclature for the description of sequence variants by the Human Genome Variation Society in 2016 (http:// varnomen.hgvs.org/), *c.*46T > A* denotes a T-to-A substitution 46 nucleotides 3′ of the translation termination codon. c.88 + 1G > T denotes the

G-to-T substitution at nucleotide +1 of an intron (in the coding DNA positioned between nucleotides 88 and 89). Initial recommendations suggested two alternative descriptions for variants in intron sequences based on a coding DNA reference sequence: the formats c.88 + 2T > G/c.89-1G > T and c.IVS2 + 2T > G/c.IVS2-1G > T. The current recommendation is that the format c. IVS2 + 2T > G/c.IVS2-1G > T should no longer be used.

The nucleotide 3′ of the translation stop codon is *1, the next *2. Therefore, in this question the appropriate nomenclature is *c.*1G > T.*

31. **A.** *TAG*, TAA, and TGA are stop codons. *TAT* and TAC are the codons for tyrosine (Tyr/Y). There is a single base-pair substitution in the 3′ downstream region of the gene. The stop codon at position 121 is replaced by a tyrosine. This is a nonstop change.

According to published nomenclature for the description of sequence variants by the Human Genome Variation Society in 2016 (http://varnomen.hgvs.org/), a no-stop change (change in stop codon, Ter/*) is a change affecting the translation termination codon (Ter, *) and is described as an extension (*p.Ter110GlnextTer17* or *p.*110Glnext*17*).

Initial recommendations suggested two alternative descriptions for variants in intron sequences based on a coding DNA reference sequence: the formats c.88 + 2T > G/c.89-1G > T and c.IVS2 + 2T > G/c.IVS2-1G > T. The current recommendation is that the format c. IVS2 + 2T > G/c.IVS2-1G > T should no longer be used.

Therefore, in this question the appropriate nomenclature is *c.365G > T(p.Ter121TyrextTer22),* or *c.365G > T(p.*121Tyrext*22),* or *c.365G > T (p.*121Yext*22).*

32. **C.** *TAG*, TAA, and TGA are stop codons. *TAT* and TAC are the codons for tyrosine (Tyr/Y). There is a single base-pair substitution in the 3′ downstream region of the gene. The stop codon at position 121 is replaced by a tyrosine. This is a no-stop change.

According to published nomenclature for the description of sequence variants by the Human Genome Variation Society in 2016 (http://varnomen.hgvs.org/), *c.76A > C* denotes that at nucleotide 76 an A is changed to a C. The protein-coding sequence ends at a translation termination codon (stop codon), described at the protein level as *"Ter"* or *"*"* (*"*"* in 1- and 3-letter amino acid code). A no-stop change (change in stop codon, Ter/*) is on that affects the translation termination

codon (Ter, *) and is described as an extension (*p. Ter110GlnextTer17* or *p.*110Glnext*17)."*

So-called silent changes can be described using p.(Leu54 =). The format p.(Leu54Leu) (or p.(L54L)) should not be used. Amino acids are described as "Trp26" or "W26," that is, with a capital first letter (not as "trp26" or "Trp26").

Therefore, in this question the appropriate nomenclature is *c.365G > T(p.Ter121TyrextTer22),* or *c.365G > T(p.*121Tyrext*22),* or *c.365G > T (p.*121Yext*22).*

33. **C.** *TAG*, TAA, and TGA are stop codons. There is a single base-pair substitution in exon 11 of the gene. It causes a silent change.

According to published nomenclature for the description of sequence variants by the Human Genome Variation Society in 2016 (http://varnomen.hgvs.org/), *c.76A > C* denotes that at nucleotide 76 an A is changed to a C. Descriptions at the protein level may be given only in addition to a description at the DNA (and RNA) level, amino acids are described as "Trp26" or "W26," that is, with capital first letter (not as "trp26" or "Trp26"), and the 3-letter amino acid code is preferred to describe the amino acid residues. The protein-coding sequence ends at a translation termination codon (stop codon), described at protein level as *"Ter"* or *"*"* (*"*"* in 1- and 3-letter amino acid code). So-called silent changes can be described using *p.(Leu54 =).* The format p. (Leu54Leu) (or p.(L54L)) should not be used.

Amino acids are described as "Trp26" or "W26," that is, with a capital first letter (not as "trp26" or "Trp26"). Initial recommendations suggested two alternative descriptions for variants in intron sequences based on a coding DNA reference sequence: the formats c.88 + 2T > G/c.89-1G > T and c.IVS2 + 2T > G/c.IVS2-1G > T. The current recommendation is that the format c. IVS2 + 2T > G/c.IVS2-1G > T should no longer be used.

Therefore, in this question the appropriate nomenclature is *c.365G > T(p.Ter121 =),* or *c.365G > T(p.*121 =).*

34. **E.** *TAG*, TAA, and *TGA* are stop codons. There is a single base-pair substitution in exon 11 of the gene. It causes a silent change.

According to published nomenclature for the description of sequence variants by the Human Genome Variation Society in 2016 (http://varnomen.hgvs.org/), *c.76A > C* denotes that at nucleotide 76 an A is changed to a C. The protein-coding sequence ends at a translation termination codon (stop codon), described at the protein level as *"Ter"* or *"*"*

("*" in 1- and 3-letter amino acid code)." So-called silent changes can be described using *p.(Leu54 =)*. The format p.(Leu54Leu) (or p.(L54L)) should not be used.

Descriptions at the protein level may be given only in addition to a description at the DNA (and RNA) level, amino acids are described as "Trp26" or "W26," that is, with a capital first letter (not as "trp26" or "Trp26"), and the 3-letter amino acid code is preferred to describe the amino acid residues.

Therefore, in this question the appropriate nomenclature is *c.365G > T(p.Ter121 =)*, or *c.365G > T(p.*121 =)*.

35. **A.** *ATG* is the start codon; it also codes for methionine (Met/M). TTA, *TTG*, CTT, CTA, CTC, and CTG code for leucine (Leu/L). There is a single base-pair substitution in exon 1 of the gene. The first codon in exon 1 is changed to Leu from Met, which activates a new initiation codon at the 5′ upstream region.

According to published nomenclature for the description of sequence variants by the Human Genome Variation Society in 2016 (http://varnomen.hgvs.org/), *c.76A > C* denotes that at nucleotide 76 an A is changed to a C. A change affecting the translation initiation codon (Met-1) introduces a new upstream initiation codon extending the N-terminus of the encoded protein described using "ext-#," where "-#" is the position of the new initiation codon (Met-#). "For example, *p.Met1ext-5*, a variant in the 5′ UTR, activates a new upstream translation initiation site starting with amino acid Met-5 (methionine-5). Another example, *p.Met1Valext-12* describes amino acid Met1 is changed to Val activating an upstream translation initiation site at position −12 (methionine-12)."

Descriptions at the protein level may be given only in addition to a description at the DNA (and RNA) level. Amino acids are described as "Trp26" or "W26," that is, with capital first letter (not as "trp26" or "Trp26"). And the 3-letter amino acid code is preferred to describe the amino acid residues.

Therefore, in this question the appropriate nomenclature is *c.1A > T(p.Met1ext-5)*, or *c.1A > T (p.Met1Leuext-5)*, or *c.1A > T(p.M1ext-5)*, or *c.1A > T (p.M1Lext-5)*.

36. **E.** *ATG* is the start codon; it also codes for methionine (Met/M). TTA, *TTG*, CTT, CTA, CTC, and CTG code for leucine (Leu/L). There is a single base-pair substitution in exon 1 of the gene. The first codon in exon 1 is changed to Leu from Met, which activates a new initiation codon at the 5′ upstream region.

According to published nomenclature for the description of sequence variants by the Human Genome Variation Society in 2016 (http://varnomen.hgvs.org/), *c.76A > C* denotes that at nucleotide 76 an A is changed to a C. A change affecting the translation initiation codon (Met-1) introduces a new upstream initiation codon extending the N-terminus of the encoded protein described using "ext-#," where "-#" is the position of the new initiation codon (Met-#). For example, *p.Met1ext-5*, a variant in the 5′ UTR, activates a new upstream translation initiation site starting with amino acid Met-5 (methionine-5). Another example, *p.Met1Valext-12* describes amino acid Met1 changing to Val, activating an upstream translation initiation site at position −12 (methionine-12).

Descriptions at the protein level may be given only in addition to a description at the DNA (and RNA) level. Amino acids are described as "Trp26" or "W26," that is, with a capital first letter (not as "trp26" or "Trp26"). And the 3-letter amino acid code is preferred to describe the amino acid residues.

Therefore, in this question the appropriate nomenclature is *c.1A > T(p.Met1ext-5)*, or *c.1A > T (p.Met1Leuext-5)*, or *c.1A > T(p.M1ext-5)*, or *c.1A > T (p.M1Lext-5)*.

37. **B.** *GCT, GCA*, GCC, and GCG code for alanine (Ala/A). There is a single base-pair deletion in the question, which causes a frameshift change at the amino acid level. Since both GCT and GCA code for alanine, the amino acid sequence at position 30 is not changed.

According to published nomenclature for the description of sequence variants by the Human Genome Variation Society in 2016 (http://varnomen.hgvs.org/), a nucleotide deletion is a sequence change in which one or more nucleotides are removed. Deletions are described using "del" after an indication of the first and last nucleotide(s) deleted, separated by a an underscore. For all descriptions, the most 3′ position possible is arbitrarily assigned to have been changed. For example, *c.76_78del* (alternatively, *c.76_78delACT*) denotes a ACT deletion from nucleotides 76 to 78. Frameshifts are described using the format *p. Arg97Glyfs*26* (alternatively, *p.Arg97GlyfsTer26*, or for short, *p.Arg97fs*), where Arg97Gly describes the change of the first amino acid affected (Arg97 replaced by a Pro residue), "fs" indicates the frameshift, and *16 gives the position of the translation termination codon (stop codon) in the new reading frame. "p.Ala30 =)" is used to describe a silent change at the amino acid level.

Descriptions at the protein level may be given only in addition to a description at the DNA (and RNA) level. Amino acids are described as "Trp26" or "W26," that is, with a capital first letter (not as "trp26" or "Trp26"), and the 3-letter amino acid code is preferred to describe the amino acid residues.

Therefore, in this question the appropriate nomenclature is *c.90del(p.A30fs)*, or *c.90delT(p. Ala30AlafsTer26)*, or *c.90delT(p.A30Afs*26)*.

38. **C.** *GCT*, GCA, GCC, and GCG code for alanine (Ala/A). GAA and *GAG* codes for glutamic acid (Glu/E). And TAA, *TAG*, and TGA are the stop codons. There is a 2-bp deletion at exon 3 of a gene in the question, which causes a frameshift change at the position 30 of amino acid sequence from alanine to glutamic acid. After the change, the third codon is TAG, a stop codon.

According to published nomenclature for the description of sequence variants by the Human Genome Variation Society in 2016 (http:// varnomen.hgvs.org/), a nucleotide deletion is a sequence change in which one or more nucleotides are removed. Deletions are described using "del" after an indication of the first and last nucleotide(s) deleted, separated by an underscore. For all descriptions the most 3′ position possible is arbitrarily assigned to have been changed. For example, *c.76_78del* (alternatively, *c.76_78delACT*) denotes an ACT deletion from nucleotides 76 to 78. Frameshifts are described using the format *p. Arg97Glyfs*26* (alternatively, *p.Arg97GlyfsTer26*, or for short, *p.Arg97fs*), where Arg97Gly describes the change of the first amino acid affected (Arg97 replaced by a Pro residue), "fs" indicates the frameshift, and *16 gives the position of the translation termination codon (stop codon) in the new reading frame.

Descriptions at the protein level may be given only in addition to a description at the DNA (and RNA) level. Amino acids are described as "Trp26" or "W26," that is, with a capital first letter (not as "trp26" or "Trp26"). The 3-letter amino acid code is preferred to describe the amino acid residues. "p.Ala30 = " is used to describe a silent change at amino acid level. p.Ala30Glu is used to describe an amino acid substitution, but not a frameshift change.

Therefore, in this question the appropriate nomenclature is *c.89_90del(p.A30fs)*, or *c.89_90del(p. Ala30)*, or *c.89_90del(p.Ala30fsTer26)*, or *c.89_90delCT(p.Ala30GlufsT*26)*, or *c.89_90delCT(p. A30Efs*26)*.

39. **D.** *GCT*, GCA, GCC, and GCG code for alanine (Ala/A). TCT, TCA, TCC, TCG, AGT, and *AGC*

code for serine (Ser/S). GGT, GGA, *GGC*, and GGG code for glycine (Gly/G). There is a 3-bp deletion at exon 3 of a gene in the question, which causes a glycine to replace the alanine at position 30 and the serine at position 31. This is an in-frame change.

According to published nomenclature for the description of sequence variants by the Human Genome Variation Society in 2016 (http:// varnomen.hgvs.org/), a nucleotide deletion is a sequence change in which one or more nucleotides are removed. Deletions are described using "del" after an indication of the first and last nucleotide(s) deleted, separated by an underscore. For all descriptions, the most 3′ position possible is arbitrarily assigned to have been changed. For example, *c.76_78del* (alternatively, *c.76_78delACT*) denotes an ACT deletion from nucleotides 76 to 78. Deletion/insertions (indels) replace one or more amino acid residues with one or more other amino acid residues. Deletion/insertions are described using "delins" as a deletion followed by an insertion after an indication of the amino acid(s) deleted separated by an underscore. For example, *p.(Cys28_Lys29delinsTrp)*, which indicates neither RNA nor protein, was analyzed, but the predicted change is a 3-bp deletion that affects the codons for cysteine-28 and lysine-29, substituting them for a codon for tryptophan.

Descriptions at the protein level may be given only in addition to a description at the DNA (and RNA) level. Amino acids are described as "Trp26" or "W26," that is, with a capital first letter (not as "trp26" or "Trp26"). The 3-letter amino acid code is preferred to describe the amino acid residues. "p.Ala30 = " is used to describe a silent change at the amino acid level. p.Ala30Gly is used to describe an amino acid substitution but not a deletion.

Therefore, in this question the appropriate nomenclature is *c.89_91del(p.A30_S31delinsG)*, or *c.89_91delCTA(p.Ala30_Ser31delinsGly)*.

40. **A.** TCT, TCA, TCC, and *TCG* code for serine (Ser/S). There is a single base-pair deletion in the question. Since RNA analysis shows the effect on splicing, the G was deleted from the end of exon 3 instead of the beginning of intron 4. This deletion causes a frameshift at the amino acid level, although the amino acid sequence at position 36 is not changed.

According to published nomenclature for the description of sequence variants by the Human Genome Variation Society in 2016 (http:// varnomen.hgvs.org/), a nucleotide deletion is a sequence change in which one or more nucleotides are removed. Deletions are described using "del" after an indication of the first and last nucleotide(s) deleted, separated by an underscore. For all descriptions, the most 3' position possible is arbitrarily assigned to have been changed. For example, *c.76_78del* (alternatively, *c.76_78delACT*) denotes an ACT deletion from nucleotides 76 to 78. Deletion/insertions (indels) replace one or more amino acid residues with one or more other amino acid residues. Deletion/insertions are described using "delins" as a deletion followed by an insertion after an indication of the amino acid(s) deleted separated by an underscore. For example, *p.(Cys28_Lys29delinsTrp)* indicates that neither RNA nor protein was analyzed, but the predicted change is a 3-bp deletion that affects the codons for cysteine-28 and lysine-29, substituting them for a codon for tryptophan. When the exon 3/intron 3 border is ..CAGgtg.. and RNA analysis shows no effect on splicing but a deletion of a G the change ..CA**Gg**tg.. to ..CA**g**tg.., it is described as *c.3delG* and not c.3 + 1delG.

Descriptions at the protein level may be given only in addition to a description at DNA (and RNA) level, amino acids are described as "Trp26" or "W26," that is, with capital first letter (not as "trp26" or "Trp26"). The 3-letter amino acid code is preferred to describe the amino acid residues. "p.Ala30 = " is used to describe a silent change at amino acid level. p.Ala30Gly is used to describe an amino acid substitution, but not a deletion.

Therefore, in this question the appropriate nomenclature is *c.108del(p.S36fs)*, or *c.108delG(p. Ser36fs)*, or *c.108delG(p.Ser36SerfsTer26)*, or *c.108delG(p.Ser36Serfs*26)*.

41. **B.** TCT, TCA, TCC, *TCG*, AGT, and AGC code for serine (Ser/S). There is a single base-pair deletion in the question. Since RNA analysis shows an effect on splicing between exon 3 and intron 4, most likely the end of exon 3 is intact. The G at the beginning of the intron 4 was deleted. This is neither an in-frame nor a frameshift change, but it may be a splicing change.

According to published nomenclature for the description of sequence variants by the Human Genome Variation Society in 2016 (http:// varnomen.hgvs.org/), a nucleotide deletion is a sequence change in which one or more nucleotides are removed. Deletions are described using "del" after an indication of the first and last nucleotide(s) deleted, separated by an underscore. For all descriptions, the most 3' position possible is arbitrarily assigned to have been changed. For example, *c.76_78del* (alternatively, *c.76_78delACT*) denotes an ACT deletion from nucleotides 76 to 78.

c.88 + 1G > T denotes the G-to-T substitution at nucleotide +1 of an intron (in the coding DNA positioned between nucleotides 88 and 89).

Since RNA analysis showed an effect on splicing, the deletion is from TCGgtt to TCGtt. Therefore, in this question the appropriate nomenclature is *c.108 + 1delG*.

42. **B.** *GGA*, GGT, GGC, and GGG code for glycine (Gly/G). There is a 3-bp insertion in the question, which adds a glycine between alanine at position 30 and serine at position 31. This is an in-frame change.

According to published nomenclature for the description of sequence variants by the Human Genome Variation Society in 2016 (http:// varnomen.hgvs.org/), insertions are designated by "ins" after an indication of the nucleotides flanking the insertion site, followed by a description of the nucleotides inserted. For example, *c.76_77insT* denotes that a T is inserted between nucleotides 76 and 77 of the coding DNA reference sequence. Insertions add one or more amino acid residues between two existing amino acids and this insertion is not a copy of a sequence immediately 5'-flanking. Insertions are described using "ins" after an indication of the amino acids flanking the insertion site, separated by an underscore and followed by a description of the amino acid(s) inserted. For example, *p.Lys2_Met3insGlnSerLys* denotes that the sequence GlnSerLys (QSK) was inserted between amino acids lysine-2 (Lys, K) and methionine-3 (Met, M), changing MKMGHQQQCC to MK**QSK**MGHQQQCC.

Deletion/insertions of two or more consecutive nucleotides (indels) are described as a deletion followed by an insertion. For example, c.112_117delinsTG (alternatively, c.112_117delAGGTCAinsTG) denotes the replacement of nucleotides 112–117 (AGGTCA) by TG. Deletion/insertions (indels) replace one or more amino acid residues with one or more other amino acid residues. Deletion/insertions are described using "delins" as a deletion followed by an insertion after an indication of the amino acid(s) deleted separated by an underscore. For example, p.(Cys28_Lys29delinsTrp) indicates that neither RNA nor protein was analyzed but the predicted change is a 3-bp deletion that affects the codons for cysteine-28 and lysine-29, substituting them for a codon for tryptophan.

Therefore, in this question the appropriate nomenclature is *c.90_91insGGA (p.A30_S31insG)*, or *c.90_91insGGA(p.Ala30_Ser31insGly)*.

43. **C.** *GCT*, GCA, GCC, and *GCG* code for alanine (Ala/A). GGA, GGT, GGC, and *GGG* code for

glycine (Gly/G). There is a 3-bp insertion in the question, which adds a glycine in/after alanine (position 30–31). This is an in-frame change.

According to published nomenclature for the description of sequence variants by the Human Genome Variation Society in 2016 (http://varnomen.hgvs.org/), insertions are designated by "ins" after an indication of the nucleotides flanking the insertion site, followed by a description of the nucleotides inserted. For example, *c.76_77insT* denotes that a T is inserted between nucleotides 76 and 77 of the coding DNA reference sequence. Deletion/insertions (indels) replace one or more amino acid residues with one or more other amino acid residues. Deletion/insertions are described using "delins" as a deletion followed by an insertion after an indication of the amino acid(s) deleted separated by an underscore. For example, *p.(Cys28_Lys29delinsTrp)* indicates that neither RNA nor protein was analyzed, but the predicted change is a 3-bp deletion that affects the codons for cysteine-28 and lysine-29, substituting them for a codon for tryptophan.

Deletion/insertions of two or more consecutive nucleotides (indels) are described as a deletion followed by an insertion. For example, c.112_117delinsTG (alternatively, c.112_117delAGGTCAinsTG) denotes the replacement of nucleotides 112–117 (AGGTCA) by TG. Insertions are described using "ins" after an indication of the amino acids flanking the insertion site, separated by an underscore and followed by a description of the amino acid(s) inserted. For example, p.Lys2_Met3insGlnSerLys denotes that the sequence GlnSerLys (QSK) was inserted between amino acids lysine-2 (Lys, K) and methionine-3 (Met, M), changing MKMGHQQQCC to MK**QSK**MGHQQQCC.

Therefore, in this question the appropriate nomenclature is *c.89_90insGGA (p.A30delinsAG)*, or *c.89_90insGGA(p.Ala30delinsAlaGly)*. Since the deletion of T does not change the amino acid at position 30, the nomenclature could also be written as *c.89_90inGGA(p.Ala30_31SerinsAsp)*.

44. **A.** *GCT*, GCA, *GCC*, and GCG code for alanine (Ala/A). *GGA*, GGT, GGC, and GGG code for glycine (Gly/G). There is a 3-bp insertion in the question, which adds a glycine in alanine (position 30). This is an in-frame change.

According to published nomenclature for the description of sequence variants by the Human Genome Variation Society in 2016 (http://varnomen.hgvs.org/), deletion/insertions of two or more consecutive nucleotides (indels) are described as a deletion followed by an insertion.

For example, *c.112_117delinsTG* (alternatively, *c.112_117delAGGTCAinsTG*) denotes the replacement of nucleotides 112–117 (AGGTCA) by TG. Deletion/insertions (indels) replace one or more amino acid residues with one or more other amino acid residues. Deletion/insertions are described using "delins" as a deletion followed by an insertion after an indication of the amino acid(s) deleted separated by an underscore. For example, *p.(Cys28_Lys29delinsTrp)* indicates the neither RNA nor protein was analyzed, but the predicted change is a 3-bp deletion that affects the codons for cysteine-28 and lysine-29, substituting them for a codon for tryptophan.

Insertions are designated by "ins" after an indication of the nucleotides flanking the insertion site, followed by a description of the nucleotides inserted. For example, c.76_77insT denotes that a T is inserted between nucleotides 76 and 77 of the coding DNA reference sequence. Insertions are described using "ins" after an indication of the amino acids flanking the insertion site, separated by an underscore and followed by a description of the amino acid(s) inserted. For example, p. Lys2_Met3insGlnSerLys denotes that the sequence GlnSerLys (QSK) was inserted between amino acids lysine-2 (Lys, K) and methionine-3 (Met, M), changing MKMGHQQQCC to MK**QSK**MGHQQQCC.

Therefore, in this question the appropriate nomenclature is *c.88_93delinsGGAGCC(p. A30_S31delinsGA)*, or *c.88_93delinsGGAGCC(p. Ala30_Ser31delinsGlyAla)*, or *c.88_93delGCTAGCinsGGAGCC(p. Ala30_Ser31delinsGlyAla)*.

45. **C.** *GCT*, GCA, *GCC*, and GCG code for alanine (Ala/A). There is a 1-bp deletion accompanied by a 4-bp insertion in the question, which did not change the alanine at the position 30, but adds an alanine between alanine (position 30) and serine (position 31). This is an in-frame change.

According to published nomenclature for the description of sequence variants by the Human Genome Variation Society in 2016 (http://varnomen.hgvs.org/), deletion/insertions of two or more consecutive nucleotides (indels) are described as a deletion followed by an insertion. For example, *c.113delinsTACTAGC* (alternatively, *c.113delGinsTACTAGC*) denotes the replacement of nucleotide 113 by 7 new nucleotides (TACTACG). Deletion/insertions (indels) replace one or more amino acid residues with one or more other amino acid residues. Deletion/insertions are described using "delins" as a deletion followed by an insertion after an indication of the amino acid(s) deleted separated by an underscore. For example, *p. Cys28delinsTrpVal* denotes a 3-bp insertion in the codon for cysteine-28, generating codons for tryptophan (Trp, W) and valine (Val, V).

Insertions are designated by "ins" after an indication of the nucleotides flanking the insertion site, followed by a description of the nucleotides inserted. For example, c.76_77insT denotes that a T is inserted between nucleotides 76 and 77 of the coding DNA reference sequence. Insertions are described using "ins" after an indication of the amino acids flanking the insertion site, separated by an underscore and followed by a description of the amino acid(s) inserted. For example, p. Lys2_Met3insGlnSerLys denotes that the sequence GlnSerLys (QSK) was inserted between amino acids lysine-2 (Lys, K) and methionine-3 (Met, M), changing MKMGHQQQCC to MK**QSK**MGHQQQCC.

Therefore, in this question the appropriate nomenclature is *c.90delinsAGCC(p.A30delinsAA)*, or *c.90delTinsAGCC(p.Ala30delinsAlaAla)*, or *c. [90T > A;90_91insGCC](p.[Al30 = ; Ala30_Ser31insAla])*. Since the deletion of T does not change the amino acid at position 30, the nomenclature could also be written as c.90delTinsAGCC(p.Ala30_Ser31insAla).

46. **C.** TCT, TCA, TCC, TCG, AGT, and *AGC* code for serine (Ser/S). There is a 3-bp deletion in the question, which deletes one of the three serines. This is an in-frame change.

According to published nomenclature for the description of sequence variants by the Human Genome Variation Society in 2016 (http://varnomen.hgvs.org/), a nucleotide deletion is a sequence change in which one or more nucleotides are removed. Deletions are described using "del" after an indication of the first and last nucleotide(s) deleted, separated by an underscore. For all descriptions *the most 3′ position possible is arbitrarily assigned to have been changed*. For example, ACT**TGTG**CC to ACT**TG**CC is described as *c6_7del (c.6_7delTG*, not as c.4_5delTG). Deletions remove one or more amino acid residues from the protein and are described using "del" after an indication of the first and last amino acid(s) deleted separated by an underscore. For example, *p.Gln8del* in the sequence MKMGH**QQQ**CC denotes a glutamine-8 (Gln, Q) deletion to MKMGH**QQ**CC.

Therefore, in this question the appropriate nomenclature is *c.22_24del(p.S8del)*, or *c.22_44del(p. Ser8del)*, or *c.22_44delAGC(p.Ser8del)*. c.16_18(p. Ser6del) and c.19_21del(Ser7del) are not correct.

47. **C.** TCT, TCA, TCC, TCG, AGT, and *AGC* code for serine (Ser/S). There is a 3-bp duplication in the question, which duplicates a serine. This is an in-frame change.

According to published nomenclature for the description of sequence variants by the Human Genome Variation Society in 2016 (http://varnomen.hgvs.org/), duplications are designated by "dup" after an indication of the first and last nucleotide(s) duplicated. It should be noted that the description "dup" may by definition be used only when the sequence copy is directly 3′-flanking the original copy. For all descriptions the most 3′ position possible is arbitrarily assigned to have been changed. For example, *g.7_8dup* (or *g.7_8dupTG*, not g.5_6dup, not g.8_9insTG) denotes a TG duplication in the TG-tandem repeat sequence changing ACTT**TGTG**CC to ACTT**TGTGTG**CC.

At the amino acid level, duplications are described using "dup" after an indication of the first and last amino acid(s) duplicated separated by an underscore. Duplicating insertions in single amino acid stretches (or short tandem repeats) are described as a duplication. And for all descriptions, the most C-terminal position possible is arbitrarily assigned to have been changed. For example, a duplicating HQ insertion in the HQ-tandem repeat sequence of MKMGH**QHQHQ**CC to MKMGH**QHQHQHQ**CC is described as *p. His7_Gln8dup* (not *p.Gln8_Cys9insHisGln*).

Therefore, in this question the appropriate nomenclature is *c.19_21dup(p.S7dup)*, or *c.19_21dup (p.Ser7dup)*, or *c.19_21dupAGC(p.Ser7dup)*.

48. **B.** There is a single base-pair insertion/duplication at intron 4 of the gene in the question. According to published nomenclature for the description of sequence variants by the Human Genome Variation Society in 2016 (http://varnomen.hgvs. org/), duplications are designated by "dup" after an indication of the first and last nucleotide(s) duplicated. It should be noted that the description "dup" may by definition be used only when the sequence copy is directly 3′-flanking the original copy. For all descriptions the most 3′ position possible is arbitrarily assigned to have been changed. For examples, *g.7dupT* (or *g.7dup*, not g.5dupT, not g.7_8insT), denotes a duplication ("insertion") of the T nucleotide at position 7 in the genomic reference sequence, changing AGAC**TTT**GTGCC to AGAC**TTTT**GTGCC.

Therefore, in this question the appropriate nomenclature is *c.108 + 3dup*, or *c.108 + 3dupT*.

49. **B.** *TAA*, TAG, and TGA are the stop codons. CCA, CCT, CCC, and *CCG* code for proline (Pro/P). The

inversion of the six base pairs in the exon 1 of this gene causes a nonsense variant at position 2 of the amino acid sequence.

According to published nomenclature for the description of sequence variants by the Human Genome Variation Society in 2016 (http://varnomen. hgvs.org/), inversions are designated by "inv" after an indication of the first and last nucleotides affected by the inversion. For example, *c.203_506inv* (or *203_506inv304*) denotes that the 304 nucleotides from position 203 to 506 have been inverted.

Descriptions at the protein level may be given only in addition to a description at the DNA (and RNA) level. "inv" is not a standard nomenclature at the amino acid level. "delins" may be used to describe the amino acid change in this situation. For example, *p.(Pro578_Lys579delinsLeuTer)* is a deletion−insertion variant resulting from the change c.1733_1735delinsTTT.

Therefore, in this question the appropriate nomenclature is *c.4_9inv(p.A2_N3delins*)*, or *c.4_9inv(p.Ala2_Asn3delinsTer)*, or *c.4_9inv(p. Ala2_Asn3delins*)*, or *c.4_9inv6(p. Ala2_Asn3delinsTer)*.

50. **B.** There is a 3-bp insertion/duplication in exon 1 of the gene in the question, which adds/duplicates an alanine. This is an in-frame change.

According to published nomenclature for the description of sequence variants by the Human Genome Variation Society in 2016 (http:// varnomen.hgvs.org/), nomenclatures should be preceded by a letter indicating the type of reference sequence used to avoid confusion in the description of a variant. Several different reference sequences can be used:

- "c." for a coding DNA sequence (like c.76G > T)
- "g." for a genomic sequence (like g.476G > T)
- "m." for a mitochondrial sequence (like m.8993T > C)
- "n" for a noncoding RNA reference sequence (gene producing an RNA transcript but not a protein)
- "r." for an RNA sequence (like r.76a > u)
- "p." for a protein sequence (like p.Lys76Asn)

DNA duplications are designated by "dup" after a description of the duplicated segment, that is, the first (and last) nucleotide(s) duplicated (even when a mononucleotide is duplicated. For example, *g.7_8dup* (or *g.7_8dupTG*, not g.5_6dup, not g.8_9insTG) denotes a TG duplication in the TG-tandem repeat sequence changing ACTT**TGTG**CC to ACTT**TGTGTG**CC.

Protein duplications are described using "dup" after an indication of the first and last amino acid(s) duplicated separated by an underscore. For

example, a duplicating HQ insertion in the HQ-tandem repeat sequence of MKMG**HQHQ**CC to MKMG**HQHQHQ**CC is described as *p. His7_Gln8dup* (not p.Gln8_Cys9insHisGln).

Therefore, in this question the appropriate nomenclature is *c.4_6dup(p.A2dup)*, or *c.4_6dup(p. Ala2dup)*, or *c.4_6dupGCC(p.Ala2dup)*.

51. **A.** There is a 3-bp deletion in exon 1 of this gene, which deletes the alanine at position 2 of the amino acid sequence. This is an in-frame change.

According to published nomenclature for the description of sequence variants by the Human Genome Variation Society in 2016 (http:// varnomen.hgvs.org/), a nucleotide deletion is a sequence change in which one or more nucleotides are removed. Deletions are described using "del" after an indication of the first and last nucleotide(s) deleted, separated by an underscore. For example, *c.76_78del* (alternatively, *c.76_78delACT*) denotes an ACT deletion from nucleotides 76 to 78. Deletions remove one or more amino acid residues from the protein and are described using "del" after an indication of the first and last amino acid(s) deleted separated by an underscore. For example, *p.Gln8del* in the sequence MKMGH**QQQ**CC denotes a glutamine-8 (Gln, Q) deletion to MKMGH**QQ**CC.

So-called silent changes can be described using p.(Leu54 =). Deletion/insertions are described using "delins" as a deletion followed by an insertion after an indication of the amino acid(s) deleted separated by an underscore. For example, p.(Cys28_Lys29delinsTrp) indicates that neither RNA nor protein was analyzed, but the predicted change is a 3-bp deletion that affects the codons for cysteine-28 and lysine-29, substituting them for a codon for tryptophan. Another example is that p.Arg97ProfsTer23 (alternatively, p. Arg97Profs*23; short p.Arg97fs) denotes a frameshift change with arginine-97 as the first affected amino acid, replacing it for a proline and creating a new reading frame ending at a stop at position 23 (counting starts with the proline as amino acid 1). Extensions are described using "ext" after a description of the change at the first amino acid affected and followed by a description of the position of the new translation initiation or termination codon. For example, p.*110Glnext*17 (alternatively p. Ter110GlnextTer17 or p.*110Qext*17) describes a variant in the stop codon (Ter/*) at position 110, changing it to a codon for glutamine (Gln, Q) and adding a tail of new amino acids to the protein's C-terminus ending at a new stop codon (Ter17/*17).

Therefore, in this question the appropriate nomenclature is *c.4_6del(p.A2del), or c.4_6del(p. Ala2del),* or *c.4_6delGCC(p.Ala2del).*

52. **D.** *AAT*, and AAC code for asparagine (Asn/N). ATT, ATA, and *ATC* code for Isoleucine (Ile/I). There is a single base-pair deletion in the exon 1 of the gene in the question, which change the amino acid sequence at position 3 from asparagine to Isoleucine. This is a frameshift change.

According to published nomenclature for the description of sequence variants by the Human Genome Variation Society in 2016 (http:// varnomen.hgvs.org/), a nucleotide deletion is a sequence change where one or more nucleotides are removed. Deletions are described using "del" after an indication of the first and last nucleotide(s) deleted, separated by an underscore. For all descriptions, the most 3′ position possible is arbitrarily assigned to have been changed. For example, *c.76_78del* (alternatively, *c.76_78delACT*) denotes an ACT deletion from nucleotides 76 to 78. Frame shifts mutation of amino acid sequence are described using the format **p.Arg97Glyfs*26** (alternatively, **p.Arg97GlyfsTer26**, or short **p. Arg97fs**), where Arg97Gly describes the change of the first amino acid affected (Arg97 replaced by a Pro residue), "fs" indicates the frameshift, and *16 gives the position of the translation termination codon (stop codon) in the new reading frame.

Therefore, in this question the appropriate nomenclature is *c.8del(p.N3fs)* or *c.8del(p.Asn3fs)* or *c.8delT(p.Asn3IlefsTer26* or *c.8delT(p.Asn3Ilefs*26).*

53. **D.** There is a single base-pair deletion in intron 11 of this gene. The variant is not a common polymorphism in general populations. This may not change the amino acid sequence.

According to published nomenclature for the description of sequence variants by the Human Genome Variation Society in 2016 (http:// varnomen.hgvs.org/), a nucleotide deletion is a sequence change in which one or more nucleotides are removed. Deletions are described using "del" after an indication of the first and last nucleotide(s) deleted, separated by an underscore. For all descriptions, the most 3′ position possible is arbitrarily assigned to have been changed. For example, ectttagGCATG to cttagGCATG in an intron is described as *c.301-3delT* (not as c.301-5delT).

Therefore, in this question the appropriate nomenclature is *c.365 + 5del* (or *c.365 + 5delT*).

54. **E.** Two base pairs in intron 11 of this gene (GA) were changed to a single base pair (C). It may not change the amino acid sequence.

According to published nomenclature for the description of sequence variants by the Human Genome Variation Society in 2016 (http:// varnomen.hgvs.org/), deletion/insertions of two or more consecutive nucleotides (indels) are described as a deletion followed by an insertion. For example, *c.112_117delinsTG* (alternatively, *c.112_117delAGGTCAinsTG*) denotes the replacement of nucleotides 112–117 (AGGTCA) by TG. Another example is *c.114_115delinsA* (alternatively, *c.[114G > A; 115delT]*).

Therefore, all the options in this question are correct.

55. **F.** There are extra two copies of TC repeats in intron 11 of this gene. So the total number of the TC repeat after the change is 4. In the question, it mentioned that this TC repeat is polymorphic in the general population. It may not change the amino acid sequence.

According to published nomenclature for the description of sequence variants by the Human Genome Variation Society in 2016 (http:// varnomen.hgvs.org/), polymorphisms are different from duplication, "dup," or insertions, "ins." For example, *g.7_8[4]* (or g.5_6[4], or *g.5TG[4]*, not g.7_10dup) is the preferred description of the addition of two extra TG's to the variable TG repeated sequence changing ACTT**TGTG**CC to ACTT**TGTGTGTG**CC.

Therefore, in this question the appropriate nomenclature is *c.365 + 2_ + 3[4]*, or *c.365 + 4_ + 5 [4]*, or *c.365 + 2TG[4]*, but not c.365 + 2_365 + 5dup.

56. **A.** There are extra two copies of TC repeats in the intron 11 of this gene. So the total number of the TC repeat is 4 after the change. In the question, it mentioned that this TC repeat is polymorphic in general populations. It may not change the amino acid sequence.

According to published nomenclature for the description of sequence variants by the Human Genome Variation Society in 2016 (http:// varnomen.hgvs.org/), polymorphisms are different from duplication, "dup," or insertions, "ins." For example, *g.7_8[4]* (or g.5_6[4], or *g.5TG[4]*, not g.7_10dup) is the preferred description of the addition of two extra TGs to the variable TG repeated sequence, changing ACTT**TGTG**CC to ACTT**TGTGTGTG**CC.

Since this repeat is a polymorphism in the general population, it is not appropriate to call it an "ins." Therefore, in this question the appropriate nomenclature is *c.365 + 2_ + 3[4]*, or *c.365 + 4_ + 5[4]*, or *c.365 + 2TG[4]*, but not c.365 + 2_365 + 5dup, c.365 + 4TC[4], c.365 + 2_365 + 3TC[4], or c.365 + 4_365 + 5TC[4].

57. C. There are extra two copies of TC repeats in intron 11 of this gene. So the total number of the TC repeat after the change is 4. In the question, it mentioned that this TC repeat is polymorphic in the general population. It may not change the amino acid sequence.

According to published nomenclature for the description of sequence variants by the Human Genome Variation Society in 2016 (http://varnomen.hgvs.org/), polymorphisms are different from duplication, "dup," or insertions, "ins." For example, *g.7_8[4]* (or g.5_6[4], or *g.5TG[4]*, not g.7_10dup) is the preferred description of the addition of two extra TGs to the variable TG repeated sequence changing ACTT**TGTG**CC to ACTT**TGTGTGTG**CC.

Therefore, in this question the appropriate nomenclature is *c.365 + 2_ + 3[4]*, or *c.365 + 4_ + 5 [4]*, or *c.365 + 2TG[4]*, but not c.365 + 2_365 + 5dup.

58. C. There are extra two copies of TC repeats in intron 11 of this gene. So the total number of TC repeats after the change is 4. In the question, it mentioned that this TC repeat is polymorphic in the general population. It may not change the amino acid sequence.

According to published nomenclature for the description of sequence variants by the Human Genome Variation Society in 2016 (http://varnomen.hgvs.org/), polymorphisms are different from duplication, "dup," or insertions, "ins." For example, *g.7_8[4]* (or g.5_6[4], or *g.5TG[4]*, not g.7_10dup) is the preferred description of the addition of two extra TG to the variable TG repeated sequence changing ACTT**TGTG**CC to ACTT**TGTGTGTG**CC.

Therefore, in this question the appropriate nomenclature is *c.365 + 2_ + 3[4]*, or *c.365 + 4_ + 5 [4]*, or *c.365 + 2TG[4]*, but not c.365 + 2_365 + 5dup.

59. C. The patient has compound heterozygous variants in the *HFE* gene for hereditary hemochromatosis. Parental tests confirmed that the C282Y was from the mother, while H63D was from the father. So the two variants are on two different chromosomes in this patient.

According to published nomenclature for the description of sequence variants by the Human Genome Variation Society in 2016 (http://varnomen.hgvs.org/), two or more changes in one individual are described by combining the changes, per chromosome (maternal and paternal), between square brackets ("[;];[;]") and using a semicolon (";") as separator: [first change maternal; second change maternal]; [first change paternal; second change paternal]. When changes are in different genes on different chromosomes a space

(" ") is used to separate the different chromosomes ("[;] [;]"). For example, *p.[Ala25Thr];[Gly28Val]* describes two changes derived from a gene on each chromosome (one paternal, one maternal); predicted change amino acid alanine-25 to threonine on one chromosome and glycine-28 to valine on the other chromosome (RNA or protein analyzed).

p.[Ala25Thr(;)Pro323Leu] describes that two changes were identified in one individual (amino acid alanine-25 to threonine and proline-323 to leucine, RNA or protein analyzed), but it is not known whether these changes are on the same chromosome (in cis) or on different chromosomes (in trans). p.[(Ala25Thr; Gly28Val)] indicates two predicted changes derived from one chromosome (RNA or protein not analyzed); amino acid alanine-25 to threonine and glycine-28 to valine.

Therefore, in this question the appropriate nomenclature is *p.[H63D];[C282Y]*.

60. D. The patient has two variants in the *HFE* gene for hereditary hemochromatosis. Parental tests have not been done. So it is not clear if the two variants are in cis (on the same chromosome) or in trans (on the two homologous chromosomes).

According to published nomenclature for the description of sequence variants by the Human Genome Variation Society in 2016 (http://varnomen.hgvs.org/), two or more changes in one individual are described by combining the changes, per chromosome (maternal and paternal), between square brackets ("[;];[;]") and using a semicolon (";") as separator: [first change maternal; second change maternal]; [first change paternal; second change paternal]. When changes are in different genes on different chromosomes a space (" ") is used to separate the different chromosomes ("[;] [;]"). For example, *p.[Ala25Thr (;)Pro323Leu]* describes that two changes were identified in one individual (amino acid alanine-25 to threonine and proline-323 to leucine, RNA or protein analyzed), but it is not known whether these changes are on the same chromosome (in cis) or on different chromosomes (in trans).

p.[Ala25Thr];[Gly28Val] describes two changes derived from a gene on each chromosome (one paternal, one maternal); predicted change amino acid alanine-25 to threonine on one chromosome. p.[(Ala25Thr; Gly28Val)] indicates two predicted changes derived from one chromosome (RNA or protein not analyzed): amino acid alanine-25 to threonine and glycine-28 to valine.

Therefore, in this question the appropriate nomenclature is *p.[H63D(;)C282Y]*.

61. B. The patient has two variants on the same chromosome (in cis) in the *HFE* gene for hereditary hemochromatosis. Parental tests confirmed that both C282Y and H63D are maternal in origin. So the two variants are on one chromosome in a haplotype.

According to published nomenclature for the description of sequence variants by the Human Genome Variation Society in 2016 (http://varnomen.hgvs.org/), two or more changes in one individual are described by combining the changes, per chromosome (maternal and paternal), between square brackets ("[;];[;]") and using a semicolon (";") as a separator: [first change maternal; second change maternal]; [first change paternal; second change paternal]. When changes are in different genes on different chromosomes a space (" ") is used to separate the different chromosomes ("[;] [;]"). For example, *p.[(Ala25Thr; Gly28Val)]* indicates two predicted changes derived from one chromosome (RNA or protein not analyzed): amino acid alanine-25 to threonine and glycine-28 to valine.

p.[Ala25Thr(;)Pro323Leu] describes that two changes were identified in one individual (amino acid alanine-25 to threonine and proline-323 to leucine, RNA or protein analyzed), but it is not known whether these changes are on the same chromosome (in cis) or on different chromosomes (in trans). p.[Ala25Thr];[Gly28Val] describes two changes derived from a gene on each chromosome (one paternal, one maternal); the predicted change is amino acid alanine-25 to threonine on one chromosome.

Therefore, in this question the appropriate nomenclature is *p.[H63D;C282Y]*.

62. B. *FMR1* gene for fragile X syndrome is located on chromosome X. A male patient has only one copy of chromosome X.

According to the ACMG Standards and Guidelines for fragile X testing published in 2013, it should be c.-129CGG(1000).

However, the HGVS also states that "in literature the Fragile-X tri-nucleotide repeat is known as the CGG-repeat, but based on the coding DNA reference sequence (GenBank NM_002024.4) and the rule that for all descriptions the most 3' position possible should be arbitrarily assigned the repeat has to be described as a GGC repeat. In addition the repeat is interrupted by GGA triplets (see, e.g., Eichler 1995) making it a complex repeat that cannot be accurately described based on sizing only. The sequence represented by the FMR1 coding DNA Reference Sequence (GenBank NM_002024.5) is c.-128GGC[9]GGA[1]GGC[10].

NOTE: based on coding DNA reference sequence NM_002024.3 this variant is described as c.-158GGC[9]GGA[1]GGC[9]GGA[1]GGC[10]. To prevent such differences the recommendation is to use the stable LRG reference sequence (Locus Reference Genomic sequence); for FMR1 LRG_762t1:c.-128GGC[9]GGA[1]GGC[10]." And "c.-128_-126[(1000)]" describes the presence of an extended GGC-repeat of about 1000 units. Brackets are used to indicate uncertainties, the description c.-128GGC[(1000)] cannot be used since the repeat is probably interrupted by one or more GGA-triplets (http://varnomen.hgvs.org/).

There are certain discrepancy between the nomenclature from ACMG guidelines and HGVS recommendations. For the purpose of this question, we use the ACMG guidelines.

Therefore, in this question the appropriate nomenclature is *c.-129(1000)*.

63. B. The patient has two variants on the same chromosome (in cis) in the *CFTR* gene for cystic fibrosis (CF). The parental tests confirmed that both of the variants were maternal origin. So the two variants are on one chromosome in a haplotype.

According to published nomenclature for the description of sequence variants by the Human Genome Variation Society in 2016 (http://varnomen.hgvs.org/), two or more changes in one individual are described by combining the changes, per chromosome (maternal and paternal), between square brackets ("[;];[;]") and using a semicolon (";") as a separator: [first change maternal; second change maternal]; [first change paternal; second change paternal]. When changes are in different genes on different chromosomes a space (" ") is used to separate the different chromosomes ("[;] [;]"). For example, *c.[76A>C; 83G>C]* describes two changes found in a gene on one chromosome; A-to-C change at nucleotide 76 and a G-to-C change at nucleotide 83.

c.[76A>C];[83G>C] describes two changes found in a gene on each chromosome (one paternal, one maternal); A-to-C change at nucleotide 76 on one chromosome and a G-to-C change at nucleotide 83 on the other chromosome. c.[76A>C(;)283G>C] denotes that two changes were identified in one individual (an A-to-C change at nucleotide 76 and a G-to-C change at nucleotide 283), but it is not known whether these changes are on the same chromosome (in cis) or on different chromosomes (in trans).

Therefore, in this question the appropriate nomenclature is *c.[350G>A;1210-12T[5]]*.

64. C. The patient has compound heterozygous variants (in trans) in the *CFTR* gene for cystic fibrosis (CF). The parental tests confirmed that R117H was maternal in origin while 5T was paternal in origin. So the two variants are on two different chromosomes in this patient.

According to published nomenclature for the description of sequence variants by the Human Genome Variation Society in 2016 (http://varnomen.hgvs.org/), two or more changes in one individual are described by combining the changes, per chromosome (maternal and paternal), between square brackets ("[;];[;]") and using a semicolon (";") as separator: [first change maternal; second change maternal]; [first change paternal; second change paternal]. When changes are in different genes on different chromosomes a space (" ") is used to separate the different chromosomes ("[;] [;]"). For example, *c.[76A > C];[83G > C]* describes two changes found in a gene on each chromosome (one paternal, one maternal); A-to-C change at nucleotide 76 on one chromosome and a G to C change at nucleotide 83 on the other chromosome.

c.[76A > C; 83G > C] describes two changes found in a gene on one chromosome; A-to-C change at nucleotide 76 and a G to C change at nucleotide 83. *c.[76A > C(;)283G > C]* denotes that two changes were identified in one individual (an A-to-C change at nucleotide 76 and a G-to-C change at nucleotide 283), but it is not known whether these changes are on the same chromosome (in cis) or on different chromosomes (in trans).

Therefore, in this question the appropriate nomenclature is *c.[350G > A];[1210-12T[5]]*.

65. A. The patient has two variants in the *CFTR* gene for cystic fibrosis (CF). The parental tests have not been done. So it is not clear if the two variants are in cis (on the same chromosome) or in trans (on the two homologous chromosomes).

According to published nomenclature for the description of sequence variants by the Human Genome Variation Society in 2016 (http://varnomen.hgvs.org/), two or more changes in one individual are described by combining the changes, per chromosome (maternal and paternal), between square brackets ("[;];[;]") and using a semicolon (";") as separator: [first change maternal; second change maternal]; [first change paternal; second change paternal]. When changes are in different genes on different chromosomes a space (" ") is used to separate the different chromosomes ("[;] [;]"). For example, *c.[76A > C(;)283G > C]* denotes that two changes were identified in one

individual (an A-to-C change at nucleotide 76 and a G to C change at nucleotide 283), but it is not known whether these changes are on the same chromosome (in cis) or on different chromosomes (in trans).

c.[76A > C];[83G > C] describes two changes found in a gene on each chromosome (one paternal, one maternal); A-to-C change at nucleotide 76 on one chromosome and a G-to-C change at nucleotide 83 on the other chromosome. *c.[76A > C; 83G > C]* describes two changes found in a gene on one chromosome; A-to-C change at nucleotide 76 and a G-to-C change at nucleotide 83.[6]

Therefore, in this question the appropriate nomenclature is *c.[350G > A(;)1210-12T[5]]*.

66. B. The patient has a homozygous *deltaF508* mutation in the *CFTR* gene for cystic fibrosis (CF). The parental tests have not been done. So it is not clear if it is a true homozygous change, or a nonamplification of the sequences analyzed on the other chromosome.

According to published nomenclature for the description of sequence variants by the Human Genome Variation Society in 2016 (http://varnomen.hgvs.org/), *c.[76A > C];[(76A > C)]* denotes a homozygous A-to-C change at nucleotide 76, not confirmed by analysis of both parents, leaving the possibility of nonamplification of the sequences analyzed on the other chromosome (e.g., due to a primer mismatch or a deletion).

c.[76A > C];[76A > C] denotes a homozygous A-to-C change at nucleotide 76. *c.[76A > C];[=]* denotes a A-to-C change at nucleotide 76 in a gene on one chromosome and a normal coding DNA reference sequence of the other chromosome. *c.[76A > C];[0]* denotes a A-to-C change at nucleotide 76 in a gene on one chromosome and the absence of the entire coding DNA reference sequence on the other chromosome.

Therefore, in this case the most appropriate nomenclature is *c.[1521_1523delCTT]; [(1521_1523delCTT)]*.

67. D. The patient has a heterozygous variant in the *CFTR* gene for cystic fibrosis (CF).

According to published nomenclature for the description of sequence variants by the Human Genome Variation Society in 2016 (http://varnomen.hgvs.org/), *c.[76A > C];[=]* denotes a A-to-C change at nucleotide 76 in a gene on one chromosome and a normal coding DNA reference sequence of the other chromosome.

c.[76A > C];[76A > C] denotes a homozygous A-to-C change at nucleotide 76. And c.[76A > C];

[(76A > C)] denotes a homozygous A-to-C change at nucleotide 76, not confirmed by analysis of both parents, leaving the possibility of nonamplification of the sequences analyzed on the other chromosome (e.g., due to a primer mismatch or a deletion). c.[76A > C];[0] denotes a A-to-C change at nucleotide 76 in a gene on one chromosome and the absence of the entire coding DNA reference sequence on the other chromosome.

Therefore, in this case the most appropriate nomenclature is *c.[1521_1523delCTT];[=]*.

68. **C.** TAA, *TAG*, and TGA are the stop codons. TCT, TCA, TCC, *TCG*, AGT, and AGC code for serine (Ser/S). There is a single base-pair substitution affecting the translation termination codon in the question, which alters termination codon (Ter/*) to serine (Ser/S). This is a nonstop change. The third codon after the change is TGA, a stop codon.

According to published nomenclature for the description of sequence variants by the Human Genome Variation Society in 2016 (http://varnomen.hgvs.org/), extensions affect either the first (start, translation initiation, N-terminus. ATG) or last codon (translation termination, stop) and as a consequence extend the protein sequence N- or C-terminally with one or more amino acids. Extensions are described using "ext" after a description of the change at the first amino acid affected and followed by a description of the position of the new translation initiation or termination codon. For example, *p.*110Glnext*17* (alternatively, *p.Ter110GlnextTer17* or *p.*110Qext*17*), which is used to describe a variant in the stop codon (Ter/*) at position 110, changing it to a codon for glutamine (Gln, Q) and adding a tail of new amino acids to the protein's C-terminus ending at a new stop codon (Ter17/*17).

Therefore, the appropriate nomenclatures in this question are *c.364A > C(p.*121Serext*3)*, *c.364A > C (p.Ter121SerextTer3)*, and *c.364A > C(p.*121Sext*3)*.

69. **D.** There is a 6-bp deletion in exon 1 of this gene, which deletes alanine (Ala/A) at position 2 and asparagine (Asn/N) at position 3. This is an in-frame change.

According to published nomenclature for the description of sequence variants by the Human Genome Variation Society in 2016 (http://varnomen.hgvs.org/), a nucleotide deletion is a sequence change in which one or more nucleotides are removed. Deletions are described using "del" after an indication of the first and last nucleotide(s) deleted, separated by an underscore. For all descriptions, the most 3' position possible is arbitrarily assigned to have been changed. For

example, *c.76_78del* (alternatively, *c.76_78delACT*) denotes an ACT deletion from nucleotides 76 to 78.

Deletions remove one or more amino acid residues from the protein and are described using "del" after an indication of the first and last amino acid(s) deleted separated by an underscore. Deletions remove either a small internal segment of the protein (in-frame deletion), part of the N-terminus of the protein (initiation codon change), or the entire C-terminal part of the protein (nonsense change). For example, *p. (Cys28_Met30del)* denotes that neither RNA nor protein was analyzed, but the predicted change is a deletion of three amino acids, from cysteine-28 to methionine-30.

Therefore, the appropriate nomenclatures in this question are *c.4_9del(p.A2_N3del)*, *c.4_9del(p. Ala2_Asn3del)*, and *c.4_9delGCCAAT(p. Ala2_Asn3del)*.

70. **C.** There is a 6-bp duplication in exon 1 of this gene, which duplicates alanine (Ala/A) at position 2 and asparagine (Asn/N) at position 3. This is an in-frame change.

According to published nomenclature for the description of sequence variants by the Human Genome Variation Society in 2016 (http://varnomen.hgvs.org/), duplications are designated by "dup" after an indication of the first and last nucleotide(s) duplicated. It should be noted that the description "dup" may by definition be used only when the sequence copy is directly 3'-flanking the original copy. For all descriptions the most 3' position possible is arbitrarily assigned to have been changed. For example, *c.77_79dup* (or *c.77_79dupCTG*) denotes that the three nucleotides 77−79 are duplicated (present twice).

For amino acid sequences, duplications are described using "dup" after an indication of the first and last amino acid(s) duplicated separated by an underscore. In-frame duplications containing a translation stop codon in the duplicated sequence are described as an insertion of a nonsense variant, not as a deletion−insertion removing the entire C-terminal amino acid sequence. For example, *p.Gly4_Gln6dup* in the sequence MKMGH<u>QQQ</u>CC denotes a duplication of amino acids glycine-4 (Gly, G) to glutamine-6 (Gln, Q) (i.e., MKMGHQGH<u>QQQ</u>CC).

Therefore, the appropriate nomenclatures in this question are *c.4_9dup(p.A2_N3dup)*, *c.4_9dup(p. Ala2_Asn3dup)*, and *c.4_9dupGCCAAT(p. Ala2_Asn3dup)*.

71. **A.** TCT, TCA, TCC, TCG, *AGT*, and AGC code for serine (Ser/S). And GGA, GGT, GGC, and *GGG* code for glycine (Gly/G). There is a 6-bp insertion

between the sixth and seventh nucleotide of exon 1, which added Ser and Gly between the second and third of the amino acid sequence. This is an in-frame change.

According to published nomenclature for the description of sequence variants by the Human Genome Variation Society in 2016 (http://varnomen.hgvs.org/), insertions are designated by "ins" after an indication of the nucleotides flanking the insertion site, followed by a description of the nucleotides inserted. Duplicating insertions should be described as duplications, not as insertions. For example, *c.76_77insT* denotes that a T is inserted between nucleotides 76 and 77 of the coding DNA reference sequence.

Amino acid sequence insertions add one or more amino acid residues between two existing amino acids, and this insertion is not a duplication of a sequence immediately 5′-flanking. Insertions are described using "ins" after an indication of the amino acids flanking the insertion site, separated by an underscore and followed by a description of the amino acid(s) inserted. For example, *p. Lys2_Met3insGlnSerLys* denotes that the sequence GlnSerLys (QSK) was inserted between the amino acids lysine-2 (Lys, K) and methionine-3 (Met, M), changing MKMGHQQQCC to MK**QSK**MGHQQQCC.

Therefore, the appropriate nomenclatures in this question are *c.6_7insAGTGGG(p.A2_N3insSG)*, and *c.6_7insAGTGGG(p.Ala2_Asn3insSerGly)*.

72. C. *CGA*, CGT, CGC, and CGG code for arginine (Arg/R). There is a 6-bp deletion, which is replaced by an insertion of three base pairs. This indel leads to Ala at the second and Asn at the third position being replaced by Arg in the amino acid sequence. This is an in-frame change.

According to published nomenclature for the description of sequence variants by the Human Genome Variation Society in 2016 (http://varnomen.hgvs.org/), deletion/insertions of two or more consecutive nucleotides (indels) are described as a deletion followed by an insertion. For example, *c.112_117delinsTG* (alternatively, *c.112_117delAGGTCAinsTG*) denotes the replacement of nucleotides 112−117 (AGGTCA) by TG.

Amino acid sequence deletion/insertions (indels) replace one or more amino acid residues with one or more other amino acid residues. Deletion/insertions are described using "delins" as a deletion followed by an insertion after an indication of the amino acid(s) deleted separated by an underscore. For example, *p.Cys28delinsTrpVal* denotes a 3-bp insertion in the codon for

cysteine-28, generating codons for tryptophan (Trp, W) and valine (Val, V).

Therefore, the appropriate nomenclatures in this question are *c.4_9delinsCGA(p.A2_N3delinsR)*, *c.4_9delinsCGA(p.Ala2_Asn3delinsArg)*, and *c.4_9delGCCAATinsCGA(p.Ala2_Asn3delinsArg)*.

73. C. The chromatograph shows a heterozygous variant, a C > T at position 268. This is an in-frame change.

According to published nomenclature for the description of sequence variants by the Human Genome Variation Society in 2016 (http://varnomen.hgvs.org/), two or more changes in one individual are described by combining the changes, per allele (chromosome) between square brackets ("[]"). Changes in different alleles (e.g., in recessive diseases) are described as "[change allele 1];[change allele 2]." Mixed descriptions like c.[76A > C];g.[91C > G] should not be used. For example, *c.[76A > C];[=]* denotes an A-to-C change at nucleotide 76 in one allele and a normal sequence in the other allele.

c.[76A > C];[76A > C] denotes a homozygous A-to-C change at nucleotide 76. c.[76A > C];[(76A > C)] denotes a homozygous A-to-C change at nucleotide 76, not confirmed by analysis of both parents, leaving the possibility of nonamplification of the second allele due to a primer mismatch or a deletion. c.[76A > C];[?] denotes an A-to-C change at nucleotide 76 in one allele and an unknown change in the other allele. c.[76A > C];[=] denotes an A-to-C change at nucleotide 76 in one allele and a normal sequence in the other allele. c.[76A > C];[0] denotes an A-to-C change at nucleotide 76 in one allele and the absence of a sequence from the other allele (e.g., for a variant in a gene on the X-chromosome in a male, where only one allele is present). Descriptions of sequence changes in different genes (e.g., for recessive diseases) are listed between square brackets, separated by a semicolon and include a reference to the sequence (gene) changed; [DMD:c.76A > C];[GJB:c.87delG].

This sample has an apparently heterozygous mutation. Therefore, the most appropriate nomenclature in this question is *c.[268C > T];[=]*.

74. D. The patient has compound heterozygous variants. The parental tests are pending. So it is not clear whether the two variants are in cis (on the same chromosome) or in trans (on the two homologous chromosomes).

According to published nomenclature for the description of sequence variants by the Human Genome Variation Society in 2016 (http://varnomen.hgvs.org/), two or more changes in one individual are described by combining the changes, per allele (chromosome) between square brackets ("[]"). Changes in different alleles (e.g., in recessive diseases) are described as "[change allele 1];[change allele 2]." Mixed descriptions like c.[76A > C];g.[91C > G] should not be used. For example, *c.[350G > A(;)1210-12T[7];[9](;) 1521_1523del]* describes a case in which variants c.350G > A, c.1210-12T[7], c.1210-12T[9] and c.1521_1523del were detected but without information on which variants are found together on one chromosome.

c.[76A > C];[76A > C] denotes a homozygous A-to-C change at nucleotide 76. c.[76A > C]; [(76A > C)] denotes a homozygous A-to-C change at nucleotide 76, not confirmed by analysis of both parents, leaving the possibility of nonamplification of the second allele due to a primer mismatch or a deletion. c.[76A > C];[?] denotes an A-to-C change at nucleotide 76 in one allele and an unknown change in the other allele. c.[76A > C];[=] denotes an A-to-C change at nucleotide 76 in one allele and a normal sequence in the other allele. c.[76A > C]; [0] denotes an A-to-C change at nucleotide 76 in one allele and the absence of a sequence from the other allele (e.g., for a variant in a gene on the X-chromosome in a male, where only one allele is present). Descriptions of sequence changes in different genes (e.g., for recessive diseases) are listed between square brackets, separated by a semicolon and include a reference to the sequence (gene) changed: [DMD:c.76A > C];[GJB:c.87delG].

Therefore, the most appropriate nomenclature in this question is *c.[268C > T(;)343C > T]*.

75. **B**. The patient has an apparently homozygous variant by the chromatograph. Targeted parent tests will be able to confirm whether the variant is in both alleles or whether there is an allelic drop due to a primer mismatch or a deletion.

According to published nomenclature for the description of sequence variants by the Human Genome Variation Society in 2016 (http:// varnomen.hgvs.org/), two or more changes in one individual are described by combining the changes, per allele (chromosome) between square brackets ("[]"). Changes in different alleles (e.g., in recessive diseases) are described as "[change allele 1];[change allele 2]." Mixed descriptions like c.[76A > C];g.[91C > G] should not be used. For example, *c.[76A > C];[(76A > C)]* denotes a homozygous A-to-C change at nucleotide 76, not confirmed by analysis of both parents, leaving the possibility of nonamplification of the second allele due to a primer mismatch or a deletion.

c.[76A > C];[76A > C] denotes a homozygous A-to-C change at nucleotide 76. c.[76A > C];[?]

denotes an A-to-C change at nucleotide 76 in one allele and an unknown change in the other allele. c.[76A > C];[=] denotes an A-to-C change at nucleotide 76 in one allele and a normal sequence in the other allele. c.[76A > C];[0] denotes an A-to-C change at nucleotide 76 in one allele and the absence of a sequence from the other allele (e.g., for a variant in a gene on the X-chromosome in a male, where only one allele is present). Descriptions of sequence changes in different genes (e.g., for recessive diseases) are listed between square brackets, separated by a semicolon and include a reference to the sequence (gene) changed: [DMD:c.76A > C];[GJB:c.87delG].

This sample has an apparently homozygous mutation, but has not been confirmed by analysis of both parents yet. Therefore, the most appropriate nomenclature in this question is *c. [268C > T];[(268C > T)]*.

76. **E**. The male patient has a hemizygous variant in a gene on chromosome X by chromatograph.

According to published nomenclature for the description of sequence variants by the Human Genome Variation Society in 2016 (http:// varnomen.hgvs.org/), *c.[76A > C];[0]* denotes a A-to-C change at nucleotide 76 in one allele and the absence of a sequence from the other allele (e.g., for a variant in a gene on the X-chromosome in a male, where only one allele is present).

c.[76A > C];[76A > C] denotes a homozygous A-to-C change at nucleotide 76. c.[76A > C];[?] denotes an A-to-C change at nucleotide 76 in one allele and an unknown change in the other allele. c.[76A > C];[=] denotes an A-to-C change at nucleotide 76 in one allele and a normal sequence in the other allele. Descriptions of sequence changes in different genes (e.g., for recessive diseases) are listed between square brackets, separated by a semicolon and include a reference to the sequence (gene) changed: [DMD:c.76A > C]; [GJB:c.87delG].

This sample has an apparently hemizygous mutation. Therefore, the most appropriate nomenclature in this question is *c.[268C > T];[0]*.

77. **F**. GCA, *GCT*, GCC, and GCG code for alanine (Ala/A). There is a 3-bp deletion in the questions, which deleted one Ala in between positions 114 and 115 at the amino acid level. This is an in-frame change.

According to published nomenclature for the description of sequence variants by the Human Genome Variation Society in 2016 (http:// varnomen.hgvs.org/), for all nomenclatures the most 3' position possible is arbitrarily assigned to have been changed regardless of the DNA or protein sequence. For example, ACTT**TGT**GCC to ACTTGCC is described as *c.5_7del (c.5_7delTGT,* not as c.4_6delTTG).

Deletions remove one or more amino acid residues from the protein and are described using "del" after an indication of the first and last amino acid(s) deleted separated by an underscore. For example, *p.Gln8del* in the sequence MKMGH**QQQ**CC denotes a glutamine-8 (Gln, Q) deletion to MKMGHQQCC.

Therefore, the most appropriate nomenclature in this question is *c.345_347del(p.A115del)* or *c.345_347del(p.Ala115del)* or *c.345_347delGCT(p.Ala115del)*.

78. **C.** GCA, *GCT*, GCC, and GCG code for alanine (Ala/A). There is a 3-bp duplication in the question, which adds an alanine into the amino acid sequence. This is an in-frame change.

According to published nomenclature for the description of sequence variants by the Human Genome Variation Society in 2016 (http://varnomen.hgvs.org/), for all nomenclatures the most 3′ position possible is arbitrarily assigned to have been changed regardless of the DNA or protein sequence. For example, *g.7dupT* (or *g.7dup,* not g.5dupT, not g.7_8insT) denotes a duplication ("insertion") of the T nucleotide at position 7 in the genomic reference sequence changing AGACTTTGTGCC to AGACTTT**T**GTGCC.

Amino acid sequence duplications are described using "dup" after an indication of the first and last amino acid(s) duplicated separated by an underscore. In-frame duplications containing a translation stop codon in the duplicated sequence are described as an insertion of a nonsense variant, not as a deletion−insertion removing the entire C-terminal amino acid sequence. For example, *p.Gly4_Gln6dup* in the sequence MKMGH**QQQ**CC denotes a duplication of amino acids glycine-4 (Gly, G) to glutamine-6 (Gln, Q) (i.e., MKMGHQGH**QQQ**CC).

Therefore, the most appropriate nomenclature in this question is *c.345dup(p.A115dup)* or *c.345dupGCT(p.Ala115dup)* or *c.345_347dup(p.Ala15dup)*.

79. **D.** There is a single base-pair substitution in the 5′ upstream sequence of the gene. This may cause a splicing change.

According to published nomenclature for the description of sequence variants by the Human Genome Variation Society in 2016 (http://varnomen.hgvs.org/), the nucleotide 5′ of the ATG-translation initiation codon is −1, the previous −2, etc. For example, in 5′ UTR of a gene, a G-to-A substitution of 12 nucleotides upstream of the ATG translation initiation codon (coding DNA-12) is expressed as c.-12G > A.

A change affecting the translation initiation codon (Met-1) introducing a new upstream initiation codon extending the N-terminus of the encoded protein described using "ext-#," where "-#" is the position of the new initiation codon (Met-#). For example, p.Met1ext-5—a variant in the 5′ UTR activates a new upstream translation initiation site starting with amino acid Met-5 (methionine-5), and p.Met1Valext-12—amino acid Met1 is changed to Val, activating an upstream translation initiation site at position −12 (methionine-12).

This change does not change the start codon. Therefore, the most appropriate nomenclature in this question is *c.-1G > A.*

80. **C.** TAT, *TAG*, and TGA are the stop codons. There is a single base-pair substitution in the 3′ downstream region of the gene. This may not change the stop codon.

According to published nomenclature for the description of sequence variants by the Human Genome Variation Society in 2016 (http://varnomen.hgvs.org/), the nucleotide 3′ of the translation stop codon is *1, the next *2, etc. For example, in the 3′ UTR of a gene a T-to-A substitution located in the 3′ UTR (70 nucleotides downstream of the termination codon) is expressed as c.*70T > A. In the 3′ gene flanking region a C-to-A substitution located 293 nucleotides downstream of the gene is expressed as *c.*293C > A.*

A change affecting the translation termination codon (Ter/*) introducing a new downstream termination codon extending the C-terminus of the encoded protein is described using "extTer#" (alternatively "ext*#") where "#" is the position of the new stop codon (Ter#/*#). For example, p.*110Glnext*17 (alternatively, p.Ter110GlnextTer17 or p.*110Qext*17) describes a variant in the stop codon (Ter/*) at position 110, changing it to a codon for glutamine (Gln, Q) and adding a tail of new amino acids to the protein's C-terminus ending at a new stop codon (Ter17/*17). p.*327Argext*? (alternatively, p.Ter327ArgextTer? or p.*327Rext*?) describes a variant in the stop codon (Ter/*) at position 327, changing it to a codon for arginine (Arg, R) and adding a tail of new amino acids of unknown length, since the shifted frame does not contain a new stop codon.

This change does not change the stop codon. Therefore, the most appropriate nomenclature in this question is *c.*1G > A.*

References

1. Povey S, et al. The HUGO Gene Nomenclature Committee (HGNC). *Hum Genet* 2001;**109**(6):678–80.

2. Eyre TA, et al. The HUGO Gene Nomenclature Database, 2006 updates. *Nucleic Acids Res* 2006;**34**(Database issue):D319–21.

3. Beaudet AL, Tsui LC. A suggested nomenclature for designating mutations. *Hum Mutat* 1993;**2**(4):245–8.

4. Reijnen MJ, et al. Hemophilia B Leyden: substitution of thymine for guanine at position-21 results in a disruption of a hepatocyte nuclear factor 4 binding site in the factor IX promoter. *Blood* 1993;**82**(1):151–8.

5. den Dunnen JT, Antonarakis SE. Mutation nomenclature extensions and suggestions to describe complex mutations: a discussion. *Hum Mutat* 2000;**15**(1):7–12.

6. den Dunnen JT, et al. HGVS recommendations for the description of sequence variants: 2016 update. *Hum Mutat* 2016;**37**(6):564–9.

7. Genetics, A.C.o.M. ACMG standards and guidelines for clinical, CF and Section G; 2011.

8. Antonarakis SE. Recommendations for a nomenclature system for human gene mutations. Nomenclature Working Group. *Hum Mutat* 1998;**11**(1):1–3.

9. Monaghan KG, et al. ACMG Standards and Guidelines for fragile X testing: a revision to the disease-specific supplements to the Standards and Guidelines for Clinical Genetics Laboratories of the American College of Medical Genetics and Genomics. *Genet Med* 2013;**15**(7):575–86.

10. Eichler EE, Hammond HA, Macpherson JN, Ward PA, Nelson DL. Population survey of the human FMR1 CGG repeat substructure suggests biased polarity for the loss of AGG interruptions. *Hum Mol Genet* 1995;**4**(12):2199–208.

11. Dalgleish R, Flicek P, Cunningham F, Astashyn A, Tully RE, Proctor G, Chen Y, McLaren WM, Larsson P, Vaughan BW, Béroud C, Dobson G, Lehväslaiho H, Taschner PE, den Dunnen JT, Devereau A, Birney E, Brookes AJ, Maglott DR, et al. Locus Reference Genomic sequences: an improved basis for describing human DNA variants. *Genome Med.* 2010;**2**(4):24 Available from: https://doi.org/10.1186/gm145.

CHAPTER

4

Disorders of Unstable Repeat Sequences

Unstable repeat sequences are part of a group of human genetic disorders caused by long and highly polymorphic tandem repeats in the noncoding or coding regions of a variety of genes. Most of these are neuromuscular disorders, such as fragile X syndrome (FXS) and Huntington disease (HD). While repeats in the coding sequence can result in the generation of toxic or malfunctioning proteins, noncoding repeats can also have significant effects, including the generation of chromosome fragility, the silencing of the genes in which they are located, the modulation of transcription and translation, and the sequestering of proteins involved in processes such as splicing and cell architecture.[1]

Anticipation: Disorders identified to date are mostly progressive, and display unusual inheritance patterns, such as anticipation. Anticipation is manifested at an earlier age at onset or a more severe phenotype in later generations of a family and can be correlated to an increased repeat expansion size. Thus, in later generations the disease onset can take place in childhood, whereas affected individuals in earlier generations had symptoms only as adults. Pediatric cases of typically adult disorders have been shown to be caused by exceptionally long repeat sequences.

Parent-of-origin effect: Gender bias in the transmission of unstable repeats from a parent to offspring is a common feature of dynamic mutations. For example, the transmission of unstable repeat sequences through males was less stable than that through females for genes involved in HD and spinocerebellar ataxia type 1 (SCA1). However, the repeats are less stable in females than males in the case of FXS and spinocerebellar ataxia type 7 (SCA7) during transmission.[2]

Somatic instability: During the past decade, somatic variations in repeat copy number have been measured in most human disorders of unstable repeat sequences, and in most mouse models for triplet diseases, including FXS, myotonic dystrophy type 1 (MD1), SCA1, and HD, among many others. For example, in HD the somatic growth of the repeat in human brain cells would be predicted to cause a more severe disease phenotype with age, since disease proteins of longer polyglutamine tracts are progressively produced. In animals, somatic expansion of the CAG tract continues progressively throughout the lifetime of animals as they develop toxic phenotypes. Evidence in human postmortem HD brains suggests that somatic expansion of the HD CAG repeat in the brain is associated with an earlier age at disease onset.[3]

The disorders coved in this chapter are:

- Huntington disease
- Friedreich ataxia
- Spinal muscular atrophy
- Spinocerebellar ataxia type 1
- Myotonic dystrophy type 1
- Myotonic dystrophy type 2
- Fragile X syndrome
- Fragile X–associated tremor/ataxia syndrome
- *FMR1*-related primary ovarian insufficiency

QUESTIONS

1. There is a class of genetic diseases due to dynamic mutations of unstable repeat sequences that change from generation to generation. Which one of the following statements regarding instability of unstable repeat sequences is correct?[4]
   A. The instability may lead to an increase or a decrease in repeat length intergenerationally or somatically.
   B. All unstable repeat disorders are autosomal dominant.
   C. All unstable repeat disorders are caused by trinucleotide repeat expansion.
   D. Expansion of unstable repeats are loss-of-function changes due to methylation
   E. None of the above.
2. Which one of the following disorders is NOT caused by the expansion of unstable repeat sequences?[4]

Self-assessment Questions for Clinical Molecular Genetics.
DOI: https://doi.org/10.1016/B978-0-12-809967-4.00004-1

A. Duchenne muscular dystrophy
B. Fragile X syndrome
C. Friedreich ataxia
D. Huntington disease
E. Myotonic dystrophy type 1
F. Myotonic dystrophy type 2

3. Which one of the following disorders is NOT caused by the expansion of trinucleotide repeat sequences?[4]
A. Fragile X syndrome
B. Friedreich ataxia
C. Huntington disease
D. Myotonic dystrophy type 1
E. Myotonic dystrophy type 2
F. All of the above
G. None of the above

4. Which one of the following disorders of unstable repeat expansion does NOT exhibit dominant inheritance patterns?
A. Fragile X syndrome
B. Friedreich ataxia
C. Huntington disease
D. Myotonic dystrophy type 1
E. Myotonic dystrophy type 2
F. All of the above
G. None of the above

5. Which one of the following disorders of unstable repeat expansion has the repeat sequence in the coding region?
A. Fragile X syndrome
B. Friedreich ataxia
C. Huntington disease
D. Myotonic dystrophy type 1
E. Myotonic dystrophy type 2
F. All of the above
G. None of the above

6. A 6-year-old boy was brought to a genetics clinic by his parents for tremor and epilepsy. His medical history was uneventful. The family history was significant for the grandfather, who was diagnosed with Huntington disease at 46 years of age; molecular testing confirmed that he had an allele with 44 copies of the CAG repeat in the HTT gene. The 27-year-old father was asymptomatic, but he carried an allele with 52 copies of the CAG repeat. The molecular test for Huntington disease detected compound heterozygous 25/66 CAG repeats in the boy. Which one of the following would be the most appropriate interpretation of the allelic difference between the grandfather, the father, and the boy?
A. Anticipation
B. Epistasis

C. Lab error with wrong specimens
D. PCR artifacts
E. Pleiotropy
F. None of the above

7. A 6-year-old boy was brought to a genetics clinic by his parents for tremor and epilepsy. The medical geneticist ordered chromosome karyotype and microarray analyses. Conventional cytogenetics detected a normal male karyotype. Chromosome microarray found a 300-kb interstitial deletion on 4p16.3 including the HTT gene, which is associated with Huntington disease. The family histories on both sides were negative for Huntington disease. And the results of trinucleotide repeats test for Huntington disease on the patient detected homozygous 25 CAG repeats. What would be the most appropriate interpretation of the chromosome microarray results?[5]
A. Normal
B. Unknown clinical significance, likely benign
C. Unknown clinical significance
D. Unknown clinical significance, likely pathogenic
E. Pathogenic

8. A 16-year-old boy was brought to a genetics clinic by his foster parents for chorea, rigidity, and gait problems. The medical history of the biological parents was not available. The doctor ordered trinucleotide repeats test for Huntington disease. The results showed that the patient had compound heterozygous 30/65 copies of CAG in the HTT gene. When a genetic counselor saw this family, she mentioned that the likelihood that the patient inherited the mutated copy from his biological father was[5,6]:
A. 10%
B. 30%
C. 50%
D. 60%
E. 90%

9. In which part of the HTT gene is the trinucleotide unstable repeat for Huntington disease is located?[5]
A. Promoter
B. 5′ UTR
C. Intron
D. Exon
E. 3′ UTR

10. Which one of the following genetic alterations in the HTT gene causes Huntington disease?[5]
A. Point mutations
B. in/del
C. (CAG)n repeats in an intron

D. (CAG)n repeats in an exon

E. (CGG)n repeat in an intron

F. (CGG)n repeat in an exon

G. (CTG)n repeat in an intron

H. (CTG)n repeat in an exon

11. Which one of the following molecular genetic assays is the most appropriate for the diagnosis of Huntington disease in clinical laboratories?[5]

A. Chromosome karyotype

B. Chromosome microarray (CMA)

C. Multiplex ligation-dependent probe amplification (MLPA)

D. PCR/capillary electrophoresis and Southern blot

E. PCR/capillary electrophoresis

F. Triplet repeat–primed PCR

12. A couple came to a genetics clinic for prenatal counseling when the wife was 6 weeks pregnant. The wife had 24/35 copies of CAG repeats in the *HTT* gene for Huntington disease (HD), which were not interrupted by CCG repeats. She was 32 years old and had no HD symptoms. Which one of the following would most likely be the risk of HD in her children?[5]

A. 0.5%

B. 30%

C. 50%

D. 80%

E. 100%

13. A couple comes to a genetics clinic for prenatal counseling when the wife is 6 weeks pregnant. The husband has 24/35 copies of the CAG repeats in the *HTT* gene for Huntington disease (HD), which are not interrupted by the CCG repeats. He is 42 years old and has no HD symptoms. Which one of the following would most likely be the risk of HD in his children?[5,7–9]

A. 0.5%

B. 10%

C. 50%

D. 80%

E. 100%

14. A couple comes to a genetics clinic for prenatal counseling when the wife is 6 weeks pregnant. The wife is apparently healthy, with an uneventful medical and family history. The husband's father died in a car accident. The husband's paternal uncle has Huntington disease (HD) and lives outside the country. The husband is 42 years old and has no symptoms of HD. A molecular test detects that he has 16/25 CAG repeats. What is the clinical significance of the results?[5]

A. The husband may not develop Huntington disease.

B. The husband does not have Huntington disease. But his children will be at risk.

C. The husband may develop Huntington disease. His children have 10% to 50% chance of having HD.

D. The husband has Huntington disease. His children have 50% chance of having HD.

E. None of the above.

15. BJ, a 32-year-old male, came to a genetics clinic for a family history of Huntington disease (HD). Physical exam did not find any symptoms associated with HD. A family history showed that his 45-year-old half-brother from the paternal side was recently diagnosed with HD. Their father died in a car accident at the age of 42. The medical geneticist ordered a molecular test for the trinucleotide repeats for Huntington disease with BJ's peripheral-blood sample. The results showed that BJ has 20/38 copies of CAG in the *HTT* gene. What would be the interpretation of this result?[5]

A. BJ had normal alleles.

B. BJ had a gray zone mutation.

C. BJ had a premutation.

D. BJ had a full mutation.

16. A couple comes to a genetics clinic for prenatal counseling when the wife is 6 weeks pregnant. The wife is apparently healthy and has an uneventful medical and family history. The husband's father died in a car crash. The husband's paternal uncle has Huntington disease (HD) and is out of contact. The husband is 42 years old and has no HD symptoms. Molecular testing shows that he has 18/34 CAG repeats. What is the clinical significance of the results?[5,8,9]

A. The husband does not have Huntington disease.

B. The husband does not have Huntington disease, but his children will be at risk.

C. The husband may develop Huntington disease, and his children have a 10%–50% chance of having HD.

D. The husband has Huntington disease, and his children have a 50% chance of having HD.

E. None of the above.

17. A couple comes to a genetics clinic for prenatal counseling when the wife is 6 weeks pregnant. The wife is apparently healthy and has an uneventful medical and family history. The husband's father died in a car crash. The husband's paternal uncle has Huntington disease (HD) and is out of contact. The husband

is 42 years old and has no HD symptoms. Molecular testing shows that he has 19/38 CAG repeats in the *HTT* gene for Huntington disease. What is the clinical significance of the results?[5]

A. The husband does not have Huntington disease.

B. The husband does not have Huntington disease, but his children will be at risk.

C. The husband may develop Huntington disease, and his children have a 10%−50% chance of having HD.

D. The husband has Huntington disease, and his children have a 50% chance of having HD.

E. None of the above.

18. A couple came to a genetics clinic for prenatal counseling when the wife was 6 weeks pregnant. The husband's father died in a car accident at age of 36. The husband's paternal uncle had Huntington disease (HD) and was out of contact. The husband was 42 years old and had no symptoms of HD. Molecular testing showed that he has 20/41 CAG repeats. What is the clinical significance of the results?[5]

A. The husband does not have Huntington disease.

B. The husband does not have Huntington disease, but his children will be at risk.

C. The husband may develop Huntington disease and his children have a 10%−50% chance of having HD.

D. The husband has Huntington disease, and his children have a 50% chance of having HD.

E. None of the above.

19. Acknowledging the technical limitations of size analysis, the American College of Medical Genetics and Genomics (ACMG) supports which one of the following acceptable ranges for alleles with less than 50 repeats with Huntington disease clinical testing and as grading criteria for the College of American Pathology (CAP)/ACMG proficiency testing survey?[5]

A. Consensus size ± 1 repeats

B. Consensus size ± 2 repeats

C. Consensus size ± 3 repeats

D. Consensus size ± 4 repeats

E. Consensus size ± 5 repeats

20. Acknowledging the technical limitations of size analysis, the American College of Medical Genetics and Genomics (ACMG) supports which one of the following acceptable ranges for alleles with 50−70 repeats with Huntington disease clinical testing and as grading criteria for the College of American Pathology (CAP)/ACMG proficiency testing survey?[5]

A. Consensus size ± 1 repeats

B. Consensus size ± 2 repeats

C. Consensus size ± 3 repeats

D. Consensus size ± 4 repeats

E. Consensus size ± 5 repeats

21. Acknowledging the technical limitations of size analysis, the American College of Medical Genetics and Genomics (ACMG) supports which one of the following acceptable ranges for the alleles with >70 repeats with Huntington disease clinical testing and as grading criteria for the College of American Pathology (CAP)/ACMG proficiency testing survey?[5]

A. Consensus size ± 1 repeats

B. Consensus size ± 2 repeats

C. Consensus size ± 3 repeats

D. Consensus size ± 4 repeats

E. Consensus size ± 5 repeats

22. The pathogenesis of Huntington disease is[4]:

A. Activating mutation

B. Loss of function

C. Novel property on the protein

D. Novel property on the RNA

E. Novel property on the DNA

F. Overexpression

23. Jordan, a healthy 26-year-old male, came to a genetics clinic for a family history of Huntington disease. He is the only child of Jessica, age 55, and Ryan, 57. Jordan is married and has no children. Jessica was diagnosed with Huntington disease at 52 years of age. Jessica's *HTT* test revealed a compound heterozygous 17/38 repeats for the (CAG)n. What would be the chance Jordan has the same condition?[4,5,7,9]

A. 1/2

B. 1/4

C. 10%

D. Up to 1%

E. Not predictable

F. None of the above

24. Jordan, the only child of Jessica, age 55, and Ryan, 57, is a healthy 28-year-old married male with a 2-year-old son. Jessica was diagnosed with Huntington disease at 52 years of age. Jessica's *HTT* test revealed a compound heterozygous 17/38 repeats for the (CAG)n. Jordan decided to be tested for Huntington's disease and found out that he has 19/38 repeats. Jordan and his wife wanted to test their son for Huntington disease.

Which one of the following actions would be the most appropriate response from the care provider?[4,5,10]

A. Ordering the molecular genetic test for Jordan's son as the couple request

B. Explaining to the couple that it is better for their son to make his own decision when he grows up, since there are no preventive measures available for HD

C. Explaining to the couple that this clinic may not provide the test to the child, and referring the couple to another clinic

D. Explaining to the couple that the genetics laboratory in the hospital provides the test only to adults and that the clinic cannot find a lab to test the son

E. Explaining to the couple that insurance will not pay to test for children and that it is better for them wait until the son grows up

25. A couple, Jenny and Scott, came to a clinic for their first prenatal care when Jenny was 6 weeks pregnant. Both of them were apparently healthy, with unremarkable medical histories. A family history revealed that Scott's mother was diagnosed with Huntington disease (HD) at 52 years of age. She had a compound heterozygous 17/42 repeats for the (CAG)n in the *HTT* gene. Scott had refused the genetic test for HD in the past. The couple was concerned about whether their unborn child could have HD. The obstetrician recommended that Scott undergo HD molecular testing first. If he does not carry an abnormal allele, the couple's unborn child would most likely not have the disease. Scott's test results showed that he had 19/42 copies of the repeat. Which one of the following would be most appropriate next step in the workup?[4,5,10]

A. Ordering a molecular genetic test with CVS sample

B. Ordering a molecular genetic test with amniocentesis sample

C. Explaining to the couple it is their unborn child's decision when he/she grow up since there are no preventative measures available for Huntington's disease

D. Explaining to the couple this clinic may not provide the test to prenatal samples, then refer the couple to another clinic

E. Explaining to the couple the genetic laboratory in this hospital only provide the test to adults, but not prenatal samples

F. Explaining to the couple the insurance won't pay if it is for prenatal diagnosis

26. Jordan, a healthy 26-year-old male, is the only child of Jessica, age 55, and Ryan, 57. Jordan is married and has no children. Jessica was diagnosed with Huntington disease at age of 53. Jessica's *HTT* test revealed a compound heterozygous 17/40 repeats for the (CAG)n. What is the chance Jordan will have the same condition?[4,5,10]

A. 1/2
B. 1/4
C. 10%
D. Up to 1%
E. Not predictable
F. None of the above

27. Zoe, a healthy 26-year-old female, is an only child of her parents. She is married and has no children. Eight years ago, Jenny's paternal uncle was diagnosed with Huntington disease (HD) with 17/37 repeats. Jenny's father had a molecular test for *HTT*, and it revealed a compound heterozygous 17/33 repeats for the (CAG)n. What is Jenny's risk for HD before the molecular test?[4,5,10]

A. 1/2
B. 1/4
C. 8%
D. Not predictable
E. None of the above

28. A couple, Jenny and Scott, came to a clinic for their first prenatal care when Jenny was 6 weeks pregnant. Both of them were apparently healthy, with unremarkable medical histories. A family history revealed that Scott's mother had been diagnosed with Huntington's disease at 2 years old. She had compound heterozygous 17/43 copies of the (CAG)n repeat in the *HTT* gene. Scott was tested and was found to have 19/43 copies of the repeat. Prenatal CVS testing was offered, and the results showed that the fetus had 17/61 copies of the repeat. Which one of the following explanations would most likely be given to Jenny and her husband?[4,5,10]

A. The baby will develop Huntington symptoms in childhood or early adulthood.

B. The baby will develop Huntington symptoms in the middle of adulthood.

C. The baby will not develop Huntington symptoms.

D. The pregnancy will most likely end in a miscarriage.

E. It is not predictable whether the baby will develop Huntington symptoms because of the high frequency of somatic mosaicism.

29. A couple came to a clinic for their first prenatal care when the wife was 6 weeks pregnant. Both of them were apparently healthy, with unremarkable medical histories. The husband had a family history of Huntington's disease (HD).

Molecular genetic testing for HD was positive with the peripheral-blood sample from the husband. Invasive prenatal diagnosis was elected. The molecular testing result with CVS sample is shown below[11–13]:

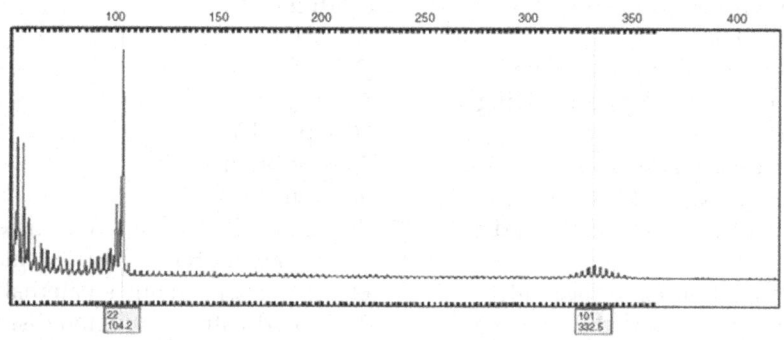

So the fetus had 22/101 copies of the repeat. Which one of the following molecular methods did the laboratory use for the assay?
A. Southern blot
B. Conventional PCR
C. Triplet repeat–primed PCR
D. Methylation study
E. Sanger sequencing

30. A couple came to a clinic for their first prenatal care when the wife was 6 weeks pregnant. They both were apparently healthy, with unremarkable medical histories. The husband had a family history of Huntington disease (HD). Molecular genetic testing of HD was positive with the peripheral-blood sample from the husband. Invasive prenatal diagnosis was elected. The test with CVS sampling is shown below[4,5,10]:

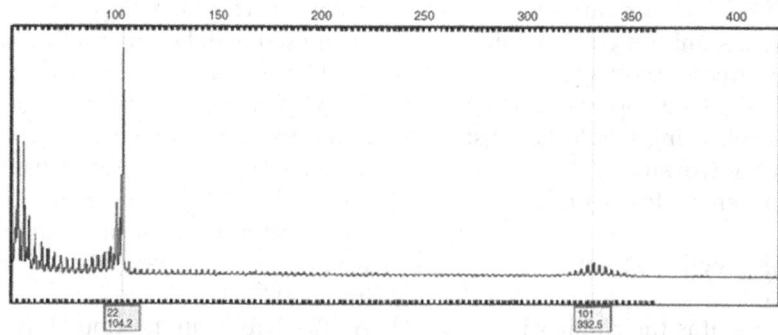

Which one of the results should be in the final report?
A. Normal allele(s)
B. Heterozygous intermediate allele
C. Heterozygous reduced-penetrance allele
D. Heterozygous full-penetrance allele
E. Heterozygous juvenile-onset allele

31. A couple came to a clinic for their first prenatal care when the wife was 6 weeks pregnant. Both

of them were apparently healthy, with unremarkable medical histories. The husband had a family history of Huntington disease (HD). Molecular genetic testing for HD was positive with the peripheral-blood sample from the husband. Invasive prenatal diagnosis was elected. The molecular testing result with the CVS sample is shown below:

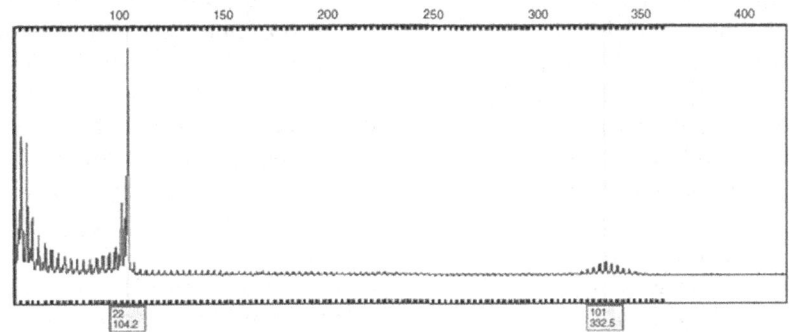

So the fetus had 22/101 copies of the repeat. Which one of the following would most likely be the predicted onset of HD symptoms if the fetus/patient develops symptoms?
A. Infancy
B. 18 years
C. 40 years
D. 60 years
E. Unclear
F. None of the above

32. Which one of the following ranges is not acceptable for Huntington clinical testing as grading criteria for the CAP/ACMG proficiency testing survey?[4,5,10]
A. Consensus size ± 2 repeats for alleles with <40 repeats
B. Consensus size ± 3 repeats for alleles with 40–50 repeats
C. Consensus size ± 3 repeats for alleles with 50–75 repeats
D. Consensus size ± 4 repeats for alleles with >75 repeats

33. Anticipation is a common phenomenon in the diseases caused by trinucleotide repeats, except in[4]:
A. Fragile X syndrome
B. Friedreich ataxia
C. Huntington disease
D. Myotonic dystrophy
E. Spinocerebellar ataxia

34. Anticipation is a common phenomenon in the diseases caused by trinucleotide repeats, except in[4]:
A. Fragile X syndrome
B. Spinal muscular atrophy
C. Huntington disease
D. Myotonic dystrophy
E. Spinocerebellar ataxia

35. The trinucleotide unstable repeat of the *FXN* gene for Friedreich ataxia is located in[14–16]:
A. Promoter
B. 5′ UTR
C. Intron
D. Exon
E. 3′ UTR

36. Which one of the following genetic changes in the *FXN* gene causes the majority of cases of Friedreich ataxia?[14–16]
A. Point mutations
B. in/del
C. (CAG)n repeats in an intron
D. (CAG)n repeats in an exon
E. (CTG)n repeats in an intron
F. (CTG)n repeats in an exon
G. (GAA)n repeat in an intron
H. (GAA)n repeat in an exon

37. BJ, a 32-year-old male, came to a genetics clinic because his 45-year-old brother had recently been diagnosed with Friedreich ataxia. Physical exam did not find any symptoms associated with Friedreich ataxia in this patient. BJ's father died in a car accident at the age of 42. What would be the risk for the development of Friedreich ataxia without further laboratory testing?
A. <1%
B. 8%
C. 25%
D. 50%
E. 75%
F. 100%
G. Cannot predict

38. BJ, a 32-year-old male, came to a genetics clinic because his 45-year-old brother had recently been diagnosed with Friedreich ataxia. Physical exam did not find any symptoms associated with

Friedreich ataxia. BJ's father died in a car accident at age of 42. The medical geneticist ordered a trinucleotide repeats test for Friedreich ataxia with BJ's peripheral-blood sample. The results showed that BJ had 11/30 copies of GAA in the *FXN* gene. Which one of the following would be the most appropriate interpretation of this molecular result?[14–16]

A. BJ had two normal alleles and would not develop symptoms for Friedreich ataxia.
B. BJ had one premutation allele, and would not develop symptoms for Friedreich ataxia.
C. BJ had one full-mutation allele and would not develop symptoms for Friedreich ataxia.
D. BJ had one full-mutation allele and would not develop symptoms for Friedreich ataxia.
E. None of the above.

39. BJ, a 32-year-old male, came to a genetics clinic because his 45-year-old brother had recently been diagnosed with Friedreich ataxia. Physical exam did not find any symptoms associated with Friedreich ataxia. BJ's father died in a car accident at age of 42. The medical geneticist ordered a trinucleotide repeats test for Friedreich ataxia with BJ's peripheral-blood sample. The results showed that BJ had 20/630 copies of GAA in the *FXN* gene. Which one of the following would be the most appropriate interpretation of this molecular result?[14–16]

A. BJ had two normal alleles and would not develop symptoms for Friedreich ataxia.
B. BJ had one premutation allele, and would not develop symptoms for Friedreich ataxia.
C. BJ had one full-mutation allele and would not develop symptoms for Friedreich ataxia.
D. BJ had one full-mutation allele and would develop symptoms for Friedreich ataxia.
E. BJ had one full-mutation allele and would develop early-onset Friedreich ataxia.
F. None of the above.

40. BJ, a 32-year-old male, came to a genetics clinic because his 45-year-old brother had recently been diagnosed with Friedreich ataxia. Physical exam did not find any symptoms associated with Friedreich ataxia. BJ's father died in a car accident at the age of 42. The medical geneticist ordered a trinucleotide repeats test for Friedreich ataxia with BJ's peripheral-blood sample. The results showed that BJ had

630/810 copies of GAA in the *FXN* gene. Which one of the following would be the most appropriate interpretation of this molecular result?[14–16]

A. BJ had two normal alleles and would not develop symptoms for Friedreich ataxia.
B. BJ had one premutation allele, and would not develop symptoms for Friedreich ataxia.
C. BJ had one full-mutation allele and would not develop symptoms for Friedreich ataxia.
D. BJ had two full-mutation alleles and would develop symptoms for Friedreich ataxia.
E. BJ had two full-mutation alleles and would develop early-onset Friedreich ataxia.
F. None of the above.

41. The pathogenesis of Friedreich ataxia is[4]:
A. Activating mutation
B. Loss of function
C. Novel property on the protein
D. Novel property on the RNA
E. Novel property on the DNA
F. Overexpression

42. Which one of following spinocerebellar ataxias is NOT caused by expansion of unstable repeat sequences?
A. Spinocerebellar ataxia type 1
B. Spinocerebellar ataxia type 2
C. Spinocerebellar ataxia type 3
D. Spinocerebellar ataxia type 4
E. All of the above
F. None of the above

43. Which one of following spinocerebellar ataxias is inherited in autosomal dominant pattern?
A. Spinocerebellar ataxia type 1
B. Spinocerebellar ataxia type 2
C. Spinocerebellar ataxia type 3
D. Spinocerebellar ataxia type 6
E. All of the above
F. None of the above

44. Which one of following spinocerebellar ataxias is caused by expansion of unstable repeat sequences?
A. Spinocerebellar ataxia type 1
B. Spinocerebellar ataxia type 3
C. Spinocerebellar ataxia type 6
D. Spinocerebellar ataxia type 7
E. All of the above
F. None of the above

45. Which one of following autosomal dominant spinocerebellar ataxias is caused by expansion of unstable repeat sequences located in an exon?
    A. Spinocerebellar ataxia type 1
    B. Spinocerebellar ataxia type 2
    C. Spinocerebellar ataxia type 6
    D. Spinocerebellar ataxia type 7
    E. All of the above
    F. None of the above

46. The trinucleotide unstable repeats of the *ATXN1* gene for autosomal dominant spinocerebellar ataxia type 1 is located in:
    A. Promoter
    B. 5′ UTR
    C. Intron
    D. Exon
    E. 3′ UTR

47. The pathogenic changes of the *ATXN1* gene for spinocerebellar ataxia type 1 is:
    A. A CGG repeat in promoter
    B. A CGG repeat in 5′ UTR
    C. A CCTG repeat in an intron
    D. A CAG repeat in an exon
    E. A CTG repeat in 3′ UTR

48. The CAG repeats of the *ATXN1* gene for autosomal dominant spinocerebellar ataxia type 1 codes for:
    A. Alanine
    B. Arginine
    C. Glutamine
    D. Histidine
    E. Proline

49. BJ, a 32-year-old male, came to a genetics clinic because his 45-year-old brother had recently been diagnosed with autosomal dominant spinocerebellar ataxia. Physical exam did not find any symptoms. BJ's father died in a car accident at age of 42. The medical geneticist ordered trinucleotide repeat tests for spinocerebellar ataxia type 1. The results showed that BJ had 20/120 copies of CAG in the *ATXN1* gene without CAT interruption. Which one of the following would be the most appropriate interpretation of this molecular result?
    A. BJ had an intermediate allele and would not develop symptoms for spinocerebellar ataxia type 1.
    B. BJ had a reduced penetrance allele, and might develop symptoms for spinocerebellar ataxia type 1.
    C. BJ had a full mutations allele, but he would not develop symptoms for spinocerebellar ataxia type 1 but is a carrier.
    D. BJ had a full mutations allele and would develop symptoms for spinocerebellar ataxia type 1.
    E. None of the above.

50. A 36-year-old female came to a clinic for inability to release a grasped object and easy fatigability. The symptoms started since she was 11 years old. Her prenatal, perinatal, and postnatal medical history were uneventful, but she had had some difficulties in primary school. She had been married for 7 years and had undergone infertility treatment over the previous 3–4 years. About 40 days ago, she had given birth to a baby girl by cesarean section. Her family history was notable for three affected brothers and three affected sisters. A muscle biopsy sample was obtained from the biceps. Light microscopic examination showed variation in fiber size characterized by hypertrophy and atrophy, angular atrophy, and muscle necrosis with myophagocytosis. A diagnosis of myotonic dystrophy was made. Which one of the following genetic assays would be the most appropriate one to confirm the diagnosis in this patient?
    A. Next-generation sequencing
    B. Sanger sequencing
    C. Targeted mutation analysis
    D. Triplet repeat–primed PCR assay
    E. None of the above

51. Which one of the following genes is associated with myotonic dystrophy type 1?
    A. *DMPK*
    B. *FXN*
    C. *FMR1*
    D. *HTT*
    E. *ZNF9*

52. The pathogenesis of myotonic dystrophy type 1 is[4]:
    A. Loss of function
    B. Novel property on the protein
    C. Novel property on the RNA
    D. Novel property on the DNA
    E. Overexpression

53. The trinucleotide unstable repeat sequence in *DM1* for myotonic dystrophy 1 is located in:
    A. Promoter
    B. 5′ UTR
    C. Intron
    D. Exon
    E. 3′ UTR

54. The pathogenic changes of the *DMPK* gene for myotonic dystrophy type 1 is:
    A. A CAA repeat
    B. A CAG repeat
    C. A CCTG repeat
    D. A CGG repeat
    E. A CTG repeat

55. OB, a 26-year-old female, comes to a genetics clinic for a family history of myotonic dystrophy type 1 (MD1). Her mother had myotonic dystrophy type 1, and died at age 56. No symptoms were found on physical exam. The medical geneticist ordered a molecular test for myotonic dystrophy type 1. The results showed that OB had 12/30 copies of CTG in the *DM1* gene. Which one of the following would be the most appropriate interpretation of this molecular result?

 A. OB had two normal alleles and would not develop symptoms for MD1.
 B. OB had a mutable normal (premutation) allele and would not develop symptoms for MD1.
 C. OB had a full-penetrance allele, but she would not develop symptoms for MD1 as a carrier.
 D. OB had a full-penetrance allele and would develop symptoms for MD1.
 E. None of the above.

56. OB, a 26-year-old female, came to a genetics clinic for a family history of myotonic dystrophy type 1. Her mother had myotonic dystrophy type 1 and died at age 56. No symptoms were found on physical exam. The medical geneticist ordered a molecular test for myotonic dystrophy type 1. The results showed that OB had 12/45 copies of CTG in the *DM1* gene. What would be the interpretation of this result?

 A. OB had two normal alleles and would not develop symptoms for MD1.
 B. OB had a mutable normal (premutation) allele and would not develop symptoms for MD1.
 C. OB had a full-penetrance allele, but she would not develop symptoms for MD1 as a carrier.
 D. OB had a full-penetrance allele and would develop symptoms for MD1.
 E. None of the above.

57. OB, a 26-year-old female, came to a genetics clinic for a family history of myotonic dystrophy type 1. Her mother had myotonic dystrophy type 1, and died at age 56. No symptoms were found on physical exam. The medical geneticist ordered a molecular test for myotonic dystrophy type 1. The results showed that OB had 24/75 copies of CTG in the *DM1* gene. What would be the interpretation of this result?

 A. OB had two normal alleles and would not develop symptoms for MD1.
 B. OB has a mutable normal (premutation) allele and would not develop symptoms for MD1.
 C. OB had a full-penetrance allele, but she would not develop symptoms for MD1 as a carrier.
 D. OB had a full-penetrance allele and would develop symptoms for MD1.
 E. None of the above.

58. A couple came to a genetics clinic for prenatal counseling when the wife was 10 weeks pregnant. The wife's father had myotonic dystrophy type 1 (MD1). The wife had the mutation for MD1 without symptoms. The husband was apparently healthy, with negative family history. The medical geneticist ordered a molecular test for MD1 on an amniotic fluid sample. The results showed that the fetus had 24/1200 copies of CTG in the *DM1* gene. What would be the interpretation of this result?[4]

 A. The fetus had two normal alleles and would not develop symptoms for MD1.
 B. The fetus had a mutable normal (premutation) allele and would not develop symptoms for MD1.
 C. The fetus had a full-penetrance allele but would not develop symptoms for MD1 as a carrier.
 D. The fetus had a full-penetrance allele and would develop symptoms for MD1.
 E. The fetus had a full-penetrance allele and would develop symptoms for MD1 early on in life.
 F. None of the above.

59. A 36-year-old female came to a clinic for prenatal care when she was 6 weeks pregnant. She had been married for 7 years and had been given infertility treatment over the previous 3–4 years. She was diagnosed with myotonic dystrophy type 1 about 1 year ago. The molecular genetic test of the *DMPK* gene revealed that she was compound heterozygosity for 12/99 repeats. CVS sampling was done and confirmed that the unborn boy had more than 1000 copies of the CTG repeats in *DMPK*. Which one of the following would best describe the estimated symptoms in the unborn boy?

 A. Reduced penetrance
 B. Mild
 C. Classic
 D. Congenital
 E. Not predictable

60. A 1-day-old boy was sent to the neonatal intensive-care unit (NICU) for severe hypotonia and respiratory distress. He died 5 days after birth from respiratory complications, even with intensive care. The molecular genetic test for MD confirmed that the newborn had 2600 copies of the CTG repeat in the *DMPK*. Both parents were apparently healthy and Caucasian. The mother was 32 years old and the father 42. Which of the following tests should be recommended as the next step in the workup?[4]

A. Maternal molecular genetic test for myotonic dystrophy type 1 followed by paternal test

B. Paternal molecular genetic test for myotonic dystrophy type 1 followed by maternal test

C. Parental molecular genetic test for myotonic dystrophy type 1

D. Maternal molecular genetic test for myotonic dystrophy type 2 followed by paternal test

E. Paternal molecular genetic test for myotonic dystrophy type 2 followed by maternal test

F. Parental molecular genetic test for myotonic dystrophy type 2

61. Which one of genes is associated with myotonic dystrophy type 2?

A. *DMPK*

B. *FXN*

C. *FMR1*

D. *HTT*

E. *ZNF9*

62. The unstable repeat sequence in the *ZNF9* (*CNBP*) gene for myotonic dystrophy type 2 is located in[4]:

A. Promoter

B. 5′ UTR

C. Intron

D. Exon

E. 3′ UTR

63. Myotonic dystrophy type 2 is characterized by myotonia and muscle dysfunction, and less commonly by cardiac conduction defects, cataracts, type 2 diabetes mellitus, and testicular failure. *ZNF9* (*CNBP*) is the only gene in which mutation is known to cause myotonic dystrophy type 2. *ZNF9* intron 1 contains a complex repeat motif, (TG)n(TCTG)n(CCTG)n. Which one of the repeat sequences is unstable and associated with Myotonic dystrophy type 2?[4]

A. CAA

B. CCTG

C. CTG

D. TCTG

E. All of the above

F. None of the above

64. A 36-year-old female came to a clinic for inability to release a grasped object and easy fatigability. The symptoms started when she was 11 years old. Her prenatal, perinatal, and postnatal medical history were uneventful, but she had had some difficulties in primary school. She had been married for 7 years, and had undergone infertility

treatment over the past 3−4 years. About 40 days ago, she had given birth to a baby girl by cesarean section. Family history was significant for three affected brothers and three affected sisters. A muscle biopsy sample was obtained from the biceps. Light microscopic examination showed variation in fiber size characterized by hypertrophy and atrophy, angular atrophy, and muscle necrosis with myophagocytosis. A diagnosis of myotonic dystrophy was made. Which one of following statements is correct?

A. The mutation for myotonic dystrophy type 1 is located in the 5′ UTR of *DMPK*.

B. The mutation for myotonic dystrophy type 2 is located in the 3′ UTR of *ZNF9* (*CNBP*).

C. Both Myotonic dystrophy type 1 and 2 are caused by trinucleotide repeat expansion.

D. Next-generation sequencing may detect 99% of mutations in both *DMPK* and *ZNF9*.

E. The baby girl will have 50% chance of developing myotonic dystrophy.

65. A 36-year-old female came to a clinic for inability to release a grasped object and easy fatigability. The symptoms started when she was 11 years old. Her prenatal, perinatal, and postnatal medical history were uneventful, but she had had some difficulties in primary school. She had been married for 7 years, and had undergone infertility treatment over the previous 3−4 years. About 40 days ago, she had given birth to a baby girl by cesarean section. Her family history was notable for three affected brothers and three affected sisters. A muscle biopsy sample was obtained from the biceps. Light microscopic examination showed variation in fiber size characterized by hypertrophy and atrophy, angular atrophy, and muscle necrosis with myophagocytosis. A diagnosis of myotonic dystrophy was made. Which one of the genetic tests would be the most appropriate to confirm the diagnosis in this patient?

A. Chromosome microarray

B. Next-generation sequencing

C. PCR/capillary electrophoresis and Southern blot

D. Sanger sequencing

E. Targeted mutation analysis

66. A 36-year-old female came to a clinic for prenatal care when she was 6 weeks pregnant. She had been married for 7 years, and had undergone infertility treatment over the previous 3−4 years. She was diagnosed with myotonic dystrophy type 1 about 1 year ago. The molecular genetic test of

the *DMPK* gene revealed that she was compound heterozygosity for 12/99 repeats. CVS testing was performed and confirmed that the unborn boy had approximately 200 copies of the CTG repeats in *DMPK*. Which one of the following would be the most appropriate interpretation for the unborn boy?

A. Reduced penetrance
B. Mild
C. Classic
D. Congenital
E. Not predictable

67. A couple came to a clinic for prenatal counseling when the wife was 6 weeks pregnant. The wife's 32-year-old brother was just diagnosed with myotonic dystrophy type 1 with 12/115 copies of the CAG repeat in the *DMPK* gene. Molecular genetic testing revealed that the wife was compound heterozygous for 12/45. Which one of the following would be the most appropriate interpretation for the wife?

A. Normal
B. Mutable normal
C. Full mutation
D. Congenital
E. None of the above

68. A 2-year-old girl was brought to a genetics clinic by her foster parents for mental retardation. The medical and family histories were unknown. Her performance IQ was 69, verbal IQ 57, and full-scale IQ 63. The most common congenital cause of mental retardation is:

A. Down syndrome
B. Fetal alcohol syndrome
C. Fragile X syndrome
D. Turner syndrome
E. None of the above

69. A 2-year-old girl was brought to a genetics clinic by her parents for mental retardation. The family history was uneventful. Her performance IQ was 69, verbal 57, and full-scale 63. The most common genetic etiology of mental retardation is:

A. Down syndrome
B. Fetal alcohol syndrome
C. Fragile X syndrome
D. Turner syndrome
E. None of the above

70. A 2-year-old boy was brought to a genetics clinic by his parents for mental retardation. The family history was significant for an older brother being "slow." The medical and family

histories were unknown. His performance IQ was 69, verbal IQ 57, and full-scale IQ 63. The most common cause of inherited mental retardation is:

A. Down syndrome
B. Fetal alcohol syndrome
C. Fragile X syndrome
D. Turner syndrome
E. None of the above

71. The unstable repeat sequence in the *FMR1* gene for fragile X syndrome is located in[17]:

A. Promoter
B. 5′ UTR
C. Intron
D. Exon
E. 3′ UTR

72. The unstable repeat sequence in the *FMR1* gene for fragile X syndrome is[17]:

A. CAA
B. CAG
C. CGG
D. CTG
E. CCTG

73. Which one of the following is the pathogenesis of fragile X syndrome?[17]

A. Loss of function
B. Novel property on the protein
C. Novel property on the RNA
D. Novel property on the DNA
E. Overexpression

74. A couple came to a genetics clinic for prenatal counseling when the wife was 6 weeks pregnant. The wife's maternal uncle had fragile X syndrome and lived outside the country. The wife was 36 years old, and apparently healthy. Molecular testing showed she had 29/189 CGG copies of the CGG repeat. Which one of the following would be the most appropriate interpretation of this molecular result?[17]

A. The wife did not have fragile X syndrome.
B. The wife did not have fragile X syndrome, but her children would be at risk for premutation.
C. The wife did not have fragile X syndrome, but she was at risk for premature ovarian failure, and her children would be at risk for fragile X syndrome.
D. The wife had fragile X syndrome.
E. None of the above.

75. A couple came to a genetics clinic for prenatal counseling when the wife was 6 weeks pregnant. The wife's maternal uncle had fragile X syndrome and lived outside the country. The wife was 36

years old, and apparently healthy. Molecular testing showed that she had 29/62 CGG copies of the CGG repeat. Which one of the following would be the most appropriate interpretation of this molecular result?[17]

A. The wife did not have fragile X syndrome.

B. The wife did not have fragile X syndrome, but her children would be at risk for premutation.

C. The wife did not have fragile X syndrome, but she was at risk for premature ovarian failure, and her children would be at risk for fragile X syndrome.

D. The wife had fragile X syndrome.

E. None of the above.

76. A couple came to a genetics clinic for prenatal counseling when the wife was 6 weeks pregnant. The wife's maternal uncle had fragile X syndrome and lived outside the country. The wife was 36 years old, and apparently healthy. Molecular testing showed that she had 29/52 copies of the CGG repeat. Which one of the following would be the most appropriate interpretation of this molecular result?[17]

A. The wife did not have fragile X syndrome.

B. The wife did not have fragile X syndrome, but her children would be at risk for premutation.

C. The wife did not have fragile X syndrome, but she was at risk for premature ovarian failure, and her children would be at risk for fragile X syndrome.

D. The wife had fragile X syndrome.

E. None of the above.

77. A couple came to a genetics clinic for prenatal counseling when the wife was 6 weeks pregnant. The wife's maternal uncle had fragile X syndrome and lived outside the country. The wife was 36 years old, and apparently healthy. Molecular testing showed that she had 29/48 copies of the CGG repeat. Which one of the following would be the most appropriate interpretation of this molecular result?[17]

A. The wife did not have fragile X syndrome.

B. The wife did not have fragile X syndrome, but her children would be at risk for premutation.

C. The wife did not have fragile X syndrome, but she was at risk for premature ovarian failure, and her children would be at risk for fragile X syndrome.

D. The wife had fragile X syndrome.

E. None of the above.

78. A couple came to a genetics clinic for prenatal counseling when the wife was 6 weeks pregnant. The wife's maternal uncle had fragile X syndrome and lived outside the country. The wife was 36

years old, and apparently healthy. Molecular testing showed that she had 29/42 CGG repeats. Which one of the following would be the most appropriate interpretation of this molecular result?

A. The wife did not have fragile X syndrome.

B. The wife did not have fragile X syndrome, but her children would be at risk for premutation.

C. The wife did not have fragile X syndrome, but she was at risk for premature ovarian failure, and her children would be at risk for fragile X syndrome.

D. The wife had fragile X syndrome.

E. None of the above.

79. A couple came to a genetics clinic for prenatal counseling when the wife was 6 weeks pregnant. The wife's maternal uncle had fragile X syndrome and lived outside the country. The wife was 21 years old. Molecular testing showed that she had 29/240 copies of the CGG repeat. Which one of the following would be the most appropriate interpretation of this molecular result?

A. The wife did not have fragile X syndrome.

B. The wife did not have fragile X syndrome, but her children would be at risk for premutation.

C. The wife did not have fragile X syndrome, but she was at risk for premature ovarian failure, and her children would be at risk for fragile X syndrome.

D. The wife had fragile X syndrome.

E. None of the above.

80. A couple came to a genetics clinic for prenatal counseling when the wife was 6 weeks pregnant. The wife's maternal uncle had fragile X syndrome and lived outside the country. The wife was 36 years old, and apparently healthy. Molecular testing showed that she had 29/180 copies of the CGG repeat. Which one of the following would be the most appropriate recommendation to the family?[17]

A. Noninvasive prenatal test (NIPT) with cell-free DNA from maternal blood

B. Prenatal diagnosis with chorionic villus sampling (CVS)

C. Prenatal diagnosis with amniotic fluid sampling

D. Since expansion usually is transmitted by the father, there is no need for prenatal diagnosis.

E. None of the above.

81. A couple came to a genetics clinic for prenatal counseling when the wife was 6 weeks pregnant. The wife's maternal uncle had fragile X syndrome and lived outside the country. The wife was 21 years old, and apparently healthy. Molecular testing showed that she had 29/240 CGG repeats. The allele with approximately 240 copies of the repeat was methylated. A CVS sample was tested

for the repeat. The results detected a single unmethylated allele with approximately 500 copies of the repeat. Which one of the following would be the clinical significance of the results?[17]

A. The unborn child would not have fragile X syndrome.

B. The unborn child would not have fragile X syndrome, but he would be at risk for fragile X–associated tremor/ataxia syndrome (FXTAS).

C. The unborn child would not have fragile X syndrome, but he would have fragile X–associated tremor/ataxia syndrome (FXTAS).

D. The unborn child would have fragile X syndrome.

E. None of the above.

82. A couple came to a genetics clinic for prenatal counseling when the wife was 6 weeks pregnant. The wife's maternal uncle had fragile X syndrome and lived outside the country. The wife was 21 years old, and apparently healthy. Molecular testing showed that she had 29/180 copies of the CGG repeat. A CVS sample was tested for the repeat. The results detected a hemizygous unmethylated allele with approximately 200 copies of the repeat. Which one of the following statements regarding this result would be the most appropriate interpretation?[17]

A. The unborn child would not have fragile X syndrome.

B. The unborn child would not have fragile X syndrome, but he would be at risk for fragile X–associated tremor/ataxia syndrome (FXTAS).

C. The unborn child would not have fragile X syndrome, but he would have fragile X–associated tremor/ataxia syndrome (FXTAS).

D. The unborn child would have fragile X syndrome.

E. The clinical implication was unclear. A follow-up amniocentesis might be required.

F. None of the above.

83. A couple came to a genetics clinic for prenatal counseling when the wife was 6 weeks pregnant. The wife's maternal uncle had fragile X syndrome and lived outside the country. The wife was 21 years old, and apparently healthy. Molecular testing showed that she had 29/150 copies of the CGG repeat. Prenatal testing with amniotic fluid detected a single unmethylated band with approximately 150 copies of the repeat. Which one of the following statements regarding this

result would be the most appropriate interpretation?[17]

A. The unborn child would not have fragile X syndrome.

B. The unborn child would not have fragile X syndrome, but he would be at risk for fragile X–associated tremor/ataxia syndrome (FXTAS).

C. The unborn child would not have fragile X syndrome, but he would have fragile X–associated tremor/ataxia syndrome (FXTAS).

D. The unborn child would have fragile X syndrome.

E. None of the above.

84. A couple came to a genetics clinic for prenatal counseling when the wife was 6 weeks pregnant. The wife's maternal uncle had fragile X syndrome and lived outside the country. The wife was 21 years old, and apparently healthy. Molecular test showed that she had 29/150 copies of the CGG repeat. Prenatal test with amniotic fluid sample detected 32/150 copies of the repeat. Which one of the following statements regarding this result would be the most appropriate interpretation?[17]

A. The unborn child would not have fragile X syndrome.

B. The unborn child would not have fragile X syndrome, but she would be at risk for FMR1-related primary ovarian insufficiency.

C. The unborn child would not have fragile X syndrome, but she would have FMR1-related primary ovarian insufficiency.

D. The unborn child would have fragile X syndrome.

E. None of the above.

85. A 26-year-old female was referred to a genetics clinic for counseling because her father had recently been diagnosed with FMR1-associated tremor/ataxia syndrome. The molecular genetic test for fragile X syndrome was ordered for her. The results came back and showed that she had 31/102 copies of the CGG repeat in the 5′ UTR region of the FMR1 gene. What was the approximate risk for her to have FMR1-related primary ovarian insufficiency?[17]

A. 1%

B. 5%

C. 20%

D. 40%

E. 60%

F. 80%

86. A couple came to a genetics clinic for prenatal counseling when the wife was 10 weeks pregnant.

She had 30/52 copies of the CGG repeat in the *FMR1* gene. Subsequent testing found that the husband had 100 copies. Prenatal ultrasound showed that the fetus was a female. What diseases would the unborn daughter be at risk to have?[17]

A. Fragile X syndrome

B. *FMR1*-associated tremor/ataxia syndrome (FXTAS)

C. *FMR1*-related primary ovarian insufficiency (POI)

D. A and B

E. B and C

F. A, B, and C

G. None of the above

87. A couple came to a genetics clinic for prenatal counseling when the wife was 10 weeks pregnant. The wife had 31/52 copies of the CGG repeat in the *FMR1* gene on Xq27.3. The husband had 30 copies. Prenatal ultrasound testing showed that the fetus was a female. What diseases would the unborn daughter be at increased risk to develop?[17]

A. Fragile X syndrome

B. *FMR1*-associated tremor/ataxia syndrome (FXTAS)

C. *FMR1*-related primary ovarian insufficiency (POI)

D. A and B

E. B and C

F. A, B, and C

G. None of the above

88. A couple came to a genetics clinic for prenatal counseling when the wife was 10 weeks pregnant. The wife had 28/30 copies of the CGG repeat in the *FMR1* gene for fragile X syndrome. The husband had approximately 100 copies. Prenatal ultrasound test results showed that the fetus was a male. What diseases would the unborn son be at increased risk to have?[17]

A. Fragile X syndrome

B. *FMR1*-associated tremor/ataxia syndrome (FXTAS)

C. *FMR1*-related primary ovarian insufficiency (POI)

D. A and B

E. B and C

F. A, B, and C

G. None of the above

89. A couple came to a genetics clinic for prenatal counseling when the wife was 10 weeks pregnant. The wife's father had recently been diagnosed with *FMR1*-associated tremor/ataxia syndrome. The physician ordered the molecular genetic test for fragile X syndrome. The wife had 30/179 copies of the CGG repeat in the *FMR1* gene. The husband had 29 copies. Prenatal ultrasound test results showed that the fetus was a male.

What disease would the unborn son be at increased risk to have?[17]

A. Fragile X syndrome

B. *FMR1*-associated tremor/ataxia syndrome (FXTAS)

C. *FMR1*-related primary ovarian insufficiency (POI)

D. A and B

E. B and C

F. None of the above

90. A 4-year-old boy was brought to a genetics clinic by his parents for mental retardation and macroorchidism. The family history showed that maternal uncle, who had passed away, had had similar problems. The doctor ordered chromosome karyotyping and microarray testing. Karyotyping showed a normal male karyotype. Microarray testing found a 1.31 Mb interstitial deletion on Xq27.3 including the *FMR1* gene. What would be the most appropriate interpretation of the microarray results?[17]

A. The boy had fragile X syndrome

B. The boy was at risk for *FMR1*-associated tremor/ataxia syndrome (FXTAS)

C. The boy was at risk for *FMR1*-related primary ovarian insufficiency (POI)

D. A and B

E. B and C

F. A, B, and C

G. None of the above

91. A couple came to a genetics clinic for prenatal counseling when the wife was 10 weeks pregnant. Family history indicated that multiple individuals from the wife's side had mild-to-moderate intellectual disability. The wife's parents passed away in a car accident when she was 8 years old. Microarray testing was ordered for the wife. The results showed that she had a 334-kb deletion in the *FMR2* gene on Xq28. The microarray on the CVS showed that the fetus was a male with the maternal inherited deletion in the *FMR2* gene. What disease would the unborn son be at increased risk to have?[17]

A. Fragile X syndrome

B. *FMR1*-associated tremor/ataxia syndrome (FXTAS)

C. *FMR1*-related primary ovarian insufficiency (POI)

D. Mental retardation, X-linked, FRAXE type

E. All of the above

F. None of the above

92. Which one of the following disorders is NOT caused by loss-of-function changes?[4]

A. Fragile X syndrome

B. Fragile X syndrome E

C. Friedreich ataxia

D. Huntington disease

E. All of the above

F. None of the above

93. Which one of the following disorders is NOT caused by gain-of-function changes?[4]

   A. Fragile X syndrome

   B. *FMR1*-associated tremor/ataxia syndrome (FXTAS)

   C. Huntington disease

   D. Myotonic dystrophy

   E. Spinocerebellar ataxia

   F. None of the above

94. Figure below shows Southern blot testing results using *Eco*R1 and *Eag*I digestion and StB12.3 probe for the CGG repeat in the *FMR1* gene. Numbers 7, 8, and 9 are the controls (7 = premutation female; 8 = full mutation female; and 9 = normal female). Which one of the male patients in the figure has fragile X syndrome?[4,17]

   A. 1

   B. 2

   C. 3

   D. 4

   E. 5

   F. 6

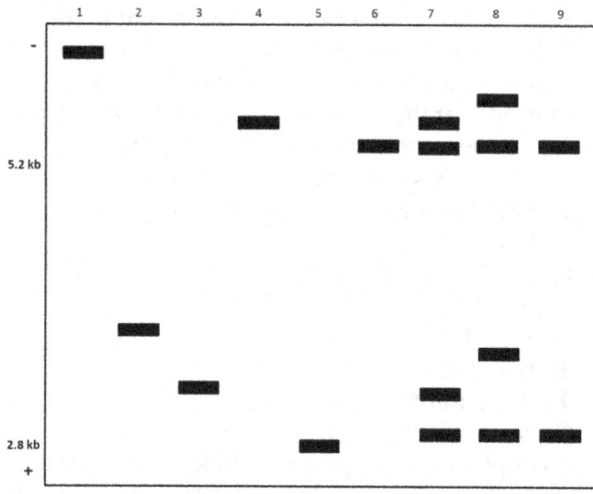

96. Figure below shows the Southern blot testing results using *Eco*R1 and *Eag*I digestion and StB12.3 probe for the CGG repeat in the *FMR1* gene. Numbers 7, 8, and 9 are the controls (7 = premutation female; 8 = full mutation female; and 9 = normal female). Which one of the male patients in the figure does not have fragile X syndrome and is not at risk for *FMR1*-associated tremor/ataxia syndrome (FXTAS)?[4,17]

   A. 1

   B. 2

   C. 3

   D. 4

   E. 5

   F. 6

95. Figure below shows the Southern blot testing results using *Eco*R1 and *Eag*I digestion and StB12.3 probe for the CGG repeat in the *FMR1* gene. Numbers 7, 8, and 9 are the controls (7 = premutation female; 8 = full mutation female; and 9 = normal female). Which one of the male patients in the figure is at risk for *FMR1*-associated tremor/ataxia syndrome (FXTAS)?[4,17]

   A. 1

   B. 2

   C. 3

   D. 4

   E. 5

   F. 6

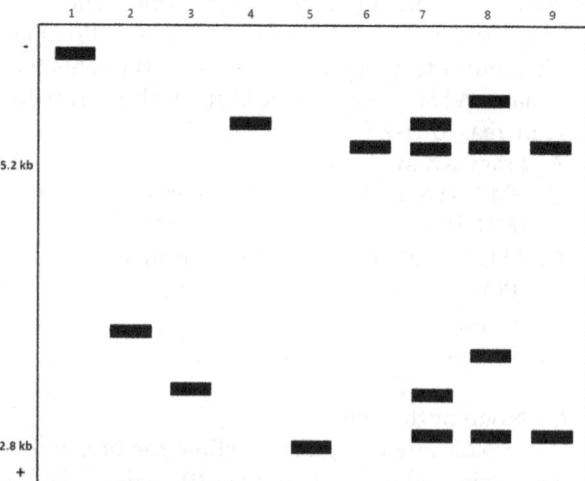

97. Figure below shows the Southern blot testing results using *Eco*R1 and *Eag*I digestion and StB12.3 probe for the CGG repeat in the *FMR1* gene. Numbers 1, 2, and 3 are the controls (1 = full mutation male;

2 = premutation male; and 3 = normal male).
Which one of the female patients in the
figure does not have fragile X syndrome, but is
at risk for *FMR1*-associated tremor/ataxia
syndrome (FXTAS) and premature ovarian
failure (POF)?[4,17]

A. 4
B. 5
C. 6
D. 7
E. 8
F. 4 and 5
G. 4 and 6
H. 4, 5, and 6
I. 5 and 7
J. 4, 5, and 7
K. All of the above
L. None of the above

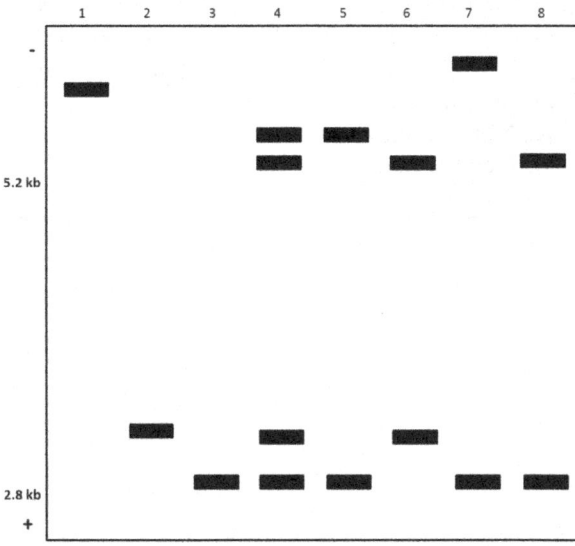

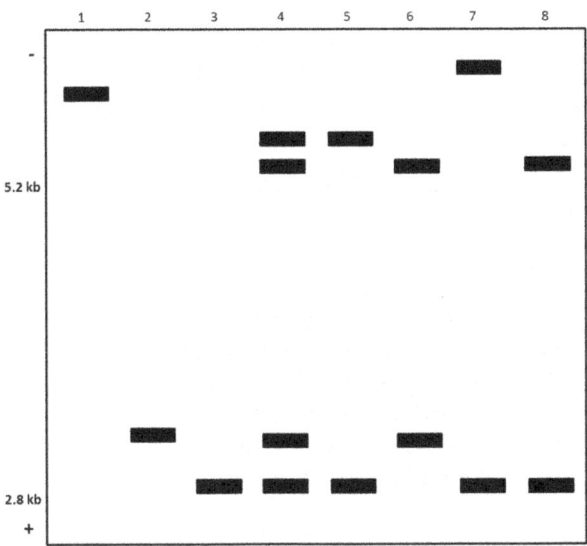

98. Figure below shows the Southern Blot
results using *Eco*R1 and *Eag*I digestion and
StB12.3 probe for the CGG repeat in the *FMR1*
gene. The number 1, 2, and 3 are the controls
(1 = full mutation male; 2 = premutation
male; and 3 = normal male). Which one of the
female patients in the figure has fragile X
syndrome?[4,17]

A. 4
B. 5
C. 6
D. 7
E. 8
F. 4 and 7
G. All of the above
H. None of the above

99. Figure below shows the Southern blot testing results
using *Eco*R1 and *Eag*I digestion and StB12.3 probe
for the CGG repeat in the *FMR1* gene. Numbers 1, 2,
and 3 are the controls (1 = full mutation male;
2 = premutation male; and 3 = normal male). Which
one of the female patients in the figure does not
have fragile X syndrome and is not at risk for *FMR1*-
associated tremor/ataxia syndrome (FXTAS), or
premature ovarian failure?[4,17]

A. 4
B. 5
C. 6
D. 7
E. 8
F. 6 and 8
G. All of the above
H. None of the above

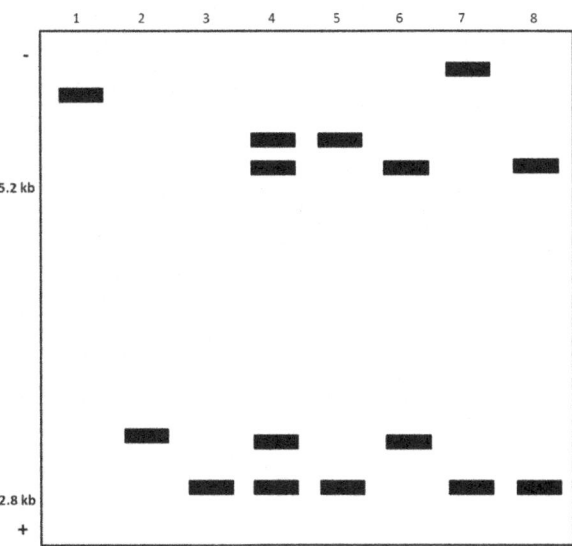

100. Figure below shows triplet repeat—primed PCR of CGG repeats in *FMR1* gene in a peripheral-blood sample. Which is the most appropriate interpretation?[4,17]
  A. Normal female
  B. Normal male
  C. Female with a gray-zone mutation
  D. Male with a gray-zone mutation
  E. Female with a premutation
  F. Male with a premutation
  G. Female with a full mutation
  H. Male with a full mutation

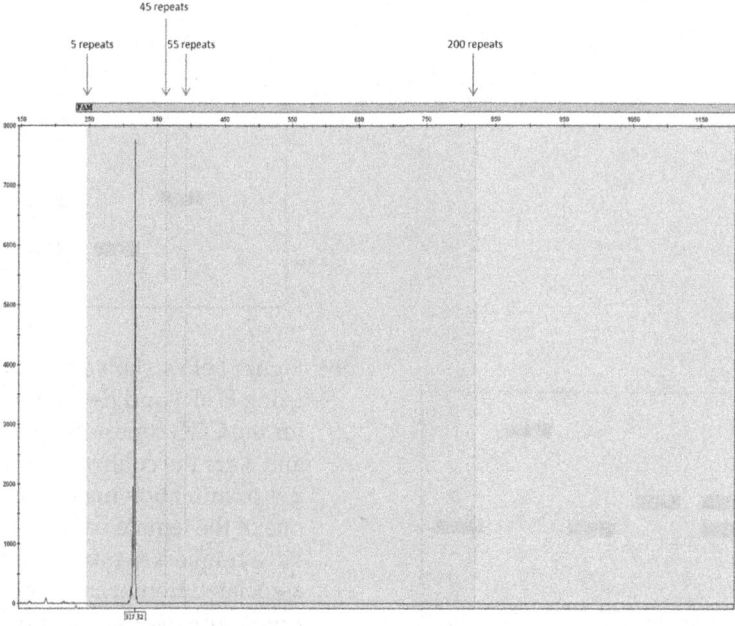

101. Figure below shows triplet repeat—primed PCR of CGG repeats in *FMR1* gene in a peripheral-blood sample. Which is the most appropriate interpretation?[4,17]
  A. Normal female
  B. Normal male
  C. Female with a gray-zone mutation
  D. Male with a gray-zone mutation
  E. Female with a premutation
  F. Male with a premutation
  G. Female with a full mutation
  H. Male with a full mutation

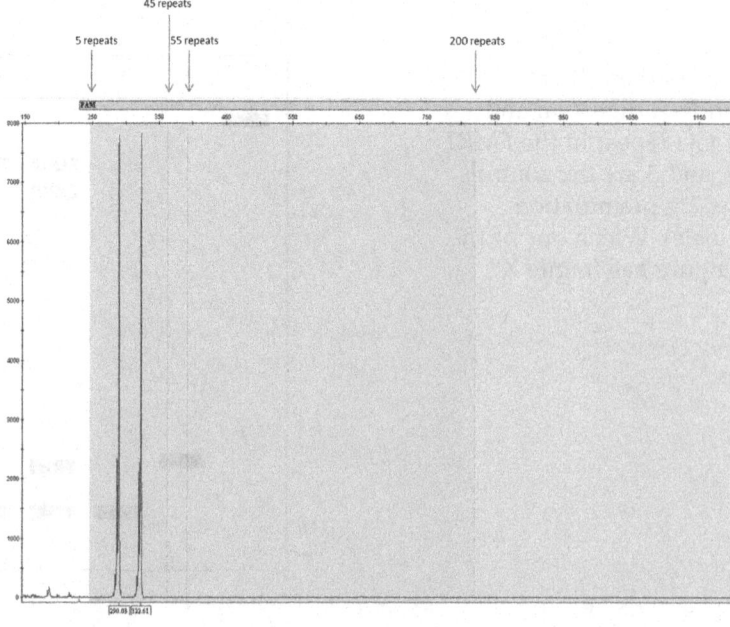

102. Figure below shows triplet repeat–primed PCR of CGG repeats in *FMR1* gene with a peripheral-blood sample. Which is the most appropriate interpretation?[4,17]
   A. Normal female
   B. Normal male
   C. Female with a gray-zone mutation
   D. Male with a gray-zone mutation
   E. Female with a premutation
   F. Male with a premutation
   G. Female with a full mutation
   H. Male with a full mutation

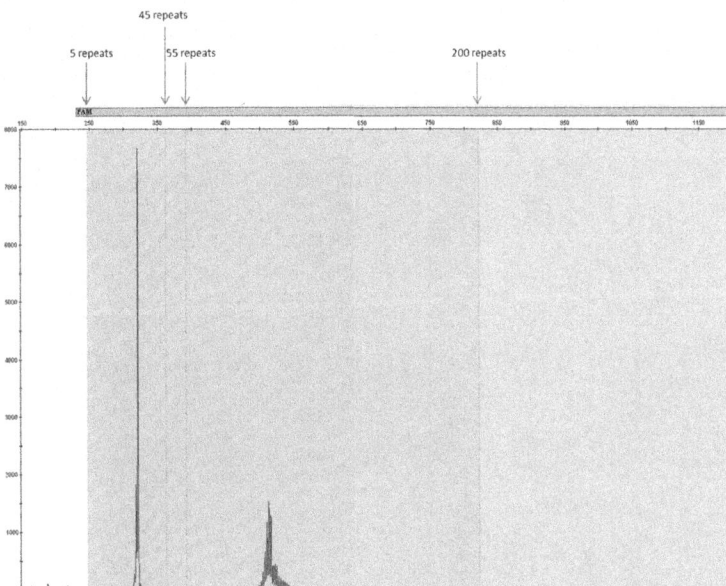

103. Figure below shows triplet repeat-primed PCR of CGG repeats in *FMR1* gene with a peripheral-blood sample. Which is the most appropriate interpretation?[4,17]
   A. Normal female
   B. Normal male
   C. Female with a gray-zone mutation
   D. Male with a gray-zone mutation
   E. Female with a premutation
   F. Male with a premutation
   G. Female with a full mutation
   H. Male with a full mutation

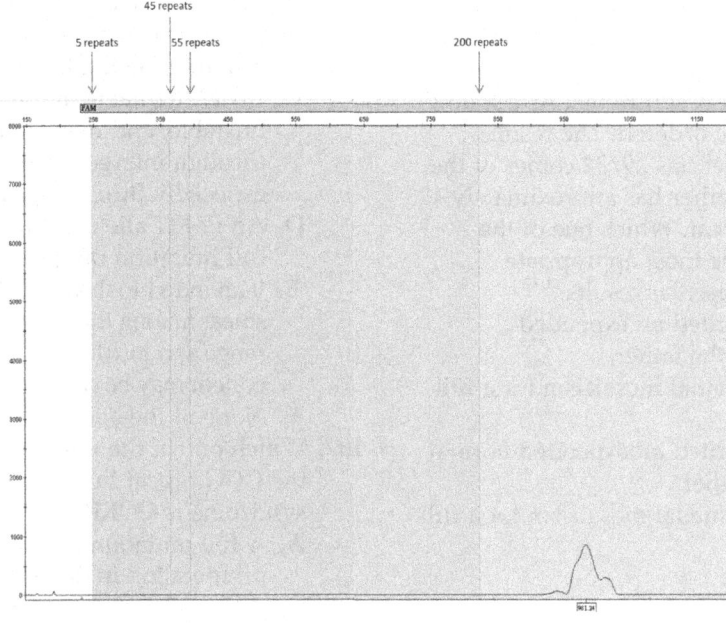

104. Figure below shows triplet repeat–primed PCR of CGG repeats in *FMR1* gene with a peripheral-blood sample. What is the most appropriate interpretation?[4,17]
  A. Normal female
  B. Normal male
  C. Female with a gray-zone mutation
  D. Male with a gray-zone mutation
  E. Female with a premutation
  F. Male with a premutation
  G. Female with a full mutation
  H. Male with a full mutation

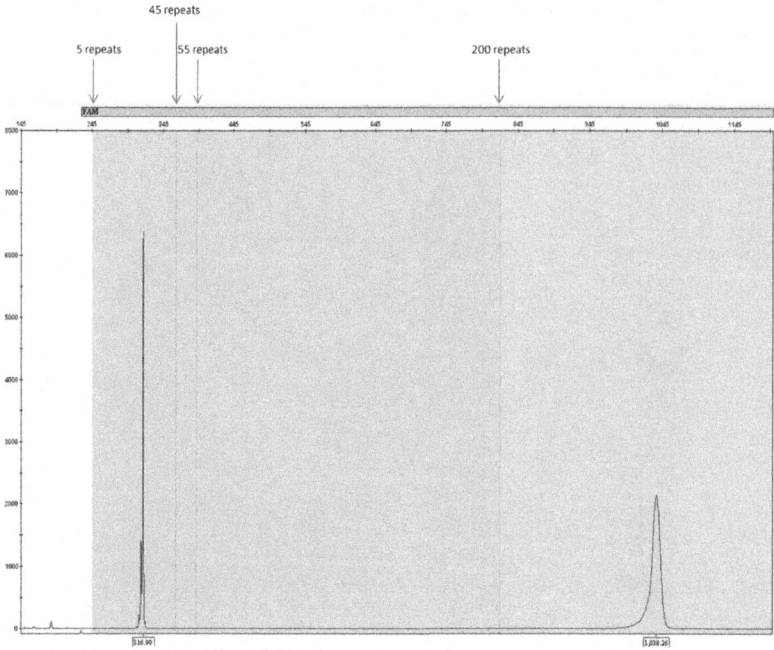

105. An apparently healthy couple gave a birth to a baby girl with intellectual disability. The family history was unremarkable on both sides. A clinical geneticist ordered chromosome, microarray, and *FMR1* tests for the infant. The chromosome and microarray results were normal. The fragile X test results showed that the baby girl has approximately 250 copies of the CGG repeat for one allele. The baby girl was diagnosed with fragile X syndrome. As a follow-up, parental tests were ordered. The results showed that the mother has 29/32 copies of the CGG repeat, but the father has approximately 125 copies of the CGG repeat. Which one of the following would be the most appropriate explanation of the molecular results?[4,17]
  A. The daughter inherited an expended permutation from the father.
  B. The father had gonadal mosaicism for a full mutation.
  C. The daughter inherited an expended normal allele from the mother.
  D. The mother had gonadal mosaicism for a full mutation.
  E. None of the above.

106. Which one of the following statements regarding the CGG repeat in the *FMR1* gene for fragile X syndrome is CORRECT?[17]
  A. Individuals, especially males, with repeats in the premutation range may expand to full mutation owing to somatic instability.
  B. Individuals, especially females, with repeats in the intermediate range may expand to full mutation owing to somatic instability.
  C. An *FMR1* allele in the premutation range is unstable, and may expand to a full mutation through intergenerational transmission, especially through a carrier female.
  D. An *FMR1* allele in the premutation range or full mutation range is usually methylated.
  E. If an individual has an allele that looks like a smear among the upper limit of the premutation range and low limit of full mutation range, the patient may be considered to have a premutation.
  F. None of the above.

107. Which one of the following statements regarding the CGG repeat in the *FMR1* gene for fragile X syndrome is CORRECT?[17]
  A. A full mutation in males may shrink to premutation in daughters during transmission.

B. Females with full mutation usually are not symptomatic.

C. Fragile X—associated tremor/ataxia syndrome (FXTAS) only appears in male premutation carriers, but not females.

D. Most of female premutation carriers develop premature ovarian failure before 40 years of age.

E. A full mutation in females may shrink to premutation during transmission.

108. Which one of the following statements regarding the CGG repeat in the *FMR1* gene for fragile X syndrome is CORRECT?[4,17]

A. An *FMR1* allele with a full mutation is hypertranscribed.

B. An *FMR1* allele with a premutation is transcriptionally silenced.

C. Fragile X is more common in the Ashkenazi Jewish population than in Caucasians.

D. The triplet-primed PCR may detect point mutations besides trinucleotide repeats.

E. The normal allele may be methylated in a female premutation carrier.

109. Jonathan, a 2-year-old male, was referred to a genetics clinic for global developmental delay and dysmorphic features. Physical examination revealed a proportionate-looking child with generalized hypotonia and dysmorphic features, including long and narrow face, high and prominent forehead, epicanthal folds, narrow and high-arched palate, posteriorly rotated ears, and a right hand with a transverse simian crease. The child was born after an uneventful full-term pregnancy. At birth, he had an undescended right testis. Combination PCR and Southern blot testing confirmed that the patient had compound heterozygous 30/243 copies of the CGG repeats. The parents were in their early 30s and were apparently health. Parental tests showed the mother (Sandy) is a carrier with 32/192. Sandy had two brothers (John and Scott), and one sister (Jenny). They were all healthy. Scott was 32 years old with 172 copies of the CGG repeat. John was 36 years old with 190 repeats. Jenny was 34 years old with 29/193 copies. Which one of the following individuals had highest risk of developing fragile X—associated tremor/ataxia syndrome?[4,17]

A. Jenny

B. John

C. Sandy

D. Scott

E. Unpredictable

110. A 2-year-old male was referred to a genetics clinic for global developmental delay and dysmorphic features. Physical examination revealed a proportionate-looking child with generalized hypotonia and dysmorphic features, including long and narrow face, high and prominent forehead, epicanthal folds, narrow and high-arched palate, posteriorly rotated ears, and a right hand with a transverse simian crease. The child was born after an uneventful full-term pregnancy. At birth, he had an undescended right testis. Chromosome microarray results were normal. Combination PCR and Southern blot testing confirmed that the patient had compound heterozygous 30/243 copies of the CGG repeats in the *FMR1* gene. Which one of the following describes the function of the *FMR1* gene product?[4]

A. Protein kinase

B. RNA-binding protein

C. Structural protein

D. Transmembrane protein

E. Zinc-finger protein

111. A couple came to a clinic for their first prenatal care when the wife was 6 weeks pregnant. Both of them were apparently healthy with unremarkable medical histories. The wife had family history of fragile X syndrome (FXS). Molecular genetic testing of the (CGG)n repeat in the *FMR1* gene showed c.-129CGG(199) with the CVS sample when the gestational age was 10 weeks. Which one of following would most likely be the physician's response to the results?[10]

A. Informing the couple that their unborn son carries a premutation allele and will be at risk for FXTAS.

B. Informing the couple that their unborn son carries an abnormal allele and will have fragile X syndrome or FXTAS.

C. Informing the couple that their unborn son carries an abnormal allele and that amniocentesis is recommended to establish the diagnosis.

D. Informing the couple that their unborn child carries an abnormal allele and will have FXS.

E. Informing the couple that their unborn child carries an abnormal allele and will have FXTAS and/or premature ovarian insufficiency (FXPOI).

112. A clinical molecular genetics laboratory plans to validate a test for fragile X syndrome with a combination of Southern blot and PCR assays for the (CGG)n repeat in the *FMR1* gene. The laboratory director put a validation plan together according to the ACMG guidelines and grading criteria for CAP proficiency testing survey. Which one of the following ranges for *FMR1* clinical testing is acceptable?

A. Consensus size ± 6 repeats for alleles with <55 repeats

B. Consensus size ± 5 repeats for alleles with <55 repeats

C. Consensus size ± 4 repeats for alleles with <55 repeats

D. Consensus size ± 3 repeats for alleles with <55 repeats

E. Consensus size ± 2 repeats for alleles with <55 repeats

F. Consensus size ± 1 repeats for alleles with <55 repeats

113. A clinical molecular genetics laboratory plans to validate a test for fragile X syndrome with combination of Southern blot and PCR assays for the (CGG)*n* repeat in the *FMR1* gene. The laboratory director put together a validation plan according to the ACMG guideline and grading criteria for CAP proficiency testing survey. Which one of the following ranges for *FMR1* clinical testing is acceptable?

A. Consensus size ± 14 repeats for alleles with 56—100 repeats

B. Consensus size ± 12 repeats for alleles with 56—100 repeats

C. Consensus size ± 10 repeats for alleles with 56—100 repeats

D. Consensus size ± 8 repeats for alleles with 56—100 repeats

E. Consensus size ± 6 repeats for alleles with 56—100 repeats

F. Consensus size ± 4 repeats for alleles with 56—100 repeats

114. A clinical molecular genetics laboratory plans to validate a test for fragile X syndrome with combination of Southern blot and PCR assays for the (CGG)*n* repeat in the *FMR1* gene. The laboratory director put together a validation plan according to the ACMG guideline and grading criteria for CAP proficiency testing survey. Which one of the following ranges for *FMR1* clinical testing is acceptable?

A. Consensus size ± 30 repeats for alleles with 56—100 repeats

B. Consensus size ± 20 repeats for alleles with 56—100 repeats

C. Consensus size ± 10 repeats for alleles with 56—100 repeats

D. Consensus size ± 1 SDs for alleles with >100 repeats

E. Consensus size ± 2 SDs for alleles with >100 repeats

F. Consensus size ± 3 SDs for alleles with >100 repeats

ANSWERS

1. **A**. The unstable repeat expansion is called a dynamic mutation because the number of tandem repeats may increase when the gene is passed from parent to offspring. The majority of unstable repeat disorders have been shown to exhibit autosomal dominant inheritance patterns. But a few exhibit autosomal recessive (Friedreich ataxia) or X-linked inheritance (fragile X syndrome) patterns. *The unstable repeats may display somatic and intergenerational instability. Sometimes, repeat length may diminish on transmission to the next generation.* For most trinucleotide repeat disorders, a high degree of somatic instability occurs early in development. Most of unstable repeat disorders are caused by expansion of trinucleotide repeats. But there are exceptions; for example, myotonic dystrophy type 2 is caused by expansion of the CCTG repeat. Fragile X syndrome is associated with a loss-of-function change by methylation if the CGG repeat number is more than 200 copies. However, Huntington disease is caused by a gain-of-function change if the CAG repeat number is more than 40 copies.

    Therefore, it is appropriate to state that the instability may lead to an increase or a decrease in repeat length intergenerationally or somatically.

2. **A**. *Duchenne muscular dystrophy is caused by point mutations, deletions, or duplications in the* DMD *gene on chromosome X.* Deletions of one or more exons account for approximately 60%—70% of pathogenic variants in individuals with Duchenne muscular dystrophy and Becker muscular dystrophy. The rest of the disorders in the question are caused by tandem nucleotide repeat sequences. Myotonic dystrophy type 2 is caused by tetranucleotide repeats (CCTG). The rest in the question are caused by trinucleotide repeats.

    Therefore, Duchenne muscular dystrophy is the only one in the list not caused by the expansion of unstable repeat sequences.

3. **E**. *Myotonic dystrophy type 2 is caused by tetranucleotide repeats (CCTG). The rest in the question are caused by trinucleotide repeats.*

4. **B**. Huntington disease, myotonic dystrophy type 1, and myotonic dystrophy type 2 exhibit autosomal dominant inheritance patterns. Fragile X syndrome exhibits X-linked dominant inheritance patterns. *Friedreich ataxia exhibits autosomal recessive inheritance patterns.*

    Therefore, Friedreich ataxia is the only one in the list that does not exhibit dominant inheritance patterns.

5. C. *The CAG repeat for Huntington disease is located in exon 1 of the HTT gene on 4p16.3.* CAG is coded for glutamine. The CGG repeat for fragile X is located in the 5′ untranslated region (UTR) of the *FMR1* gene on chromosome X. The CTG repeat for myotonic dystrophy type 1 is located in the 3′ untranslated region (UTR) of *DMPK* on 19q13.32. The CCTG repeat for myotonic dystrophy type 2 is located in intron 1 of *CNBP(ZNF9)* on 3q21.3. The GAA repeat for Friedreich ataxia is located in intron 1 of *FXN* on 9q21.11.

Therefore, Huntington disease is the only one in the list that has the repeat sequence in the coding region.

6. A. The unstable repeat expansion is called a dynamic mutation because the number of tandem repeats may increase when the gene is passed from parent to offspring. So the condition may worsen or have an earlier onset from generation to generation, which is called "genetic anticipation."

Epistasis is a phenomenon that consists of the effect of one gene being dependent on the presence of one or more "modifier genes" (genetic background). *Pleiotropy* means that one gene may cause multiple phenotypic expressions or disorders. For example, phenylketonuria (PKU) affects multiple organ systems but is caused by one gene defect, *PAH* (http://ghr.nlm.nih.gov). Lab error with wrong specimens is possible, but the possibility is low. PCR artifacts cannot explain the intergenerational size change.

Therefore, anticipation would be the most appropriate interpretation of the allelic difference between the grandfather, the father, and the boy.

7. C. Huntington disease is an autosomal dominant neurodegenerative genetic disorder. Adult-onset Huntington disease, the most common form of this disorder, usually appears when a person is in their 30s or 40s. Many people with Huntington disease develop involuntary jerking or twitching movements known as chorea (http://ghr.nlm.nih.gov). The *HTT* gene for Huntington disease is located on 4p16.3. The CAG repeat coded for glutamine is located in the first exon of the *HTT* gene. The mutant proteins with expanded polyglutamine sequences are novel property mutants. The expanded tract confers novel features on the protein that damage specific populations of neurons and produce neurodegeneration by a unique toxic mechanism. A normal allele is 6−26 repeats; a gray zone allele 26−35; a reduced penetrance allele 36−39; and a full mutation ≥ 40. A deletion of the *HTT* gene is a loss-of-function change instead of a gain-of-function change.

Therefore, the clinical significance of this change would be unknown in this patient.

8. E. Juvenile Huntington disease (HD) is defined by the onset of symptoms before age 20 years and accounts for 5%−10% of HD cases. Severe mental deterioration, prominent motor and cerebellar symptoms, speech and language delay, and rapid decline are also characteristic of juvenile HD. Individuals with juvenile HD usually have an *HTT* allele with CAG repeats greater than 60. And most often, these children inherit the expanded allele from their fathers (around 90%), although on occasion they inherit it from their mothers.

Therefore, there was an approximately 90% chance that this child with juvenile HD inherited the mutated copy of the *HTT* gene from his biological father.

9. D. The trinucleotide unstable repeat for Huntington disease is located in *exon 1* of the *HTT* gene.

10. D. Huntington disease is an autosomal dominant neurodegenerative genetic disorder. *The CAG repeat* coded for glutamine is located in exon 1 of the *HTT* gene for Huntington disease. The mutant proteins with expanded polyglutamine sequences are novel property mutants. The expanded tract confers novel features on the protein that damage specific populations of neurons and produce neurodegeneration by a unique toxic mechanism.

Therefore, (CAG)n repeats in an exon of the *HTT* gene causes Huntington disease.

11. D. The CAG repeat coded for glutamine is located in exon 1 of the *HTT* gene for Huntington disease. If an individual has more than 150 of the CAG repeat, the standard PCR method may not able to detect it. So the person's results may be interpreted as homozygous for the normal allele instead of compound heterozygous for a juvenile HD allele and a normal allele.

Multiplex Ligation-dependent Probe Amplification (MLPA) is a technology to detect in/del and single base-pair mutations, such as alpha-thalassemia. PCR/capillary electrophoresis and Southern blot is a technology that has been used to detect both large (> 1000 bp with Southern blot) and to genotype small trinucleotide repeats (<1000 bp with PCR/capillary electrophoresis) accurately, such as clinical diagnosis of fragile X syndrome. Triplet repeat−primed PCR is a relatively new technology used to diagnosis fragile X syndrome to replace Southern blotting. It may be used to diagnose other diseases, too, such as myotonic dystrophy. PCR/capillary electrophoresis is used to tell the size differences of DNA fragments, especially for fragments less than 1000 bp, such as the *FLT3*-ITD for myeloid disorders.

Therefore, PCR/capillary electrophoresis and Southern blotting is the most appropriate for the diagnosis of Huntington disease in clinical laboratories as compared with the others choices.

12. **A**. Huntington disease (HD) is an autosomal dominant neurodegenerative genetic disorder. The CAG repeat coded for glutamine is located in the first exon of the *HTT* gene for HD. A normal allele is 6–26 repeats; a gray zone (intermediate) allele 27–35; a reduced penetrance (premutation) allele 36–39; and a full mutation ≥40. The wife is heterozygous for a gray zone allele. It is possible that anticipation will happen during miosis. However, *anticipation occurs more commonly in paternal transmission of the mutated allele. There has never been a documented case of maternal gray zone allele expansion into the full mutation range.* Expanded intermediate alleles are preferentially transmitted by males with advanced paternal age.

Therefore, 0.5% would a good estimation of the risk of HD in the patient's children.

13. **B**. Huntington disease is an autosomal dominant neurodegenerative genetic disorder. The CAG repeat coded for glutamine is located in the first exon of the *HTT* gene for HD. A normal allele is 6–26 repeats; a gray zone (intermediate) allele 27–35; a reduced penetrance (premutation) allele 36–39; and a full mutation ≥40.

The husband is heterozygous for a gray zone (intermediate) allele. The likelihood that transmission of an allele in the gray zone range will expand into an HD full mutation depends on several factors, including the sex of the transmitting individual, the size of the allele, the molecular configuration of the region surrounding the CAG repeats, and its haplotype. Anticipation occurs more commonly in paternal transmission of the mutated allele. *This risk may be as high as 6%–10% for paternal alleles carrying a CAG repeat of 35.*

Therefore, 10% would a good estimation of the risk of HD in the patient's children.

14. **A**. Huntington disease is an autosomal dominant neurodegenerative genetic disorder. The CAG repeat coded for glutamine is located in the first exon of the *HTT* gene for HD. *A normal allele is 6–26 repeats;* a gray zone (intermediate) allele 27–35; a reduced penetrance (premutation) allele 36–39; and a full mutation ≥40.

The husband has two normal alleles (16/25). Therefore, the husband may not develop Huntington disease, and his children won't inherit an abnormal allele from him.

15. **C**. Huntington disease is an autosomal dominant neurodegenerative genetic disorder. The CAG repeat coded for glutamine is located in the first

exon of the *HTT* gene for HD. A normal allele is 6–26 repeats; a gray zone (intermediate) allele 27–35; a *reduced penetrance (premutation) allele 36–39;* and a full mutation ≥40.

Therefore, BJ had one premutation allele (38).

16. **B**. Huntington disease is an autosomal dominant neurodegenerative genetic disorder. The CAG repeat coded for glutamine is located in the first exon of the *HTT* gene for HD. A normal allele is 6–26 repeats; a *gray zone (intermediate) allele 27–35;* a reduced penetrance (premutation) allele 36–39; and a full mutation ≥40.

The husband has one gray zone (intermediate) allele (34). Therefore, he does not have and will not develop Huntington disease, but his offspring will be at risk.

17. **D**. Huntington disease is an autosomal dominant neurodegenerative genetic disorder. The CAG repeat coded for glutamine is located in the first exon of the *HTT* gene for HD. A normal allele is 6–26 repeats; a gray zone (intermediate) allele 27–35; *a reduced penetrance (premutation) allele 36–39;* and a full mutation ≥40.

The husband has one premutation allele (reduced penetrance allele 38). Therefore, he may develop Huntington disease, and his offspring will be at risk of having Huntington disease, too, especially considering that anticipation occurs more commonly in paternal transmission of the mutated allele.

18. **D**. Huntington disease is an autosomal dominant neurodegenerative genetic disorder. The CAG repeat coded for glutamine is located in the first exon of the *HTT* gene for HD. A normal allele is 6–26 repeats; a gray zone (intermediate) allele 27–35; a reduced penetrance (premutation) allele 36–39; and a *full mutation ≥40.*

The husband has one full-mutation allele (41). Therefore, he has Huntington disease, and his children will have a 50% chance of inheriting the full-mutation allele for Huntington disease.

19. **B**. Based on the analysis of previous College of American Pathology (CAP)/American College of Medical Genetics and Genomics (ACMG) proficiency testing survey results for Huntington disease, the acceptable range for sizing CAG repeats was revised in 2012. As grading criteria for the CAP/ACMG proficiency testing survey: *consensus size ± 2 repeats for alleles with <50 repeats.*

20. **C**. Based on the analysis of previous College of American Pathology (CAP)/American College of Medical Genetics and Genomics (ACMG) proficiency testing survey results for Huntington disease, the acceptable range for sizing CAG repeats was revised in 2012. As grading criteria for the

CAP/ACMG proficiency testing survey: *consensus size ± 3 repeats for alleles with 50–75 repeats.*

21. **D.** Based on the analysis of previous College of American Pathology (CAP)/American College of Medical Genetics and Genomics (ACMG) proficiency testing survey results for Huntington disease, the acceptable range for sizing CAG repeats was revised in 2012. As grading criteria for the CAP/ACMG proficiency testing survey: *consensus size ± 4 repeats for alleles with >75 repeats.*

22. **C.** In Huntington disease, the expanded tract of polyglutamine confers *novel features on the protein* that damage specific populations of neurons and produce neurodegeneration by a unique toxic mechanism.

    An activating mutation may activate the existing function of the gene product without normal regulation in cells, such as *BRAF* V600E in metastasized melanoma. Loss-of-function mutations, also called inactivating mutations, result in the gene product having less or no function (being partially or wholly inactivated). Disorders associated with such mutations are most often recessive, such as cystic fibrosis (CF). The majority of metabolic disorders caused by enzyme inactivation are autosomal recessive disorders with homozygous or compound heterozygous functional mutations. It is not unreasonable to assume that the majority of autosomal recessive disorders has loss-of-function mutations (http://ghr.nlm.nih.gov).

    Therefore, gain of novel property on the protein is the pathogenesis of Huntington disease.

23. **E.** An abnormal CAG repeat may expand, contract, or be stably transmitted when passed from parent to child. Although small expansions and contractions are common in maternal and paternal transmission of abnormal alleles, large expansions occur only in paternal transmissions. Allele sizes of 36–39 CAG repeats have been reported in both clinically affected and clinically unaffected individuals.

    Therefore, it is *not possible to predict* the chance Jordan had the same condition as Jessica.

24. **B.** Huntington disease (HD) is a midlife-onset neurodegenerative disease that produces choreic movements and cognitive decline, often accompanied by psychiatric changes. The symptoms result from the selective loss of neurons, most notably in the caudate nucleus and putamen. Currently there is no effective treatment. It is an autosomal dominant disease caused by expansion of a polymorphic trinucleotide (CAG) repeat in the *HTT* gene.

    Testing of asymptomatic individuals younger than age 18 years who are at risk for adult-onset disorders for which no treatment exists is not considered appropriate, primarily because it negates the autonomy of the child with no compelling benefit. Further, concern exists regarding the potential unhealthy adverse effects that such information may have on family dynamics, the risk of discrimination and stigmatization in the future, and the anxiety that such information may cause. Although testing is appropriate to consider in symptomatic individuals in a family with an established diagnosis of HD regardless of age.

    In the ACMG Standards and Guidelines for Huntington disease, published in 2014, it clearly states: *"It is strongly suggested that predictive testing not be offered to individuals until they are at least 18 years old"* (https://www.acmg.net).

    Therefore, it would be appropriate to explain to the couple it is better for their son to make his own decision when he grows up, since there are no preventive measures available for Huntington disease.

25. **A.** Huntington disease (HD) is a midlife-onset neurodegenerative disease with no effective treatment. Testing of asymptomatic individuals younger than age 18 years who are at risk for adult-onset disorders for which no treatment exists is not considered appropriate. Prenatal testing can be used for diagnosis in amniotic fluid cells and in chorionic villus samples. This will help the couple to make an informed decision about this pregnancy. CVS is done in the first trimester, and amniocentesis is done in the second trimester. The wife was 6 weeks pregnant. Therefore, CVS is the preferred test to get the results earlier in order to make a decision.

26. **A.** Huntington disease is an autosomal dominant midlife-onset neurodegenerative disease caused by expansion of a polymorphic trinucleotide (CAG) repeat in the *HTT* gene. Jessica has a full mutation.

    Therefore, Jordan, Jessica's son, has a *50% chance to inherit the full-mutation allele from Jessica.*

27. **C.** Huntington disease is an autosomal-dominant midlife-onset neurodegenerative disease caused by expansion of a polymorphic trinucleotide (CAG) repeat in the *HTT* gene. Normal alleles have 26 or fewer CAG repeats; intermediate alleles 27–35; reduced-penetrance HD-causing alleles 36–39; and full-penetrance HD-causing alleles ≥ 40.

    Jenny's father has an intermediate (gray zone) allele of the CAG repeat. Jenny has a 50% chance of inheriting the abnormal allele. If Jenny inherited the abnormal allele without anticipation, she is not going to be symptomatic, since gray zone mutations have yet to be convincingly associated with an HD phenotype. But gray zone mutations can be meiotically unstable in sperm. Pathologic expansion of paternally derived alleles in this size range has been described. The likelihood that transmission of a mutable normal allele will expand into an HD allele depends on several factors, including the sex of the transmitting individual, the size of the allele, the molecular configuration of the region surrounding the CAG repeat, and the its haplotype. There have been no reports of maternally transmitted alleles in this range producing offspring with affected alleles. *This risk may be as high as 6%–10% for paternal alleles carrying a CAG repeat of 35.*

Therefore, Jenny has a 6%–10% chance of inheriting an expanded paternal allele and to have HD.

28. **A**. *The fetus has an HTT allele with more than 60 CAG repeats, which is usually associated with juvenile onset of symptoms.* Juvenile Huntington disease (HD) is defined by the onset of symptoms before age 20 years and accounts for 5%–10% of HD cases. Severe mental deterioration, prominent motor and cerebellar symptoms, speech and language delay, and rapid decline are also characteristic of juvenile HD (http://www.ncbi. nlm.nih.gov/books/NBK1305/).

Therefore, the baby will develop Huntington symptoms in childhood or early adulthood.

29. **C**. *Triplet repeat—primed PCR (TP PCR)* refers to amplify the CAG(n) repeat region in *HTT* for Huntington disease (HD) by PCR using three primers: a fluorescence-labeled forward primer, located upstream of the CAG(n) region, a chimeric

reverse primer located partially within the CAG(n) region, and a reverse primer located downstream of the repeat region. The chimeric reverse primer hybridizes to multiple locations within the CAG (n) repeat region, creating PCR products of varying sizes. Reactions are separated by capillary electrophoresis. TP PCR provides a characteristic ladder on the fluorescence trace, enabling the rapid identification of large pathogenic repeats that cannot be amplified using flanking primers. Because the 5′ end of the reverse chimeric primer exactly matches the sequence 3′ of the CAG(n) region, this product is preferentially amplified. The true alleles are therefore distinguished as the highest peaks. Stutter peaks extending from the smaller allele and terminating with the larger allele represent products from the reverse primer hybridizing within the CAG(n) region. When an allele is too large to be amplified by this assay, a stutter peak of decreasing amplitude extends to the end of the electropherogram. Results are evaluated for the presence of this distinct stutter pattern extending into the expanded allele range. Positive control, negative control, and no template control should be included on each run. Post-PCR detection of the alleles can be achieved by fragment-length analysis.

The traditional way of molecular test for HD is PCR/capillary electrophoresis and Southern blot. This triplet-repeat primed PCR simplifies testing for HD.

Therefore, did the laboratory used triplet-repeat primed PCR method for the assay.

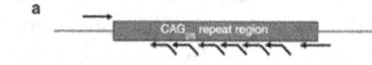

a

CAG repeat region

b

GATGAAGGCCTTCGAGTCCCTCAAGTCCTTCCAGCAGCAGCAGCAGCAGCAGCAGCAGCAGCAGCAGCAGCAGC
AGCAGCAGCAGCAGCAGCAACAGCCGCCACCGCCGCCGCCGCCGCCGCCGCCTCCTCAGCTTCCTCAGCCGC
CGCG

HD chimeric primer F: 5′ 6-FAM-*ATG AAG GCC TTC GAG TCC CTC AAG TCC* 3′
HD chimeric primer R: 5′ *CGG TGG CGG CTG TTG CTG CTG CTG CTG CTG*_3′

Schematic representation of Huntington disease (HD) chimeric assay. (a) HD chimeric assay primers. **(b)** HD chimeric primer sequences.

30. **E**. Normal alleles have 26 or fewer CAG repeats; intermediate alleles 27–35; reduced-penetrance HD-causing alleles 36–39; full-penetrance HD-causing alleles ≥ 40; and juvenile-onset alleles ≥ 60.

Therefore, the fetus was heterozygous for a juvenile-onset allele.

31. **B**. Huntington disease is an autosomal dominant neurodegenerative genetic disorder. Adult-onset Huntington disease, the most common form of

this disorder, usually appears in a person's 30s or 40s. *Juvenile Huntington disease (HD) is defined by the onset of symptoms before age 20 years and accounts for 5%–10% of HD cases.* Severe mental deterioration, prominent motor and cerebellar symptoms, speech and language delay, and rapid decline are also characteristic of juvenile HD. Individuals with juvenile HD *usually have an HTT allele with CAG repeats >60.*

Therefore, it would be most likely the fetus/patient would develop HD symptoms in his/her late childhood or young adulthood, such as at 18 years of age.

32. **B.** Since 1998, it has been the intent of the College of American Pathology (CAP)/American College of Medical Genetics and Genomics (ACMG) Biochemical and Molecular Genetics Resource Committee to standardize the accuracy of CAG repeat quantitation for Huntington disease (HD). Based on the analysis of previous CAP/ACMG proficiency testing survey results for HD, the acceptable range for sizing CAG repeats was revised in 2012. Acknowledging the technical limitations of size analysis, the ACMG supports the following acceptable ranges for HD clinical testing and as grading criteria for the CAP/ACMG proficiency testing survey: *consensus size ± 2 repeats for alleles with less than 50 repeats*; consensus size ± 3 repeats for alleles with 50–75 repeats; and consensus size ± 4 repeats for alleles with >75 repeats.

    Therefore, "consensus size ± 3 repeats for alleles with 40-50 repeats" is an incorrect statement.

33. **B.** *Friedreich ataxia* (FRDA) is inherited in an autosomal recessive manner. Anticipation is not observed because the disease is typically not observed in more than one generation. Fragile X syndrome (FXS), Huntington disease (HD), myotonic dystrophy (MD), and spinocerebellar ataxia (SCA) are all autosomal dominant genetic disorders caused by expansion of unstable repeat sequences. Anticipation is one of characteristics of these disorders.

    Therefore, anticipation is a common phenomenon in the diseases caused by trinucleotide repeats, but not in Friedreich ataxia.

34. **B.** *Spinal muscular atrophy* (SMA) does not caused by trinucleotide repeat expansion. Therefore, anticipation is not observed in this disease. Fragile X syndrome (FXS), Huntington disease (HD), myotonic dystrophy (MD), and spinocerebellar ataxia (SCA) are all autosomal dominant genetic disorders caused by expansion of unstable repeat sequences. Anticipation is one of characteristics of these disorders.

    Therefore, nnticipation is a common phenomenon in the diseases caused by trinucleotide repeats, but not in spinal muscular atrophy.

35. **C.** Friedreich ataxia is a genetic condition that affects the nervous system and causes movement problems. People with this condition develop ataxia, which worsens over time. Other features of this condition include the gradual loss of strength and sensation in the arms and legs, muscle stiffness, and impaired speech (http://ghr.nlm.nih.gov). The most common type of mutation, which is observed on both alleles in more than 90% of individuals with Friedreich ataxia, is an abnormally expanded GAA repeat in *intron 1 of the* FXN *gene*. (http://www.ncbi.nlm.nih.gov/books/NBK1281/).

    Therefore, the trinucleotide unstable repeat of the *FXN* gene for FRDA is located in intron 1 of the *FXN* gene.

36. **G.** Friedreich ataxia is a genetic condition that affects the nervous system and causes movement problems. The most common type of mutation, which is observed on both alleles in more than 90% of individuals with Friedreich ataxia, *is an abnormally expanded GAA repeat in intron 1 of the FXN gene* (http://www.ncbi.nlm.nih.gov/books/NBK1281/).

    Therefore, (GAA)n repeat in an intron of the *FXN* gene causes majority cases of Friedreich ataxia.

37. **C.** Friedreich ataxia is *an autosomal recessive genetic condition* that affects the nervous system and causes movement problems. Therefore, BJ had a 25% chance to be affected, since his parents were obligate carriers.

38. **A.** For Friedreich ataxia the exact demarcation between normal and full-penetrance alleles remains poorly defined. Four classes of alleles are recognized for the GAA repeat sequence in intron 1 of *FXN*: *normal allele, 5–33;* mutable normal (premutation) allele, 34–65; borderline allele, 44–66; and full-penetrance allele 66–1700 (http://www.ncbi.nlm.nih.gov/books/NBK1281/).

    Therefore, BJ has two normal alleles, and he will not develop symptoms for FRDA.

39. **C.** Friedreich ataxia is an *autosomal recessive* genetic condition that affects the nervous system and causes movement problems. The most common type of mutation, which is observed on both alleles in more than 90% of individuals with Friedreich ataxia, is an abnormally expanded GAA repeat in intron 1 of the *FXN* gene. The exact demarcation between normal and full-penetrance alleles remains poorly defined. Four classes of alleles are recognized for the GAA repeat sequence in intron 1 of *FXN*: normal allele, 5–33; mutable normal (premutation) allele, 34–65; borderline allele, 44–66; and *full-penetrance allele 66–1700* (http://www.ncbi.nlm.nih.gov/books/NBK1281/).

    Therefore, BJ was a carrier of Friedreich ataxia, and he would not develop symptoms for Friedreich ataxia himself.

40. **D.** Friedreich ataxia is an autosomal recessive genetic condition that affects the nervous system and causes movement problems. The most common type of mutation, which is observed on both alleles in more than 90% of individuals with Friedreich ataxia, is an abnormally expanded GAA repeat in intron 1 of the *FXN* gene. The exact demarcation between normal and full-penetrance alleles remains poorly defined. Four classes of alleles are recognized for the GAA repeat sequence in intron 1 of *FXN*: normal allele, 5−33; mutable normal (premutation) allele, 34−65; borderline allele, 44−66; and *full-penetrance allele 66−1700.* (http://www.ncbi.nlm.nih.gov/books/NBK1281/).

    Therefore, BJ had two full-mutation alleles, and would develop symptoms for Friedreich ataxia, but not early onset, as he was 32-year-old man without symptoms.

41. **A.** The molecular pathogenesis of Friedreich ataxia reflects *the loss of the normal functions* of the affected protein, frataxin.

    An activating mutation may activate the existing function of the gene product without normal regulation in cells, such as *BRAF* V600E in metastasized melanoma. Loss-of-function mutations, also called "inactivating mutations," result in the gene product having less or no function (being partially or wholly inactivated). Disorders associated with such mutations are most often recessive, such as cystic fibrosis (CF). The majority of metabolic disorders caused by enzyme inactivation are autosomal recessive disorders with homozygous or compound heterozygous functional mutations. It is not unreasonable to assume that the majority of autosomal recessive disorders has loss-of-function mutations. In Huntington disease, the expanded tract of polyglutamine confers novel features on the protein that damage specific populations of neurons and produce neurodegeneration by a unique toxic mechanism (http://ghr.nlm.nih.gov).

    Therefore, Friedreich ataxia is caused by loss of function mutation.

42. **D.** Expansion of the CAG repeats in the *ATXN1* gene causes spinocerebellar ataxia type 1 (SCA1). Expansion of the CAG repeats in the *ATXN2* gene causes spinocerebellar ataxia type 2 (SCA2). Expansion of the CAG repeats in the *ATXN3* gene causes spinocerebellar ataxia type 3 (SCA3). *The gene responsible for SCA4 has been located on 1p36, but has not been identified* (http://omim.org).

    Therefore, it is not clear whether SCA4 is NOT caused by expansion of unstable repeat sequences.

43. **E.** The hereditary ataxias can be inherited in an autosomal dominant, autosomal recessive, or X-linked manner. *Spinocerebellar ataxia (SCA) types 1, 2, 3, 4, 6, and 7 are inherited in autosomal dominant pattern.*

    Therefore, all types of the spinocerebellar ataxia listed in the question are inherited in autosomal dominant pattern.

44. **E.** Expansion of the CAG repeats in the *ATXN1* gene causes autosomal dominant spinocerebellar ataxia type 1 (SCA1). Expansion of the CAG repeats in the *ATXN3* gene causes autosomal dominant spinocerebellar ataxia type 3 (SCA3). Expansion of the CAG repeats in the *CACNA1A* gene causes autosomal dominant spinocerebellar ataxia type 6 (SCA6). Expansion of the CAG repeats in one of the exons in the *ATXN7* gene causes autosomal dominant spinocerebellar ataxia type 7 (SCA7) (http://omim.org) (http://www.ncbi.nlm.nih.gov/books/NBK1138/).

    Therefore, choice E is correct.

45. **E.** Expansion of the CAG repeats in one of exons of the *ATXN1* gene causes autosomal dominant spinocerebellar ataxia type 1 (SCA1). Expansion of the CAG repeats in one of the exons the *ATXN2* gene causes autosomal dominant spinocerebellar ataxia type 2 (SCA2). Expansion of the CAG repeats in one of the exons in the *CACNA1A* gene causes autosomal dominant spinocerebellar ataxia type 6 (SCA6). Expansion of the CAG repeats in one of the exons in the *ATXN7* gene causes autosomal dominant spinocerebellar ataxia type 7 (SCA7). (http://omim.org; http://www.ncbi.nlm.nih.gov/books/NBK1138/).

    Therefore, choice E is correct.

46. **D.** The trinucleotide unstable repeats *in one of the exons of the ATXN1 gene* causes autosomal dominant spinocerebellar ataxia type 1 (SCA1) (http://www.ncbi.nlm.nih.gov/books/NBK1184/).

    Therefore, the trinucleotide unstable repeats of the *ATXN1* gene for autosomal dominant Spinocerebellar ataxia type 1 is located in an exon.

47. **D.** *The CAG repeats in one of exons of the* ATXN1 *gene* causes autosomal dominant spinocerebellar ataxia type 1 (SCA1) (http://www.ncbi.nlm.nih.gov/books/NBK1184/).

    Therefore, a CAG repeat in an exon of the *ATXN1* gene causes spinocerebellar ataxia type 1.

48. **C.** Spinocerebellar ataxia type 1 (SCA1) is characterized by progressive cerebellar ataxia, dysarthria, and eventual deterioration of bulbar functions. The CAGs are translated to

polyglutamine in the amino acid sequence, which induces neurologic disease in SCA1 (http://www.ncbi.nlm.nih.gov/books/NBK1184/).

Therefore, the CAG repeats of the *ATXN1* gene codes for glutamine.

49. **D**. The CAG repeats in one of exons of the *ATXN1* gene causes autosomal dominant spinocerebellar ataxia type 1 (SCA1). An allele with 39 CAG repeats without the CAT repeat interruptions has the lowest number of repeats to be associated with symptoms. However, 39–44 CAG repeat alleles have to be uninterrupted by CAT repeats to be considered abnormal and likely to be associated with symptoms. There is an inverse correlation between the size of the expansion and the age at onset. Complex alleles may occur; one individual has been reported with symptomatic SCA1 with a 58-CAG-repeat sequence interrupted by two CAT repeats; however, this person had an uninterrupted 45-CAT-repeat stretch. More recently, additional pathogenic alleles carrying 46–70 uninterrupted CAG repeats but with CAT interruptions have been reported. In the case of such interrupted alleles, correlation with age at onset may be more appropriate if the uninterrupted CAG stretch alone is considered (http://www.ncbi.nlm.nih.gov/books/NBK1184/).

Therefore, in this case, BJ has a full-mutation allele (120 copies of CAG without CAT interruption), and will develop symptoms for autosomal dominant spinocerebellar ataxia type 1.

50. **D**. Myotonic dystrophy (MD) is the most common form of adult-onset muscular dystrophy. It is characterized by progressive muscle wasting and weakness. People with this disorder often have myotonia and are not able to relax certain muscles after use. Also, affected people may have slurred speech or temporary locking of their jaw. The features of this disorder often develop during a person's 20s or 30s, although they can occur at any age. There are two major types of myotonic dystrophy: type 1 and type 2. Their signs and symptoms overlap, although type 2 tends to be milder than type 1. The muscle weakness associated with type 1 particularly affects the lower legs, hands, neck, and face. Muscle weakness in type 2 primarily involves the muscles of the neck, shoulders, elbows, and hips. Both type 1 and type 2 are caused by expansion of unstable repeats (http://ghr.nlm.nih.gov/condition/myotonic-dystrophy).

Triplet repeat—primed PCR assay, also called PCR repeat-primed assay, involves a forward primer unique to a sequence near the repeat and a reverse primer composed of several repeat units that can bind anywhere in the repeat region, thus creating amplicons of varying sizes. The reverse primer is used in lower concentrations and is exhausted in a few cycles, after which an anchor primer takes over as the reverse primer. Repeat expansions produce a characteristic sawtooth pattern with a 3-bp periodicity. This approach reduces the number of Southern blot analyses, which are time consuming and labor-intensive.

Next-generation sequencing (NGS) is often referred to as massively parallel sequencing. Using NGS, some clinical relevant genes could be sequenced all at once in a single test. This clearly has the potential to provide information on lots of genes all at once. However, sequencing such as Sanger sequencing through the repeat region, including unstable short tandem repeats, such as trinucleotide repeats or tetranucleotide repeats is still a challenge for this technology. Targeted mutation analysis is an efficient way to detect point mutations, such as C282Y in the *HFE* gene for hereditary hemochromatosis.

Therefore, triplet repeat—primed PCR assay would be the most appropriate genetic assay to confirm the diagnosis in this patient.

51. **A**. *Myotonic dystrophy type 1 (DM1) is inherited in an autosomal dominant manner and is caused by expansion of an unstable repeat in the* DMPK *gen on 19p13.3* (http://www.ncbi.nlm.nih.gov/books/NBK1165/).

Mutations in *FXN* are associated with autosomal recessive FRDA. Mutations in *FMR1* are associated with X-linked fragile X syndrome, fragile X—associated tremor/ataxia syndrome (FXTAS), and *FMR1*-related primary ovarian insufficiency (POI). Mutations in *HTT* are associated autosomal dominant Huntington disease. Mutations in *ZNF9* (*CBNBP*) are associated autosomal dominant Myotonic dystrophy type 2. All these disorders are caused by expansion of unstable repeat sequences in the majority of patients.

Therefore, *DMPK* is associated with myotonic dystrophy type 1.

52. **C**. *The pathogenesis of myotonic dystrophy 1 (DM1) appears to results from the binding of the CUG repeats to RNA-binding proteins*. Many of the RNA-binding proteins "quenched" by the excessive number of CUG repeats are regulators of splicing. More than a dozen distinct pre-mRNAs have been shown to have splicing alterations in MD1, including cardiac troponin T and insulin receptor.

Therefore, the CAG expansion creates novel property on the RNA (choice C).

53. **E.** The trinucleotide unstable repeat for myotonic dystrophy 1 is located *in the 3′ UTR of the* DMPK *gene* (http://www.ncbi.nlm.nih.gov/books/NBK1165/).

54. **E.** *Myotonic dystrophy 1 is caused by expansion of a CTG trinucleotide repeat in the 3′ noncoding region of* DMPK (http://www.ncbi.nlm.nih.gov/books/NBK1165/).

Fragile X syndrome is caused by a (CGG)*n* repeat located in the 5′UTR of the *FMR1* gene on chromosome X. Myotonic dystrophy 2 is caused by a (CCTG)*n* repeat located in an intron of the *DM2* gene. Huntington disease is caused by a (CAG) repeat located in one of the exons of the *HTT* gene.

Therefore, the pathogenic changes of the *DMPK* gene for myotonic dystrophy type 1 is a CTG repeat.

55. **A.** Myotonic dystrophy 1 is an autosomal dominant disease caused by expansion of a CTG trinucleotide repeat in the 3′ noncoding region of *DMPK*. OB had *two normal alleles* of the CTG repeat in *DMPK*.

Therefore, she would NOT develop symptoms for myotonic dystrophy type 1.

56. **B.** Myotonic dystrophy 1 is an autosomal dominant disease caused by expansion of a CTG trinucleotide repeat in the 3′ noncoding region of *DMPK*. OB had one normal allele and *one mutable normal (premutation) allele* of the CTG repeat in *DMPK*.

Therefore, she would NOT develop symptoms for myotonic dystrophy type 1. But her offspring will be at risk to have this disease owing to anticipation.

57. **D.** Myotonic dystrophy 1 (MD1) is an autosomal dominant disease, caused by expansion of a CTG trinucleotide repeat in the 3′ noncoding region of *DMPK*. OB had one normal allele and *one full-penetrance allele* of the CTG repeat in *DMPK*.

Therefore, she would develop symptoms for myotonic dystrophy type 1, and her children will have a 50% chance of inheriting the full-penetrance allele and to be affected.

58. **E.** Myotonic dystrophy 1 (MD1) is an autosomal dominant disease caused by expansion of a CTG trinucleotide repeat in the 3′ noncoding region of *DMPK*. In general, longer CTG repeat expansions correlate with an earlier age at onset and more severe disease. However, abnormal test results do not predict the age at onset or severity of the disease because of the overlap of CTG repeat length associated with the three phenotypes and the possibility of somatic mosaicism for the size

of the CTG expansion. Regardless, CTG repeat lengths of 730−1000 or greater are more likely to be associated with congenital myotonic dystrophy 1.

The fetus had one normal allele and *one full-penetrance allele associated with congenital MD1.* Therefore, he/she would develop symptoms for congenital MD1.

59. **D.** Myotonic dystrophy 1 (MD1) is an autosomal dominant disease caused by expansion of a CTG trinucleotide repeat in the 3′ noncoding region of *DMPK. When a patient has more than 1000 copies of the repeat, he/she usually has congenital MD1* (http://www.ncbi.nlm.nih.gov/books/NBK1165/).

Therefore, the unborn child would have congenital MD1.

60. **A.** Myotonic dystrophy type 1 (MD1) is an autosomal dominant disease caused by expansion of a CTG trinucleotide repeat in the 3′ noncoding region of *DMPK*. The diagnosis of MD1 is suspected in individuals with characteristic muscle weakness and is confirmed by molecular genetic testing of *DMPK*. CTG repeat length exceeding 34 repeats is abnormal. Molecular genetic testing detects pathogenic variants in nearly 100% of affected individuals: normal allele 5−34; mutable normal (premutation) 35−49; full-penetrance allele >50. When a patient has more than 1000 copies of the repeat, he/she usually has congenital MD1. Although repeat expansions occur through both maternal and paternal transmissions, *the larger repeat expansions observed in congenital cases are almost exclusively due to maternal transmission* (http://www.ncbi.nlm.nih.gov/books/NBK1165/).

This newborn boy had 2600 copies of the CTG repeat. He had congenital MD1.

Therefore, it better to test the mother first for this autosomal dominant condition. If the mother's result is normal, then test the father.

61. **E.** *Myotonic dystrophy type 2 (MD2) is inherited in an autosomal dominant manner and is caused by expansion of an unstable repeat in the ZNF9 (CBNBP) gene* (http://www.ncbi.nlm.nih.gov/books/NBK1466/).

Mutations in *DMPK* are associated autosomal dominant myotonic dystrophy type 1. Mutations in *FXN* are associated autosomal recessive Friedreich ataxia. Mutations in *FMR1* are associated X-linked fragile X syndrome, fragile X−associated tremor/ataxia syndrome (FXTAS), and *FMR1*-related primary ovarian insufficiency (POI). Mutations in *HTT* are associated with autosomal dominant Huntington disease. All these disorders are caused by expansion of unstable repeat sequences in the majority of patients.

Therefore, *ZNF9* is associated with myotonic dystrophy type 2.

62. **C.** The unstable repeats for myotonic dystrophy type 2 (MD2) is located *in intron 1 of the ZNF9 (CBNBP) gene* (http://www.ncbi.nlm.nih.gov/books/NBK1466/).

63. **B.** *ZNF9* (*CBNBP*) is the only gene in which mutation is known to cause myotonic dystrophy type 2 (MD2). *ZNF9* intron 1 contains a complex repeat motif, (TG)*n*(TCTG)*n*(CCTG)*n*. *Expansion of the CCTG repeat causes MD2. The number of CCTG repeats in expanded alleles ranges from approximately 75 to more than 11,000, with a mean of approximately 5000 repeats* (http://www.ncbi.nlm.nih.gov/books/NBK1466/).

Therefore, (CCTG)n in the *ZNF9* gene is unstable and associated with Myotonic dystrophy type 2.

64. **E.** Myotonic dystrophy (MD) is the most common form of adult-onset muscular dystrophy. It is characterized by progressive muscle wasting and weakness. People with this disorder often have myotonia and are not able to relax certain muscles after use. Affected people may also have slurred speech or temporary locking of their jaw. The features of this disorder often develop during a person's 20s or 30s, although they can occur at any age. There are two major types of myotonic dystrophy: type 1 and type 2. Their signs and symptoms overlap, although type 2 tends to be milder than type 1. The muscle weakness associated with type 1 particularly affects the lower legs, hands, neck, and face. Muscle weakness in type 2 primarily involves the muscles of the neck, shoulders, elbows, and hips. Type 1 is caused by trinucleotide repeat expansion in the 3′ UTR of the *DMPK* gene. Type 2 is caused by tetranucleotide repeat expansion in one of introns of *ZNF9* (*CBNBP*) (http://ghr.nlm.nih.gov/condition/myotonic-dystrophy) (http://www.ncbi.nlm.nih.gov/books/NBK1165/).

Next-generation sequencing (NGS) is often referred to as massively parallel sequencing. Using NGS, some clinically relevant genes could be sequenced all at once in a single test. This clearly has the potential to provide information on lots of genes all at once. However, sequencing through repeat region including unstable short tandem repeats, such as trinucleotide repeats or tetranucleotide repeats is still a challenge for this technology.

Therefore, *the patient's baby girl will have a 50% chance of developing myotonic dystrophy since both*

myotonic dystrophy type 1 and type 2 are autosomal dominant disorders.

65. **C.** Myotonic dystrophy (MD) is the most common form of adult-onset muscular dystrophy. It is characterized by progressive muscle wasting and weakness. People with this disorder often have myotonia and are not able to relax certain muscles after use. Also, affected people may have slurred speech or temporary locking of their jaw. The features of this disorder often develop during a person's 20s or 30s, although they can occur at any age. There are two major types of myotonic dystrophy: type 1 and type 2. Their signs and symptoms overlap, although type 2 tends to be milder than type 1. The muscle weakness associated with type 1 particularly affects the lower legs, hands, neck, and face. Muscle weakness in type 2 primarily involves the muscles of the neck, shoulders, elbows, and hips. Both type 1 and type 2 are caused by expansion of unstable repeats (http://ghr.nlm.nih.gov/condition/myotonic-dystrophy).

Conventional PCR amplification techniques are successful only for normal and small premutation alleles and are not informative for homozygous female repeat alleles. Southern blot analysis for categorization and sizing is very laborious and time consuming and involves large amounts of high-quality DNA, which are not always available. The combination of *Southern blot and polymerase chain reaction/capillary electrophoresis* provides an accurate means of identifying patients affected by myotonic dystrophy. Southern blotting is used to detect large repeat fragments. And polymerase chain reaction/capillary electrophoresis is used to detect small repeat fragments.

Next-generation sequencing (NGS) is often referred to as massively parallel sequencing. Using NGS, some clinically relevant genes could be sequenced all at once in a single test. This clearly has the potential to provide information on lots of genes all at once. However, sequencing including Sanger sequencing through repeat regions including unstable short tandem repeats, such as trinucleotide repeats or tetranucleotide repeats is still a challenge for this technology. Targeted mutation analysis is an efficient way to detect point mutations, such as C282Y in the *HFE* gene for hereditary hemochromatosis.

Therefore, PCR/capillary electrophoresis and Southern blotting would be the most appropriate genetic assay to confirm the diagnosis in this patient.

66. **C**. Myotonic dystrophy 1 (MD1) is an autosomal dominant disease caused by expansion of a CTG trinucleotide repeat in the 3' noncoding region of *DMPK*. *A full-penetrance allele has >50 of the CTG repeats* (http://www.ncbi.nlm.nih.gov/books/NBK1165/).

Therefore, the unborn child would have classic myotonic dystrophy 1.

67. **B**. Myotonic dystrophy 1 (MD1) is an autosomal dominant disease caused by expansion of a CTG trinucleotide repeat in the 3' noncoding region of *DMPK*. The diagnosis of MD1 is suspected in individuals with characteristic muscle weakness and is confirmed by molecular genetic testing of *DMPK*. CTG repeat lengths exceeding 34 repeats is abnormal. Molecular genetic testing detects pathogenic variants in nearly 100% of affected individuals: normal allele 5–34 repeats; mutable normal (premutation) allele 35–49; and full-penetrance allele: >50. When a patient has more than 1000 copies of the repeat, he/she usually has congenital myotonic dystrophy 1 (http://www.ncbi.nlm.nih.gov/books/NBK1165/).

The wife had 12/45 copies of the CTG repeat. Therefore, she had a mutable normal allele without symptoms.

68. **B**. There are many causes of mental retardation (MR), including genetic disorders, infections during pregnancy, drug and alcohol use during pregnancy, problems with the birth or delivery, prematurity, and low family IQ in general. The American Psychiatric Association defines MR as the combination of: (1) tested IQ at or under 70, (2) problems with learning and social adaptation, and (3) symptoms that begin before 18 years of age. MR is further subdivided into two categories: mild (IQ 50–70) and moderate to severe (IQ under 50).

Fetal alcohol syndrome is the most common congenital cause of MR.

69. **A**. There are many causes of mental retardation (MR) including genetic disorders, infections during pregnancy, drug and alcohol use during pregnancy, problems with the birth or delivery, prematurity, and low family IQ in general. The American Psychiatric Association defines MR as the combination of: (1) tested IQ at or under 70, (2) problems with learning and social adaptation, and (3) symptoms that begin before 18 years of age. MR is further subdivided into two categories: mild (IQ 50–70) and moderate to severe (IQ under 50).

Fetal alcohol syndrome is the most common congenital cause of MR. *Down syndrome is the common genetic etiology of MR.*

70. **C**. Mental retardation (MR) is also called "intellectual disability." There are many causes of MR, including genetic disorders, infections during pregnancy, drug and alcohol use during pregnancy, problems with the birth or delivery, prematurity, and low family IQ in general. The American Psychiatric Association defines MR as the combination of: (1) tested IQ at or under 70, (2) problems with learning and social adaptation, and (3) symptoms that begin before 18 years of age. MR is further subdivided into two categories: mild (IQ 50–70) and moderate to severe (IQ under 50).

Fetal alcohol syndrome is the most common congenital cause of MR. Down syndrome is the common genetic etiology of MR. *Fragile X is the most common cause of inherited MR.*

71. **B**. Fragile X syndrome is nearly always characterized by moderate intellectual disability in affected males and mild intellectual disability in affected females. The diagnosis of fragile X syndrome rests on the detection of an alteration in *FMR1*. More than 99% of individuals with fragile X syndrome have a mutation in *FMR1* caused by expansion of trinucleotide repeats (typically >200) accompanied by aberrant methylation of *FMR1*. The trinucleotide repeat for fragile X is located in the *5' UTR of the* FMR1 *gene* (http://www.ncbi.nlm.nih.gov/books/NBK1384/).

72. **C**. Fragile X syndrome is caused by *expansion of the CGG trinucleotide repeats (typically >200) accompanied by aberrant methylation of* FMR1 (http://www.ncbi.nlm.nih.gov/books/NBK1384/).

73. **A**. Fragile X syndrome is caused by a *loss-of-function* mutation in *FMR1*, which is an expansion of the CGG trinucleotide repeats (typically >200) accompanied by aberrant methylation of *FMR1*. Other mutations within *FMR1* that cause fragile X syndrome include deletions and point mutations (http://www.ncbi.nlm.nih.gov/books/NBK1384/).

74. **C**. Fragile X syndrome is nearly always characterized by moderate intellectual disability in affected males and mild intellectual disability in affected females. The diagnosis of fragile X syndrome rests on the detection of an alteration in *FMR1*. For the CGG repeat in the *FMR1* gene on Xq27.3, the normal allele has 5–44 copies of the repeat, the intermediate allele (gray zone, inconclusive, borderline) allele 45–54 copies, the *premutation 55–200 copies;* and the full-mutation allele more than 200 repeats. In typical fragile X families, the mutation is a multistep expansion occurring over one or more generations in a

region of CGG repeats in the 5′ untranslated region of the gene. Females with premutation have *increased an risk of having premature ovarian failure and fragile X—associated tremor/ataxia syndrome.* Because of potential repeat instability upon transmission of premutation alleles, women with alleles in this range are considered to be *at risk of having children affected with fragile X syndrome* (http://www.ncbi.nlm.nih.gov/books/NBK1384/).

The wife has 29/189 copies of the CGG repeat. Therefore, she had a premutation allele. She did not have fragile X syndrome, but she was at risk for premature ovarian failure, and her children would be at risk for fragile X syndrome.

75. **C.** Fragile X syndrome is nearly always characterized by moderate intellectual disability in affected males and mild intellectual disability in affected females. The diagnosis of fragile X syndrome rests on the detection of an alteration in *FMR1.* For the CGG repeat in the *FMR1* gene on Xq27.3, the normal allele has 5—44 copies of the repeat, the intermediate allele (gray zone, inconclusive, borderline) 45—54 copies, the *premutation allele 55—200 copies;* and the full-mutation allele more than 200 repeats. In typical fragile X families, the mutation is a multistep expansion occurring over one or more generations in a region of CGG repeats in the 5′ untranslated region of the gene. Females with premutation have *increased risk to have premature ovarian failure and fragile X—associated tremor/ataxia syndrome.* Because of potential repeat instability upon transmission of premutation alleles, women with alleles in this range are considered to be *at risk of having children affected with fragile X syndrome* (http://www.ncbi.nlm.nih.gov/books/NBK1384/).

The wife has 29/62 copies of the CGG repeat. Therefore, she had a premutation allele. She did not have fragile X syndrome, but she was at risk for premature ovarian failure, and her children would be at risk for fragile X syndrome.

76. **B.** Fragile X syndrome is nearly always characterized by moderate intellectual disability in affected males and mild intellectual disability in affected females. The diagnosis of fragile X syndrome rests on the detection of an alteration in *FMR1.* For the CGG repeat in the *FMR1* gene on Xq27.3, the normal allele has 5—44 copies of the repeat, the *intermediate allele (gray zone, inconclusive, borderline) 45—54 copies,* the premutation allele 55—200 copies; and the full—mutation allele more than 200 repeats. In typical fragile X families, the mutation is a

multistep expansion occurring over one or more generations in a region of CGG repeats in the 5′ untranslated region of the gene. *Females with the intermediate allele do not have fragile X symptoms.* The rate of expansions of intermediate alleles is not well understood. Minor increases and decreases in repeat number can occur when alleles of this size are passed on, but there is no measurable risk of a child with fragile X syndrome in the next generation. Alleles of this size may be associated with fragile X syndrome in future generations or in distant relatives. *A gray-zone allele of 52 repeats was reported to expand to a premutation allele of 56 repeats in one generation,* which subsequently expanded to a full-mutation allele in the next generation. Testing at-risk relatives of individuals with an intermediate allele may determine the stability of the allele in the family (http://www.ncbi.nlm.nih.gov/books/NBK1384/).

The wife has 29/52 copies of the CGG repeat. Therefore, she did not have fragile X syndrome, but her children would be at risk for premutation.

77. **B.** Fragile X syndrome is nearly always characterized by moderate intellectual disability in affected males and mild intellectual disability in affected females. The diagnosis of fragile X syndrome rests on the detection of an alteration in *FMR1.* For the CGG repeat in the *FMR1* gene on Xq27.3, the normal allele has 5—44 copies of the repeat, the *intermediate allele (gray zone, inconclusive, borderline) 45—54 copies,* the premutation allele 55—200 copies; and the full-mutation allele more than 200 repeats. In typical fragile X families, the mutation is a multistep expansion occurring over one or more generations in a region of CGG repeats in the 5′ untranslated region of the gene. *Females with the intermediate allele do not have fragile X symptoms.* The rate of expansions of intermediate alleles is not well understood. Minor increases and decreases in repeat number can occur when alleles of this size are passed on, but there is no measurable risk of a child with fragile X syndrome in the next generation. Alleles of this size may be associated with fragile X syndrome in future generations or in distant relatives. *A gray-zone allele of 52 repeats was reported to expand to a premutation allele of 56 repeats in one generation,* which subsequently expanded to a full-mutation allele in the next generation. Testing at-risk relatives of individuals with an intermediate allele may determine the stability of the allele in the family (http://www.ncbi.nlm.nih.gov/books/NBK1384/).

The wife has 29/48 copies of the CGG repeat. Therefore, she did not have Fragile X syndrome, but her children would be at risk for premutation.

78. **A**. The wife had 29/42 copies of the CGG repeat. Therefore, she had two normal stable alleles (5–44). She would not develop fragile X syndrome and her children were not at risk for fragile X syndrome.

79. **D**. The wife had 29/240 copies of the CGG repeat. Therefore, she had a full-mutation allele (>200). She would develop mild fragile X symptoms. Her sons would be at 50% risk for classical fragile X syndrome.

80. **C**. The wife had 29/180 CGG repeats. So she had a premutation allele (55–200 copies). There was 50% chance that her unborn child would inherit the abnormal allele from her. The risk of anticipation could not be estimated in this family. It was possible that the unborn child would inherit a premutation allele or a full-mutation allele (>200). A prenatal diagnostic test should be offered to the family instead of a screening test. A methylation study would be crucial for the diagnosis of this unborn child.

A noninvasive prenatal test (NIPT) with cell-free DNA from maternal blood may be used for prenatal screening test, but not diagnosis. Chorionic villus sampling (CVS) and amniotic fluid can be used for prenatal diagnostic testing. But because methylation is not fully established at the time of CVS, the appearance of full mutations examined by a methylation-specific method may vary in CVS as compared with blood and amniocytes. So it is an acceptable option to omit methylation analysis entirely when testing CVS specimens. In the minor fraction of CVS cases with a result that is ambiguous between a large premutation and a small full mutation by size criteria alone, a follow-up amniocentesis may be required.

Therefore, prenatal diagnosis with amniotic fluid sample would be the most appropriate test for the family.

81. **D**. Hypermethylation is typically present on most or all copies, with the exception of DNA extracted from CVS. This test can be used for prenatal diagnosis in cells obtained from amniocentesis and chorionic villus sampling (CVS). Because methylation is not fully established at the time of CVS, the appearance of full mutations examined by a methylation-specific method may vary in CVS as compared with blood and amniocytes.

The fetus had a hemizygous unmethylated allele with approximately 500 repeat. So the unborn child was a male, since the CGG repeat

for fragile X is located in the *FMR1* gene on Xq27.3. He had a full mutation (>200). The unmethylation of the full mutation may be explained by the source of the sample.

Therefore, the unborn child would have fragile X symptoms.

82. **E**. Hypermethylation is typically present on most or all copies, with the exception of DNA extracted from CVS. This test can be used for prenatal diagnosis in cells obtained from amniocentesis and chorionic villus sampling (CVS). Because methylation is not fully established at the time of CVS, the appearance of full mutations examined by a methylation-specific method may vary in CVS as compared with blood and amniocytes. So it is an acceptable option to omit methylation analysis entirely when testing CVS specimens. In the minor fraction of CVS cases with a result that is ambiguous between a large premutation and a small full mutation by size criteria alone, a follow-up amniocentesis may be required.

The fetus had a hemizygous unmethylated allele with approximately 200 repeat (full mutation: >200), which is at the borderline of premutation and full mutation. So the unborn child was a male, since the CGG repeat for fragile X is located in the *FMR1* gene on Xq27.3. He had a premutation (55–200 copies) or a full mutation (>200) allele. It was unclear if the unmethylation of the abnormal allele was due to the source of the sample, or it was a premutation. If he has a premutation, he will be at risk for fragile X–associated tremor/ataxia syndrome. If he has a full mutation, he will have fragile X syndrome.

Therefore, the clinical implication of the fragile X test with the CVS sample in this patient was unclear. A follow-up amniocentesis might be required.

83. **B**. The fetus had a hemizygous unmethylated allele with approximately 150 repeats. So the unborn child was a male, since the CGG repeat for fragile X is located in the *FMR1* gene on Xq27.3. He had a premutation allele (55–200 copies).

Fragile X–associated tremor/ataxia syndrome (FXTAS) is characterized by late-onset progressive cerebellar ataxia and intention tremor in individuals who have an *FMR1* premutation. Other neurologic symptoms include short-term memory loss, executive-function deficits, cognitive decline, dementia, parkinsonism, peripheral neuropathy, lower-limb proximal muscle weakness, and autonomic dysfunction. Both males and females with a premutation are at increased risk for FXTAS. The prevalence of

FXTAS is estimated at approximately 40%–45% overall for males with a premutation who are older than age 50 years. Penetrance in males is age-related. FXTAS occurs in both male and female premutation carriers, but the penetrance in individuals older than age 50 years is lower in females (16.5%) than in males (45.5%) (http://www.ncbi.nlm.nih.gov/books/NBK1384/).

Therefore, the unborn child would not have fragile X syndrome, but he would be at risk for fragile X–associated tremor/ataxia syndrome (FXTAS).

84. **B.** The fetus had compound heterozygous 32/150 copies of the CGG repeat. So the unborn child was a girl, since the CGG repeat for fragile X is located in the *FMR1* gene on Xq27.3. She had a premutation allele (55–200 copies).

POI is characterize by cessation of menses before age 40 years, and has been observed in carriers of premutation alleles of the CGG repeat in *FMR1*. The risk for POI was 21% (estimates range from 15% to 27% in various studies) in premutation carriers, as compared with a 1% background risk (http://www.ncbi.nlm.nih.gov/books/NBK1384/).

Therefore, the unborn child would not have fragile X syndrome, but she would be at risk for *FMR1*-related primary ovarian insufficiency.

85. **C.** The woman had a compound heterozygous 31/102 copies of the CGG repeat. So she had a premutation allele (55–200 copies) and would be at risk for *FMR1*-related primary ovarian insufficiency (POI). POI is characterize by cessation of menses before age 40 years, and it has been observed in carriers of premutation alleles. *FMR1*-related primary ovarian insufficiency (age at cessation of menses, <40 years) occurs in approximately 20% of females who have an *FMR1* premutation.

Therefore, the woman had an approximately 20% risk of having FMR1-related primary ovarian insufficiency.

86. **E.** The wife had a compound heterozygous 30/52 copies of the CGG repeat. So she had an intermediate allele (gray zone, inconclusive, borderline) (45–54 copies), and would be not be symptomatic. Anticipation may happen when she passed on her abnormal allele to the next generation. The husband had 100 copies of the repeat, so he had a premutation allele (55–200 copies) and would be at risk for fragile X–associated tremor/ataxia syndrome.

The daughter will inherit one copy of the *FMR1* gene from the mother (either the normal or the intermediate allele) and the premutation allele (100 copies of the CGG repeat) from the father. Although anticipations occur through both maternal and paternal transmissions, it observed much more often in maternal transmissions (http://www.ncbi.nlm.nih.gov/books/NBK1384/).

Therefore, it would be most likely that the future daughter would have a premutation allele, and she would be at risk for both *premature ovarian failure* and *fragile X–associated tremor/ataxia syndrome.*

87. **E.** The wife had a compound heterozygous 31/52 copies of the CGG repeat. The husband had 30 copies of the repeat (normal allele, 5–44 copies). So the wife had an intermediate allele (gray zone, inconclusive, borderline) (45–54 copies). Intermediate alleles do not cause fragile X syndrome. However, about 14% of intermediate alleles are unstable and may expand into the premutation range when transmitted by the mother. They are not known to expand to full mutations. So her unborn daughter would be at risk for a premutation allele (55–200 copies). Females with a premutation are at risk for premature ovarian failure and fragile X–associated tremor/ataxia syndrome. (http://www.ncbi.nlm.nih.gov/books/NBK1384/).

Therefore, the daughter would be at increased risk to develop premature ovarian failure and fragile X–associated tremor/ataxia syndrome.

88. **G.** Fragile X is an X-linked disorder. The wife had a compound heterozygous 28/30 copies of the CGG repeat in the *FMR1* gene on Xq27.3, so she had two normal alleles (5–44 copies). The husband had approximately 100 of the repeat (premutation, 55–200 copies). The son will inherit one of the normal alleles from the mother and none from the father (http://www.ncbi.nlm.nih.gov/books/NBK1384/).

Therefore, the son would not be at increased risk to have fragile X syndrome, or to develop premature ovarian failure and fragile X–associated tremor/ataxia syndrome.

89. **D.** The wife had a compound heterozygous 30/179 copies of the CGG repeat in the *FMR1* gene on Xq27.3, so she had a premutation allele (55–200 copies). The husband had 29 copies (normal allele, 5–44 copies) (http://www.ncbi.nlm.nih.gov/books/NBK1384/). The son will inherit one copy of the *FMR1* gene from the mother (either the normal or the premutation allele). Because of potential repeat instability upon transmission of premutation alleles, women with alleles in this range are considered to be at risk of having children affected with fragile X

syndrome. *FMR1*-related primary ovarian insufficiency (POI) is characterized by the cessation of menses before age 40 years, and has been observed in female carriers of premutation alleles of the CGG repeat in *FMR1*.

Therefore, the unborn son would be at risk for fragile X syndrome, or fragile X−associated tremor/ataxia syndrome. (http://www.ncbi.nlm. nih.gov/books/NBK1384/).

90. **A**. More than 99% of patients with *fragile X syndrome* have full mutation of the CGG repeats in the *FRM1* gene. Fewer than 1% of individuals with fragile X syndrome have a partial or full deletion of *FMR1*. The abnormalities of the *FMR1* gene cause a loss-of-protein function. The protein is an RNA-binding protein that associates with polyribosomes to suppress the translation of proteins from its RNA targets. These targets appear to be involved in cytoskeletal structure, synaptic transmission, and neuronal maturation. The disruption of these processes is likely to underlie the mental retardation and learning abnormalities seen in fragile X patients (http:// www.ncbi.nlm.nih.gov/books/NBK1384/).

Therefore, the boy had fragile X syndrome.

91. **D**. Mutations in the *FMR1* gene (X27.3) are associated with fragile X syndrome, fragile X−associated tremor/ataxia syndrome, and premature ovarian insufficiency. The *FMR2* gene is located on Xq28, which lies approximately 150−600 kb distal to the *FMR1* gene and is folate-sensitive. *The* FMR2 *gene is associated with mental retardation, X-linked, FRAXE type*, instead of fragile X syndrome (http://www.ncbi.nlm.nih.gov/ books/NBK1384/).

Therefore, the unborn son would have mental retardation, X-linked, FRAXE type.

92. **D**. *Huntington disease* is caused by gain of a novel property in the mutated *HTT* gene product, which damages specific populations of neurons and produce neurodegeneration by a unique toxic mechanism. The rest of the disorder choices are caused by loss-of-function changes.

93. **A**. *Fragile X syndrome* is caused by a loss-of-protein function of the *FRM1* gene product. The rest of the disorders choices are caused by gain-of-function changes.

94. **A**. The *FMR1* gene for fragile X syndrome is located on Xq27.3. Males have only one allele, while females have two alleles. X inactivation (methylation of *FMR1*) is random. *Full-mutation alleles usually have more than 200 CGG repeats with several hundred to several thousand repeats being typical and associated with aberrant hypermethylation of the* FMR1 *promoter in males and females. If the*

CGG repeat is in the normal to premutation range, the methylation is random in females. Males have only one copy of the X chromosome and the *FMR1* gene usually is not methylated if the CGG repeat is in the normal to premutation range.

1 = full mutation male (methylated); 2 = invalid signal pattern (full-mutation alleles should be methylated in males and females); 3 = premutation male (unmethylated); 4 = invalid signal pattern (premutation alleles in male should not be methylated); 5 = normal male (unmethylated); 6 = invalid signal pattern (normal alleles should be unmethylated in male); 7 = premutation female (the premutation and normal alleles should be methylated randomly); 8 = full mutation female (full-mutation allele is methylated in females); 9 = normal female (two normal alleles are methylated randomly).

Therefore, the first patient in the figure is a male with fragile X syndrome.

95. **C**. The *FMR1* gene for fragile X syndrome is located on Xq27.3. Males have only one allele, while females have two alleles. X inactivation (methylation of *FMR1*) is random. Full-mutation alleles usually have more than 200 CGG repeats with several hundred to several thousand repeats being typical and associated with aberrant hypermethylation of the *FMR1* promoter in males and females. If the CGG repeat is in normal to premutation range, the methylation is random in female. *Males have only one copy of X chromosome, the* FMR1 *gene usually is not methylated if the CGG repeat is in normal to premutation range.*

1 = full mutation male (methylated); 2 = invalid signal pattern (full-mutation alleles should be methylated in males and females); 3 = *premutation male (unmethylated)*; 4 = invalid signal pattern (premutation alleles in male should not be methylated); 5 = normal male (unmethylated); 6 = invalid signal pattern (normal alleles should be unmethylated in male); 7 = premutation female (the premutation and normal alleles should be methylated randomly); 8 = full mutation female (full-mutation allele is methylated in females); 9 = normal female (two normal alleles are methylated randomly).

Therefore, the individual 3 in the figure is at risk for *FMR1*-associated tremor/ataxia syndrome (FXTAS).

96. **E**. The *FMR1* gene for fragile X syndrome is located on Xq27.3. Males have only one allele, while females have two alleles. X inactivation (methylation of *FMR1*) is random. Full-mutation alleles usually have more than 200 CGG repeats

with several hundred to several thousand repeats being typical and associated with aberrant hypermethylation of the *FMR1* promoter in males and females. If the CGG repeat is in the normal to premutation range, the methylation is random in female. *Males have only one copy of the X chromosome and the* FMR1 *gene usually is not methylated if the CGG repeat is in the normal to premutation range.*

1 = full mutation male (methylated); 2 = invalid signal pattern (full-mutation alleles should be methylated in males and females); 3 = premutation male (unmethylated); 4 = invalid signal pattern (premutation alleles in male should not be methylated); 5 = *normal male (unmethylated)*; 6 = invalid signal pattern (normal alleles should be unmethylated in male); 7 = premutation female (the premutation and normal alleles should be methylated randomly); 8 = full mutation female (full-mutation allele is methylated in females); 9 = normal female (two normal alleles are methylated randomly).

Therefore, the individual 5 in the figure does not have Fragile X, and is not at risk for *FMR1*-associated tremor/ataxia syndrome (FXTAS).

97. **H**. The *FMR1* gene for fragile X syndrome is located on Xq27.3. Males have only one allele, while females have two alleles. X inactivation (methylation of *FMR1*) is random. Full-mutation alleles usually have more than 200 CGG repeats with several hundred to several thousand repeats being typical and associated with aberrant hypermethylation of the *FMR1* promoter in males and females. If the CGG repeat is in the normal to premutation range, the methylation is random in females. Males have only one copy of the X chromosome and the *FMR1* gene usually is not methylated if the CGG repeat is in normal to premutation range.

1 = full mutation male (methylated); 2 = premutation male (unmethylated); 3 = normal male (unmethylated); 4 = *premutation female (the premutation and normal alleles are methylated randomly)*; 5 = *premutation female (the premutation alleles are methylated due to skewed X inactivation)*; 6 = *premutation female (the normal allele is methylated due to skewed X inactivation)*; 7 = full mutation female (full-mutation allele is methylated in females); 8 = normal female (two normal alleles are methylated randomly).

Therefore, the individuals 4, 5, and 6 in the figure do not have Fragile X, but is at risk for *FMR1*-associated tremor/ataxia syndrome (FXTAS) and premature ovarian failure (POF).

98. **D**. The *FMR1* gene for fragile X syndrome is located on Xq27.3. Males have only one allele, while females have two alleles. X inactivation (methylation of *FMR1*) is random. Full-mutation alleles usually have more than 200 CGG repeats with several hundred to several thousand repeats being typical and associated with aberrant hypermethylation of the *FMR1* promoter in males and females. If the CGG repeat is in normal to premutation range, the methylation is random in female. Males have only one copy of X chromosome and the *FMR1* gene usually is not methylated if the CGG repeat is in normal to premutation range.

1 = full mutation male (methylated); 2 = premutation male (unmethylated); 3 = normal male (unmethylated); 4 = premutation female (the premutation and normal alleles are methylated randomly); 5 = premutation female (the premutation alleles are methylated due to skewed X inactivation); 6 = premutation female (the normal allele is methylated due to skewed X inactivation); 7 = *full mutation female (full-mutation allele is methylated in females)*; 8 = normal female (two normal alleles are methylated randomly).

Therefore, the individual 7 in the figure has Fragile X syndrome.

99. **F**. The *FMR1* gene for fragile X syndrome is located on Xq27.3. Males have only one allele, while females have two alleles. X inactivation (methylation of *FMR1*) is random. Full-mutation alleles usually have more than 200 CGG repeats with several hundred to several thousand repeats being typical and associated with aberrant hypermethylation of the *FMR1* promoter in males and females. If the CGG repeat is in the normal to premutation range, the methylation is random in female. Males have only one copy of the X chromosome and the *FMR1* gene usually is not methylated if the CGG repeat is in normal to premutation range.

1 = full mutation male (methylated); 2 = premutation male (unmethylated); 3 = normal male (unmethylated); 4 = premutation female (the premutation and normal alleles are methylated randomly); 5 = premutation female (the premutation alleles are methylated due to skewed X inactivation); 6 = premutation female (the normal allele is methylated due to skewed X inactivation); 7 = full mutation female (full-mutation allele is methylated in females); 8 = *normal female (two normal alleles are methylated randomly)*.

Therefore, the individuals 6 and 8 in the figure do not have Fragile X, and not at risk for FMR1-associated tremor/ataxia syndrome (FXTAS), or premature ovarian failure.

100. **B.** For the CGG repeat in the *FMR1* gene on Xq27.3, a normal allele has 5–44 copies of the repeat, an intermediate (gray zone, inconclusive, borderline) allele has 45–54 copies, a premutation has 55–200 copies, and a full mutation has more than 200 repeats.

This patient has one allele in the normal range (5–44). Therefore, this is a normal male patient.

101. **A.** For the CGG repeat in the *FMR1* gene on Xq27.3, a normal allele has 5–44 copies of the repeat, an intermediate (gray zone, inconclusive, borderline) allele has 45–54 copies, a premutation has 55–200 copies, and a full mutation has more than 200 repeats.

This patient has two alleles in the normal range (5–44). Therefore, this is a normal female patient.

102. **E.** For the CGG repeat in the *FMR1* gene on Xq27.3, a normal allele has 5–44 copies of the repeat, an intermediate (gray zone, inconclusive, borderline) allele has 45–54 copies, a premutation has 55–200 copies, and a full mutation has more than 200 repeats.

This patient has two alleles. One is in the normal range (5–44). Another one has more than 55 repeats, but less than 200, which is in the premutation range. Therefore, this is a female patient with a premutation.

103. **H.** For the CGG repeat in the *FMR1* gene on Xq27.3, a normal allele has 5–44 copies of the repeat, an intermediate (gray zone, inconclusive, borderline) allele has 45–54 copies, a premutation has 55–200 copies, and a full mutation has more than 200 repeats.

This patient has one allele. It has more than 200 repeats. Therefore, this is a male patient with a full mutation.

104. **G.** For the CGG repeat in the *FMR1* gene on Xq27.3, a normal allele has 5–44 copies of the repeat, an intermediate (gray zone, inconclusive, borderline) allele has 45–54 copies, a premutation has 55–200 copies, and a full mutation has more than 200 repeats.

This patient has two alleles. One is in the normal range (5–44). Another has more than 200 repeats, which is in the full-mutation range. Therefore, this is a female patient with a full mutation.

105. **B.** The mother had two normal alleles (5–4 copies). The father had a premutation allele (55–200 copies). The daughter had one normal allele and one full-mutation allele (>200 copies).

To date, there have been no reports of male or female with normal alleles or carriers of intermediate alleles having offspring with an *FMR1* allele in the full-mutation range. All fragile X males and the overwhelming majority of affected females inherited their mutations from their mother. Men with a premutation will almost always pass the premutation to all of their daughters. *An extremely rare phenomenon involves unaffected males with a premutation who have had affected daughters, apparently by gonadal mosaicism for full mutations.*

Therefore, in this scenario, most likely the father had gonadal mosaicism for the full mutation, since a premutation was detected in his peripheral-blood sample.

106. **C.** Full mutations lead to transcriptional silencing of the *FMR1* gene owing to methylation of CpG islands upstream of the repeat region. A full-mutation male may have a combination of a predominant band with a diffuse smear, as does a premutation. Smear of expansions extending from premutation to full mutation results from somatic instability of larger repeats. Expansion of a premutation is usually not associated with methylation and transcriptional silencing of the *FMR1* gene. Therefore, it is important to test the methylation status of the allele in order to differentiate a full mutation from a premutation.

Premutation alleles are unstable and may expand to full mutations in future generations. Premutation carrier males typically transmit the CGG repeat region to their progeny with small changes in repeat numbers. *When the premutation is transmitted by a carrier female, there is an increased probability of expansion of the CGG repeat region to a full-mutation allele (anticipation), leading to mental retardation in most male offspring and 50% of female offspring (as a result of unfavorable lyonization of the X chromosome)* (http://www.ncbi.nlm.nih.gov/books/NBK1384/).

Therefore, a *FMR1* allele in the premutation range is unstable, and may expand to a full mutation through intergenerational transmission, especially through a carrier female.

107. **A.** Fragile X syndrome occurs in individuals with an *FMR1* full mutation or other loss-of-function mutation. Full mutations lead to transcriptional silencing of the *FMR1* gene owing to methylation of CpG islands upstream of the repeat region. *A full mutation in males may shrink to premutation in daughters during transmission* (http://www.ncbi.nlm.nih.gov/books/NBK1384/).

Premutation alleles are usually not associated with methylation and transcriptional silencing of the *FMR1* gene. But they are unstable and may expand to full mutations in future generations. Premutation carrier males typically transmit the CGG repeat region to their progeny with small changes in repeat numbers. When the premutation is transmitted by a carrier female, there is an increased probability of expansion of the CGG repeat region to a full-mutation allele (anticipation), leading to mental retardation in most male offspring and 50% of female offspring as a result of unfavorable lyonization of the X chromosome. Female carriers of premutation are at 20% risk of premature ovarian failure. Male premutation carriers, and more rarely female premutation carriers, are at risk of a late-onset fragile X−associated tremor/ataxia syndrome (FXTAS) (http://www.ncbi.nlm.nih.gov/books/NBK1384/).

Therefore, a full mutation in males may shrink to premutation in daughters during transmission.

108. **D**. Fragile X syndrome is caused by transcriptional silencing of the *FMR1* gene owing to full mutations, but the pathogenesis of the disease is not fully understood. Premutation alleles are usually not associated with methylation and transcriptional silencing of the *FMR1* gene. But they are unstable and may expand to full mutations in future generations. Evidence suggests that FXTAS results from the twofold to fivefold increased levels of the *FMR1* mRNA in these patients. A female premutation carrier has a 50% of chance of having a methylated normal allele or a methylated premutation allele as a result of unfavorable lyonization of the X chromosome (http://www.ncbi.nlm.nih.gov/books/NBK1384/).

Triplet repeat−primed PCR (TP PCR) allows rapid detection of PCR products formed by a chimeric primer binding inside a triplet-repeat region. In TRP PCR for fragile X syndrome, one primer is anchored completely outside the CGG repeat region, whereas the other overlaps the CGG repeat and the adjacent nonrepeated sequence. A third primer can be anchored outside the CGG region that, when paired with the opposite anchored primer, will amplify "over" the CGG repeat. This will increase the amount of full-length product from the largest CGG-repeat allele and in some assays enables accurate sizing of alleles up to 200 CGG repeats. From the chimeric primer annealing at each CGG repeat, multiple amplicons are made, forming products each with a length differing by three bases (http://www.ncbi.nlm.nih.gov/books/NBK1384/).

Therefore, the triplet-primed PCR may detect copy-number changes of trinucleotide repeats, but not point mutations.

109. **B**. Mutations in the *FMR1* gene are associated with fragile X syndrome, fragile X−associated tremor/ataxia syndrome (FXTAS), and premature ovarian insufficiency. FXTAS is a late-onset, progressive development of intention tremor and ataxia often accompanied by progressive cognitive and behavioral difficulties including memory loss, anxiety, reclusive behavior, deficits of executive function, and dementia. *The risk for FXTAS is higher in males who carry a premutation as compared with females. The penetrance of FXTAS increases with age and with premutation repeat length.*

Therefore, John has higher risk for FXTAS than his siblings.

110. **B**. The gene product is fragile X mental retardation protein (FMRP), a widely expressed *RNA-binding protein*. The fragile X syndrome is caused by a loss of the FMRP. FMRP is a selective RNA-binding protein that can form a messenger ribonucleoprotein complex that can associate with polysomes. FMRP has been shown to behave in vitro as an inhibitor of protein translation (http://www.ncbi.nlm.nih.gov/books/NBK1384/).

Therefore, the *FMR1* gene product is a RNA-binding protein.

111. **C**. The FMR1 gene is located on chromosome X. Since only one allele of FMR1 was seen in this CVS specimen, it is likely the fetus is a male. Older males and females with premutations are at risk for fragile X−associated tremor/ataxia syndrome (FXTAS). FXTAS is a late-onset, progressive development of intention tremor and ataxia often accompanied by progressive cognitive and behavioral difficulties, including memory loss, anxiety, reclusive behavior, deficits of executive function, and dementia. The risk for FXTAS is higher in males who carry a premutation as compared with females. The penetrance of FXTAS increases with age and with premutation repeat length. A premutation (55−200 repeats) is also associated with premature ovarian insufficiency (FXPOI) in females.

The molecular test of the (CGG)n repeats can be used for prenatal diagnosis in cells obtained from amniocentesis and CVS. In this case, c.-129CGG (199) indicated that Southern blotting was used to characterize the CGG repeat in this chorionic villus sampling (CVS) sample and that the exact size of the repeat cannot be determined, which may be a premutation (55−200), or a full mutation (>200). A methylation study would be helpful to determine whether the fetus had a premutation or a full mutation. Because methylation is not fully established at the time of CVS, follow-up amniocentesis would be appropriate to establish the diagnosis in this fetus (http://www.ncbi.nlm.nih.gov/books/NBK1384/).

Therefore, in this case a follow-up amniocentesis should be recommended.

112. **B.** It has been the intent of the College of American Pathology (CAP)/American College of Medical Genetics and Genomics (ACMG) Biochemical and Molecular Genetics Resource Committee to standardize the accuracy of CGG-repeat quantitation. The acceptable range for sizing CGG repeats is based on the analysis of CAP/ACMG proficiency testing survey results for fragile X. Acknowledging the technical limitations of size analysis, the ACMG supports the following acceptable ranges for *FMR1* clinical testing and/or as grading criteria for the CAP/ACMG proficiency testing survey: *consensus size ± 5 repeats for alleles with <55 repeats* (https://www.acmg.net/).

113. **C.** It has been the intent of the College of American Pathology (CAP)/American College of Medical Genetics and Genomics (ACMG) Biochemical and Molecular Genetics Resource Committee to standardize the accuracy of CGG-repeat quantitation. The acceptable range for sizing CGG repeats is based on the analysis of CAP/ACMG proficiency testing survey results for fragile X. Acknowledging the technical limitations of size analysis, the ACMG supports the following acceptable ranges for *FMR1* clinical testing and/or as grading criteria for the CAP/ACMG proficiency testing survey: *consensus size ± 10 repeats for alleles with 56−100 repeats* (https://www.acmg.net/).

114. **E.** It has been the intent of the College of American Pathology (CAP)/American College of Medical Genetics and Genomics (ACMG) Biochemical and Molecular Genetics Resource Committee to standardize the accuracy of CGG-repeat quantitation. The acceptable range for sizing CGG repeats is based on the analysis of CAP/ACMG proficiency testing survey results for fragile X. Acknowledging the technical limitations of size analysis, the ACMG supports the following acceptable ranges for *FMR1* clinical testing and/or as grading criteria for the CAP/ACMG proficiency testing survey: *consensus size ± 2 SDs for alleles with >100 repeats* (https://www.acmg.net/).

References

1. Siwach P, Ganesh S. Tandem repeats in human disorders: mechanisms and evolution. *Front Biosci* 2008;**13**:4467−84.
2. Budworth H, McMurray CT. A brief history of triplet repeat diseases. *Methods Mol Biol* 2013;**1010**:3−17.
3. Swami M, et al. Somatic expansion of the Huntington's disease CAG repeat in the brain is associated with an earlier age of disease onset. *Hum Mol Genet* 2009;**18**(16):3039−47.
4. Nussbaum RL, McInnes RR, Willard HF. 8th ed. *Thompson & Thompsongenetics in medicine*, xi. Philadelphia: Elsevier; 2016. p. 546.
5. ACMG/ASHG statement. Laboratory guidelines for Huntington disease genetic testing. The American College of Medical Genetics/American Society of Human Genetics Huntington Disease Genetic Testing Working Group. *Am J Hum Genet* 1998;**62**(5):1243−7.
6. Nahhas FA, et al. Juvenile onset Huntington disease resulting from a very large maternal expansion. *Am J Med Genet A* 2005;**137A**(3):328−31.
7. Ha AD, Jankovic J. Exploring the correlates of intermediate CAG repeats in Huntington disease. *Postgrad Med* 2011;**123**(5):116−21.
8. Aziz NA, et al. CAG repeat expansion in Huntington disease determines age at onset in a fully dominant fashion. *Neurology* 2012;**79**(9):952 author reply 952-3.
9. Semaka A, et al. CAG size-specific risk estimates for intermediate allele repeat instability in Huntington disease. *J Med Genet* 2013;**50**(10):696−703.
10. Scuffham TM, MacMillan JC. Huntington disease: who seeks presymptomatic genetic testing, why and what are the outcomes? *J Genet Couns* 2014;**23**(5):754−61.
11. Chen L, et al. An information-rich CGG repeat primed PCR that detects the full range of fragile X expanded alleles and minimizes the need for southern blot analysis. *J Mol Diagn* 2010;**12**(5):589−600.
12. Jama M, et al. Triplet repeat primed PCR simplifies testing for Huntington disease. *J Mol Diagn* 2013;**15**(2):255−62.
13. Bean L, Bayrak-Toydemir P. American College of Medical Genetics and Genomics Standards and Guidelines for Clinical Genetics Laboratories, 2014 edition: technical standards and guidelines for Huntington disease. *Genet Med* 2014;**16**(12):e2.
14. Pandolfo M. Molecular genetics and pathogenesis of Friedreich ataxia. *Neuromuscul Disord* 1998;**8**(6):409−15.
15. Holloway TP, et al. Detection of interruptions in the GAA trinucleotide repeat expansion in the FXN gene of Friedreich ataxia. *Biotechniques* 2011;**50**(3):182−6.
16. Nachbauer W, et al. Friedreich ataxia: executive control is related to disease onset and GAA repeat length. *Cerebellum* 2014;**13**(1):9−16.
17. Monaghan KG, et al. ACMG Standards and Guidelines for fragile X testing: a revision to the disease-specific supplements to the Standards and Guidelines for Clinical Genetics Laboratories of the American College of Medical Genetics and Genomics. *Genet Med* 2013;**15**(7):575−86.

Further Reading

- Cure SMA (www.curesma.org/)
- FRAXA (www.fraxa.org/)
- Friedreich's Ataxia News (www.friedreichsataxianews.com/)
- Huntington's NSW ACT (www.huntingtonsnsw.org.au/)
- Huntington Association (www.hda.org.uk/)
- Muscular Dystrophy Association (www.mda.org/)
- Myotonic Dystrophy Foundation (www.myotonic.org/)
- National Ataxia Foundation (www.ataxia.org/)
- National Fragile X Foundation (www.fragilex.org)
- Orphanet (www.orpha.net/)
- SMA Foundation (http://www.smafoundation.org/)
- SMA News Today (www.smanewstoday.com/)
- The fragile X Association of Australia (www.fragilex.org.au/)

CHAPTER

5

Cystic Fibrosis

Cystic fibrosis (CF) is an autosomal recessive disorder, characterized by severe damage to the lungs, digestive system, and other organs. It is caused by variants in *CFTR*, which was discovered in 1989. The *CFTR* genotype determines total CFTR activity at the cell surface. In general, the presence of biallelic variants that produce little to no CFTR activity are associated with early onset of symptoms and progression. The presence of variants associated with residual CFTR activity may be related to delayed onset. Other influencing factors may include modifier genes, such as *MBL2* and *TGF-ß1*, affecting lung function and disease course, and environmental factors, such as nutritional status, cigarette smoking, age at onset of lung infection, and socioeconomic status.

Approximately 2000 variants in the *CFTR* gene have been identified to date, although the majority are extremely rare, and not all *CFTR* variants are pathogenic. To date, only 242 *CFTR* variants have been confirmed to be disease-causing. F508del is the most common CFTR pathogenic variant worldwide. Up to 92% of patients with CF have at least one F508del allele.

Carrier frequencies vary significantly among races and ethnicities. On average, about 1 in every 31 Americans is a symptomless carrier of a deleterious *CFTR* allele. One of 29 Caucasian Americans are CF carriers, as are 1 of 46 Hispanic Americans, 1 of 65 African Americans, and 1 of 90 Asian Americans. In Ashkenazi Jews, the carrier frequency is 1 in 24. Because of the high carrier frequencies in certain populations, carrier screen and newborn screen became important and widely available in the United Staets.[1,2]

Treatment of manifestations has been used to manage CF-related symptoms, which significantly improve the quality of patient's life. The recent approvals of ivacaftor and lumacaftor represent a new era of precision medicine in the treatment of this disorder.[3]

We assigned one chapter to this disease because it is highly prevalent in the United States and is associated with significantly shorter life spans. Genetic testing plays an important role in carrier and newborn screening and provides guidance for targeted therapy in some patients.

QUESTIONS

1. Cystic fibrosis (CF) is one of the most common autosomal recessive disorders in North America. Approximately 1 in 2500 liveborn children in the United States has CF. Which one of following defects causes multisystem symptoms in patients with CF?[5]
   A. Transmembrane sodium channel
   B. Transmembrane chloride channel
   C. Transmembrane cation channel
   D. Transmembrane calcium channel
   E. Transmembrane ion channel

2. Cystic fibrosis (CF) is a genetic disease that causes changes in secretions of the body. Mutations in the cystic fibrosis transmembrane conductance regulator (*CFTR*) gene cause CF. The CFTR protein regulates chloride transport that is important for the function of the lungs, upper respiratory tract, pancreas, liver, sweat glands, and genitourinary tract. Over 1500 mutations have been described in *CFTR*. Which one of the following describes the functional changes of the mutations in CF?[5]
   A. Dominant negative
   B. Gain of function
   C. Loss of function
   D. Not sure
   E. None of the above

3. How frequently do patients with congenital bilateral absence of the vas deferens (CBAVD) have at least one variant in the *CFTR* gene including the 5T variant?[6]
   A. 20%
   B. 35%
   C. 50%
   D. 75%
   E. 95%

4. How frequently do patients with congenital bilateral absence of the vas deferens (CBAVD) have two variants in the *CFTR* gene including the 5T variant?[6]
   A. 20%
   B. 35%
   C. 50%
   D. 75%
   E. 95%

5. Cystic fibrosis (CF) is a genetic disease that causes changes in secretions of the body. Mutations in the cystic fibrosis transmembrane conductance regulator (*CFTR*) gene cause CF. The CFTR protein regulates chloride transport that is important for function of the lungs, upper respiratory tract, pancreas, liver, sweat glands, and genitourinary tract. Over 1500 mutations have been described in *CFTR*. In April 2001, the American College of Medical Genetics and Genomics (ACMG) Cystic Fibrosis (CF) Carrier Screening Working Group recommended a panel of mutations and variants that should be tested to determine carrier status within the *CFTR* gene as a part of population screening programs.[4] The panel was updated in 2004.[5] How many mutations/ variants are in the updated minimum mutation panel recommended by ACMG in 2004 for CF (not counting the reflex test)?[7]
   A. 15
   B. 23
   C. 25
   D. 60
   E. 139

6. What is the carrier frequency of cystic fibrosis (CF) in Ashkenazi Jews?[8]
   A. 1/16
   B. 1/24
   C. 1/33
   D. 1/58
   E. 1/61
   F. 1/94

7. What is the carrier frequency of cystic fibrosis (CF) in Caucasians?[8]
   A. 1/17
   B. 1/25
   C. 1/33
   D. 1/42
   E. 1/60
   F. 1/94

8. Which one of the populations below has the lowest cystic fibrosis carrier frequency?[8]
   A. Ashkenazi Jewish
   B. European Caucasian
   C. Hispanic American
   D. African American
   E. Asian American
   F. None of the above

9. Which individual below has the lowest risk of being a cystic fibrosis (CF) carrier, assuming that she/he does NOT have a family history of CF and is apparently healthy?[8]
   A. Descendant of Ashkenazi Jewish/European Caucasians
   B. Descendant of European Caucasian/Hispanic Americans
   C. Descendant of African American/Hispanic Americans
   D. Descendant of African American/Asian Americans
   E. Descendant of Hispanic American/Asian Americans
   F. None of the above

10. Which of the following orders is the correct one for cystic fibrosis carrier frequency (from highest to the lowest)?[8]
    A. Ashkenazi Jewish > European Caucasian > Hispanic American > African American > Asian American
    B. Ashkenazi Jewish > European Caucasian > African American > Hispanic American > Asian American
    C. Ashkenazi Jewish > European Caucasian > African American > Asian American > Hispanic American
    D. Ashkenazi Jewish > European Caucasian > Hispanic American > Asian American > African American
    E. Ashkenazi Jewish > European Caucasian > Asian American > African American > Hispanic American
    F. None of the above

11. Which one of the following is the approximate analytical sensitivity of the ACMG-recommended cystic fibrosis (CF) carrier test panel with 23 mutations in Ashkenazi Jews?[8]
    A. 95%
    B. 90%
    C. 80%
    D. 70%
    E. 60%

12. Which one of the following is the approximate analytical sensitivity of the ACMG-recommended cystic fibrosis (CF) carrier test panel with 23 mutations in non-Hispanic Caucasians?[8]
    A. 95%
    B. 90%
    C. 80%
    D. 70%
    E. 60%

13. A laboratory director tried to design allele-specific oligonucleotide probes for a cystic fibrosis (CF) carrier test. The mutation that needs to be detected

is ATTTGGTTCTCACCTGA[a/g]
CAGCGGCTCACAGTTGATGA. Which pair of
probes would she pick as the probes for this
mutation?

A. TGGTTCTCACCTGA**a**CAGCGGCTCACAGTT
and TGGTTCTCACCTGA**g**CAGCGGCTCACA
GTT

B. AACTGTGAGCCGCTGt**t**TCAGGTGAGAACCA
and TGGTTCTCACCTGA**g**CAGCGGCTCACA
GTT

C. TGGTTCTCACCTGA**t**CAGCGGCTCACAGTT
and AACTGTGAGCCGCTG**c**TCAGGTGAGAA
CCA

D. AACTGTGAGCCGCTG**a**TCAGGTGAGAACCA
and AACTGTGAGCCGCTG**c**TCAGGTGAGAA
CCA

14. Which one of the following assays has better
analytical sensitivity than the others to detect
patients with cystic fibrosis (CF)?[8,9]

A. ACMG-recommended 23-mutation panel
B. *CFTR* gene Sanger sequencing
C. Immunoreactive trypsinogen (IRT)-IRT
D. Sweat chloride test
E. None of the above

15. A European Caucasian couple comes to a clinic for
their preconception counseling. They both are
apparently healthy, with no remarkable medical
history. The wife's family history was uneventful.
The husband's brother died of cystic fibrosis (CF)
at 15 years of age. The husband did not have a
molecular genetic test for CF. What is the risk that
the couple's firstborn child will have CF?

A. 1/54
B. 1/150
C. 1/200
D. 3/400
E. None of the above

16. An Ashkenazi Jewish couple comes to a clinic for
their preconception counseling. They both are
apparently healthy, with no remarkable medical
history. The wife's brother died of cystic
fibrosis (CF) at 16 years of age. The wife has not
had a molecular genetic test for CF. The
husband's family history was uneventful. What is
the risk that the couple's firstborn child
will have CF?

A. 1/54
B. 1/150
C. 1/200
D. 3/400
E. None of the above

17. A European Caucasian couple came to a clinic for
their first prenatal checkup when the wife was 6

weeks pregnant. They both are apparently healthy
with no remarkable medical history. This was their
first pregnancy. The wife's brother died of cystic
fibrosis (CF) at 19 years of age. Molecular testing
in the family confirmed that the wife carried a
copy of the familial *CFTR* mutation from her
mother's side. The husband's family history was
negative. The husband had not had a molecular
CFTR test. What was the risk that their firstborn
child would have CF?

A. 1/25
B. 1/50
C. 1/100
D. 1/200
E. None of the above

18. A couple came to a clinic for their first prenatal
checkup when the wife was 6 weeks pregnant.
The wife was a Ashkenazi Jewish and the
husband was a Hispanic American. They both are
apparently healthy, with no remarkable medical
history. This was their first pregnancy. The
physician ordered the ACMG-recommended 23-
mutation panel for cystic fibrosis (CF) with the
wife's peripheral-blood sample. The detection rate
of the panel was 94% in Ashkenazi Jews. The test
results were negative. The reflex molecular test
with the husband's blood sample for the same
panel was pending. What was the wife's residual
risk to be a CF carrier?[10]

A. 1/24
B. 1/192
C. 1/384
D. 1/768
E. 1/1534
F. None of the above

19. A European Caucasian couple came to a clinic for
their first prenatal checkup when the wife was 6
weeks pregnant. They both are apparently healthy,
with no remarkable medical history. They have
two healthy children. This is their third pregnancy.
The wife's brother died of cystic fibrosis (CF) when
he was 19 years old. The wife carries a copy of the
familial *CFTR* mutation from her mother's side.
The family history on the husband side was
negative. The husband had not had molecular
CFTR test yet. What was the risk that their third
child would have CF?[10]

A. 1/100
B. 1/385
C. 1/770
D. 1/1540
E. 1/3080
F. None of the above

20. Which one of the following methods has been widely used as the first- tier cystic fibrosis (CF) test in newborn screening (NBS) programs in the United States?[9]
    A. *CFTR* gene Sanger sequencing
    B. High-performance liquid chromatography (HPLC)
    C. Immunoreactive trypsinogen (IRT)
    D. Mass spectrometry (MS)
    E. Sweat sodium chloride test
    F. None of the above

21. An African couple moved to United States 2 weeks before their baby, Johnny, was born. The newborn screening (NBS) test for cystic fibrosis (CF) was positive. And Johnny had meconium ileus. Which one of the following findings may lead to the positive NBS CF report?[9]
    A. High value of immunoreactive trypsinogen (IRT)
    B. Low value of immunoreactive trypsinogen (IRT)
    C. High value of sweat chloride
    D. Low value of sweat chloride
    E. None of the above

22. The newborn screening program (NBS) in Massachusetts (MA) referred a newborn boy, Johnny, with a p.F508del variant to a Cystic Fibrosis (CF) Foundation—accredited care center for further evaluation and diagnostic testing. Which one of the following assays would be the most appropriate to confirm the diagnosis in Johnny after the positive CF screening?[9]
    A. *CFTR* gene Sanger sequencing
    B. High-performance liquid chromatography (HPLC)
    C. Immunoreactive trypsinogen (IRT)
    D. Mass spectrometry (MS)
    E. Sweat sodium chloride test
    F. None of the above

23. An African couple moved to the United States 2 weeks before their baby, Johnny, was born. The newborn screening test (NBS) showed elevated immunoreactive trypsinogen (IRT), and a p. F508del mutation was found with the DNA test. Follow-up sweat chloride testing showed a level of 22 mmol/L at 16 days of age. Which one of the following would be the most appropriate interpretation of the sweat chloride test results?[9]
    A. Normal
    B. Intermediate
    C. Abnormal
    D. Not sure
    E. None of the above

24. An African couple moved to the United States 2 weeks before their baby, Johnny, was born. The newborn screening test (NBS) showed elevated immunoreactive trypsinogen (IRT), and a p. F508del mutation was found with the DNA test. Follow-up sweat chloride testing showed 45 mmol/L at 16 days of age. Which one of the following would be the most appropriate interpretation of the sweat chloride test results?[9]
    A. Normal
    B. Intermediate
    C. Abnormal
    D. Not sure
    E. None of the above

25. An African couple moved to the United States 2 weeks before their baby, Johnny, was born. The newborn screening test (NBS) showed elevated immunoreactive trypsinogen (IRT), and a p.F508del mutation was found with the DNA test. Follow-up sweat chloride testing showed 62 mmol/L at 16 days of age. Which one of the following would be the most appropriate interpretation of the sweat chloride test results?[5]
    A. Normal
    B. Intermediate
    C. Abnormal
    D. Not sure
    E. None of the above

26. Which one of the following mutations in the *CFTR* gene is the most common for cystic fibrosis (CF) worldwide?[5]
    A. p.F508del
    B. p.R117H
    C. p.G551D
    D. c.1210-12T[5]
    E. p.G542X

27. Which one of the following mutations is NOT included in the revised American College of Medical Genetics and Genomics (ACMG) cystic fibrosis (CF) carrier screening panel published in 2004, but is in the recommended reflex test?[4,5]
    A. p.F508del
    B. p.R117H
    C. p.G551D
    D. c.1210-12T[5]
    E. 5T/7T/9T

28. A couple came to a clinic for prenatal care when the wife was 6 weeks pregnant. The wife was a 23-year-old Caucasian. The husband was a 26-year-old African American. Family history was unremarkable on both sides. Carrier screening tests for cystic fibrosis (CF) with the American College of Medical Genetics and Genomics (ACMG)—recommended 23 mutations were offered to the wife first. The results showed that the wife was a carrier of the R117H mutation. Which one of the following mutations/variants

should also be tested for the wife to interpret this molecular result according to the ACMG recommendation?[4,5]

A. 5T/7T/9T

B. TH11/TG12/TG13

C. I507V

D. F508C

E. None of the above

29. A couple came to a clinic for prenatal care when the wife was 6 weeks pregnant. The wife was a 23-year-old Caucasian. The husband was a 26-year-old African American. Family history was unremarkable on both sides. Carrier screening tests for cystic fibrosis (CF) with the American College of Medical Genetics and Genomics (ACMG)—recommended 23 mutations were offered to the couple. The results showed that the wife was compound heterozygous for R117H and 7T in intron 8. The husband's test detected a heterozygous p.F508del mutation. What was the risk that their firstborn child would have CF?[10]

A. 1/4

B. 1/16

C. 1/482

D. 1/964

E. 1/1928

F. Not clear

G. None of the above

30. A couple came to a clinic for prenatal care when the wife was 6 weeks pregnant. The wife was a 23-year-old Caucasian. The husband was a 26-year-old African American. Family history was unremarkable on both sides. Carrier screening tests for cystic fibrosis (CF) with the American College of Medical Genetics and Genomics (ACMG)—recommended 23 mutations were offered to the wife first. The results showed that the wife was compound heterozygous for R117H and 5T in intron 8. Subsequently, the husband's test detected a heterozygous p.F508del mutation. What was the risk that their firstborn child would have CF?[4,5]

A. 1/4

B. 1/16

C. 1/482

D. 1/964

E. 1/1928

F. Not clear

G. None of the above

31. The R117H mutation in *CFTR* is modified by the 5T/7T/9T polymorphism in intron 8. Which one of the following mechanisms explains how 5T/7T/9T modifies phenotypes in patients with R117H?[5]

A. The polymorphism affects splicing function.

B. The polymorphism affects the modification of mRNA with the polyadenylation at the 3′ end.

C. The polymorphism affects the promoter function at the 5′ end.

D. The polymorphism affects the enhancer function.

E. The polymorphism maps to a locus other than *CFTR*.

F. Unclear.

G. None of the above.

32. A newlywed, apparently healthy Caucasian couple came to a clinic for preconception counseling. Family history was unremarkable on both sides. Carrier screening tests for cystic fibrosis (CF) with the American College of Medical Genetics and Genomics (ACMG)—recommended 23 mutations were offered to the wife first. The results showed that the wife was a carrier of the F508del mutation. Subsequently, the husband's test results indicated that he was a carrier of the R117H mutation, and the reflex test found 5T. For which one of the following medical problems would the husband be at risk?[4-6]

A. Heart failure

B. Infertility

C. Obesity

D. Sudden death

E. All of the above

F. None of the above

33. A couple came to a clinic for prenatal care when the wife was 6 weeks pregnant. The wife was a 23-year-old Caucasian. The husband was a 26-year-old African American. Family history was unremarkable on both sides. Carrier screening tests for cystic fibrosis (CF) with the American College of Medical Genetics and Genomics (ACMG)—recommended 23 mutations were offered to the wife first. The results showed that the wife was a carrier of the R117H mutation, and the reflex test detected 5T. The husband's test detected a heterozygous p.F508del mutation. Which one of the following statements is the most appropriate one?[4,5]

A. The wife is a CF patient with mild symptoms.

B. The wife is not a CF carrier.

C. The fetus will have 25% chance of having CF.

D. Not sure.

E. None of the above.

34. A couple came to a clinic for prenatal care when the wife was 6 weeks pregnant. The wife was a 23-year-old Caucasian. The husband was a 26-year-old African American. Family history is unremarkable on both sides. Carrier screening tests for cystic fibrosis (CF) with the American College

of Medical Genetics and Genomics (ACMG)—recommended 23 mutations were offered to the wife first. The results showed that the wife was a carrier of the R117H mutation, and the reflex test detected 5T. Subsequently, the husband's test results turned out to be negative. Which one of the following statements is appropriate?[4-6]

A. The child is not at risk for CF.
B. The child still has significant risk for CF.
C. The child is at risk for infertility if it is a male.
D. All of the above.
E. None of the above.

35. A Caucasian couple came to a clinic for prenatal care when the wife was 6 weeks pregnant. They were apparently healthy, with uneventful medical histories. Neither of them had a family history of cystic fibrosis. This is their first pregnancy. Carrier screening tests for cystic fibrosis (CF) with the American College of Medical Genetics and Genomics (ACMG)—recommended 23 mutations were offered to the couple. The results showed that the wife was a carrier of the R117H mutation, and the reflex test detected 7T. The husband's test results turned out to be negative. What was the residual risk that their firstborn child would have CF?[4,5,10]

A. 1/4
B. 1/50
C. 1/964
D. >1/3856
E. None of the above

36. A Caucasian couple came to a clinic for prenatal care when the wife was 6 weeks pregnant. They were apparently healthy, with uneventful medical histories. Neither of them had a family history of cystic fibrosis (CF). Carrier screening tests for CF with the ACMG-recommended 23 mutations in the CFTR gene were ordered for the wife first. The results showed that the wife was a carrier of the R117H mutation and 5T. Which one of the following would be the most appropriate next step in the workup?[4,5]

A. Test the husband with the same CF mutation panel.
B. State in the report that the wife is not a carrier.
C. Recommend prenatal CF diagnostic testing to the couple.
D. Recommend CF testing to the wife's parents and/or other family members.
E. The posttest risk is significantly decreased. There is no need for follow-up.

37. A Caucasian couple came to a clinic for prenatal care when the wife was 6 weeks pregnant. They were apparently healthy, with uneventful medical histories. Neither of them had a family history of

cystic fibrosis (CF). Carrier screening tests for CF with the ACMG-recommended 23 mutations in the CFTR gene were ordered for the couple. The results showed that the wife was a carrier of the R117H mutation and 5T. The husband's test detected a heterozygous p.F508del mutation. Which one of the following would be the most appropriate next step in the workup?[4,5]

A. Test the husband with the same CF mutation panel.
B. State in the report that the wife is not a carrier.
C. Recommend prenatal CF diagnostic testing to the couple.
D. Recommend CF testing to the wife's parents and/or other family members.
E. The posttest risk is significantly decreased. There is no need for follow-up.

38. A 23-year-old African American woman was 14 weeks pregnant. She and her Caucasian husband came for prenatal care. Ultrasound showed that the fetus had an echogenic bowel. Neither of them had a family history of cystic fibrosis (CF). Amniocentesis was offered. The chromosome results were normal. The CF 23-mutation panel test showed that the fetus was homozygous for the p.F508del. Which one of the following would be the most appropriate next step in the workup?[4,5]

A. Test the wife and the husband with the same CF mutation panel.
B. State that the fetus will be a CF patient with homozygous F508del.
C. Sequence the CFTR gene reflex to del/dup with the amniotic fluid sample.
D. Sequence the CFTR gene reflex to del/dup with the wife and husband's peripheral-blood samples.
E. Sequence the CFTR gene reflex to del/dup after birth.

39. An African American couple moved to the United States 2 weeks before their baby, Johnny, was born. The newborn screening test showed elevated immunoreactive trypsinogen (IRT), and a p.F508del mutation was found with the DNA test. Follow-up sweat chloride testing showed 45 mmol/L at 10 days of age. Sanger sequencing for cystic fibrosis (CF) found that Johnny was heterozygous for p.F508del and 5T in the CFTR gene. Which one of the following symptoms would Johnny be at risk for?[6]

A. Heart failure
B. Infertility
C. Obesity
D. Sudden death
E. All of the above
F. None of the above

40. A 23-year-old African American woman was 14 weeks pregnant. She and her Caucasian husband came for prenatal care. Ultrasound showed that the fetus had an echogenic bowel. Neither of the couple had a family history of cystic fibrosis. Amniocentesis was offered. The chromosome results were normal. The CF panel test for the 23 mutations showed that the fetus was homozygous for the F508del. Which one of the following tests should NOT be included in the reflex test?[4,5]
    A. IVS8(T)n
    B. I506V
    C. I507V
    D. F508C

41. An African American couple moved to the United States 2 weeks after their baby, Johnny, was born. Johnny had meconium ileus. Neither of the parents has a family history of cystic fibrosis (CF). What would be the most appropriate test to rule out CF?[9]
    A. Sequence the *CFTR* gene reflex to del/dup to Johnny
    B. Sweat chloride test
    C. The 23-mutation panel recommended by ACMG
    D. The 60-mutation panel in the *CFTR* gene
    E. The 139-mutation panel in the *CFTR* gene

42. An African American couple moved to the United States 2 weeks after their baby, Johnny, was born. Johnny had meconium ileus. A sweat chloride test was positive. Cystic fibrosis (CF) molecular testing found that Johnny was homozygous for one mutation in the *CFTR* gene. The physician offered ivacaftor for the targeted therapy. Which one of the following mutations would Johnny most likely have?[7]
    A. F508del
    B. G542X
    C. G551D
    D. $621 + 1G > T$
    E. W1282X
    F. N1303K

43. An African American couple moved to the United States 2 weeks after their baby, Johnny, was born. Johnny had meconium ileus. Sweat chloride test showed a borderline result (59 mmol/L). Sanger sequencing of the *CFTR* gene for cystic fibrosis (CF) detected that Johnny had three changes, p. F508del, p.R117H, and 5T. Which one of the following would be the most appropriate next step in the workup?[4,5]
    A. Classify the patient as a CF carrier.
    B. Diagnose the patient as having CBAVD.
    C. Diagnose the patient as having CF.
    D. Perform a parental targeted molecular test.
    E. None of the above.

44. Which one of the following assays should NOT be offered to a couple during pregnancy as a routine cystic fibrosis (CF) carrier screening?[4,5,9]
    A. Sanger sequencing
    B. The 23-mutation panel
    C. The 60-mutation panel
    D. The 139-mutation panel
    E. None of the above

45. Newborn screening (NBS) programs referred a newborn boy, Johnny, to a Cystic Fibrosis (CF) Foundation—accredited care center for further evaluation and diagnostic test because his immunoreactive trypsinogen (IRT)/IRT test was positive. The follow-up sweat test in the care center was 45 mmol/L. The DNA test revealed that the infant has G551D, R117H, and 5T variants. The parental targeted molecular genetic test revealed that the R117H and 5T variants in the infant is in *cis*. Which one of the following would be the most appropriate interpretation?[4,5]
    A. The patient does not have CF, so there is no need for follow-up.
    B. The patient has CF, and treatment should be started right away.
    C. The patient may have congenital absence of the vas deferens.
    D. The patient is a CF carrier, and he may develop mild symptoms.
    E. None of the above.

46. Newborn screening (NBS) programs referred a 2-day old boy, Johnny, to a Cystic Fibrosis (CF) Foundation—accredited care center for further evaluation and diagnostic testing because his immunoreactive trypsinogen (IRT)/IRT test was positive. The patient was asymptomatic. The family history was uneventful. The parents were apparently healthy. The boy has two sisters and one brother. The follow-up sweat test in the care center was 68 mmol/L. The DNA test revealed that the infant has F508del and G551D variants. The physician started the treatment immediately. Which would be the most appropriate next step in the workup for the family?
    A. Recommending targeted molecular genetic testing to the parents
    B. Recommending targeted molecular genetic testing for the siblings
    C. Recommending sweat sodium chloride testing to the parents
    D. Recommending sweat sodium chloride testing for the siblings
    E. None of the above

47. A molecular genetic laboratory receives about 60 samples per week for the cystic fibrosis (CF) carrier test. Which one of the following would be

the most common clinical indication for the CF carrier test in this laboratory?

A. Prenatal diagnosis
B. Postnatal diagnosis
C. Diagnostic confirmation after newborn screening
D. Family-based testing after proband identification
E. Reducing the risk of affected newborns in at-risk populations
F. None of the above

48. An Ashkenazi Jewish couple comes to a clinic for their first prenatal counseling when the wife is 6 weeks pregnant. One of the wife's brothers died of cystic fibrosis (CF) when he was 24 years old. The parents of the wife are healthy and live in Israel. The wife has two apparently healthy brothers in the United States. The wife and her siblings have not been tested for CF. The husband is a carrier of p.F508del in *CFTR* found by population-based screening. What is the risk that the couple's firstborn child will have CF?

A. 1/4
B. 1/6
C. 1/16
D. 1/964
E. 1/1928
F. Not clear
G. None of the above

49. An Ashkenazi Jewish couple comes to a clinic for their first prenatal counseling when the wife is 6 weeks pregnant. One of the wife's brothers died of cystic fibrosis (CF) when he was 24 years old. The parents of the wife are healthy and live in Israel. The wife has two apparently healthy brothers in the United States. The wife and her siblings have not been tested for CF. The husband is a carrier of p.F508del in *CFTR* found by population-based screening. Which test will be the most appropriate for this family as the next step in the workup?[9]

A. The ACMG 23-mutation panel with the peripheral-blood sample from the wife
B. The ACMG 23-mutation panel with the chorionic villus sampling (CVS)
C. The ACMG 23-mutation panel with the amniocentesis sample
D. Sanger sequencing analysis of the chorionic villus sampling (CVS)
E. Sanger sequencing analysis of the amniocentesis sample
F. None of the above

50. An Ashkenazi Jewish couple comes to a clinic in for preconception counseling. One of the wife's brothers died of cystic fibrosis (CF) at 24 years of age. The parents of the wife are healthy and live in Israel. The wife has two apparently healthy brothers in the United States. The wife and her siblings have not been tested for CF. The husband is a carrier of p.F508del in *CFTR* found by population-based screening. Which test should be done first for this family?

A. The ACMG 23-mutation panel with the peripheral-blood sample from the wife
B. The ACMG 23-mutation panel with the chorionic villus sampling (CVS)
C. The ACMG 23-mutation panel with the amniocentesis sample
D. Sanger sequencing analysis of the chorionic villus sampling (CVS)
E. Sanger sequencing analysis of the amniocentesis sample
F. None of the above

51. An Ashkenazi Jewish couple came to a clinic in for preconception counseling. One of the wife's brothers died of cystic fibrosis (CF) at 24 years of age. The parents of the wife were healthy and live in Israel. The wife had two apparently healthy brothers in the United States. The wife and her siblings had not been tested for CF. The husband was a carrier of p.F508del in *CFTR* found by population-based screening. The ACMG 23-mutation panel was offered to the wife, and the results was negative. What is the residual risk that the couple's firstborn child will have CF?[10]

A. 1/4
B. 1/6
C. 1/44
D. 1/385
E. 1/1540
F. Not clear
G. None of the above

52. An Italian couple came to a clinic for preconception counseling. The wife's brother died of cystic fibrosis (CF) when he was 19 years old. The wife carries the familial *CFTR* mutation, F508del. The family history on the husband's side was negative. The husband was tested using a mutation panel, and the results were negative. At 16 weeks' gestation, prenatal ultrasound identified an echogenic bowel abnormality. The follow-up sequencing of the amniotic fluid sample predicted that the fetus would have CF with a compound heterozygous mutations of F508del and c.91C > T (p.R31C). Which one of the following may explain the results?

A. It was a laboratory error. The tube was mislabeled.

B. The c.91C > T(p.R31C) mutation may be not included in the initial carrier screening mutation panel.

C. The c.91C > T(p.R31C) mutation may be a false negative results in the husband because of a genetic variant under the primer and/or probe.

D. Based on the mutations identified in the fetus, it was not possible to determine which parent carried the c.91C > T(p.R31C) mutation.

E. All of the above.

F. None of the above.

ANSWERS

1. **B**. Cystic fibrosis (CF) is a genetic disease that causes severe damage to the lungs and digestive system. An estimated 30,000 children and adults in the United States (70,000 worldwide) have CF (http://www.cff.org). Improvements in screening and treatment allows most patients with CF to live into their 20s and 30s, and some are living into their 40s and 50s.

   CFTR is the only gene associated with CF. The CFTR protein is a chloride channel that transports negatively charged chloride ions into and out of cells. Mutations in the *CFTR* gene disrupt the function of *the chloride channels,* preventing them from regulating the flow of chloride ions and water across cell membranes. As a result, mucus produced along the passageways of the lungs, pancreas, and other organs is unusually thick and sticky. This mucus clogs the airways and various ducts, causing the characteristic signs and symptoms of cystic fibrosis (http://ghr.nlm.nih.gov/).

   Therefore, transmembrane chloride channel defects cause multiorgan/multisystem symptoms in patients with CF.

2. **C**. Cystic fibrosis (CF) is an autosomal recessive (AR) genetic disease. *CFTR* is the only gene associated with CF. Mutations in the *CFTR* gene cause *loss of function* of the chloride channels, preventing them from regulating the flow of chloride ions and water across cell membranes.

   Dominant negative mutation is used to describe a mutation whose gene product adversely affects the normal, wild-type gene product within the same cell, usually by dimerizing/polymerizing with it. Dominant negative mutations are often more deleterious than mutations causing the production of no gene product (null alleles)—for example, osteogenesis imperfecta (OI) caused by mutations in *COL1A1* and *COL1A2* for collagen. Gain-of-function mutations, also called "activating mutations," change the gene product such that its effect gets stronger (enhanced activation) or even is superseded by a different and abnormal function. Most gain-of-function mutations are inherited in dominant mode. But autosomal dominant (AD) disorders may be caused by haploinsufficiency instead of gain-of-function mutations. *Loss-of-function mutations*, also called "inactivating mutations," result in the gene product having less or no function (being partially or wholly inactivated). Disorders associated with such mutations are most often recessive. The majority of metabolic disorders caused by enzyme inactivation are AR disorders with homozygous or compound heterozygous functional mutations. It is not unreasonable to assume that the majority of AR disorders has loss-of-function mutations. For example, lactose intolerance is usually the result of a loss/reduction of function in alleles for lactase (http://ghr.nlm.nih.gov).

   Therefore, CF patients have loss-of-function mutations in the *CFTR* gene.

3. **D**. Congenital bilateral absence of the vas deferens (CBAVD) is one of the causes of male infertility. Among these patients, *78% had at least one* CFTR *mutation.* So males with mutations in *CFTR* are at high risk for infertility.

   Therefore, about 75% of patients with congenital bilateral absence of the vas deferens (CBAVD) have at least one variant in the *CFTR* gene including the 5T variant.

4. **C**. Congenital bilateral absence of the vas deferens (CBAVD) is one of the causes of male infertility. Among congenital bilateral absence of the vas deferens (CBAVD) patients, *46% had two* CFTR *mutations.* So males with mutations in *CFTR* are at high risk for infertility.

   Therefore, abut 50% of patients with congenital bilateral absence of the vas deferens (CBAVD) have two variants in the *CFTR* gene including the 5T variant.

5. **B**. In April 2001, the American College of Medical Genetics (ACMG) Cystic Fibrosis (CF) Carrier Screening Working Group recommended a panel of 25 mutations and variants that should be tested to determine carrier status within the *CFTR* gene as a part of population screening programs. In 2004, the panel was reduced to *23 mutations* by the removal of 1078delT and I148T. The current panel of 23 mutations recommended by the ACMG, represents only 1.2% of all mutations (over 1800 in total) reported in the *CFTR* gene, but accounts for approximately 85% of mutations occurring in CF patients and covers both affected alleles in 72% of patients.

   Therefore, 23 mutations/variants are in the updated minimum mutation panel recommended by ACMG in 2004 for CF (not counting the reflex test).

6. B. The cystic fibrosis (CF) carrier frequency is variable in populations. The detection rate of carrier screening tests with the ACMG-recommended 23 mutations is variable based on the carrier frequencies in the populations. *In Ashkenazi Jewish population, the carrier frequency is 1/24 and the detection rate of the ACMG-recommended 23 mutations is 94% (see the table below).*

Therefore, the carrier frequency of Cystic Fibrosis (CF) is about 1/24 in Ashkenazi Jewish.

Cystic Fibrosis (CF) Deletion Rates, Carrier Frequencies, and Residual Risk After Negative Testing Result With the ACMG Recommended 23 Mutations in Populations.

Ethnicities in the United States	Detection rate	Carrier frequency	Residual risk after negative testing
Jewish	94%	*1/24*	1/380
Caucasian	88%	1/25	1/200
Hispanic	72%	1/58	1/200
African	64%	1/61	1/170
Asian	49%	1/94	1/180

Modified from the American College of Medical Genetics. Technical standards and genetics for CFTR mutation testing, 2006 edition. Genet Med 2002 Sep–Oct;4 (5):379–91. PMID: 12394352.

7. B. The cystic fibrosis (CF) carrier frequency is variable in populations. The detection rate of carrier screening tests with the ACMG-recommended 23 mutations is variable based on the carrier frequencies in the populations. *In the European Caucasian population, the carrier frequency is 1/25 and the detection rate of the ACMG 23 mutations is 88% (see the table below).*

Therefore, the carrier frequency of Cystic Fibrosis (CF) is about 1/25 in Caucasian.

Cystic Fibrosis (CF) Deletion Rates, Carrier Frequencies, and Residual Risk After Negative Testing Result With the ACMG Recommended 23 Mutations in Populations.

Ethnicities in the United States	Detection rate	Carrier frequency	Residual risk after negative testing
Jewish	94%	*1/24*	1/380
Caucasian	88%	1/25	1/200
Hispanic	72%	1/58	1/200
African	64%	1/61	1/170
Asian	49%	1/94	1/180

Modified from the American College of Medical Genetics. Technical standards and genetics for CFTR mutation testing, 2006 edition. Genet Med 2002 Sep–Oct;4 (5):379–91. PMID: 12394352.

8. E. The cystic fibrosis (CF) carrier frequency is variable in populations. The detection rate of carrier

screening test with the ACMG- recommended 23 mutations is variable based on the carrier frequencies in the populations. In Ashkenazi Jews the carrier frequency is 1/24, in European Caucasians 1/25, in Hispanic Americans 1/58, in African Americans 1/61, and in *Asian Americans 1/94* (see the table below).

Therefore, the carrier frequency of cystic fibrosis (CF) in Asian Americans is lower than that in the other populations listed.

Cystic Fibrosis (CF) Deletion Rates, Carrier Frequencies, and Residual Risk After Negative Testing Result With the ACMG Recommended 23 Mutations in Populations.

Ethnicities in the United States	Detection rate	Carrier frequency	Residual risk after negative testing
Jewish	94%	*1/24*	1/380
Caucasian	88%	1/25	1/200
Hispanic	72%	1/58	1/200
African	64%	1/61	1/170
Asian	49%	1/94	1/180

Modified from the American College of Medical Genetics. Technical standards and genetics for CFTR mutation testing, 2006 edition. Genet Med 2002 Sep–Oct;4 (5):379–91. PMID: 12394352.

9. D. The cystic fibrosis (CF) carrier frequency is variable in populations. The detection rate of carrier screening tests with the ACMG-recommended 23 mutations is variable based on the carrier frequencies in the populations. In Ashkenazi Jews the carrier frequency is 1/24, in European Caucasians 1/25, in Hispanic Americans 1/58, in African Americans 1/61, and in Asian American 1/94 (see the table below). Therefore, choice D is correct.

Cystic Fibrosis (CF) Deletion Rates, Carrier Frequencies, and Residual Risk After Negative Testing Result With the ACMG Recommended 23 Mutations in Populations.

Ethnicities in the United States	Detection rate	Carrier frequency	Residual risk after negative testing
Jewish	94%	*1/24*	1/380
Caucasian	88%	1/25	1/200
Hispanic	72%	1/58	1/200
African	64%	1/61	1/170
Asian	49%	1/94	1/180

Modified from the American College of Medical Genetics. Technical standards and genetics for CFTR mutation testing, 2006 edition. Genet Med 2002 Sep–Oct;4 (5):379–91. PMID: 12394352.

10. A. The cystic fibrosis (CF) carrier frequency is variable in populations. The detection rate of carrier screening tests with the ACMG-recommended 23 mutations is variable based on the carrier frequencies in the populations. In

Ashkenazi Jews the carrier frequency is 1/24, in European Caucasians 1/25, in Hispanic Americans 1/58, in African Americans 1/61, and in Asian Americans 1/94.

If a couple is of Ashkenazi Jewish/European Caucasian descent, their child(ren) will have $1/24 \times 1/25 \times 1/4 = 1/2400$ chance of being a CF patient.

If a couple is of European Caucasian/Hispanic American descent, their child(ren) will have $1/25 \times 1/58 \times 1/4 = 5800$ chance of being a CF patient.

If a couple is of African American/Hispanic American descent, their child(ren) will have $1/61 \times 1/58 \times 1/4 = 1/14,152$ chance of being a CF patient.

If a couple is of African American/Asian American descent, their child(ren) will have $1/61 \times 1/94 \times 1/4 = 1/22,936$ chance of being a CF patient.

If a couple is of Hispanic American/Asian American descent, their child(ren) will have $1/58 \times 1/94 \times 1/4 = 1/21,808$ chance of being a CF patient.

Therefore, the correct one for Cystic Fibrosis carrier frequency (from highest to the lowest) is Ashkenazi Jewish > European Caucasian > Hispanic American > African American > Asian American (see the table below).

Cystic Fibrosis (CF) Deletion Rates, Carrier Frequencies, and Residual Risk After Negative Testing Result With the ACMG Recommended 23 Mutations in Populations.

Ethnicities in the United States	Detection rate	Carrier frequency	Residual risk after negative testing
Jewish	94%	1/24	1/380
Caucasian	88%	1/25	1/200
Hispanic	72%	1/58	1/200
African	64%	1/61	1/170
Asian	49%	1/94	1/180

Modified from the American College of Medical Genetics. Technical standards and genetics for CFTR mutation testing, 2006 edition. Genet Med 2002 Sep–Oct;4 (5):379–91. PMID: 12394352.

11. A. The detection rate of carrier screening tests with the ACMG-recommended 23 mutations is variable based on the carrier frequencies in the populations. *In Ashkenazi Jews the detection rate is 94%*, in European Caucasians 88%, in Hispanic Americans 72%, in African Americans 64%, and in Asian Americans 49%. Therefore, the ACMG-recommended cystic fibrosis (CF) carrier test panel with 23 mutations has 95% analytical sensitivity to detect carriers in Ashkenazi Jews.

Therefore, the analytical sensitivity of the ACMG recommended cystic fibrosis (CF) carrier test panel with 23 mutations is approximate 95% in Ashkenazi Jewish (see the table below).

Cystic Fibrosis (CF) Deletion Rates, Carrier Frequencies, and Residual Risk After Negative Testing Result With the ACMG Recommended 23 Mutations in Populations.

Ethnicities in the United States	Detection rate	Carrier frequency	Residual risk after negative testing
Jewish	94%	1/24	1/380
Caucasian	88%	1/25	1/200
Hispanic	72%	1/58	1/200
African	64%	1/61	1/170
Asian	49%	1/94	1/180

Modified from the American College of Medical Genetics. Technical standards and genetics for CFTR mutation testing, 2006 edition. Genet Med 2002 Sep–Oct;4 (5):379–91. PMID: 12394352.

12. B. The detection rate of carrier screening tests with the ACMG-recommended 23 mutations is variable based on the carrier frequencies in the populations. In Ashkenazi Jews the detection rate is 94%, *in European Caucasians 88%*, in Hispanic Americans 72%, in African Americans 64%, and in Asian Americans 49%. Therefore, the ACMG-recommended cystic fibrosis (CF) carrier test panel with 23 mutations has 95% analytical sensitivity to detect carriers in non-Hispanic Caucasian.

Therefore, the analytical sensitivity of the ACMG recommended cystic fibrosis (CF) carrier test panel with 23 mutations is approximate 90% in non-Hispanic Caucasian (see the table below).

Cystic Fibrosis (CF) Deletion Rates, Carrier Frequencies, and Residual Risk After Negative Testing Result With the ACMG Recommended 23 Mutations in Populations.

Ethnicities in the United States	Detection rate	Carrier frequency	Residual risk after negative testing
Jewish	94%	1/24	1/380
Caucasian	88%	1/25	1/200
Hispanic	72%	1/58	1/200
African	64%	1/61	1/170
Asian	49%	1/94	1/180

Modified from the American College of Medical Genetics. Technical standards and genetics for CFTR mutation testing, 2006 edition. Genet Med 2002 Sep–Oct;4 (5):379–91. PMID: 12394352.

13. A. Allele-specific oligonucleotide (ASO) hybridization is one of the early methods used to discriminate between two alleles for single-nucleotide polymorphisms (SNPs). Two ASO probes are required, one specific for each allele.

Stringency conditions are employed such that a single-base mismatch is sufficient to prevent hybridization of the nonmatching probe.

Therefore, choice A is correct.

14. **C.** *The immunoreactive trypsinogen (IRT) screening test for cystic fibrosis (CF) has a high sensitivity but is not very specific, resulting in a large number of screened positive infants found to have a normal sweat test (low positive predictive value, high false positive rate).* So IRT is used as initial screening test for CF in newborn screening (NBS) programs, and tandem ITD–TD is used some states to increase the specificity of NBS.

The primary test to confirm the diagnosis of CF is the sweat chloride test. Sweat chloride testing is positive in more than 90% of individuals with CF.

Sequencing of all exons, intron–exon borders, promoter regions, and specific intronic regions detects more than 98% of *CFTR* mutations. However, since the cost for Sanger sequencing is higher than that for sweat chloride testing, most of the time Sanger sequencing is used only to confirm the diagnosis.

Over 1800 mutations have been described in *CFTR* for CF. The ACMG-recommended 23 mutations in the *CFTR* gene have been used as a screening test to identify asymptomatic carriers.

Therefore, *immunoreactive trypsinogen (IRT) is the most sensitive assay to detect patients with CF.*

15. **B.** Cystic fibrosis (CF) is an autosomal recessive disease. The carrier frequency is 1/25 in European Caucasians. Since the husband's brother died of CF, the parents of the husband are obligate carriers. The husband is not an obligate carrier, but he has a 2/3 chance to be a carrier and a 1/3 of chance of having two normal alleles.

Therefore, the risk of the couple having a CF child is $2/3 \times 1/25 \times 1/4 = 1/150$.

16. **B.** Cystic fibrosis (CF) is an autosomal recessive disease. The carrier frequency is 1/24 in Ashkenazi Jews. Since the wife's brother died of CF, the parents of the wife are obligate carriers. The wife is not an obligate carrier. But she has a 2/3 chance to be a carrier and a 1/3 chance to have two normal alleles.

Therefore, the risk of the couple's firstborn child having CF is $2/3 \times 1/25 \times 1/4 = 1/150$.

17. **C.** Cystic fibrosis (CF) is an autosomal recessive disease. The carrier frequency is 1/25 in European Caucasians. The wife is a carrier of a heterozygous mutation in the *CFTR* gene. Therefore, the risk of the couple's firstborn child having CF was $1/25 \times 1/4 = 1/100$.

18. **C.** Bayesian probability theory provides a mathematical framework for performing inference or reasoning using probability.

Probability	Husband is a carrier	Husband is not a carrier
Prior probability	1/24	$(1 - 1/24) = 23/24$
Conditional probability	$(1 - 94\%) = 6/100 = 3/50$	1
Joint probability	$1/24 \times 3/50 = 3/1200$	$23/24 \times 1 = 1150/1200$
Posterior probability	$\dfrac{3/1200}{3/1200 + 1150/1200}$	$= 3/1153 = 1/384$

Therefore, the residual risk of the wife of the being a CF carrier was 1/384.

19. **D.** Bayesian probability theory provides a mathematical framework for performing inference or reasoning using probability.

Probability	Husband is a carrier	Husband is not a carrier
Prior probability	$1 \times 1/25$	$(1 - 1/25) = 24/25$
Conditional probability	$(1/4)^2 = 1/16$	1
Joint probability	$1/25 \times 1/16 = 1/400$	$24/25 \times 1 = 384/400$
Posterior probability	$\dfrac{1/400}{1/400 + 384/400}$	$= 1/385$

Therefore, the risk of the couple's third born child would have CF was $1/385 \times 1 \times 1/4 = 1/1540$.

20. **C.** Newborn screening (NBS) for cystic fibrosis (CF) depends on the initial identification of *high values of immunoreactive trypsinogen (IRT)* in the blood of the newborn. After an abnormal IRT value is identified, most NBS programs perform a DNA test to identify known *CFTR* gene mutations (IRT/DNA strategy), while other programs repeat the IRT measurement in a second blood sample obtained from the infant at approximately 2 weeks of age (IRT/IRT strategy). Both strategies have been reported to provide approximately 90%–95% sensitivity, and both identify newborns at risk for a wide spectrum of disease severity. If the NBS is positive then a diagnostic test for CF should be done. It is either a sweat test or a molecular test for gene mutations. High-performance liquid chromatography (HPLC) and/or mass spectrometry (MS) have been used to test for fatty acid oxidation disorders, but not CF.

Therefore, IRT is usually used as the first-tier CF test in NBS programs in the United States.

21. **A.** Newborn screening (NBS) for cystic fibrosis (CF) depends on the initial identification of *high values of immunoreactive trypsinogen (IRT)* in the blood of the newborn. After an abnormal IRT value is identified, most NBS programs perform a DNA test to identify known *CFTR* gene mutations (IRT/DNA strategy), while other programs repeat the IRT measurement in a second blood sample obtained from the infant at approximately 2 weeks of age (IRT/IRT strategy). Both strategies have been reported to provide approximately 90%–95% sensitivity, and both identify newborns at risk for a wide spectrum of disease severity. A positive screening result must be followed by referral for direct diagnostic testing. It is either a sweat test or a molecular test for gene mutations.

Usually an elevated sweat chloride level is used to diagnose CF. Molecular tests are used to confirm the diagnosis and provide genetic information for the family-based test to others.

Therefore, elevated IRT may lead to the positive NBS CF report.

22. **E.** Newborn screening (NBS) for cystic fibrosis (CF) usually use immunoreactive trypsinogen (IRT) followed by DNA testing to identify known *CFTR* gene mutations (IRT/DNA strategy) or tandem IRT/IRT strategy in the blood of the newborn. Both strategies have been reported to provide approximately 90%–95% sensitivity, and both identify newborns at risk for a wide spectrum of disease severity.

If the NBS is positive then a diagnostic test for CF should be done. It is either a sweat test or a molecular test for gene mutations. *Usually sweat chloride testing is done for diagnosis.* Molecular testing is used to confirm the diagnosis and provide genetic information for the family-based test to others because of high cost.

Therefore, sweat chloride testing would be the most appropriate method to confirm the diagnosis in Johnny after the positive CF screening.

23. **A.** Based on the available data on sweat chloride test results in healthy and cystic fibrosis (CF)–affected infants, the consensus committee from the Cystic Fibrosis Foundation recommends the following sweat chloride reference ranges for infants up to age 6 months: ≤ 29 mmol/L, *CF unlikely;* 30–59 mmol/L, intermediate; ≥ 60 mmol/L, indicative of CF.

Therefore, it would be unlikely that Johnny had CF.

24. **B.** Based on the available data on sweat chloride test results in healthy and CF-affected infants, the consensus committee from the Cystic Fibrosis Foundation recommends the following sweat chloride reference ranges for infants up to age 6 months: ≤ 29 mmol/L, CF unlikely; *30–59 mmol/L, intermediate;* ≥ 60 mmol/L, indicative of CF.

Therefore, Johnny had intermediate sweat chloride test results.

25. **C.** Based on the available data on sweat chloride test results in healthy and CF-affected infants, the consensus committee from the Cystic Fibrosis Foundation recommends the following sweat chloride reference ranges for infants up to age 6 months: ≤ 29 mmol/L, CF unlikely; 30–59 mmol/L, intermediate; *≥ 60 mmol/L, indicative of CF.*

Therefore, the sweat chloride test results indicated that Johnny had CF.

26. **A.** Cystic fibrosis (CF) is characterized by the buildup of thick, sticky mucus that can progressively damage the respiratory system and cause chronic digestive system problems. The most common mutation is *p.F508del (ΔF508)* in the *CFTR* gene. It accounts for approximately 70% of all mutant *CFTR* alleles worldwide.

Therefore, p.F508del is the most common one in the *CFTR* gene for Cystic Fibrosis (CF) worldwide.

27. **E.** In April 2001, the American College of Medical Genetics (ACMG) Cystic Fibrosis (CF) Carrier Screening Working Group recommended a panel of 25 mutations and variants that should be tested to determine carrier status within the *CFTR* gene as a part of population screening programs. In 2004, the panel was reduced to 23 mutations by removing 1078delT and I148T. All the mutations in the question are in the revised panel except *5T/7T/9T.*

The poly-T tract in intron 8 of the *CFTR* gene has been demonstrated to impact CFTR function by aberrant splicing of exon 9. The Poly-T tract in the splice acceptor region occurs in three forms: 5T, 7T, and 9T. Both 7T and 9T alleles are considered polymorphic variants, but 5T alleles are considered variably penetrant mutations that are thought to decrease the efficiency of intron 8 splicing. Because the frequency of R117H/5T is appreciable, *the Working Group recommends retaining R117H, whereas emphasizing the need to perform a screening test for 5T only as a reflex when R117H is present.*

Therefore, 5T/7T/9T in intron 8 is not in the ACMG-recommended 23-mutation panel, but is in the reflex test.

28. **A.** *CFTR*-related disorders include cystic fibrosis (CF) and congenital bilateral absence of the vas deferens (CBAVD). *The phenotype associated with the R117H mutation in the* CFTR *gene is influenced by the 5T/7T/9T polymorphism in intron 8.* This polymorphism affects whether exon 9 is included in

the transcript. The 5T variant paired (in *trans*) with a CF mutation has been found in men with CBAVD. And R117H mutation is considered to be pathogenic for classic CF when in *cis* with 5T (http://www.ncbi.nlm.nih.gov/books/NBK1250/).

Therefore, the 5T/7T/9T polymorphism in intron 8 of the *CFTR* gene should also be tested for the wife to interpret this molecular result according to the ACMG recommendation.

29. **D.** *The phenotype associated with the R117H mutation in the* CFTR *gene is influenced by the 5T/7T/9T polymorphism in intron 8.* This polymorphism affects whether exon 9 is included in the transcript. Both 7T and 9T alleles are considered polymorphic variants, but 5T alleles are considered variably penetrant mutations thought to decrease the efficiency of intron 8 splicing. So compound heterozygous R117H mutation and T7 are considered benign. Bayesian probability theory provides a mathematical framework for performing inference or reasoning using probability. In this case we need calculate the residual risk for the wife first:

Probability	Wife is a carrier	Wife is not a carrier
Prior probability	$1 \times 1/25$	$(1-1/25)=24/25$
Conditional probability	$(1\%-88\%) \approx 1/10$	1
Joint probability	$1/25 \times 1/10 = 1/250$	$24/25 \times 1 = 240/250$
Posterior probability	$\dfrac{1/250}{1/250 + 240/250}$	$= 1/241$

Therefore, the risk of the couple's third born child would have CF was $1/241 \times 1 \times 1/4 = 1/964$.

30. **F.** The phenotype associated with the R117H mutation in the *CFTR* gene is influenced by the 5T/7T/9T polymorphism in intron 8. This polymorphism affects whether exon 9 is included in the transcript. Both 7T and 9T alleles are considered polymorphic variants, but 5T alleles are considered variably penetrant mutations that are thought to decrease the efficiency of intron 8 splicing. So compound heterozygous R117H mutation and T5 are considered pathogenic if they are in *cis*.

Therefore, the risk, that their firstborn child would have CF was unclear.

31. **A.** The phenotype associated with the R117H mutation in the *CFTR* gene is influenced by the 5T/ 7T/9T polymorphism in intron 8, which *affects whether exon 9 is included in the transcript (splicing change).* The Working Group recommends performing a screening test for 5T only as a reflex

when R117H is present. 7T in *cis* can modify the R117H phenotype or alone can contribute to CBAVD. The 5T variant paired (in *trans*) with a CF mutation has been found in men with CBAVD. And R117H mutation is considered to be pathogenic for classic CF when in *cis* with 5T (http://www.ncbi.nlm.nih.gov/books/NBK1250/).

Therefore, the phenotypic effect of R117H is modified by 5T/7T/9T, which affects splicing.

32. **B.** *CFTR* R117H mutation is present in 0.3% of the Caucasian population, leading to a range of cystic fibrosis (CF) clinical presentations from congenital bilateral absence of the vas deferens (CBAVD) to classic CF. The 5T/7T/9T polymorphism in intron 8 influences phenotypes associated with the R117H mutation in the *CFTR* gene. Both 7T and 9T alleles are considered polymorphic variants, but 5T alleles are considered variably penetrant mutations thought to decrease the efficiency of intron 8 splicing. Since about 5% of the US population has the 5T polymorphism, the 5T/7T/9T analysis is performed only as a reflex test for those with R117H positive results.

R117H/7T is associated with milder forms of CF such as CBAVD, while *R117H/5T alleles may be associated with classic CF or CBAVD. The 5T allele by itself has also been associated with male infertility due to CBAVD, with or without mild or atypical symptoms of CF.* There is no known clinical significance of 5T in females (http://www.ncbi.nlm.nih.gov/books/ NBK1250/). And among CBAVD patients, 78% had at least one *CFTR* mutation and 46% had two.

Therefore, in this case the husband is at risk for infertility owing to CBAVD.

33. **D.** The phenotype associated with the R117H mutation in the *CFTR* gene is influenced by the 5T/7T/9T polymorphism in intron 8, which affects whether exon 9 is included in the transcript. 5T/ 7T/9T analysis is performed only as a reflex test for R117H positive results, since about 5% of the US population has the 5T polymorphism. If positive for 5T, the laboratory will request peripheral-blood specimens from the parents to determine whether the 5T polymorphism is in *cis* or *trans* with the R117H allele in order to provide additional information for genetic counseling. If R117H and 5T are in *cis*, they may be considered as one pathogenic allele (http://www.ncbi.nlm. nih.gov/books/NBK1250/).

In this case, the phase of R117H and 5T in the wife was not clear. Therefore, *the wife might or might not be a CF carrier.* Testing the wife's parents would help to interpret this result in the wife.

34. **C.** *CFTR*-related disorders include cystic fibrosis (CF) and congenital bilateral absence of the vas

deferens (CBAVD). The phenotype associated with the R117H mutation in the *CFTR* gene is influenced by the 5T/7T/9T polymorphism in intron 8, which affects whether exon 9 is included in the transcript. 5T/7T/9T analysis is performed only as a reflex test for R117H positive results, since about 5% of the US population has the 5T polymorphism. If positive for 5T, the laboratory will request appropriate specimens from family members to determine whether the 5T polymorphism is in *cis* or *trans* with the R117H allele in order to provide additional information for genetic counseling (http://www.ncbi.nlm.nih.gov/books/NBK1250/). And among CBAVD patients, 78% had at least one *CFTR* mutation and 46% had two.

In this case, the wife was not considered a carrier of CF. The fetus would be at low risk for CF. Since the 23-mutation panel is a screening test, the residential risk exists. If the fetus were a male, he would be *at risk for CBAVD (male infertility)*.

Therefore, the unborn child is at risk for infertility if it is a male.

35. **D.** *The phenotype associated with the R117H mutation in the* CFTR *gene is influenced by the 5T/7T/9T polymorphism in intron 8*. This polymorphism affects whether exon 9 is included in the transcript. Both 7T and 9T alleles are considered polymorphic variants, but 5T alleles are considered variably penetrant mutations that are thought to decrease the efficiency of intron 8 splicing. So compound heterozygous R117H mutation and T7 are considered benign. Bayesian probability theory provides a mathematical framework for performing inference or reasoning using probability. In this case, we need to calculate the residual risk for the wife first:

Probability	Wife is a carrier	Wife is not a carrier
Prior probability	$1 \times 1/25$	$(1 - 1/25) = 24/25$
Conditional probability	$(1\% - 88\%) \approx 1/10$	1
Joint probability	$1/25 \times 1/10 = 1/250$	$24/25 \times 1 = 240/250$
Posterior probability	$\dfrac{1/250}{1/250 + 240/250}$	$= 1/241$

Therefore, the risk of the couple's third born child would have CF was $1/241 \times 1/241 \times 1/4 = 1/232,324$.

36. **A.** The phenotype associated with the R117H mutation in the *CFTR* gene is influenced by the 5T/7T/9T polymorphism in intron 8, which affects whether exon 9 is included in the transcript. The

5T variant paired (in *trans*) with a CF mutation has been found in men with CBAVD. And R117H mutation can also cause classic CF when in *cis* with 5T (http://www.ncbi.nlm.nih.gov/books/NBK1250/).

In this case, the wife may be a carrier. But a definitive conclusion cannot be made until the wife's parents are tested. Since the wife was pregnant, the first priority is to evaluate the risk of CF for the fetus. Therefore, *the next step in the workup should be testing the husband for the carrier status*. If the husband were a carrier, the fetus would have a significant risk for CF. Prenatal diagnostic testing should be offered at that point. The wife's parents may be tested later for the benefit of other family members.

37. **C.** The phenotype associated with the R117H mutation in the *CFTR* gene is influenced by the 5T/7T/9T polymorphism in intron 8, which affects whether exon 9 is included in the transcript. The 5T variant paired (in *trans*) with a CF mutation has been found in men with CBAVD. And R117H mutation can also cause classic CF when in *cis* with 5T (http://www.ncbi.nlm.nih.gov/books/NBK1250/).

In this case, the wife may be a carrier, but the definitive conclusion cannot be made until the wife's parents are tested. Since the wife was pregnant, the first priority is to evaluate the risk of CF for the fetus. Since the husband was a carrier, the fetus would have a significant risk for CF. Therefore, *the next step in the workup should be prenatal diagnostic testing*. The wife's parents may be tested later for the benefit of the family members.

38. **C.** Noncystic fibrosis (CF)−causing variants at codons 506, 507, and 508 can cause a false positive result when certain test methods are employed. If the individual is a carrier for I507del, or F508del, and also has the I506V, I507V, or F508C variant on the other chromosome, this situation may lead to a false positive test for homozygosity for the I507del or F508del mutation. The I506V and I507V mutations do not produce a phenotype, while F508C has been associated with congenital bilateral absence of the vas deferens (CBAVD). A male who carries F508del or I507del paired with F508C should be counseled regarding the association of this genotype with male infertility (http://www.ncbi.nlm.nih.gov/books/NBK1250/).

Sequencing the *CFTR* gene reflex to del/dup with the amniotic fluid sample might confirm the genotype in order to rule in/rule out the diagnosis.

It was plausible to test the parents for the F508del mutation. However, the wife was 6 weeks pregnant. Early diagnosis is critical for the family to make an informed decision. Therefore, *sequencing the CFTR gene reflex to del/dup with the amniotic fluid sample is the most appropriate choice in this case.*

39. **B.** F508del/5T and F508del/R117H are the two most common kinds of compound heterozygote in men with Congenital Bilateral Absence of vas deferens (CBAVD).

Therefore, Johnny is at risk for *male infertility* due to CBAVD.

40. **A.** Noncystic fibrosis (CF)—causing variants at codons 506, 507, and 508 can cause a false positive result when certain test methods are employed. If the individual is a carrier for I507del or F508del, and also has the I506V, I507V, or F508C variant on the other chromosome, this situation may lead to a false positive test for homozygosity for the I507del or F508del mutation. The I506V and I507V mutations do not produce a phenotype, while F508C has been associated with Congenital Bilateral Absence of vas deferens (CBAVD). A male who carries F508del or I507del paired with F508C should be counseled regarding the association of this genotype with male infertility. IVS8(T)n, also called 5T/7T/9T, modifies the phenotypic effect of R117H, but not F508del (http://www.ncbi.nlm.nih.gov/books/NBK1250/).

Therefore, *IVS8(T) should not be included as a reflex test when the homozygous mutation for F508del was found.*

41. **B.** Meconium ileus is obstruction of the terminal ileum by abnormally tenacious meconium. It is almost always an early manifestation of cystic fibrosis (CF), which causes GI secretions to be extremely viscid and adherent to the intestinal mucosa. Meconium ileus occurs at birth in 15%—20% of newborns with CF.

The first-line diagnosis assay for CF is the *sweat chloride test.* To deliver the medication through the skin, iontophoresis is used to, whereby one electrode is placed onto the applied medication and an electric current is passed to a separate electrode on the skin. The resultant sweat is then collected on filter paper or in a capillary tube and analyzed for abnormal amounts of sodium and chloride. People with CF have increased amounts of sodium and chloride in their sweat. In contrast, people with CF have less thiocyanate and hypothiocyanite in their saliva and mucus.

CF can also be diagnosed by identification of mutations in the *CFTR* gene. A targeted mutation test with 23 mutations in *CFTR* can detect only

64% of mutations in the African American population. Sequence the *CFTR* gene reflex to del/dup may detect more than 98% of CFTR mutations. However, it is more expensive than the sweat test.

Therefore, sweat chloride testing would be the most appropriate test for Johnny to rule out CF.

42. **C.** Cystic fibrosis (CF) is caused by defects in cystic fibrosis transmembrane conductance regulator (CFTR), which regulates fluid flow within cells and affects the components of sweat, digestive fluids, and mucus. *G551D* is by far the commonest gating mutation worldwide and to date. In the cases of G551D mutation, the protein is trafficked to the correct area, the epithelial cell surface. But the protein cannot transport chloride through the channel.

Ivacaftor, trade name Kalydeco from Vertex Pharmaceuticals, is a *CFTR* potentiator. It has been designed to target class 3, so-called gating mutations, as a result of which CFTR reaches the cell surface but fails to open. It binds to the channels directly to induce a nonconventional mode of gating, which in turn increases the probability that the channel is open. *Ivacaftor is Food and Drug Administration (FDA)—approved for patients with G551D mutation, which accounts for 4%—5% of cases of CF.* Later Ivacaftor was found to be effective for patients with G1244E, G1349D, G178R, G551S, S1251N, S1255P, S549N, or S549R also.

Therefore, Johnny would most likely have G551D in the *CFTR* gene.

43. **D.** p.F508del is the most common mutation in the *CFTR* gene for cystic fibrosis (CF) worldwide. 5T/7T/9T analysis is performed only as a reflex test for R117H positive results. The 5T variant paired (in *trans*) with a CF mutation has been found in men with CBAVD. And R117H mutation can also cause classical CF when in *cis* with 5T (http://www.ncbi.nlm.nih.gov/books/NBK1250/). Therefore, the ACMG charged the Accreditation of Genetic Services Committee recommended that the R117H mutation be included in the test panel for CF. Reflex testing for the 5T/7T/9T variant is recommended only when the R117H mutation is positive. If a patient is positive for R117H and 5T, the laboratory will request appropriate specimens from family members to determine whether the 5T polymorphism is in *cis* or *trans* with the R117H allele in order to provide additional information for genetic counseling (http://www.ncbi.nlm.nih.gov/books/NBK1250/).

Therefore, in this case *the parental test* is the most appropriate next step in the workup.

44. **A.** *Complete analysis of the CFTR gene by DNA sequencing is not appropriate for routine carrier screening.* Complete sequencing is reserved for: (1) patients with CF, (2) patients with a family history of CF, (3) males with congenital bilateral absence of the vas deferens and (4) newborns with a positive NBS when mutation testing with the standard 23-mutation panel has a negative result (http://www.ncbi.nlm.nih.gov/books/NBK1250/).

Therefore, Sanger sequencing is not an appropriate test to identify CF carriers.

45. **B.** Cystic fibrosis (CF) is an autosomal recessive disease. R117T in *CFTR* is not a pathogenic variant by itself. 5T/7T/9T variant in intron 8 may modify the phenotype if an individual has a heterozygous R117H variant. 7T in *cis* can modify the R117H phenotype or alone can contribute to Congenital Bilateral Absence of vas deferens (CBAVD). The 5T variant paired (in *trans*) with a CF mutation has been found in men with CBAVD. *And R117H mutation can also cause classic CF when in cis with 5T* (http://www.ncbi.nlm.nih.gov/books/NBK1250/).

Therefore, *Johnny has CF, and treatment should be started right away.*

46. **D.** The parents are the obligate carriers. Carriers usually don't have symptoms. If the siblings have CF, they need to be treated as soon as possible.

Therefore, the siblings should be tested for CF with *sweat sodium chloride test* to rule out CF before testing the parents to confirm carrier status.

47. **E.** To have cystic fibrosis (CF), a child must inherit one copy of a CF gene mutation from each parent. *Carrier testing* allows parents and families to find out what their chances of having a child with CF are in order to help make important family planning decisions.

Therefore, most likely in this laboratory, the majority of the CF carrier testing was to reduce the risk of affected newborns in at-risk populations.

48. **B.** Cystic fibrosis (CF) is an autosomal recessive disease. The carrier frequency is 1 of 24 in Ashkenazi Jews. Since the wife's brother died from CF, the parents of the wife are obligate carriers. The wife is not an obligate carrier, but she has a 2/3 of chance of being a carrier and a 1/3 of chance of having two normal alleles, since she is apparently healthy. The husband is a silent carrier of CF.

Therefore, the fetus has $2/3 \times 1 \times 1/4 = 1/6$ *chance* to have CF.

49. **D.** The fetus has $2/3 \times 1 \times 1/4 = 1/6$ chance of having CF, since the wife has a 2/3 of chance of being a carrier. *With such a high risk, it is it is better*

to test the fetus to establish a diagnosis. The residual risk of the fetus having CF is still about 1/100 if the result is negative with the 23-mutation panel recommended by the ACMG. So sequencing test will be considered to be diagnostic in this family.

Prenatal testing is possible by analysis of DNA extracted from fetal cells obtained by chorionic villus sampling (CVS) at approximately 10–12 weeks' gestation or by amniocentesis usually performed at approximately 15–18 weeks' gestation.

Therefore, *sequencing analysis of the CVS sample* will be appropriate, since the wife is 6 weeks pregnant.

50. **A.** Cystic fibrosis (CF) is an autosomal recessive disease. The carrier frequency is 1 of 24 in Ashkenazi Jews. Since the wife's brother died from CF, the parents of the wife are obligate carriers. The wife is not an obligate carrier, but she has a 2/3 chance of being a carrier and a 1/3 chance of having two normal alleles, since she is apparently healthy. Because this is preconception counseling, the 23-mutation panel may be offered first as the most cost-effective assay to decrease the carrier risk in the wife. If the result is negative, the risk for the couple to have a child with CF is significantly reduced.

Therefore, the wife should be tested first in the family for the ACMG 23 mutation panel with a peripheral blood sample.

51. **C.** Bayesian probability theory provides a mathematical framework for performing inference or reasoning using probability. In this case, we need to calculate the residual risk for the wife first:

Probability	Wife is a carrier	Wife is not a carrier
Prior probability	2/3	1/3
Conditional probability	$(1\%–94\%) \approx 1/20$	1
Joint probability	$2/3 \times 1/20 = 1/30$	$1/3 \times 1 = 10/30$
Posterior probability	$\dfrac{1/30}{1/30 + 10/30}$	$= 1/11$

Therefore, the risk of the couple's third born child would have CF was $1/11 \times 1 \times 1/4 = 1/44$.

52. **E.** Echogenic bowel can be seen in normal fetuses, in fetuses with CF, or in fetuses with other conditions, such as trisomy 21 and intrauterine growth retardation (IUGR) (http://www.ncbi.nlm.nih.gov/books/NBK1250/). It was most likely that the c.91C > T(p.R31C) mutation was not included in the initial carrier screening mutation panel. However, it was also possible that there was a

technical error in the initial carrier screening panel that led to a false negative result, such as a genetic variant under the primer/probe or a mislabeled tube. Based on the mutation identified in the fetus, it was not possible to determine which parent carried the c.91C > T mutation, although most likely the husband carried it. To definitively answer the question of the origin of the mutation and to interpret the fetal results, it was necessary to phase the mutations by testing the parents.

Therefore, all the choices in the question may explain the results.

References

1. Committee on Genetics. Committee Opinion No. 691: carrier screening for genetic conditions. *Obstet Gynecol* 2017;**129**(3):e41−55.
2. Committee on Genetics. Committee Opinion No. 691 summary: carrier screening for genetic conditions. *Obstet Gynecol* 2017;**129**(3):597−9.
3. Quon BS, Rowe SM. New and emerging targeted therapies for cystic fibrosis. *BMJ* 2016;**352**:i859.
4. Gilbert F. Cystic fibrosis carrier screening: steps in the development of a mutation panel. *Genet Test* 2001;**5**(3):223−7.
5. Watson MS, et al. Cystic fibrosis population carrier screening: 2004 revision of American College of Medical Genetics mutation panel. *Genet Med* 2004;**6**(5):387−91.
6. Yu J, et al. CFTR mutations in men with congenital bilateral absence of the vas deferens (CBAVD): a systemic review and meta-analysis. *Hum Reprod* 2012;**27**(1):25−35.
7. Pabary R, Thursfield R, Davies JC. Highlights of the North American Cystic Fibrosis Conference 2011. *J R Soc Med* 2012;**105**(Suppl. 2):S9−13.
8. American College of Obstetricians and Gynecologists Committee. ACOG Committee Opinion No. 486: update on carrier screening for cystic fibrosis. *Obstet Gynecol* 2011;**117**(4):1028−31.
9. Farrell PM, et al. Guidelines for diagnosis of cystic fibrosis in newborns through older adults: cystic fibrosis foundation consensus report. *J Pediatr* 2008;**153**(2):S4−14.
10. Ogino S, et al. Bayesian analysis for cystic fibrosis risks in prenatal and carrier screening. *Genet Med* 2004;**6**(5):439−49.

Additional Resources

- American Lung Association (http://www.lung.org/)
- CFTR.info (http://www.cftr.info/)
- CFTR Science (https://www.cftrscience.com/)
- Cystic Fibrosis (http://cysticfibrosis.com/)
- Cystic Fibrosis Foundation (https://www.cff.org/)
- Cystic Fibrosis Mutation Database (http://www.genet.sickkids.on.ca/app)
- Cystic Fibrosis Research Inc (http://cfri.org/)
- Cystic Fibrosis Source (https://www.cfsource.com/)
- Jewish Genetic Disease Consortium (https://www.jewishgeneticdiseases.org/)
- Kids Health (https://kidshealth.org/)
- National Heart, Lung, and Blood Institute (https://www.nhlbi.nih.gov/)
- Orphanet (https://www.orpha.net/)

Nonneoplastic Hematological Disorders

Human blood is made up of red blood cells (RBCs), white blood cells (WBCs), platelets, and plasma. Hematopoietic stem cells are stored in bone marrow. Some stem cells stay in the marrow to mature and others travel to the lymph nodes, spleen, and liver for differentiation, production, and destruction (extramedullary hematopoiesis).

The hematopoietic systems are affected by a wide spectrum of diseases. One way to organize these disorders is based on whether they are malignant. Neoplastic hematological disorders (see Chapter 8: Oncology—Acquired) accounted for 56% of the cases and nonneoplastic hematological disorders (this chapter) for 44%. Among the nonneoplastic hematological disorders (Fig. 6.1), 45.3% were iron deficiency anemia and 17.5% were immunogenic thrombocytopenic purpura.[1]

Another way to organize these disorders is based on whether they primarily affect RBCs, WBCs, or the hemostatic system, which includes platelets and clotting factors in plasma. The primary function of RBCs, or erythrocytes, is to carry oxygen from the lungs to other tissues and carbon dioxide, as a waste product,

away from the tissues and back to the lungs. Hemoglobins (Hbs) are important proteins in the RBCs that carry oxygen from the lungs to all parts of our body. Nonneoplastic genetic disorders related to RBCs include (but are not limited to) hemoglobinopathies, such as sickle cell disease, thalassemia, and other genetic defects affecting the hemoglobin chains within RBCs; hereditary spherocytosis, hereditary elliptocytosis; abetalipoproteinemia; 6-phosphate dehydrogenase deficiency, and glutathione synthetase deficiency (see Chapter 11: Prenatal Care, Newborn Screen, and Metabolic Disorders).

The primary function of WBCs, or leukocytes, is to fight infections. The most important types of WBCs for protecting the body from infections and foreign cells include the neutrophils, monocytes, lymphocytes, eosinophils, and basophils. Each type has its own role in fighting bacterial, viral, fungal, and parasitic infections. Nonneoplastic genetic disorders related to WBCs include (but are not limited to) primary immunodeficiencies such as immunodysregulation, polyendocrinopathy, enteropathy, X-linked (IPEX) syndrome;

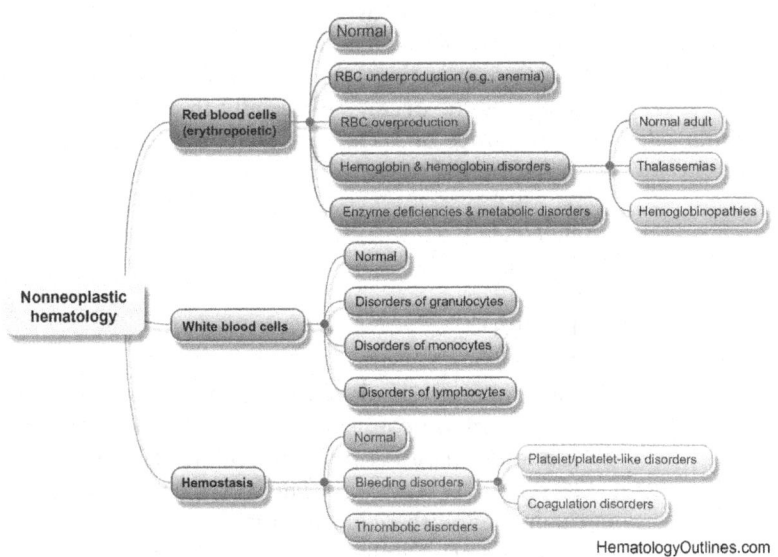

FIGURE 6.1 Classification of nonneoplastic hematological disorders. *Source: From Dr. Hooman H. Rashidi: HematologyOutlines.com*

Self-assessment Questions for Clinical Molecular Genetics.
DOI: https://doi.org/10.1016/B978-0-12-809967-4.00006-5

253

autoimmune lymphoproliferative syndrome (ALPS); X-linked lymphoproliferative disease (XLP); ataxia telangiectasia; Wiskott–Aldrich syndrome (WAS) (see Chapter 12: Other Common Genetic Syndromes); Chediak–Higashi syndrome; combined immunodeficiency; common variable immunodeficiency; DiGeorge syndrome; hypogammaglobulinemia; and hyper-IgA/IgE deficiencies.

The primary function of platelets, or thrombocytes, is blood clotting. Deriving from megakaryocytes in the bone marrow, platelets initiate the clotting sequence and protect the integrity of vasculatures. Nonneoplastic genetic disorders related to platelets include (but are not limited to) thrombocytopathies, such as adenosine 5'-diphosphate (ADP) receptor defects, Bernard–Soulier syndrome, Glanzmann thrombasthenia, and gray platelet syndrome; thrombocytopenias, such as congenital amegakaryocytic thrombocytopenia, thrombocytopenia-absent radius (TAR) syndrome, thrombocytopenic purpuras; and hemolytic uremic syndrome.

Plasma carries blood cells, nutrients, waste products, antibodies, clotting factors, chemical messengers such as hormones, and proteins that help maintain the body's fluid balance. Nonneoplastic genetic disorders related to plasma include (but are not limited to) bleeding disorders, such as von Willebrand disease and hemophilia A and B; thrombophilias, such as factor V Leiden and protein deficiencies; iron overload syndromes, such as hereditary hemochromatosis; and nonthrombocytopenic purpuras.

QUESTIONS

1. Which one of the following types of hemoglobins has $\alpha^2\beta^2$?
   A. Hemoglobin A (HbA)
   B. Hemoglobin F (HbF)
   C. Hemoglobin A2 (HbA2)
   D. Hemoglobin S (HbS)
   E. None of the above

2. Which one of the following types of hemoglobins has $\alpha^2\gamma^2$?
   A. Hemoglobin A (HbA)
   B. Hemoglobin F (HbF)
   C. Hemoglobin A2 (HbA2)
   D. Hemoglobin S (HbS)
   E. None of the above

3. Which one of the following types of hemoglobins has $\alpha^2\delta^2$?
   A. Hemoglobin A (HbA)
   B. Hemoglobin F (HbF)
   C. Hemoglobin A2 (HbA2)
   D. Hemoglobin S (HbS)
   E. None of the above

4. Sickle cell disease (SCD) is characterized by intermittent vaso-occlusive events and chronic hemolytic anemia. Vaso-occlusive events result in tissue ischemia, leading to acute and chronic pain as well as damage to any organ in the body, including the bones, lungs, liver, kidneys, brain, eyes, and joints. SCD is most common in:
   A. African Americans
   B. Asian Indians
   C. Hispanic Americans
   D. Middle Easterners
   E. Native Americans
   F. Northern Europeans

5. Newborn screening (NBS) for sickle cell disease (SCD) is now done in all states. A blood spot from a prick on a baby's heel is used to screen for a number of different genetic conditions. The initial NBS test determines the amount of normal hemoglobin in the blood spot. If too little normal hemoglobin is found on the initial NBS, another test is performed. If the second test is also abnormal, the parents are notified and the child is referred to a specialist for an evaluation. Which one of the following assays is NOT used as the test of choice for SCD in the NBS in the United States?
   A. Electrophoresis
   B. High-performance liquid chromatography (HPLC)
   C. Isoelectric focusing (IEF) electrophoresis
   D. Sanger sequencing of *HBB*
   E. None of the above

6. Sickle cell disease (SCD) is an inherited hematological disorder caused by abnormal hemoglobins. Abnormal sickle-shaped hemoglobins cannot deliver enough oxygen to the body. This causes individuals with SCD to experience episodes of pain and hemolytic anemia. Over time, the lack of oxygen damages the organs, especially the spleen, brain, lungs and kidneys. SCD is caused by a mutation in:
   A. *HBA1*
   B. *HBA2*
   C. *HBA*
   D. *HBB1*
   E. *HBB2*
   F. *HBB*

7. An apparently healthy couple came to a clinic for preconception counseling. The wife was a 23-year-old African American. The husband was a 26-year-old Caucasian. The wife's brother was diagnosed with sickle cell disease (SCD) at 5 years of age. The husband's family history was

negative. Neither spouse had been tested for SCD. What would be the risk of their firstborn child having SCD?

A. 100%

B. 50%

C. 25%

D. <1%

E. Can't predict

8. Which one of the following is the most common pattern of hemoglobins identified by high-performance liquid chromatography (HPLC) in patients with sickle cell disease (SCD) by age 6 weeks?

A. HbS, HbA2, HbF, and HbA

B. HbS, HbF, and HbA

C. HbS, HbA2, and HbF

D. HbS and HbF

E. HbS, HbF, and HbC

F. None of the above

9. A 5-year-old boy was brought to an emergency department by his parents for an episode of sickle crisis. The medical history showed that the patient had HbSβ°. Which one of the followings following would most likely be the pattern of hemoglobins identified by high-performance liquid chromatography (HPLC) in this patient's peripheral-blood sample?

A. HbS, HbA2, HbF, and HbA

B. HbS, HbF, and HbA

C. HbS, HbA2, and HbF

D. HbS and HbF

E. HbS, HbF, and HbC

F. None of the above

10. A 5-year-old boy was brought to an emergency department by his parents for an episode of sickle crisis. The medical history showed that the patient had HbSS. Which one of the following would most likely be the pattern of hemoglobins identified by high-performance liquid chromatography (HPLC) in this patient's peripheral-blood sample?

A. HbS, HbA2, HbF, and HbA

B. HbS, HbF, and HbA

C. HbS, HbA2, and HbF

D. HbS and HbF

E. HbS

F. None of the above

11. A 5-year-old boy was brought to a clinic by his parents for an annual physical exam. The medical history showed the patient had HbSβ$^+$. Which one of the following would most likely be the pattern of hemoglobins identified by high-performance liquid chromatography (HPLC) in this patient's peripheral-blood sample?

A. HbS, HbF, and HbA2

B. HbS, HbF, and HbC

C. HbS, HbF, and HbA

D. HbS and HbF

E. HbS

F. None of the above

12. A 5-year-old boy was brought to a clinic by his parents for an annual physical exam. Medical history showed the patient had HbSC. Which one of the following would most likely be the pattern of hemoglobins identified by high-performance liquid chromatography (HPLC) in this patient's peripheral-blood sample?

A. HbS, HbF, and HbA2

B. HbS, HbF, and HbC

C. HbS, HbF, and HbA

D. HbS and HbF

E. HbS

F. None of the above

13. A 17-year-old male from Algeria was brought to the emergency department in a local hospital for the acute onset (3 hours) of left hemiparesis. Noncontrast-enhanced computed tomography (CT) of the brain showed an acute right MCA infarct. The patient has a medical history of sickle cell disease (SCD), but no history of thromboembolic disease, no family history of venous or arterial thrombosis, and no atherosclerotic risk factors for stroke. His CBC at the time showed a hemoglobin of 87 g/dL, hematocrit 0.240, MCV 89.0 fL, platelet count 650,000/μL, white-blood-cell count 11,200 μL^{-1}, and ANC 9800/μL. If he was homozygous for HbS, which one of the hemoglobins would the patient most likely do NOT have by isoelectric focusing electrophoresis (IFE)?

A. HbA

B. HbA2

C. HbF

D. None of the above

14. A medical geneticist received an abnormal newborn screening (NBS) result from the state laboratory. The patient had FSA for hemoglobin by isoelectric focusing electrophoresis (IFE). Which one of the following would most likely be the clinical diagnosis?

A. Sickle cell anemia (HbSS)

B. Sickle hemoglobin C disease (HbSC)

C. HbSβ$^+$ thalassemia

D. HbSβ° thalassemia

E. None of the above

15. A medical geneticist received an abnormal newborn screening (NBS) result for hemoglobin from the state laboratory. The patient had FS by isoelectric focusing electrophoresis (IFE). Which

one of the following would most likely be the follow-up molecular genetic test results?

A. Homozygous p.Glu6Val mutation in *HBA*
B. Homozygous p.Glu6Lys mutation in *HBA*
C. Compound heterozygous p.Glu26Lys and p.Glu6Lys mutation in *HBA*
D. Homozygous p.Glu6Val mutation in *HBB*
E. Homozygous p.Glu6Lys mutation in *HBB*
F. Compound heterozygous p.Glu26Lys and p.Glu6Lys mutation in *HBB*

16. A medical geneticist received an abnormal newborn screening (NBS) result for hemoglobin from the state laboratory. The patient had FS by isoelectric focusing electrophoresis (IFE). Which one of the following would most likely be the follow-up molecular genetic test results?

A. Homozygous p.Glu6Lys mutation in *HBB*
B. Homozygous p.Glu6Val mutation in *HBB*
C. Homozygous p.Glu26Lys mutation in *HBB*
D. Homozygous p.Glu121Lys mutation in *HBB*
E. None of the above

17. A medical geneticist received an abnormal newborn screening (NBS) result for hemoglobin from the state laboratory. The patient had FSC by isoelectric focusing electrophoresis (IEF). Which one of the following would most likely be the follow-up molecular genetic test results?

A. Compound heterozygous p.Glu6Lys in *HBA* and p.Glu6Val in *HBB*
B. Compound heterozygous p.Glu6Val in *HBA* and p.Glu6Lys in *HBB*
C. Compound heterozygous p.Glu6Val and p.Glu6Lys in *HBA*
D. Compound heterozygous p.Glu6Val and p.Glu6Lys in *HBB*
E. None of the above

18. A medical geneticist received an abnormal newborn screening (NBS) result for hemoglobin from the state laboratory. The patient had FSC by isoelectric focusing electrophoresis (IEF). Which one of the following would most likely be the follow-up molecular genetic test results?

A. Compound heterozygous p.Glu6Val and p.Glu6Lys in *HBA*
B. Compound heterozygous p.Glu6Val and p.Glu6Lys in *HBB*
C. Compound heterozygous p.Glu6Lys and p.Glu26Lys in *HBA*
D. Compound heterozygous p.Glu6Lys and p.Glu26Lys in *HBB*
E. Compound heterozygous p.Glu6Val and p.Glu26Lys in *HBA*
F. Compound heterozygous p.Glu6Val and p.Glu26Lys in *HBB*
G. None of the above

19. A medical geneticist received an abnormal newborn screening (NBS) result for hemoglobin from the state laboratory. The patient had FSE by isoelectric focusing electrophoresis (IFE). Which one of the following would most likely be the follow-up molecular genetic test results?

A. Compound heterozygous p.Glu6Val and p.Glu6Lys in *HBA*
B. Compound heterozygous p.Glu6Val and p.Glu6Lys in *HBB*
C. Compound heterozygous p.Glu6Lys and p.Glu26Lys in *HBA*
D. Compound heterozygous p.Glu6Lys and p.Glu26Lys in *HBB*
E. Compound heterozygous p.Glu6Val and p.Glu26Lys in *HBA*
F. Compound heterozygous p.Glu6Val and p.Glu26Lys in *HBB*
G. None of the above

20. A medical geneticist received an abnormal newborn screening (NBS) result for hemoglobin from the state laboratory. The patient had FCE by isoelectric focusing electrophoresis (IFE). Which one of the following would most likely be the follow-up molecular genetic test results?

A. Compound heterozygous p.Glu6Val and p.Glu6Lys in *HBA*
B. Compound heterozygous p.Glu6Val and p.Glu6Lys in *HBB*
C. Compound heterozygous p.Glu6Lys and p.Glu26Lys in *HBA*
D. Compound heterozygous p.Glu6Lys and p.Glu26Lys in *HBB*
E. Compound heterozygous p.Glu6Val and p.Glu26Lys in *HBA*
F. Compound heterozygous p.Glu6Val and p.Glu26Lys in *HBB*
G. None of the above

21. A medical geneticist received an abnormal newborn screening (NBS) result for hemoglobin from the state laboratory. The patient had FSE by isoelectric focusing electrophoresis (IFE). When should the test be confirmed with a complementary method?

A. Within 2 weeks
B. Within 4 weeks
C. Within 6 weeks
D. Within 8 weeks
E. Within 2 months
F. Within 1 year

22. A medical geneticist received an abnormal newborn screening (NBS) result for hemoglobin from the state laboratory. The patient had FS by isoelectric focusing electrophoresis (IFE). At 6 weeks, an HPLC assay confirmed that the patient

had more HbF than HbS. Which one of the following would most likely be the next step in the workup for a diagnosis?

A. No more steps, diagnose the patient with sickle cell disease clinically.

B. Molecular genetic analysis of *HBB*.

C. Molecular genetic analysis of *HBA*.

D. No more steps, diagnose the patient with alpha thalassemia clinically.

E. None of the above.

23. A medical geneticist received an abnormal newborn screening (NBS) result for hemoglobin from the state laboratory. The patient had FS by isoelectric focusing electrophoresis (IFE). Molecular genetic studies further confirmed that the patient had sickle cell disease (SCD) with two copies of the p.Glu6Val variant in *HBB*. When should be the patient's next follow-up appointment if there were no acute symptoms?

A. 6 months

B. 1 year

C. 2 years

D. 6 years

E. None of the above

24. A 17-year-old male from Sudan came to a clinic for jaundice, normocytic anemia, and recurrent acute bone pains. A complete blood count (CBC) revealed that the hemoglobin was 6.6 g/dL, MCV 82.4 fL, platelet count 463,000/μL, white-blood-cell count 9900/μL, absolute neutrophil count 8400/μL, reticulocyte count 7.1%, and bilirubin 84 mg/dL. Blood film revealed numerous sickle cells. The sickle solubility test was positive. The physician prescribed a medicine for the patient that might increase the hemoglobin level. Which type of hemoglobins would most likely be induced pharmacologically to treat sickle cell disease in this adolescent?

A. HbA

B. HbA2

C. HbF

D. HbH

E. None of the above

25. A 17-year-old male from Libya came to a clinic for jaundice, normocytic anemia, and recurrent acute bone pains. A complete blood count (CBC) revealed that the hemoglobin was 6.4 g/dL, MCV 82.2 fL, platelet count 462,000/μL, white-blood-cell count 9800/μL, absolute neutrophil count 8400/μL, reticulocyte count 6.9%, and bilirubin 84 mg/dL. Blood film revealed numerous sickle cells. The sickle solubility test was positive. The physician prescribed a medicine for the patient that might increase the hemoglobin level. Which type of hemoglobins would most likely be

induced pharmacologically to treat sickle cell disease in this adolescent?

A. $\alpha^2\beta^2$

B. $\alpha^2\delta^2$

C. $\alpha^2\gamma^2$

D. $\varsigma^2\gamma^2$

E. None of the above

26. A 17-year-old male from Libya came to a clinic for jaundice, normocytic anemia, and recurrent acute bone pains. A complete blood count (CBC) revealed that the hemoglobin was 6.3 g/dL, MCV 82.1 fL, platelet count 460,000/μL, white-blood-cell count 9800/μL, absolute neutrophil count 8600 μL^{-1}, reticulocyte count 6.9%, and bilirubin 84 mg/dL. Blood film revealed numerous sickle cells. The sickle solubility test was positive. The physician prescribed a medicine for the patient that might increase the HbF level. Which one of the following medicines did the physician prescribe for this patient?

A. All-*trans* retinoic acid (ATRA)

B. Gleevec (imatinib)

C. Hydroxyurea

D. Zelboraf (vemurafenib)

E. None of the above

27. Sickle cell disease (SCD) is caused by a variant of the beta globin gene called sickle hemoglobin (HbS). Inherited autosomal recessively, either two copies of HbS or one copy of HbS plus another beta-globin variant (such as HbC) are required for disease expression. Which one of the following homozygous or compound heterozygous conditions causes the most severe type of SCD?

A. Hemoglobins S and S

B. Hemoglobins S and C

C. Hemoglobins S and E

D. Hemoglobin S and β^+ thalassemia

E. None of the above

28. Sickle cell disease (SCD) is caused by a variant of the beta-globin gene called sickle hemoglobin (HbS). Inherited autosomal recessively, either two copies of HbS or one copy of HbS plus another beta-globin variant (such as HbC) are required for disease expression. Which one of the following homozygous or compound heterozygous conditions causes the most severe type of SCD?

A. Hemoglobins S and C

B. Hemoglobins S and E

C. Hemoglobin S and β^+ thalassemia

D. HbS and $\beta°$ thalassemia

E. None of the above

29. Sickle cell disease (SCD) is caused by a variant of the beta-globin gene called sickle hemoglobin (HbS). Inherited autosomal recessively, either two copies of HbS or one copy of HbS plus another

beta-globin variant (such as HbC) are required for disease expression. Which one of the following homozygous or compound heterozygous conditions causes the most severe type of SCD comparing with others?

A. Hemoglobins S and S

B. Hemoglobins S and C with α-thalassemia trait

C. Hemoglobins S and E

D. Hemoglobin S and β^+ thalassemia with α-thalassemia trait

E. Hemoglobin S and $\beta°$ thalassemia with α-thalassemia trait

F. None of the above

30. A 6-day-old African American girl was brought to a genetics clinic by her parents for positive newborn screening (NBS) for sickle cell disease (SCD). Before preconception, the screening test revealed that the father was negative, and the mother was positive for the sickle cell trait. They were told that the chance for them to have a child with SCD was low. The parents were confused and angry. Which one of the following hematological abnormalities would most likely present in the father accounting for the child's SCD?

A. Glucose-6-phosphate dehydrogenase (G6PD) deficiency

B. Alpha-thalassemia trait

C. Beta-thalassemia trait

D. Hereditary elliptocytosis

E. Hemoglobin Constant Spring trait

F. None of the above

31. A 5-year-old Asian girl was brought to a clinic by her parents for an annual physical exam. Her medical history was significant for alpha thalassemia. Which one of the following hemoglobins would most likely increase significantly in this patient?

A. HbA

B. HbA2

C. HbF

D. HbH

E. Hb Barts

F. None of the above

32. A 5-year-old Asian girl was brought to a clinic by her parents for an annual physical exam. Her medical history was significant for beta thalassemia. Which one of the following hemoglobins would most likely increase significantly in this patient?

A. HbA

B. HbA2

C. HbF

D. HbH

E. Hb Bart

F. None of the above

33. An African American couple came to a genetics clinic for preconception counseling. Both the husband and wife had siblings who died from infection in childhood due to sickle cell disease (SCD). The couple had three healthy boys who were 8, 6, and 3 years old. In African Americans, the carrier frequency of SCD is 1/14. Which one of the following would be the risk that their next child had SCD?

A. 1/11

B. 1/81

C. 1/324

D. 1/4356

E. 1/16,900

34. A 4-year-old recent immigrant girl from South African was brought to a clinic for a physical examination. She was short for her age (−1.7 SD), sleepy, and pale and had a big belly. The physical examination showed that she was jaundiced and had hepatosplenomegaly. Her upper jaw and forehead were prominent. Her medical history was unclear, but the mother mentioned that the girl was like "a bacterial bag"—always catching cold—and that it usually took a longer time for her to recover than her friends. The physician ordered a blood test, which showed that the patient had mild microcytic hypochromic anemia. A targeted molecular assay for alpha thalassemia was ordered as a follow-up test. Which one of the following assays would most likely be used for this alpha thalassemia test in this patient?

A. Chromosomal microarray analysis (CMA)

B. Multiplex ligation-dependent probe amplification (MLPA)

C. Next-generation sequencing

D. Sanger sequencing

E. None of the above

35. An African American couple came to a genetics clinic for preconception counseling. Both the husband and wife had siblings who died in childhood of infection due to sickle cell disease (SCD). Which one of the following type of pathogenic variants would most likely cause SCD in both families?

A. Missense

B. Nonsense

C. Frameshift mutation

D. Splice-site mutation

E. Nonstop mutation

36. Sickle cell disease (SCD) is caused by a variant of the beta-globin gene called sickle hemoglobin (HbS). Inherited autosomal recessively, either two copies of HbS or one copy of HbS plus another beta-globin variant (such as HbC) are required for disease expression. HbS carriers are protected

from malaria infection, and this protection probably led to the high frequency of HbS in individuals of African and Mediterranean ancestry. Despite this advantage, individuals with SCD exhibit significant morbidity and mortality. Symptoms include chronic anemia, acute chest syndrome, stroke, splenic and renal dysfunction, pain crises, and susceptibility to bacterial infections. Which one of the following explains the structural abnormality of globin HbS?

A. A missense mutation leads to decreased elasticity of red blood cells.

B. A missense mutation leads to expression of an unstable globin in red blood cells.

C. A nonsense mutation leads to a premature truncation of the hemoglobin in red blood cells.

D. A splicing site mutation leads to expression of a longer than normal β^E globin.

E. None of the above.

37. How many copies of alpha-globin chains are NOT functional in patients with α^+ thalassemia?

A. 1 of alpha

B. 2 of alpha

C. 3 of alpha

D. 4 of alpha

E. None of the above

38. How many copies of alpha-globin chains are NOT functional in patients with α° thalassemia?

A. 1 of alpha

B. 2 of alpha

C. 3 of alpha

D. 4 of alpha

E. None of the above

39. How many copies of alpha-globin chains are NOT functional in patients with HbH disease?

A. 1 of alpha

B. 2 of alpha

C. 3 of alpha

D. 4 of alpha

E. 1 of beta

F. 2 of beta

G. 3 of beta

H. 4 of beta

40. How many copies of alpha globin chains are NOT functional in patients with Hb Barts disease?

A. 1 of alpha

B. 2 of alpha

C. 3 of alpha

D. 4 of alpha

E. 1 of beta

F. 2 of beta

G. 3 of beta

H. 4 of beta

41. Alpha thalassemia is a nonneoplastic hematological disorder involving *HBA1* and *HBA2* on 16p and is due to impaired production of alpha chains leading to a relative excess of beta-globin chains. Alpha thalassemia is common in sub-Saharan Africa, Mediterranean Basin, Middle East, South Asia, and Southeast Asia. Which one of following types of pathogenic variants is most common in patients with alpha thalassemia?

A. Deletion

B. Duplication

C. Inversion

D. Short tandem duplication

E. Single nucleotide mutation

42. An Asian American couple came to a genetics clinic for preconception counseling. The wife's brother had alpha thalassemia. The wife was an $-\alpha^{3.7}$ carrier. How many copies of alpha-globin chains were deleted in the wife?

A. 1

B. 2

C. 3

D. 4

E. Not sure

43. An Asian American couple came to a genetics clinic for preconception counseling. The wife's brother had alpha thalassemia. The wife was an $-\alpha^{4.2}$ carrier. How many copies of alpha-globin chains were deleted in the wife?

A. 1

B. 2

C. 3

D. 4

E. Not sure

44. An Asian American couple came to a genetics clinic for prenatal counseling. The wife's brother had alpha thalassemia. The wife was an $--\alpha^{THAI}$ carrier. The husband's family history was unremarkable. But a molecular genetic test found the husband had an $-\alpha^{4.2}$ allele. What would be the risk that their first child had Hb Bart?

A. > 99%

B. 50%

C. 25%

D. < 1%

E. Not sure

45. An Asian American couple came to a genetics clinic for prenatal counseling. The wife's brother had alpha thalassemia. The wife was an $--\alpha^{SEA}$ carrier. The husband's family history was unremarkable. But a molecular genetic test

found the husband had an $-\alpha^{4.2}$ allele. What would be the risk that their first child had HbH?

A. $>99\%$
B. 50%
C. 25%
D. $<1\%$
E. Not sure

46. Hemoglobin Constant Spring (HB$^{\text{Constant Spring}}$, Hb^{CS}), which causes thalassemia-like disease is common in Southeast Asia. Which one of following describes the pathogenic variant of Hb^{CS} most appropriately?

A. Missense
B. Nonsense
C. Frameshift mutation
D. Splice-site mutation
E. Nonstop mutation
F. Deletion

47. Hemoglobin Constant Spring (HB$^{\text{Constant Spring}}$, Hb^{CS}), (c.427T > C), which causes thalassemia-like disease, is common in Southeast Asia, which causes thalassemia like disease. It is a pathogenic variant in:

A. *HBA1*
B. *HBA2*
C. *HBZ*
D. *HBB*
E. None of the above

48. Beta thalassemia is a nonneoplastic hematological disorder involving *HBB* on 11p due to impaired production of beta chains leading to a relative excess of alpha-globin chains. Beta thalassemia is a fairly common blood disorder worldwide. It occurs most frequently in people from Mediterranean countries, North Africa, the Middle East, India, Central Asia, and Southeast Asia. Which one of following type of pathogenic variants is most common in patients with beta thalassemia?

A. Deletion
B. Duplication
C. Inversion
D. Short tandem duplication
E. Single nucleotide mutation

49. A 5-year-old girl was brought to a clinic by her legal guardians for her first physical examination after being adopted from Thailand. The girl was apparently healthy. The physical examination revealed that she had mild hepatosplenomegaly without jaundice. Regular blood testing showed microcytic hypochromic anemia. Her HbA and HbF were in the normal range. Which one of the following disorders would be in the differential list for the diagnosis in this patient?

A. Hb^{CS}/Hb^{CS}
B. HbS
C. β° thalassemia
D. β^{+} thalassemia
E. None of the above

50. A 5-year-old girl was brought to a clinic by her legal guardians for her first physical examination after being adopted from Thailand. The girl was apparently healthy. The physical examination revealed that she had mild hepatosplenomegaly without jaundice. Regular blood testing showed microcytic hypochromic anemia. Her HbF was elevated. In which one of the following disorders does HbF increase more than in the others?

A. HbH
B. HbSC
C. $\beta^{\circ}/\beta^{\circ}$
D. β^{+}/β^{+}
E. None of the above

51. Which one of the hemoglobinopathies has the earliest onset and the worst prognosis?

A. Hb Barts
B. HbH
C. HbSS
D. $\beta^{\circ}/\beta^{\circ}$ thalassemia
E. β^{+}/β^{+} thalassemia
F. None of the above

52. A 4-year-old black girl from Nigeria recently was adopted by a US couple. She was brought to a clinic for a physical examination. She was short for her age (-1.7 SD), sleepy, and pale and had a big belly. The physical examination revealed that she was jaundiced and had hepatosplenomegaly. Her upper jaw and forehead were prominent. Her medical history was not clear. But the mother mentioned that the girl seemed to catch cold easily. The physician ordered blood tests, which showed that the patient had mild microcytic hypochromic anemia. The doctor ordered a molecular test for thalassemias. The results showed that the patient was homozygous for one of the most common mutations in *HBA* genes in the African population. Which one of the following pathogenic variants would this girl most likely have?

A. $-\alpha^{3.7}$
B. $--\alpha^{\text{SEA}}$
C. c.427T > C in *HBA2*
D. 20-Mb terminal deletion of 16p
E. None of the above

53. A couple comes to a clinic for preconception consultation. The husband is from Nigeria, and the wife is from Thailand. The husband is a carrier of α^{+} thalassemia (α-thalassemia silent carrier). The wife is a carrier of α° thalassemia

(α-thalassemia trait). What is the risk that their firstborn child will have hemoglobin H (HbH) disease?

A. <1%
B. 25%
C. 50%
D. 99%
E. None of the above

54. A couple comes to a clinic for a preconception consultation. The husband is from Nigeria, and the wife is from Thailand. The husband is a carrier of α^+ thalassemia (α-thalassemia silent carrier). The wife is a carrier of α° thalassemia (α-thalassemia trait). What is the risk that their firstborn child will have Hb Barts syndrome?

A. <1%
B. 25%
C. 50%
D. 99%
E. None of the above

55. An Asian couple came to a clinic for their first prenatal care when the wife was 6 weeks pregnant. A carrier test confirmed that the husband was a carrier of α^+ thalassemia (α-thalassemia silent carrier). The wife was a carrier of α° thalassemia (α-thalassemia trait). Molecular diagnostic tests of a CVS sample was ordered, and results showed that the fetus carried both paternal and maternal mutant alleles. Which one of the following hemoglobins would most likely be increased in this child by 2 years of age?

A. HbA
B. HbA2
C. Hb Barts
D. HbF
E. None of the above

56. An Asian couple came to a clinic for their first prenatal care when the wife was 6 weeks pregnant. A carrier test confirmed that the husband was a carrier of α^+ thalassemia (α-thalassemia silent carrier). The wife was a carrier of α° thalassemia (α-thalassemia trait). Molecular diagnostic test of a CVS sample was ordered, and results showed that the fetus carried both paternal and maternal mutant alleles. Which one of the following hemoglobins would most likely be decreased in this child by 2 years of age?

A. HbA
B. HbA2
C. Hb Barts
D. HbF
E. None of the above

57. An Asian couple came to a clinic for their first prenatal care when the wife was 6 weeks pregnant. A carrier test confirmed that the husband was a carrier of α^+ thalassemia (α-thalassemia silent carrier). The wife was a carrier of α° thalassemia (α-thalassemia trait). Molecular diagnostic testing of a CVS sample was ordered; the results showed that the fetus carried both paternal and maternal mutant alleles. Which one of the following hemoglobins would most likely be stable in this child by 2 years of age?

A. HbA
B. HbA2
C. Hb Barts
D. HbH
E. None of the above

58. An Asian couple came to a clinic for their first prenatal care when the wife was 6 weeks pregnant. A carrier test confirmed that the husband was a carrier of α^+ thalassemia (α-thalassemia silent carrier). The wife was a carrier of α° thalassemia (α-thalassemia trait). Molecular diagnostic testing of a CVS sample was ordered; the results showed that the fetus carried both paternal and maternal mutant alleles. Which one of the following hemoglobins would most likely be stable in this child by 2 years of age?

A. HbA
B. Hb Barts
C. HbF
D. HbH
E. None of the above

59. An Asian couple came to a clinic for their first prenatal care when the wife was 6 weeks pregnant. A carrier test confirmed that both the husband and the wife were carriers of α° thalassemia (α-thalassemia trait). Molecular diagnostic testing of a CVS sample was ordered; the results showed that the fetus carried both paternal and maternal mutant alleles. Which one of the hemoglobins would this child have at birth?

A. HbA
B. Hb Barts
C. HbF
D. HbH
E. All of the above
F. None of the above

60. Which one of the following statements regarding thalassemia is correct?

A. α^+ thalassemia is symptomatic.
B. α° thalassemia is symptomatic.
C. HbH is symptomatic.
D. Hb Barts is a type of β thalassemia.
E. HbH is a type of β thalassemia.

61. Alpha thalassemia is often identifiable in utero. But beta thalassemia usually presents only after birth. Which one of the following may be the reason?
    A. Delta hemoglobin tetramers transport oxygen during fetal development.
    B. Fetal hemoglobin is sufficient to meet oxygen needs prenatally, but not after birth.
    C. In utero, all oxygen requirements are provided by maternal red blood cells.
    D. Prenatally, alpha-globin tetramers are capable of supplying oxygen to the fetus.
    E. None of the above.

62. An individual with beta thalassemia has an increased level of:
    A. HbA
    B. Hb Bart
    C. HbF
    D. HbH
    E. None of the above

63. An individual with beta thalassemia has a decreased level of:
    A. HbA
    B. HbA2
    C. Hb Barts
    D. HbH
    E. None of the above

64. Hemoglobin Constant Spring (Hb^{CS}) is the most common nondeletional alpha-thalassemia mutation and is an important cause of HbH-like disease in Southeast Asia. Patients with Hb^{CS} variants have almost normal mean cell volumes (MCVs), and the anemia is more severe than that in with other alpha-thalassemia variants. Which of the following explains the pathogenesis of Hb^{CS}?
    A. A missense mutation
    B. A nonsense mutation
    C. A stop codon mutation
    D. A splice-site mutation
    E. None of the above

65. Hemoglobin Constant Spring (Hb^{CS}) is the most common nondeletional alpha-thalassemia mutation and is an important cause of HbH-like disease in Southeast Asia. Patients with Hb^{CS} variants have almost normal mean cell volumes (MCVs), and the anemia is more severe than that in other alpha-thalassemia variants. Hb^{CS} is caused by a mutation in:
    A. *HBA1*
    B. *HBA2*
    C. *HBA3*
    D. *HBB1*
    E. *HBB2*
    F. None of the above

66. A couple comes to a clinic for their preconception counseling. They moved from Thailand to the United States 1 year ago. They both are carriers of α° thalassemia (α-thalassemia trait). Molecular genetic studies reveal that they both are heterozygous for a deletion involving *HBA1*, *HBA2*, and *HBZ*. For which of the following problems will the couple be at risk?
    A. Multiple miscarriages
    B. Offspring with Hb Barts disease
    C. Offspring with hemoglobin H (HbH) disease
    D. Offspring with β thalassemia
    E. All of the above
    F. None of the above

67. A couple comes to a clinic for preconception counseling. They moved from the Philippines to the United States 1 year ago. They both are carriers of α° thalassemia (α-thalassemia trait). Molecular genetic studies reveal that the husband is heterozygous for a deletion involving both *HBA1* and *HBA2*, while the wife is heterozygous for a deletion involving *HBA1*, *HBA2*, and *HBZ*. For which of the following will the couple be at risk?
    A. Infertility
    B. Conceiving a fetus with Hb Bart hydrops fetalis syndrome
    C. Conceiving a fetus with hemoglobin H (HbH) disease
    D. Conceiving a fetus with β thalassemia
    E. All of the above
    F. None of the above

68. A couple comes to a clinic for preconception counseling. They just moved from Saudi Arabia to the United States. The husband carries α° thalassemia (α-thalassemia trait), while the wife carries α$^+$ thalassemia (α-thalassemia silent carrier). For which one of the following will the couple be at risk?
    A. Infertility
    B. Offspring with Hb Barts hydrops fetalis syndrome
    C. Offspring with hemoglobin H (HbH) disease
    D. Offspring with β thalassemia
    E. All of the above
    F. None of the above

69. A couple comes to a clinic for preconception counseling. They moved from India to the United States 1 year ago. Both of them are carriers of α° thalassemia (α-thalassemia trait). Molecular genetic studies reveal that both of them are heterozygous for a deletion involving both *HBA1* and *HBA2*, leaving the *HBZ* gene intact. For which of the following will the couple be at risk?

A. Conceiving a fetus with Hb Barts hydrops fetalis syndrome

B. Conceiving a fetus with hemoglobin H (HbH) disease

C. Conceiving a fetus with β thalassemia

D. Infertility

E. All of the above

F. None of the above

70. A couple comes to a clinic for preconception counseling. They moved from Papua New Guinea to the United States 1 year ago. The wife has a positive family history of thalassemia. Molecular genetic studies reveal that she has a 3.7-kb deletion on 16p13.3. Which of the following genes is most likely deleted in the wife?

A. *HS40*

B. *HBA1*

C. *HBA2*

D. *HBZ*

E. *HBB*

F. *HBD*

G. *HBG*

71. A couple comes to a clinic for preconception counseling. They moved from Egypt to the United States 1 year ago. The wife has positive family history of thalassemia. Molecular genetic studies reveal that she has a 4.2-kb deletion on 16p13.3. Which of the following genes is most likely deleted in the wife?

A. *HS40*

B. *HBA1*

C. *HBA2*

D. *HBZ*

E. *HBB*

F. *HBD*

G. *HBG*

72. A couple from Philippine comes to a genetics clinic for preconception counseling. The family history is positive for alpha thalassemia on both sides. A targeted molecular assay is ordered to rule out alpha thalassemia. Both of them are negative for six common deletions. What is the detection rate of the targeted deletion analysis for alpha thalassemia?[16]

A. 90%

B. 50%

C. 30%

D. 10%

E. 1%

73. A Chinese couple comes to a genetics clinic for preconception counseling. The family history is positive for alpha thalassemia on both sides. A targeted molecular assay is ordered to rule out alpha thalassemia. Both of them are negative for six common deletions for alpha thalassemia. What is the residual risk that this couple's firstborn child will have alpha thalassemia?

A. 1/4

B. 1/40

C. 1/400

D. 1/4000

E. 1/40,000

74. Which one of the following variants in the *HBA1/HBA2* gene(s) may be predicted to be associated with relative milder symptoms in patients with alpha thalassemia than others if the effect from the expression of *HBB* and the extra copies of *HBA1/HBA2* are not considered?

A. $-\alpha^{3.7}$

B. p.Leu126Pro in *HBA2*

C. Hb$^{\text{Constant Spring}}$

D. $--^{\text{SEA}}$

E. p.Asp75Gly in *HBA1*

75. Which one of the following variants in the *HBA1/HBA2* gene(s) may be predicted to be associated with more severe symptoms in patients with alpha thalassemia than others if the effect from the expression of *HBB* and the extra copies of *HBA1/HBA2* are not considered?

A. $-\alpha^{3.7}$

B. $-\alpha^{4.2}$

C. Hb$^{\text{Constant Spring}}$

D. p.Asp75Gly in *HBA1*

E. Not clear

76. Which one of the following variants in the *HBA1/HBA2* gene(s) may be associated with more severe symptoms in patients with alpha thalassemia than in others if the effect from the expression of *HBB* and the extra copies of *HBA1/HBA2* are not considered?

A. $-\alpha^{3.7}$

B. $-\alpha^{4.2}$

C. Hb$^{\text{Constant Spring}}$

D. $--^{\text{SEA}}$

E. p.Asp75Gly in *HBA1*

77. A Turkish couple came to a genetics clinic for counseling. Their firstborn son died 2 days after delivery from generalized edema, ascites, and pleural and pericardial effusions. They had three miscarriages before this one. Otherwise, their medical history and physical examination were negative. The family history was unremarkable

on the husband's side. The wife's sister had a pregnancy complicated with fetal death due to hydrops fetalis. Molecular genetic tests of alpha thalassemia were ordered for the couple. Which of the following genotypes would the wife most likely have?

A. αα/αα
B. -α/αα
C. -α/-α
D. --/αα
E. --/-α

78. A Nepalese couple came to a genetics clinic for counseling. Their 6-year-old firstborn son was diagnosed with hemoglobin H (HbH) disease. They had two miscarriages before this child was born. Otherwise, their medical history and physical examination were negative. The family history was unremarkable on the husband's side. The wife's sister had a pregnancy complicated with fetal death due to hydrops fetalis. Molecular genetic tests of alpha thalassemia were ordered for the couple. Which of the following genotypes would the wife most likely have?

A. αα/αα
B. -α/αα
C. -α/-α
D. --/αα
E. --/-α

79. An Egyptian couple came to a genetics clinic for counseling. Their 6-year-old firstborn son was diagnosed with hemoglobin H (HbH) disease. They had two miscarriages before this child was born. Otherwise, their medical history and physical examination were negative. The family history was unremarkable on the husband's side. The wife's sister had a pregnancy complicated with fetal death due to hydrops fetalis. Molecular genetic tests of alpha thalassemia were ordered for the couple. Which of the following genotypes would the husband most likely have?

A. αα/αα
B. -α/αα
C. -α/-α
D. --/αα
E. --/-α

80. A couple comes to a clinic for preconception counseling. They moved from Malaysia to the United States 1 year ago. The wife has positive family history of thalassemia. Molecular genetic studies reveal that she has a nonsense mutation in one of the hemoglobin genes on 11p15.4. Which of the following genes is most likely mutated in the wife?

A. *HS40*
B. *HBA1*
C. *HBA2*
D. *HBB*
E. *HBD*
F. *HBG*
G. *HBZ*

81. BJ, a 1-year-old girl, was pale and in the 10th percentile for height and weight. Her parents brought BJ from their homeland in Greece to the United States when she was 3 months old. A blood smear revealed microcytic and hypochromic RBCs of distinctly variable size, shape, and density. Her hemoglobin was 5.6 g/dL, mean corpuscular volume (MCV) 56 fl, red-cell distribution width (RDW) 26%, and reticulocyte count slightly increased. Her hemoglobin isoelectric focusing (IEF) electrophoresis pattern showed predominantly hemoglobins E and F with no hemoglobin A. High-performance liquid chromatography (HPLC) found 55% hemoglobin E and 45% hemoglobin F. These findings, along with her clinical presentation, were determined to be consistent with a diagnosis of hemoglobin E/beta thalassemia. Which one of the following molecular findings would most likely be consistent with BJ's diagnosis?

A. Compound heterozygous p.Glu6Lys and p.Lys8ValfsTer13 in *HBB*
B. Compound heterozygous p.Glu6Lys and p.Ser9ValfsTer13 in *HBB*
C. Compound heterozygous p.Glu6Val and p.Lys8ValfsTer13 in *HBB*
D. Compound heterozygous p.Ser9ValfsTer13 and p.Glu26Lys in *HBB*
E. Compound heterozygous p.Lys8ValfsTer13 and p.Ser9ValfsTer13 in *HBB*
F. None of the above

82. Marina, a 7-year-old girl, was pale and in the 10th percentile for height and weight. Her parents brought Marina from their homeland in Greece to the United States when she was 1 year old. A blood smear revealed microcytic and hypochromic red cells of distinctly variable size, shape, and density. Her hemoglobin was 5.6 g/dL, MCV 56 fl, RDW 26%, and reticulocyte count slightly increased. Her hemoglobin isoelectric focusing (IEF) electrophoresis pattern showed predominantly hemoglobin F and no hemoglobin A. High-performance liquid chromatography (HPLC) found 98% hemoglobin F. These findings, along with her clinical presentation, were determined to be consistent with a diagnosis of beta thalassemia major.

Which one of the following molecular findings would most likely be consistent with Marina's diagnosis?

A. Compound heterozygous p.Glu6Lys and p.Lys8ValfsTer13 in *HBB*

B. Compound heterozygous p.Glu6Lys and p.Ser9ValfsTer13 in *HBB*

C. Compound heterozygous p.Glu6Val and p.Lys8ValfsTer13 in *HBB*

D. Compound heterozygous p.Ser9ValfsTer13 and p.Glu26Lys in *HBB*

E. Compound heterozygous p.Lys8ValfsTer13 and p.Ser9ValfsTer13 in *HBB*

F. None of the above

83. Marina, a 7-year-old girl, was pale and in the 10th percentile for height and weight. Her parents brought Marina from their homeland in Greece to the United States when she was 1 year old. A blood smear revealed microcytic and hypochromic red cells of distinctly variable size, shape, and density. Her hemoglobin was 5.6 g/dL, MCV 56 fl, RDW 26%, and reticulocyte count slightly increased. Her hemoglobin isoelectric focusing (IEF) electrophoresis pattern showed predominantly hemoglobin F and no hemoglobin A. High-performance liquid chromatography (HPLC) found 98% hemoglobin F, and 2% of others. These findings, along with his clinical presentation, were determined to be consistent with a diagnosis of beta thalassemia major. Which one of the following molecular findings would most likely be consistent with Marina's diagnosis?

A. Compound heterozygous c.-138C > A and p.Ala27Ser in *HBB*

B. Compound heterozygous c.91 + 6T > C and c.*6C > G in *HBB*

C. Compound heterozygous p.Glu26Lys and p.Ser9ValfsTer13 in *HBB*

D. Compound heterozygous p.Glu6Lys and p.Glu6Val in *HBB*

E. Compound heterozygous p.Lys8ValfsTer13 and p.Ser9ValfsTer13 in *HBB*

F. None of the above

84. Marina, a 7-year-old girl, was pale and in the 10th percentile for height and weight. Her parents brought Marina from their homeland in Greece to the United States when she was 1 year old. A blood smear revealed microcytic and hypochromic red cells of distinctly variable size, shape, and density. Her hemoglobin was 5.6 g/dL, MCV 56 fl, RDW 26%, and reticulocyte count

slightly increased. Her hemoglobin isoelectric focusing (IEF) electrophoresis pattern showed predominantly hemoglobin F and no hemoglobin A. High-performance liquid chromatography (HPLC) found 98% hemoglobin F, and 2% of others. Molecular tests identified compound heterozygous p.Lys8ValfsTer13 and p.Ser9ValfsTer13 in *HBB*. Which one of the following diagnoses would be most appropriate for Marina?

A. β thalassemia major

B. β thalassemia minor

C. HbH

D. Hb Barts

E. None of the above

85. A 12-month-old female with Hawaiian and Chinese ethnicities is noted to have Hb of 9.1 g/dL with an MCV of 58 on a routine CBC screen at her 1-year well-child checkup. She is apparently healthy. A physical exam reveals that she has pallor and is otherwise healthy. Her hemoglobin isoelectric focusing (IEF) electrophoresis pattern shows predominantly hemoglobins F and A. High-performance liquid chromatography (HPLC) finds 65% hemoglobin F and 35% A. Which one of the following molecular findings is most likely consistent with the diagnosis in this patient?

A. Compound heterozygous c.-138C > A and c.-81A > G in *HBB*

B. Compound heterozygous p.Glu6Val and p.Lys8ValfsTer13 in *HBB*

C. Compound heterozygous p.Glu26Lys and p.Ser9ValfsTer13 in *HBB*

D. Compound heterozygous p.Glu6Lys and p.Glu6Val in *HBB*

E. Compound heterozygous p.Lys8ValfsTer13 and p.Ser9ValfsTer13 in *HBB*

F. None of the above

86. A 12-month-old female of Hawaiian, Chinese, and Portuguese ethnicities is noted to have Hb of 9.1 g/dL with an MCV of 58 on a routine CBC screen at her 1-year well-child checkup. She is apparently healthy and has no symptoms. A physical examination reveals that she has pallor, and otherwise healthy. Her hemoglobin isoelectric focusing (IEF) electrophoresis pattern shows predominantly hemoglobins F and A. High-performance liquid chromatography (HPLC) finds 65% hemoglobin F and 35% hemoglobin A. These findings are determined to be consistent with a diagnosis of beta thalassemia minor.

Which one of the following molecular findings is most likely consistent with the diagnosis in this patient?

A. Compound heterozygous c.-138C > A and p.Ala27Ser in *HBB*

B. Compound heterozygous p.Glu6Val and p.Lys8ValfsTer13 in *HBB*

C. Compound heterozygous p.Glu26Lys and p.Ser9ValfsTer13 in *HBB*

D. Compound heterozygous p.Glu6Lys and p.Glu6Val in *HBB*

E. Compound heterozygous p.Lys8ValfsTer13 and p.Ser9ValfsTer13 in *HBB*

F. None of the above

87. A 12-month-old female of Hawaiian, Chinese, and Portuguese ethnicities is noted to have Hb of 9.1 g/dL with an MCV of 58 on a routine CBC screen at her 1-year regular checkup. She is apparently healthy and has no symptoms. A physical examination reveals that she has pallor and is otherwise. Her hemoglobin isoelectric focusing (IEF) electrophoresis pattern showed predominantly hemoglobins F and A. High-performance liquid chromatography (HPLC) found 65% hemoglobin F and 35% hemoglobin A. A molecular test identified compound heterozygous c.-138C > A and c.-81A > G in *HBB*. Which one of the following diagnoses is the most appropriate in this patient?

A. β thalassemia major

B. β thalassemia minor

C. HbH

D. Hb Barts

E. None of the above

88. A 1-month-old boy was brought to a local hospital to follow up on a positive newborn hemoglobinopathy screening. He had only hemoglobin (Hb) F at 24 hours and 1 week of age. The pregnancy and delivery were unremarkable. The boy was apparently healthy and thriving. The parents were second cousins from Pakistan. Which one of the following genetic abnormalities would the patient most likely have?

A. Heterozygous Hb^{CS}

B. Homozygous -α$^{20.5}$

C. Homozygous p.Glu6Val in *HBB*

D. Homozygous p.Gln39Ter in *HBB*

E. None of the above

89. Hemoglobin E (HbE) is an abnormal hemoglobin with a single point mutation at the amino acid position 26 in the *HBB* gene for the β chain (p. Glu26Lys); it is very common in Southeast Asians but has a low frequency among other ethnicities. *HBB* with the HbE mutation produces only small amounts of anomalous β-globin mRNA with the mutation. Which one of the following explains the quantitative reduction in the synthesis of the structurally abnormal HbE?[2]

A. The β^E globin is not stable.

B. The β^E mutation disrupts a promoter sequence.

C. The β^E globin only forms homotetramers.

D. The β^E mutation creates an abnormal cryptic splice site.

E. The β^E globin competes the binding sites on α globin with normal β globin.

90. A 23-year-old male came to a clinic for vomiting blood. A physical examination and laboratory test confirmed that the patient had jaundice, tremor, esophageal varices, hepatosplenomegaly, and Kayser—Fleischer rings in both eyes. Which one of the following genes would most likely be sequenced in order to confirm the diagnosis in this patient?

A. *ATP7A*

B. *ATP7B*

C. *ATP8A*

D. *ATP8B*

E. *HFE*

91. A research project was given a grant to study the potential utility of exome sequencing for newborn screening (NBS). Compound heterozygous c.2333G > T(p.Arg778Leu) and c.3207C > A(p. His1069Gln) mutations in *ATP7B* were found in a newborn. Which one of the following disorders would this newborn most likely develop in his/her lifetime?

A. Hereditary hemochromatosis

B. Menkes disease

C. Wilson disease

D. Not sure

E. None of the above

92. A 23-year-old female came to the emergency department of a hospital for vomiting blood. A physical examination and laboratory test revealed the patient had jaundice, tremor, esophageal varices, hepatosplenomegaly, and Kayser—Fleischer rings in both eyes. The patient had a 12-year-old full sister who was apparently healthy. What would be the risk that this female patient's sister had the same disease?

A. <1%

B. 1/4

C. 1/2

D. 2/3

E. 99%

F. None of the above

93. A 23-year-old female came to the emergency department of a hospital for vomiting blood. A physical examination and laboratory test revealed

that the patient had jaundice, tremor, esophageal varices, hepatosplenomegaly, and Kayser–Fleischer rings in both eyes. The patient had a 12-year-old full sister who was apparently healthy. What would be the risk that this female patient's sister was a silent carrier of the disease?

A. <1%
B. 1/4
C. 1/2
D. 2/3
E. 99%
F. None of the above

94. A 23-year-old female came to the emergency department of a hospital for vomiting blood. A physical examination and laboratory test revealed that the patient had jaundice, tremor, esophageal varices, hepatosplenomegaly, and Kayser–Fleischer rings in both eyes. The patient had a 12-year-old full sister who did not have an elevated copper level. What would be the risk that this female patient's sister was a silent carrier of the disease?

A. <1%
B. 1/4
C. 1/2
D. 2/3
E. 99%
F. None of the above

95. A research project was given a grant to study the potential utility of exome sequencing for newborn screening (NBS). A p.Ser637Leu mutation was identified in *ATP7A* in a newborn boy. Which one of the following disorders does this newborn most likely have?

A. Hereditary hemochromatosis
B. Menkes disease
C. Wilson disease
D. Not sure
E. None of the above

96. A 7-month-old male infant was brought to a genetics clinic by his parents for gradual onset of hypotonia and seizures. He was born at term to healthy and nonconsanguineous parents. He was the first child in the family. His early development was age-appropriate for 3 months, and then regressed. At 5 months of age, myoclonic jerks were noted. His physical examination at 7 months revealed a cherubic appearance, with a depressed nasal bridge, and brittle, scattered, and hypopigmented scalp hairs. He had no eye contact and no head control. Laboratory tests revealed low serum copper (16 μg/dL; reference range, 70–154 μg/dL) and low serum ceruloplasmin (57 mg/L; reference range, 187–321 mg/L). A CT scan of the head demonstrated cerebral atrophy and subdural

effusion. Which one of the following genes would most likely be sequenced in order to confirm the diagnosis in this patient?

A. *ATP7A*
B. *ATP7B*
C. *ATP8A*
D. *ATP8B*
E. *HFE*

97. A 55-year-old male presents to a clinic for hypogonadism and glucose intolerance. He has iron overload with a transferrin saturation of 99% and a ferritin level of 4000 ng/mL. His parents are first cousins once removed and apparently healthy. His older brother was diagnosed with hemochromatosis 5 years ago. Which one of the following genes most likely harbors germline pathogenic variant(s) in this patient?

A. *HAMP*
B. *HFE*
C. *HJV*
D. *SLC40A1*
E. *TFR2*

98. A 55-year-old male presents to a clinic for hypogonadism and glucose intolerance. He has iron overload with a percent transferrin saturation of 99% and a ferritin of 4000 ng/mL. His parents are first cousins once removed and apparently healthy. His older brother was diagnosed with hemochromatosis 5 years ago. Which one of the following genes LEAST likely harbors germline pathogenic variant(s) in this patient?

A. *HJV*
B. *HAMP*
C. *HFE*
D. *TFR2*
E. *SLC40A1*

99. A 21-year-old man presents with new-onset dyspnea. He had been well until 3 weeks ago. He has no known medical conditions and no family history of premature heart disease. He does not smoke, drink alcohol, or use illicit drugs. He has not had any recent viral illness. An ECG identifies a globally dilated heart with a left ventricular ejection fraction of 25%. In the evaluation of his heart failure, he is found to have a serum iron of 297, total iron capacity of 342, and ferritin of 2172 ng/mL. Which one of the following genes most likely harbors germline pathogenic variant(s) in this patient?

A. *HFE*
B. *TFR2*
C. *HJV*
D. *HAMP*
E. *SLC40A1*
F. None of the above

100. A 35-year-old Irish American male, Jon, presented to a genetics clinic because his brother was recently diagnosed with hemochromatosis. Jon's medical history and physical history were unremarkable. His lab test revealed serum ferritin was 600 ng/mL, transferrin saturation (fasting) 80%, hemoglobin 14.5, and hematocrit 44%. He was diagnosed with hereditary hemochromatosis biochemically even though his physical examination was unremarkable. He was married and had four beers every day. A molecular test was ordered to confirm the diagnosis. Which one of the following would most likely be Jon's molecular test result?
   A. Homozygous p.Cys282Tyr in *HFE*
   B. Homozygous p.His63Asp in *HFE*
   C. Homozygous p.Ser65Cys in *HFE*
   D. Compound heterozygous p.Cys282Tyr and p.His63Asp in *HFE*
   E. Compound heterozygous p.His63Asp and p.Ser65Cys in *HFE*
   F. None of the above

101. A 35-year-old Caucasian male presented to a genetics clinic because his father was diagnosed with cirrhosis 1 month ago. His medical history and physical examination were unremarkable. A molecular test confirmed that the patient was homozygous for the *HFE* C282Y mutation, as was his father. He was married and drank 4 beers every day. What would be his risk of having clinical symptoms of hemochromatosis in his lifetime?[3]
   A. About 0.5%
   B. Up to 6%
   C. 1/4
   D. 1/2
   E. 100%
   F. None of the above

102. Jon was a 36-year-old British descent with no symptoms. He recently completed an annual physical examination as required by his employer. Blood collected for screening purposes revealed elevated transferrin saturation (83%). Jon's medical history and family history were unremarkable. The physical examination did not yield positive findings. Further blood work revealed a serum ferritin level of 600 ng/mL, transferrin saturation (fasting) of 80%, hemoglobin 14.5, and hematocrit of 44%. AST and ALT were normal. A molecular test identified compound heterozygous p.Cys282Tyr and p.His63Asp variants in *HFE*. What would be

his risk of having clinical symptoms of hemochromatosis in his lifetime?[3]
   A. About 0.5%
   B. Up to 6%
   C. 1/4
   D. 1/2
   E. 100%
   F. None of the above

103. A 47-year-old German male with a history of hereditary hemochromatosis presents with fatigue, weakness, erectile dysfunction, and bilateral knee arthralgias. He also has noted darkening of his skin. There is no history of diabetes, heart failure, or arrhythmias. His physical examination is significant for increased skin pigmentation, mild hepatomegaly, and small effusions in both knees. Pertinent laboratory data reveals a serum ferritin of 750 ng/mL, transferrin saturation of 80%, and normal liver function. The fasting blood sugar is 100 mg/dL. What most likely is the *HFE* genotype in this patient?
   A. C282Y/C282Y
   B. C282Y/WT (wild type)
   C. H63D/C282Y
   D. H63D/H63D
   E. H63D/WT
   F. None of the above

104. An otherwise healthy newborn boy was brought to a clinic for prolonged bleeding after circumcision. Coagulation testing revealed an increased PTT in the context of normal PT and bleeding time. Coagulation factor assays revealed that the factor VIII clotting activity was lower than 1% with a normal and functional von Willebrand factor level. Molecular genetic tests confirmed the diagnosis and found that the mother carried the same variant. What would be the risk that the couple's next child would have the same disease?
   A. <1%
   B. 1/4
   C. 1/2
   D. 2/3
   E. 99%
   F. None of the above

105. An otherwise healthy newborn boy was brought to a clinic for prolonged bleeding after circumcision. Coagulation testing revealed an increased PTT in the context of a normal PT and bleeding time. Coagulation factor assays revealed that the factor VIII clotting activity was lower than 1% with a normal and functional von Willebrand factor level. Molecular genetic tests confirmed the diagnosis and found that the mother carried the same variant. What would be the risk of the couple's next son having the same disease?

A. <1%
B. 1/4
C. 1/2
D. 2/3
E. 99%
F. None of the above

106. An otherwise healthy newborn boy was brought to a clinic for prolonged bleeding after circumcision. Coagulation testing revealed an increased PTT in the context of a normal PT and bleeding time. Coagulation factor assays revealed that the factor VIII clotting activity was lower than 1% with a normal and functional von Willebrand factor level. Molecular genetic tests of *F8* confirmed the diagnosis. Which one of the following statements would be most appropriate?

A. The patient has hemophilia B.
B. The symptoms would be mild in this patient.
C. The patient did not need therapy.
D. It is an X-linked recessive disease.
E. In most patients the mutation is de novo.

107. An otherwise healthy newborn boy was brought to a clinic for prolonged bleeding after circumcision. Coagulation testing revealed an increased PTT in the context of a normal PT and bleeding time. Coagulation factor assays revealed that the factor IX clotting activity was lower than 1% with a normal and functional von Willebrand factor level. Molecular genetic tests of *F9* confirmed the diagnosis. The mother carried the same variant. Which one of the following statements would be the most appropriate?

A. The patient had hemophilia A.
B. The future siblings would have a 25% of being affected, too.
C. The disease is self-limited; there is no need for therapy.
D. This is the most common form of hemophilia.
E. In most patients the mutation is de novo.

108. An otherwise healthy newborn boy was brought to a clinic for prolonged bleeding after circumcision. Coagulation testing revealed an increased PTT in the context of a normal PT and bleeding time. Coagulation factor assays revealed the factor VIII clotting activity was lower than 1% with a normal and functional von Willebrand factor level. The family history was positive for hemophilia A in multiple members. Which one of the following types of variants would most likely be detected in this patient?

A. Deletion
B. Insertion
C. Inversion
D. Short tandem repeats (STRs)
E. Single-nucleotide polymorphisms (SNPs)
F. Translocation

109. An otherwise healthy newborn boy was brought to a clinic for prolonged bleeding after circumcision. Coagulation testing revealed an increased PTT in the context of a normal PT and bleeding time. Coagulation factor assays revealed the factor VIII clotting activity was lower than 1% with a normal and functional von Willebrand factor level. The family history was positive for hemophilia A in multiple members. And a nonsense mutation in the *F8* was identified in a maternal uncle. A molecular genetic test was ordered for the targeted mutation analysis on this patient. Which one of the molecular techniques would be most appropriate for the targeted mutation analysis?

A. Multiplex ligation-dependent probe amplification (MLPA)
B. Next-generation targeted mutation panel in *F8*
C. Quantitative PCR
D. Sanger sequencing
E. None of the above

110. An otherwise healthy newborn boy was brought to a clinic for prolonged bleeding after circumcision. Coagulation testing revealed an increased PTT in the context of a normal PT and bleeding time. Coagulation factor assays revealed that the factor VIII clotting activity was lower than 1% with a normal and functional von Willebrand factor level. A molecular genetic test was ordered to confirm the diagnosis. Which one of the following molecular techniques would most likely be used as the first-line test in order to confirm the diagnosis in this patient?[14]

A. Denaturing high-performance liquid chromatography (dHPLC)
B. PCR
C. Sequence analysis of the exons of *F8*
D. TaqMan genotype assays
E. None of the above

111. A couple came to a clinic for their first prenatal care. The wife stated that her biological brother had a bleeding problem. Diagnostic tests were done. The physician found that the wife was a carrier of a mutation in *F8*, which leads to a new stop codon at exon 10. The fetus had the same mutation in *F8* according to amniocentesis, and was a normal male according to chromosome karyotype. How

severe would the symptoms be if the fetus had hemophilia A?

- A. Severe
- B. Moderate
- C. Mild
- D. None of the above

112. A couple came to a clinic for their first prenatal care. The wife's maternal uncle had died in childhood from bleeding problems (see the pedigree below). Her brother had

bleeding problems when he was a child, but they resolved during adolescence. Which gene was most likely mutated in this family?[4]

- A. *F8*
- B. *F9*
- C. *F11*
- D. *F13A*
- E. *F13B*
- F. *vWF*

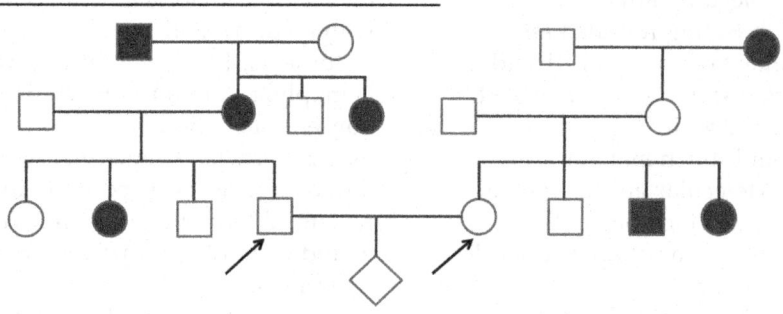

113. A couple came to a clinic for their first prenatal care. The wife had been adopted at 8 years of age. She stated that her biological brother had bleeding problems. Tests were done. The physician found that the wife was a carrier of a mutation in *F9*. The fetus had the same mutation according to amniocentesis and was a normal male according to chromosome karyotyping. The genetic counselor described the potential symptoms after birth, potential management plan, local support groups, and recurrent risk. She also mentioned that the unborn child's symptoms might become milder after puberty. Which one of the following mutations would the mother/fetus most likely have?[4]

- A. c.-6G > A
- B. Intron 22-A inversion
- C. Intron 1 inversion
- D. p.Glu117*
- E. None of the above

114. A couple came to a clinic for their first prenatal care. The wife's maternal uncle had died in childhood from bleeding problems (see the pedigree below). The wife's brother had also had bleeding problems when he was a child, but they resolved during adolescence. Which one of the following tests would be the most appropriate first step for the prenatal diagnosis?

- A. Amniocentesis to test the fetus
- B. CVS to test the fetus
- C. NIPT
- D. Test the mother for carrier status
- E. Test the mother's affected brother for molecular diagnosis
- F. Test the husband and wife for carrier status

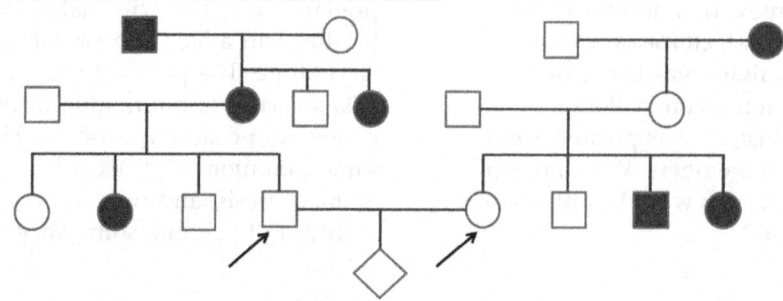

115. A couple brought their 8-year-old boy to a genetics clinic for bleeding problems (see the pedigree below). Molecular results from the boy revealed a point mutation in the promoter region of *F8*. Which one of following statements would be correct if the mutation was from the maternal side?[5]

   A. Most likely the grandfather passed on the mutation to the mother owing to a new mutation.

   B. Most likely the grandfather is a carrier of the mutation.

   C. Most likely the grandmother passed on the mutation to the mother owing to a new mutation.

   D. Most likely the grandmother is a carrier of the mutation.

   E. Most likely the mother passed on the mutation to the boy owing to a new mutation.

   F. All of the above.

   G. None of the above.

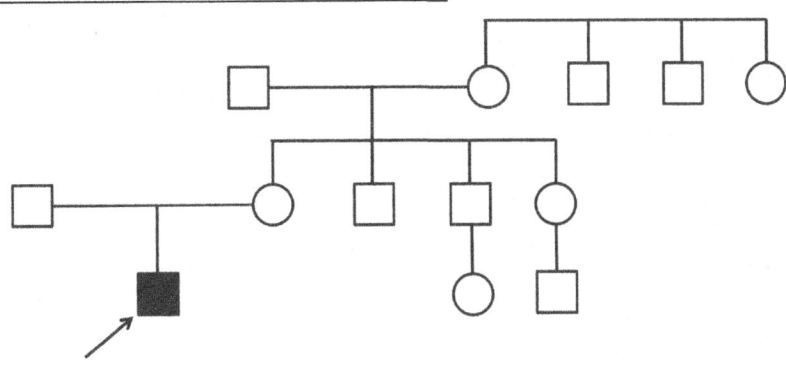

116. A couple brought their 8-year-old boy to a genetics clinic for bleeding problems (see the pedigree below). Results of a molecular test revealed that the boy had a deletion in the *F8* gene. Which one of following statements would be correct if the mutation was from the maternal side?[5]

   A. The mother was an obligate carrier of the mutation.

   B. Most likely the mother was a carrier of the mutation.

   C. Most likely the grandfather passed on the mutation to the mother owing to a new mutation.

   D. Most likely the grandfather was a carrier, too.

   E. Most likely the grandmother passed on the mutation to the mother owing to a new mutation.

   F. Most likely the grandmother was a carrier, too.

   G. Most likely the mother passed on the mutation to the boy owing to a new mutation.

   H. E and G.

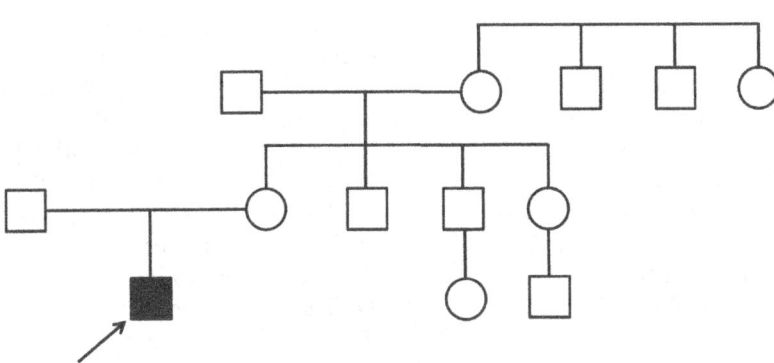

117. A couple brought their 8-year-old boy to a genetics clinic for bleeding problems (see the pedigree below). Results of a molecular test showed that the boy had an inversion in the *F8* gene. Which one of following statements would be correct if the mutation was from the maternal side?[5]
   A. Most likely the grandfather passed on the mutation to the mother owing to a new mutation.
   B. Most likely the grandfather is a carrier of the mutation.

C. Most likely the grandmother passed on the mutation to the mother owing to a new mutation.
D. Most likely the grandmother is a carrier of the mutation.
E. Most likely the mother passed on the mutation to the boy owing to a new mutation.
F. All of the above.

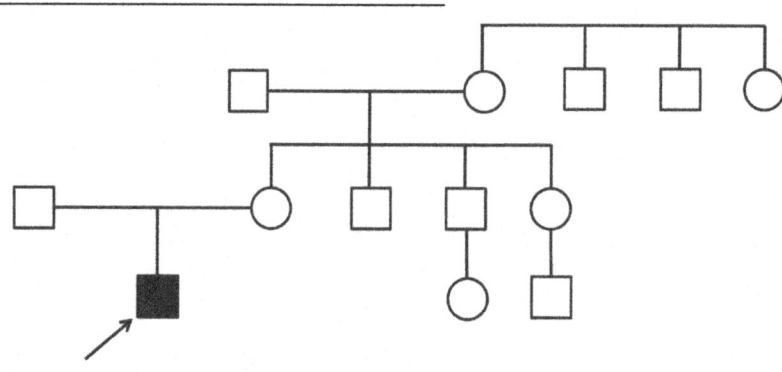

118. A couple came to a clinic for their first prenatal care when the wife was 6 weeks pregnant. The couple was apparently healthy. The wife's maternal uncle had died in childhood of hemophilia. The husband's family history was unremarkable. Which one of following genes would most likely harbor a germline pathogenic variant in the family?
   A. *F8*
   B. *F9*
   C. *F11*
   D. *F13A*
   E. *F13B*
   F. *vWF*

119. A couple came to a clinic for their first prenatal care when the wife was 6 weeks pregnant. The couple was apparently healthy. The wife's maternal uncle had died in childhood of hemophilia. The husband's family history was unremarkable. A molecular NGS panel was ordered. Which one of the following genes would most likely NOT be in this panel?

   A. *F2*
   B. *F8*
   C. *F9*
   D. *F11*
   E. *F13A*
   F. *F13B*
   G. None of the above

120. A couple came to a clinic for their first prenatal care when the wife was 6 weeks pregnant. This was their first pregnancy. They had unremarkable medical history. A family history revealed that the wife's maternal uncle had hemophilia B. And several males on her mother's side of the family might have been affected. The wife's two brothers were apparently healthy. The molecular test of *F9* in the wife did not identify pathogenic mutation(s) in the exon regions. However, the wife was a heterozygote for a rare SNP in linkage with *F9*. Who should be evaluated next for the SNP in this family?
   A. The wife's mother
   B. The wife's father
   C. The wife's brother
   D. The wife's uncle
   E. None of the above

121. A 26-year-old pregnant female is evaluated for a possible coagulation disorder, and her factor VIII activity is approximately 50% of normal. Molecular genetic analysis reveals a 5-bp deletion 250 bp upstream of the first exon of *F8*. Which one of the following mechanisms most likely is the molecular basis of the factor VIII deficiency in this patient if the 5-bp deletion is pathogenic?
    A. Alteration of the splicing of the factor VIII mRNA
    B. Alteration of the transcriptional activity of factor VIII mRNA
    C. Dominant negative activity of the mutant factor VIII protein
    D. Leading to a truncated factor VIII protein
    E. None of the above

122. An otherwise healthy 6-day-old French boy was brought to a clinic for prolonged bleeding after circumcision. He was hemodynamically stable, and the acute bleeding had been controlled with cautery, local hemostatic agents, and dressing. The infant was the couple's first child. The mother was 29 years old, and apparently healthy. Her maternal uncle had "some kind of bleeding disorder." The father was 32 years old and had no personal or family history of abnormal bleeding. Evaluation of the boy revealed a normal complete blood count. Coagulation testing revealed an increased PTT in the context of a normal PT and bleeding time. Coagulation factor assays revealed a normal and functional von Willebrand factor level. Which one of the following genes would most likely harbor a germline pathogenic variant in this patient?
    A. *F8*
    B. *F9*
    C. *F11*
    D. *F13A*
    E. *F13B*
    F. *vWF*

123. An otherwise healthy 6-day-old Ashkenazi Jewish boy was brought to a clinic for prolonged bleeding after circumcision. He was hemodynamically stable, and the acute bleeding had been controlled with cautery, local hemostatic agents, and dressing. The infant was the couple's first child. Both of the parents were apparently healthy and had no family history of abnormal bleeding. Evaluation of the infant revealed a normal complete blood count. Coagulation testing revealed an increased PTT in

the context of a normal PT and bleeding time. Coagulation factor assays revealed a normal and functional von Willebrand factor level. Which of the following genes would most likely harbor a germline pathogenic variant in this patient?
    A. *F8*
    B. *F9*
    C. *F11*
    D. *F13A*
    E. *F13B*
    F. *vWF*

124. A 32-day-old boy is brought to an emergency department for seizure. He does not have a fever. A physical examination reveals minor bruising. Lumbar puncture shows erythrocytes in the spinal fluid. A head CT scan reveals bilateral parenchymal hemorrhages. There is no family history of unusual bleeding on both sides. The boy did not bleed at circumcision, but there was delayed detachment of the umbilical cord with subsequent bleeding of the umbilical stump that lasted for several days. Prothrombin time, partial thromboplastin time, and thrombin time are normal. Coagulation factor assays reveal a normal and functional von Willebrand factor level. Which one of the following genes most likely harbors a germline pathogenic variant in this patient?
    A. *F8*
    B. *F9*
    C. *F11*
    D. *F13A*
    E. *F13B*
    F. *vWF*

125. A 26-year-old pregnant female is evaluated for a possible coagulation disorder, and her protein C is approximately 50% of normal. A molecular genetic analysis reveals a single base pair mutation in exon 3 of *PROC*. It changes a codon from TAT to TAG. Which one of the following mechanisms most likely describes the molecular basis of the protein C deficiency in this patient?
    A. Alteration of the splicing of the protein C mRNA
    B. Alteration of the transcriptional activity of protein C
    C. Dominant negative activity of a missense mutation
    D. Leading to a truncated protein C
    E. None of the above

126. A 26-year-old pregnant female is evaluated for a possible coagulation disorder, and her protein C

is approximately 50% of normal. A molecular genetic analysis reveals a single base-pair mutation in exon 3 of *PROC*. It changes a codon from TAT to TGA. Which one of the following mechanisms most likely describes the molecular basis of the protein C deficiency in this patient?
- A. Alteration of the transcriptional activity of protein C
- B. Dominant negative activity of a missense mutation
- C. Alteration of the splicing of the protein C mRNA
- D. Leading to a truncated protein C
- E. None of the above

127. A 26-year-old pregnant female is evaluated for a possible coagulation disorder, and her protein C is approximately 50% of normal. A molecular genetic analysis reveals a single base-pair mutation in exon 3 of *PROC*. It changes a codon from TAT to TAA. Which one of the following mechanism does most likely describe the molecular basis of the protein C deficiency in this patient?
- A. Alteration of the transcriptional activity of protein C
- B. Dominant negative activity of a missense mutation
- C. Alteration of the splicing of the protein C mRNA
- D. Leading to a truncated protein C
- E. None of the above

128. Methylenetetrahydrofolate reductase (MTHFR) is the rate-limiting enzyme in the methyl cycle, and it is encoded by the *MTHFR* gene. Homozygous *MTHFR* C677T polymorphism is associated with an increased risk for[6]:
- A. Depression
- B. Homocystinuria
- C. Hypertension
- D. Schizophrenia
- E. Thrombosis

129. The *MTHFR* gene provides instructions for making the enzyme methylenetetrahydrofolate reductase. This enzyme plays a role in processing amino acids and building blocks of proteins. Methylenetetrahydrofolate reductase is important for a chemical reactions involving forms of the vitamin folate (vitamin B_9). Which one of the following statements regarding the *MTHFR* molecular genetic test is correct[6]:

- A. The ACMG recommends ordering *MTHFR* polymorphism genotyping as part of the clinical evaluation for thrombophilia or recurrent pregnancy loss.
- B. The ACMG recommends ordering *MTHFR* polymorphism genotyping for thrombophilia to at-risk family members.
- C. A clinical geneticist should ensure that a patient with an *MTHFR* polymorphism(s) has received a thorough and appropriate evaluation for his or her thrombophilia symptoms.
- D. *MTHFR* status changes the recommendation that women of childbearing age should take the standard dose of folic acid supplementation to reduce the risk of neural-tube defects.
- E. If a patient is homozygous for the "thermolabile" variant c.665C > T, the lab report should recommend long-term follow-up for the increased risk for venous thrombosis.

130. The *MTHFR* gene provides instructions for making enzyme methylenetetrahydrofolate reductase. This enzyme plays a role in processing amino acids and building blocks of proteins. Methylenetetrahydrofolate reductase is important for a chemical reaction involving forms of the vitamin folate (vitamin B_9). Which one of the following statements regarding *MTHFR* molecular genetic test is correct?[6]
- A. Patients who are homozygous for the "thermolabile" variant with normal plasma homocysteine still have increased risk for venous thrombosis related to their *MTHFR* status.
- B. Patients who are homozygous for the c.665C > T "thermolabile" variant and also have elevated homocysteine have increased mortality from cardiovascular disease.
- C. In individuals who are homozygous for factor V Leiden, homozygosity for the "thermolabile" variant increases the thrombotic risk to a clinically significant degree.
- D. If the patient is homozygous for the "thermolabile" variant c.665C > T, the geneticist may order a fasting total plasma homocysteine, if not previously ordered, to provide more accurate counseling.
- E. Total homocysteine levels decrease with age and are higher in the pregnant population.

131. Two weeks after a left ankle fracture, a 46-year-old male suffered a proximal left leg deep vein thrombosis (DVT). After the initial treatment, he was referred to a genetics clinic for homozygous C677T *MTHFR* polymorphism. The remaining thrombophilia workup was negative. Which one of the following statements regarding the C677T *MTHFR* polymorphism would most likely be correct?[6]
   A. Most individuals with homozygous C677T *MTHFR* polymorphism will develop DVT at some point in their lifetime.
   B. Most individuals with homozygous C677T *MTHFR* polymorphism will not develop DVT in their lifetime.
   C. Individuals with homozygous C677T *MTHFR* polymorphism have a markedly increased risk for recurrent DVT.
   D. Testing of other family members for the *MTHFR* polymorphism was indicated.
   E. This patient was at high risk to have recurrent thromboses.

132. A laboratory workup of a 36-year-old female with newly diagnosed unprovoked pulmonary embolism demonstrates no thrombophilia. But she is heterozygous for the G20210A mutation in *F2*. Which one of the following statements regarding a heterozygous factor II mutation is correct?
   A. Most individuals with a heterozygous *F2* G20210A mutation will develop a venous thromboembolism at some point in their lifetime.
   B. Individuals with a heterozygous *F2* G20210A mutation are at markedly increased risk for arterial thromboembolism.
   C. Most individuals with a heterozygous *F2* G20210A mutation will not develop a venous thromboembolism at some point in their lifetime.
   D. All offspring of individuals with a heterozygous *F2* G20210A mutation will also be heterozygous for factor II G20210A mutation.
   E. Individuals with a heterozygous *F2* G20210A mutation are at high risk to have recurrent thromboses.

133. A 32-year-old pregnant regional sale representative of a large pharmaceutical company had been traveling around the country for the past 2 weeks. On the flight home, she experienced pain, swelling, and redness in her right lower leg. In a local emergency department, her vital signs were stable. She was afebrile. A clinical diagnosis of deep-vein thrombosis was made. After the initial treatment,

she was referred to a genetics clinic for follow-up. She was not on any medicine while visiting the clinic. Laboratory analysis did not demonstrate thrombophilia. Molecular genetic testing revealed that she was heterozygous for factor V Leiden. Which one of the following statements regarding the heterozygous factor V Leiden is correct?
   A. Most individuals with a heterozygous factor V Leiden will develop a venous thromboembolism at some point in their lifetime.
   B. Individuals with a heterozygous factor V Leiden have a markedly increased risk for arterial thromboembolism.
   C. Most individuals with a heterozygous factor V Leiden will not develop a venous thromboembolism in their lifetime.
   D. This patient was at high risk to have recurrent thromboses.
   E. All offspring of individuals with a heterozygous factor V Leiden will also be heterozygous for factor V Leiden.

134. A 66-year-old otherwise healthy male is seen in a clinic for a follow-up 5 weeks after completing 6 months of warfarin therapy for the first episode of unprovoked femoral-vein thrombosis. Plasma D-dimer testing performed 30 days after stopping warfarin is normal. The patient is heterozygous for the p.C677T mutation for methylenetetrahydrofolate reductase (*MTHFR*), the c.20210 G > A mutation for prothrombin, and the c.1691 G > A mutation for factor V Leiden. A thrombophilia workup has been otherwise negative. The family history is significant for an unprovoked pulmonary embolism in the patient's sister at age 61. Which one of the following factors increases this patient's risk for recurrent thrombosis?
   A. A heterozygous c.1691 G > A mutation in *F5*
   B. A heterozygous c.C677T mutation in *MTHFR*
   C. A heterozygous 20210 mutation in *F2*
   D. All of the above
   E. None of the above

135. A 66-year-old otherwise healthy male is seen in a clinic for a follow-up 5 weeks after completing 6 months of warfarin therapy for the first episode of unprovoked femoral-vein thrombosis. Plasma D-dimer testing performed 30 days after stopping warfarin is normal. The patient is heterozygous for the p.C677T mutation for methylenetetrahydrofolate reductase (*MTHFR*), 20210 G > A (c.*96C > T) for prothrombin, and the c.1691 G > A(p.Arg506Gln) mutation for factor V Leiden. A thrombophilia workup has been otherwise negative. The family history is

significant for an unprovoked pulmonary embolism in the patient's sister at age 61. Which one of the following factors does NOT increase this patient's risk for recurrent thrombosis?

A. Male sex

B. A heterozygous c.1691 G > A mutation in *F5*

C. A heterozygous c.C677T mutation in *MTHFR*

D. All of the above

E. None of the above

136. A patient underwent factor V Leiden testing; results showed a heterozygous mutation for c.1691 G > A(p.Arg506Gln). What would be her increased risk for venous thrombosis comparing with individuals without the mutation?

A. 1-Fold

B. 5-Fold

C. 20-Fold

D. 40-Fold

E. 80-Fold

137. A patient underwent factor V Leiden testing; results showed a homozygous mutation for c.1691 G > A(p.Arg506Gln). What would be her increased risk for venous thrombosis as compared with individuals without the mutation?

A. 1-Fold

B. 5-Fold

C. 20-Fold

D. 40-Fold

E. 80-Fold

138. A patient had *F2* mutation test using a TaqMan assay, and results showed a heterozygous mutation for 20210 G > A (c.*96C > T). What would be her increased risk for venous thrombosis as compared with individuals without the mutation?[7]

A. 1-Fold

B. 3-Fold

C. 20-Fold

D. 40-Fold

E. 80-Fold

139. A patient carries a heterozygous factor V Leiden allele, c.1691 G > A(p.Arg506Gln) and a heterozygous factor II 20210G > A (c.*96C > T) mutation. What would be her increased risk for venous thrombosis as compared with individuals without the two mutations?[8]

A. 1-Fold

B. 3-Fold

C. 20-Fold

D. 40-Fold

E. 80-Fold

140. The factor V Leiden allele contains a G-to-A substitution at nucleotide 1691, producing a missense mutation that substitutes glutamine for arginine at amino acid residue 506 (p.R506Q) in the protein product. Which one of the following protein's action sites is activated in patients with the factor V Leiden allele?

A. Protein A

B. Protein B

C. Protein C

D. Protein S

E. Prothrombin

141. Clotting factor II, or prothrombin, is a vitamin K−dependent proenzyme that functions in the blood coagulation cascade. Factor II deficiency is a rare, inherited or acquired bleeding disorder. Which one of the following statements regarding *F2* 20210G > A mutation is correct?

A. The prothrombin 20210G > A mutation is located in the 5′ untranslated region of the factor II gene.

B. The prothrombin 20210G > A mutation represents a loss-of-function mutation.

C. The prothrombin 20210G > A mutation is more common in Asians than in Caucasians.

D. The clinical sensitivity of the prothrombin 20210G > A mutation is about 90%.

E. Low penetrance of the prothrombin 20210G > A mutation is the main reason why clinical specificity is less than 100%.

142. Factor V is a protein in the coagulation pathway. It is primarily made in liver. The protein circulates in the bloodstream in an inactive form until the coagulation system is activated by an injury that damages blood vessels. What is the function of activated factor V?

A. Inhibits the activity of protein C

B. Inhibits the activity of protein S

C. Cleaves prothrombin (II) to thrombin (IIa)

D. Cleaves factor X to Xa

E. Cleaves factor VIII to VIIIa

143. Factor V Leiden thrombophilia is an inherited disorder of blood clotting with a specific gene mutation, which has an increased tendency to form abnormal blood clots that can block blood vessels. Which one of the following statements regarding the factor V Leiden allele is correct?

A. The factor V Leiden allele is more common in African Americans than in Caucasians.

B. The factor V Leiden allele is located in the 5′ untranslated region of the factor V gene.

C. Factor V Leiden accounts for at least 80% or 90%−95% of cases of activated protein S (APS) resistance.

D. Overall, the clinical sensitivity of the factor V Leiden mutation is between 70% and 90%.

E. Factor V Leiden testing is recommended for diagnostic purposes in individuals with recurrent pregnancy loss.

144. Factor V Leiden thrombophilia is an inherited disorder of blood clotting with a specific gene mutation, which has an increased tendency to form abnormal blood clots that can block blood vessels. Which one of the following statements regarding the factor V Leiden test is correct?
   A. Factor V Leiden testing is recommended for patients with a personal or family history of arterial thrombotic disorders.
   B. Factor V Leiden testing is recommended for diagnostic purposes in individuals with recurrent pregnancy loss.
   C. Factor V Leiden testing is recommended as a predictive test in asymptomatic individuals for venous thrombosis.
   D. Factor V Leiden testing is recommended as a predictive test in relatives of the proband.
   E. Factor V Leiden testing is recommended as a screening test to all pregnant women.

145. Factor V Leiden thrombophilia is an inherited disorder of blood clotting with a specific gene mutation. Patients with thrombophilia have an increased tendency to form abnormal blood clots that can block blood vessels. However, an individual with positive result of a factor V Leiden test may not develop venous thrombosis in their lifetime. Which one of the following is the primary reason for the low specificity?
   A. Variable express
   B. Incomplete penetrance
   C. Other alleles at the primers or probe region mislead the genotype
   D. Individuals with a heterozygous Leiden allele do not have increased risk for venous thrombosis.
   E. Accident happens before venous thrombosis.

146. A 46-year-old Caucasian businessman suddenly developed shortness of breath on the way home after an intercontinental trip. His leg was swollen and warm. Subsequent studies identified a thrombus in the popliteal and iliac veins, and a pulmonary embolus. Both of the parents had a similar medical history. Which one of the following gene analyses would most likely NOT be a part of the genetic evaluation for this patient?[5]
   A. *FII*
   B. *FV*
   C. *FVIII*
   D. *PROC1*
   E. *PROS1*
   F. *SERPINC1*

147. Factor V Leiden thrombophilia is an inherited disorder of blood clotting with a specific gene mutation. People with factor V Leiden thrombophilia have a higher-than-average risk of developing a deep venous thrombosis (DVT). However, not everyone with factor V Leiden mutation will develop thrombosis in his/her lifetime. In which one of the following ethnic populations is the factor V Leiden mutation most common?[5]
   A. African American
   B. Asian
   C. Caucasian
   D. Latino
   E. Native American

148. Factor V Leiden thrombophilia is an inherited disorder of blood clotting with a specific gene mutation. People with factor V Leiden thrombophilia have a higher than average risk of developing a deep venous thrombosis (DVT). The risk for thrombophilia is higher in individuals with a homozygous factor V Leiden allele than in those with a heterozygous allele. Which one of the following is correct with regard to the factor V Leiden mutation?[5]
   A. Loss of function
   B. Gain of function
   C. Dominant negative
   D. Complete penetrance
   E. None of the above

149. Protein C deficiency is a congenital or acquired condition that leads to increased risk for thrombosis. The risk for thrombosis is higher in individuals with homozygous protein C mutations than in those with heterozygous mutations. Which one of the following is correct with regard to the mutations in protein C?[5]
   A. Loss of function
   B. Gain of function
   C. Dominant negative
   D. Complete penetrance
   E. None of the above

150. A 28-year-old female presents to a clinic for consultation. She has no current symptoms but is concerned because her father has acute intermittent porphyria (AIP) and she is 6 weeks pregnant. The patient has no abnormalities identified on physical examination. She has no episodes. Her urine porphobilinogen (PBG) is 6.2 μmol/L (normal range, 0–8.8) and her urine 5-aminolevulinic acid (ALA) 23 μmol/L (normal, 0–35). Her erythrocytic porphobilinogen

deaminase level is 1.2 mU/g (normal range, 2.1−4.3). Which one of the following statements is most appropriate?

A. Her child will have an approximately 90% chance of being healthy with AIP symptoms.

B. Her child will have a 50% risk of having AIP symptoms.

C. She will have increased risk to develop renal cancer.

D. Acute attack is more common in men than in women.

E. Molecular genetic testing of *HMBS* is commonly used to confirm the diagnosis.

151. A 35-year-old female presents to a clinic for an initial visit. She has no current symptoms but is concerned because her father has acute intermittent porphyria (AIP). She and her father have the same heterozygous mutation in *HMBS*. The patient has no abnormalities identified on physical examination. She has been apparently healthy, without episodes. What is her risk of having episodes in her lifetime?[9-11]

A. Up to 20%

B. 1/4

C. 1/2

D. 100%

E. None of the above

152. A 35-year-old female presents to a clinic for an initial visit. She has no current symptoms but is concerned because her father has acute intermittent porphyria (AIP). She and her father have the same heterozygous mutation in *HMBS*. The patient has no abnormalities identified on physical examination. She has been apparently healthy, without episodes. For which of the following malignancies is she at increased risk of having in her lifetime?

A. Renal-cell carcinoma

B. Stomach cancer

C. Colorectal cancer

D. Hepatocellular carcinoma

E. None of the above

153. A 25-year-old PhD student came to the emergency department of a local hospital for severe abdominal pain around the umbilicus; the pain was stabbing in character and radiated toward the back and had persisted for about 3 weeks. She went to a friend's college graduation party before the episodes. After the pain subsided, she developed acute-onset, rapidly progressive weakness in all four limbs and was bedridden for 4−5 days. Then she gradually improved over a period of 1 month. She remained

asymptomatic for approximately 3 months before she had second episode of similar abdominal pain, which persisted for about 2 weeks. Then she developed rapidly progressive weakness starting in the right upper limb followed by the left upper limb and gradually affecting both lower limbs in a week, then progressing to her being bedridden. She had dark-colored urine during both of the episodes. Her total leukocyte count was 8900/mm^3, with a differential count of neutrophils 60%, lymphocytes 36%, and erythrocytes 4%. Her hemoglobin was 12 g/dL and ESR, 35 mm in the first hour. Urine had elevated level of porphobilinogen (PBG) and delta aminolevulinic acid (ALA). The total fecal porphyrin concentration and coproporphyrin isomer ratio were normal, and a plasma porphyrin fluorescence emission scan was normal. Which one of the following molecular genetic tests would most likely be positive in this patient?

A. *HMBS*

B. *UROD*

C. *PPOX*

D. *CPOX*

E. *GATA1*

F. *UROS*

154. A 25-year-old female came to the emergency department of a local hospital twice in the past 6 months for severe abdominal pain, which resolved in about 2 weeks. A high level of porphobilinogen (PBG) and delta-aminolevulinic acid (ALA) were detected in her urine during both episodes. The physician suspected the patient had porphyria, and ordered a next-generation sequencing (NGS) panel for porphyrias. Which one of the following genes would most likely NOT be in this NGS panel?

A. *HMBS*

B. *UROD*

C. *FXN*

D. *CPOX*

E. *GATA1*

F. *UROS*

155. In May, while the family was having their first vacation after the birth of a 1-year-old boy, he was brought to an emergency department in Florida for swelling, burning, itching, and redness of the skin on the sun-exposed areas. Markedly increased free erythrocyte protoporphyrin and zinc-chelated erythrocyte protoporphyrin were found in his blood sample. One of his maternal uncles and a maternal granduncle have had similar episodes throughout their lives. The

physician suspected that the infant had porphyria. Which one of the following would most likely be the recurrent risk in this family?

A. 100%
B. 50%
C. 25%
D. <1%
E. None of the above

156. In May, while the family was having their first vacation after the birth of a 1-year-old boy, he was brought to an emergency department in Florida for swelling, burning, itching, and redness of the skin on the sun-exposed areas. Markedly increased free erythrocyte protoporphyrin and zinc-chelated erythrocyte protoporphyrin were found in the blood sample. One of his maternal uncles and a maternal granduncle have had similar episodes throughout their life. The physician suspected the infant had porphyria, and ordered a molecular test. What kind of pathogenic mutations would the patient most likely have?

A. Deficient enzyme activity
B. Haploinsufficiency
C. Epigenetic modification
D. Overexpression
E. None of the above

157. A 68-year-old female was referred to a genetics clinic for purpuric, punctate, and tiny macules on the fingertips of both hands and the tongue for 50 years. She had numerous episodes of mild-to-severe nasal bleeding of unknown cause. She had been treated for epistaxis with electrocauterization therapy several times. She had a history of admissions to gastroenterology clinics owing to exacerbations of anemia and melena 2 years ago. A physical examination revealed that she had pallor and that telangiectasias discolored the oral mucosa and tongue. The family history was significant for recurrent epistaxis and telangiectatic lesions in her mother and two sisters. No abnormalities were detected by chest X-ray. Laboratory workups revealed a WBC count of $2500/mm^3$, platelet count $207,000/mm^3$, hemoglobin 6.5 g/dL, ferritin 3.72 ng/mL (normal range, 13−150), and serum iron 34 μg/dL (normal range, 50−150). Other laboratory findings were normal, including bleeding time, coagulation time, prothrombin time (PT), activated partial thromboplastin time (aPTT), and stool occult blood. Endoscopy of the upper digestive tract indicated multiple gastric angiodysplasias of the fundus and body of stomach. The histopathological examination of the biopsy

revealed dilated capillaries lined by flat endothelial cells in the papillary dermis. The medical geneticist suspected that the patient had a genetic condition. Which one of the following genetic conditions would this patient most likely have if she had one?[12]

A. Ataxia telangiectasia
B. Hemophilia A
C. Hereditary hemochromatosis
D. Hereditary hemorrhagic telangiectasia
E. None of the above

158. A 68-year-old female was referred to a genetics clinic for purpuric, punctate, and tiny macules on the fingertips of both hands and the tongue for 50 years. She had numerous episodes of mild-to-severe nasal bleeding of unknown cause. She had been treated for epistaxis with electrocauterization therapy several times. She had a history of admissions to gastroenterology clinics owing to exacerbations of anemia and melena 2 years ago. A physical examination revealed that she had pallor and that telangiectasias discolored the oral mucosa and tongue. The family history was significant for recurrent epistaxis and telangiectatic lesions in her mother and two sisters. No abnormalities were detected by chest X-ray. Laboratory workups revealed a WBC count of $2500/mm^3$, platelet count $207,000/mm^3$, hemoglobin 6.5 g/dL, ferritin 3.72 (13−150 ng/mL), and serum iron 34 μg/dL (normal range, 50−150). Other laboratory findings were normal including bleeding time, coagulation time, prothrombin time (PT), activated partial thromboplastin time (aPTT), and stool occult blood. Endoscopy of the upper digestive tract indicated multiple gastric angiodysplasias of the fundus and body of stomach. The histopathological examination of the biopsy revealed dilated capillaries lined by flat endothelial cells in the papillary dermis. The medical geneticist suspected the that patient had a genetic condition and ordered a sequencing assay for the patient. Which one of the following genes would most likely be included in the sequencing assay for this patient?[12]

A. *ATM*
B. *F8*
C. *HFE*
D. *ENG*
E. None of the above

159. A 68-year-old female was referred to a genetics clinic for purpuric, punctate, and tiny macules on the fingertips of both hands and the tongue for 50 years. She had numerous episodes of mild-to-severe nasal bleeding of unknown cause. She had

been treated for epistaxis with electrocauterization therapy several times. She had a history of admissions to gastroenterology clinics owing to exacerbations of anemia and melena 2 years ago. A physical examination revealed that she had pallor and that telangiectasias discolored the oral mucosa and tongue. The family history was significant for recurrent epistaxis and telangiectatic lesions in her mother and two sisters. No abnormalities were detected on chest X-ray. Laboratory workups revealed a WBC count of 2500/mm^3, platelet count 207,000/mm^3, hemoglobin 6.5 g/dL, ferritin 3.72 ng/mL (normal range, 13–150), and serum iron 34 μg/dL (normal range, 50–150). Other laboratory findings were normal, including bleeding time, coagulation time, prothrombin time (PT), activated partial thromboplastin time (aPTT), and stool occult blood. Endoscopy of the upper digestive tract indicated multiple gastric angiodysplasias of the fundus and body of the stomach. The histopathological examination of the biopsy revealed dilated capillaries lined by flat endothelial cells in the papillary dermis. The medical geneticist suspected that the patient had a genetic condition and ordered a sequencing assay. Which one of the following genes would most likely be included in the sequencing assay ordered for this patient?[12]

A. ATM
B. F8
C. HFE
D. SMAD4
E. None of the above

160. A 31-year-old pregnant female presented to a clinic for a 2-week history of pleuritic chest pain at a gestational age of 20 weeks. Her medical and family history was unremarkable before the pregnancy. During the pregnancy, she began to experience mild episodes of spontaneous epistaxis and also noted the development of cutaneous telangiectasias on her fingertips, lips, and chest. As she entered her second trimester, she noticed the onset of exertional dyspnea but attributed this to her gravid uterus. Dyspnea gradually worsened over the subsequent weeks, and 2 weeks prior to her visit, she experienced the onset of bilateral pleuritic chest pain. Her chest X-ray revealed bilateral nodular densities. And chest CT demonstrated a 2-cm arteriovenous malformation (AVM) in the right upper lobe and a 4-cm AVM in the lingula, both of which were abutting the pleurae, in addition to multiple smaller AVMs in both lungs. The physician suspected that the patient has a genetic condition.

After consulting with a medical geneticist, the physician ordered a genetic test for the patient. Which one of the following assays would most likely be used for this genetic test?

A. Chromosome breakage study
B. Chromosome microarray
C. Methylation study
D. Multiplex ligation-dependent probe amplification (MLPA)
E. Next-generation sequencing analysis
F. Sanger sequencing analysis
G. Targeted mutation analysis
H. None of the above

161. A 31-year-old pregnant female presented to a clinic for a 2-week history of pleuritic chest pain at a gestational age of 20 weeks. She had a known family history of hereditary hemorrhagic telangiectasia (HHT). Her mother and one of her sisters had undergone genetic tests and a deletion in the ENG gene for HHT was identified in both of them. The patient herself had been asymptomatic and was never screened for the familial deletion in the ENG gene before this pregnancy. During the pregnancy, she began to experience mild episodes of spontaneous epistaxis and also noted the development of cutaneous telangiectasias on her fingertips, lips, and chest. As she entered her second trimester, she noticed the onset of exertional dyspnea but attributed this to her gravid uterus. Dyspnea gradually worsened over the subsequent weeks, and 2 weeks prior to her visit she experienced onset of bilateral pleuritic chest pain. Her chest X-ray revealed bilateral nodular densities. And chest CT demonstrated a 2-cm arteriovenous malformation (AVM) in the right upper lobe and a 4-cm AVM in the lingula, both of which were abutting the pleurae, in addition to multiple smaller AVMs in both lungs. A genetic test confirmed that she had the familial deletion in ENG. What would be her unborn child's risk for HHT?

A. 99%
B. 1/2
C. 1/4
D. 1/8
E. 1/12
F. <1%

162. A 2-year-old boy was born from the first normal pregnancy of a couple; his weight was 3420 g. His family history was positive for two maternal uncles who died before the age of 3 years with severe infections, diarrhea, erythroderma, and elevated immunoglobulins class E (IgEs). Since his first month of life, this patient had suffered

from septicemia, pneumonias, pyelonephritis, and meningitis accompanied by eczematous dermatitis and IgEs up to 4000 IU/L. At the age of 17 months, he developed type 1 diabetes mellitus (T1DM). He was underweight (−3.42 SDs) and had phenotypic features such as coarse face, muscle hypotonia, joint hyperextensibility, eczematous dermatitis, and subcutaneous cold abscesses. Autoimmune thyroiditis and celiac disease were excluded. Lately, intermittent watery diarrhea appeared, with progression to the severe intractable form. Finally, aggravating symptoms of nephritis, cachexia, and respiratory insufficiency were the cause for his death at the age of 2 years 3 months. A sequencing analysis identified a pathogenic variant, c.1010G < A(p. Arg337Gln), at exon 10 of the *FOXP3* gene. Which one of the following diseases did this deceased patient most likely have?

A. Autoimmune lymphoproliferative syndrome
B. Immune dysregulation, polyendocrinopathy, enteropathy X-linked (IPEX) syndrome
C. von Willebrand disease
D. Wiskott−Aldrich syndrome
E. X-linked lymphoproliferative disease
F. None of the above

163. A 2-year-old boy was born from the first normal pregnancy of a couple; his weight was 3420 g. His family history was positive for two maternal uncles who died before the age of 3 years with severe infections, diarrhea, erythroderma, and elevated immunoglobulins class E (IgEs). Since his first month of life, this patient had suffered from septicemia, pneumonias, pyelonephritis, and meningitis accompanied by eczematous dermatitis and IgEs up to 4000 IU/L. At the age of 17 months, he developed type 1 diabetes mellitus (T1DM). He was underweight (−3.42 SDs) and had phenotypic features such as coarse face, muscle hypotonia, joint hyperextensibility, eczematous dermatitis, and subcutaneous cold abscesses. Autoimmune thyroiditis and celiac disease were excluded. Lately, intermittent watery diarrhea appeared, with progression to the severe intractable form. Finally, aggravating symptoms of nephritis, cachexia, and respiratory insufficiency were the cause for his death at the age of 2 years 3 months. A sequencing analysis identified a pathogenic variant, c.1010G < A(p. Arg337Gln), at exon 10 of the *FOXP3* gene, which confirmed immune dysregulation, polyendocrinopathy, enteropathy X-linked (IPEX) syndrome. Subsequent testing revealed that the patient's mother and his unborn sister (the mother was 23 weeks pregnant with a girl) had

the same pathogenic variant. Which one of the following statements would most appropriately describe the likelihood that the unborn sister of the proband would develop symptoms of IPEX?

A. She would not have any symptoms.
B. Most likely she would not have any symptoms.
C. She would have similar symptoms.
D. Most likely she would have symptoms.
E. Unknown.

164. A 14-year-old male was admitted to a local hospital for diabetic ketoacidosis. He was diagnosed with polyendocrine autoimmune association diabetes mellitus type 1, autoimmune thyroiditis, and hypogonadotropic hypogonadism. This patient had celiac disease, which was characterized by recurrent diarrhea, positive IgA antitissue transglutaminase antibodies, and total villous atrophy on intestinal biopsy sample. He also presented with recurrent eczematous dermatitis associated with elevated serum concentrations of immunoglobulin E. The family history was positive for unexplained early deaths of the patient's maternal uncles. A diagnosis of immune dysregulation, polyendocrinopathy, enteropathy, X-linked (IPEX) syndrome was sustained. Which one of the following genes would most likely harbor a germline pathogenic variant for IPEX syndrome in this patient?

A. *CASP10*
B. *FAS*
C. *FASLG*
D. *FOXP3*
E. All of the above
F. None of the above

165. A 14-year-old male was admitted to a local hospital for diabetic ketoacidosis. He was diagnosed with polyendocrine autoimmune association diabetes mellitus type 1, autoimmune thyroiditis, and hypogonadotropic hypogonadism. The patient had celiac disease that was characterized by recurrent diarrhea, positive IgA antitissue transglutaminase antibodies, and total villous atrophy on an intestinal biopsy sample. He also presented with recurrent eczematous dermatitis associated with elevated serum concentration of immunoglobulin E. His family history was positive for unexplained early deaths of the his maternal uncles. A diagnosis of immune dysregulation, polyendocrinopathy, enteropathy, X-linked (IPEX) syndrome was sustained, and Sanger sequencing analysis of the *FOXP3* gene was ordered. What

would be the likelihood that Sanger sequencing analysis of *FOXP3* would confirm the diagnosis of IPEX in this patient?[13]

A. < 10%

B. 25%

C. 50%

D. 75%

E. 99%

166. A 22-month-old Hispanic boy was brought to a clinic for pallor, fatigue and "swelling" since 8 months of age. A physical examination revealed bilateral cervical, axillary, and inguinal lymphadenopathy and splenomegaly. Lab tests revealed hypergammaglobulinemia (IgG, 2300 mg/dL; normal range, 400−1000), CD5 + B cells, and CD3 + but CD4−, CD8−, and CD7− (17%) T cells. IHC stains of lymph nodes identified a "virgin" T-cell immunophenotype (CD45RA + and CD45RO−) stain pattern. A diagnosis of autoimmune lymphoproliferative syndrome (ALPS) was sustained, and a molecular test was ordered. Which one of the following genes would most likely harbor a pathogenic variant in this patient?

A. *CASP10*

B. *FAS*

C. *FASLG*

D. *FOXP3*

E. None of the above

167. A 22-month-old Hispanic boy was brought to a clinic for pallor, fatigue and "swelling" since 8 months of age. A physical examination revealed bilateral cervical, axillary and inguinal lymphadenopathy, and splenomegaly. Lab tests revealed hypergammaglobulinemia (IgG, 2300 mg/dL; normal range, 400−1000), CD5 + B cells, and CD3 + but CD4−, CD8−, and CD7− (17%) T cells. IHC stains of lymph nodes identified a "virgin" T-cell immunophenotype (CD45RA + and CD45RO−) stain pattern. A diagnosis of autoimmune lymphoproliferative syndrome (ALPS) was sustained, and a molecular test was ordered. Which one of the following genes would NOT likely harbor a pathogenic variant in this patient?

A. *CASP10*

B. *FAS*

C. *FASLG*

D. *FOXP3*

E. None of the above

168. A 22-month-old Hispanic boy was brought to a clinic for pallor, fatigue and "swelling" since 8 months of age. A physical examination revealed bilateral cervical, axillary, and inguinal lymphadenopathy and splenomegaly. Lab tests

revealed hypergammaglobulinemia (IgG, 2300 mg/dL; normal range, 400−1000), CD5 + B cells, and CD3 + but CD4−, CD8−, and CD7− (17%) T cells. IHC stains of lymph nodes identified a "virgin" T-cell immunophenotype (CD45RA + and CD45RO−) stain pattern. A diagnosis of autoimmune lymphoproliferative syndrome (ALPS) was sustained, and a molecular test was ordered. What would be the likelihood that Sanger sequencing analysis of the three genes for ALPS would confirm the diagnosis in this patient?

A. < 10%

B. 25%

C. 50%

D. 75%

E. 99%

169. A 22-month-old Hispanic boy was brought to a clinic for pallor, fatigue and "swelling" since 8 months of age. A physical examination revealed bilateral cervical, axillary, and inguinal lymphadenopathy and splenomegaly. Lab tests revealed hypergammaglobulinemia (IgG, 2300 mg/dL; normal range, 400−1000), CD5 + B cells, and CD3 + but CD4−, CD8−, and CD7− (17%) T cells. IHC stains of lymph nodes identified a "virgin" T-cell immunophenotype (CD45RA + and CD45RO−) stain pattern. A heterozygous pathogenic variant, c.721A > C(p. Thr241Pro), in the *FAS* gene was identified in the peripheral-blood sample from this patient. Which one of the following diseases did the deceased patient most likely have?

A. Autoimmune lymphoproliferative syndrome

B. Immune dysregulation, polyendocrinopathy, enteropathy X-linked (IPEX) syndrome

C. von Willebrand disease

D. Wiskott−Aldrich syndrome

E. X-linked lymphoproliferative disease

F. None of the above

170. A 22-month-old Hispanic boy was brought to a clinic for pallor, fatigue and "swelling" since 8 months of age. His perinatal medical history and family history were unremarkable (the mother was adopted). A physical examination revealed bilateral cervical, axillary, and inguinal lymphadenopathy and splenomegaly. Lab tests revealed hypergammaglobulinemia (IgG, 2300 mg/dL; normal range, 400−1000), CD5 + B cells, and CD3 + but CD4−, CD8−, and CD7− (17%) T cells. IHC stains of lymph nodes identified a "virgin" T-cell immunophenotype (CD45RA + and CD45RO−) stain pattern. A diagnosis of autoimmune lymphoproliferative syndrome (ALPS) was sustained, and a molecular

test was ordered. A heterozygous pathogenic variant, c.721A > C(p.Thr241Pro), in the *FAS* gene was identified in the peripheral-blood sample from this patient. Subsequent testing revealed that the patient's mother and his unborn sister (the mother was 23 weeks pregnant with a girl) had the same mutation. Which one of the following statements most appropriately describes the likelihood that the unborn sister would develop ALPS symptoms?

A. She would not have any symptoms.

B. Most likely she would not have any symptoms.

C. She would have similar symptoms.

D. Most likely she would have symptoms.

E. Unknown.

171. A 2-year-old boy was brought to an emergency department with epistaxis and fever. A physical examination revealed ecchymotic spots all over the body, with bruises found on the lips and buccal cavity. The platelet count on admission was 22,000/mm³. The patient started having coffee-grounds vomitus. Medical history was significant for skin rashes, recurrent infections, and episodes of bloody stools. Perinatal history was uneventful. Family history revealed that one of the mother's brothers had died with similar symptoms at the age of 4 and that no clear diagnosis was made at that time. Bone marrow biopsy results were negative. Blood urea, creatinine, and urine were normal. The immunoglobulin profile showed high immunoglobulin A (IgA), low immunoglobulin M (IgM), high immunoglobulin E (IgE), and normal immunoglobulin G (IgG). A diagnosis of Wiskott–Aldrich syndrome (WAS) was sustained, and a molecular test was ordered. A missense mutation, c.167C > T(p.Ala56Val), in the *WAS* gene was identified in the peripheral-blood sample from this patient. Subsequent testing revealed that the patient's mother and his unborn sister (the mother was 23 weeks pregnant with a girl) had the same mutation. Which one of the following statements most appropriately describes the likelihood that the unborn sister would develop WAS symptoms?

A. She would not have any symptoms.

B. Most likely she would not have any symptoms.

C. She would have similar symptoms.

D. Most likely she would have symptoms.

E. Unknown.

172. A 2-year-old boy was brought to an emergency department with epistaxis and fever. A physical examination revealed ecchymotic spots all over

the body, with bruises found on the lips and buccal cavity. The platelet count on admission was 22,000/mm³. The patient started having coffee-grounds vomitus. Medical history was significant for skin rashes, recurrent infections, and episodes of bloody stools. His prenatal and postnatal history was uneventful. His family history revealed that one of the mother's brothers had died with similar symptoms at the age of 4 and that no clear diagnosis was made at that time. Bone marrow biopsy results were negative. Blood urea, creatinine, and urine were normal. The immunoglobulin profile showed high immunoglobulin A (IgA), low immunoglobulin M (IgM), high immunoglobulin E (IgE), and normal immunoglobulin G (IgG). A diagnosis of Wiskott–Aldrich syndrome (WAS) was sustained, and a molecular test was ordered. What would be the likelihood that Sanger sequencing analysis and del/dup analysis of the *WAS* gene would confirm the diagnosis in this patient?

A. < 10%

B. 25%

C. 50%

D. 75%

E. > 99%

173. In the late 1970s, the world witnessed the heart-wrenching tale of David Vetter, the "bubble boy." Born with X-linked SCID (XSCID), a complete deficiency of T cells and NK cells, David lived his entire life inside a plastic bubble, deprived of all human contact. Sadly, David Vetter died in 1984 as a result of complications following an allogeneic bone marrow transplantation designed to cure his disease. Nearly 10 years later, the genetic defect responsible for XSCID was identified by genetic linkage analyses. Which one of the following genes is responsible for XSCID, according to the publication in *Cell* in 1993?[15]

A. *FAS*

B. *IL1RG*

C. *IL2RG*

D. *FOXP3*

E. None of the above

174. In the late 1970s, the world witnessed the heart-wrenching tale of David Vetter, the "bubble boy." Born with X-linked SCID (XSCID), a complete deficiency of T cells and NK cells, David lived his entire life inside a plastic bubble, deprived of all human contact. Sadly, David Vetter died in 1984 as a result of complications following an allogeneic bone marrow transplantation designed to cure his disease. Nearly 10 years later, the genetic defect responsible for XSCID was

identified by genetic linkage analyses. Which type of cells is NOT decreased in patients with XSCID?

A. B cells
B. T cells
C. NK cells
D. All of the above
E. None of the above

175. X-linked severe combined immunodeficiency (XSCID) is caused by mutations in the common cytokine receptor γ chain, resulting in disruption of development of T lymphocytes and natural killer cells. B-lymphocyte function is also intrinsically compromised. Gene therapy for XSCID is a highly effective strategy for restoration of functional cellular and humoral immunity. However, there are clinically significant adverse effects. Which one of the following adverse effects do patients with XSCID intend to develop after gene therapy?

A. Osteosarcoma
B. T-cell leukemia
C. Infections
D. Renal-cell carcinoma
E. None of the above

176. Gene therapy is a promising treatment option for a number of diseases, including inherited disorders, some types of cancer, and certain viral infections. However, the technique remains risky and is still under study to make sure that it will be safe and effective. Gene therapy is currently being tested only for the treatment of diseases that have no other cures. Which one of the following diseases was treated with gene therapy for the first time in 1990?

A. Adenosine deaminase deficiency
B. Adrenoleukodystrophy
C. Cystic fibrosis
D. Gaucher disease
E. X-linked severe combined immunodeficiency
F. None of the above

ANSWERS

1. **A.** Hemoglobin is the protein molecule in red blood cells that carries oxygen from the lungs to the body's tissues and returns carbon dioxide from the tissues back to the lungs. Hemoglobin is made up of four globin chains that are connected together. The normal adult hemoglobin (Hb) contains two alpha-globin chains and two beta-globin chains (HbA, $\alpha^2\beta^2$). In fetuses and infants, beta-globin chains are not common and the hemoglobin is made up of two alpha chains and

two gamma chains (HbF, $\alpha^2\gamma^2$). As the infant grows, the gamma chains are gradually replaced by beta chains, forming the adult hemoglobin structure. Each globin chain contains an important iron-containing porphyrin compound termed heme. Embedded within the heme compound is an iron atom that is vital in transporting oxygen and carbon dioxide in our blood. The iron contained in hemoglobin is also responsible for the red color of blood. Hemoglobin also plays an important role in maintaining the shape of the red blood cells.

Hemoglobin A2 (HbA2, $\alpha^2\delta^2$) is a normal variant of hemoglobin A that consists of two alpha and two delta chains and is found at low levels in normal human blood. Hemoglobin A2 may be increased in beta thalassemia or in people who are heterozygous for the beta thalassemia gene.

Therefore, hemoglobin A has $\alpha^2\beta^2$.

2. **B.** Hemoglobin is the protein molecule in red blood cells that carries oxygen from the lungs to the body's tissues and returns carbon dioxide from the tissues back to the lungs. Hemoglobin is made up of four globin chains that are connected together. The normal adult hemoglobin (Hb) contains two alpha-globin chains and two beta-globin chains (HbA: $\alpha^2\beta^2$). In fetuses and infants, beta chains are not common and the hemoglobin is made up of two alpha chains and two gamma chains (HbF, $\alpha^2\gamma^2$). As the infant grows, the gamma chains are gradually replaced by beta chains, forming the adult hemoglobin structure. Each globin chain contains an important iron-containing porphyrin compound called "heme." Embedded within the heme compound is an iron atom that is vital in transporting oxygen and carbon dioxide in the blood. The iron contained in hemoglobin is also responsible for the red color of blood. Hemoglobin also plays an important role in maintaining the shape of the red blood cells.

Hemoglobin A2 (HbA2, $\alpha^2\delta^2$) is a normal variant of hemoglobin A that consists of two alpha and two delta chains and is found at low levels in normal human blood. Hemoglobin A2 may be increased in beta thalassemia or in people who are heterozygous for the beta thalassemia gene.

Therefore, hemoglobin F has $\alpha^2\gamma^2$.

3. **C.** Hemoglobin is the protein molecule in red blood cells that carries oxygen from the lungs to the body's tissues and returns carbon dioxide from the tissues back to the lungs. Hemoglobin is made up of four globin chains that are connected together. The normal adult hemoglobin (Hb)

contains two alpha-globin chains and two beta-globin chains (HbA, $\alpha^2\beta^2$). In fetuses and infants, beta chains are not common and the hemoglobin molecule is made up of two alpha chains and two gamma chains (HbF, $\alpha^2\gamma^2$). As the infant grows, the gamma chains are gradually replaced by beta chains, forming the adult hemoglobin structure. Each globin chain contains an important iron-containing porphyrin compound called "heme." Embedded within the heme compound is an iron atom that is vital in transporting oxygen and carbon dioxide in our blood. The iron contained in hemoglobin is also responsible for the red color of blood. Hemoglobin also plays an important role in maintaining the shape of the red blood cells.

Hemoglobin A2 (HbA2, $\alpha^2\delta^2$) is a normal variant of hemoglobin A that consists of two alpha and two delta chains and is found at low levels in normal human blood. Hemoglobin A2 may be increased in beta thalassemia or in people who are heterozygous for the beta-thalassemia gene.

Therefore, hemoglobin A2 has $\alpha^2\delta^2$.

4. **A.** Sickle cell anemia is more common in certain populations and ethnicities. *It is most common in people of African descent.* It affects 1 of every 375 African American infants. And it is also common in people whose families come from South or Central America (especially Panama), the Caribbean islands, Mediterranean countries (such as Turkey, Greece, and Italy), India, and Saudi Arabia.

Therefore, sickle cell disease is more common in African Americans than in the other populations in the list.

5. **D.** All 50 U.S. states provide universal newborn screening (NBS) for sickle cell disease (SCD) because of its high morbidity and mortality rates. The primary purpose of screening is to identify infants with SCD, the most prevalent disorder included in neonatal screening panels. Screening also identifies infants with other hemoglobinopathies, hemoglobinopathy carriers, and in some states, infants with alpha-thalassemia syndromes.

The majority of NBS programs perform isoelectric focusing electrophoresis (IFE) of an eluate of dried blood spots. A few programs use HPLC, DNA testing, or cellulose acetate electrophoresis as the initial screening method. Specimens with abnormal screening results are retested using a second, complementary electrophoretic technique, HPLC, citrate agar, IEF,

or DNA-based assays (not Sanger sequencing). Infants with hemoglobins that suggest SCD or other clinically significant hemoglobinopathies require confirmatory testing of a separate blood sample by age 6 weeks. The sensitivity and specificity of current screening method is excellent, and 99% of U.S. infants at highest risk for sickle cell disease are born in states with universal screening (http://www.ncbi.nlm.nih.gov/books/NBK1377/).

Sanger sequencing is a relatively more expensive and time-consuming test compared with IFE, HPLC, and others mentioned in the question.

Therefore, Sanger sequencing may be used to confirm the diagnosis, but not used as a screening test.

6. **F.** In the human genome, there are two copies of hemoglobin alpha (*HBA1* and *HBA2*), and one copy of hemoglobin beta (*HBB*). Sickle cell disease (SCD) is a group of autosomal recessive nonneoplastic hematological disorders associated with pathogenic variants in *HBB* and defined by the presence of predominantly hemoglobin S (HbS), or HbS along with other Hb variants that allow for HbS polymerization. Normal adult human hemoglobin is a heterotetramer composed of two α-hemoglobin chains and two β-hemoglobin chains. *Hemoglobin S results from a single nucleotide variant in HBB, changing the sixth amino acid in the β-hemoglobin chain from glutamic acid to valine (Glu6Val).*

Sickle cell anemia (homozygous HbSS) accounts for 60%−70% of SCD in the United States. Other forms of SCD result from coinheritance of HbS with other abnormal β-globin chain variants, the most common forms being sickle hemoglobin C disease (HbSC) and two types of sickle β thalassemia (HbSβ + thalassemia and HbS$\beta°$ thalassemia). Rarer forms result from coinheritance of other Hb variants such as D-Punjab, O-Arab, and E. The diagnosis of SCD is established by demonstrating the presence of significant quantities of HbS by isoelectric focusing (IEF), cellulose acetate electrophoresis, high-performance liquid chromatography (HPLC), or (less commonly) DNA analysis. Targeted mutation analysis is used to identify the common pathogenic variants of *HBB* associated with hemoglobin S, hemoglobin C, and additional rarer pathogenic variants. *HBB* sequence analysis may be used to detect pathogenic variants associated with β-thalassemia hemoglobin variants. Gel electrophoresis or HPLC can differentiate these disorders from heterozygous carriers of the HbS pathogenic variant (HbAS) (http://www.ncbi.nlm.nih.gov/books/NBK1377/).

Therefore, SCD is caused by a mutation in the *HBB* gene.

7. **D**. Sickle cell disease (SCD) is an inherited autosomal recessive disorder. Since the wife's brother had SCD, the wife had a 2/3 chance of being a carrier. SCD is most common in people of African descent, and affects 1 of every 375 African American infants. And it is also common in people whose families come from South or Central America (especially Panama), the Caribbean islands, Mediterranean countries (such as Turkey, Greece, and Italy), India, and Saudi Arabia. But it is not common in European Caucasians.

Therefore, the chance of the husband being a carrier would be very low (<1%). And the chance of the couple's firstborn child having SCD would be less than 1% even though the wife had a 2/3 chance of being a carrier.

8. **D**. Fetal hemoglobin (hemoglobin F, HbF, $\alpha^2\gamma^2$) is the main oxygen-transporting protein in the human fetus during the last 7 months of development in the uterus and persists in the newborn until roughly 6 months of age. HbF differs most from adult hemoglobin (HbA) in that it is able to bind oxygen with greater affinity than HbA, giving the developing fetus better access to oxygen from the maternal bloodstream. When fetal hemoglobin production is switched off after birth, normal children begin producing HbA. Children with sickle cell disease (SCD) instead begin producing a defective form of hemoglobin, hemoglobin S (HbS). The defective red blood cells have a greater tendency to lead to vaso-occlusive episodes. Since HbF remains the predominant form of hemoglobin after birth, the number of painful episodes decreases in patients with SCD.

In older infants the amount of HbS will increase as HbF decreases. By 2 years of age, the amount of HbS and HbF stabilizes. *By high-performance liquid chromatography (HPLC), most patients with SCD will have HbS and HbF, but no HbA.* Hemoglobin A2 (HbA2) is a normal variant of hemoglobin A that consists of two alpha and two delta chains ($\alpha^2\delta^2$) and is found at low levels in normal human blood (1.5%–3.1% of all Hb molecules in adults) and is increased in people with SCD.

It is also known that homozygous HbS accounts for 60%–70% of SCD in the United States. Other forms of SCD result from coinheritance of HbS with other abnormal

β-globin-chain variants, the most common forms being sickle hemoglobin C disease (HbSC) and two types of sickle β thalassemia (HbSβ$^+$ thalassemia and HbSβ$^\circ$ thalassemia). Rarer forms result from coinheritance of other Hb variants such as D-Punjab, O-Arab, and E (http://www.ncbi.nlm.nih.gov/books/NBK1377/).

Therefore, HbS and HbF are the most common hemoglobins detectable by HPLC in infants with HBSS, but others may appear (HbA2 is not identifiable because of its very low concentration in patients' blood).

9. **D**. Fetal hemoglobin (hemoglobin F, HbF, or $\alpha^2\gamma^2$) is the main oxygen-transporting protein in the human fetus during the last 7 months of development in the uterus and persists in the newborn until roughly 6 months old. HbF differs most from adult hemoglobin (HbA) in that it is able to bind oxygen with greater affinity than HbA, giving the developing fetus better access to oxygen from the maternal bloodstream. When fetal hemoglobin production is switched off after birth, normal children begin producing HbA. Children with sickle cell disease (SCD) instead begin producing a defective form of hemoglobin, hemoglobin S (HbS). The defective red blood cells have a greater tendency to lead to vaso-occlusive episodes. Since HbF remains the predominant form of hemoglobin after birth, the number of painful episodes decreases in patients with SCD.

In older infants, the amount of HbS will increase as HbF decreases. Hemoglobin A2 (HbA2) is a normal variant of hemoglobin A that consists of two alpha and two delta chains ($\alpha^2\delta^2$) and is found at low levels in normal human blood (1.5%–3.1% of all hemoglobin molecules in adults) and is increased in people with SCD (http://www.ncbi.nlm.nih.gov/books/NBK1377/).

Since this patient had sickle β$^\circ$-thalassemia (HbSβ-thalassemia), he did not have beta chain to synthesize HbA.

Therefore, it would be most likely that he only had HbS and HbF in his blood (HbA2 is not identifiable because of its very low concentration in patients' blood).

10. **D**. Fetal hemoglobin (hemoglobin F, HbF, or $\alpha^2\gamma^2$) is the main oxygen-transporting protein in the human fetus during the last seven 7 months of development in the uterus and persists in the newborn until roughly 6 months of age. HbF differs most from adult hemoglobin (HbA) in that it is able to bind oxygen with greater affinity than HbA, giving the developing fetus better access to oxygen from the maternal bloodstream. When fetal hemoglobin production is switched off after

birth, normal children begin producing HbA. Children with sickle cell disease (SCD) instead begin producing a defective form of hemoglobin, hemoglobin S (HbS). The defective red blood cells have a greater tendency to lead to vaso-occlusive episodes. Since HbF remains the predominant form of hemoglobin after birth, the number of painful episodes decreases in patients with SCD.

In older infants, the amount of HbS will increase as HbF decreases. Hemoglobin A2 (HbA2) is a normal variant of hemoglobin A that consists of two alpha and two delta chains ($\alpha^2\delta^2$) and is found at low levels in normal human blood (1.5%−3.1% of all hemoglobin molecules in adults) and is increased in people with SCD (http://www.ncbi.nlm.nih.gov/books/NBK1377/).

Since this patient had homozygous HbS, he did not beta chain to synthesize HbA.

Therefore, it would be most likely that he only had HbS and HbF in his blood (HbA2 is not identifiable because of its very low concentration in patients' blood).

11. **C.** Fetal hemoglobin (hemoglobin F, HbF, or $\alpha^2\gamma^2$) is the main oxygen-transporting protein in the human fetus during the last 7 months of development in the uterus and persists in the newborn until roughly 6 months of age. HbF differs most from adult hemoglobin (HbA) in that it is able to bind oxygen with greater affinity than HbA, giving the developing fetus better access to oxygen from the maternal bloodstream. When fetal hemoglobin production is switched off after birth, normal children begin producing HbA. Children with sickle cell disease (SCD) instead begin producing a defective form of hemoglobin, hemoglobin S (HbS). The defective red blood cells have a greater tendency to lead to vaso-occlusive episodes. Since HbF remains the predominant form of hemoglobin after birth, the number of painful episodes decreases in patients with SCD.

In older infants, the amount of HbS will increase as HbF decreases. Hemoglobin A2 (HbA2) is a normal variant of hemoglobin A that consists of two alpha and two delta chains ($\alpha^2\delta^2$) and is found at low levels in normal human blood (1.5%−3.1% of all hemoglobin molecules in adults) and is increased in people with SCD (http://www.ncbi.nlm.nih.gov/books/NBK1377/).

Since this patient had sickle β^+-thalassemia (HbSβ^+-thalassemia), he had some beta chains to synthesize HbA.

Therefore, it would be most likely that he had HbS, HbF and HbA in his blood (HbA2 is not identifiable because of its very low concentration in patients' blood).

12. **B.** Fetal hemoglobin (hemoglobin F, HbF, or $\alpha^2\gamma^2$) is the main oxygen-transporting protein in the human fetus during the last 7 months of development in the uterus and persists in the newborn until roughly 6 months of age. HbF differs most from adult hemoglobin (HbA) in that it is able to bind oxygen with greater affinity than HbA, giving the developing fetus better access to oxygen from the maternal bloodstream. When fetal hemoglobin production is switched off after birth, normal children begin producing HbA. Children with sickle cell disease (SCD) instead begin producing a defective form of hemoglobin, hemoglobin S (HbS). The defective red blood cells have a greater tendency to lead to vaso-occlusive episodes. Since HbF remains the predominant form of hemoglobin after birth, the number of painful episodes decreases in patients with SCD.

In older infants, the amount of HbS will increase as HbF decreases. Hemoglobin A2 (HbA2) is a normal variant of hemoglobin A that consists of two alpha and two delta chains ($\alpha^2\delta^2$) and is found at low levels in normal human blood (1.5%−3.1% of all hemoglobin molecules in adults) and is increased in people with SCD (http://www.ncbi.nlm.nih.gov/books/NBK1377/).

Since this patient had sickle hemoglobin C disease (HbSC), he did not have beta chains to synthesize HbA. Therefore, it would be most like that he had HbS, HbF and HbC in his blood (HbA2 is not identifiable because of its very low concentration in patients' blood).

13. **A.** Sickle cell disease (SCD) is characterized by intermittent vaso-occlusive events and chronic hemolytic anemia. Vaso-occlusive events result in tissue ischemia, leading to acute and chronic pain as well as damage to any organ in the body, including the bones, lungs, liver, kidneys, brain, eyes, and joints. Dactylitis (pain and/or swelling of the hands or feet) in infants and young children is often the earliest manifestation of SCD.

SCD is an autosomal recessive disorder encompassing a group of symptomatic diseases associated with pathogenic variants in the *HBB* gene on 11p15.4 and defined by the presence of predominantly hemoglobin S (HbS), or HbS along with other Hb variants that allow for HbS polymerization. Normal adult hemoglobin is a heterotetramer composed of two α-hemoglobin chains and two β-hemoglobin chains (HbA, $\alpha^2\beta^2$). HbS results from a single nucleotide variant in *HBB*, p.Glu6Val. Sickle cell anemia (homozygous HbSS) accounts for 60%−70% of SCD in the United States. Other forms of SCD result from coinheritance of HbS with other abnormal β-globin chain variants, the most common forms being sickle hemoglobin C and two types of sickle β thalassemia (HbSβ$^+$ thalassemia and HbSβ° thalassemia) (http://www.ncbi.nlm.nih.gov/books/NBK1377/).

If a patient has two copies of HbS, he/she does not have normal hemoglobin B protein products. Therefore, no HbA ($\alpha^2\beta^2$) can be synthesized in this patient.

14. **C.** Sickle cell disease (SCD) is characterized by intermittent vaso-occlusive events and chronic hemolytic anemia. Vaso-occlusive events result in tissue ischemia, leading to acute and chronic pain as well as organ damage that can affect any organ in the body, including the bones, lungs, liver, kidneys, brain, eyes, and joints. Dactylitis (pain and/or swelling of the hands or feet) in infants and young children is often the earliest manifestation of SCD.

SCD is an autosomal recessive disorder encompassing a group of symptomatic diseases associated with pathogenic variants in the *HBB* gene on 11p15.4 and defined by the presence of predominantly hemoglobin S (HbS), or HbS along with other Hb variants that allow for HbS polymerization. Normal adult hemoglobin is a heterotetramer composed of two α-hemoglobin chains and two β-hemoglobin chains (HbA, $\alpha^2\beta^2$). HbS results from a single nucleotide variant in *HBB*, p.Glu6Val. Sickle cell anemia (homozygous HbSS) accounts for 60%−70% of SCD in the United States. Other forms of SCD result from coinheritance of HbS with other abnormal β-globin chain variants, the most common forms being sickle hemoglobin C disease (HbSC) and two types of sickle β thalassemia (HbSβ$^+$ thalassemia and HbSβ° thalassemia). *Patients with β$^+$ thalassemia have reduced levels of normal β-globin chains. Patients with β° thalassemia have no β-globin chain synthesis* (http://www.ncbi.nlm.nih.gov/books/NBK1377/).

Therefore, the newborn in this question would most likely have HbSβ$^+$ thalassemia since he/she had HbF, HbS, and HbA.

15. **D.** *Sickle cell disease (SCD) is an autosomal recessive disease encompassing a group of symptomatic disorders associated with pathogenic variants in the* HBB *gene on 11p15.4 and defined by the presence of predominantly hemoglobin S (HbS), or HbS along with other Hb variants that allow for HbS polymerization. Normal adult hemoglobin is a heterotetramer composed of two α-hemoglobin chains and two β-hemoglobin chains (HbA, $\alpha^2\beta^2$).* HbS results from a single nucleotide variant in HBB, p. Glu6Val. *Sickle cell anemia (homozygous HbSS) accounts for 60%−70% of SCD in the United*

States. Other forms of SCD result from coinheritance of HbS with other abnormal β-globin chain variants, the most common forms being sickle hemoglobin C disease (HbSC) and two types of sickle β thalassemia (HbSβ$^+$ thalassemia and HbSβ° thalassemia). Patients with β$^+$ thalassemia have reduced levels of normal β-globin chains. Patients with β° thalassemia have no β-globin-chain synthesis (http://www.ncbi.nlm.nih.gov/books/NBK1377/).

This newborn in this question had only HbF and HbS, so that he might have sickle cell anemia (homozygous HbS), or sickle β° thalassemia. The p.Glu6Lys variant in the *HBB* gene results in HbC. The p.Glu26Lys variant in the *HBB* gene results in HbE. Therefore, it would be most likely that he/she was homozygous for the p.Glu6Val variant related to HbS in *HBB*.

16. **B.** *Sickle cell disease (SCD) is an autosomal recessive disease encompassing a group of symptomatic disorders associated with pathogenic variants in the* HBB *gene on 11p15.4 and defined by the presence of predominantly hemoglobin S (HbS), or HbS along with other Hb variants that allow for HbS polymerization. Normal adult hemoglobin is a heterotetramer composed of two α-hemoglobin chains and two β-hemoglobin chains (HbA, $\alpha^2\beta^2$).* HbS results from a single nucleotide variant in HBB, p. Glu6Val. *Sickle cell anemia (homozygous HbSS) accounts for 60%−70% of SCD in the United States.* Other forms of SCD result from coinheritance of HbS with other abnormal β-globin chain variants, the most common forms being sickle hemoglobin C disease (HbSC) and two types of sickle β thalassemia (HbSβ$^+$ thalassemia and HbSβ° thalassemia). Patients with β$^+$ thalassemia have reduced levels of normal β-globin chains. Patients with β° thalassemia have no β-globin chain synthesis (http://www.ncbi.nlm.nih.gov/books/NBK1377/).

The newborn in this question had only HbF and HbS, so he might have sickle cell anemia (homozygous HbSS), or sickle β° thalassemia. The p.Glu6Lys variant results in HbC. The p.Glu26Lys variant results in HbE. The p.Glu121Lys variant results in HbO. Therefore, it would be most likely that he/she was homozygous for the p.Glu6Val variant in *HBB*.

17. **D.** *Sickle cell disease (SCD) is an autosomal recessive disease encompassing a group of symptomatic disorders associated with pathogenic variants in the* HBB *gene on 11p15.4 and defined by the presence of predominantly hemoglobin S (HbS), or HbS along with other Hb variants that allow for HbS polymerization. Normal adult hemoglobin is a*

heterotetramer composed of two α hemoglobin chains and two β hemoglobin chains (HbA, α²β²). *HbS results from a single nucleotide variant in* HBB, *p. Glu6Val.* Sickle cell anemia (homozygous HbSS) accounts for 60% to 70% of SCD in the United States. Other forms of SCD result from coinheritance of HbS with other abnormal β-globin chain variants, the most common forms being sickle hemoglobin C disease (HbSC) and two types of sickle β-thalassemia (HbSβ⁺ thalassemia and HbSβ° thalassemia). Patients with β⁺ thalassemia have reduced levels of normal β-globin chains. Patients with β° thalassemia have no β-globin chain synthesis (http://www.ncbi.nlm.nih.gov/books/NBK1377/).

This newborn had HbF, HbS, and HbC so that he has sickle hemoglobin C disease (HbSC). *The p. Glu6Lys variant results in HbC.* Therefore, it would be most likely that he/she had compound heterozygous p.Glu6Val and p.Glu6Lys variants in *HBB.*

18. **B**. *Sickle cell disease (SCD) is an autosomal recessive disease encompassing a group of symptomatic disorders associated with pathogenic variants in the* HBB *gene on 11p15.4 and defined by the presence of predominantly hemoglobin S (HbS), or HbS along with other Hb variants that allow for HbS polymerization.* Normal adult hemoglobin is a heterotetramer composed of two α-hemoglobin chains and two β-hemoglobin chains (HbA, α²β²). *HbS results from a single nucleotide variant in* HBB, *p. Glu6Val.* Sickle cell anemia (homozygous HbSS) accounts for 60%–70% of SCD in the United States. Other forms of SCD result from coinheritance of HbS with other abnormal β-globin chain variants, the most common forms being sickle hemoglobin C disease (HbSC) and two types of sickle β thalassemia (HbSβ⁺ thalassemia and HbSβ° thalassemia). Patients with β⁺ thalassemia have reduced levels of normal β-globin chains. Patients with β° thalassemia have no β-globin chain synthesis (http://www.ncbi.nlm.nih.gov/books/NBK1377/).

This newborn had HbF, HbS, and HbC, so he has sickle hemoglobin C disease (HbSC). *The p. Glu6Lys variant results in HbC.* The p.Glu26Lys variant results in HbE. Therefore, it would be most likely that he/she had compound heterozygous p.Glu6Val and p.Glu6Lys variants in *HBB.*

19. **F**. *Sickle cell disease (SCD) is an autosomal recessive disease encompassing a group of symptomatic disorders associated with pathogenic variants in the* HBB *gene on 11p15.4 and defined by the presence of predominantly hemoglobin S (HbS), or HbS along with other Hb variants that allow for HbS*

polymerization. Normal adult hemoglobin is a heterotetramer composed of two α-hemoglobin chains and two β-hemoglobin chains (HbA, α²β²). *HbS results from a single nucleotide variant in* HBB, *p. Glu6Val.* Sickle cell anemia (homozygous HbSS) accounts for 60%–70% of SCD in the United States. Other forms of SCD result from coinheritance of HbS with other abnormal β-globin chain variants, the most common forms being sickle hemoglobin C disease (HbSC) and two types of sickle β thalassemia (HbSβ⁺ thalassemia and HbSβ° thalassemia). Patients with β⁺ thalassemia have reduced levels of normal β-globin chains. Patients with β° thalassemia have no β-globin chain synthesis (http://www.ncbi.nlm.nih.gov/books/NBK1377/). Most SCD results from the following variants:

Hemoglobin S (Glu6Val pathogenic variant)
Hemoglobin C (HbC; Glu6Lys pathogenic variant)
Hemoglobin D (D-Punjab; Glu121Gln pathogenic variant)
Hemoglobin E (HbE; Glu26Lys pathogenic variant)
Hemoglobin O (O-Arab; Glu121Lys pathogenic variant)

This newborn had only HbF, HbS, and HbE so that he has sickle hemoglobin E disease (HbSE). Therefore, it would be most likely that he/she had compound heterozygous p.Glu6Val and p. Glu26Lys variants in *HBB.*

20. **D**. *Sickle cell disease (SCD) is an autosomal recessive disease encompassing a group of symptomatic disorders associated with pathogenic variants in the* HBB *gene on 11p15.4 and defined by the presence of predominantly hemoglobin S (HbS), or HbS along with other Hb variants that allow for HbS polymerization.* Normal adult hemoglobin is a heterotetramer composed of two α-hemoglobin chains and two β-hemoglobin chains (HbA, α²β²). HbS results from a single nucleotide variant in *HBB*, p.Glu6Val. Sickle cell anemia (homozygous HbSS) accounts for 60%–70% SCD in the United States. Other forms of SCD result from coinheritance of HbS with other abnormal β-globin chain variants, the most common forms being sickle hemoglobin C disease (HbSC) and two types of sickle β thalassemia (HbSβ⁺ thalassemia and HbSβ° thalassemia). Patients with β⁺ thalassemia have reduced levels of normal β-globin chains. Patients with β° thalassemia have no β-globin chain synthesis (http://www.ncbi.nlm.nih.gov/books/NBK1377/). Most of SCD results from the following variants:

Hemoglobin S (HbC; Glu6Val pathogenic variant)
Hemoglobin C (HbC; Glu6Lys pathogenic variant)

Hemoglobin D (D-Punjab; Glu121Gln pathogenic variant)

Hemoglobin E (HbE; Glu26Lys pathogenic variant)
Hemoglobin O (O-Arab; Glu121Lys pathogenic variant)

This newborn had only HbF, HbC, and HbE so that he has sickle hemoglobin E disease (HbSE). Therefore, it would be most likely that he/she had compound heterozygous p.Glu6Lys and p. Glu26Lys variants in *HBB*.

21. **C.** All 50 U.S. states provide universal newborn screening (NBS) for sickle cell disease (SCD) to identify infants with SCD because of the high morbidity and mortality rate. Screening also identifies infants with other hemoglobinopathies, hemoglobinopathy carriers, and in some states, infants with alpha-thalassemia syndromes.

The majority of NBS programs perform isoelectric focusing (IEF) of an eluate of dried blood spots. A few programs use high-performance liquid chromatography (HPLC), DNA testing, or cellulose acetate electrophoresis as the initial screening method. Specimens with abnormal screening results are retested using a second, complementary electrophoretic technique, HPLC, citrate agar, IEF, or DNA-based assay. Infants with hemoglobins that suggest SCD or other clinically significant hemoglobinopathies require confirmatory testing of a separate blood sample *within 6 weeks.* The sensitivity and specificity of current NBS methods is excellent, and 99% of U.S. infants at highest risk for SCD are born in states with universal screening (http://www.ncbi.nlm.nih.gov/books/NBK1377/).

Therefore, it would be most likely that the complementary test was done within in 6 weeks.

22. **B.** Sickle cell disease (SCD) is an autosomal recessive disease encompassing a group of symptomatic disorders associated with pathogenic variants in the *HBB* gene on 11p15.4 and defined by the presence of predominantly hemoglobin S (HbS), or HbS along with other Hb variants that allow for HbS polymerization. Normal adult hemoglobin is a heterotetramer composed of two α-hemoglobin chains and two β-hemoglobin chains (HbA, $\alpha^2\beta^2$). HbS results from a single nucleotide variant in *HBB*, p. Glu6Val. Sickle cell anemia (homozygous HbSS) accounts for 60%−70% of SCD in the United States. *Patients with sickle cell anemia (homozygous HbSS) have no β-globin chain synthesis.* Other forms of SCD result from coinheritance of HbS with other abnormal β-globin chain variants, the most common forms being sickle hemoglobin C disease (HbSC) and two types of sickle β thalassemia

(HbSβ⁺ thalassemia and HbSβ° thalassemia). Patients with β⁺ thalassemia have reduced levels of normal β-globin chains. *Patients with β° thalassemia have no β-globin chain synthesis* (http://www.ncbi.nlm.nih.gov/books/NBK1377/).

This newborn has only HbF and HbS, so may have sickle cell anemia (homozygous HbS), or sickle β° thalassemia. Therefore, it would be most likely that he was offered a molecular genetic study for the *HBB* gene to distinguish sickle cell anemia (homozygous HbS) from sickle β° thalassemia as the next step in the workup for a diagnosis.

23. **B.** Sickle cell disease (SCD) is an autosomal recessive disease encompassing a group of symptomatic disorders associated with pathogenic variants in the *HBB* gene on 11p15.4 and defined by the presence of predominantly hemoglobin S (HbS), or HbS along with other Hb variants that allow for HbS polymerization. Normal adult hemoglobin is a heterotetramer composed of two α-hemoglobin chains and two β-hemoglobin chains (HbA, $\alpha^2\beta^2$). HbS results from a single nucleotide variant in *HBB*, p.Glu6Val. Sickle cell anemia (homozygous HbS) accounts for 60%−70% of SCD in the United States. Patients with sickle cell anemia (homozygous HbS) have no β-globin chain synthesis. Other forms of SCD result from coinheritance of HbS with other abnormal β-globin chain variants, the most common forms being sickle hemoglobin C disease (HbSC) and two types of sickle β thalassemia (HbSβ⁺ thalassemia and HbSβ° thalassemia). Patients with β⁺ thalassemia have reduced levels of normal β-globin chains. Patients with β° thalassemia have no β-globin chain synthesis (http://www.ncbi.nlm.nih.gov/books/NBK1377/).

Regardless of the outcome of testing in the newborn period, additional testing that should be done at about age 1 year (once HbF levels have fallen) includes a CBC, reticulocyte count, some type of electrophoresis or high-performance liquid chromatography (HPLC), a measure of iron status, and inclusion body preparation with BCB (brilliant cresyl blue) stain. Together, these help to determine whether there is a coexisting thalassemia component, and if so, if it is α thalassemia or β thalassemia. This is important for genetic counseling and for providing insight into disease-specific outcomes.

Therefore, it is appropriate for this patient to have a checkup at 1 year if there were no acute symptoms.

24. **C.** Fetal hemoglobin (HbF, $\alpha^2\gamma^2$) is the main oxygen-transporting protein in the human fetus

during the last 7 months of development in the uterus and persists in the newborn until roughly 6 months of age. Functionally, HbF differs most from adult hemoglobin (HbA, $\alpha^2\beta^2$) in that it is able to bind oxygen with greater affinity than the adult form, giving the developing fetus better access to oxygen from the mother's bloodstream. In newborns, HbF ($\alpha^2\gamma^2$) is nearly completely replaced by HbA ($\alpha^2\beta^2$) by approximately 6 months after birth, except in a few thalassemia cases, in which there may be a delay in cessation of HbF production until 3–5 years of age. *In adults, HbF ($\alpha^2\gamma^2$) production can be reactivated pharmacologically by hydroxycarbamide (Hydrea), which is useful in the treatment of diseases such as sickle cell disease (SCD). It is the only FDA-approved therapy for sickle cell disease.*

Hemoglobin A2 (HbA2, $\alpha^2\delta^2$) is a normal variant of HbA that consists of two alpha and two delta chains and is found at low levels in normal human blood. HbA2 may be increased in beta thalassemia or in people who are heterozygous for the beta-thalassemia gene. HbA2 exists in small amounts in all adult humans (1.5%–3.1% of all hemoglobin molecules) and is increased in people with SCD. Hemoglobin Portland (Hb Portland, $\zeta^2\gamma^2$) exists at low levels during embryonic and fetal life and is composed of two zeta chains and two gamma chains.

Therefore, it would be most likely that HbF was induced pharmacologically to treat SCD in this adolescent.

25. **C.** Fetal hemoglobin (HbF, $\alpha^2\gamma^2$) is the main oxygen-transporting protein in the human fetus during the last 7 months of development in the uterus and persists in the newborn until roughly 6 months of age. Functionally, HbF differs most from adult hemoglobin (HbA, $\alpha^2\beta^2$) in that it is able to bind oxygen with greater affinity than the adult form, giving the developing fetus better access to oxygen from the mother's bloodstream. In newborns, HbF ($\alpha^2\gamma^2$) is nearly completely replaced by HbA ($\alpha^2\beta^2$) by approximately 6 months postnatally, except in a few thalassemia cases in which there may be a delay in cessation of HbF production until 3–5 years of age. *In adults, HbF ($\alpha^2\gamma^2$) production can be reactivated pharmacologically by hydroxycarbamide (Hydrea), which is useful in the treatment of diseases such as sickle cell disease (SCD). It is the only FDA-approved therapy for sickle cell disease.*

Hemoglobin A2 (HbA2, $\alpha^2\delta^2$) is a normal variant of HbA that consists of two alpha and two delta chains and is found at low levels in normal human blood. HbA2 may be increased in beta thalassemia or in people who are heterozygous

for the beta-thalassemia gene. HbA2 exists in small amounts in all adult humans (1.5%–3.1% of all Hb molecules) and is increased in people with SCD. Hemoglobin Portland (Hb Portland, $\zeta^2\gamma^2$) exists at low levels during embryonic and fetal life and is composed of two zeta chains and two gamma chains.

Therefore, it would be most likely that $\alpha^2\gamma^2$ was induced pharmacologically to treat SCD in this adolescent.

26. **C.** Fetal hemoglobin (HbF, $\alpha^2\gamma^2$) is the main oxygen-transporting protein in the human fetus during the last 7 months of development in the uterus and persists in the newborn until roughly 6 months of age. Functionally, HbF differs most from adult hemoglobin (HbA, $\alpha^2\beta^2$) in that it is able to bind oxygen with greater affinity than the adult form, giving the developing fetus better access to oxygen from the mother's bloodstream. In newborns, HbF is nearly completely replaced by HbA ($\alpha^2\beta^2$) by approximately 6 months after birth, except in a few thalassemia cases in which there may be a delay in cessation of HbF production until 3–5 years of age. *In adults, HbF ($\alpha^2\gamma^2$) production can be reactivated pharmacologically by hydroxycarbamide (Hydrea), which is useful in the treatment of diseases such as sickle cell disease (SCD). It is the only FDA-approved therapy for sickle cell disease.*

all-*trans* retinoic acid (ATRA) is the first-line drug for patients with acute promyelocytic leukemia (APML, APL). Vemurafenib (Zelboraf) and dabrafenib (Tafinlar) are drugs for patients with *BRAF* V600E mutation−positive metastatic melanoma, thyroid cancer, lung cancer, and so forth. Gleevec (imatinib) is the medicine for patients with t(9;22) positive chronic myeloid leukemia (CML).

Therefore, it would be most likely that the physician prescribed hydroxyurea to treat SCD in this adolescent.

27. **A.** Sickle cell disease (SCD) encompasses a group of symptomatic disorders associated with pathogenic variants in *HBB* and is defined by the presence of predominantly hemoglobin S (HbS), or HbS along with other Hb variants that allow for HbS polymerization. Normal human hemoglobin is a heterotetramer composed of two α-hemoglobin chains and two β-hemoglobin chains. Hemoglobin S results from a single nucleotide variant in *HBB*, resulting in the sixth amino acid in the β-hemoglobin chain changing from glutamic acid to valine (p.Glu6Val).

Hemoglobin SS disease is the predominant hemoglobin in people with SCD. The alpha chain is normal. The disease-causing mutation exists in the beta chain, giving the molecule the structure, $\alpha^2\beta^{S2}$. Patients with hemoglobin SS disease have no β-globin chain synthesis.

Hemoglobin SC disease is caused by a copy of hemoglobin S gene inherited from one parent, and a hemoglobin C gene inherited from the other. The hemoglobin C molecule disturbs the red-cell metabolism only slightly. However, the disturbance is enough to allow the deleterious effects of the hemoglobin S to be manifested. On average, patients with hemoglobin SC disease have milder symptoms than do those with hemoglobin SS disease, and have more severe symptoms than do those with homozygous hemoglobin C disease.

A number of other syndromes exist that involve a hemoglobin S compound heterozygous state. They are less common than hemoglobin SC disease. Hemoglobin SE disease is caused by a copy of hemoglobin S gene inherited from one parent and a copy of hemoglobin E gene inherited from the other. People with hemoglobin E disease have a mild hemolytic anemia and mild splenomegaly. Hemoglobin E trait is benign. Hemoglobin E is extremely common in Southeast Asia and in some areas equals hemoglobin A in frequency. The expression of a single hemoglobin S gene normally produces no problem (e.g., sickle cell trait).

Sickle/beta thalassemia causes by a copy of hemoglobin S gene inherited from one parent and a copy of beta thalassemia gene inherited from the other. The severity of the condition is determined to a large extent by the quantity of normal hemoglobin produced by the beta-thalassemia gene. If the gene produces no normal hemoglobin (β° thalassemia), the condition is virtually identical to SCD. Patients with sickle/β° thalassemia have no β-globin chain synthesis. Some patients have a gene that produces a small amount of normal hemoglobin, called β⁺ thalassemia. Patients with sickle/β⁺ thalassemia have an amount of hemoglobin A that depends on the level of function of the β⁺-thalassemia gene. The severity of the condition is dampened when significant quantities of normal hemoglobin are produced by the β⁺-thalassemia gene. Sickle/beta thalassemia is the most common sickle syndrome seen in people of Mediterranean descent (Italian, Greek, and Turkish). Beta thalassemia is quite common in this region, and the sickle cell mutation occurs in some sections of these countries (http://www.ncbi.nlm. nih.gov/books/NBK1377/).

Therefore, HbS and HbS is the most severe form of SCD in the list.

28. D. Sickle cell disease (SCD) encompasses a group of symptomatic disorders associated with pathogenic variants in *HBB* and defined by the presence of predominantly hemoglobin S (HbS), or HbS along with other Hb variants that allow for HbS polymerization. Normal human hemoglobin is a heterotetramer composed of two α-hemoglobin chains and two β-hemoglobin chains. Hemoglobin S results from a single nucleotide variant in *HBB*, resulting in the sixth amino acid in the β-hemoglobin chain changing from glutamic acid to valine (p.Glu6Val).

Hemoglobin SS disease is the predominant hemoglobin in people with SCD. The alpha chain is normal. The disease causing mutation exists in the beta chain, giving the molecule the structure, $\alpha^2\beta^{S2}$. *Patients with hemoglobin SS disease have no β-globin chain synthesis.*

Hemoglobin SC disease is caused by a copy of the hemoglobin S gene inherited from one parent and a hemoglobin C gene inherited from the other. The hemoglobin C molecule disturbs the red-cell metabolism only slightly. However, the disturbance is enough to allow the deleterious effects of the hemoglobin S to be manifested. On average, patients with hemoglobin SC disease have milder symptoms than do those with hemoglobin SS disease and have more severe symptoms than do those with homozygous hemoglobin C disease.

A number of other syndromes exist that involve a hemoglobin S compound heterozygous state. They are less common than hemoglobin SC disease. Hemoglobin SE disease is caused by a copy of the hemoglobin S gene inherited from one parent and a copy of the hemoglobin E gene inherited from the other. People with hemoglobin E disease have a mild hemolytic anemia and mild splenomegaly. Hemoglobin E trait is benign. Hemoglobin E is extremely common in Southeast Asia and in some areas equals hemoglobin A in frequency. The expression of a single hemoglobin S gene normally produces no problem (for example sickle cell trait).

Sickle/beta thalassemia causes by a copy of hemoglobin S gene inherited from one parent and a copy of the beta-thalassemia gene inherited from the other. The severity of the condition is determined to a large extent by the quantity of normal hemoglobin produced by the beta-thalassemia gene. If the gene produces no normal hemoglobin (β° thalassemia), the condition is virtually identical to SCD. *Patients with sickle/β° thalassemia have no β-globin chain synthesis.* Some patients have a gene that produces a small amount of normal hemoglobin, called β⁺ thalassemia. Patients with sickle/β⁺ thalassemia have an amount of hemoglobin A that depends on the level of function of the β^+-thalassemia gene. The severity of the condition is dampened when significant quantities of normal hemoglobin are produced by the β^+-thalassemia gene. Sickle/beta thalassemia is the most common sickle syndrome seen in people of Mediterranean descent (Italian, Greek, and Turkish). Beta thalassemia is quite common in this region, and the sickle cell mutation occurs in some sections of these countries (http://www.ncbi.nlm.nih.gov/books/NBK1377/).

Therefore, hemoglobin S and β° thalassemia (Hbβ°) is the most severe form of SCD in the list.

29. **A.** Sickle cell disease encompasses a group of symptomatic disorders associated with pathogenic variants in *HBB* and defined by the presence of predominantly hemoglobin S (HbS), or HbS along with other Hb variants that allow for HbS polymerization. Normal human hemoglobin is a heterotetramer composed of two α-hemoglobin chains and two β-hemoglobin chains. Hemoglobin S results from a single nucleotide variant in *HBB*, resulting in the sixth amino acid in the β-hemoglobin chain changing from glutamic acid to valine (p.Glu6Val).

Hemoglobin SS disease is the predominant hemoglobin in people with SCD. The alpha chain is normal. The disease-producing mutation exists in the beta chain, giving the molecule the structure, $\alpha^2\beta^{S2}$. Patients with hemoglobin SS disease have no β-globin-chain synthesis.

Hemoglobin SC disease is caused by a copy of the hemoglobin S gene inherited from one parent and a hemoglobin C gene inherited from the other. The hemoglobin C molecule disturbs the red-cell metabolism only slightly. However, the disturbance is enough to allow the deleterious effects of hemoglobin S to be manifested. On average, patients with hemoglobin SC disease have milder symptoms than do those with hemoglobin SS disease and have more severe symptoms than do those with homozygous hemoglobin C disease.

A number of other syndromes exist that involve a hemoglobin S compound heterozygous state. They are less common than hemoglobin SC disease. Hemoglobin SE disease is caused by a copy of the hemoglobin S gene inherited from one parent and a copy of the hemoglobin E gene inherited from the other. People with hemoglobin E disease have a mild hemolytic anemia and mild splenomegaly. Hemoglobin E trait is benign. Hemoglobin E is extremely common in Southeast Asia and in some areas equals hemoglobin A in frequency. The expression of a single hemoglobin S gene normally produces no problem (e.g., sickle cell trait).

Sickle/beta thalassemia is caused by a copy of the hemoglobin S gene inherited from one parent and a copy of the beta-thalassemia gene inherited from the other. The severity of the condition is determined to a large extent by the quantity of normal hemoglobin produced by the beta-thalassemia gene. If the gene produces no normal hemoglobin (β° thalassemia), the condition is virtually identical to SCD. Patients with sickle/β° thalassemia have no β-globin-chain synthesis. Some patients have a gene that produces a small amount of normal hemoglobin, called β^+ thalassemia. Patients with sickle/β^+ thalassemia have an amount of hemoglobin A that depends on the level of function of the β^+-thalassemia gene. The severity of the condition is dampened when significant quantities of normal hemoglobin are produced by the β^+-thalassemia gene. *On average, patients with hemoglobin S and β° thalassemia with α-thalassemia trait have reduced clinical severity as compared with patients with hemoglobin S and β° thalassemia due to less of an imbalance between alpha and beta hemoglobins* (http://www.ncbi.nlm.nih.gov/books/NBK1377/).

Therefore, hemoglobin S and S (HbSS) is the most severe form of SCD in the list.

30. **C.** Sickle cell disease (SCD) encompasses a group of symptomatic disorders associated with pathogenic variants in *HBB* and defined by the presence of predominantly hemoglobin S (HbS), or HbS along with other Hb variants that allow for HbS polymerization. Normal adult human hemoglobin is a heterotetramer composed of two α-hemoglobin chains and two β-hemoglobin chains. Hemoglobin S results from a single nucleotide variant in *HBB*, resulting in the sixth amino acid in the β-hemoglobin chain changing from glutamic acid to valine (p.Glu6Val). Sickle cell anemia (homozygous HbS) accounts for 60%–70% of sickle cell disease in the United States. Other forms of sickle cell disease result from coinheritance of HbS with other abnormal β-globin chain variants, the most common forms being sickle hemoglobin C disease (HbC) and two types of sickle β thalassemia (HbSβ^+ thalassemia and HbSβ° thalassemia) (http://www.ncbi.nlm.nih.gov/books/NBK1377/).

Even when only one parent has the sickle cell trait, a couple still may have children with SCD. They can have children with compound heterozygous forms of SCD, such as hemoglobin SC disease (HbSC), sickle/beta thalassemia (HbSβ° or HbSβ^+), and hemoglobin SE disease (HbSE). In this case, a negative test for the presence of *HBB* Glu6Val mutation for HbS does not exclude the presence of other abnormal beta hemoglobins, which may lead to an asymptomatic thalassemia trait in the father.

A glucose 6-phosphate dehydrogenase (G6PD) deficiency and hereditary elliptocytosis are both common among African Americans. But they are not caused mutations in hemoglobin genes. The alpha-thalassemia trait and Hemoglobin Constant Spring (Hb^{CS}) trait are both abnormalities of the alpha-globin, rather than the beta-globin, locus. *Among the possible answers, only the beta-thalassemia trait is an abnormality of the beta globin.*

Therefore, it would most likely that the father had beta-thalassemia trait so that the child in question had sickle/beta thalassemia.

31. **D.** Alpha thalassemia (α thalassemia) has two clinically significant forms: hemoglobin Barts hydrops fetalis (Hb Barts) syndrome and hemoglobin H (HbH) disease (see the table below). Hb Barts syndrome is the more severe form. Death usually occurs in the neonatal period. A 5-year-old patient with alpha thalassemia most likely has HbH disease. Hemoglobin patterns in HbH disease are as shown in the table.

Hemoglobin type	Structure	Normal, birth	Normal, adult	HbH disease	Hydrops fetalis
HbA	$\alpha_2\beta_2$	20%−25%	96%−98%	60%−90%	NA
HbF	$\alpha_2\gamma_2$	75%−80%	<1%	<1.0%	NA
HbA$_2$	$\alpha_2\delta_2$	0.5%	2%−3%	<2.0%	NA
HbH	β_4	NA	NA	5%−30%, *adult* 20%−40%, *birth*	NA
Hb Bart	γ_4	NA	NA	2%−5%	100%

(https://www.cdc.gov/ncbddd/sicklecell/documents/nbs_hemoglobinopathy-testing_122015.pdf).

Therefore, it would be most likely that HbH increased significantly in this patient.

32. **C.** Beta thalassemia (β thalassemia) is characterized by reduced synthesis of the hemoglobin subunit beta resulting in microcytic hypochromic anemia. Patients with β thalassemia have decreased amounts of HbA and *increased amounts of hemoglobin F (HbF)* in peripheral-blood samples after age 12 months (http://www.ncbi.nlm.nih.gov/books/NBK1426/).

Therefore, it would be most likely that HbF increased significantly in this patient.

33. **C.** Both of the parents had a 2/3 chance to be a carrier of sickle cell disease (SCD), since they had siblings with SCD. The prior probability of the couple having a SCD child is $2/3 \times 2/3 = 4/9$. Bayesian analysis for the carrier probability of both parents being carriers is 1/81 (see the table below). Therefore, the risk of their next child with SCD would be $1/81 \times 1/4 = 1/324$.

	Carrier	Noncarrier
Prior probability	$2/3 \times 2/3 = 4/9$	$1 - (2/3 \times 2/3) = 5/9$
Conditional probability	$(1/4)^3 = 1/64$	1
Joint probability	$4/9 \times 1/64 = 1/144$	$5/9 \times 1 = 80/144$
Posterior probability	$\dfrac{1/144}{1/144 + 80/144}$	$= 1/81$

34. **B.** Alpha thalassemia is a nonneoplastic hematological disorder that reduces the production of hemoglobin because of the impaired production of 1, 2, 3, or 4 alpha-globin chains, leading to a relative excess of beta-globin chains. The degree of impairment is based on which clinical phenotype is present (how many chains are affected). Testing for α thalassemia includes hematological testing of red-blood-cell indices, peripheral-blood smear, supravital staining to detect RBC inclusion bodies, and qualitative and quantitative hemoglobin analysis. *HBA1*, the gene encoding α1-globin, and *HBA2*, the gene encoding α2-globin, are the two genes most commonly associated with α thalassemia. *Molecular genetic testing of HBA1 and HBA2 detects deletions in about 90% and point mutations in about 10% of affected individuals.*

Chromosome microarray analysis (CMA) is the first-line test for individuals with multiple congenital anomalies, developmental delay, intellectual disability, and autism; it is used to detect copy-number gain or loss. The ACMG has recommended CMA as the first-line test for individuals with multiple congenital anomalies, developmental delay, intellectual disability, and autism. Multiplex ligation-dependent probe amplification (MLPA) is a time-efficient technique to detect genomic deletions and insertions bigger than single-nucleotide variants and in/dels, but smaller than what CMA can detect. Next-generation sequencing (NGS) is a high-throughput test to sequence multiple genes at the same time. It is an appropriate test for Fanconi anemia, hearing loss, and other disorders. Sanger sequencing is the most appropriate molecular test for single-gene disorders when the most pathogenic variants are single nucleotide variants and in/dels. It is an appropriate test for Gaucher disease, Wiskott—Aldrich syndrome (WAS), and other disorders.

Exonic and whole-gene deletions/duplications in *HBA1* and *HBA2* are not readily detectable by sequence analysis of the coding and flanking intronic regions of genomic DNA. The most common form of alpha (+) thalassemia seen in the

United States is due to the $-\alpha^{3.7}$ deletion, which is too small to be detected by CMA. Therefore, MLPA would most likely be used for the alpha-thalassemia test in this patient.

35. **A.** *Sickle cell disease (SCD) is an autosomal recessive disorder of hemoglobin in which β-subunit genes have a missense mutation that substitutes valine for glutamic acid at amino acid 6 (p.Glu6Val).* The p.Glu6Val mutation in β globin decreases the solubility of deoxygenated hemoglobin and causes it to form a gelatinous network of stiff fibrous polymers that distort red blood cells, giving them a sickle shape (http://www.ncbi.nlm.nih.gov/books/NBK1377/).

    Therefore, in patients with SCD, the missense p.Glu6Val mutation is responsible for the unique properties of HbS.

36. **A.** Sickle cell disease (SCD) encompasses a group of symptomatic disorders associated with pathogenic variants in *HBB* and defined by the presence of predominantly hemoglobin S (Hb S), or HbS along with other Hb variants that allow for HbS polymerization. Normal human hemoglobin is a heterotetramer composed of two α-hemoglobin chains and two β-hemoglobin chains. Hemoglobin S results from a single nucleotide variant in *HBB*, changing the sixth amino acid in the β-hemoglobin chain from glutamic acid to valine (p.Glu6Val).

    In deoxygenated sickle hemoglobin, an interaction between the p.Glu6Val residue and the complementary regions on adjacent molecules can result in the formation of highly ordered insoluble molecular polymers that aggregate and distort the shape of the red blood cells, making them brittle and poorly deformable, increasing adherence to the endothelium. This can lead to veno-occlusion and potentially decreased tissue perfusion and ischemia (http://www.ncbi.nlm.nih.gov/books/NBK1377/).

    Therefore, a missense mutation in *HBB* leads to decreased elasticity of red blood cells in globin Hb S.

37. **A.** All four alpha-globin alleles are deleted or inactivated in Hb Barts syndrome. Deletion or dysfunction of three alleles results in HbH disease. Alpha° thalassemia results from deletion or dysfunction of two alleles, and *α^{+} thalassemia results from deletion or dysfunction of one allele* (http://www.ncbi.nlm.nih.gov/books/NBK1377/).

    Therefore, 1 out of 4 alpha alleles in *HBA1* and *HBA2* is not functional in patients with α^{+} thalassemia.

38. **B.** All four alpha-globin alleles are deleted or inactivated in Hb Barts syndrome. Deletion or dysfunction of three alleles results in HbH disease (3/4). *Alpha° thalassemia results from*

deletion or dysfunction of two alleles (2/4), and α^{+} thalassemia results from deletion or dysfunction of one allele (1/4) (http://www.ncbi.nlm.nih.gov/books/NBK1377/).

    Therefore, 2 out of 4 alpha alleles in *HBA1* and *HBA2* is not functional in patients with α° thalassemia.

39. **C.** All four α globin alleles are deleted or inactivated in Hb Bart syndrome (4/4). *Deletion or dysfunction of three alleles results in HbH disease (3/4).* thalassemia results from deletion or dysfunction of two alleles, and α^{+} thalassemia results from deletion or dysfunction of one allele (http://www.ncbi.nlm.nih.gov/books/NBK1377/).

    Therefore, 3 out of 4 alpha alleles in *HBA1* and *HBA2* are not functional in patients with Hb H disease.

40. **D.** *All four α-globin alleles are deleted or inactivated in Hb Barts syndrome.* Deletion or dysfunction of three alleles results in HbH disease (3/4). Alpha°-thalassemia results from deletion or dysfunction of two alleles, and α^{+}-thalassemia results from deletion or dysfunction of one allele (http://www.ncbi.nlm.nih.gov/books/NBK1377/).

    Therefore, all 4 alpha alleles in *HBA1* and *HBA2* are not functional in patients with Hb Bart disease.

41. **A.** *HBA1*, encoding α1-globin, and *HBA2*, encoding α2-globin, are the two genes associated with α thalassemia. They are localized to the telomeric region of chromosome 1613.3 in a cluster containing the embryonically expressed *HBZ* encoding ζ globin and a *cis*-acting regulatory element, HS-40, located 40 kb upstream of *HBZ* (see Fig. 6.2).

    The most common cause of alpha thalassemia is deletions. The most common form of alpha thalassemia seen in the United States is due to the $\alpha^{3.7}$ deletion and is present in approximately 30% of African Americans (http://www.ncbi.nlm.nih.gov/books/NBK1377/). Therefore, deletion is most common in patients with alpha thalassemia in comparison with other types of variants.

42. **A.** Alpha thalassemia is a nonneoplastic hematological disorder involving the genes *HBA1* and *HBA2*. *HBA1*, encoding α1-globin, and *HBA2*, encoding α2-globin, are localized to the telomeric region of chromosome 16p13.3 in a cluster. Molecular genetic testing of *HBA1* and *HBA2* detects deletions in about 90% and point mutations in about 10% of affected individuals. The most common deletions for alpha thalassemia remove *one* ($-\alpha^{3.7}$ and $-\alpha^{4.2}$) or both ($--^{Med}$ and $--^{SEA}$) of the α genes, as do the unusual deletions

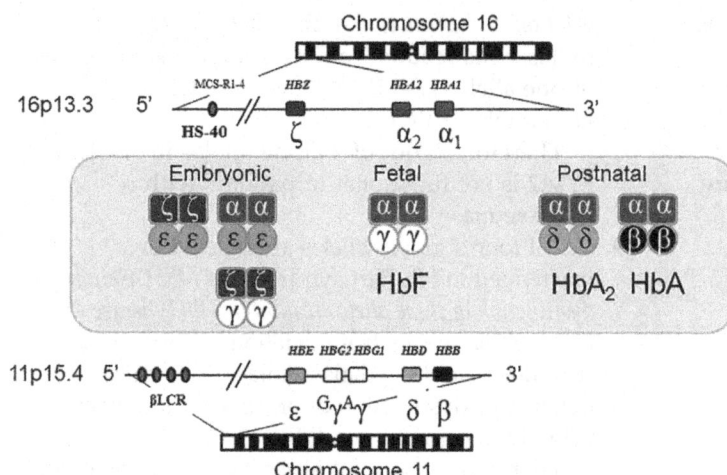

FIGURE 6.2 Schematic presentation of the chromosomal location of the α- and β-globin gene clusters on 16p and 11p respectively. The embryonic and foetal genes are indicated as open boxes. The genes which remain active throughout postnatal life in grey and black. The different hemoglobins expressed during the embryonic period are shown, from left to right Hb Gower-1 (ζ2ε2), Hb Gower-2 (α2ε2) and Hb Portland (ζ2γ2), foetal period (HbF) and postnatal period (HbA and HbA2). *Source: Farashi S, Harteveld CL. Molecular basis of α-thalassemia. Blood Cells Mol Dis. 2018 May;70:43–53. http://dx.doi.org/10.1016/j.bcmd.2017.09.004.*

α-^{ZF} and $(\alpha\alpha)^{TM}$ (http://www.ncbi.nlm.nih.gov/books/NBK1377/).

Therefore, one of four copies of alpha-globin chains was deleted in the wife, since she was an -$\alpha^{3.7}$ carrier.

43. A. Alpha thalassemia is a nonneoplastic hematological disorder involving the genes *HBA1* and *HBA2*. *HBA1*, encoding α1 globin, and *HBA2*, encoding α2-globin, are localized to the telomeric region of chromosome 16p in a cluster. Molecular genetic testing of *HBA1* and *HBA2* detects deletions in about 90% and point mutations in about 10% of affected individuals. The most common deletions for α thalassemia remove *one* (-$\alpha^{3.7}$ *and* -$\alpha^{4.2}$) or both (--^{Med} and --^{SEA}) of the α genes, as do the unusual deletions α-^{ZF} and $(\alpha\alpha)^{TM}$ (http://www.ncbi.nlm.nih.gov/books/NBK1377/).

Therefore, one of four copies of alpha globin chains were deleted in the wife, since she was an -$\alpha^{4.2}$ carrier.

44. D. Alpha thalassemia (α thalassemia) is a nonneoplastic hematological disorder involving the genes *HBA1* and *HBA2*. *HBA1*, encoding α1 globin, and *HBA2*, encoding α2 globin, are localized to the telomeric region of chromosome 16p13.3 in a cluster. Molecular genetic testing of *HBA1* and *HBA2* detects deletions in about 90% and point mutations in about 10% of affected individuals. The most common deletions for α thalassemia remove one (-$\alpha^{3.7}$ and -$\alpha^{4.2}$) or both (--^{Med}, --^{SEA}, --^{FIL}, and --^{THAI}) α genes, as do the unusual deletions α-^{ZF} and $(\alpha\alpha)^{TM}$. All four α alleles are deleted or dysfunctional (inactivated) in patients with Hb Barts hydrops fetalis syndrome. Hemoglobin H (HbH) disease is a result of deletion or dysfunction of three of four α-globin alleles.

Two of four copies of alpha-globin chains were deleted in the wife, since she was an --α^{THAI} carrier. And one of four copies of alpha-globin chains was deleted in the husband, since he was an -$\alpha^{4.2}$ carrier. Therefore, the couple's firstborn child would have 25% chance to have HbH, but not Hb Barts (<1%).

45. C. Alpha thalassemia is a nonneoplastic hematological disorder involving the genes *HBA1* and *HBA2*. *HBA1*, encoding α1 globin, and *HBA2*, encoding α2 globin, are localized to the telomeric region of chromosome 16p in a cluster. Molecular genetic testing of HbA1 and HbA2 detects deletions in about 90% and point mutations in about 10% of affected individuals. The most common deletions for α thalassemia remove one (-$\alpha^{3.7}$ and -$\alpha^{4.2}$) or both (--^{Med}, --^{SEA}, --^{FIL}, and --^{THAI}) α genes, as do the unusual deletions α-^{ZF} and $(\alpha\alpha)^{TM}$. All four α alleles are deleted or dysfunctional (inactivated) in patients with hemoglobin Bart hydrops fetalis syndrome. Hemoglobin H (HbH) disease is a result of deletion or dysfunction of three of four alpha-globin alleles.

Two of four copies of alpha-globin chains were deleted in the wife since she was an --α^{THAI} carrier. And one out of four copies of alpha-globin chains was deleted in the husband since he was an -$\alpha^{4.2}$ carrier. Therefore, the couple's firstborn child would have a 25% chance of having HbH, but not Hb Barts (<1%).

46. E. *HBA1*, encoding α1 globin, and *HBA2*, encoding α2 globin, are the two genes associated with α thalassemia. They are localized to the telomeric region of chromosome 16p in a cluster containing the embryonically expressed *HBZ* encoding ζ globin and a *cis*-acting regulatory element, HS-40, located 40 kb upstream of *HBZ* (see Fig. 6.2).

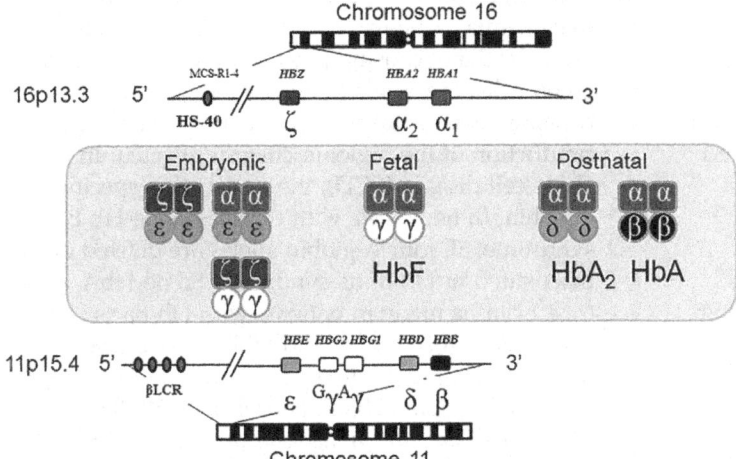

Diagram of the alpha-globin gene cluster on 16p13.3. In order from telomere to centromere, the genes are HS-40, ζ2, ψζ1, ψα2, ψα1, α2 (*HBA2*), and α1 (*HBA1*). HS-40 is a *cis*-acting regulatory element located 40 kb upstream of ζ2. ζ2 (*HBZ*) and encodes ζ2 globulin. The ψα1, ψα2, and ψζ1 are pseudogenes. Alpha 1 and 2 encoded α1 and α2 globulins, respectively. X, Y, and Z are homologous regions separated by nonhomologous DNA regions. During meiosis, misalignment of chromosome homologs followed by reciprocal recombination at X, Y, or Z results in deletion or duplication events, such as the loss of a single α-globin gene on one chromosome and the triplication of α-globin genes on the other chromosome. *From GeneReviews: http://www.genereviews.org/, and copyright:* © *1993–2016 University of Washington.*

The most common nondeletion mutation, which is frequently seen in Southeast Asia, is Hb^Constant Spring (Hb^CS, c.427T > C). *It is a missense mutation of the termination codon of HBA2, leading to an elongated protein chain.* This mutation leads to the production of an α-globin chain elongated by 31 amino acids. Hb^CS is produced in very small amounts because its mRNA is unstable. Heterozygotes for Hb^CS and other rare elongated variants, along with the presence of the Hb variant, produce the α°-thalassemia phenotype (http://www.ncbi.nlm.nih.gov/books/NBK1435/).

Therefore, Hb^CS is a nonstop mutation.

47. **B.** *HBA1*, encoding α1 globin, and *HBA2*, encoding α2 globin, are the two genes associated with α thalassemia. They are localized to the telomeric region of chromosome 16p in a cluster containing the embryonically expressed *HBZ* encoding ζ globin and a *cis*-acting regulatory element, HS-40, located 40 kb upstream of *HBZ* (see Fig. 6.2).

The most common nondeletion mutation, which is frequently seen in Southeast Asia, is Hb^CS (c.427T > C). *It is a missense mutation of the termination codon of HBA2, leading to an elongated protein chain.* This mutation leads to the production of an α-globin chain elongated by 31 amino acids. Hb^CS is produced in very small amounts because its mRNA is unstable. Heterozygotes for Hb^CS and other rare elongated variants, along with the presence of the Hb variant, produce the α° thalassemia phenotype (http://www.ncbi.nlm.nih.gov/books/NBK1435/).

Hemoglobin gamma (*HBG*), hemoglobin delta (*HBD*), and hemoglobin beta (*HBB*) are located on 11p15.4 from terminal to proximal, respectively. Mutations in *HBB* are more common in beta (β) thalassemia than deletions. So sequence analysis may detect 99% of the pathogenic mutations in *HBB* for β thalassemia (http://www.ncbi.nlm.nih.gov/books/NBK1426/).

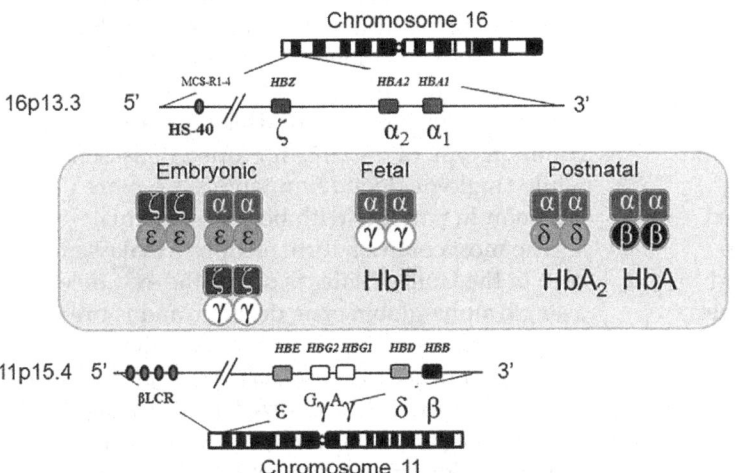

Diagram of the alpha-globin gene cluster on 16p13.3. In order from telomere to centromere, the genes are HS-40, ζ2, ψζ1, ψα2, ψα1, α2 (*HBA2*), and α1 (*HBA1*). HS-40 is a *cis*-acting regulatory element located 40 kb upstream of ζ2. ζ2 (*HBZ*) and encodes ζ2 globulin. The ψα1, ψα2, and ψζ1 are pseudogenes. Alpha 1 and 2 encoded α1 and α2 globulins, respectively. X, Y, and Z are homologous regions separated by nonhomologous DNA regions. During meiosis, misalignment of chromosome homologs followed by reciprocal recombination at X, Y, or Z results in deletion or duplication events, such as the loss of a single α-globin gene on one chromosome and the triplication of α-globin genes on the other chromosome. *From GeneReviews: http://www.genereviews.org/, and copyright:* © *1993–2016 University of Washington.*

Therefore, Hb^{CS} is a mutation in *HBA2*.

48. **E.** Beta thalassemia (β thalassemia) is characterized by reduced synthesis of the hemoglobin subunit beta (hemoglobin beta chain) that results in microcytic hypochromic anemia, an abnormal peripheral-blood smear with nucleated red blood cells, and reduced amounts of hemoglobin A (HbA) on hemoglobin analysis. Individuals with beta thalassemia major have severe anemia and hepatosplenomegaly. They usually come to medical attention within the first 2 years of life. Beta thalassemias are inherited in an autosomal recessive manner. *Most patients have single-nucleotide mutations (SNPs) in HBB.* Sequencing analysis of *HBB* may identify 99% of pathogenic variants (http://www.ncbi.nlm.nih.gov/books/NBK1377/).

    Therefore, single nucleotide mutation is most common in patients with beta thalassemia in comparison with other types of variants.

49. **A.** $Hb^{Constant\ Spring}$ (Hb^{CS}) is the most common nondeletion mutation in Southeast Asia. It is a missense mutation of the termination codon of *HBA2*, c.427T > C, which leads to an elongated protein chain. This mutation leads to the production of an α-globin chain elongated by 31 amino acids. Hb^{CS} is produced in very small amounts because its mRNA is unstable (http://www.ncbi.nlm.nih.gov/books/NBK1435/).

    HbF increases in patients with beta thalassemia, or disorders caused by mutations in *HBB*, such as sickle cell disease (SCD). But *in patients with alpha thalassemia, such as Hb^{CS}/Hb^{CS}, HbF does not increase* (http://www.ncbi.nlm.nih.gov/books/NBK1377/).

    Therefore, Hb^{CS}/Hb^{CS} would be in the differential list for the diagnosis in this patient, since her HbA and HbF were in the normal range.

50. **C.** In fetuses and infants, the hemoglobin is made up of two alpha chains and two gamma chains (HbF: $\alpha^2\gamma^2$). As the infant grows, the gamma chains are gradually replaced by beta chains, forming the adult hemoglobin HbA ($\alpha^2\beta^2$). HbF increases in diseases associated with mutations in the *HBB* gene, such as beta thalassemia (β°/β°, β°/β⁺, β⁺/β⁺), and sickle cell disease (SCD), but not in alpha thalassemia. The absence of beta globin is referred to as beta zero (β°) thalassemia. Other *HBB* gene mutations allow some beta globin to be produced but in reduced amounts. A reduced amount of beta globin is called beta plus (β⁺) thalassemia (http://www.ncbi.nlm.nih.gov/books/NBK1435/).

    Therefore, β°/β° is associated with a more significant HbF increase than in the others.

51. **A.** Normally, the majority of adult hemoglobin (HbA) is composed of two α-globin and two β-globin chains arranged into a heterotetramer. In thalassemia, patients have defects in either the α- or β-globin chain, causing production of abnormal red blood cells. In α thalassemias, production of the α-globin chain is affected, while in β thalassemia, production of the β-globin chain is affected. In sickle cell disease (SCD), the mutation is specific to β globin. In newborns with α thalassemia Hb Barts syndrome, all four α-globin alleles are deleted or inactivated in Hb Barts syndrome. So no HbA ($\alpha^2\beta^2$) can be made in patients with Hb Barts syndrome. HbA2 ($\alpha^2\delta^2$) and HbF ($\alpha^2\gamma^2$) cannot increase to compensate for the lack of HbA owing to lack of α-globin chain. *Patients with Hb Barts syndrome usually die in the neonatal period* (http://www.ncbi.nlm.nih.gov/books/NBK1435/).

    Beta thalassemias are due to mutations in the *HBB* gene on chromosome 11. The severity of the disease depends on the nature of the mutation. Mutations are characterized as β° or β thalassemia major if they prevent any formation of β chains. Otherwise, they are characterized as either β⁺ or β thalassemia intermedia if they allow some β-chain formation. In patients with mutations in the *HBB* gene, such as beta thalassemia (β°/β°, β°/β⁺, β⁺/β⁺), and SCD, HbF increases, but not in alpha thalassemia. The increased HbF results in relatively milder symptoms in β thalassemia than in α thalassemia (http://www.ncbi.nlm.nih.gov/books/NBK1426/).

    Therefore, Hb Barts has the earliest onset and the worst prognosis among all the hemoglobinopathies listed.

52. **A.** Thalassemia syndromes are the commonest monogenic diseases in the world. The worldwide distribution of inherited alpha thalassemia corresponds to areas of malaria exposure. Alpha thalassemia is common in sub-Saharan Africa, the Mediterranean Basin, the Middle East, South Asia, and Southeast Asia, and different genetic subtypes have variable frequencies in each of these areas. The epidemiology of alpha thalassemia in the United States reflects this global distribution pattern. Deletions are the most common type of variants for alpha thalassemia, while single-nucleotide mutations are more common in patients with beta thalassemia.

    The most common form of alpha⁺ thalassemia seen in the United States is due to the $-\alpha^{3.7}$ deletion, a single alpha-globin gene deletion, and is present in approximately 30% of African Americans. *The highest frequency (0.30−0.40) of the $-\alpha^{3.7}$ allele (causing α^+ thalassemia) has been observed in the equatorial belt, including Nigeria, Ivory Coast, and Kenya. And $--\alpha^{SEA}$ is one of common deletions of HBA1 and HBA2 in Southeast Asia, as the name indicates.*

Hemoglobin Constant Spring (Hb^{CS}) is an unstable α-globin variant causing α-thalassemia phenotypes. Sequence variant Hb$^{Constant\ Spring}$ (Hb^{CS}, c.427T > C) is a missense mutation of the termination codon of *HBA2*, leading to an elongated protein chain. It is the most common nondeletion in the genes for alpha globin and alpha thalassemia.

Alpha thalassemia retardation-16 (ATR-16) syndrome, a contiguous-gene deletion syndrome, results from a large deletion on the short arm of chromosome 16 from band 16p13.3 to the terminus, which removes *HBA1* and *HBA2* together with other flanking genes. Among the few reported individuals with deletion of 16p, microcephaly and short stature were variable; IQ ranged from 53 to 76. Facial features are distinctive; talipes equinovarus (club foot) is common, as are hypospadias and cryptorchidism in males. Typically, hematological features are those of the α-thalassemia trait reflecting deletion of *HBA1* and *HBA2* in cis configuration, such as --/αα. The deletion may be de novo or inherited from a parent who carries a balanced chromosome rearrangement. Worldwide, it is not as common as alpha thalassemia (http://www. ncbi.nlm.nih.gov/books/NBK1435/).

Therefore, it would be most likely that the patient had the -α$^{3.7}$ allele for alpha thalassemia.

53. **B.** Alpha thalassemia typically results from deletions involving the *HBA1* and *HBA2* genes. They are localized to the telomeric region of chromosome 16p in a cluster with *HBZ* and HS-40. Alpha-thalassemia silent carrier (α$^+$ thalassemia) results from a deletion or nondeletion mutation that inactivates one of the two α-globin genes (*HBA1* or *HBA2*) on one chromosome (1/4). Alpha-thalassemia trait results from deletion or inactivation of two α-globin alleles (--/αα in *cis* configuration or -α/-α in *trans* configuration) (2/4). Alpha thalassemia is usually inherited in an autosomal recessive manner. HbH disease results from the deletion or inactivation of three α-globin alleles (3/4), usually as a result of a compound heterozygous state for α° thalassemia and α$^+$ thalassemia (http://www. ncbi.nlm.nih.gov/books/NBK1435/).

Therefore, the couple's firstborn child will have a 25% chance of having HbH disease, a 25% chance of having α° thalassemia, a 25% chance of having α$^+$ thalassemia, and a 25% chance of being unaffected and not a carrier. Once an at-risk child is known to be unaffected, the risk of his/ her having either α° thalassemia or α$^+$ thalassemia is 2/3.

54. **A.** Alpha thalassemia typically results from deletions involving the *HBA1* and *HBA2* genes. They are localized to the telomeric region of chromosome 16p in a cluster with *HBZ* and HS-40. Alpha-thalassemia silent carrier (α$^+$ thalassemia) results from a deletion or nondeletion mutation that inactivates one of the two α-globin genes (*HBA1* or *HBA2*) on one chromosome (1/4). Alpha-thalassemia trait (α° thalassemia) results from the deletion or inactivation of two α-globin alleles (--/αα in *cis* configuration or -α/-α in *trans* configuration) (2/4) (http://www.ncbi.nlm.nih.gov/books/ NBK1435/). Alpha thalassemia is usually inherited in an autosomal recessive manner. All four α-globin alleles are deleted or inactivated in Hb Barts syndrome as a result of deletion or inactivation of all four α-globin alleles (4/4).

The couple's child would have 25% chance of having Hb Barts disease, a 25% chance of having α° thalassemia, a 25% chance of having α$^+$ thalassemia, and a 25% chance of being unaffected and not a carrier. If an at-risk child is known to be unaffected, he/her has 2/3 risk to have either α° or α$^+$ thalassemia is 2/3. Therefore, the couple's firstborn child will have a <1% chance of having Hb Barts syndrome.

55. **C.** Alpha thalassemia typically results from deletions involving the *HBA1* and *HBA2* genes. *HBA1* and *HBA2* are localized to the telomeric region of chromosome 16p in a cluster with *HBZ* and HS-40. Hemoglobin H (HbH) disease results from deletion or inactivation of three α-globin alleles, usually as a result of a compound heterozygous state for α° thalassemia and α$^+$ thalassemia (3/4). *Patients with HbH disease usually have decreased HbA, increased Hb Barts and HbH, normal percentages of HbA2 and HbF, and RBC inclusion bodies* (http://www.ncbi.nlm.nih.gov/ books/NBK1435/).

Therefore this child would most likely have an increased chance of having Hb Barts by 2 years of age.

56. **A.** Alpha thalassemia typically results from deletions involving the *HBA1* and *HBA2* genes. *HBA1* and *HBA2* are localized to the telomeric region of chromosome 16p in a cluster with *HBZ* and HS-40. Hemoglobin H (HbH) disease results from deletion or inactivation of three α-globin alleles, usually as a result of a compound heterozygous state for α° thalassemia and α$^+$ thalassemia (3/4). *Patients with HbH disease usually have decreased HbA, increased Hb Barts and HbH, normal percentages of HbA2 and HbF, and RBC*

inclusion bodies (http://www.ncbi.nlm.nih.gov/books/NBK1435/).

Therefore, this child most likely would have decreased HbA by 2 years of age.

57. **B.** Alpha thalassemia typically results from deletions involving the *HBA1* and *HBA2* genes. *HBA1* and *HBA2* are localized to the telomeric region of chromosome 16p in a cluster with *HBZ* and HS-40. HbH disease results from deletion or inactivation of three α-globin alleles, usually as a result of a compound heterozygous state for α° thalassemia and α$^+$ thalassemia (3/4). *Patients with HbH disease usually have decreased HbA, increased Hb Barts and HbH, normal percentages of HbA2 and HbF, and RBC inclusion bodies* (http://www.ncbi.nlm.nih.gov/books/NBK1435/).

Therefore, this child would most likely have stable HbA2 by 2 years of age.

58. **C.** Alpha thalassemia typically results from deletions involving the *HBA1* and *HBA2* genes. *HBA1* and *HBA2* are localized to the telomeric region of chromosome 16p in a cluster with *HBZ* and HS-40. HbH disease results from deletion or inactivation of three α-globin alleles, usually as a result of a compound heterozygous state for α° thalassemia and α$^+$ thalassemia (3/4). *Patients with HbH disease usually have decreased HbA, increased Hb Barts and HbH, normal percentages of HbA2 and HbF, and RBC inclusion bodies* (http://www.ncbi.nlm.nih.gov/books/NBK1435/).

Therefore, this child would most likely have stable HbF by 2 years of age.

59. **B.** Alpha thalassemia typically results from deletions involving the *HBA1* and *HBA2* genes. *HBA1* and *HBA2* are localized to the telomeric region of chromosome 16p in a cluster with *HBZ* and HS-40. α°-Thalassemia trait carriers have two copies of dysfunctional α-globin chains due to deletion(s) and/or mutation(s). If a fetus has four dysfunctional (inactivated) α-globin chains, he/she has Hb Barts hydrops fetalis syndrome, which is the most severe clinical form of α thalassemia. Affected fetuses are either stillborn or die soon after birth. Red cells with Hb Barts have an extremely high oxygen affinity and are incapable of effective tissue oxygen delivery. The clinical features are severe anemia, marked hepatosplenomegaly, diffuse edema, heart failure, and extramedullary erythropoiesis. *Patients with Hb Barts syndrome have only Hb Barts.*

Therefore, this future child would most likely have Hb Bart sat birth.

60. **C.** Alpha thalassemia typically results from deletions involving the *HBA1* and *HBA2* genes localized to the telomeric region of chromosome

16p in a cluster with *HBZ* encoding ζ globin and a *cis*-acting regulatory element, HS-40, located 40 kb upstream of *HBZ*.

Alpha-thalassemia silent carrier (α$^+$ thalassemia) results from a deletion or nondeletion mutation that inactivates one of the two copies of α globin alleles (*HBA1* or *HBA2*) on one chromosome (1/4 alleles). Carriers of α$^+$ thalassemia may have a completely silent hematologic phenotype or may present with a moderate, thalassemia-like hematologic picture, such as reduced MCV and MCH, but normal HbA2 and HbF.

Alpha thalassemia trait (α° thalassemia) results from deletion or inactivation of two α-globin alleles (--/αα in *cis* configuration or -α/-α in *trans* configuration) (2/4 allele). Carriers of α° thalassemia show microcytosis (low MCV), hypochromia (low MCH), normal percentages of HbA2 and HbF, and RBC inclusion bodies. Patients are considered to be α-thalassemia carriers without symptoms.

HbH disease results from deletion or inactivation of three α-globin alleles, usually as a result of a compound heterozygous state for α° thalassemia and α° thalassemia (3/4 alleles). Patients with HbH disease (chronic microcytic, hypochromic hemolytic anemia of variable severity) usually are symptomatic.

Hemoglobin Barts hydrops fetalis (Hb Barts) syndrome, the most severe form of α thalassemia, is characterized by fetal onset of generalized edema, ascites, pleural and pericardial effusions, and severe hypochromic anemia, in the absence of ABO or Rh blood group incompatibility. It is usually detected by ultrasonography at 22–28 weeks' gestation and can be suspected in an at-risk pregnancy at 13–14 weeks' gestation when increased nuchal thickness, possible placental thickness, increased cerebral media artery velocity and increased cardiothoracic ratio are present. Death in the neonatal period is almost inevitable. All four α-globin alleles are deleted or dysfunctional (inactivated, 4/4 alleles) (http://www.ncbi.nlm.nih.gov/books/NBK1435/).

Therefore, patients with HbH usually are symptomatic.

61. **B.** Fetal hemoglobin ($\alpha^2\gamma^2$), composed of two alpha and two gamma subunits, is the primary hemoglobin present during fetal development. Around the time of birth, gamma expression is diminished as β-globin expression is increased. Individuals with alpha thalassemia have deletions/mutations that impair α-globin production. Fetal hemoglobin ($\alpha^2\gamma^2$) cannot be produced effectively, which affects fetal

development significantly. Therefore, alpha thalassemia is identifiable in utero.

Individuals with beta thalassemia have mutations that impair beta-globin production. Production of fetal hemoglobin ($\alpha^2\gamma^2$) is not affected by inactivation of the beta-globin gene. However, production of adult hemoglobin HbA ($\alpha^2\beta^2$) is impaired by the inactivation of beta globin gene. Therefore, individuals with beta thalassemia begin to show symptoms as the proportion of fetal hemoglobin HbF drops without a concomitant rise in adult hemoglobin HbA ($\alpha^2\beta^2$) after birth.

62. **C.** Beta thalassemia (β thalassemia) is caused by mutations in the *HBB* gene on the short arm of chromosome 11 (11p15.4), and is inherited in an autosomal recessive fashion. The severity of the disease depends on the nature of the mutation. *HBB* blockage over time leads to decreased beta-chain synthesis. *The body's inability to construct new beta chains leads to the underproduction of HbA, secondary to the increased production of HbF.* (http://www.ncbi.nlm.nih.gov/books/NBK1426/).

Therefore, an individual with beta thalassemia has an increased level of HbF.

63. **A.** Beta thalassemia (β thalassemia) is caused by mutations in the *HBB* gene on the short arm of chromosome 11 (11p15.4) and is inherited in an autosomal recessive fashion. The severity of the disease depends on the nature of the mutation. *HBB* blockage over time leads to decreased beta-chain synthesis. *The body's inability to construct new beta chains leads to the underproduction of HbA, secondary to the increased production of HbF* (http://www.ncbi.nlm.nih.gov/books/NBK1426/).

Therefore, an individual with beta thalassemia has a decreased level of HbA.

64. **C.** *Hb^{CS} is caused by a mutation in the stop codon of the α2-globin gene, HBA2, that results in poor expression (1% of normal) of an α globin, which has 31 additional amino acids.* Hemoglobin Constant Spring (Hb^{CS}) is the most common nondeletional α-thalassemia mutation and is an important cause of HbH-like disease in Southeast Asia. The quantity of hemoglobin in the cells is low for two reasons. First, the messenger RNA for hemoglobin Constant Spring is unstable; some is degraded prior to protein synthesis. Second, the Constant Spring alpha-chain protein is itself unstable. The result is a thalassemic phenotype. The designation Constant Spring derives from the isolation of the hemoglobin variant in a family of ethnic Chinese background from the Constant Spring district of Jamaica (http://www.ncbi.nlm.nih.gov/books/NBK1435/).

Therefore, Hb^{CS} is a stop codon mutation in *HBA2*.

65. **B.** *Hb^{CS} is caused by a mutation in the stop codon of the α2-globin gene, HBA2, that results in poor expression (1% of normal) of an α globin, which has 31 additional amino acids. Hemoglobin Constant Spring (Hb^{CS}) is the most common nondeletional α-thalassemia mutation and is an important cause of HbH-like disease in Southeast Asia.* There are two copies of the α-globin gene, *HBA1* and *HBA2*, tandemly located on the short arm of chromosome 16. There is no *HBA3* in the human genome.

Beta thalassemia (β thalassemia) is caused by mutations in the *HBB* gene on chromosome 11 and is inherited in an autosomal recessive fashion. There is only one *HBB* gene in humans.

Therefore, Hb^{CS} is a stop codon mutation in *HBA2*.

66. **A.** If the couple are both carriers of the α°-thalassemia deletion mutation in which both *HBA1* and *HBA2* as well as *HBZ* are deleted (such as $\alpha\alpha/--^{FIL}$ or genotype of $\alpha\alpha/--^{THAI}$), *they are not at risk of having offspring with Hb Barts hydrops fetalis syndrome because homozygotes for such mutations are lost shortly after conception as a miscarriage* (http://www.ncbi.nlm.nih.gov/books/NBK1435/).

Therefore, this couple will be at risk for multiple miscarriages.

67. **B.** If the couple are both carriers of a deletion involving both *HBA1* and *HBA2*, but only one of them has a deletion that extends into *HBZ* (such as $\alpha\alpha/--^{SEA}$ and $\alpha\alpha/--^{FIL}$), *the couple is at risk of having offspring with Hb Barts hydrops fetalis syndrome* because the single *HBZ* in the fetus produces sufficient ζ globin for fetal development (http://www.ncbi.nlm.nih.gov/books/NBK1435/).

Therefore, this couple will be at risk for having offspring with Hb Barts hydrops fetalis syndrome.

68. **C.** Two tandem genes for alpha globin (*HBA1* and *HBA2*) are located on the short arm of chromosome 16 (16p13.3). *Hemoglobin H (HbH) disease results from deletion or inactivation of three out of four α globin alleles, usually as a result of a compound heterozygous state for α° thalassemia (α-/α-, or $\alpha\alpha/--$) and α^+ thalassemia ($\alpha\alpha/\alpha$-).* HbH disease is characterized by chronic microcytic, hypochromic hemolytic anemia. The severity mainly correlates with the severity of the α° thalassemia. *Patients with HbH disease usually have decreased HbA, increased Hb Barts and HbH, normal percentages of HbA2 and HbF, and RBC inclusion bodies* (http://www.ncbi.nlm.nih.gov/books/NBK1435/).

Therefore, this couple will be at risk for having offspring with HbH disease.

69. **A.** Two tandem genes for alpha globin (*HBA1* and *HBA2*) are located on the short arm of chromosome 16 (16p13.3) with *HBZ*. If a couple are both carriers of an α° thalassemia deletion

mutation ($\alpha\alpha$/--), *each of their offspring has a 1/4 risk of having Hb Barts hydrops fetalis syndrome* (http://www.ncbi.nlm.nih.gov/books/NBK1435/).

Therefore, this couple will be at risk for having offspring with Hb Barts hydrops fetalis syndrome.

70. C. Alpha thalassemia is a nonneoplastic hematological disorder that reduces the production of hemoglobin. Hemoglobin is the

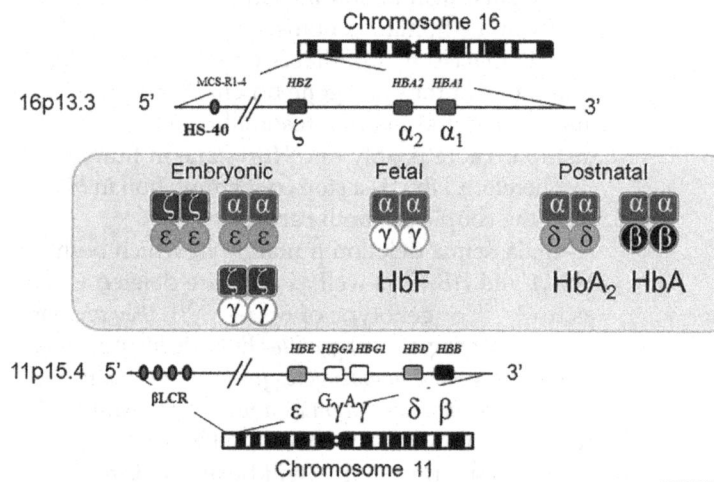

nih.gov/books/NBK1435/). Therefore, the *HBA2* gene is most likely deleted in the wife.

71. C. Alpha thalassemia is a nonneoplastic hematological disorder that reduces the production of hemoglobin. Hemoglobin is the protein in red blood cells that carries oxygen to cells throughout the body. Alpha thalassemia typically results from deletions involving the *HBA1* and *HBA2* genes on

Schematic presentation of the chromosomal location of the α- and β-globin gene clusters on 16p and 11p respectively. The embryonic and foetal genes are indicated as open boxes. The genes which remain active throughout postnatal life in grey and black. The different hemoglobins expressed during the embryonic period are shown, from left to right Hb Gower-1 ($\zeta2\epsilon2$), Hb Gower-2 ($\alpha2\epsilon2$) and Hb Portland ($\zeta2\gamma2$), foetal period (HbF) and postnatal period (HbA and HbA2) *Source: Farashi S, Harteveld CL. Molecular basis of α-thalassemia. Blood Cells Mol Dis. 2018 May;70:43–53. http://dx.doi.org/10.1016/j.bcmd.2017.09.004.*

protein in red blood cells that carries oxygen to cells throughout the body. Alpha thalassemia typically results from deletions involving the *HBA1* and *HBA2* genes on 16p13.3 (see the figure below). The mRNAs produced by *HBA1* and *HBA2* have identical coding regions and can be distinguished only by their 3' UTR.

Reciprocal recombination between the Z boxes, which are 3.7 kb apart, or between the X boxes, 4.2 kb apart, gives rise to chromosomes with a single α-globin gene. The two resulting α-thalassemia mutations are referred to as the 3.7-kb rightward deletion ($-\alpha^{3.7}$) and the 4.2-kb leftward deletion ($-\alpha^{4.2}$), respectively (see Fig. 6.2) (http://www.ncbi.nlm.

16p13.3 (see the figure below). The mRNAs produced by *HBA1* and *HBA2* have identical coding regions and can be distinguished only by their 3' UTR.

Reciprocal recombination between the Z boxes, which are 3.7 kb apart, or between the X boxes, 4.2 kb apart, gives rise to chromosomes with a single α-globin gene. The two resulting α-thalassemia mutations are referred to, respectively, as the 3.7-kb rightward deletion ($-\alpha^{3.7}$) and the 4.2-kb leftward deletion ($-\alpha^{4.2}$) (see Fig. 6.2) (http://www.ncbi.nlm.nih.gov/books/NBK1435/).

Therefore, the *HBA2* gene is most likely deleted in the wife.

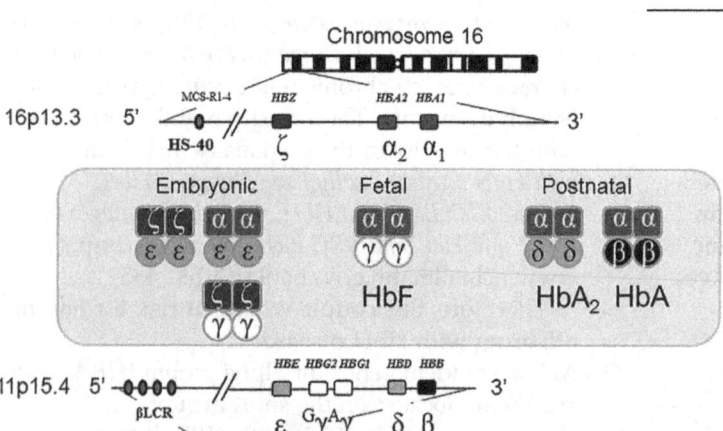

Schematic presentation of the chromosomal location of the α- and β-globin gene clusters on 16p and 11p respectively. The embryonic and foetal genes are indicated as open boxes. The genes which remain active throughout postnatal life in grey and black. The different hemoglobins expressed during the embryonic period are shown, from left to right Hb Gower-1 ($\zeta2\epsilon2$), Hb Gower-2 ($\alpha2\epsilon2$) and Hb Portland ($\zeta2\gamma2$), foetal period (HbF) and postnatal period (HbA and HbA2). *Source: Farashi S, Harteveld CL. Molecular basis of α-thalassemia. Blood Cells Mol Dis. 2018 May;70:43–53. http://dx.doi.org/10.1016/j.bcmd.2017.09.004.*

72. A. Alpha thalassemia (α thalassemia) is an autosomal recessive disease with two clinically significant forms: hemoglobin Barts hydrops fetalis (Hb Bart) syndrome and hemoglobin H (HbH) disease. *HBA1*, the gene encoding α1-globin, and *HBA2*, the gene encoding α2-globin, are the two genes associated with α thalassemia. *Molecular genetic testing of HBA1 and HBA2 detects deletions in about 90% and point mutations in about 10% of affected individuals.* The six common deletions are $-\alpha^{3.7}$, $-\alpha^{4.2}$, $- -^{SEA}$, $- -^{FIL}$, $- -^{MED}$, and $- -^{THAI}$ (http://www.ncbi.nlm.nih.gov/books/NBK1435/).

Therefore, the detection rate of the six common deletions is approximately 90%.

73. C. Alpha thalassemia (α thalassemia) is an autosomal recessive disease with two clinically significant forms: hemoglobin Bart hydrops fetalis (Hb Barts) syndrome and hemoglobin H (HbH) disease. *HBA1*, the gene encoding α1 globin, and *HBA2*, the gene encoding α2-globin, are the two genes associated with α thalassemia. Molecular genetic testing of *HBA1* and *HBA2* detects deletions in about 90% and point mutations in about 10% of affected individuals. The six common deletions are $-\alpha^{3.7}$, $-\alpha^{4.2}$, $- -^{SEA}$, $- -^{FIL}$, $- -^{MED}$, and $- -^{THAI}$ (http://www.ncbi.nlm.nih.gov/books/NBK1435/).

Therefore, the residual risk for this couple having a child with α thalassemia is: $1/10 \times 1/10 \times 1/4 = 1/400$.

74. E. The clinical manifestations of alpha thalassemia (α thalassemia) depend on the degree of α-globin chain deficiency relative to β-globin production. The different α-thalassemia mutations vary widely in severity. *The most and least severe (respectively) are nondeletion HBA2, -α³·⁷ (because of a compensatory increase of the α-globin gene output from the remaining HBA1), and nondeletion HBA1.* For the $-\alpha^{4.2}$ deletion, evidence is inconclusive for a compensatory increase in the expression of the remaining α gene. The most common nondeletion mutation, which is frequently seen in Southeast Asia, is Hb$^{Constant\ Spring}$ (Hb^{CS}, c.427T > C). It is a missense mutation of the termination codon of *HBA2* leading to an elongated protein chain. This mutation leads to the production of an α-globin chain elongated by 31 amino acids. Hb^{CS} is produced in very small amounts because its mRNA is unstable. The phenotype α thalassemia may be modified by triplication or quadruplication of the α-globin genes on one chromosome.

Therefore, p.Asp75Gly in *HBA1* may be predicted to have milder symptoms than the remaining choices if the effect from the expression of *HBB* and the extra copies of *HBA1/HBA2* are not considered.

75. C. The clinical manifestations of alpha thalassemia (α thalassemia) depend on the degree of α-globin chain deficiency relative to β-globin production. The different α-thalassemia mutations vary widely in severity. *The most and least severe (respectively) are nondeletion HBA2, -α³·⁷ (because of a compensatory increase of the α-globin gene output from the remaining HBA1), and nondeletion HBA1.* For the -α⁴·² deletion, evidence is inconclusive for a compensatory increase in the expression of the remaining α gene. The most common nondeletion mutation, which is frequently seen in Southeast Asia, is Hb$^{Constant\ Spring}$ (Hb^{CS}, c.427T > C). It is a missense mutation of the termination codon of *HBA2*, leading to an elongated protein chain. This mutation leads to the production of an α-globin chain elongated by 31 amino acids. Hb^{CS} is produced in very small amounts because its mRNA is unstable. The phenotype of α thalassemia may be modified by triplication or quadruplication of the α-globin genes on one chromosome.

Therefore, Hb$^{Constant\ Spring}$ may be predicted to have more severe symptoms than the remaining choices in the question if the effect from the expression of *HBB* and the extra copies of *HBA1/HBA2* are not considered.

76. D. The clinical manifestations of alpha thalassemia (α thalassemia) depend on the degree of α-globin chain deficiency relative to β-globin production. The six most common deletions for α thalassemia are $-\alpha^{3.7}$, $-\alpha^{4.2}$, $- -^{SEA}$, $- -^{FIL}$, $- -^{MED}$, and $- -^{THAI}$. The -α⁴·² removes the entire *HBA2*. The -α³·⁷ gives rise to a hybrid *HBA2/HBA1* gene. *The rest of the four common deletions involve both HBA1 and HBA2 and HBZ at the terminal sides of HBA1 and HBA2* ($- -^{SEA}$, $- -^{FIL}$, $- -^{MED}$, and $- -^{THAI}$).

The different α-thalassemia mutations vary widely in severity. The most and least severe (respectively) are nondeletion *HBA2*, -α³·⁷ (because of compensatory increase of the α-globin gene output from the remaining *HBA1*), and nondeletion *HBA1*. For the -α⁴·² deletion, evidence is inconclusive for a compensatory increase in the expression of the remaining α-globin gene. The most common nondeletion mutation, which is frequently seen in Southeast Asia, is Hb$^{Constant\ Spring}$ (Hb^{CS}, c.427T > C). It is a missense mutation of the termination codon of *HBA2*, leading to an elongated protein chain. This mutation leads to the production of an α-globin chain elongated by 31 amino acids. Hb^{CS} is produced in very small amounts because its mRNA is unstable. The phenotype of α thalassemia may be modified by triplication or quadruplication of the α-globin genes on one chromosome.

Therefore, − −^{SEA} may be predicted to have more severe symptoms than the remaining choices if the effect from the expression of *HBB* and the extra copies of *HBA1*/*HBA2* are not considered.

77. D. Alpha thalassemia is an autosomal recessive nonneoplastic hematological disorder characterized by a reduced production of hemoglobin. Hemoglobin is the protein in red blood cells that carries oxygen to cells throughout the body. Alpha thalassemia typically results from deletions involving the *HBA1* and *HBA2* genes. *HBA1*, encoding α1-globin, and *HBA2*, encoding α2-globin, are the two genes associated with α thalassemia. They are localized to the telomeric region of chromosome 16p in a cluster containing the embryonically expressed *HBZ* encoding ζ globin and a *cis*-acting regulatory element, HS-40, located 40 kb upstream of *HBZ*.

Hemoglobin Barts hydrops fetalis (Hb Barts) syndrome is characterized by fetal onset of generalized edema, ascites, pleural and pericardial effusions, and severe hypochromic anemia, in the absence of ABO or Rh blood group incompatibility. It is usually detected by ultrasonography at 22−28 weeks' gestation and can be suspected in an at-risk pregnancy at 13−14 weeks' gestation when increased nuchal thickness, possible placental thickness, increased cerebral media artery velocity, and increased cardiothoracic ratio are present. Death in the neonatal period is almost inevitable. Patients with Hb Barts syndrome have only hemoglobin Barts (Hb Barts). All four α-hemoglobins alleles are deleted (−−/−−) or dysfunctional (inactivated) (http://www.ncbi.nlm.nih.gov/books/NBK1435/).

The newborn in this question had hemoglobin Barts hydrops fetalis (Hb Barts) syndrome (−−/−−). The mother was apparently healthy. Therefore, it would be most likely the genotype of the mother was −−/αα.

78. D. Alpha thalassemia is an autosomal recessive nonneoplastic hematological disorder characterized by reduced production of hemoglobin. Hemoglobin is the protein in red blood cells that carries oxygen to cells throughout the body. Alpha thalassemia typically results from deletions involving the *HBA1* and *HBA2* genes. *HBA1*, encoding α1-globin, and *HBA2*, encoding α2-globin, are the two genes associated with α thalassemia. They are localized to the telomeric region of chromosome 16p in a cluster containing the embryonically expressed *HBZ* encoding ζ globin and a *cis*-acting regulatory element, HS-40, located 40 kb upstream of *HBZ*.

Hemoglobin H (HbH) disease results from deletion or inactivation of three of four α-globin

alleles, usually as a result of a compound heterozygous state for α° thalassemia (−−/αα) and α⁺ thalassemia (-α/αα). Hb Barts syndrome results from deletion or inactivation of all four α-globin alleles (−−/−−), usually as a result of the homozygous state for α° thalassemia (−−/αα). In Southeast Asian (in particular) and Mediterranean populations, HbH disease and hemoglobin Barts (γ4) are common because of the frequent coinheritance of an allele lacking both alpha-globin genes (−−/αα) and another allele lacking one alpha-globin gene (-α/αα) (http://www.ncbi.nlm.nih.gov/books/NBK1435/).

The child in this question had hemoglobin H (HbH) disease (−−/-α). Therefore, most likely the mother carried the familial −−/αα alleles because her sister's unborn child had the −−/−− alleles. And the husband has the -α/αα allele, since he is apparently healthy with no history of thalassemia.

79. B. Alpha thalassemia is an autosomal recessive nonneoplastic hematological disorder characterized by reduced production of hemoglobin. Hemoglobin is the protein in red blood cells that carries oxygen to cells throughout the body. Alpha thalassemia typically results from deletions involving the *HBA1* and *HBA2* genes. *HBA1*, encoding α1-globin, and *HBA2*, encoding α2-globin, are the two genes associated with α thalassemia. They are localized to the telomeric region of chromosome 16p in a cluster containing the embryonically expressed *HBZ* encoding ζ globin and a *cis*-acting regulatory element, HS-40, located 40 kb upstream of *HBZ*.

Hemoglobin H (HbH) disease results from deletion or inactivation of three of four α-globin alleles, usually as a result of a compound heterozygous state for α° thalassemia (−−/αα) and α⁺ thalassemia (-α/αα). Hb Barts syndrome results from the deletion or inactivation of all four α-globin alleles (−−/−−), usually as a result of the homozygous state for α° thalassemia (−−/αα). In Southeast Asian (in particular) and Mediterranean populations, HbH disease and hemoglobin Barts (γ4) are common because of the frequent coinheritance of an allele lacking both α-globin genes (−−/αα) and another allele lacking 1 α-globin gene (-α/αα) (http://www.ncbi.nlm.nih.gov/books/NBK1435/).

The child in this question has hemoglobin H (HbH) disease (−−/-α). Therefore, most likely the mother carried the familial −−/αα alleles because her sister's unborn child had the −−/−− alleles. And the husband has the -α/αα allele, since he is apparently healthy with no history of thalassemia.

80. D. Thalassemia is a nonneoplastic hematological disorder that reduces the production of hemoglobin. Hemoglobin is the protein in red blood cells that carries oxygen to cells throughout the body. Alpha thalassemia typically results from deletions involving the *HBA1* and *HBA2* genes. *HBA1*, encoding α1-globin, and *HBA2*, encoding α2-globin, are the two genes associated with α thalassemia. They are localized to the telomeric region of chromosome 16p (16p13.3) in a cluster containing the embryonically expressed *HBZ* encoding ζ globin and a *cis*-acting regulatory element, HS-40, located 40 kb upstream of *HBZ* (http://www.ncbi.nlm.nih.gov/books/NBK1435/).

Hemoglobin gamma (HBG), hemoglobin delta (HBD), and hemoglobin beta (HBB) are located on the short arm of chromosome 11 (11p15.4) from terminal to proximal, respectively. Beta thalassemia is more common than thalassemias due to variants in *HBG* and *HBD*. Mutations in *HBB* are more common than deletions in beta (β) thalassemia. Sequence analysis may detect 99% of the pathogenic mutations in *HBB* for β thalassemia. Alpha or beta thalassemias are more common than delta or gamma thalassemias (http://www. ncbi.nlm.nih.gov/books/NBK1426/).

Therefore, it is most likely that *HBB* is mutated in the wife.

81. **D.** Beta thalassemia (β thalassemia) is characterized by reduced synthesis of the hemoglobin subunit beta that results in microcytic hypochromic anemia, an abnormal peripheral-blood smear with nucleated red blood cells, and reduced amounts of hemoglobin A (HbA) on hemoglobin analysis. Beta thalassemia is an autosomal recessive disease results from the variants in the *HBB* gene on 11p15.4. Some of variants in *HBB* may cause hemoglobinopathy other than β thalassemia, such as:
Hemoglobin S (HbC; Glu6Val pathogenic variant)
Hemoglobin C (HbC; Glu6Lys pathogenic variant)
Hemoglobin D (D-Punjab; Glu121Gln pathogenic variant)
Hemoglobin O (O-Arab; Glu121Lys pathogenic variant)
Hemoglobin E (HbE; Glu26Lys pathogenic variant)
The p.Lys8ValfsTer13 and p.Ser9ValfsTer13 mutations are nonsense variants in HBB for β thalassemia. Therefore, in this case it would be most likely that BJ had compound heterozygous p.Ser9ValfsTer13 and p.Glu26Lys, which results in hemoglobin E/β thalassemia.

82. **E.** Beta thalassemia (β thalassemia) is characterized by reduced synthesis of the hemoglobin subunit beta that results in microcytic hypochromic anemia, an abnormal peripheral-blood smear with nucleated red blood cells, and reduced amounts of hemoglobin A (HbA) on hemoglobin analysis. Beta thalassemia, an autosomal recessive disease, results from the variants in the *HBB* gene on 11p15.4. Some variants in *HBB* may cause hemoglobinopathy other than β thalassemia, such as:
Hemoglobin S (HbC; Glu6Val pathogenic variant)
Hemoglobin C (HbC; Glu6Lys pathogenic variant)
Hemoglobin D (D-Punjab; Glu121Gln pathogenic variant)
Hemoglobin O (O-Arab; Glu121Lys pathogenic variant)
Hemoglobin E (HbE; Glu26Lys pathogenic variant)
The p.Lys8ValfsTer13 and p.Ser9ValfsTer13 mutations are nonsense variants in HBB for β thalassemia. Therefore, in this case it would be most likely that Marina had compound heterozygous p.Lys8ValfsTer13 and p. Ser9ValfsTer13, which results in β thalassemia major.

83. **E.** Beta thalassemia (β thalassemia) is characterized by reduced synthesis of the hemoglobin subunit beta that results in microcytic hypochromic anemia, an abnormal peripheral-blood smear with nucleated red blood cells, and reduced amounts of hemoglobin A (HbA) on hemoglobin analysis. Beta thalassemia is an autosomal recessive disease, results from the variants in the *HBB* gene on 11p15.4. Some variants in *HBB* may cause hemoglobinopathy other than β thalassemia, such as:
Hemoglobin S (HbC; Glu6Val pathogenic variant)
Hemoglobin C (HbC; Glu6Lys pathogenic variant)
Hemoglobin D (D-Punjab; Glu121Gln pathogenic variant)
Hemoglobin O (O-Arab; Glu121Lys pathogenic variant)
Hemoglobin E (HbE; Glu26Lys pathogenic variant)
Nonsense, frameshift, or sometimes splicing mutations usually result in β° thalassemia alleles (complete absence of hemoglobin subunit beta production). Pathogenic variants in the promoter area (either the CACCC or the TATA box), the polyadenylation signal, or the 5′−3′ untranslated region, or by splicing abnormalities usually results in β^{+} thalassemia alleles (residual output of globin beta chains). c.-138C > A is a transcriptional mutant in the proximal CACC box of the promoter region. c.91 + 6T > C and p. Ala27Ser are splicing variants, mild or silent *HBB* pathogenic variants for β thalassemia. The c.*6C > G mutation is a mild pathogenic variant

in 3′ UTR of *HBB*. The p.Lys8ValfsTer13 and p. Ser9ValfsTer13 mutations are nonsense variants in *HBB*.

Therefore, in this case it would be most likely that Marina had compound heterozygous p. Lys8ValfsTer13 and p.Ser9ValfsTer13, resulting in β thalassemia major.

84. **A.** Beta thalassemia (β thalassemia) is characterized by reduced synthesis of the hemoglobin subunit beta that results in microcytic hypochromic anemia, an abnormal peripheral-blood smear with nucleated red blood cells, and reduced amounts of hemoglobin A (HbA) on hemoglobin analysis. Beta thalassemia, an autosomal recessive disease, results from the variants in the *HBB* gene on 11p15.4.

β thalassemia may be divided into thalassemia major and thalassemia minor. Individuals with thalassemia major have severe anemia and hepatosplenomegaly; they usually come to medical attention within the first 2 years of life. Without treatment, affected children have severe failure to thrive and shortened life expectancy. Individuals with thalassemia intermedia or minor present later and have milder anemia that only rarely requires transfusion. *Nonsense, frameshift, or sometimes splicing mutations usually result in β° thalassemia alleles (complete absence of hemoglobin subunit beta production).* Pathogenic variants in the promoter area (either the CACCC or the TATA box), the polyadenylation signal, or the 5′ or 3′ untranslated region, or by splicing abnormalities usually results in β⁺ thalassemia alleles (residual output of globin beta chains). The p. Lys8ValfsTer13 and p.Ser9ValfsTer13 mutations are nonsense variants in *HBB*. HbH and Hb Barts are different forms of α thalassemia.

Therefore, it would be most likely that this patient had β thalassemia major.

85. **A.** Beta thalassemia (β thalassemia) is characterized by reduced synthesis of the hemoglobin subunit beta that results in microcytic hypochromic anemia, an abnormal peripheral-blood smear with nucleated red blood cells, and reduced amounts of hemoglobin A (HbA) on hemoglobin analysis. Beta thalassemia is an autosomal recessive disease that results from the variants in the *HBB* gene on 11p15.4. Some variants in *HBB* may cause hemoglobinopathy other than β thalassemia, such as:
Hemoglobin S (HbC; Glu6Val pathogenic variant)
Hemoglobin C (HbC; Glu6Lys pathogenic variant)
Hemoglobin D (D-Punjab; Glu121Gln pathogenic variant)

Hemoglobin O (O-Arab; Glu121Lys pathogenic variant)
Hemoglobin E (HbE; Glu26Lys pathogenic variant)

β thalassemia may be divided into thalassemia major and thalassemia minor. Individuals with thalassemia major have severe anemia and hepatosplenomegaly; they usually come to medical attention within the first 2 years of life. Without treatment, affected children have severe failure to thrive and shortened life expectancy. Individuals with thalassemia intermedia or minor present later and have milder anemia that only rarely requires transfusion.

Nonsense, frameshift, or sometimes splicing mutations usually result in β° thalassemia alleles (complete absence of hemoglobin subunit beta production). *Pathogenic variants in the promoter area (either the CACCC or the TATA box), the polyadenylation signal, or the 5′ or 3′ untranslated region, or by splicing abnormalities usually results in β⁺ thalassemia alleles (residual output of globin beta chains).* The c.-138C > A mutation is a transcriptional mutant in the proximal CACC box of the promoter region. And the c.-81A > G mutation is a mild pathogenic variant in the TATA box. The p.Lys8ValfsTer13 and p. Ser9ValfsTer13 mutations are nonsense variants in *HBB*.

In this case the patient has β thalassemia minor since she had HbA (rule out HbS, HbC, HbD, and HbE, also). Therefore, it is most like that the patient has compound heterozygous c.-138C > A and c.-81A > G, which results in β thalassemia minor.

86. **A.** Beta thalassemia (β thalassemia) is characterized by reduced synthesis of the hemoglobin subunit beta that results in microcytic hypochromic anemia, an abnormal peripheral-blood smear with nucleated red blood cells, and reduced amounts of hemoglobin A (HbA) on hemoglobin analysis. Beta thalassemia is an autosomal recessive disease results from the variants in the *HBB* gene on 11p15.4. Some of variants in *HBB* may cause hemoglobinopathy other than β thalassemia, such as:
Hemoglobin S (HbC; Glu6Val pathogenic variant)
Hemoglobin C (HbC; Glu6Lys pathogenic variant)
Hemoglobin D (D-Punjab; Glu121Gln pathogenic variant)
Hemoglobin E (HbE; Glu26Lys pathogenic variant)
Hemoglobin O (O-Arab; Glu121Lys pathogenic variant)

Nonsense, frameshift, or sometimes splicing mutations usually results in β° thalassemia alleles (complete absence of hemoglobin subunit beta production). *Pathogenic variants in the promoter area (either the CACCC or the TATA box), the polyadenylation signal, or the 5' or 3' untranslated region, or by splicing abnormalities usually results in β⁺ thalassemia alleles (residual output of beta-globin chains).* The p.Ala27Ser mutation is a splicing variant, a mild or silent *HBB* pathogenic variant for β thalassemia. The c.-138C > A mutation is a transcriptional mutant in the proximal CACC box of the promoter region. The p.Lys8ValfsTer13 and p.Ser9ValfsTer13 mutations are nonsense variants in *HBB*.

In this case, the patient has β thalassemia minor with 30% residual HbA. Therefore, it is most like that the patient has compound heterozygous c.-138C > A and p.Ala27Ser, which results in β thalassemia minor.

87. **B.** Beta thalassemia (β thalassemia) is characterized by reduced synthesis of the hemoglobin subunit beta that results in microcytic hypochromic anemia, an abnormal peripheral-blood smear with nucleated red blood cells, and reduced amounts of hemoglobin A (HbA) on hemoglobin analysis. Beta thalassemia is an autosomal recessive disease results from the variants in the *HBB* gene on 11p15.4.

β thalassemia may be divided into thalassemia major and thalassemia minor. Individuals with thalassemia major have severe anemia and hepatosplenomegaly; they usually come to medical attention within the first 2 years of life. Without treatment, affected children have severe failure to thrive and shortened life expectancy. Individuals with thalassemia intermedia or minor present later and have milder anemia that only rarely requires transfusion. Nonsense, frameshift, or sometimes splicing mutations usually result in β° thalassemia alleles (complete absence of hemoglobin subunit beta production). *Pathogenic variants in the promoter area (either the CACCC or the TATA box), the polyadenylation signal, or the 5' or 3' untranslated region, or by splicing abnormalities usually result in β⁺ thalassemia alleles (residual output of beta-globin chains).* The c.-138C > A mutation is a transcriptional mutant in the proximal CACC box of the promoter region. The c.-81A > G mutation is a mild pathogenic variant in the TATA box. HbH and Hb Barts are different forms of α thalassemia associated with pathogenic variants in *HBA1* and/or *HBA2*.

This patient has 35% residual HbA, and she has compound heterozygous mutations in the promoter regions of *HBB* for β thalassemia. Therefore, β thalassemia minor is the most appropriate diagnosis in this patient.

88. **D.** Beta thalassemia major causes patients to have no HbA ($\alpha^2\beta^2$), but persistent HbF ($\alpha^2\gamma^2$). Fetal hemoglobin (HbF, $\alpha^2\gamma^2$) is the main oxygen transport protein in the human fetus during the last 7 months of development in the uterus and persists in the newborn until roughly 6 months old. It constitutes approximately 60%−80% of total hemoglobin in the full-term newborn, then gradually is replaced by HbA. Hemoglobin A (HbA, $\alpha^2\beta^2$) is the most common human hemoglobin tetramer in adults comprising over 97% of the total red-blood-cell hemoglobin. Homozygous p.Glu6Val in *HBB* results in sickle cell disease. (http://www.ncbi.nlm.nih.gov/books/NBK1426/).

Hemoglobin Constant Spring (Hb^{CS}) is a variant in which a mutation in *HBA2* produces an alpha-globin chain that is abnormally long. HB-$\alpha^{20.5}$ removes *HBA2* and part of *HBA1* and produce α° thalassemia.

This full-term Pakistanian patient had alpha globin due to the presence of HbF ($\alpha^2\gamma^2$). The absence of any adult hemoglobin (HbA) in him likely indicates beta thalassemia major because of homozygous mutations in *HBB*, which leads to two null beta alleles. *β° thalassemia (complete absence of hemoglobin subunit beta production) alleles result from nonsense, frameshift, or (sometimes) splicing mutations.* Therefore, it would be most likely that this patient had beta thalassemia major with homozygous p.Gln39Ter in *HBB*.

89. **D.** Hemoglobin E (HbE) results from a thalassemic structural variant in *HBB*. It is characterized by the presence of an abnormal structure as well as a biosynthetic defect. *The nucleotide substitution at codon 26, producing the HbE variant ($\alpha^2\beta^2$, p.Glu26Lys), activates a potential cryptic RNA splice region, resulting in alternative splicing at this position.* Because the normal donor site has to compete with this new site, the level of normally spliced β messenger RNA with the HbE mutation is reduced, resulting in the clinical phenotype of a mild form of β thalassemia. A homozygous state for Hb E results in a mild hemolytic microcytic anemia. Compound heterozygosities for β thalassemia and Hb E result in a wide range of often severe but sometimes mild or even clinically asymptomatic clinical phenotypes (http://www.ncbi.nlm.nih.gov/books/NBK1426/).

Therefore, the β^E mutation reduces the quantity of the synthesized structurally abnormal Hb E by creating an abnormal cryptic splice site.

90. **B.** Wilson disease is a disorder of copper metabolism that can present with hepatic, neurologic, or psychiatric disturbances or a combination of these, in individuals ranging from 3 to over 50 years of age. Kayser–Fleischer rings, frequently present as a result of copper deposition in Descemet's membrane of the cornea and reflect a high degree of copper storage in the body. *Wilson disease, an autosomal recessive disease, results from mutations in the* ATP7B *gene* (http://www.ncbi.nlm.nih.gov/books/NBK1512/)

Variants in *ATP7A* result in X-linked recessive Menkes disease. Variants in *HFE* are associated with hereditary hemochromatosis. *ATP8A* and *ATP8B* are not recognized genes in *Homo sapiens*.

Therefore, *ATP7B* would most likely be sequenced in order to confirm the diagnosis in this patient.

91. **C.** Hereditary hemochromatosis, Menkes disease, and Wilson disease are all caused by dysfunction of metal metabolism. Menkes disease is an X-linked recessive disorder, while hereditary hemochromatosis and Wilson disease are autosomal recessive disorders. Germline pathogenic variants in *ATP7B* result in Wilson's disease. Germline pathogenic variants in *ATP7A* results in Menkes disease. Germline pathogenic variants in *HFE* result in hereditary hemochromatosis (http://www.ncbi.nlm.nih.gov/books/NBK1512/).

The c.3207C > A(p.His1069Gln) mutation is the common mutation in *ATP7B* in populations of European origin and is associated with neurologic or hepatic disease, and a mean age at onset of about 20 years. The c.2333G > T(p.Arg778Leu) mutation in exon 8 is the most common mutation in the Asian population, found at a high frequency in all Chinese and ethnically related populations studies.

Therefore, *compound heterozygous c.2333G > T(p. Arg778Leu) and c.3207C > A(p.His1069Gln) mutations in* ATP7B *result in Wilson disease.*

92. **B.** Wilson disease is a disorder of copper metabolism that can present with hepatic, neurologic, or psychiatric disturbances, or a combination of these, in individuals ranging from 3 to over 50 years of age. Kayser–Fleischer rings, frequently present, result from copper deposition in Descemet's membrane of the cornea and reflect a high degree of copper storage in the body. *Wilson disease is an autosomal recessive disease results from mutations in the* ATP7B *gene* (http://www.ncbi.nlm.nih.gov/books/NBK1512/).

This patient's parents were obligate carriers. Therefore, this female patient's sister had a 25% (1/4) risk of being affected, too.

93. **C.** Wilson disease is a disorder of copper metabolism that can present with hepatic, neurologic, or psychiatric disturbances, or a combination of these, in individuals ranging from 3 to over 50 years of age. Kayser–Fleischer rings, frequently present, result from copper deposition in Descemet's membrane of the cornea and reflect a high degree of copper storage in the body. *Wilson disease is an autosomal recessive disease results from mutations in the* ATP7B *gene* (http://www.ncbi.nlm.nih.gov/books/NBK1512/).

This patient's parents were obligate carriers. The 12-year-old sister did not have symptoms, but her copper level was not tested. An elevated copper level could not be ruled out, but she remained asymptomatic. Therefore, this female patient's sister had a 50% (1/2) chance of being a silent carrier.

94. **D.** Wilson disease is a disorder of copper metabolism that can present with hepatic, neurologic, or psychiatric disturbances, or a combination of these, in individuals ranging from 3 to over 50 years of age. Kayser–Fleischer rings, frequently present, result from copper deposition in Descemet's membrane of the cornea and reflect a high degree of copper storage in the body. *Wilson disease, an autosomal recessive disease, results from mutations in the* ATP7B *gene* (http://www.ncbi.nlm.nih.gov/books/NBK1512/).

This patient's parents were obligate carriers. The 12-year-old sister did not have symptoms and did not have an elevated copper level. So there was no indication that the sister had Wilson disease. Therefore, this female patient's sister had 2/3 chances to be a silent carrier, since she did not have Wilson disease.

95. **B.** Hereditary hemochromatosis, Menkes disease, and Wilson disease are all caused by dysfunction of metal metabolism. *Menkes disease is X-linked recessive,* while hereditary hemochromatosis and Wilson disease are autosomal recessive disorders. *Germline pathogenic variants in* ATP7A *results in Menkes disease.* Germline pathogenic variants in *ATP7B* result in Wilson disease. Germline pathogenic variants in *HFE* result in hereditary hemochromatosis.

Therefore, it would be most likely that this newborn boy had Menkes disease caused by p.Ser637Leu mutation in *ATP7A*.

96. **A.** Infants with classic Menkes disease appear healthy until age 2–3 months, when loss of developmental milestones, hypotonia, seizures,

and failure to thrive occur. The diagnosis is usually suspected when infants exhibit typical neurological changes and concomitant characteristic changes of the hair (short, sparse, coarse, twisted, and often lightly pigmented). Temperature instability and hypoglycemia may be present in the neonatal period. Death usually occurs by age 3 years. *Menkes disease, an X-linked recessive disease, results from mutations in the* ATP7A *gene* (http://www.ncbi.nlm.nih.gov/books/NBK1413/).

Germline pathogenic variants in *ATP7B* result in autosomal recessive Wilson disease. Germline pathogenic variants in *HFE* are associated with hereditary hemochromatosis. *ATP8A* and *ATP8B* are not recognized as genes in *Homo sapiens*.

Therefore, *ATP7A* would most likely be sequenced in order to confirm the diagnosis in this patient.

97. **B.** Hemochromatosis is a group of nonneoplastic hematological disorders classified by the age at onset and other factors, such as genetic cause and mode of inheritance. HFE-*associated hereditary hemochromatosis (HFE-HH) is the most common form of the disorder.* Ferroportin-related hereditary hemochromatosis is an adult-onset disorder. Men with these two types typically develop symptoms between the ages of 40 and 60, and women usually develop symptoms after menopause.

HFE-HH is an autosomal recessive disease characterized by excessive storage of iron in the liver, skin, pancreas, heart, joints, and testes. In untreated individuals, early symptoms may include abdominal pain, weakness, lethargy, and weight loss. The risk of cirrhosis is significantly increased when the serum ferritin is higher than 1000 ng/mL. Other findings may include a progressive increase in skin pigmentation, diabetes mellitus, congestive heart failure and/or arrhythmias, arthritis, and hypogonadism. Clinical *HFE*-HH is more common in men than in women. The diagnosis of clinical *HFE*-HH in individuals with clinical findings consistent with *HFE*-HH and the diagnosis of biochemical *HFE*-HH are typically based on findings of an elevated transferrin-iron saturation of 45% or higher and a serum ferritin concentration above the upper limit of normal, such as >300 ng/mL in men and >200 ng/mL in women, and two *HFE*-HH causing mutations on confirmatory *HFE* molecular genetic testing (http://www.ncbi.nlm.nih.gov/books/NBK1440/).

Juvenile hereditary hemochromatosis is a juvenile-onset autosomal recessive disease. Iron accumulation begins early in life, and symptoms may begin to appear in childhood. By age 20, decreased or absent secretion of sex hormones is evident. Females usually begin menstruation in a normal manner, but menses stop after a few years. Males may experience delayed puberty or sex hormone deficiency symptoms such as impotence. If the disorder is untreated, heart disease is evident by age 30. Variants in two genes, *HJV* and *HAMP*, result in juvenile hemochromatosis. *HJV* (HFE2) (locus name HFE2A) encoding hemojuvelin accounts for more than 90% of cases. *HAMP* (HEPC) (locus name HFE2B) encoding hepcidin accounts for fewer than 10% of cases (http://www.ncbi.nlm.nih.gov/books/NBK1170/).

TFR2-related hereditary hemochromatosis (*TFR2*-HH) is an autosomal recessive disease. Onset of *TFR2*-HH is usually intermediate between *HFE*-HH and juvenile hereditary hemochromatosis. Symptoms of *TFR2*-HH generally begin before age 30. *TFR2*-HH is characterized by increased intestinal iron absorption resulting in iron accumulation in the liver, heart, pancreas, and endocrine organs. The age at onset is earlier than in *HFE*-associated HH. Some individuals present in the second decade and others present as adults with fatigue and arthralgia and/or organ involvement, including liver cirrhosis, diabetes mellitus, and arthropathy. In other individuals, *TFR2*-HH may not be progressive even if untreated (http://www.ncbi.nlm.nih.gov/books/NBK1349/).

Ferroportin-related hereditary hemochromatosis is an autosomal dominant late-onset iron overload disorder. Iron storage affects reticuloendothelial rather than parenchymal cells. It is caused by mutations in *SLC40A1* encoding ferroportin.

This patient and his brother are diagnosed in their 50s. The disease seems to be inherited in autosomal recessive manner since the parents are related and are apparently healthy. Therefore, *HFE* most likely harbors germline pathogenic variant(s) in this patient.

98. **E.** Hemochromatosis is a group of nonneoplastic hematological disorders classified by the age at onset and other factors such as genetic cause and mode of inheritance. *HFE*-associated hereditary hemochromatosis (*HFE*-HH) is the most common form of the disorder. Ferroportin-related hereditary hemochromatosis is an adult-onset disorder. Men with these two types typically develop symptoms between the ages of 40 and 60, and women usually develop symptoms after menopause.

HFE-HH is an autosomal recessive disease characterized by excessive storage of iron in the liver, skin, pancreas, heart, joints, and testes. In untreated individuals, early symptoms may include abdominal pain, weakness, lethargy, and weight loss. The risk of cirrhosis is significantly increased when the serum ferritin is higher than 1000 ng/mL. Other findings may include progressive increase in skin pigmentation, diabetes mellitus, congestive heart failure and/or arrhythmias, arthritis, and hypogonadism. Clinical *HFE*-HH is more common in men than in women. The diagnosis of clinical *HFE*-HH in individuals with clinical findings consistent with *HFE*-HH and the diagnosis of biochemical *HFE*-HH are typically based on finding elevated transferrin-iron saturations of 45% or higher and serum ferritin concentration above the upper limit of normal (i.e., >300 ng/mL in men and >200 ng/mL in women) and two *HFE*-HH causing mutations on confirmatory *HFE* molecular genetic testing (http://www.ncbi.nlm. nih.gov/books/NBK1440/).

Juvenile hereditary hemochromatosis is an juvenile-onset autosomal recessive disease. Iron accumulation begins early in life, and symptoms may begin to appear in childhood. By age 20, decreased or absent secretion of sex hormones is evident. Females usually begin menstruation in a normal manner, but menses stop after a few years. Males may experience delayed puberty or sex hormone deficiency symptoms such as impotence. If the disorder is untreated, heart disease is evident by age 30. Variants in two genes, *HJV* and *HAMP*, result in juvenile hemochromatosis. *HJV* (HFE2) (locus name HFE2A) encoding hemojuvelin accounts for more than 90% of cases. *HAMP* (HEPC) (locus name HFE2B) encoding hepcidin accounts for fewer than 10% of cases (http://www.ncbi.nlm.nih. gov/books/NBK1170/).

TFR2-related hereditary hemochromatosis (*TFR2*-HH) is an autosomal recessive disease. Onset of *TFR2*-HH usually intermediate between *HFE*-HH and juvenile hereditary hemochromatosis. Symptoms of *TFR2*-HH generally begin before age 30. *TFR2*-HH is characterized by increased intestinal iron absorption resulting in iron accumulation in the liver, heart, pancreas, and endocrine organs. The age at onset is earlier than in *HFE*-associated HH. Some individuals present in the second decade and others present as adults with fatigue and arthralgia and/or organ involvement including liver cirrhosis, diabetes mellitus, and arthropathy.

In other individuals, *TFR2*-HH may not be progressive even if untreated (http://www.ncbi. nlm.nih.gov/books/NBK1349/).

Ferroportin-related hereditary hemochromatosis is an autosomal dominant late-onset iron overload disorder. Iron storage affects reticuloendothelial rather than parenchymal cells. *It is caused by mutations in* SLC40A1 *encoding ferroportin.*

This patient and his brother are diagnosed in their 50s. The disease seems to be inherited in an autosomal recessive manner, since the parents are related and are apparently healthy. Therefore, *SLC40A1* for autosomal dominant hemochromatosis LEAST likely harbors germline pathogenic variant(s) in this patient.

99. **C.** Juvenile hemochromatosis is characterized by onset of severe iron overload occurring typically in the first to third decades of life. Prominent clinical features include hypogonadotropic hypogonadism, cardiomyopathy, arthropathy, and liver fibrosis or cirrhosis. Juvenile hemochromatosis is inherited in an autosomal recessive manner. The two genes in which mutations are known to cause juvenile hemochromatosis are *HJV* encoding hemojuvelin, accounting for more than 90% of cases, and *HAMP* encoding hepcidin, accounting for fewer than 10% of cases (http://www.ncbi.nlm.nih. gov/books/NBK1170/).

Clinically serious iron loading, resulting in congestive heart failure at age 21 is most likely to be seen in juvenile hemochromatosis. The more common hereditary hemochromatosis, *HFE*-associated hereditary hemochromatosis, does not generally result in major clinical manifestations until at least the fourth decade of life. Ferroportin-related hereditary hemochromatosis is an adulthood-onset disease. It can result in severe iron loading manifestations, but it is autosomal dominant and often the transferrin saturation is normal despite substantial iron overload. *TFR2*-related hereditary hemochromatosis has a similar presentation to *HFE*-HH. The age at onset is earlier and progression is slower than in juvenile HH. It is caused by homozygous/compound heterozygous mutations in *TFR2*, which encodes transferrin receptor 2.

Therefore, *HJV* for juvenile hemochromatosis most likely harbors germline pathogenic variant(s) in this patient.

100. **A.** *HFE*-associated hereditary hemochromatosis (*HFE*-HH) is an autosomal recessive nonneoplastic hematological disorder characterized by excessive storage of iron in the

liver, skin, pancreas, heart, joints, and testes. In untreated individuals, early symptoms may include abdominal pain, weakness, lethargy, and weight loss. The risk of cirrhosis is significantly increased when the serum ferritin is higher than 1000 ng/mL. Other findings may include a progressive increase in skin pigmentation, diabetes mellitus, congestive heart failure and/or arrhythmias, arthritis, and hypogonadism. Clinical *HFE*-HH is more common in men than in women. The diagnosis of clinical *HFE*-HH in individuals with clinical findings consistent with *HFE*-HH and the diagnosis of biochemical *HFE*-HH are typically based on finding elevated transferrin-iron saturations of 45% or higher and serum ferritin concentrations above the upper limit of normal (>300 ng/mL in men and >200 ng/mL in women) and two *HFE*-HH causing mutations on confirmatory *HFE* molecular genetic testing (http://www.ncbi.nlm.nih.gov/books/NBK1440/).

At least 28 distinct pathogenic variants in *HFE* have been reported. Two missense variants account for the vast majority of disease causing alleles in the population are p.Cys282Tyr and p.His63Asp. In addition, p.Ser65Cys has been seen in combination with p.Cys282Tyr in individuals with iron overload. *Homozygous p.Cys282Tyr is in 60%–90% of individuals with HFE-HH.* Compound heterozygous p.Cys282Tyr and p.His63Asp are in 3%–8% (http://www.ncbi.nlm.nih.gov/books/NBK1440/).

Therefore, homozygous p.Cys282Tyr would most likely be Jon's molecular test result.

101. **B.** Approximately 87% of individuals of European origin with *HFE*-hereditary hemochromatosis (*HFE*-HH) are either homozygous for the p.Cys282Tyr mutation or compound heterozygous for p.Cys282Tyr and p.His63Asp mutations. Three phenotypes of *HFE*-HH are now recognized:
- Clinical *HFE*-HH (individuals with end-organ damage [e.g., advanced cirrhosis, cardiac failure, skin pigment changes, or diabetes] secondary to iron storage). Alcohol consumption worsens the symptoms in *HFE*-HH.
- Biochemical *HFE*-HH (individuals with evidence of iron overload as determined by transferrin-iron saturation and serum ferritin concentration only).
- Nonexpressing p.Cys282Tyr homozygotes (p.Cys282Tyr homozygotes without clinical or biochemical evidence of iron overload, such as normal serum ferritin concentration).

Several large-scale screening studies in general populations have demonstrated that most individuals homozygous for the p.Cys282Tyr mutation do not have clinical *HFE*-HH. However, a significant proportion of individuals with this genotype (especially males) have biochemical *HFE*-HH, but not everyone. *In the absence of unbiased data, penetrance of clinical end points of iron overload was reported to be as low as 2% in a large study.* Currently, no test can predict whether an individual homozygous for p.Cys282Tyr will develop clinical *HFE*-HH. The penetrance for p.Cys282Tyr/p.His63Asp compound heterozygotes is lower; only approximately 0.5%–2.0% of such individuals develop clinical evidence of iron overload (http://www.ncbi.nlm.nih.gov/books/NBK1440/).

Therefore, this patient had up to 6% of risk developing clinical symptom of hemochromatosis in his lifetime.

102. **A.** Approximately 87% of individuals of European origin with *HFE*-hereditary hemochromatosis (*HFE*-HH) are either homozygous for the p.Cys282Tyr mutation or compound heterozygous p.Cys282Tyr and p.His63Asp mutations. Three phenotypes of *HFE*-HH are now recognized:
- Clinical *HFE*-HH (individuals with end-organ damage [e.g., advanced cirrhosis, cardiac failure, skin pigment changes, or diabetes] secondary to iron storage). Alcohol consumption worsens the symptoms in *HFE*-HH.
- Biochemical *HFE*-HH (individuals with evidence of iron overload as determined by transferrin-iron saturation and serum ferritin concentration only).
- Nonexpressing p.Cys282Tyr homozygotes (p.Cys282Tyr homozygotes without clinical or biochemical evidence of iron overload, such as normal serum ferritin concentration).

Several large-scale screening studies in the general population have demonstrated that most individuals homozygous for the p.Cys282Tyr mutation do not have clinical *HFE*-HH. However, a significant proportion of individuals with this genotype (especially males) have biochemical *HFE*-HH, but not everyone. In the absence of unbiased data, penetrance of clinical end points of iron overload was reported to be as low as 2% in a large study. Currently, no test can predict whether an individual homozygous for p.Cys282Tyr will develop clinical *HFE*-HH. *The penetrance for p.Cys282Tyr/p.His63Asp compound heterozygotes is lower; only approximately*

0.5%—2.0% of such individuals develop clinical evidence of iron overload (http://www.ncbi.nlm.nih.gov/books/NBK1440/).

Therefore, this patient had about 0.5% risk of developing clinical symptoms of hemochromatosis in his lifetime.

103. **A.** *HFE*-associated hereditary hemochromatosis (*HFE*-HH) is characterized by inappropriately high absorption of iron by the gastrointestinal mucosa. Clinical symptoms of *HFE*-HH are related to excessive storage of iron in the liver, skin, pancreas, heart, joints, and testes. In untreated individuals, early symptoms may include abdominal pain, weakness, lethargy, and weight loss. The risk of cirrhosis is significantly increased when the serum ferritin is higher than 1000 ng/mL. Other findings may include progressive increase in skin pigmentation, diabetes mellitus, congestive heart failure and/or arrhythmias, arthritis, and hypogonadism. Clinical *HFE*-HH is more common in men than in women. *HFE*-HH is inherited in an autosomal recessive manner (http://www.ncbi.nlm.nih.gov/books/NBK1440/).

Approximately 87% of individuals of European origin with *HFE*-HH are either homozygous for the p.Cys282Tyr (C282Y) mutation or compound heterozygous p.Cys282Tyr and p.His63Asp (H63D) mutations. *Homozygotes for p.Cys282Tyr have a greater risk for iron overload than p.Cys282Tyr/p.His63Asp compound heterozygotes.*

Therefore, it is most likely the patient is homozygous for p.Cys282Tyr.

104. **B.** Hemophilia A is an X-linked recessive nonneoplastic hematological disorder characterized by a deficiency in factor VIII clotting activity that results in prolonged oozing after injuries, tooth extractions, or surgery and delayed or recurrent bleeding prior to complete wound healing. The diagnosis is established in individuals with low factor VIII clotting activity in the presence of a normal von Willebrand factor (VWF) level. Severe hemophilia A is indicated by active factor VIII levels <1 or 2%. Carrier females most likely are asymptomatic but have a 50% chance of transmitting the *F8* pathogenic variant in each pregnancy. Sons who inherit the pathogenic variant will be affected. Daughters who inherit the pathogenic variant will be carriers (http://www.ncbi.nlm.nih.gov/books/NBK1404/).

Therefore, the couple's next child would have $1/2 \times 1/2 = 1/4$ risk of having hemophilia A, since the mother is a carrier.

105. **C.** Hemophilia A is an X-linked recessive nonneoplastic hematological disorder

characterized by deficiency in factor VIII clotting activity that results in prolonged oozing after injuries, tooth extractions, or surgery and delayed or recurrent bleeding prior to complete wound healing. The diagnosis is established in individuals with low factor VIII clotting activity in the presence of a normal von Willebrand factor (VWF) level. Severe hemophilia A is indicated by active factor VIII levels <1 or 2%. Carrier females most likely are asymptomatic, but have a 50% chance of transmitting the *F8* pathogenic variant in each pregnancy. Sons who inherit the pathogenic variant will be affected. Daughters who inherit the pathogenic variant will be carriers (http://www.ncbi.nlm.nih.gov/books/NBK1404/).

Therefore, the couple's next son would have a 1/2 risk of having hemophilia A, since the mother is a carrier.

106. **D.** *Hemophilia A is an X-linked recessive nonneoplastic hematological disorder* characterized by a deficiency in factor VIII clotting activity that results in prolonged oozing after injuries, tooth extractions, or surgery and delayed or recurrent bleeding prior to complete wound healing. The diagnosis is established in individuals with low factor VIII clotting activity in the presence of a normal von Willebrand factor (VWF) level. Severe hemophilia A is indicated by active factor VIII levels <1 or 2%. *F8* is the only gene in which pathogenic variants are known to cause hemophilia A. One-third to one-half of affected males have no family history of hemophilia, which may due to a de novo variant in the affected male or his mother. In this case, the nature of the variant is not revealed, so we may not predict symptoms. Immediate treatment of bleeding or prophylaxis is always necessary for patients with hemophilia A (http://www.ncbi.nlm.nih.gov/books/NBK1404/). Hemophilia B is an X-linked recessive disorder of factor IX due to variants in *F9*.

Therefore, choice D is correct.

107. **B.** *Hemophilia B is an X-linked recessive disorder* characterized by deficiency in factor IX clotting activity that results in prolonged oozing after injuries, tooth extractions, or surgery and delayed or recurrent bleeding prior to complete wound healing. The diagnosis is established in individuals with low factor IX clotting activity in the presence of a normal von Willebrand factor (VWF) level. Severe hemophilia B is indicated by active factor IX levels <1 or 2%. Molecular genetic testing of *F9*, the gene encoding factor IX, identifies pathogenic variants in more than 99% of individuals with hemophilia B. Approximately

50% of affected males have no family history of hemophilia B. Hemophilia B is not a self-limited disease. Immediate treatment of bleeding or prophylaxis is always necessary (http://www.ncbi.nlm.nih.gov/books/NBK1495/). Hemophilia A is an X-linked recessive disorder of factor VIII due to variants in *F8*.

In this case, both the patient and the mother carried the same variant in *F9*. *Siblings of the patient would have 25% chances to be affected.* Therefore, choice B is correct.

108. **C.** Hemophilia A is an X-linked recessive disorder of factor VIII due to variants in *F8*. *An F8 intron 22-A inversion is identified in nearly half of families with severe hemophilia A. An intron 1 inversion is identified in 2%−5% of individuals with severe hemophilia A* (http://www.ncbi.nlm.nih.gov/books/NBK1495/).

Therefore, an inversion would most likely be detected in this patient.

109. **D.** Sanger sequencing by capillary electrophoresis, a chain-termination method of DNA sequencing, has been a powerful technique in molecular biology. DNA is replicated in the presence of dideoxynucleotides (ddNPTs). These bases stop the replication process when they are incorporated into the growing strand of DNA, resulting in varying lengths of short DNA. These short DNA strands are ordered by size; by reading the end letters from the shortest to the longest piece, the whole sequence of the original DNA is revealed. *Sanger sequencing of target region in F8 may reveal whether a specific single-nucleotide variant, such as a nonsense mutation in this case, is in an individual.*

Next-generation sequencing (NGS) refers to non-Sanger-based high-throughput DNA sequencing technologies. Millions or billions of DNA strands can be sequenced in parallel, yielding substantially more throughput. It parallelizes the sequencing process, producing thousands or millions of sequences concurrently while lowering the cost of DNA sequencing beyond what is possible with standard dye-terminator methods. NGS may be used to detect SNPs and very small in/dels, such as a 5-bp deletion. But it cannot detect deletion or duplication of one or more exons or the entire gene. It is not the test of choice to detect a known single-nucleotide variant, such as a nonsense mutation, in family members.

A real-time polymerase chain reaction is a laboratory technique of molecular biology based on the polymerase chain reaction (PCR). It monitors the amplification of a targeted DNA molecule at each cycle of PCR. When the DNA is in the log-linear phase of amplification, the amount of fluorescence increases above the background. Quantitative PCR may be used to quantify gene expression.

Multiplex ligation-dependent probe amplification (MLPA) permits multiple targets to be amplified with only a single primer pair. Each probe consists of two oligonucleotides that recognize adjacent target sites on the DNA. One probe oligonucleotide contains the sequence recognized by the forward primer, the other the sequence is recognized by the reverse primer. Only when both probe oligonucleotides are hybridized to their respective targets can they be ligated into a complete probe. The advantage of splitting the probe into two parts is that the ligated oligonucleotides but not the unbound probe oligonucleotides are amplified. If the probes were not split in this way, the primer sequences at either end would cause the probes to be amplified regardless of their hybridization to the template DNA, and the amplification product would not be dependent on the number of target sites present in the sample DNA. Each complete probe has a unique length, so its resulting amplicons can be separated and identified by (capillary) electrophoresis. Because the forward primer used for probe amplification is fluorescently labeled, each amplicon generates a fluorescent peak that can be detected by a capillary sequencer. Comparing the peak pattern obtained on a given sample with that obtained on various reference samples, the relative quantity of each amplicon can be determined. This ratio is a measure for the ratio in which the target sequence is present in the sample DNA. MLPA may be used to detect SNPs and CNV, such as diagnosing patients with Duchenne muscular dystrophy.

This patient's factor VIII clot activity was lower than 1% with a normal and functional von Willebrand factor level. So he had a severe form of hemophilia A (factor VIII deficiency). Hemophilia A is an X-linked disease resulting from variants in *F8* on Xq28.

Therefore, Sanger sequencing would be the test of choice for targeted test of the nonsense mutation in family members.

110. **B.** Hemophilia A is an X-linked disease that results from variants in the *F8* gene for factor VIII on Xq28. *An intron 22-A inversion (14−20 kb) is identified in nearly half of families with severe hemophilia A, but it is not identified in families with moderate or mild hemophilia A. This*

inversion can be detected by multiple techniques (e.g., long-range PCR, inverse PCR). An intron 1 inversion (1 kB) is identified in 2%–5% of individuals with severe hemophilia A and has not been described in families with moderate or mild hemophilia A. The mutation detection rate in individuals with hemophilia A who do not have one of the two common inversions varies from 75% to 98%, depending on the testing methods used. In the severe form of the disease the mutation detection rate is even lower, about 55%. A factor VIII level less than 1% of normal is classified as severe hemophilia A. For individuals with severe hemophilia A, a targeted molecular genetic testing is generally performed to identify the intron 22 or intron 1 inversion. The incidence of intron 22 inversion is approximately 50% in severe HA patients, and without a significant ethnic difference. The intron 22 inversion is also a high-risk factor for inhibitor formation. Thus, it has drawn special attention as a hotspot of F8 mutation. In a previous report, HA patients with intron 22 inversion exhibited an inhibitor prevalence of >22%. For this reason, tests for the intron 22 inversion have been the primary step of F8 mutation profiling. If the inversion test is negative, sequence analysis of the 26 exons in *F8* is performed. Deletion/duplication analyses are considered last (http://www.ncbi.nlm.nih.gov/books/NBK1495/).

This patient's factor VIII clotting activity was lower than 1% with a normal and functional von Willebrand factor level. So he had a severe form of hemophilia A (factor VIII deficiency). Therefore, PCR would most likely be used as the first-line test to detect inversions in order to confirm the diagnosis in this patient.

111. **A.** Hemophilia A is characterized by prolonged oozing after injuries, tooth extractions, or surgery and delayed or recurrent bleeding prior to complete wound healing. The diagnosis is established in individuals with low factor VIII clotting activity in the presence of a normal von Willebrand factor (VWF) level. Severe hemophilia A is indicated by active factor VIII levels <1 or 2%. Hemophilia A is inherited in an X-linked manner. Carrier females have a 50% chance of transmitting the *F8* pathogenic variant in each pregnancy. Sons who inherit the pathogenic variant will be affected. Daughters who inherit

the pathogenic variant will be carriers. *F8* is located on Xq28 with 26 exons. *Single-nucleotide variants leading to new stop codons are essentially all associated with a severe phenotype, as are most frameshift mutations* (http://www.ncbi.nlm.nih.gov/books/NBK1495/).

Therefore, the unborn boy would most likely have severe hemophilia A.

112. **B.** All the genes listed in the question are associated with hemophilia. The family had X-linked hemophilia, which narrows it down to *F8* and *F9*. Factor IX Leyden is an unusual *F9* variant caused by point mutations in the *F9* promoter. *It is associated with very low levels of factor IX and severe hemophilia during childhood, but spontaneous resolution at puberty as factor IX levels nearly normalize.*

Therefore, it would be most likely that *F9* was mutated in the family.

113. **A.** Hemophilia B is a very heterogeneous disease both in clinical severity and at the molecular level. Point mutations, particularly missense mutations of *F9* are the most frequent changes that affect the *F9* gene. Missense mutations in the promoter region possibly disrupt the recognition sequences for several specific gene regulatory proteins and result in the reduced transcription of coagulation factor IX. This situation gives rise to a specific hemophilia B phenotype—*hemophilia B Leyden*. If there is a mutation in the hepatocyte nuclear factor 4 (HNF-4) binding site in the 5′ UTR, an unidentified protein presumably binds to this site and an androgen-responsive element exerts its effect through this protein–protein interaction. So at puberty, during which androgen levels increase, the phenotype severity decreases to a mild level. Research has supported that other transcription factors may contribute to the recovery of hemophilia at puberty.

The intron 22-A inversion and intron 1 inversion of *F8* are the common pathogenic variants for hemophilia A. p.Glu117stop of *F11* is a common pathogenic variants for hemophilia C in Ashkenazi Jews.

Therefore, it would be most likely that the mother/fetus had c.-6G > A in the 5′ UTR region of *F9*.

114. **E.** The hemophilia is in the maternal family. The mother most likely is a carrier because of the positive family history. The husband may carry a

mutation, too, but the likelihood is as much as for any male in general population. Predictive testing and testing isolated carriers are difficult.

Therefore, the brother of the mother should be tested first in order to detect the familial mutation, since he was the proband (index case) of this family for hemophilia.

115. **A.** If a mother has a son with hemophilia, but no other affected relatives, her prior risk for being a carrier depends on the type of mutation. *Point mutations and the common F8 inversions almost always arise in male meiosis. As a result, 98% of mothers of a male with one of these mutations carry a new mutation derived from their father (the maternal grandfather of the affected male).* In contrast, deletion mutations usually arise during female meiosis.

Therefore, most likely the grandfather passed on the mutation to the mother owing to a new mutation.

116. **G.** If a mother has a son with hemophilia, but no other affected relatives, her prior risk for being a carrier depends on the type of mutation. Point mutations and the common *F8* inversions almost always arise in male meiosis. As a result, 98% of mothers of a male with one of these mutations carry the mutation owing to a new mutation in their father (the maternal grandfather of the affected male). In contrast, *deletion mutations usually arise during female meiosis.*

Therefore, in this case it would be most likely the mother passed on the mutation to the boy owing to a new mutation.

117. **A.** If a mother has a son with hemophilia, but no other affected relatives, her prior risk for being a carrier depends on the type of mutation. *Point mutations and the common F8 inversions almost always arise in male meiosis. As a result, 98% of mothers of a male with one of these mutations carry the mutation owing to a new mutation in their father (the maternal grandfather of the affected male).* In contrast, deletion mutations usually arise during female meiosis.

Therefore, it would be most likely the grandfather passed on the mutation to the mother owing to a new mutation.

118. **A.** All the genes listed in the question are associated with hemophilia. *F8*-associated hemophilia A is the most common type of hemophilia, and it is inherited in an X-linked recessive manner. Hemophilia B, caused by variants in *F9*, is an X-linked recessive disease, too. But the prevalence/incidence of hemophilia B is not as much as that for hemophilia A. *F13*, *F13B*, and *vWF* are associated autosomal recessive hemophilia.

Therefore, it would be most likely that *F8* harbors a germline pathogenic variant in the family.

119. **A.** *F8, F9, F11, F13, F13B*, and *vWF* are all associated with hemophilia, but not *F2*. *F2* is associated with thrombophilia. Therefore, it is most likely that *F2* was not in this NGS panel for hemophilia.

120. **D.** Hemophilia B is an X-linked recessive disease. The diagnosis of hemophilia B is established in individuals with low factor IX clotting activity. Molecular genetic testing of *F9*, the gene encoding factor IX, identifies pathogenic variants in more than 99% of individuals with hemophilia B. Linkage analysis is possibly appropriate if no mutation detected by sequencing and deletion/duplication analysis of *F9*. It may be used to track an unidentified *F9* disease causing allele in a family and to identify the person in whom the de novo mutation originated (http://www.ncbi.nlm.nih.gov/books/NBK1495/).

In this case, it was important to know whether the wife's uncle, the affected member, had the SNP. If the wife's maternal uncle did not have the SNP, the SNP did not in link with hemophilia B phenotype in this family.

Therefore, the wife's uncle, the affected member, should be evaluated next for the SNP in this family.

121. **B.** Promoters are usually located upstream of the transcription start sites of genes on the DNA, which can be about 100–1000 bp long. *Promoters initiate transcription of a particular gene.* A variant at the exon–intron boundary most likely changes splicing. Dominant negative effect usually is caused by a variant in an exon. Truncating variant usually is caused by variants in exons also.

Therefore, most likely the 5-bp deletion in a promoter region alters transcriptional activity of factor VIII mRNA, which causes the factor VIII deficiency in this patient, if it is pathogenic.

122. **A.** Hemophilia A is the second most common form of hereditary coagulopathy, which is caused by deficiency in factor VIII (*F8*) clotting activity. The diagnosis of hemophilia A is established in individuals with low factor VIII clotting activity in the presence of a normal von Willebrand factor (VWF) level. Hemophilia A results from variants in *F8* on X chromosome. Molecular genetic testing of *F8* identifies pathogenic variants in as many as 98% of individuals with hemophilia A. The birth prevalence of hemophilia A is approximately 1:4000–1:5000 live male births worldwide.

von Willebrand disease (VWD) is the most common form of hereditary coagulopathy, which is caused by deficient or defective plasma von Willebrand factor (VWF), a large multimeric glycoprotein that plays a pivotal role in primary hemostasis by mediating platelet hemostatic function and stabilizing blood coagulation factor VIII (*F8*). Bleeding history may become more apparent with increasing age. The infant had an increased PTT in the context of a normal PT and bleeding time, and a normal and functional von Willebrand factor level which rule out the diagnosis of VWD. VWD affects 0.1%–1% of the population. One in 10,000 seeks tertiary care referral.

Hemophilia B is the third most common form of hereditary coagulopathy, which is caused by deficiency in factor IX (*F9*) clotting activity. The diagnosis of hemophilia B is established in individuals with low factor IX clotting activity. Hemophilia B results from variants in *F9* on the X chromosome. Molecular genetic testing of *F9* identifies pathogenic variants in more than 99% of individuals with hemophilia B. The birth prevalence of hemophilia B is approximately 1 in 20,000 live male births worldwide.

Hemophilia C is a rare form of hereditary coagulopathy that is caused by deficiency in factor XI (*F11*) clotting activity. It predominantly occurs in Jews of Ashkenazi descent. It is the fourth most common coagulation disorder after von Willebrand disease and hemophilias A and B. Hemophilia C is inherited in an autosomal recessive manner. It is distinguished from hemophilia A and B by the fact it does not lead to bleeding into the joints. The diagnosis of hemophilia C is established in individuals with low factor XI (*F11*) clotting activity. Hemophilia C was described first in two sisters and a maternal uncle of an American Jewish family. All three bled after dental extractions, and the sisters also bled after tonsillectomy. In the United States, it is thought to affect 1 in 100,000 of the adult population, a rate that makes hemophilia A 10 times more common than hemophilia C. In Israel, the estimated rate for heterozygosity is 8%.

Factor XIII deficiency occurs exceedingly rarely; it causes a severe bleeding tendency. Most are due to mutations in the A subunit gene (located on chromosome 6p25-p24). Umbilical cord bleeding is common in factor XIII deficiency, reported in almost 80% of cases. Up to 30% of patients sustain a spontaneous intracranial hemorrhage. The diagnosis is established in individuals with low factor XIII (*F13*) clotting

activity. The mutation of *F13* is inherited in an autosomal recessive manner. The birth prevalence of factor XIII deficiency is approximately 1 in 5 million live births worldwide (https://ghr.nlm.nih.gov/condition/hemophilia).

This patient was a male infant. He had an increased PTT in the context of a normal PT and bleeding time, which ruled out factor XIII deficiency. Coagulation factor assays ruled out VWD because his vWF activity was normal. A male relative from his mother's side had "bleeding problems," too, and his mother was apparently healthy without bleeding history. This raises suspicion for X-linked coagulopathy. Therefore, it would be most likely that this patient had hemophilia A caused by a germline pathogenic variant in *F8*, since hemophilia A is the second most common form of hereditary coagulopathy.

123. **C**. *Hemophilia C is a rare form of hereditary coagulopathy, which is caused by deficiency in factor XI (F11) clotting activity. It predominantly occurs in Jews of Ashkenazi descent.* It is the fourth most common coagulation disorder after von Willebrand disease and hemophilia A and B. Hemophilia C is inherited in an autosomal recessive manner. It is distinguished from hemophilia A and B by the fact that it does not lead to bleeding into the joints. The diagnosis of hemophilia C is established in individuals with low factor XI (*F11*) clotting activity. Hemophilia C was described first in two sisters and a maternal uncle of an American Jewish family. All three bled after dental extractions, and the sisters also bled after tonsillectomy. In the United States, it is thought to affect 1 in 100,000 of the adult population, a rate that makes hemophilia A 10 times more common than hemophilia C. In Israel, the estimated rate for heterozygosity is 8%.

von Willebrand disease (VWD) is the most common form of hereditary coagulopathy; it is caused by deficient or defective plasma von Willebrand factor (VWF), a large multimeric glycoprotein that plays a pivotal role in primary hemostasis by mediating platelet hemostatic function and stabilizing blood coagulation factor VIII (*F8*). Bleeding history may become more apparent with increasing age. The infant had an increased PTT in the context of a normal PT and bleeding time and a normal and functional von Willebrand factor level; this rules out the diagnosis of VWD. VWD affects 0.1%–1% of the population. One in 10,000 seeks tertiary care referral.

Hemophilia A is the second most common form of hereditary coagulopathy, which is caused by deficiency in factor VIII (*F8*) clotting activity. The diagnosis of hemophilia A is established in individuals with low factor VIII clotting activity in the presence of a normal von Willebrand factor (VWF) level. Hemophilia A results from variants in the *F8* gene on chromosome X. Molecular genetic testing of *F8* identifies pathogenic variants in as many as 98% of individuals with hemophilia A. The birth prevalence of hemophilia A is approximately 1:4000−1:5000 of live male births worldwide.

Hemophilia B is the third most common form of hereditary coagulopathy, which is caused by deficiency in factor IX (*F9*) clotting activity. The diagnosis of hemophilia B is established in individuals with low factor IX clotting activity. Hemophilia B results from variants in *F9* on X chromosome. Molecular genetic testing of *F9* identifies pathogenic variants in more than 99% of individuals with hemophilia B. The birth prevalence of hemophilia B is approximately 1 in 20,000 live male births worldwide.

Factor XIII deficiency occurs exceedingly rarely, causing a severe bleeding tendency. Most are due to mutations in the A subunit gene (located on chromosome 6p25-p24). Umbilical cord bleeding is common in factor XIII deficiency, reported in almost 80% of cases. Up to 30% of patients sustain a spontaneous intracranial hemorrhage. The diagnosis is established in individuals with low factor XIII (*F13*) clotting activity. The mutation of *F13* is inherited in an autosomal recessive manner. The birth prevalence of factor XIII deficiency is approximately 1 in 5 million live births worldwide (https://ghr.nlm.nih.gov/condition/hemophilia).

This patient was the only person in the family who had the bleeding problem. He had an increased PTT in the context of a normal PT and bleeding time, which ruled out factor XIII deficiency. Coagulation factor assays ruled out VWD because his VWF activity was normal. He was of Ashkenazi Jewish descendent. Therefore, it would be most likely that he had hemophilia C caused by mutations in *F11*, since the estimated prevalence is 6.4/1000 among Ashkenazi Jewish.

124. **D.** Factor XIII deficiency occurs exceedingly rarely; it causes a tendency for severe bleeding. Most of these deficiencies are due to mutations in the A subunit gene (located on chromosome 6p25-p24). *Umbilical cord bleeding is common in factor XIII deficiency, reported in almost 80% of cases.* Up to 30% of patients sustain a spontaneous

intracranial hemorrhage. The diagnosis is established in individuals with low factor XIII (*F13*) clotting activity. *The mutation of F13 is inherited in an autosomal recessive manner.* The birth prevalence of factor XIII deficiency is approximately 1 in 5 million live births worldwide. It is extremely important to diagnose of factor XIII deficiency because these patients tend to develop intracranial hemorrhages.

von Willebrand disease (VWD) is the most common form of hereditary coagulopathy, which is caused by deficient or defective plasma von Willebrand factor (VWF), a large multimeric glycoprotein that plays a pivotal role in primary hemostasis by mediating platelet hemostatic function and stabilizing blood coagulation factor VIII (*F8*). A bleeding history may become more apparent with increasing age. The infant had an increased PTT in the context of a normal PT and bleeding time and a normal and functional von Willebrand factor level, which rules out the diagnosis of VWD. VWD affects 0.1%−1% of the population. One in 10,000 seeks tertiary care referral.

Hemophilia A is the second most common form of hereditary coagulopathy, which is caused by a deficiency in factor VIII (*F8*) clotting activity. The diagnosis of hemophilia A is established in individuals with low factor VIII clotting activity in the presence of a normal von Willebrand factor (VWF) level. Hemophilia A results from variants in the *F8* gene on chromosome X. Molecular genetic testing of *F8* identifies pathogenic variants in as many as 98% of individuals with hemophilia A. The birth prevalence of hemophilia A is approximately 1:4000−1:5000 of live male births worldwide.

Hemophilia B is the third most common form of hereditary coagulopathy, which is caused by deficiency in factor IX (*F9*) clotting activity. The diagnosis of hemophilia B is established in individuals with low factor IX clotting activity. Hemophilia B results from variants in *F9* on the X chromosome. Molecular genetic testing of *F9* identifies pathogenic variants in more than 99% of individuals with hemophilia B. The birth prevalence of hemophilia B is approximately 1 in 20,000 live male births worldwide.

Hemophilia C is a rare form of hereditary coagulopathy, which is caused by a deficiency in factor XI (*F11*) clotting activity. It predominantly occurs in Jews of Ashkenazi descent. It is the fourth most common coagulation disorder after von Willebrand disease and hemophilia A and B. Hemophilia C is inherited in an autosomal recessive manner. It is distinguished from hemophilia A and B by the fact it does not lead to bleeding into the joints. The diagnosis of hemophilia C is established in individuals with low factor XI (*F11*) clotting activity. Hemophilia C was described first in two sisters and a maternal uncle of an American Jewish family. All three bled after dental extractions, and the sisters also bled after tonsillectomy. In the United States, it is thought to affect 1 in 100,000 of the adult population, a rate that makes hemophilia A 10 times more common than hemophilia C. In Israel, the estimated rate for heterozygosity is 8% (https://ghr.nlm.nih.gov/condition/hemophilia).

This patient is the only personal in the family has the bleeding problem. His prothrombin time, partial thromboplastin time, and thrombin time are all normal, which ruled out factor VIII, and factor XI deficiencies. Coagulation factor assays ruled out VWD because his vWF activity is normal. Therefore, it is most likely that the patient in this question has factor XIII deficiency.

125. **D.** *TAT* codes for cystine. *TAG, TAA,* and *TGA* code for the stop codon. Therefore, *the single-nucleotide variant most likely leads to a truncated protein C in this patient*, which stops the translation prematurely.

Therefore, the variant in *PROC* leads to a truncated protein C, which results in protein C deficiency in this patient.

126. **D.** *TAT* codes for cystine. TAG, TAA, and *TGA* code for stop codons. Therefore, *the single-nucleotide variant most likely leads to a truncated protein C in this patient*, which stops the translation prematurely.

Therefore, the variant in *PROC* leads to a truncated protein C, which results in protein C deficiency in this patient.

127. **D.** *TAT* codes for cystine. TAG, *TAA*, and TGA code for stop codons. Therefore, *the single-nucleotide variant most likely leads to a truncated protein C in this patient*, which stops the translation prematurely.

Therefore, the variant in *PROC* leads to a truncated protein C, which results in protein C deficiency in this patient.

128. **B.** There are two commonly recognized polymorphic variants in the *MTHFR* gene (coded for methylenetetrahydrofolate reductase): the "thermolabile" variant c.665C > T(p.Ala222Val), historically more commonly referred to as C677T, and the c.1286A > C(p.Glu429Ala) variant. Both are missense variants known to decrease enzyme activity (https://ghr.nlm.nih.gov/gene/MTHFR).

Reduced enzyme activity of MTHFR is a genetic risk factor for hyperhomocysteinemia, especially in the presence of low serum folate levels. Mild-to-moderate hyperhomocysteinemia has been identified as a risk factor for venous thrombosis and has been associated with other cardiovascular diseases, such as coronary artery disease. Hyperhomocysteinemia is multifactorial, involving a combination of genetic, physiological, and environmental factors. Several enzymes with vitamin B cofactors—including vitamin B_6, vitamin B_{12}, and folate—are involved in regulating homocysteine levels. Individuals who are *MTHFR* polymorphism homozygotes may have hyperhomocysteinemia, usually to a mild or moderate degree of uncertain clinical significance. Because *MTHFR* polymorphism is only one of many factors contributing to the overall clinical picture, the utility of this testing in thromboembolic disease is currently ambiguous.

The American Congress of Obstetricians and Gynecologists does not recommend the measurement of homocysteine or *MTHFR* polymorphisms in the evaluation of the etiology of venous thromboembolism.

Therefore, Homozygous *MTHFR* C677T polymorphism is associated with increased risk for homocystinuria, but not others listed in the question.

129. **C.** There are two commonly recognized polymorphic variants in the *MTHFR* gene (coded for methylenetetrahydrofolate reductase): the "thermolabile" variant c.665C > T(p.Ala222Val), historically more commonly referred to as C677T, and the c.1286A > C(p.Glu429Ala) variant; both are missense changes that are known to decrease enzyme activity (https://ghr.nlm.nih.gov/gene/MTHFR).

Reduced enzyme activity of *MTHFR* is a genetic risk factor for hyperhomocysteinemia, especially in the presence of low serum folate levels. Hyperhomocysteinemia is multifactorial, involving a combination of genetic, physiological, and environmental factors. Individuals who are *MTHFR* polymorphism homozygotes may have hyperhomocysteinemia, usually to a mild or moderate degree of uncertain clinical significance. Mild-to-moderate hyperhomocysteinemia has been identified as a risk factor for venous thrombosis and has been associated with other cardiovascular diseases, such as coronary artery disease.

However, there is growing evidence that *MTHFR* polymorphism testing has minimal clinical utility and, therefore, should not be ordered as a part of a routine evaluation for thrombophilia. The American Congress of Obstetricians and Gynecologists does not recommend the measurement of homocysteine or *MTHFR* polymorphisms in the evaluation of the etiology of venous thromboembolism.

In its practice guidelines, the ACMG recommends:

- "*MTHFR* polymorphism genotyping should not be ordered as part of the clinical evaluation for thrombophilia or recurrent pregnancy loss.
- *MTHFR* polymorphism genotyping should not be ordered for at-risk family member.
- *A clinical geneticist who serves as a consultant for a patient in whom an MTHFR polymorphism(s) has ensured a thorough and appropriate evaluation for his or her symptoms.*
- If the patient is homozygous for the "thermolabile" variant c.665C > T, the geneticist may order a fasting total plasma homocysteine, if not previously ordered, to provide more accurate counseling.
- *MTHFR* status does not change the recommendation that women of childbearing age should take the standard dose of folic acid supplementation to reduce the risk of neural tube defects as per the general population guidelines.

Therefore, a clinical geneticist should ensure that a patient with an *MTHFR* polymorphism(s) has received a thorough and appropriate evaluation for his or her thrombophilia symptoms according to the ACMG recommendation.

130. **D.** In its practice guidelines, the ACMG recommends:

- "*MTHFR* polymorphism genotyping should not be ordered as part of the clinical evaluation for thrombophilia or recurrent pregnancy loss.
- *MTHFR* polymorphism genotyping should not be ordered for at-risk family members.
- A clinical geneticist who serves as a consultant for a patient in whom an *MTHFR* polymorphism(s) has received a thorough and appropriate evaluation for his or her symptoms.
- If the patient is homozygous for the "thermolabile" variant c.665C > T, the geneticist may order a fasting total plasma homocysteine, if not previously ordered, to provide more accurate counseling.
- *MTHFR* status does not changes the recommendation that women of childbearing age should take the standard dose of folic acid supplementation to reduce the risk of neural

tube defects as per the general population guidelines."

In the ACMG guideline it also states "*A fasting total plasma homocysteine level may be obtained in any patient who is homozygous for the 'thermolabile' variant, in order to provide more information for counseling.* For the purpose of laboratory interpretation, it should be noted that total homocysteine levels increase with age and are lower in the pregnant population."

"Patients who are homozygous for the 'thermolabile' variant with normal plasma homocysteine can be reassured that there is currently no evidence of increased risk for venous thromboembolism or recurrent pregnancy loss related to their *MTHFR* status, common reasons for which clinical testing is done. A patient who is homozygous for the c.665C < T 'thermolabile' variant but also has elevated homocysteine, however, may be at mildly increased risk for both of these events (venous thromboembolism odds ratio, 1.27; recurrent pregnancy loss pooled risk, 2.7). The patient can also be reassured that there is no evidence of any association with *MTHFR* 'thermolabile' variant homozygosity and mortality, from cardiovascular disease or otherwise."

"In individuals who have a known thrombophilia, such as factor V Leiden or prothrombin c.*97G > A, most available studies support the contention that *MTHFR* genotype status does not alter their thrombotic risk to a clinically significant degree."

Therefore, if the patient is homozygous for the "thermolabile" variant c.665C > T, the geneticist may order a fasting total plasma homocysteine, if not previously ordered, to provide more accurate counseling according to the ACMG recommendation.

131. **B.** *Homozygosity for the* MTHFR C677T *polymorphism can be associated with elevated homocysteine levels but, by itself, is not a risk factor for deep-vein thrombosis (DVT).* Therefore, there was no clinical indication for testing the *MTHFR* polymorphism in this patient's family members.

In 2013, the American College of Medical Genetics (ACMG) published a practice guideline regarding clinical *MTHFR* test. It states, "*MTHFR* polymorphism testing is frequently ordered by physicians as part of the clinical evaluation for thrombophilia. It was previously hypothesized that reduced enzyme activity of MTHFR led to mild hyperhomocysteinemia which led to an increased risk for venous thromboembolism, coronary heart disease, and recurrent pregnancy loss. Recent meta-analyses have disproven an association between hyperhomocysteinemia and risk for coronary heart disease and between *MTHFR* polymorphism status and risk for venous thromboembolism. *There is growing evidence that* MTHFR *polymorphism testing has minimal clinical utility and, therefore should not be ordered as a part of a routine evaluation for thrombophilia.*"

Therefore, most individuals with homozygous *MTHFR* C677T polymorphism will not develop a DVT in their lifetime.

132. **C.** Prothrombin-related thrombophilia (factor II deficiency) is an autosomal dominant disorder characterized by venous thromboembolism (VTE) that manifest most commonly in adults as deep vein thrombosis (DVT) in the legs or pulmonary embolism. The clinical expression of prothrombin-related thrombophilia is variable. *Many individuals heterozygous or homozygous for the 20210G > A (G20210A or c.*97G > A) allele in* F2 *never develop thrombosis. The relative risk for DVT in adults heterozygous for the 20210G > A allele is increased 2- to 5-fold.* In children, the relative risk for thrombosis is increased 3- to 4-fold. A 20210G > A heterozygosity has at most a modest effect on recurrence risk after a first episode. Homozygosities for this allele confer a higher risk for thrombosis than heterozygosities, although the magnitude is not well defined. Whereas 20210G > A homozygotes may develop thrombosis more frequently and at a younger age, the risk is much lower than that associated with homozygous protein C deficiency or homozygous protein S deficiency. Numerous reports of asymptomatic 20210G > A homozygotes emphasize the contribution of other genetic and acquired risk factors to thrombosis (http://www.ncbi.nlm.nih.gov/books/NBK1148/).

Current evidence suggests that a 20210G > A heterozygosity has at most a modest effect on recurrence risk after initial treatment of a first VTE. Although the data are conflicting, the majority of more recent studies found no increase in risk. *An evidence review by the Evaluation of Genomic Applications in Practice and Prevention (EGAPP) concluded that a 20210G > A heterozygosity is not predictive of VTE recurrence* (http://www.egappreviews.org). The clinical circumstances of the first event (provoked or unprovoked), individual characteristics such as male sex, and global hemostasis tests (e.g., D-dimer) are more important determinants of recurrence.

Therefore, most individuals with a heterozygous *F2* G20210A mutation will not develop a venous thromboembolism at some point of their lifetime.

133. **C.** *The risk for VTE deep-vein thrombosis (DVT) is increased 3- to 8-fold in factor V Leiden heterozygotes and 9- to 80-fold in homozygotes. Current evidence suggests that a heterozygous factor V Leiden mutation has at most a modest effect on recurrence risk after initial treatment of a first VTE* (http://www.ncbi.nlm.nih.gov/books/NBK1368/).

Therefore, most individuals with a heterozygous factor V Leiden will not develop a venous thromboembolism in their lifetime.

134. **A.** In this patient with a first episode of unprovoked VTE, male sex is an important consideration in determining the need for long-term anticoagulation. Other risk factors for recurrent VTE are a positive D-dimer test while on vitamin K antagonists and a positive D-dimer test 4 weeks after discontinuation of vitamin K antagonists. *Current evidence suggests that a heterozygous factor V Leiden mutation (c.1691G > A) has a modest effect on recurrence risk after initial treatment of a first VTE.* MTHFR *and prothrombin (factor II) c.20210G > A mutations are not associated with an increased risk for recurrent VTE.*

Therefore, a heterozygous c.1691 G > A mutation in *F5* increases this patient's risk for recurrent thrombosis.

135. **C.** In this patient with a first episode of unprovoked VTE, male sex is an important consideration in determining the need for long-term anticoagulation. Other risk factors for recurrent VTE are a positive D-dimer test while on vitamin K antagonists and a positive D-dimer test 4 weeks after discontinuation of vitamin K antagonists. Current evidence suggests that a heterozygous factor V Leiden mutation (c.1691G > A, p.Arg506Gln) has a modest effect on recurrence risk after initial treatment of a first VTE. MTHFR *and prothrombin (factor II) 20210G > A (c.*96G > A) mutations are not associated with an increased risk for recurrent VTE.* Although a history of VTE in a first-degree relative increases the likelihood of a first VTE in patients, a positive family history has never been independently associated with a greater chance of recurrence.

Therefore, a heterozygous c.C677T mutation in *MTHFR* does NOT increase this patient's risk for recurrent thrombosis.

136. **B.** Both the factor V Leiden mutation and the prothrombin 20210G > A mutation exhibit semidominant expression in that both heterozygotes and homozygotes are at increased risk of occurrence/recurrence of venous

thrombosis. *The relative risk for venous thrombosis associated with the factor V Leiden mutation in the absence of other acquired or environmental predispositions is approximately 4- to 7-fold for heterozygotes and 80-fold for homozygotes.* The relative risk for venous thrombosis associated with the prothrombin 20210G > A mutation in the absence of other acquired or environmental predispositions is approximately 2- to 4-fold for heterozygotes (https://www.acmg.net).

Therefore, this patient would have 5-fold increased risk for venous thrombosis as compared with individuals without the mutation.

137. **E.** Both the factor V Leiden mutation and the prothrombin 20210G > A mutation exhibit semidominant expression in that both heterozygotes and homozygotes are at increased risk of occurrence/recurrence of venous thrombosis. *The relative risk for venous thrombosis associated with the factor V Leiden mutation in the absence of other acquired or environmental predispositions is approximately 4- to 7-fold for heterozygotes and 80-fold for homozygotes.* The relative risk for venous thrombosis associated with the prothrombin 20210G > A mutation in the absence of other acquired or environmental predispositions is approximately 2- to 4-fold for heterozygotes (https://www.acmg.net).

Therefore, this patient would have an 80-fold increased risk for venous thrombosis as compared with individuals without the mutation.

138. **B.** The relative risk for venous thromboembolism (VTE) is increased 2- to 5-fold in 20210G > A (c.*96C > T) heterozygotes. In a meta-analysis of 79 studies, *a 20210G > A heterozygosity in F2 was associated with a 3-fold increased risk for VTE* (http://www.ncbi.nlm.nih.gov/books/NBK1148/).

Therefore, this patient would have 3-fold increased risk for venous thrombosis as compared with individuals without the mutation.

139. **C.** *Individuals with a heterozygous factor V Leiden variant and a heterozygous prothrombin 20210G > A mutation have a 20-fold increased risk of having a venous thrombosis as compared with individuals without either mutation.* Between 1% and 10% of symptomatic carriers of the factor V Leiden mutation also carry the prothrombin 20210G > A mutation. These individuals have a 50- to 80-fold relative risk of thrombosis as compared to homozygotes for the factor V Leiden mutation (https://www.acmg.net/Pages/ACMG_Activities/stds-2002/fv-pt.htm). A prothrombin 20210G > A allele was 4- to 5-fold more common in symptomatic factor V Leiden

homozygotes with VTE than in controls with no thrombotic history.

Therefore, this patient would have 20-fold increased risk for venous thrombosis comparing with individuals without the two mutations.

140. **C.** The Leiden allele of the factor V gene contains a G-to-A substitution at nucleotide 1691, producing a missense mutation that substitutes glutamine for arginine at amino acid residue 506 (p.R506Q) in the protein product. *The R506Q site is one of the activated protein C (APC) cleavage sites in the factor Va molecule* (https://www.acmg.net).

Therefore, Protein C's activation sites is cleavage and activated in patients with the factor V Leiden allele.

141. **E.** The prothrombin 20210G > A mutation is located in the 3′ untranslated region of the factor II gene. It represents a gain-of-function mutation, causing increased cleavage-site recognition, increased 3′ end processing, and increased mRNA accumulation and protein synthesis. The 20210G > A mutation is reported to be present in about 2% of the general population, with an increased frequency (3.0%) in southern Europeans and a decreased frequency (1.7%) in northern Europeans. It is very rare among those of Asian and African descent.

Clinical sensitivity can be defined as the proportion of individuals who have had (or will have) deep-vein thrombosis and who have at least one prothrombin 20210G > A mutation. The clinical sensitivity of the prothrombin 20210G > A mutation varies between 5% and 19%.

Clinical specificity can be defined as the proportion of individuals who do not have or will not develop deep-vein thrombosis and do not have any known mutations in the prothrombin gene. *Low penetrance of the prothrombin 20210G > A mutation is the main reason why clinical specificity is less than 100%.* Analytic error is possible, but likely to be a much smaller factor in clinical false positive test results (https://www.acmg.net/Pages/ACMG_Activities/stds-2002/fv-pt.htm).

Therefore, low penetrance of the prothrombin 20210G > A mutation is the main reason why clinical specificity is less than 100% according to ACMG recommendation.

142. **C.** Factor V is a protein of the coagulation cascade. It is synthesized primarily in the liver. The protein circulates in the bloodstream in an inactive form until the coagulation system is activated by an injury that damages blood vessels. When coagulation factor V is activated, it interacts with coagulation factor X. *The active forms of these two coagulation factors (factor Va and*

factor Xa) form a complex that converts the important coagulation protein prothrombin (factor II) to its active form, thrombin. Thrombin then converts the protein fibrinogen into fibrin, which is the material that forms the clot (https://ghr.nlm.nih.gov/gene/F5).

Therefore, the activated Factor V cleavages prothrombin (II) to thrombin (IIa).

143. E. The factor V Leiden allele contains a G > A substitution at nucleotide 1691 (c.1691G > a), producing a missense mutation that substitutes glutamine for arginine at amino acid residue 506 (p.R506Q) in the protein product. The p.R506Q site is one of the activated protein C (APC) cleavage sites in the factor Va molecule. Factor V Leiden accounts for at least 80% or 90%−95% of cases of APC resistance. Protein S is a cofactor to protein C in the inactivation of factor Va and VIIIa, but protein S does not interact with factor Va directly.

The factor V Leiden mutation is most prevalent in the United States and European Caucasian populations. The factor V Leiden mutation is found in 5.27% of Caucasian Americans and is progressively less common in Hispanic Americans (2.21% heterozygotes), Native Americans (1.25% heterozygotes), African Americans (1.23% heterozygotes), and Asian Americans (0.45% heterozygotes).

Clinical sensitivity can be defined as the proportion of individuals who have had (or will have) deep vein thrombi and who have at least one factor V Leiden. Clinical sensitivity is equivalent to the detection rate. Overall, the clinical sensitivity of the factor V Leiden mutation is between 20% and 50%.

In the ACMG Consensus Statement on Factor V Leiden Mutation Testing, *factor V Leiden testing is predominantly used and recommended for diagnostic purposes in individuals with clinical symptoms of venous thrombosis or with recurrent pregnancy loss. While predictive testing in asymptomatic individuals and in relatives of known factor V Leiden carriers is technically possible, its clinical utility for that purpose is markedly hampered by the low penetrance of the mutations and the appreciable risks inherent in prophylactic anticoagulant therapy* (https://www.acmg.net).

Therefore, the factor V Leiden testing is recommended for diagnostic purposes in individuals with recurrent pregnancy loss according to the Consensus Statement.

144. B. In the ACMG Consensus Statement on Factor V Leiden Mutation Testing, *factor V Leiden testing is predominantly used and recommended for diagnostic purposes in individuals with clinical symptoms of venous thrombosis or with recurrent pregnancy loss. While predictive testing in asymptomatic individuals and in relatives of known factor V Leiden or prothrombin 20210G > A carriers is technically possible, its clinical utility for that purpose is markedly hampered by the low penetrance of the mutations and the appreciable risks inherent in prophylactic anticoagulant therapy.*

Routine testing is not recommended for patients with a personal or family history of arterial thrombotic disorders (e.g., acute coronary syndromes or stroke) except for the special situation of myocardial infarction in young female smokers. Testing may be worthwhile for young patients (<50 years of age) who develop acute arterial thrombosis in the absence of other risk factors for atherosclerotic arterial occlusive disease (https://www.acmg.net).

Therefore, the factor V Leiden testing is recommended for diagnostic purposes in individuals with recurrent pregnancy loss according to the Consensus Statement.

145. B. Both the factor V Leiden mutation (c.1691G > A, p.R506Q) and the prothrombin 20210G > A (c.*96C > T) mutation exhibit semidominant expression in that both heterozygotes and homozygotes are at increased risk of occurrence/recurrence of venous thrombosis. The relative risk for venous thrombosis associated with the factor V Leiden mutation in the absence of other acquired or environmental predispositions is approximately 4- to 7-fold for heterozygotes and 80-fold for homozygotes. The relative risk for venous thrombosis associated with the prothrombin 20210G > A mutation in the absence of other acquired or environmental predispositions is approximately 2- to 4-fold for heterozygotes.

Data from several studies strongly suggest that the pathogenesis of venous thromboembolism is multifactorial and requires interactions between both inherited and acquired risk factors. Heterozygosities for the factor V Leiden or prothrombin 20210G > A mutations alone may be a relatively weak risk factor unless a second genetic risk factor or an acquired factor, such as older age, also exists (https://www.acmg.net).

Therefore, the penetrance of the factor V Leiden mutation and the prothrombin 20210G > A mutation are low for venous thromboembolism (incomplete penetrance: most individuals with a mutation will not develop a venous thrombosis).

146. **C.** Venous thrombosis is a panethnic multifactorial disorder. Identifiable genetic factors are present in 25% of unselected patients, including defects in coagulation factor inhibition and impaired clot lysis. Factor V (*F5*) Leiden occurs in 12%–14% of patients with VTE, prothrombin (*F2*) mutations in 6%–18%, and deficiency of antithrombin III (*SERPINC1*) or protein C (*PROC1*) or protein S (*PROS1*) in 5%–15%. Factor VIII (*F8*) is associated with hemophilia but not thrombosis.

    Therefore, factor VIII (*F8*) would most likely NOT be a part of the genetic evaluation for thrombosis in this patient.

147. **C.** *The factor V Leiden (c.1691G > A, p.Arg506Gln) mutation has a prevalence of 2%–15% in general Caucasian populations,* but it is rare in Hispanic American (2.2%), Asians (0.45%), Africans (1.2%), and Native Americans (1.25%).

    Therefore, the FV Leiden mutation is more common in Caucasian than in other ethnics listed in the question.

148. **B.** The factor V Leiden (c.1691G > A, p. Arg506Gln) mutation removes the preferred site for protein C proteolysis of activated factor V. Slowing inactivation of activated factor V predisposes carriers to thrombophilia. The risk is higher for individuals with homozygous *FV* Leiden mutations.

    Therefore, *F5* Leiden mutation is a gain-of-function mutation.

149. **A.** The activated form of protein C is proteolytically inactivating factor V. Mutations in protein C (*PROC1*) slow inactivation of factor V, which predisposes carriers to thrombophilia.

    Therefore, mutations in *PROC1* are loss-of-function mutations.

150. **A.** Acute intermittent porphyria (AIP) is inherited in *an autosomal dominant manner*, is caused by mutations in the *HMBS* gene. All individuals with AIP have an approximately 50% reduction in PBG deaminase enzymatic activity. Therefore, the woman's child will have 50% chance of inheriting the *HMBS* mutation from her. However, most likely her child will not have any episodes throughout his/her lifetime, which is called *clinically latent, appearing in 90% of patients.* Her child has a 10% chance of having clinically manifestations, according to the population data. Acute attacks, which may be provoked by certain drugs, alcoholic beverages, endocrine factors, calorie restriction, stress, and infections, usually resolve within 2 weeks. Attacks, which are very rare before puberty, are more common in women than men. The main use of molecular genetic testing of an individual with biochemically proven AIP is to identify a pathogenic variant for the molecular investigation of the individual's family (i.e., cascade screening).

    Therefore, the child will have approximately 90% chance of being healthy with two normal copies of *HMBS* or one normal copy of *HMBS*.

151. **A.** Acute intermittent porphyria (AIP) is inherited in an autosomal dominant manner. About 1% of probands may have a de novo mutation. Sibs and offspring of individuals with an *HMBS* pathogenic variant are at 50% risk of inheriting the *HMBS* pathogenic variant. However, because penetrance is low, the likelihood of an individual with an inherited *HMBS* pathogenic variant having an acute attack is small. The penetrance for clinical manifestations of an *HMBS* disease-causing mutation is not accurately known.

    In one study, 52% of relatives ascertained through cascade screening were found to have "typical" clinical symptoms with increased ALA and PBG and decreased HMBS activity in Swiss patients. However, *most reviews written by experienced porphyria specialists quote a penetrance of 10%–20%, by which they imply an acute attack (acute abdominal pain ± associated autonomic, motor, or CNS symptoms) leading to a hospital admission for medical management.* Population surveys suggest a lower figure. The minimum prevalence of disease specific *HMBS* mutations in France is 597 per million inhabitants. The prevalence of overt AIP in France was recently reported as 5.5 in 1 million, indicating a penetrance of about 1% (http://www.ncbi.nlm.nih.gov/books/NBK1193/).

    Therefore, it is fair to estimate that this patient's risk of having episodes in her lifetime is up to 20%.

152. **D.** Acute intermittent porphyria (AIP) is an autosomal dominant nonneoplastic hematological disorder resulting from half-normal activity of the enzyme hydroxymethylbilane synthase (HMBS). The long-term complications are chronic renal failure, *hepatocellular carcinoma* (HCC), and hypertension. Therefore, this patient is at risk for hepatocellular carcinoma.

153. **A.** Porphyrias are a group of rare inherited or acquired disorders of certain enzymes that normally participate in the production of porphyrins and heme. They manifest with either neurological complications or skin problems or occasionally both. *This PhD student has autosomal dominant acute intermittent porphyria (AIP) resulting from variants in the HMBS gene, which lead to*

deficiency of hydroxymethylbilane synthase (HMBS).
AIP is characterized clinically by life-threatening acute neurovisceral attacks of severe abdominal pain without peritoneal signs, often accompanied by nausea, vomiting, tachycardia, and hypertension. Attacks may be complicated by hyponatremia and neurological findings, such as mental changes, convulsions, and peripheral neuropathy, that may progress to respiratory paralysis. Acute attacks, which may be provoked by certain drugs, alcoholic beverages, endocrine factors, calorie restriction, stress, and infections, usually resolve within 2 weeks. Acute attacks of porphyria are associated with an increased urinary concentration of porphobilinogen (PBG) and delta aminolevulinic acid (ALA). The total fecal porphyrin concentration and coproporphyrin isomer ratio are normal. Plasma porphyrin fluorescence emission scanning either shows a peak around 619 nm or is normal. Most individuals with AIP have one or a few attacks in their life time; the majority will remain asymptomatic throughout their lives. About 5% (mainly women) have recurrent attacks (defined as >4 attacks/year) that may persist for years. Other long-term complications are chronic renal failure, hepatocellular carcinoma (HCC), and hypertension. Attacks, which are very rare before puberty, are more common in women than in men. All individuals with a heterozygous genetic change in *HMBS* are at risk of developing acute attacks. However, most never have symptoms and are said to have latent (or presymptomatic) AIP.

A germline heterozygous *UROD* pathogenic variant results in type II porphyria cutanea tarda (type II PCT) characterized by blistering over the dorsal aspects of the hands and other sun-exposed areas of skin, skin friability after minor trauma, facial hypertrichosis and hyperpigmentation, severe thickening of affected skin areas (pseudoscleroderma), and increased risk for hepatocellular carcinoma (HCC). A germline heterozygous pathogenic variant in *PPOX*, encoding the mitochondrial enzyme protoporphyrinogen oxidase (PPOX), results in variegate porphyria (VP) characterized by a cutaneous porphyria with chronic blistering skin lesions and an acute porphyria with severe episodic neurovisceral symptoms. Identification of gain-of-function germline pathogenic variants in *ALAS2* on the X chromosome, the gene encoding erythroid-specific 5-aminolevulinate synthase 2, is diagnostic for X-linked protoporphyria characterized in affected males by

cutaneous photosensitivity (usually beginning in infancy or childhood) that results in tingling, burning, pain, and itching within minutes of sun/light exposure and may be accompanied by swelling and redness. Vesicular lesions are uncommon. Pain, which may seem out of proportion to the visible skin lesions, may persist for hours or days after the initial phototoxic reaction. Photosensitivity usually remains for life. Identification of a germline heterozygous pathogenic variant in *CPOX* (encoding the enzyme coproporphyringen-III oxidase) is diagnostic for hereditary coproporphyria (HCP) characterized by low-grade pain starting in the abdomen and slowly increasing over a period of days (not hours), with nausea progressing to vomiting. Biallelic *UROS* germline pathogenic variants, or on rare occasion a hemizygous germline pathogenic variant in the X-linked gene *GATA1*, result in congenital erythropoietic porphyria (CEP), which is characterized in most individuals by severe cutaneous photosensitivity at birth or in early infancy with blistering and increased friability of the skin over light-exposed areas (http://www.ncbi.nlm.nih.gov/books).

Therefore, a molecular genetic test of *HMBS* would most likely be positive in this patient.

154. **C.** Porphyrias are a group of rare inherited or acquired disorders of certain enzymes that normally participate in the production of porphyrins and heme. They manifest with either neurological complications or skin problems or occasionally both. Acute intermittent porphyria (AIP) results from germline heterozygous pathogenic variants in *HMBS*. Type II porphyria cutanea tarda (type II PCT) results heterozygous pathogenic variants in *UROD*. X-linked protoporphyria (XLP) results from pathogenic gain-of-function variants in *ALAS2*. Hereditary coproporphyria (HCP) results from heterozygous germline pathogenic variants in *CPOX*. Congenital erythropoietic porphyria (CEP) results from biallelic germline pathogenic variants in *UROS* or hemizygous pathogenic variants in the X-linked gene *GATA1*.

The (GAA)n repeat sequence in the intron 1 of the FXN gene is associated with autosomal recessive Friedreich ataxia, but not porphyrias. Therefore, it would be most likely that *FXN* was not in the next-generation sequencing (NGS) panel for porphyrias.

155. **C.** X-linked protoporphyria (XLP) is characterized in affected males by cutaneous photosensitivity (usually beginning in infancy or childhood) that results in tingling, burning, pain, and itching

within minutes of sun/light exposure and may be accompanied by swelling and redness. Vesicular lesions are uncommon. Pain may persist for hours or days after the initial phototoxic reaction. Photosensitivity usually remains for life. The phenotype in heterozygous females ranges from asymptomatic to as severe as affected males. *Detection of markedly increased free erythrocyte protoporphyrin and zinc-chelated erythrocyte protoporphyrin is the most sensitive biochemical diagnostic test for XLP.* (http://www.ncbi.nlm.nih.gov/books/NBK121284/).

Identification of gain-of-function germline pathogenic variants in *ALAS2*, the gene encoding erythroid specific 5-aminolevulinate synthase 2, confirmed the diagnosis. The mother was an obligate carrier. Therefore, the recurrent rate in this family would be 1/2 (the risk of inherited the mutated chromosome X) $\times$ 1/2 (the risk from being a boy) = 1/4, or 25%.

156. D. X-linked protoporphyria (XLP) is characterized by cutaneous photosensitivity (usually beginning in infancy or childhood) that results in tingling, burning, pain, and itching within minutes of sun/light exposure and may be accompanied by swelling and redness in affected males. Vesicular lesions are uncommon. Pain may persist for hours or days after the initial phototoxic reaction. Photosensitivity usually remains for life. The phenotype in heterozygous females ranges from asymptomatic to as severe as affected males. Detection of markedly increased free erythrocyte protoporphyrin and zinc-chelated erythrocyte protoporphyrin is the most sensitive biochemical diagnostic test for XLP. (http://www.ncbi.nlm.nih.gov/books/NBK121284/).

X-linked protoporphyria is caused by mutations of the *ALAS2* gene and is inherited as an X-linked dominant trait. Males often develop a severe form of the disorder while females may not develop any symptoms (asymptomatic) or may develop a form as severe as that seen in males. The *ALAS2* gene is located on the short arm of the X chromosome (Xp11.21). The gene encodes a protein known as erythroid-specific 5-aminolevulinate synthase 2. Mutations of the *ALAS2* gene lead to the overproduction of this enzyme, which, in turn, results in elevated levels of the chemical protoporphyrin. Protoporphyrin abnormally accumulates in certain tissues of the body, especially the blood, liver, and skin. The symptoms of X-linked protoporphyria develop because of this abnormal accumulation of protoporphyrin. For example, when protoporphyrins absorb energy from sunlight,

they enter an excited state (photoactivation), and this abnormal activation results in the characteristic damage to the skin. Accumulation of protoporphyrins in the liver causes toxic damage to the liver and may contribute to the formation of gallstones. Protoporphyrin is formed within red blood cells in the bone marrow and then enters the blood plasma, which carries it to the skin, where it can be photoactivated by sunlight and cause damage (https://rarediseases.org).

Therefore, it would be most likely that the patient had a gain-of-function germline pathogenic variant in *ALAS2*, the gene encoding erythroid specific 5-aminolevulinate synthase 2.

157. D. *Hereditary hemorrhagic telangiectasia (HHT)* is an autosomal dominant condition characterized by the presence of multiple arteriovenous malformations (AVMs) that lack intervening capillaries and result in direct connections between arteries and veins. Although HHT is a developmental disorder and infants are occasionally severely affected, in most people the features are age-dependent and the diagnosis is not suspected until adolescence or later. Small AVMs (or telangiectases) close to the surface of the skin and mucous membranes often rupture and bleed after slight trauma. The most common clinical manifestation is spontaneous and recurrent nosebleeds (epistaxis) beginning on average at age 12 years. Approximately 25% of individuals with HHT have GI bleeding, which most commonly begins after age 50 years. Large AVMs often cause symptoms when they occur in the brain, liver, or lungs; complications from bleeding or shunting may be sudden and catastrophic. Germline pathogenic variants in the *ENG*, *ACVRL1* (*ALK1*), *SMAD4*, and *GDF2* genes are associated with HHT. Molecular genetic testing of all four genes may detect pathogenic variants in approximately 80%–90% of individuals who meet unequivocal clinical diagnostic criteria for HHT (http://www.ncbi.nlm.nih.gov/books/NBK1351/).

Ataxia telangiectasia (AT) is an autosomal recessive chromosomal breakage syndrome characterized by progressive cerebellar gait beginning between ages 1 and 4 years, oculomotor apraxia, choreoathetosis, telangiectasias of the conjunctivae, immunodeficiency, frequent infections, and an increased risk for malignancy, particularly leukemia and lymphoma. Patients with AT are hypersensitive to ionizing radiation and have an increased susceptibility to cancer, usually leukemia or lymphoma (http://www.ncbi.nlm. nih.gov/books/NBK26468/). Hemophilia A is an X-linked recessive nonneoplastic hematological disorder characterized by a deficiency in factor VIII clotting activity that results in prolonged oozing after injuries, tooth extractions, or surgery and delayed or recurrent bleeding prior to complete wound healing. *HFE*-hereditary hemochromatosis is an autosomal recessive disease characterized by excessive storage of iron in the liver, skin, pancreas, heart, joints, and testes. In untreated individuals, early symptoms may include abdominal pain, weakness, lethargy, and weight loss.

Therefore, it would be most likely this patient had HHT if she had a genetic condition.

158. **D.** Hereditary hemorrhagic telangiectasia (HHT) is an autosomal dominant condition characterized by the presence of multiple arteriovenous malformations (AVMs) that lack intervening capillaries and result in direct connections between arteries and veins. Although HHT is a developmental disorder and infants are occasionally severely affected, in most people the features are age-dependent and the diagnosis is not suspected until adolescence or later. Small AVMs (or telangiectases) close to the surface of the skin and mucous membranes often rupture and bleed after slight trauma. The most common clinical manifestation is spontaneous and recurrent nosebleeds (epistaxis) beginning on average at age 12 years. Approximately 25% of individuals with HHT have GI bleeding, which most commonly begins after age 50 years. Large AVMs often cause symptoms when they occur in the brain, liver, or lungs; complications from bleeding or shunting may be sudden and catastrophic. *Germline pathogenic variants in the* ENG, ACVRL1 (ALK1), SMAD4, *and* GDF2 *genes are associated with HHT*. Molecular genetic testing of all four genes may detect pathogenic variants in approximately 80%–90% of individuals who meet unequivocal clinical diagnostic criteria for HHT (http://www.ncbi.nlm.nih.gov/books/ NBK1351/).

Ataxia telangiectasia (AT) is an autosomal recessive chromosomal breakage syndrome characterized by progressive cerebellar gait beginning between ages 1 and 4 years, oculomotor apraxia, choreoathetosis, telangiectasias of the conjunctivae, immunodeficiency, frequent infections, and an increased risk for malignancy, particularly leukemia and lymphoma. Patients with AT are hypersensitive to ionizing radiation and have an

increased susceptibility to cancer, usually leukemia or lymphoma. Germline pathogenic variants in the *ATM* gene are associated with AT (http://www.ncbi.nlm.nih.gov/books/ NBK26468/). Hemophilia A is an X-linked recessive nonneoplastic hematological disorder characterized by deficiency in factor VIII clotting activity that results in prolonged oozing after injuries, tooth extractions, or surgery and delayed or recurrent bleeding prior to complete wound healing. Germline pathogenic variants in the *F8* gene are associated with hemophilia A. *HFE*-hereditary hemochromatosis is an autosomal recessive disease characterized by excessive storage of iron in the liver, skin, pancreas, heart, joints, and testes. In untreated individuals, early symptoms may include abdominal pain, weakness, lethargy, and weight loss. Germline pathogenic variants in the *HFE* gene are associated with *HFE*-hereditary hemochromatosis.

Therefore, the *ENG* gene would most likely be included in the sequencing assay ordered for this patient in order to rule out genetic etiologies.

159. **D.** Hereditary hemorrhagic telangiectasia (HHT) is an autosomal dominant condition characterized by the presence of multiple arteriovenous malformations (AVMs) that lack intervening capillaries and result in direct connections between arteries and veins. Although HHT is a developmental disorder and infants are occasionally severely affected, in most people the features are age-dependent and the diagnosis is not suspected until adolescence or later. Small AVMs (or telangiectases) close to the surface of the skin and mucous membranes often rupture and bleed after slight trauma. The most common clinical manifestation is spontaneous and recurrent nosebleeds (epistaxis) beginning on average at age 12 years. Approximately 25% of individuals with HHT have GI bleeding, which most commonly begins after age 50 years. Large AVMs often cause symptoms when they occur in the brain, liver, or lungs; complications from bleeding or shunting may be sudden and catastrophic. *Germline pathogenic variants in the* ENG, ACVRL1 (ALK1), SMAD4, *and* GDF2 *genes are associated with HHT*. Molecular genetic testing of all four genes may detect pathogenic variants in approximately 80%–90% of individuals who meet unequivocal clinical diagnostic criteria for HHT (http://www.ncbi.nlm.nih.gov/books/ NBK1351/).

Ataxia telangiectasia (AT) is an autosomal recessive chromosomal breakage syndrome characterized by progressive cerebellar gait beginning between ages 1 and 4 years, oculomotor apraxia, choreoathetosis, telangiectasias of the conjunctivae, immunodeficiency, frequent infections, and an increased risk for malignancy, particularly leukemia and lymphoma. Patients with AT are hypersensitive to ionizing radiation with an increased susceptibility to cancer, usually leukemia or lymphoma. Germline pathogenic variants in the ATM gene are associated with AT (http://www.ncbi.nlm.nih.gov/books/NBK26468/). Hemophilia A is an X-linked recessive nonneoplastic hematological disorder characterized by a deficiency in factor VIII clotting activity that results in prolonged oozing after injuries, tooth extractions, or surgery and delayed or recurrent bleeding prior to complete wound healing. Germline pathogenic variants in the F8 gene are associated with hemophilia A. HFE-hereditary hemochromatosis is an autosomal recessive disease characterized by excessive storage of iron in the liver, skin, pancreas, heart, joints, and testes. In untreated individuals, early symptoms may include abdominal pain, weakness, lethargy, and weight loss. Germline pathogenic variants in the HFE gene are associated with hemophilia A.

Therefore, the SMAD4 gene would most likely be included in the sequencing assay ordered for this patient in order to rule out genetic etiologies.

160. E. Hereditary hemorrhagic telangiectasia (HHT) is an autosomal dominant condition characterized by the presence of multiple arteriovenous malformations (AVMs) that lack intervening capillaries and result in direct connections between arteries and veins. Although HHT is a developmental disorder and infants are occasionally severely affected, in most people the features are age-dependent and the diagnosis is not suspected until adolescence or later. Small AVMs (or telangiectases) close to the surface of the skin and mucous membranes often rupture and bleed after slight trauma. The most common clinical manifestation is spontaneous and recurrent nosebleeds (epistaxis) beginning on average at age 12 years. Approximately 25% of individuals with HHT have GI bleeding, which most commonly begins after age 50 years. Large AVMs often cause symptoms when they occur in the brain, liver, or lungs; complications from bleeding or shunting may be sudden and catastrophic. Germline pathogenic variants in the ENG, ACVRL1 (ALK1), SMAD4, and GDF2 genes are associated with HHT. Molecular genetic testing

of all four genes may detect pathogenic variants in approximately 80%−90% of individuals who meet unequivocal clinical diagnostic criteria for HHT (http://www.ncbi.nlm.nih.gov/books/NBK1351/).

Chromosome breakage study is the diagnostic test for Fanconi anemia. Chromosome microarray analysis (CMA) is the first-line test for individuals with multiple congenital anomalies, developmental delay, intellectual disability, and autism. CMA study is used to detect copy-number gains or losses. The ACMG recommends CMA as the first-line test for individuals with multiple congenital anomalies, developmental delay, intellectual disability, and autism. Methylation study is used to identify epigenetic changes in the genome, such as methylation study for Prader−Willi/Angelman syndromes. Multiplex ligation-dependent probe amplification (MLPA) is a time-efficient technique to detect genomic deletions and insertions bigger than single-nucleotide variants and in/dels, but smaller than what CMA can detect. Next-generation sequencing (NGS) is a high-throughput test to sequence multiple genes at the same time. It is an appropriate test for Fanconi anemia, hearing loss, and other conditions. Sanger sequencing is the most appropriate molecular test for single-gene disorders when the most pathogenic variants are single-nucleotide variants and in/dels. It is an appropriate test for Gaucher disease, Wiskott−Aldrich syndrome, and other conditions. Targeted mutation analysis is used to identify specific mutations, which is a cost-effective test when there is founder effect in a population. Targeted mutation analysis is also commonly used to diagnose family members after the mutation is identified in the proband. It is an appropriate test for carrier test of cystic fibrosis (CF).

Therefore, a next-generation sequencing (NGS) assay including at least the four genes would most likely be used for the genetic test ordered for this patient in order to rule out HHT.

161. B. *Hereditary hemorrhagic telangiectasia (HHT) is an autosomal dominant condition* characterized by the presence of multiple arteriovenous malformations (AVMs) that lack intervening capillaries and result in direct connections between arteries and veins. Although HHT is a developmental disorder and infants are occasionally severely affected, in most people the features are age-dependent and the diagnosis is not suspected until adolescence or later. Small AVMs (or telangiectases) close to the surface of the skin and mucous membranes

often rupture and bleed after slight trauma. The most common clinical manifestation is spontaneous and recurrent nosebleeds (epistaxis) beginning on average at age 12 years. Approximately 25% of individuals with HHT have GI bleeding, which most commonly begins after age 50 years. Large AVMs often cause symptoms when they occur in the brain, liver, or lungs; complications from bleeding or shunting may be sudden and catastrophic. Germline pathogenic variants in the *ENG*, *ACVRL1* (*ALK1*), *SMAD4*, and *GDF2* genes are associated with HHT. Molecular genetic testing of all four genes may detect pathogenic variants in approximately 80%−90% of individuals who meet unequivocal clinical diagnostic criteria for HHT (http://www.ncbi.nlm.nih.gov/books/NBK1351/).

Therefore, the patient's unborn child would have a 1/2 chance to inherit the familial deletion in the *ENG* gene for HHT.

162. **B.** Immune dysregulation, polyendocrinopathy, enteropathy, X-linked (IPEX) syndrome, autoimmune lymphoproliferative syndrome (ALPS), X-linked lymphoproliferative disease (XLP), and Wiskott−Aldrich syndrome (WAS) are all congenital nonneoplastic hematological disorders characterized by immunodeficiency. Von Willebrand disease (vWD) is the most common hereditary coagulation abnormality described in humans that is caused by pathogenic variants in *vWF* on 12p13.2.

IPEX is characterized by systemic autoimmunity, typically beginning in the first year of life. Presentation is most commonly the clinical triad of watery diarrhea, eczematous dermatitis, and endocrinopathy (most commonly insulin-dependent diabetes mellitus). Most children have other autoimmune phenomena including Coombs-positive anemia, autoimmune thrombocytopenia, autoimmune neutropenia, and tubular nephropathy. Without aggressive immunosuppression or bone marrow transplantation, the majority of affected males die within the first 1−2 years of life from metabolic derangements or sepsis. A few with a milder phenotype have survived into the second or third decade of life. There are no specific laboratory tests to confirm the diagnosis. Molecular analysis of the *FOXP3* gene on Xp11.23 is required for the diagnosis. *FOXP3* is the only gene in which germline pathogenic variants are known to cause IPEX syndrome (http://www.ncbi.nlm.nih.gov/books/NBK1118/).

ALPS, caused by defective lymphocyte homeostasis, is characterized by nonmalignant lymphoproliferation such as lymphadenopathy, hepatosplenomegaly with or without hypersplenism, autoimmune disease mostly directed toward blood cells, and lifelong increased risk for both Hodgkin and non-Hodgkin lymphoma. Heterozygous or homozygous (compound heterozygous) germline pathogenic variants in *FAS*, *FASLG*, and *CASP10* result in ALPS (http://www.ncbi.nlm.nih.gov/books/NBK1406/).

XLP is caused by germline pathogenic variants in *SH2D1A* and *XIAP* (*BIRC4*). The three most commonly recognized phenotypes of *SH2D1A*-related XLP are hemophagocytic lymphohistiocytosis (HLH) associated with Epstein−Barr virus (EBV) infection (58% of individuals), dysgammaglobulinemia (31%), and lymphoproliferative disorders (malignant lymphoma) (30%). Manifestations of *SH2D1A*-related XLP can also occur in the absence of EBV. *XIAP*-related XLP also presents with HLH (often associated with EBV) or dysgammaglobulinemia, but no cases of lymphoma have been described to date (http://www.ncbi.nlm.nih.gov/books/NBK1406/).

Wiskott−Aldrich syndrome (WAS) is an X-linked disorder caused by germline pathogenic variants in *WAS* on Xp11.23, which is characterized by thrombocytopenia, eczema, and combined immunodeficiency.

Therefore, it was most likely that this deceased patient had had IPEX.

163. **B.** *FOXP3* is the only gene in which germline pathogenic variants are known to cause immune dysregulation, polyendocrinopathy, enteropathy, X-linked (IPEX) syndrome. Male patients usually have neonatal enteropathy and neonatal polyendocrinopathy. *Female carriers of FOXP3 pathogenic variants are generally healthy.* But there are occasionally reported female carriers with mild symptoms due to the pattern of X inactivation.

Therefore, the unborn sister of the patient in this question would most likely not have any symptoms even if she inherited the familial pathogenic variant.

164. **D.** Immune dysregulation, polyendocrinopathy, enteropathy, X-linked (IPEX) syndrome is characterized by systemic autoimmunity, typically beginning in the first year of life. Presentation is most commonly the clinical triad of watery diarrhea, eczematous dermatitis, and endocrinopathy (most commonly insulin-dependent diabetes mellitus). Most children have other autoimmune phenomena, including

Coombs-positive anemia, autoimmune thrombocytopenia, autoimmune neutropenia, and tubular nephropathy. Without aggressive immunosuppression or bone marrow transplantation, the majority of affected males die within the first 1–2 years of life from metabolic derangements or sepsis; a few with a milder phenotype have survived into the second or third decade of life. There are no specific laboratory tests to confirm the diagnosis. *FOXP3 is the only gene in which mutations are known to cause IPEX syndrome.* Molecular analysis of the *FOXP3* gene on Xp11.23 is required for the diagnosis (http://www.ncbi.nlm.nih.gov/books/NBK1118/).

Heterozygous or homozygous (compound heterozygous) pathogenic variants in *FAS*, *FASLG*, and *CASP10* result in autoimmune lymphoproliferative syndrome (ALPS). ALPS, which is caused by defective lymphocyte homeostasis characterized by nonmalignant lymphoproliferation such as lymphadenopathy, hepatosplenomegaly with or without hypersplenism, autoimmune disease, mostly directed toward blood cells, and a lifelong increased risk for both Hodgkin and non-Hodgkin lymphoma (http://www.ncbi.nlm.nih.gov/books/NBK1406/).

This patient had late-onset IPEX syndrome presenting a severe phenotype with aggressive autoimmune-associated symptoms, which led to his death. Therefore, *FOXP3* would most likely harbor a germline pathogenic variant for IPEX syndrome in this patient.

165. **B.** Immune dysregulation, polyendocrinopathy, enteropathy, X-linked (IPEX) syndrome is characterized by systemic autoimmunity, typically beginning in the first year of life. Presentation is most commonly the clinical triad of watery diarrhea, eczematous dermatitis, and endocrinopathy (most commonly insulin-dependent diabetes mellitus). Most children have other autoimmune phenomena, including Coombs-positive anemia, autoimmune thrombocytopenia, autoimmune neutropenia, and tubular nephropathy. Without aggressive immunosuppression or bone marrow transplantation, the majority of affected males die within the first 1–2 years of life from metabolic derangements or sepsis; a few with a milder phenotype have survived into the second or third decade of life (http://www.ncbi.nlm.nih.gov/books/NBK1118/).

There are no specific laboratory tests to confirm the diagnosis. *FOXP3* is the only gene in which mutations are known to cause IPEX

syndrome. Molecular analysis of the *FOXP3* gene on Xp11.23 is required for the diagnosis. *Sanger sequencing analysis of all exons, exon–intron boundaries, and the first polyadenylation site of FOXP3 detects mutations in approximately 25% of males with a clinical symptoms suggestive of IPEX syndrome.* Research has suggested the possibility of an additional autosomal locus. Among the males who lack *FOXP3* mutations, approximately half have low *FOXP3* mRNA expression levels and low numbers of *FOXP3*-expressing cells in peripheral blood, suggesting that defects in other genes or gene products, possibly in the same pathway as *FOXP3*, may cause a similar phenotype.

This patient had late-onset IPEX syndrome, presenting with a severe phenotype with aggressive autoimmune-associated symptoms, which led to his death. Therefore, there was a 25% chance that Sanger sequencing analysis of *FOXP3* would confirm the diagnosis in this patient.

166. **B.** Autoimmune lymphoproliferative syndrome (ALPS), caused by defective lymphocyte homeostasis, is characterized by nonmalignant lymphoproliferation such as lymphadenopathy, hepatosplenomegaly with or without hypersplenism, autoimmune disease mostly directed toward blood cells, and lifelong increased risk for both Hodgkin and non-Hodgkin lymphoma. Heterozygous or homozygous (compound heterozygous) germline pathogenic variants in *FAS*, *FASLG*, and *CASP10* result in ALPS. *ALPS-FAS is the most common and best-characterized type of ALPS, which is caused by heterozygous germline mutations in* FAS (http://www.ncbi.nlm.nih.gov/books/NBK1406/).

Therefore, *FAS* would most likely harbor a pathogenic variant in this patient.

167. **D.** Autoimmune lymphoproliferative syndrome (ALPS), caused by defective lymphocyte homeostasis, is characterized by nonmalignant lymphoproliferation such as lymphadenopathy, hepatosplenomegaly with or without hypersplenism, autoimmune disease mostly directed toward blood cells, and lifelong increased risk for both Hodgkin and non-Hodgkin lymphoma. *Heterozygous or homozygous (compound heterozygous) germline pathogenic variants in FAS, FASLG, and CASP10 result in ALPS.* ALPS-*FAS* is the most common and best-characterized type of ALPS, which is caused by heterozygous germline mutations in *FAS* (http://www.ncbi.nlm.nih.gov/books/NBK1406/).

Immune dysregulation, polyendocrinopathy, enteropathy, X-linked (IPEX) syndrome is characterized by systemic autoimmunity, typically beginning in the first year of life. Presentation is most commonly the clinical triad of watery diarrhea, eczematous dermatitis, and endocrinopathy (most commonly insulin-dependent diabetes mellitus). Molecular analysis of the *FOXP3* gene on Xp11.23 is required for the diagnosis. *FOXP3* is the only gene in which germline pathogenic variants are known to cause IPEX syndrome (http://www.ncbi.nlm.nih.gov/books/NBK1118/).

Therefore, it would be most likely that *FOXP3* did not harbor a pathogenic variant in this patient.

168. **D.** Autoimmune lymphoproliferative syndrome (ALPS), caused by defective lymphocyte homeostasis, is characterized by nonmalignant lymphoproliferation such as lymphadenopathy, hepatosplenomegaly with or without hypersplenism, autoimmune disease mostly directed toward blood cells, and lifelong increased risk for both Hodgkin and non-Hodgkin lymphoma. Heterozygous or homozygous (compound heterozygous) pathogenic variants in *FAS*, *FASLG*, and *CASP10* result in ALPS. ALPS-*FAS* is the most common and best-characterized type of ALPS, associated with heterozygous germline mutations in *FAS*. *Approximately 20%–25% of individuals with ALPS currently lack a genetic diagnosis* (http://www.ncbi.nlm.nih.gov/books/NBK1406/).

Therefore, there was a 75% chance that Sanger sequencing analysis of *FAS*, *FASLG*, and *CASP10* would confirm the diagnosis in this patient.

169. **A.** Immune dysregulation, polyendocrinopathy, enteropathy, X-linked (IPEX) syndrome, autoimmune lymphoproliferative syndrome (ALPS), X-linked lymphoproliferative disease (XLP), and Wiskott–Aldrich syndrome (WAS) are all congenital nonneoplastic hematological disorders characterized by immunodeficiency. Von Willebrand disease (vWD) is the most common hereditary coagulation abnormality described in humans that is caused by pathogenic variants in *vWF* on 12p13.2.

ALPS, caused by defective lymphocyte homeostasis, is characterized by nonmalignant lymphoproliferations such as lymphadenopathy, hepatosplenomegaly with or without hypersplenism, autoimmune disease mostly directed toward blood cells, and lifelong increased risk for both Hodgkin and non-

Hodgkin lymphoma. *Heterozygous or homozygous (compound heterozygous) germline pathogenic variants in FAS, FASLG, and CASP10 result in ALPS* (http://www.ncbi.nlm.nih.gov/books/NBK1406/).

IPEX is characterized by systemic autoimmunity, typically beginning in the first year of life. Presentation is most commonly the clinical triad of watery diarrhea, eczematous dermatitis, and endocrinopathy (most commonly insulin-dependent diabetes mellitus). Most children have other autoimmune phenomena, including Coombs-positive anemia, autoimmune thrombocytopenia, autoimmune neutropenia, and tubular nephropathy. There are no specific laboratory tests to confirm the diagnosis. *FOXP3* is the only gene in which mutations are known to cause IPEX syndrome. Molecular analysis of the *FOXP3* gene on Xp11.23 is required for the diagnosis (http://www.ncbi.nlm.nih.gov/books/NBK1118/).

XLP is caused by mutations in *SH2D1A* and *XIAP* (*BIRC4*). The three most commonly recognized phenotypes of *SH2D1A*-related XLP are hemophagocytic lymphohistiocytosis (HLH) associated with Epstein–Barr virus (EBV) infection (58% of individuals), dysgammaglobulinemia (31%), and lymphoproliferative disorders (malignant lymphoma) (30%). Manifestations of *SH2D1A*-related XLP can also occur in the absence of EBV. *XIAP*-related XLP also presents with HLH (often associated with EBV) or dysgammaglobulinemia, but no cases of lymphoma have been described to date (http://www.ncbi.nlm.nih.gov/books/NBK1406/).

Wiskott–Aldrich syndrome (WAS) is an X-linked disorder caused by pathogenic variants in *WAS* on Xp11.23, which is characterized by thrombocytopenia, eczema, and combined immunodeficiency.

Therefore, it was most likely that the deceased patient had ALPS.

170. **E.** Autoimmune lymphoproliferative syndrome (ALPS), caused by defective lymphocyte homeostasis, is characterized by nonmalignant lymphoproliferation such as lymphadenopathy, hepatosplenomegaly with or without hypersplenism, autoimmune disease mostly directed toward blood cells, and lifelong increased risk for both Hodgkin and non-Hodgkin lymphoma. Heterozygous or homozygous (compound heterozygous) germline pathogenic variants in *FAS*, *FASLG*, and *CASP10* result in ALPS. In general, ALPS is an autosomal dominant disorder, however, patients with biallelic germline

pathogenic variants have been seen (http://www.ncbi.nlm.nih.gov/books/NBK1406/).

The patient in this question had a heterozygous pathogenic variant in *FAS*, which resulted in symptoms related to ALPS. His mother, who had the same familial pathogenic variant was asymptomatic. *The risk of developing ALPS-related complications in the unborn sister depends on the nature of the mutation, as well as the presence of other as-yet incompletely understood genetic or environmental factors.* Therefore, it was unclear if the unborn sister of the proband would develop symptoms.

171. **B.** Wiskott–Aldrich syndrome (WAS) is an X-linked recessive immunodeficiency characterized by thrombocytopenia, eczema, and recurrent infections. *WAS* on Xp11.23 is the only gene associated with WAS. *Female carriers of a WAS pathogenic variant rarely have significant clinical symptoms and generally have no immunologic or biochemical markers of the disorder; however, mild thrombocytopenia is noted in a small proportion* (http://www.ncbi.nlm.nih.gov/books/NBK1178/)

Therefore, it was most likely the unborn sister of the proband would not develop WAS symptoms.

172. **E.** Wiskott–Aldrich syndrome (WAS) is an X-linked recessive immunodeficiency characterized by thrombocytopenia, eczema, and recurrent infections. *WAS* on Xp11.23 is the only gene in which pathogenic variants are known to cause WAS. *Sanger sequencing of WAS may identify approximately 95% of pathogenic variants, and del/dup may identify about 5% of pathogenic variants.*

Therefore, there was more than a 99% chance that Sanger sequencing analysis and del/dup analysis of the *WAS* gene would confirm the diagnosis in this patient.

173. **C.** *X-linked severe combined immunodeficiency (XSCID) is a combined cellular and humoral immunodeficiency caused by pathogenic variants in IL2RG.* Germline pathogenic variants in *FAS* result in autoimmune lymphoproliferative syndrome (ALPS). Germline pathogenic variants in *FOXP3* result in immune dysregulation, polyendocrinopathy, enteropathy, X-linked (IPEX) syndrome. *IL1RG* is not a known gene.

Therefore, *IL2RG* is responsible for XSCID according to the publication in Cells in 1993.

174. **A.** X-linked severe combined immunodeficiency (XSCID) is an immunodeficiency disorder in which the body produces very few T cells and NK cells. *In the absence of T cell help, B cells become defective.* Therefore, the number of B cells does not decrease in patients with XSCID.

175. **B.** X-linked severe combined immunodeficiency (XSCID) is a combined cellular and humoral immunodeficiency caused by pathogenic variants in *IL2RG*. If the DNA is integrated in a sensitive spot in the genome, for example—in a tumor suppressor gene—the therapy could induce a tumor. This has occurred in clinical trials for XSCID patients, in which hematopoietic stem cells were transduced with a corrective transgene using a retrovirus, and *this led to the development of T-cell leukemia in 3 of 20 patients.* Insertion of the *IL2RG* gene near the *LMO2* gene may activate the *LMO2* gene, which is a known oncogene. The activation of *LMO2* in the development of T-cell leukemia is unclear.

Therefore, patients with XSCID tend to develop T-cell leukemia after gene therapy.

176. **A.** *Adenosine deaminase (ADA) deficiency is one form of an autosomal recessive SCID (severe combined immunodeficiency), a disorder that affects the immune system.* ADA deficiency is very rare, but very dangerous, because a malfunctioning immune system leaves the body open to infection from bacteria and viruses. Gene therapy attempts to treat genetic diseases at the molecular level by correcting what is wrong with defective genes. A 4-year-old girl with ADA deficiency became the first gene therapy patient on September 14, 1990, at the NIH Clinical Center. White blood cells were taken from her, and the normal genes for making adenosine deaminase were inserted into them. The corrected cells were injected into her. Dr. W. French Anderson helped develop this landmark clinical trial when he worked at the National Heart, Lung, and Blood Institute.

Therefore, adenosine deaminase deficiency was treated with gene therapy for the first time in 1990.

References

1. Ariizumi H, Maeda T, Nakashima H, Hattori N, Yanagisawa K, Saito B, et al. A descriptive epidemiological study of hematological disorders in showa university hospital. *J Showa Univ Soc* 2013;73(3):8.
2. Fucharoen S, Weatherall DJ. The hemoglobin E thalassemias. *Cold Spring Harb Perspect Med* 2012;2(8):a011734.
3. Canavese C, et al. Clinical relevance of hemochromatosis-related HFE C282Y/H63D gene mutations in patients on chronic dialysis. *Clin Nephrol* 2002;58(6):438–44.
4. Reijnen MJ, et al. Hemophilia B Leyden: substitution of thymine for guanine at position-21 results in a disruption of a hepatocyte nuclear factor 4 binding site in the factor IX promoter. *Blood* 1993;82(1):151–8.
5. Nussbaum RL, McInnes RR, Willard HF. *Thompson & Thompson genetics in medicine.* 8th ed. Philadelphia: Elsevier; 2016. xi, 546 pp.

6. Hickey SE, Curry CJ, Toriello HV. ACMG Practice Guideline: lack of evidence for MTHFR polymorphism testing. *Genet Med* 2013;**15**(2):153–6.

7. Gohil R, Peck G, Sharma P. The genetics of venous thromboembolism. A meta-analysis involving approximately 120,000 cases and 180,000 controls. *Thromb Haemost* 2009;**102**(2):360–70.

8. Ehrenforth S, et al. Impact of environmental and hereditary risk factors on the clinical manifestation of thrombophilia in homozygous carriers of factor V:G1691A. *J Thromb Haemost* 2004;**2**(3):430–6.

9. Schuurmans MM, et al. Influence of age and gender on the clinical expression of acute intermittent porphyria based on molecular study of porphobilinogen deaminase gene among Swiss patients. *Mol Med* 2001;**7**(8):535–42.

10. Gregor A, et al. Molecular study of the hydroxymethylbilane synthase gene (HMBS) among Polish patients with acute intermittent porphyria. *Hum Mutat* 2002;**19**(3):310.

11. Martinez di Montemuros F, et al. Molecular analysis of the hydroxymethylbilane synthase (HMBS) gene in Italian patients with acute intermittent porphyria: report of four novel mutations. *Hum Mutat* 2000;**15**(5):480.

12. Lee HE, et al. A case of hereditary hemorrhagic telangiectasia. *Ann Dermatol* 2009;**21**(2):206–8.

13. Owen CJ, et al. Mutational analysis of the FOXP3 gene and evidence for genetic heterogeneity in the immunodysregulation, polyendocrinopathy, enteropathy syndrome. *J Clin Endocrinol Metab* 2003;**88**(12):6034–9.

14. Margaglione M, Castaman G, Morfini M, Rocino A, Santagostino E, Tagariello G, et al. The Italian AICE-Genetics hemophilia A database: results and correlation with clinicalphenotype. *Haematologica* 2008;**93**(5):722–8 Available from: https://doi.org/10.3324/haematol.12427.

15. Noguchi M, Yi H, Rosenblatt HM, Filipovich AH, Adelstein S, Modi WS, et al. Interleukin-2 receptor gamma chain mutation results in X-linked severe combined immunodeficiency in humans. *Cell* 1993;**73**(12):147–57.

16. Farashi S, Harteveld CL. Molecular basis of α-thalassemia. *Blood Cells Mol Dis.* 2008 May;**70**:43–53 Available from: http://dx.doi.org/10.1016/j.bcmd.2017.09.004.

7

Oncology—Constitutional

Genetic changes in malignancies may be constitutional (this chapter) or acquired (see Chapter 8: Oncology—Acquired). Germline pathogenic variants play a major role in about 5%–10% of all cancers. There are more than 50 recognized hereditary cancer predisposition syndromes. Genetic tests can answer the question of whether an individual with positive family history has the familial mutation. These test results guide an individual's future medical decision, and help asymptomatic family members take proactive measures to prevent cancers from happening.

PROTO-ONCOGENES VERSUS TUMOR SUPPRESSOR GENES

Two classes of regulatory genes are directly involved in carcinogenesis regardless of constitutional or acquired: proto-oncogenes and tumor suppressor genes. Proto-oncogenes stimulate cell proliferation, often through signal transduction and execution of mitogenic signals. Upon activation, a proto-oncogene becomes a tumor-inducing oncogene, such as *RAS*, *WNT*, *MYC*, *ERK*, or *TRK*. So activating mutation in proto-oncogenes usually have a dominant effect. One mutated copy in a cell is enough to turn a normal cell into a malignant one.

Tumor suppressor genes restrain inappropriate cell growth and division, as well as stimulating cell death to keep our cells in proper balance. In addition, some of these genes are involved in DNA repair processes, preventing the accumulation of mutations in cancer-related genes. Deactivation of tumor suppressor genes accelerates cell proliferation without or with limited error checking. So loss-of-function mutations in tumor suppressor genes are usually recessive in nature. In order for a particular cell to become cancerous, both copies of the cell's tumor suppressor genes must be mutated. The examples are *TP53* for Li–Fraumeni syndrome, and *BRCA1/BRCA2* for breast and ovarian cancers.

The exceptions are Cockayne syndrome, cardiofaciocutaneous syndrome, and progeria, which are caused by proto-oncogenes and/or tumor suppressor genes but are not associated with an increased risk for malignancies.

HEREDITARY CANCER PREDISPOSITION SYNDROME AND KNUDSON'S TWO-HIT HYPOTHESIS

The majority of hereditary cancer predisposition syndromes (HCPSs) are autosomal dominant conditions with incomplete penetrance caused by pathogenic variants in tumor suppressor genes. Knudson's two-hit hypothesis has provided extremely important insights into the pathogenesis of tumors in HCPSs. An individual with an autosomal dominant HCPS must be born with one hit (mutation) already in the germline and later acquire a second, tumor-activating hit. This hypothesis explains why patients with the hereditary forms of cancer tend to have earlier onset than the ones with sporadic forms, such as retinoblastoma. Again, using retinoblastoma as an example, children born with a mutation in the *RB1* gene usually develop bilateral and/or multifocal retinoblastoma, with a higher risk of developing cancers in other areas as well. On the other hand, children with sporadic retinoblastoma usually develop only one tumor in one eye at a later age than those with the hereditary form.

CHROMOSOME BREAKAGE SYNDROMES

Chromosome breakage syndromes are a group of autosomal recessive genetic conditions associated with chromosomal instability and breakage. They are characterized by defects in DNA repair mechanisms or genomic instabilities, and they often lead to an increased tendency to develop certain types of malignancies. The examples are ataxia telangiectasia, bloom syndrome, Fanconi anemia, and Nijmegen breakage syndrome.

FOUNDER EFFECT IN ASHKENAZI JEWISH

A founder effect can result either from a true founder event (the establishment of a new population from individuals derived from a much larger population) or from an extreme reduction in population size (a bottleneck in size). Both founder effect and heterozygous advantage have been invoked to account for several disease-associated alleles in the Ashkenazi Jewish population.

The disorders covered in this chapter are:

- Ataxia telangiectasia
- Beckwith Wiedemann syndrome
- Birt Hogg Dubé syndrome
- Bloom syndrome
- Cardiofaciocutaneous syndrome (CFC)
- Cockayne syndrome
- Costello syndrome
- Cowden syndrome
- Denys Drash syndrome (DDS)
- *DICER1* syndrome
- Familial adenomatous polyposis (FAP)
- Fanconi anemia
- Frasier syndrome
- Gorlin syndrome
- Hereditary breast and ovarian cancer
- Hereditary diffuse gastric cancer
- Hereditary nonpolyposis colorectal cancer (HNPCC)
- Hereditary telangiectasia
- Juvenile Polyposis syndrome
- Li Fraumeni
- Lynch syndrome
- Multiple endocrine neoplasia (MEN1)
- Multiple endocrine neoplasia type 2 (MEN 2)
- *MYH*-associated polyposis
- Neurofibromatosis type 1
- Neurofibromatosis type 2
- Nijmegen breakage syndrome
- Noonan syndrome
- *PTEN* hamartomatous syndrome
- Peutz Jeghers syndrome
- Simpson Golabi Behmel syndrome (SGBS)
- Tuberous sclerosis
- von Hippel Lindau disease
- Xeroderma pigmentosum (XP)
- Waardenburg syndrome
- WAGR syndrome

QUESTIONS

1. The Amsterdam criteria are a set of diagnostic criteria used to help identify families with Lynch syndrome, also known as hereditary nonpolyposis colorectal cancer (HNPCC). The original criteria were published in 1990, and they were revised in 1999. What is the detection sensitivity of the revised Amsterdam criteria (Amsterdam II criteria) to the clinical diagnosis of Lynch syndrome?
   A. 60%
   B. 70%
   C. 80%
   D. 90%
   E. 100%
   F. None of the above

2. A couple came to a clinic for their first prenatal care when the wife was 6 weeks pregnant. The wife's brother had just had a proactive colectomy because of familial adenomatous polyposis (FAP). The couple wanted to find out the risk of their first unborn child developing FAP. What should be the next step in the workup be to estimate the risk in this family?
   A. Testing the wife for the *APC* gene
   B. Recommending CVS to test the fetus for the *APC* gene
   C. Testing the wife's brother for the *APC* gene
   D. Recommending that the couple test the child after he/she is born
   E. Recommending amniocentesis to test the fetus for the *APC* gene

3. A couple came to a clinic for their first prenatal care when the wife was 6 weeks pregnant. The wife's maternal uncle died of colorectal cancer (CRC) when he was 42 years old. He had "some kind of familial polyposis disease." The couple wanted to find out the risk of their first unborn child developing colorectal cancer. Which one of the following assays would most likely be used for the genetic test to establish/rule out genetic etiologies in this family?
   A. Chromosome microarray
   B. Denaturing high-performance liquid chromatography (dHPLC) analysis of the *APC* gene
   C. Exome sequencing
   D. Multiplex ligation-dependent probe amplification (MLPA) analysis of the *APC* gene
   E. Next-generation sequencing for hereditary colorectal cancers
   F. Sequence analysis of the *APC* gene

4. A 48-year-old male was diagnosed with colon cancer. The family history was uneventful. Which one of the following hereditary cancer syndromes should be ruled out in this patient even with the negative family history?[1]
   A. Familial adenomatous polyposis (FAP)
   B. Juvenile polyposis syndrome

C. Lynch syndrome

D. *MYH*-associated polyposis

E. Peutz—Jeghers syndrome

5. A 35-year-old female came to a genetics clinic because recently her 38-year-old brother was diagnosed with Lynch syndrome with a pathogenetic variant in the *MLH1* gene. The medical geneticist ordered a targeted molecular test for this female patient, and the results were positive. Which one of the following cancers would this female patient *NOT* have an increased risk of developing?[1]

A. Endometrial cancer

B. Hepatobiliary tract cancer

C. Lung cancer

D. Ovarian cancer

E. Stomach cancer

6. A 35-year-old female came to a genetics clinic because recently her 38-year-old brother was diagnosed with Lynch syndrome with a pathogenetic variant in the *MLH1* gene. The medical geneticist ordered a targeted molecular test for this female patient, and the results were positive. Which one of the following cancers would this female patient *NOT* have an increased risk of developing?[1]

A. Breast cancer

B. Endometrial cancer

C. Hepatobiliary tract cancer

D. Ovarian cancer

E. Stomach cancer

7. A 48-year-old male was recently diagnosed with colorectal cancer (CRC). Microsatellite instability (MSI) analyses of the tumor sample showed a high level of MSI. What would be the most likely diagnosis for this patient?

A. Familial adenomatous polyposis (FAP)

B. Lynch syndrome

C. *MYH*-associated polyposis

D. Sporadic colon cancer

E. None of the above

8. A 48-year-old male was recently diagnosed with colorectal cancer (CRC). Microsatellite instability (MSI) analyses of the tumor sample demonstrated MSI in 40% of markers. What would be the most likely diagnosis for this patient?

A. Familial adenomatous polyposis (FAP)

B. Lynch syndrome

C. *MYH*-associated polyposis

D. Sporadic colon cancer

E. None of the above

9. A 48-year-old male was recently diagnosed with colorectal cancer (CRC). Microsatellite instability (MSI) analyses were ordered to rule out Lynch syndrome. Which one of the following specimens would be most appropriate for the MSI test in this patient?

A. Buccal swab

B. Peripheral-blood sample

C. Resected tumor tissue

D. Skin tissue

E. Urine sample

F. None of the above

10. A 48-year-old male was recently diagnosed with colorectal cancer (CRC). Microsatellite instability (MSI) analyses of the tumor sample showed a high level of MSI. Which one of the following microsatellites would most likely demonstrate instability if the patient had Lynch syndrome?

A. A mononucleotide polymorphism

B. A trinucleotide polymorphism

C. A pentanucleotide polymorphism

D. A single-nucleotide polymorphism

E. Unclear

11. A 48-year-old male was recently diagnosed with colorectal cancer (CRC). Microsatellite instability (MSI) analyses of the tumor sample showed a high level of MSI. What percentage (or more) of the repeats would be unstable if an MSI-high profile was reported?

A. 20%

B. 40%

C. 60%

D. 80%

E. 100%

12. Which one of the following type of malignancies, besides colon cancer, has a high incidence of microsatellite instability (MSI)?

A. Cervical cancer

B. Endometrial carcinoma

C. Intestinal cancer

D. Ovarian cancer

E. Stomach cancer

13. Some endometrial cancers exhibit microsatellite instability (MSI) as the result of somatic *MLH11* promoter methylation. How frequently is MSI seen in patients with endometrial carcinoma?

A. <1%

B. 5%—10%

C. 20%—30%

D. 40%—50%

E. >90%

14. Microsatellites are particularly susceptible to acquire errors in patients with Lynch syndrome when the function of mismatch repair genes is impaired. Therefore, microsatellite instability (MSI) testing is used to identify tumors caused by defective mismatch repair with a panel of microsatellite markers. How frequently is microsatellite instability (MSI) seen in patients with colorectal carcinoma (CRC) due to Lynch syndrome?

A. <1%

B. 5%—10%

C. 20%–30%

D. 40%–50%

E. >99%

15. A 46-year-old female was diagnosed with endometrial adenocarcinoma 2 weeks ago. The oncologist contacted the pathologist to request microsatellite instability (MSI) analysis to rule out Lynch syndrome. The results showed three of five mononucleotide polymorphisms were unstable. However, it also showed that one of the control pentanucleotide polymorphisms had allele 20/20 in the tumor tissue, while it had alleles 20/24 in the peripheral-blood sample from the patient. Which one of the following statements would be the most appropriate reaction to this result?

A. The molecular MSI test did not work; immunohistochemistry staining for MSI is recommended.

B. Repeat the test with the same specimens.

C. Report out as MSI-high profile in the tumor sample with loss of heterozygosity (LOH).

D. Second tumor and peripheral-blood specimens from the same patient should be requested in order to run the test again.

E. The personal identification test should be run on both the tumor and peripheral-blood specimens to confirm that they are from same patient.

16. A 48-year-old Caucasian female came to a genetics clinic owing to her history of colon cancer at age 44. Her medical history was uneventful except for the colon cancer. Her family history was significant for a brother diagnosed with colon cancer at age 45 and her mother diagnosed with endometrial cancer at age 50. She also had one unaffected sister. The physical examination was unremarkable. Of which one of the following hereditary cancer syndromes should we be suspicious in this family?

A. Cowden syndrome

B. Li–Fraumeni syndrome

C. Lynch syndrome

D. Multiple endocrine neoplasia type 1 (MEN1)

E. von Hippel–Lindau disease

17. A 48-year-old Caucasian female came to a genetics clinic to rule out genetic etiologies for her newly diagnosed colon cancer. Her medical history was uneventful except for the colon cancer. Her family history was uneventful. The physical examination was unremarkable. Which one of the following genetic tests should be done first to rule out genetic etiologies, according to ACMG Technical Standard and Guidelines for Genetic Testings for Inherited CRC, 2014?[1]

A. *APC, MUTYH*

B. *BRAF* gene p.V600E mutation

C. Exome sequencing

D. MSI

E. NGS with *BMPR1A, SMAD2, STK11*, and *PTEN*

F. NGS with *MLH1, MSH2, MSH6, PMS2*, and *PSM6*

18. A 48-year-old Caucasian female came to a genetics clinic to rule out a genetic etiologies for her newly diagnosed colon cancer. Her medical history was significant only for the colon cancer. Her family history was uneventful. The physical examination was unremarkable. Microsatellite instability (MSI) testing revealed a high level of MSI. Which one of the following genetic tests should be done next to further rule out genetic etiologies, according to the ACMG Technical Standard and Guidelines for Genetic Testings for Inherited CRC, 2014?[1]

A. *APC, MUTYH*

B. *BRAF* gene p.V600E mutation

C. Exome sequencing

D. Microsatellite instability test

E. NGS with *BMPR1A, SMAD2, STK11*, and *PTEN*

F. NGS with *MLH1, MSH2, MSH6, PMS2*, and *PSM6*

19. A 48-year-old Caucasian female came to a genetics clinic because of her history of colon cancer at age 44. Her medical history was significant only for the colon cancer. Her family history was positive for a brother diagnosed with colon cancer at age 45 and her mother diagnosed with endometrial cancer at age 50. She also had one unaffected sister. The physical examination was unremarkable. Which one of following assays would be appropriate for this family in order to rule out genetic etiologies?

A. Chromosome microarray

B. Multiplex ligation-dependent probe amplification (MLPA)

C. NGS with *BMPR1A, SMAD2, STK11*, and *PTEN*

D. NGS with *MLH1, MSH2, MSH6, PMS2*, and *PSM6*

E. No need for genetic tests

20. A 34-year-old female came to a clinic for her first prenatal care. Her personal medical history was unremarkable. Family history revealed that her sister was diagnosed with colon cancer at age 49 and her maternal grandmother died of stomach cancer at the age of 62. The genetic counselor explained to the patient the possibility of hereditary cancer syndromes and ordered a molecular test for the patient. The results

demonstrated that the patient had a deleterious pathogenic variant in the *PMS2* gene. Which one of following hereditary cancer syndromes did the patient have?

A. Familial adenomatous polyposis
B. Juvenile polyposis syndrome
C. Lynch syndrome
D. *MYH*-associated polyposis
E. Peutz–Jeghers syndrome

21. Lynch syndrome (LS) is the most common cause of inherited colorectal cancer (CRC), characterized by a significantly increased risk for CRC and endometrial cancer as well as a risk of several other malignancies. Most individuals with LS have a germline pathogenic variant in one of the DNA mismatch repair genes. Which one of following genes is *NOT* a mismatch repair gene?

A. *APC*
B. *MLH1*
C. *MLH3*
D. *MSH6*
E. *PMS1*
F. *PMS2*

22. Lynch syndrome (LS) is the most common cause of inherited colorectal cancer (CRC), characterized by a significantly increased risk for CRC and endometrial cancer as well as a risk of several other malignancies. Most individuals with LS have a germline pathogenic variant in one of the DNA mismatch repair genes. Which one of following genes is associated with Lynch syndrome, but is *NOT* a mismatch repair gene?

A. *EpCAM*
B. *MLH1*
C. *MLH3*
D. *MSH6*
E. *PMS1*
F. *PMS2*

23. A 34-year-old female came to a clinic for her first prenatal care. Her personal medical history was unremarkable. Her family history revealed that her sister was diagnosed with colon cancer at age 49 and her maternal grandmother died of stomach cancer at the age of 62. The genetic counselor explained to the patient the possibility of hereditary cancer syndromes, and ordered a molecular test for her. The results demonstrated the patient had a deletion in the *EpCAM* gene. Which one of following microsatellite instability (MSI) findings would this patient most likely have?

A. MSI-high
B. MSI-low
C. MSI-stable
D. Not sure
E. None of the above

24. A 34-year-old female came to a clinic for her first prenatal care. Her personal medical history was unremarkable. Her family history revealed that her sister was diagnosed with colon cancer at age 49 and her maternal grandmother died of stomach cancer at the age of 62. The genetic counselor explained to the patient the possibility of hereditary cancer syndromes and ordered a molecular test for her. The results demonstrated the patient had a deletion in the *EpCAM* gene. Which one of following immunohistochemistry (IHC) findings would this patient have?

A. Loss expression of *MLH1* and *MSH2*
B. Loss expression of *MLH1* and *PMS2*
C. Loss expression of *MSH2* and *MSH6*
D. Loss expression of *MSH2* and *PMS2*
E. None of the above

25. A 26-year-old female came to a genetics clinic because of a positive family history of colon cancer. Her medical history was uneventful. Her family history was significant because her father died of colon cancer at the age of 56 and one of her paternal aunts was diagnosed with endometrial cancer at the age of 42. The physical examination was unremarkable. Which one of the following genes would most likely *NOT* provide information to confirm or rule out genetic etiologies in this patient?

A. *MLH1*
B. *MSH2*
C. *MSH3*
D. *MSH6*
E. *PMS2*

26. A 66-year-old male was diagnosed with colorectal carcinoma (CRC) 2 weeks ago. The oncologist contacted the pathologist to request microsatellite instability (MSI) analysis to rule out Lynch syndrome. The results showed that three of five mononucleotide polymorphisms were unstable. Immunohistochemistry (IHC) stains for *MLH1*, *MSH2*, *PMS2*, and *MSH6* were done with the tumor tissue. The results showed no staining for *MHL1* and *PMS2*, but staining for *MSH2* and *MSH6*. A *BRAF* mutation test was positive for the V600E mutation. Which one of the following mutations is most likely detectable in tumor?

A. p.Arg134Ter in *PMS2*
B. Promoter hypermethylation in *PMS2*
C. p.Pro622Leu in *MSH2*
D. Promoter hypermethylation in *MSH2*
E. p.Ser252Ter in *MHL1*
F. Promoter hypermethylation in *MHL1*

27. Lynch syndrome is the most common cause of inherited colorectal cancer (CRC), characterized by a significantly increased risk for CRC and endometrial cancer as well as a risk of several

other malignancies. Lynch syndrome refers to patients and families with a germline pathogenic variant in one of the DNA mismatch repair genes (*MLH1, MSH2, MSH6, PMS2*) or the *EpCAM* gene. Testing tumors for evidence of defective DNA mismatch repair has been used to identify individuals at risk for Lynch syndrome. However, microsatellite instability has been seen in significant amount of individuals with sporadic CRCs. Which one of the following DNA mismatch repair genes tends to be hypermethylated in individuals with sporadic CRCs?

A. *MLH1*
B. *MLH3*
C. *MSH6*
D. *PMS1*
E. *PMS2*

28. A 26-year-old female came to a genetics clinic because of a positive family history of colon cancer. Her medical history was uneventful. The family history was significant because the father died of colon cancer at the age of 56 and one of her paternal aunts was diagnosed with colon cancer at age 42. The physical examination was unremarkable. A molecular test confirmed that the patient had a pathogenic variant in the *MSH2* gene. Which one of the following malignancies would this patient have the highest risk of developing in her lifetime?

A. Cervical cancer
B. Endometrial carcinoma
C. Hepatocellular carcinoma
D. Ovarian cancer
E. Stomach cancer

29. A 26-year-old female came to a genetics clinic because of a positive family history of colon cancer. Her medical history was uneventful. The family history was significant because the father died of colon cancer at the age of 56 and one of her paternal aunts was diagnosed with colon cancer at age 42. The physical examination was unremarkable. A molecular test confirmed the patient had a pathogenic variant in the *MSH2* gene. What would be this patient's risk of developing colorectal cancer in her lifetime?

A. 20%
B. 40%
C. 60%
D. 80%
E. >99%

30. A 26-year-old female came to a genetics clinic because of a positive family history of colon cancer. Her medical history was uneventful. The family history was significant because the father

died of colon cancer at the age of 56 and one of her paternal aunts was diagnosed with colon cancer at age 42. The physical examination was unremarkable. A molecular test confirmed the patient had a pathogenic variant in the *MSH2* gene. What would be this patient's risk of developing endometrial carcinoma in her lifetime?

A. 20%
B. 40%
C. 60%
D. 80%
E. >99%

31. A 46-year-old female was diagnosed with endometrial adenocarcinoma 2 weeks ago. The oncologist contacted the pathologist to request microsatellite instability (MSI) analysis to rule out Lynch syndrome. The results showed that three of five mononucleotide polymorphisms were unstable. Immunohistochemistry (IHC) stains for *MLH1, MSH2, PMS2,* and *MSH6* were done with the tumor tissue. The results showed no staining for *MHL1* and *PMS2*, but staining for *MSH2* and *MSH6*. Which one of the following would be appropriate next step in the workup for this patient?

A. *BRAF* mutation analysis
B. Diagnosing the patient with endometrial adenocarcinoma without genetic etiology
C. Diagnosing the patient with Lynch syndrome
D. Performing next-generation sequencing for all the genes for hereditary colon cancer
E. Performing sequencing analysis of *MLH1* and *PMS1*
F. Performing sequencing analysis of *MSH2* and *MSH6*

32. A 59-year-old male was referred to a genetics clinic for a recent diagnosis of colon cancer. The family history was positive because his father died of colon cancer at the age of 68 and his sister was diagnosed with endometrial cancer at age 51. He was tested for microsatellite instability (MSI) with microsatellite markers and expression of *MLH1* and *MSH2* by immunohistochemistry (IHC) stains. The results showed MSI in three of six markers, loss of expression of *MSH2*, and normal expression of *MLH1*. Molecular genetic tests of both *MSH2* and *MSH6* were negative. Which one of the following tests might be the next step in the workup to further rule out Lynch syndrome in this patient?

A. A larger next-generation sequencing panel for hereditary colon cancer syndromes
B. *BRAF* gene p.V600E mutation test
C. *EpCAM* gene 3′ deletion test
D. *MLH1* promoter methylation study

E. *MLH1* and *PMS2* gene-mutation test

33. A 59-year-old male was referred to a genetics clinic for a recent diagnosis of colon cancer. The family history was positive because his father died of colon cancer at the age of 68 and his sister was diagnosed with endometrial cancer at the age of 51. He was tested for microsatellite instability (MSI) with microsatellite markers and expression of *MLH1* and *MSH2* by immunohistochemistry (IHC) stains. The results showed MSI in three of six markers, loss of expression of *MSH2*, and normal expression of *MLH1*. Molecular genetic tests of both *MSH2* and *MSH6* were negative. To further rule out Lynch syndrome in this patient, the medical geneticist ordered a molecular test on the *EpCAM* gene, and the results turned out to be positive. Which one of the following changes in *EpCAM* would most likely be detected in this patient?
    A. Deletion
    B. Frameshift mutation
    C. Insertion
    D. Missense mutation
    E. Nonsense mutation

34. A 59-year-old male was referred to a genetics clinic for a recent diagnosis of colon cancer. The family history was positive because his father died of colon cancer at the age of 68 and his sister was diagnosed with endometrial cancer at the age of 51. He was tested for microsatellite instability (MSI) with microsatellite markers and expression of *MLH1* and *MSH2* by immunohistochemistry (IHC) stains. The results showed MSI in three of six markers, loss of expression of *MSH2*, and normal expression of *MLH1*. Molecular genetic tests of both *MSH2* and *MSH6* were negative. To further rule out Lynch syndrome in this patient, the medical geneticist ordered a molecular test on the *EpCAM* gene, and a deletion on the 3′ end of the gene was detected. How would the deletion in *EpCAM* cause Lynch syndrome in this patient?
    A. It causes somatic hypermethylation of *MLH1*.
    B. It causes somatic hypermethylation of *MSH2*.
    C. It causes somatic hypermethylation of *MSH6*.
    D. It causes somatic hypermethylation of *PMS2*.
    E. None of the above.

35. A 62-year-old male was diagnosed with colon cancer. His medical and family histories were uneventful. The physical examination was unremarkable. He was tested for microsatellite instability (MSI) with microsatellite markers and expression of *MLH1* and *MSH2* by immunohistochemistry (IHC) stains. The results showed a high level of MSI, loss of expression of *MLH1*, and normal expression of *MSH2*. Predictably, which one of the following genes lose

expression, too, in the tumor tissue from this patient?
    A. *BRAF*
    B. *MSH6*
    C. *PMS2*
    D. All of the above
    E. None of the above

36. A 62-year-old male was diagnosed with colon cancer. His medical and family histories were uneventful. The physical examination was unremarkable. He was tested for microsatellite instability (MSI) with microsatellite markers and expression of *MLH1* and *MSH2* by immunohistochemistry (IHC) stains. The results showed high level of MSI, loss of expression of *MSH2*, and normal expression of *MLH1*. Predictably which one of the following genes would lose expression, too, in the tumor tissue from this patient?
    A. *BRAF*
    B. *MSH6*
    C. *PMS2*
    D. All of the above
    E. None of the above

37. A 62-year-old male was diagnosed with colon cancer. His medical and family histories were uneventful. The physical examination was unremarkable. He was tested for microsatellite instability (MSI) with microsatellite markers and expression of *MLH1*, and *MSH2* by immunohistochemistry (IHC) stains. The results showed 50% of MSI, loss of expression of *MLH1*, and normal expression of *MSH2*. What would be the next step in the workup according to ACMG Technical Standard and Guidelines for Genetic Testing for Inherited CRC, 2014?[1]
    A. *BRAF* p.V600E test
    B. *BRAF* p.V600K test
    C. *BRAF* sequence
    D. *MLH1* and *MSH2* sequence
    E. *MLH1* and *MSH6* sequence
    F. *MLH1* and *PMS2* sequence

38. A 63-year-old male was diagnosed with colon cancer. His medical and family histories were uneventful. The physical examination was unremarkable. He was tested for microsatellite instability (MSI) with STR markers and expression of the mismatch repair (MMR) genes by immunohistochemistry (IHC) stains. The results showed MSI in three of six markers and loss of expression of *MSH2* and *MSH6*. What would be the next step in the workup according to ACMG Technical Standard and Guidelines for Genetic Testing for Inherited CRC, 2014?[1]
    A. *BRAF* p.V600E mutation test
    B. *BRAF* p.V600K test
    C. *BRAF* sequence

D. *MSH2* sequence

E. *MSH6* gene-mutation test

F. *MSH2* and *MSH6* gene-mutation test

39. A 48-year-old man was diagnosed with colorectal cancer (CRC) 1 month ago. He was referred to a genetics clinic to rule out genetic etiologies for his CRC. A colonoscopy at the time of diagnosis showed >100 adenomatous polyps throughout the colon. His family history was negative for polyposis and/or CRC. What would be the most appropriate molecular test as the next step in the workup to rule out genetic etiologies in this patient?

A. Sequence the *APC* gene with reflex to *APC* del/dup analysis

B. Sequence the *MUTYH* gene with reflex to *MUTYH* del/dup analysis

C. Sequence the *MLH1* gene with reflex to *MLH1* del/dup analysis

D. Sequence the *MSH2* gene with reflex to *MSH2* del/dup analysis

E. Sequence the *APC* and *MUTYH* genes with reflex to *APC* and *MUTYH* del/dup analysis

F. Sequence the *MLH1* and *MSH2* genes with reflex to *MLH1* and *MSH2* del/dup analysis

40. All of the following tumors are consistent with Lynch syndrome, EXCEPT:

A. *BRAF* mutation–negative, *MLH1* methylation negative, MSI-high colorectal cancer

B. MLH1 immunohistochemistry (IHC)–negative, *BRAF* mutation–positive colorectal cancer

C. MSH2 and MSH6 immunohistochemistry (IHC)–negative endometrial adenocarcinoma

D. MSI-high, *MLH1* methylation–negative endometrial adenocarcinoma

E. MSI-high, MLH1 immunohistochemistry (IHC)–negative endometrial adenocarcinoma with three first-degree relatives for either colorectal cancer or endometrial adenocarcinoma

41. A 48-year-old woman was diagnosed with colorectal cancer (CRC) 1 month ago. She was referred to a genetics clinic to rule out genetic etiologies for her CRC. A colonoscopy at the time of diagnosis showed >100 adenomatous polyps throughout the colon. The family history was negative for polyposis and/or CRC. A *KRAS* mutation analysis showed that the patient had a somatic c.34G > T mutation. Which one of the hereditary cancer predisposition syndromes would this patient most likely have if she had one?

A. Familial adenomatous polyposis

B. Lynch syndrome

C. *MYH*-associated polyposis

D. Peutz–Jeghers syndrome

E. *PTEN* hamartomatous syndrome

42. A 16-year-old male was referred to a genetics clinic for mild cognitive impairment with >1000 colorectal adenomatous polyps. Genetic evaluations uncovered that he also had mild dysmorphic features. The family history was unremarkable on both sides. The medical geneticist ordered a test to rule out genetic etiologies. Which one of the following genetic tests would be most appropriate for this patient?

A. Chromosome microarray

B. Methylation study of the *APC* gene

C. Sequence the *APC* gene

D. Sequence the *MUTYH* gene

E. Sequence *APC* and *MUTYH* genes

F. None of the above

43. BJ, a 47-year-old female, was referred to a genetics clinic for counseling because of a medical history of endometrial carcinoma at age 46. Her family history was positive for her mother diagnosed with endometrial carcinoma at the age of 51 and her brother diagnosed with colon cancer in his 40s. The physical examination was unremarkable. The medical geneticist offered BJ a hereditary colorectal cancer (CRC) next-generation sequencing (NGS) panel to rule out Lynch syndrome. Which one of the following genes associated with Lynch syndrome has more pseudogenes than the others?

A. *BRAF*

B. *EpCAM*

C. *MLH1*

D. *MSH2*

E. *MUTYH*

F. *PMS2*

44. A 46-year-old male was diagnosed with colorectal carcinoma (CRC) 2 weeks ago. The oncologist contacted the pathologist to request microsatellite instability (MSI) analysis to rule out Lynch syndrome. The results showed that one of five mononucleotide polymorphisms were unstable. Immunohistochemistry (IHC) stains for *MLH1, MSH2, PMS2,* and *MSH6* were done with the tumor tissue. The results showed staining for all four proteins. His family history was positive for CRC in one sister and one maternal uncle and for endometrial carcinoma in one maternal aunt. The patient met the clinical diagnosis for Lynch syndrome based on Amsterdam II Criteria. Which one of the following genes would most likely harbor a pathogenic variant in this patient?

A. *BRAF*

B. *MLH1*

C. *MSH2*

D. *MSH6*

E. *PMS2*

45. A 16-year-old female patient was referred to a genetics clinic for a 1-year history of bloody mucoid diarrhea. The physical examination revealed that she had clinodactyly, and her weight was 2 SD below the mean. Laboratory tests showed hypochromic microcytic anemia. Her upper gastrointestinal endoscopy and colonoscopy showed polyps from the fundus to the cecum with variable sizes and irregular surfaces. Histological studies indicated the presence of typical hamartomatous polyps without dysplasia. Clinical diagnosis of juvenile polyposis was made. The medical geneticist ordered a molecular test for this patient. Which gene(s) listed would most likely be included in the genetic evaluations for this patient?

A. *APC*
B. *BMPR1A*
C. *APC* and *BMPR1A*
D. *SMAD4*
E. *BMPR1A* and *SMAD4*
F. *STK11*
G. *APC* and *STK11*

46. A 13-year-old male patient was referred to a genetics clinic to rule out genetic etiologies for his recurrent GI bleeding, mucocutaneous telangiectases, and pulmonary arteriovenous malformations. His pediatric gastroenterologist found and had been able to control the polyps in the stomach and colon by upper endoscopy and colonoscopy. Histopathological evaluations of the lesions in the upper duodenum demonstrated high-grade dysplasia. Which one of the following analyses would most likely be used for the genetic evaluation to rule out genetic etiologies in this patient?

A. Chromosome karyotype
B. Microarray copy-number analysis
C. *APC* sequencing
D. *BMPR1A* sequencing
E. *SMAD4* sequencing
F. *STK11* sequencing

47. A 13-year-old male patient was referred to a genetics clinic to rule out genetic etiologies for his recurrent GI bleeding due to polyp development in his duodenum. His pediatric gastroenterologist found and had been able to control the polyps in the stomach and colon by upper gastrointestinal endoscopy. Colonoscopy showed polyps from the fundus to the cecum with variable sizes and irregular surfaces. Histopathological evaluations of the lesions indicated the presence of typical hamartomatous polyps with high-grade dysplasia. The physical examination revealed the patient had developmental delay and macrocephaly (> 2 SD above the mean). Which

one of the following analyses would most likely be used for the genetic evaluation to rule out genetic etiologies in this patient?

A. Chromosome karyotype
B. Microarray copy-number analysis
C. *APC* sequencing
D. *BMPR1A* sequencing
E. *SMAD4* sequencing
F. *PTEN* sequencing

48. A 16-year-old high school student comes to a genetics clinic about his risk for cancers. His father passed away at the age of 9 because of complications of colorectal cancer (CRC). His paternal uncle also died of CRC at the age of 55. His paternal grandmother died of breast cancer at the age of 61. Several of his cousins either have died of or been diagnosed with various types of cancers. Physical examination reveals freckling on his buccal mucosa. The patient states he had many more freckles around his mouth and on his hands and feet, but they have faded as he has gotten older. The rest of the physical examination is normal. The fecal occult blood test is positive. What one of the following hereditary cancer predisposition syndromes may this patient have if he has one?

A. Familial adenomatous polyposis
B. Lynch syndrome
C. *MYH*-associated polyposis
D. Peutz−Jeghers syndrome
E. *PTEN* hamartomatous syndrome

49. A 17-year-old female was admitted to a hospital because of sharp and intermittent abdominal pain around the periumbilical region. The patient reported blackening of the stool for 5 days. Her medical history was significant for several episodes of nonbilious and nonbloody vomiting. The physical examination revealed multiple, black-pigmented lesions on the face, lower lip, and buccal mucosa, which the patient had had since childhood. Laboratory tests revealed hypochromic microcytic anemia (hemoglobin, 8.2 g/dL; normal range, 12−16). A barium examination of the small bowel and abdominal ultrasonography (US) suggested intussusception of the jejunum. The patient underwent an exploratory laparotomy. A small bowel segment was resected. Histopathological examinations revealed hamartomatous polyps consistent with a clinical diagnosis of Peutz−Jeghers syndrome (PJS). Which gene(s) listed below would most likely be included in the genetic test for this patient?

A. *APC*
B. *BMPR1A*
C. *APC* and *BMPR1A*

D. *SMAD4*
E. *BMPR1A* and *SMAD4*
F. *STK11*
G. *APC* and *STK11*

50. A 17-year-old female was admitted to a hospital because of sharp and intermittent abdominal pain around the periumbilical region. The patient reported blackening of the stool for 5 days. Her medical history was significant for several episodes of nonbilious and nonbloody vomiting. The physical examination revealed multiple, black-pigmented lesions on the face, lower lip, and buccal mucosa, which the patient had had since childhood. Laboratory tests revealed hypochromic microcytic anemia (hemoglobin, 8.2 g/dL; normal range, 12–16). A barium examination of the small bowel and abdominal ultrasonography (US) suggested intussusception of the jejunum. The patient underwent an exploratory laparotomy. A small bowel segment was resected. Histopathological examinations revealed hamartomatous polyps consistent with a clinical diagnosis of Peutz–Jeghers syndrome (PJS). Which one of the following represents the approximate detection rate of sequencing analysis of the *STK11* gene in patients diagnosed with PJS clinically?
   A. 25%
   B. 50%
   C. 75%
   D. 99%
   E. Unknown

51. A 52-year-old female presented to a clinic for intermittent abdominal pain and diarrhea for 3 years. Her medical history revealed that she had had more than 30 polyps in the small intestine and colorectum, which had been resected under the guidance of enteroscopy and colonoscopy. Histopathological examinations of the resected polyps revealed that they were hamartomatous. Her family history was unremarkable. The physical examination of the patient was negative except for pigmentation on her lips and extremities, which had been there all her life. Molecular genetic tests detected a heterozygous pathogenic variant in the *STK11* gene. A diagnosis of Peutz–Jeghers syndrome was made. Which one of the following cancers would the patient have highest risk of developing in her lifetime?
   A. Brain tumor
   B. Breast cancer
   C. Cervical cancer
   D. Melanoma
   E. None of the above

52. A microarray copy-number analysis was ordered for a 4-year-old girl with autism. The results revealed a 324-kb deletion on 19p13.3, including the *STK11* gene. What would be the clinical significance of this finding?
   A. Pathogenic
   B. Unknown clinical significance, likely pathogenic
   C. Unknown clinical significance
   D. Unknown clinical significance, likely benign
   E. Benign

53. A 43-year-old woman was referred to a genetics clinic by her gynecologist because of a recent diagnosis of primary bilateral breast cancer. Her medical history was unremarkable. The physical examination revealed that the patient had mild intellectual disability and that her head size was greater than the 98th percentile of the mean. Her family history was positive on the maternal side. Her maternal aunt was diagnosed with endometrial cancer at age 62. Her maternal uncle was diagnosed with renal cell carcinoma in his 60s. Her maternal granduncle died of "a disease in his neck" when he was in his early 40s. Which one of the following hereditary cancer predisposition syndromes would this patient most likely have if she had one?
   A. Familial adenomatous polyposis
   B. Lynch syndrome
   C. *MYH*-associated polyposis
   D. Peutz–Jeghers syndrome
   E. *PTEN* hamartomatous tumor syndrome

54. A 43-year-old woman was referred to a genetics clinic by her gynecologist because of a recent diagnosis of a primary bilateral breast cancer. Her medical history was unremarkable. The physical examination showed that the patient had mild intellectual disability and that her head size was greater than the 98th percentile of the mean. Her family history was positive on the maternal side. Her maternal aunt had endometrial cancer at age 62. Her maternal uncle was diagnosed with renal cell carcinoma in his 60s. Her maternal granduncle died of a "disease in his neck" when he was in his early 40s. Which one of the following gene-sequencing tests would be the most appropriate first-tier genetic evaluation for this patient?
   A. *BRAC1*
   B. *BRAC2*
   C. *BRAC1* and *BRAC2*
   D. *CDH1*
   E. *PTEN*
   F. *STK11*
   G. *VHL*

55. A 17-year-old female was admitted to a hospital because of sharp and intermittent abdominal pain around the periumbilical region. The patient reported blackening of the stool for 5 days. Her medical history was significant for several episodes of nonbilious and nonbloody vomiting. Laboratory tests revealed hypochromic microcytic anemia (hemoglobin, 8.2 g/dL; normal range, 12−16). A barium examination of the small bowel and abdominal ultrasonography (US) suggested intussusception of the jejunum. The patient underwent an exploratory laparotomy. A small-bowel segment was resected. Histopathological examinations revealed hamartomatous polyps. The family history was negative for both polyposis and cancers. A medical geneticist was called for consultation. Which one of the following genes would most likely *NOT* be sequenced in this patient to rule out genetic etiologies?

A. *APC*

B. *BMPR1A*

C. *SMAD4*

D. *STK11*

E. *PTEN*

56. A 17-year-old female was admitted to a hospital because of sharp and intermittent abdominal pain around the periumbilical region. The patient reported blackening of the stool for 6 days. Her medical history was significant for several episodes of nonbilious and nonbloody vomiting. Laboratory tests revealed hypochromic microcytic anemia (hemoglobin, 8.2 g/dL; normal range, 12−16). A barium examination of the small bowel and abdominal ultrasonography (US) suggested intussusception of the jejunum. The patient underwent an exploratory laparotomy. A small-bowel segment was resected. Histopathological examinations revealed hamartomatous polyps. The family history was negative for both polyposis and cancers. A medical geneticist was called for consultation. Which one of the following gene panels would be the most appropriate first-tier genetic evaluation for this patient?

A. *APC, MUTYH*

B. *BMPR1A, SMAD2, STK11, PTEN*

C. *MLH1, MSH2, MSH6, PMS2, PSM6*

D. *MUTYH, STK11, PTEN*

E. All of the above

F. None of the above

57. A 10-year-old boy was brought to a clinic by her parents for bloody stool and significant growth retardation. His family history was significant for familial adenomatous polyposis (FAP). The maternal grandfather, maternal aunt, and two cousins had been diagnosed with FAP. The

physical examination revealed that the patient was small for his age (below the 5th percentile) and had multiple small polyps detected on rectal exam. Laboratory tests demonstrated hypochromic microcytic anemia. A colonoscopy revealed multiple and diffuse polyps, supporting the diagnosis of FAP. Which one of the following gene-sequencing tests would be the most appropriate first-tier genetic evaluation for this patient?

A. *APC*

B. *BMPR1A*

C. *MLH1*

D. *MUTYH*

E. None of the above

58. A 59-year-old male was referred to a genetics clinic for cancer risk assessment because of a personal history of polyposis and colorectal cancer (CRC). The medical history revealed adenomatous polyposis at the age of 40 and CRC at the age of 56. His family history was unremarkable on both sides. The *APC* gene was sequenced, and the results were negative. Which one of the following gene-sequencing tests would be the most appropriate next step in the genetic evaluation for this patient?

A. *BMPR1A*

B. *MLH1*

C. *MUTYH*

D. *SMAD4*

E. *PTEN*

F. None of the above

59. A 10-year-old boy was diagnosed with adenomatous polyposis of the small intestine 2 weeks ago. A colonoscopy detected hundreds of polyposis. Histopathological examinations revealed adenomatous polyps. The family history was negative for both polyposis and cancers. A clinical geneticist was called for consultation. Which one of the following gene panels would be the most appropriate first genetic evaluation for this patient?

A. *APC, MUTYH*

B. *BMPR1A, SMAD2, STK11, PTEN*

C. *MLH1, MSH2, MSH6, PMS2, PSM6*

D. *MUTYH, STK11, PTEN*

E. All of the above

F. None of the above

60. How frequently do patients with breast cancer(s) have predisposition mutations in the *BRCA1* or *BRCA2* gene?

A. <1%

B. 5%−10%

C. 15%

D. 20%−25%

E. 40%

61. How frequently do patients with hereditary breast cancer(s) have predisposition mutations in the *BRCA1* or *BRCA2* gene?
- **A.** <1%
- **B.** 5%–10%
- **C.** 15%
- **D.** 20%–25%
- **E.** 40%

62. A 58-year-old Caucasian female was diagnosed with triple-negative multifocal breast cancer. Her medical history was significant for ovarian cancer diagnosed at age 52. Which one of the following genetic tests would be appropriate for this patient?
- **A.** *BRCA2* sequencing
- **B.** *BRCA1* sequencing
- **C.** *BRCA1* and *BRCA2* sequencing
- **D.** *HER2* FISH
- **E.** *STK11* sequencing
- **F.** *PTEN* sequencing

63. A 28-year-old Caucasian female was diagnosed with triple-positive right breast cancer. Which one of the following genetic tests would be appropriate in this patient?
- **A.** *BRCA2* sequencing
- **B.** *BRCA1* sequencing
- **C.** *BRCA1* and *BRCA2* sequencing
- **D.** *HER2* FISH
- **E.** *HER2* sequencing
- **F.** *PTEN* sequencing

64. A 28-year-old female presents with a 1-month history of a palpable mass in her right breast. The initial mammogram revealed an asymmetric retroareolar mass with circumscribed borders and

with breast cancer at age 36. *BRCA1* and *BRCA2* tests were ordered for this patient, and the result was negative. Which one of the following genes will *NOT* be considered in the next step in the workup to rule out genetic etiologies?
- **A.** *ATM*
- **B.** *CDH1*
- **C.** *CHEK2*
- **D.** *PALB2*
- **E.** *PTEN*
- **F.** *STK11*
- **G.** *TP53*
- **H.** *VHL*
- **I.** All of the above
- **J.** None of the above

65. An Ashkenazi Jewish couple was transferred to a clinic for prenatal care when the wife was 6 months pregnant. They were both apparently healthy, with unremarkable medical histories. Their family history was significant for breast cancers on both sides (see the figure below). Targeted molecular tests were ordered and pathogenic variants in the *BRCA2* gene were detected on both. Which one of the following disorders would the couple's children be at risk of developing besides breast cancer?
- **A.** Ataxia telangiectasia
- **B.** Bloom syndrome
- **C.** Fanconi anemia
- **D.** Hereditary telangiectasia
- **E.** Nijmegen breakage syndrome
- **F.** All of the above
- **G.** None of the above

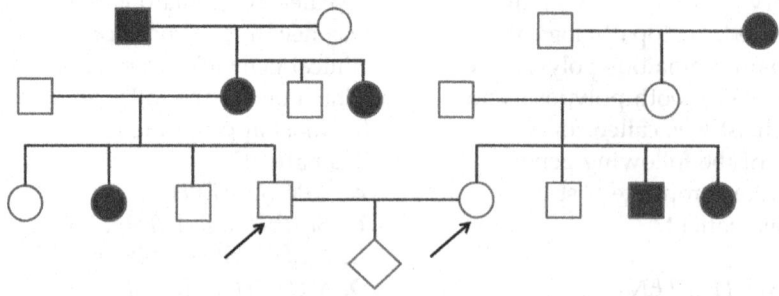

no associated calcifications. Also noted on the mammogram was an enlarged axillary node. A biopsy of the breast mass confirmed the diagnosis of triple-negative breast cancer. The family history was positive for a paternal aunt who died of breast cancer and a cousin who was diagnosed

66. An Ashkenazi Jewish couple was transferred to a clinic for prenatal care when the wife was 6 months pregnant. They were both apparently healthy. Their medical histories were unremarkable. The family history was significant for breast cancers on both sides (see the figure below). Targeted molecular tests were ordered and pathogenic variants in the *BRCA2* gene were detected in both the husband and the wife. If their firstborn child developed Fanconi anemia, which one of the following genes would most likely harbor a pathogenic variant in both parents?

A. *BRCA1*
B. *BRCA2*
C. *PTEN*
D. *TP53*
E. *VHL*

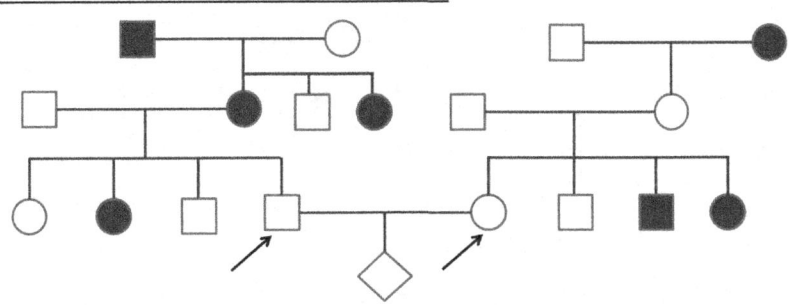

67. A couple came to a clinic for preconception counseling. They both were apparently healthy. Their medical history was unremarkable. The family history was significant for breast cancers on both sides (see the figure below). Molecular tests were ordered, and pathogenic variants in the *BRCA1* gene were detected in both the husband and the wife. Which one of the following disorders would the couple's children be at risk of developing besides breast cancer?

A. Ataxia telangiectasia
B. Bloom syndrome
C. Fanconi anemia
D. Hereditary telangiectasia
E. Nijmegen breakage syndrome

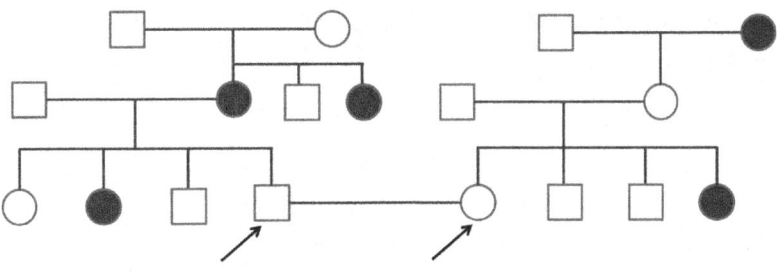

68. A 52-year-old Ashkenazi Jewish male was diagnosed with breast cancer 2 weeks ago. He was referred to a genetics clinic to rule out genetic etiologies. Aside from the breast cancer, his medical history was unremarkable. The physical examination was uneventful. His family history was significant for his sister being diagnosed with ovarian cancer at age 48 and his paternal uncle dying of breast cancer at age 62. Which one of the following genes should be tested first to rule out genetic etiologies in this patient?

A. *BRCA1*
B. *BRCA2*
C. *CDH1*
D. *STK11*
E. *PTEN*

69. Joanne, a 43-year-old female, came to a genetics clinic to find out her risk for malignancies. Her medical history was unremarkable. The physical examination was uneventful. However, her older sister, Lily, was diagnosed with ovarian cancer at the age of 53 (see the figure below for pedigree). Her mother, Lisa, died of breast cancer at the age

of 68. Her maternal uncle, Jeffrey, had breast
cancer. Her maternal grandfather, Tom, had
breast cancer. Which one of the following
individuals in this family should be tested first
for a potential genetic etiology?

A. Joanne
B. John
C. Joey
D. Lily
E. Suanne

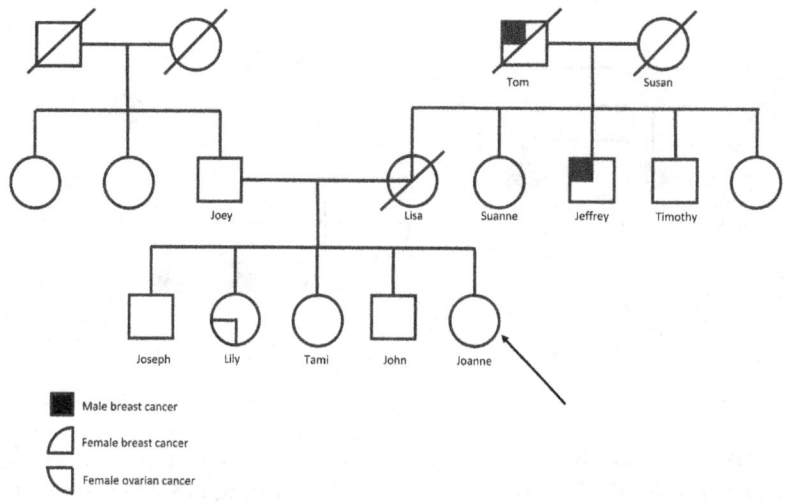

70. Joanne, a 43-year-old female, came to a genetics
clinic to find out her risk for malignancies. Her
medical history was unremarkable. The physical
examination was negative. However, her older
sister, Lily, was diagnosed with ovarian cancer at
the age of 53 (see the figure below for pedigree).
Her mother, Lisa, died of breast cancer at the age
of 68. Her maternal uncle, Jeffrey, had breast
cancer. Her maternal grandfather, Tom, had

breast cancer. Which one of the following genes
most like harbored a pathogenic variant in this
family?

A. *BRCA1*
B. *BRCA2*
C. *PTEN*
D. *TP53*
E. *VHL*

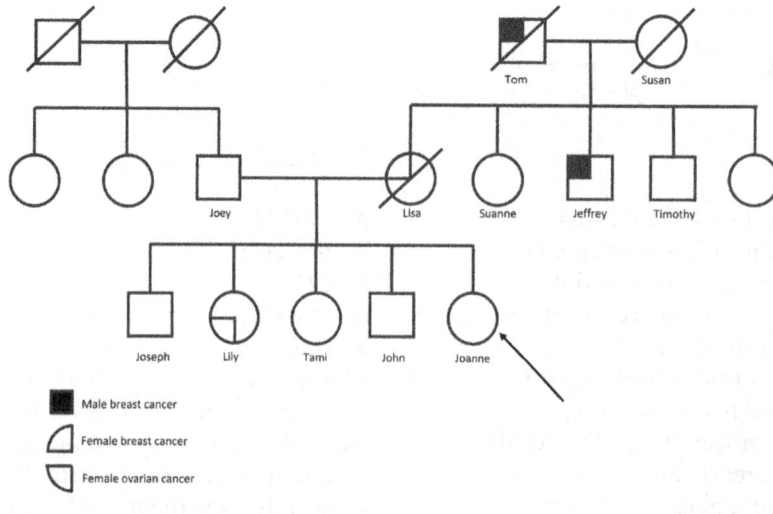

71. A 38-year-old Ashkenazi Jewish female was diagnosed with breast cancer 2 weeks ago. She was referred to a genetics clinic because her paternal grandmother had died from breast cancer at the age of 58 and an uncle from her father's side was diagnosed with prostate cancer at the age of 45. No other family members had been diagnosed with cancers. She was not married and was a secretary at a small company. Her insurance reimburses only 20% of the cost of genetic tests. She was willing to pay out of her own pocket for genetic tests. Which one of the following tests would be the most cost-effective first step in the workup to rule out genetic etiologies in this patient?

   A. Target mutation analysis of *BRCA1* and *BRCA2*
   B. Target mutation analysis of *BRCA1*
   C. Target mutation analysis of *BRCA2*
   D. Sequencing analysis of *BRCA1* and *BRCA2*
   E. Sequencing analysis of *BRCA1*
   F. Sequencing analysis of *BRCA2*

72. A 30-year-old Ashkenazi Jewish woman was diagnosed with multifocal breast cancer. A left breast core biopsy revealed a high-grade ductal carcinoma in situ. She was referred to a genetics clinic because of a positive family history. Her mother was diagnosed with breast cancer at the age of 41. Her maternal aunt was diagnosed with breast cancer at the age of 42 and ovarian cancer at the age of 62. Her maternal grandmother was diagnosed with ovarian cancer at the age of 58. Which one of the following mutations in the *BRCA1/2* genes would most likely be detected in this patient?

   A. c.68_69delAG in *BRCA1*
   B. c.68_69delAG in *BRCA2*
   C. c.999del5 in *BRCA1*
   D. c.999del5 in *BRCA2*
   E. All of the above
   F. None of the above

73. A 30-year-old Ashkenazi Jewish was diagnosed with multifocal breast cancer. A left breast core biopsy revealed a high-grade ductal carcinoma in situ. She was referred to a genetics clinic because of a positive family history. Her mother was diagnosed with breast cancer at the age of 41. Her maternal aunt was diagnosed with breast cancer at the age of 42 and ovarian cancer at the age of 62. Her maternal grandmother was diagnosed with ovarian cancer at the age of 58. Which one of the following mutations in the *BRCA1/2* genes would most likely be detected in this patient?

   A. c.5946delT in *BRCA1*
   B. c.5946delT in *BRCA2*
   C. A large deletion within *BRCA1* detected using Southern blot analysis
   D. A large deletion within *BRCA2* detected using Southern blot analysis
   E. All of the above
   F. None of the above

74. A 30-year-old Ashkenazi Jewish woman was diagnosed with multifocal breast cancer. A left breast core biopsy revealed a high-grade ductal carcinoma in situ. She was referred to a genetics clinic because of a positive family history. Her mother was diagnosed with breast cancer at the age of 41. Her maternal aunt was diagnosed with breast cancer at the age of 42 and ovarian cancer at the age of 62. Her maternal grandmother was diagnosed with ovarian cancer at the age of 58. Which one of the following mutations in the *BRCA1/2* genes would most likely be detected in this patient?

   A. c.5266dupC in *BRCA1*
   B. c.5266dupC in *BRCA2*
   C. c.5966del5 in *BRCA1*
   D. c.5966del5 in *BRCA2*
   E. All of the above
   F. None of the above

75. The prevalence of *BRCA1* and *BRCA2* deleterious mutations is higher in those of Ashkenazi Jewish descent than in those of Western European descent in the United States. Which one of the following genetic terms is most appropriate to describe this phenomenon?[2,3]

   A. Founder effect
   B. Genetic drift
   C. Genetic heterogeneity
   D. Incomplete penetrance
   E. Variable expression

76. As with other hereditary cancer predisposition syndromes, *BRCA1* and *BRCA2* hereditary breast and ovarian cancer is inherited in an autosomal dominant matter. Individuals carrying a pathogenic variant in *BRCA1* or *BRCA2* have an increased lifetime risk of developing breast cancer and ovarian cancer. But not everyone with a pathogenic variant in *BRCA1* or *BRCA2* will develop malignancies in her/his lifetime. Which one of the following genetic terms is most appropriate to describe this phenomenon?[2,3]

   A. Founder effect
   B. Genetic heterogeneity
   C. Heterozygous advantage
   D. Incomplete penetrance
   E. Variable expression

77. Which one of the following genetic alterations is *NOT* associated with increased risks for breast cancer?
    A. *BRCA1*
    B. *BRCA2*
    C. *PALB2*
    D. *PTEN*
    E. *STK11*
    F. *VHL*

78. A number of models have been developed to assess a woman's risk of having breast cancer, with varying degrees of validation. Which one of the following situations is suitable for the Gail model?[4,21]
    A. An individual with a personal history of breast cancer(s) and/or ovarian cancer(s)
    B. An individual with a family history of breast cancer(s) and/or ovarian cancer(s)
    C. An individual without a personal history of breast cancer(s) and limited information on family history
    D. An individual with personal and family histories of breast cancer(s) and/or ovarian cancer(s)
    E. An individual or family member(s) with a *BRCA1* or *BRCA 2* mutation
    F. None of the above

79. A number of models have been developed to assess a woman's risk of having breast cancer with varying degrees of validation. Which one of the following situations is suitable for the Claus model?[4]
    A. An individual with a personal history of breast cancer(s) and/or ovarian cancer(s)
    B. An individual with a family history of breast cancer(s) and/or ovarian cancer(s)
    C. An individual without a personal history of breast cancer(s) and limited information on family history
    D. An individual with personal and family histories of breast cancer(s) and/or ovarian cancer(s)
    E. An individual or family member(s) with a *BRCA1* or *BRCA2* mutation
    F. All of the above
    G. None of the above

80. A number of models have been developed to assess a woman's risk of having breast cancer with varying degrees of validation. Which one of the following situations is suitable for the BRCAPRO model?[4]

A. An individual with personal history of breast cancer(s) and/or ovarian cancer(s)
B. An individual with family history of breast cancer(s) and/or ovarian cancer(s)
C. An individual without personal history of breast cancer(s), and limited information on family history
D. An individual with personal and family history of breast cancer(s) and/or ovarian cancer(s)
E. All of the above
F. None of the above

81. A number of models have been developed to assess a woman's risk of having breast cancer, with varying degrees of validation. Which one of the following situations is suitable for the use of the Tyrer–Cuzick model?[4]
    A. An individual with personal history of breast cancer(s) and/or ovarian cancer(s)
    B. An individual with family history of breast cancer(s) and/or ovarian cancer(s)
    C. An individual without personal history of breast cancer(s), and limited information on family history
    D. An individual with personal and family history of breast cancer(s) and/or ovarian cancer(s)
    E. An individual or family member(s) with a *BRCA1* or *BRCA 2* mutation
    F. All of the above
    G. None of the above

82. A 28-year-old female was diagnosed with a bilateral breast cancer. Biopsy results showed that the tumor was estrogen-, progesterone-, and Her2/neu-negative. Which one of the following tests would be most appropriate for this patient to rule out genetic etiologies?
    A. Sequencing reflex to del/dup analysis of *BRCA1* and *BRCA2*
    B. Sequencing reflex to del/dup analysis of *PALB2*
    C. Sequencing reflex to del/dup analysis of *STK11*
    D. Sequencing reflex to del/dup analysis of *TP53*
    E. All of the above
    F. None of the above

83. A 3-year-old girl was referred to a genetics clinic for a personal history of adrenocortical carcinoma diagnosed at the age of 18 month and rhabdomyosarcoma diagnosed at age 2½. Her parents were apparently healthy. However, her

maternal grandfather was diagnosed with renal cell carcinoma at the age of 45 and died at the age of 60. Her great grandmother had osteosarcoma diagnosed at the age of 44. Which one of the following hereditary cancer predisposition syndromes would this patient most likely have, if she had one?
A. Hereditary diffuse gastric cancer
B. Li−Fraumeni syndrome
C. Lynch syndrome
D. *PTEN* hamartomatous syndrome
E. von Hippel−Lindau syndrome

84. A 3-year-old Ashkenazi Jewish girl was referred to a genetics clinic for a personal history of adrenocortical carcinoma diagnosed at the age 18 months and rhabdomyosarcoma diagnosed at the age of $2^{1}/_{2}$. Her parents were apparently healthy. However, her maternal grandfather was diagnosed with renal cell carcinoma at the age of 45 and died at the age of 60. Her great grandmother had osteosarcoma diagnosed at the age of 44. The physician suspected that the patient had Li−Fraumeni syndrome. Which one of the following assays would most likely be used for the genetic evaluation to confirm the diagnosis in this patient?
A. Chromosome breakage study
B. Chromosome karyotype
C. Chromosome microarray
D. Methylation study
E. Multicolor flow cytometry FISH (flow-FISH)
F. Sequencing
G. Targeted-mutation analysis
H. None of the above

85. A 3-year-old Ashkenazi Jewish girl was referred to a genetics clinic for a personal history of adrenocortical carcinoma diagnosed at the age 18 months and rhabdomyosarcoma diagnosed at the age of $2^{1}/_{2}$. Her parents were apparently healthy. However, her maternal grandfather was diagnosed with renal cell carcinoma at the age of 45 and died at the age of 60. Her great grandmother had osteosarcoma diagnosed at the age of 44. The physician suspected that the patient had one of the hereditary cancer predisposition syndromes. Which one of the following genes would most likely be tested to establish the diagnosis?
A. *CDH1*
B. *MLH1*
C. *SMAD4*
D. *PTEN*
E. *TP53*

86. A 28-year-old female was diagnosed with multifocal breast cancer. Biopsy results showed that the tumor was estrogen-, progesterone-, and Her2/neu-positive. A mastectomy was performed. Her medical history revealed that she had had another surgery to remove rhabdomyosarcomas when she was 5 years old. Which one of the following tests would be most appropriate for this patient to rule out genetic etiologies?
A. Sequencing reflex to del/dup analysis of *BRCA1* and *BRCA2*
B. Sequencing reflex to del/dup analysis of *PALB2*
C. Sequencing reflex to del/dup analysis of *STK11*
D. Sequencing reflex to del/dup analysis of *TP53*
E. All of the above
F. None of the above

87. A 3-year-old girl was diagnosed with rhabdomyosarcoma. Her past medical and family histories were unremarkable. Which one of the following tests would be most appropriate for this patient to rule out genetic etiologies?
A. Sequencing reflex to del/dup analysis of *RB1*
B. Sequencing reflex to del/dup analysis of *VHL*
C. Sequencing reflex to del/dup analysis of *WT1*
D. Sequencing reflex to del/dup analysis of *TP53*
E. All of the above
F. None of the above

88. An 8-year-old boy was diagnosed with adrenocortical carcinomas (ACC). His past medical and family histories were unremarkable. Which one of the following genetic tests would be most appropriate for this patient to rule out genetic etiologies?
A. Sequencing reflex to del/dup analysis of *RB1*
B. Sequencing reflex to del/dup analysis of *VHL*
C. Sequencing reflex to del/dup analysis of *WT1*
D. Sequencing reflex to del/dup analysis of *TP53*
E. All of the above
F. None of the above

89. A 3-year-old girl was diagnosed with choroid plexus tumor. Her past medical and family histories were unremarkable. Which one of the following genetic tests would be most appropriate for this patient to rule out genetic etiologies?
A. Sequencing reflex to del/dup analysis of *RB1*
B. Sequencing reflex to del/dup analysis of *VHL*
C. Sequencing reflex to del/dup analysis of *WT1*
D. Sequencing reflex to del/dup analysis of *TP53*
E. All of the above
F. None of the above

90. Joanne, a 43-year-old female came to a genetics clinic because she was recently diagnosed with breast cancer. Her family history was significant for adrenocortical carcinoma, breast cancer, and osteosarcoma (see the pedigree below). Lily, her older sister, was diagnosed with adrenocortical carcinoma at the age of 42. Lisa, her mother, was diagnosed with breast cancer at the age of 52. Her maternal grandfather, Tom, died from osteosarcoma at the age of 56. Which one of the following genetic conditions would most likely be consistent with the clinical presentations in this family?

A. Cowden syndrome
B. Hereditary breast and ovarian cancer
C. Li–Fraumeni syndrome
D. Multiple endocrine neoplasia type 1 (MEN1)
E. Multiple endocrine neoplasia type 2 (MEN2)
F. von Hippel–Lindau

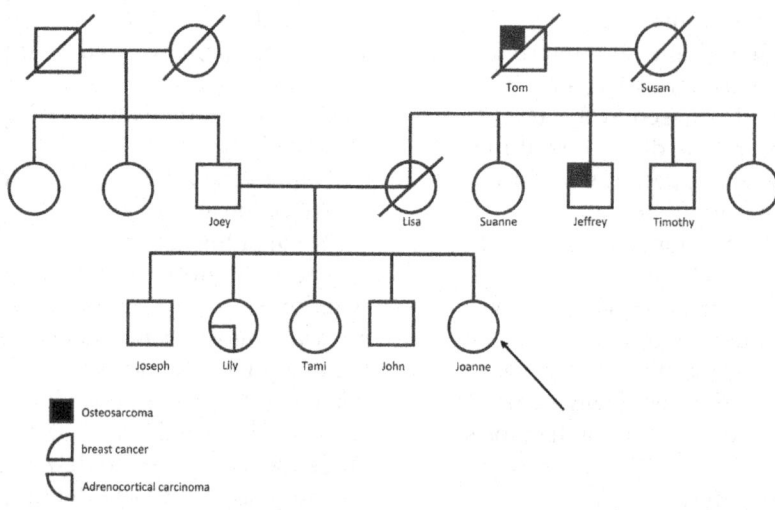

91. Joanne, a 36-year-old female came to a genetics clinic because she was recently diagnosed with breast cancer. Her family history was significant for adrenocortical carcinoma, breast cancer, and osteosarcoma (see the pedigree below). Lily, her older sister, was diagnosed with adrenocortical carcinoma at the age of 42. Lisa, her mother, was diagnosed with breast cancer at the age of 52. Her maternal grandfather, Tom, died from osteosarcoma at the age of 56. Which one of the following genes should be analyzed first to confirm/rule out genetic etiologies in this family?

A. *BRCA1*
B. *BRCA2*
C. *PTEN*
D. *TP53*
E. *VHL*

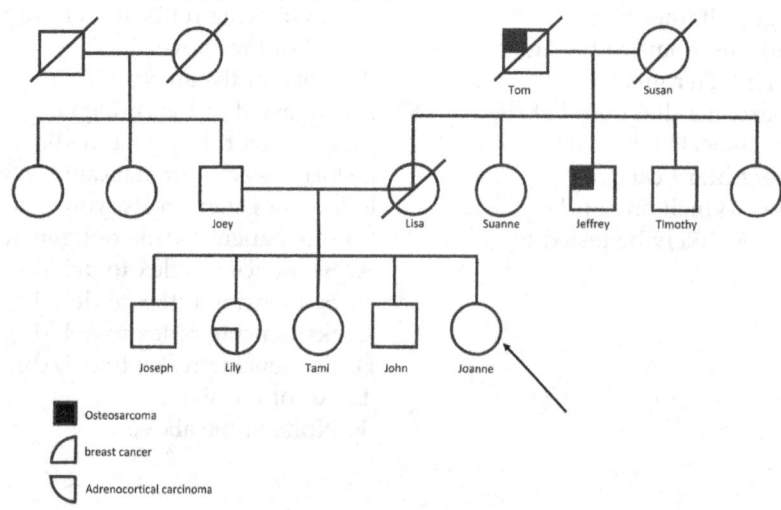

92. A 15-year-old male was diagnosed with pheochromocytoma. The physical examination was negative. His medical history was remarkable because he had had a surgery to remove the left kidney for multiple focal clear-cell renal-cell carcinomas at age 10. The family history was unremarkable. Which one of the following genetic tests would be most appropriate for this patient to rule out genetic etiologies?

A. Sequencing reflex to del/dup analysis of *RET*
B. Sequencing reflex to del/dup analysis of *SDHB*
C. Sequencing reflex to del/dup analysis of *SDHD*
D. Sequencing reflex to del/dup analysis of *VHL*
E. None of the above

93. A 17-year-old male was diagnosed with multifocal pheochromocytoma. The medical and family history was unremarkable. Which one of the following genetic tests would *NOT* be appropriate for this patient to rule out genetic etiologies?

A. Sequencing reflex to del/dup analysis of *RET*
B. Sequencing reflex to del/dup analysis of *SDHB*
C. Sequencing reflex to del/dup analysis of *SDHD*
D. Sequencing reflex to del/dup analysis of *TP53*
E. Sequencing reflex to del/dup analysis of *VHL*

94. Joanne, a 36-year-old female, came to a genetics clinic because she was recently diagnosed with clear-cell renal-cell carcinoma. Her family history was significant for cerebellar hemangioblastomas, renal-cell carcinoma, and pheochromocytoma. Lily, her older sister, was diagnosed with pheochromocytoma at the age of 43. Lisa, her mother, was diagnosed with renal-cell carcinoma at the age of 46. Her maternal grandfather, Tom, died from cerebellar hemangioblastomas at the age of 56. Which one of the following genetic conditions would most likely be consistent with the clinical presentations in this family?

A. Cowden syndrome
B. Hereditary breast and ovarian cancer
C. Li–Fraumeni syndrome
D. Multiple endocrine neoplasia type 1 (MEN1)
E. Multiple endocrine neoplasia type 2 (MEN2)
F. von Hippel–Lindau

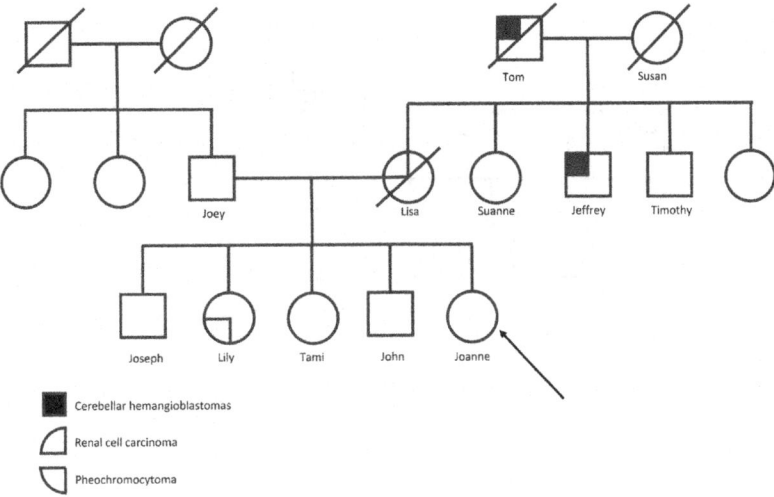

95. A 20-year-old female came to an emergency department with symptoms of paroxysmal attacks of palpitation, dizziness, blurring of vision, and headache for the past 6 months. The attacks were irregular and occurred once within 2–3 days to two to three times a day. Each attack persisted for few minutes to half an hour. Physical examination was unremarkable except for high blood pressure during a paroxysmal attack (systolic, 140–210 mmHg; diastolic, 100–140 mmHg). The physician suspected that the patient had secondary hypertension due to adrenal pheochromocytoma. After consulting a medical geneticist, the physician ordered a next-generation sequencing (NGS) panel for pheochromocytoma. Which one of the following genes would *NOT* be expected in the NGS panel for this patient?

A. NF1
B. RET
C. SDHD
D. TP53
E. VHL
F. None of the above

96. Joanne, a 36-year-old female came to a genetics clinic because she was recently diagnosed with clear-cell renal-cell carcinoma. Her family history was significant for cerebellar hemangioblastomas, renal-cell carcinoma, and pheochromocytoma (see the pedigree below). Lily, her older sister, was diagnosed with pheochromocytoma at the age of 43. Lisa, her mother, was diagnosed with renal-cell carcinoma at the age of 46. Her maternal grandfather, Tom, died from cerebellar hemangioblastomas at the age of 56. Which one of the following genes should be analyzed first to confirm/rule out genetic etiologies in this family?

A. BRCA1
B. BRCA2
C. PTEN
D. TP53
E. VHL

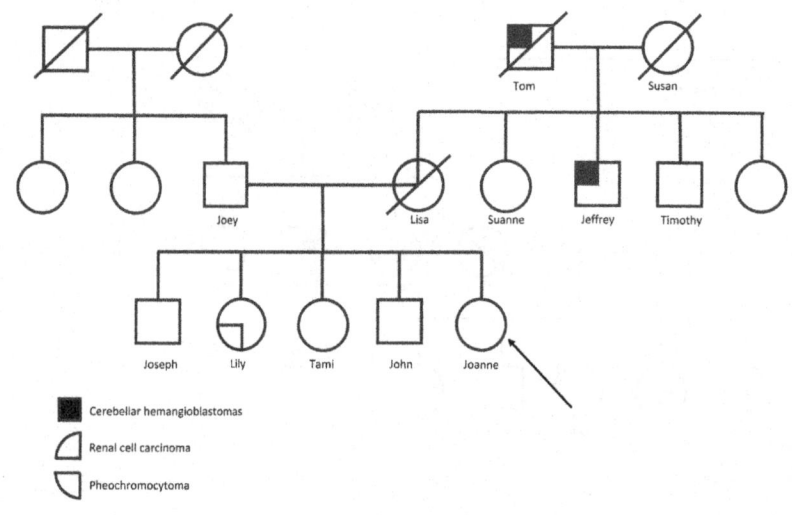

97. Joanne, a 38-year-old female came to a genetics clinic because she was recently diagnosed with breast cancer. Her family history was significant for thyroid cancer, breast cancer, and endometrial carcinoma (see the pedigree below). Lily, her older sister, was diagnosed with endometrial carcinoma at the age of 48. Lisa, her mother, was diagnosed with breast cancer at the age of 52. Her maternal grandfather, Tom, died from thyroid cancer at the age of 52. Which one of the following genetic conditions would most likely be consistent with the clinical presentations in this family?

A. Cowden syndrome
B. Hereditary breast and ovarian cancer
C. Li–Fraumeni syndrome
D. Multiple endocrine neoplasia type 1 (MEN1)
E. Multiple endocrine neoplasia type 2 (MEN2)
F. von Hippel–Lindau disease

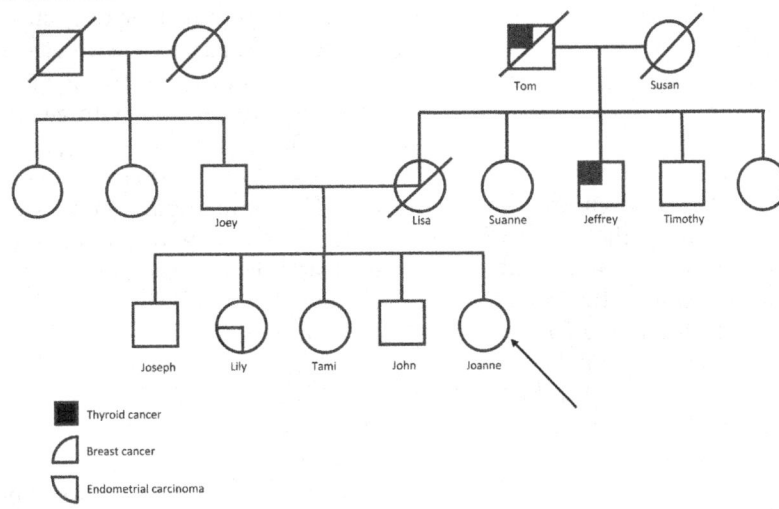

98. Joanne, a 38-year-old female, came to a genetics clinic because she was recently diagnosed with breast cancer. Her family history was significant for thyroid cancer, breast cancer, and endometrial carcinoma (see the pedigree below). Lily, her older sister, was diagnosed with endometrial carcinoma at the age of 48. Lisa, her mother, was diagnosed with breast cancer at the age of 52. Her maternal grandfather died from thyroid cancer at the age of 52. Which one of the following genes should be analyzed first to rule out genetic etiologies in this family?

A. *BRCA1*
B. *BRCA2*
C. *PTEN*
D. *TP53*
E. *VHL*

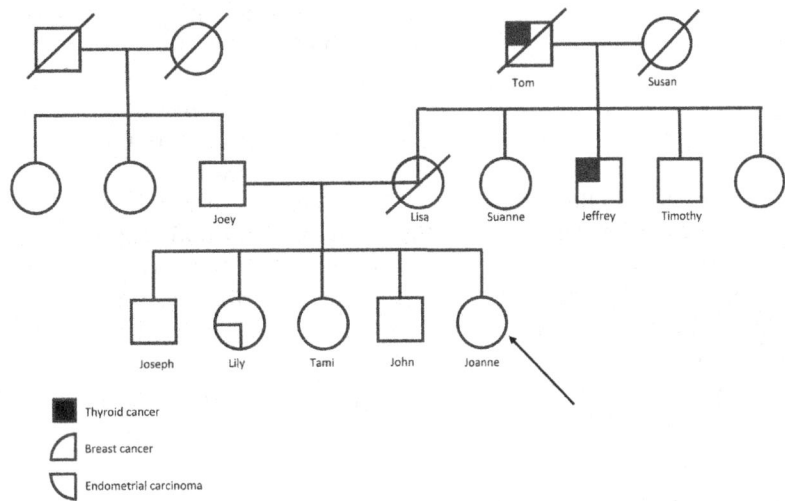

99. A 48-year-old female presented to a genetics clinic for a personal history of two synchronous primary breast cancers diagnosed at the age of 47 and a family history of thyroid cancer and renal-cell carcinoma on the maternal side of the family. A pathogenic variant was detected in the *PTEN* gene, which was known to cause the *PTEN* hamartoma tumor syndrome (PHTS). Which one of thyroid cancers would most likely the members of this family have?
  A. Anaplastic thyroid cancer
  B. Follicular thyroid cancer
  C. Medullary thyroid cancer
  D. Papillary thyroid cancer
  E. None of the above

100. A 48-year-old female presented to a genetics clinic for a personal history of two synchronous primary breast cancers diagnosed at the age of 47 and a family history of thyroid cancer and renal-cell carcinoma on the maternal side of the family. A pathogenic variant was detected in the *PTEN* gene, which was known to cause the *PTEN* hamartomatous tumor syndrome (PHTS). Which one of thyroid cancers would most likely the members of this family *NOT* have?
  A. Anaplastic thyroid cancer
  B. Follicular thyroid cancer
  C. Medullary thyroid cancer
  D. Papillary thyroid cancer
  E. None of the above

101. A molecular geneticist teaches a course for genetic counseling students. The current presentation is on hereditary cancer predisposition syndromes. One of the students asks which malignancy is the most common in individuals with Cowden syndrome. Which one of the following would be your answer for this question?
  A. Breast cancers
  B. Colorectal cancers
  C. Endometrial cancers
  D. Kidney tumors
  E. Melanomas
  F. Thyroid cancers

102. A 38-year-old male came to a genetics clinic for a positive family history of gastric cancer. His father was diagnosed with gastric cancer at the age of 39 and died at the age of 56. His paternal uncle was diagnosed with gastric cancer at the age of 36 and died at the age of 48. His brother had undergone a gastrectomy 2 years ago.

The familial pathogenic variant had not been tested. Which one of the following genetic conditions would be consistent with the clinical presentations in this family?
  A. Cowden syndrome
  B. Hereditary diffuse gastric cancer
  C. Li—Fraumeni syndrome
  D. Multiple endocrine neoplasia type 1 (MEN1)
  E. Multiple endocrine neoplasia type 2 (MEN2)
  F. von Hippel—Lindau

103. A 38-year-old male came to a genetics clinic for a positive family history of gastric cancer. His father was diagnosed with gastric cancer at the age of 39 and died at the age of 56. His paternal uncle was diagnosed with gastric cancer at the age of 36 and died at the age of 48. His brother had undergone a proactive gastrectomy 2 years ago. The familial pathogenic variant had not been tested. Which one of the following genes should be tested first to rule out genetic etiologies in this family?[5]
  A. *CDH1*
  B. *MLH1*
  C. *SMAD4*
  D. *PTEN*
  E. *TP53*

104. A 38-year-old male came to a genetics clinic for a positive family history of gastric cancer. His father was diagnosed with gastric cancer at the age of 39 and died at the age of 56. His paternal uncle was diagnosed with gastric cancer at the age of 36 and died at the age of 48. His brother had undergone a proactive gastrectomy 2 years ago. The familial pathogenic variant had not been tested. The medical geneticist ordered a sequencing test on the *CDH1* gene for this patient, and a pathogenic variant in exon 3 of the gene was detected. Which one of the following malignancies would this patient have an increased risk of developing besides a gastric cancer?[6]
  A. Breast cancer
  B. Colorectal cancer
  C. Endometrial carcinoma
  D. Osteosarcoma
  E. Renal-cell carcinoma

105. A 38-year-old male came to a genetics clinic for a positive family history of gastric cancer. His father was diagnosed with gastric cancer at the age of 39 and died at the age of 56. His paternal uncle was diagnosed with gastric cancer at the age of 36 and died at the age of 48. His brother had undergone a proactive gastrectomy 2 years ago. The familial pathogenic variant had not been tested. Which one of the following populations has higher risk of developing diffuse gastric cancer if they carry a pathogenic variant in the *CDH1* gene?

A. Male

B. Female

C. Equal in male and female

D. Unknown

106. A 32-year-old female came to a clinic for an elective gastrectomy because she had a familial *CDH1* mutation, c.2398delC, inherited from her mother. Her mother died of gastric cancer at the age of 42. Her 36-year-old brother had the familial pathogenic variant in *CDH1*, too, and he had an elective gastrectomy at the age of 35. Which one of the following malignancies, in addition to gastric cancer, would the patient also have an increased risk of developing in her lifetime?

A. Cervical cancer

B. Colon cancer

C. Lobular breast cancer

D. Ovarian cancer

E. All of the above

F. None of the above

107. A 32-year-old female came to a clinic for an elective gastrectomy because she had a familial *CDH1* mutation, c.2398delC, inherited from her

mother. Her mother died of gastric cancer at the age of 42. Her 36-year-old brother had the familial pathogenic variant in *CDH1*, too, and he had an elective gastrectomy at the age of 35. What would be the patient's lifetime risk of developing diffused gastric cancer if she did not undergo elective gastrectomy?

A. 20%

B. 40%

C. 60%

D. 80%

E. >99%

108. Joseph, an 8-year-old boy, was brought to a clinic for fatigue and multiple infections, including two pneumonias in 1 month. The physical examination revealed that his height was less than 2.5 SD below the mean. He had two café au lait spots and malformation of his left thumb. A CBC showed pancytopenia. Chromosome breakage studies were ordered, and the results were positive. Then a Fanconi anemia next-generation sequencing (NGS) panel was ordered. The result showed that the patient had a pathogenic mutation in the *FANCB* gene. Which one of the following individuals should also be tested for the risk of Fanconi anemia in this family (see the pedigree below)?

A. Joanne

B. John

C. Lily

D. Tami

E. All of the above

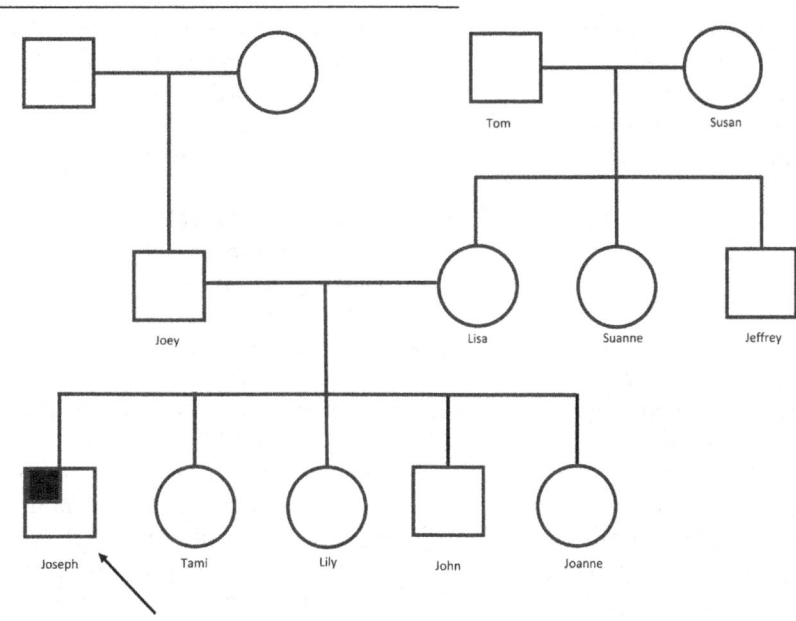

109. An 8-year-old boy was brought to a clinic for fatigue and multiple infections, including two pneumonias in 1 month. The physical examination revealed that his height was less than 2.5 SD below the mean, and he had two café au lait spots and malformation of his left thumb. A CBC showed pancytopenia. Chromosome breakage studies were ordered, and the results were positive. Then a Fanconi anemia next-generation sequencing (NGS) panel was ordered, and the result was positive, too. The parents were tested for carrier status. After receiving the parental results, the medical geneticist and the genetic counselor counseled the mother for the increased risk for breast cancer and ovarian cancer. Which one of the following genes is most likely to be mutated in the mother than the others?

- **A.** *FANCA*
- **B.** *FANCB*
- **C.** *FANCC*
- **D.** *FANCD1*
- **E.** *FACND2*

110. A 7-year-old girl was brought to a clinic for fatigue and multiple infections, including two pneumonias in 1 month. The physical examination revealed that her height was less than 2.5 SD below the mean, and she had two café au lait spots and malformation of her left thumb. A CBC showed leukopenia. Chromosome breakage studies were ordered, and the results were positive. Then a Fanconi anemia next-generation sequencing (NGS) panel was ordered, and the result was positive, too. The parents were tested for carrier status. After receiving the parental results, the medical geneticist and the genetic counselor counseled the mother for the increased risk for breast cancer. Which one of the following genes would most likely be mutated in the mother?

- **A.** *FANCF*
- **B.** *FANCI*
- **C.** *FANCL*
- **D.** *FANCN*
- **E.** None of the above

111. A 6-year-old boy was brought to a clinic for fatigue and multiple infections, including two pneumonias in 1 month. The physical examination revealed that his height was less than 2.5 SD below the mean, and he had two café au lait spots and a hypoplastic left thumb. A CBC showed pancytopenia. Chromosome breakage studies were ordered, and the results were positive. Then a Fanconi anemia next-generation sequencing (NGS) panel was ordered, and the

result was positive, too. The parents were tested for carrier status. After receiving the parental results, the medical geneticist and the genetic counselor counseled the mother for the increased risk for breast and ovarian cancer. Which one of the following genes would most likely be mutated in the mother?

- **A.** *FANCE*
- **B.** *FANCG*
- **C.** *FANCI*
- **D.** *FANCJ*
- **E.** *FANCL*

112. A 7-year-old Ashkenazi Jewish girl is brought to a genetics clinic for fatigue and multiple infections, including two pneumonias in 1 month. The physical examination reveals that her height is less than 2.5 SD below the mean, and she has two café au lait spots and absence of the left thumb. A CBC shows pancytopenia. Chromosome breakage studies are positive. A Fanconi anemia next-generation sequencing (NGS) panel is ordered. Which one of the following genes is most likely mutated in this girl?

- **A.** *FANCA*
- **B.** *FANCB*
- **C.** *FANCC*
- **D.** *FANCG*
- **E.** *FANCN*

113. A 23-year-old Ashkenazi Jewish male was diagnosed with acute myeloid leukemia (AML) 1 week ago. The physical examination revealed that he had two café au lait spots and absence of the left thumb. Chromosome breakage studies confirmed the diagnosis of Fanconi anemia. A hematopoietic stem-cell transplantation (HSCT) was administrated. For which one of the following conditions would the patient still be at high risk even after HSCT?

- **A.** Bone-marrow failure
- **B.** Relapse
- **C.** Secondary myelodysplastic syndrome (MDS)
- **D.** Solid tumor
- **E.** All of the above
- **F.** None of the above

114. A 16-year-old boy was brought to a clinic for fatigue and being prone to infections. The physical examination revealed that his height was 2.5 SD below the mean. He had three café au lait spots and a hypoplastic right thumb. A CBC showed pancytopenia. The family history was negative. The father was 6 ft. 2 in., and the mother was 5 ft. 8 in. Chromosome breakage studies were ordered. The results with a peripheral-blood sample were inconclusive. Which one of the following tests would be most appropriate to establish diagnosis if mosaicism was suspected in this patient?

A. Chromosome breakage study with fibroblast cells

B. Complementary study

C. Diagnose the patient clinically without further tests

D. Fanconi anemia next-generation sequencing panel

E. None of the above

115. A 16-year-old man with hearing loss came to a clinic for fatigue and being prone to infections. A CBC showed pancytopenia. He was diagnosed with bone-marrow failure. Chromosome breakage studies confirmed that the patient had Fanconi anemia. Androgen was administrated. The genetic counselor mentioned the increase risk of one disease because of the androgen therapy. For which one of the following disorders would this patient be at increased because of the androgen therapy?

A. Infertility

B. Liver tumors

C. MDS/AML

D. Relapse

E. All of the above

F. None of the above

116. An Ashkenazi Jewish couple came to a clinic for preconception counseling. The past medical histories on both sides were unremarkable. The husband's mother died of bone-marrow failure due to Fanconi anemia (FA). The wife's family history was uneventful. The physical examination was negative. What would be their first child's risk for FA?

A. 1/4

B. 1/8

C. 1/200

D. 1/400

E. 1/800

117. A 2-year-old Ashkenazi Jewish boy was brought to a clinic for genetic counseling. The physical examination revealed three café au lait spots on his back. His medical history was unremarkable. The family history was significant for the mother's uncle dying of esophageal squamous-cell carcinoma. The mother remembered that her uncle's left thumb looked "funny" and "maybe shorter." The physician offered a genetic test for the boy to rule out Fanconi anemia (FA). Which one of the following tests would the physician most likely have ordered for this patient?

A. Chromosome breakage study of the peripheral-blood sample

B. Complementary study

C. Next-generation sequencing of all 15 FA genes

D. Target mutation analysis of the *FANCC* gene

E. Target mutation analysis of the *FANCA*, *FANCC*, and *FANCD1* genes

F. None of the above

118. A 6-year-old girl was brought to a clinic for fatigue and multiple infections, including two pneumonias in 1 month. The physical examination revealed that her height was less than 2.5 SD below the mean. She had two café au lait spots and a hypoplastic right thumb. A CBC showed pancytopenia. Chromosome breakage studies were positive. A Fanconi anemia next-generation sequencing (NGS) panel was ordered, and the result was positive, too. Which one of the following sequence changes would most likely be the pathogenic variant detected in this patient?

A. p.S849Ffs*40 in *FANCA*

B. c.710-12A > G in *FANCA*

C. p.L717G in *FANCB*

D. p.F713F in *FANCB*

E. c.-490G > T in *FANCG*

F. Not sure

119. A 6-year-old boy was brought to a clinic by his mother for fatigue and multiple infections, including two pneumonias in 1 month. The physical examination revealed that his height was less than 2.5 SD below the mean. He had two café au lait spots and a hypoplastic left thumb. A CBC showed pancytopenia. His father had been in the same hospital for bone-marrow failure. Chromosome breakage studies were ordered, and the results were positive. Then a Fanconi anemia next-generation sequencing (NGS) panel detected a pathogenic variant in the *FANCB* gene. The mother had been pregnant for 6 weeks (calculated from the first day of her last period), and she asked about the risk of the fetus having the same condition. What would be the unborn child's risk for Fanconi anemia?

A. 1/2

B. 1/4

C. 1/8

D. 1/200

E. 1/400

F. 1/800

120. A 12-year-old girl was referred to a genetics clinic by her pediatrician for progressive neck swelling and fever for 1 month and unsteady gait and

seizures for 2 years. She presented to the clinic in a wheelchair. Her medical history was significant for recurrent respiratory tract infection. Her unsteady gait had increased progressively, leading her to be wheelchair-bound. These symptoms were associated with difficulty in swallowing and speech. The family history was remarkable because her youngest brother and maternal uncle had a similar illness. Her maternal uncle had seizures and was wheelchair-bound at the age of 12 and died at the age of 35 from respiratory tract infection. Her paternal grandfather died of myocardial infarction at the age of 45. She also had a healthy brother. The parents were second-degree relatives. The physical examination revealed that the girl was small for her age and had gray hairs. She had telangiectasia over the bulbar conjunctivae. Her cervical and axillary lymph nodes were enlarged bilaterally. Pes cavus was noted. Features of cerebellar dysfunction such as cerebellar ataxia, dyssynergia, dysarthria, and intentional tremors were present. Deep tendon reflexes were diminished, and plantar responses were flexor. Which one of the following disorders would this patient most likely have if she had a genetic condition?[7]

A. Ataxia telangiectasia
B. Bloom syndrome
C. Fanconi anemia
D. Nijmegen breakage syndrome
E. All of the above
F. None of the above

121. A 12-year-old girl was referred to a genetics clinic by her pediatrician for progressive neck swelling and fever for 1 month and unsteady gait and seizures for 2 years. She presented to the clinic in a wheelchair. Her medical history was significant for recurrent respiratory tract infection. Her unsteady gait had increased progressively, leading her to be wheelchair-bound. These symptoms were associated with difficulty in swallowing and speech. The family history was remarkable because her youngest brother and maternal uncle had a similar illness. Her maternal uncle had seizures and was wheelchair-bound at the age of 12 and died at the age of 35 from respiratory tract infection. Her paternal grandfather died of myocardial infarction at the age of 45. She also had a healthy brother. The parents were second-degree relatives. The physical examination revealed that the girl was small for her age, with gray hairs. She had telangiectasia over the bulbar conjunctivae. Her cervical and axillary lymph nodes were enlarged

bilaterally. Pes cavus was noted. Features of cerebellar dysfunction such as cerebellar ataxia, dyssynergia, dysarthria, and intentional tremors were present. Deep tendon reflexes were diminished, and plantar responses were flexor. The medical geneticist suspected that the patient had ataxia telangiectasia. Which one of the following genes would most likely be mutated in this girl?[7]

A. *ATM*
B. *BLM*
C. *BRIP1*
D. *NBN*
E. None of the above

122. A 6-year-old boy was brought to a clinic for progressive gait and truncal ataxia starting at 2 years old, progressively slurred speech, and oculocutaneous telangiectasia. Immunoblotting for ATM protein was positive. A clinical diagnosis of ataxia telangiectasia was made. The *ATM* gene was sequenced and showed compound heterozygous mutations in the gene. Parental tests confirmed that one was from the father and one from the mother. Which one of the following diseases would the mother have an increased risk of developing in her lifetime?

A. Breast cancer
B. Cervical cancer
C. Endometrial carcinoma
D. Insulin-resistant diabetes mellitus
E. Leukemia/lymphoma

123. A 6-year-old boy was brought to a clinic for progressive gait and truncal ataxia starting at 2 years old, progressively slurred speech, and oculocutaneous telangiectasia. Immunoblotting for ATM protein was positive. A clinical diagnosis of ataxia telangiectasia was made. The mother had been pregnant for 6 weeks (calculated from the first day of her last period), and she asked about the risk of the fetus having the same condition. What would be the unborn child's risk for ataxia telangiectasia?

A. 1/2
B. 1/4
C. 1/8
D. 1/12
E. 1/16

124. A 10-year-old girl was referred to a genetics clinic for short stature. She was the second child of a marriage between first cousins. She had a slender body build, short stature, and microcephaly. Her face was long and narrow with a prominent nose. There was sun-sensitive erythema affecting the butterfly area of the face. Spots of hyperpigmentation and hypopigmentation were

observed on the trunk and limbs. Telangiectatic spots were observed in some areas of the trunk. Additionally, generalized hirsutism was present in the whole body. Her bone age was 2 years deficient of her chronological age. The medical geneticist suspected that the patient had Bloom syndrome. Which one of the following assays would most likely be used to diagnose Bloom syndrome in this patient?

A. Chromosome breakage study
B. Chromosome karyotype
C. Methylation study
D. Multiplex ligation-dependent probe amplification (MLPA)
E. Sister chromatid exchanges
F. None of the above

125. A 10-year-old girl was referred to a genetics clinic for short stature. She was the second child of a marriage between first cousins. She had a slender body build, short stature, and microcephaly. Her face was long and narrow with a prominent nose. There was sun-sensitive erythema affecting the butterfly area of the face. Spots of hyperpigmentation and hypopigmentation were observed on the trunk and limbs. Telangiectatic spots were observed in some areas of the limbs. Additionally, generalized hirsutism was present in the whole body. Her bone age was 2 years deficient of her chronological age. Her family history was unremarkable. Chromosome studies revealed increased sister chromatid exchange. Which one of the following disorders would this patient most likely have?

A. Ataxia telangiectasia
B. Bloom syndrome
C. Fanconi anemia
D. Nijmegen breakage syndrome
E. All of the above
F. None of the above

126. A 10-year-old girl was referred to a genetics clinic for short stature. She was the second child of a marriage between first cousins. She had a slender body build, short stature, and microcephaly. Her face was long and narrow with a prominent nose. There was sun-sensitive erythema affecting the butterfly area of the face. Spots of hyperpigmentation and hypopigmentation were observed on the trunk and limbs. Telangiectatic spots were observed in some areas of the limbs. Additionally, generalized hirsutism was present in the whole body. Her bone age was 2 years deficient of her chronological age. Her family

history was unremarkable. The medical geneticist suspected that the patient had Bloom syndrome. Chromosome studies revealed increased sister chromatid exchange. Which one of the following genes would most likely be mutated in this girl?

A. ATM
B. BLM
C. BRIP1
D. NBN
E. None of the above

127. A 10-year-old girl was referred to a genetics clinic for short stature. She was the second child of a marriage between first cousins. She had a slender body build, short stature, and microcephaly. Her face was long and narrow with a prominent nose. There was sun-sensitive erythema affecting the butterfly area of the face. Spots of hyperpigmentation and hypopigmentation were observed on the trunk and limbs. Telangiectatic spots were observed on some areas of the limbs. Additionally, generalized hirsutism was present in the whole body. Her bone age was 2 years deficient of her chronological age. Her family history was unremarkable. Chromosome studies revealed increased sister chromatid exchange. The mother had been pregnant for 6 weeks (calculated from the first day of her last period), and asked about the risk of the fetus having the same condition. What would be the unborn child's risk of having ataxia telangiectasia?

A. 1/2
B. 1/4
C. 1/8
D. 1/12
E. 1/16

128. A 10-year-old Ashkenazi Jewish girl was referred to a genetics clinic for short stature. She was the second child of a nonconsanguineous marriage after normal delivery. She had a slender body build, short stature, and microcephaly. Her face was long and narrow with a prominent nose. There was sun-sensitive erythema affecting the butterfly area of the face. The spots of hyperpigmentation and hypopigmentation were observed on the trunk and limbs. Telangiectatic spots were observed on some areas of the limbs. Additionally, generalized hirsutism was present in the whole body. Her bone age was 2 years deficient of her chronological age. Her family history was unremarkable. The medical geneticist suspected that the patient had Bloom syndrome. Which one of the following assays would be the

most cost-effective initial genetic workups to confirm the diagnosis in this patient?

A. Chromosome breakage study
B. Chromosome karyotype
C. Methylation study
D. Multiplex ligation-dependent probe amplification (MLPA)
E. Sequencing analysis
F. Targeted-mutation analysis
G. None of the above

129. An Ashkenazi Jewish couple came to a clinic for preconception counseling. The past medical histories on both sides were unremarkable. The physical examination was negative. The wife's maternal grandmother died of pulmonary failure due to Bloom syndrome. The family history of the father's side was negative. What would be their first child's risk for Bloom syndrome?

A. 1/8
B. 1/200
C. 1/400
D. 1/800
E. 1/1000

130. Bloom syndrome is an inherited disorder characterized by short stature, a skin rash that develops after exposure to the sun, and a greatly increased risk of cancer. It occurs rarely in all national and ethnic groups but is relatively less rare in Ashkenazi Jews. Which one of the following pathogenic variants in the *BLM* gene is referred as blm^{Ash} because it appears in 1/100 of the Ashkenazi Jewish population?

A. 657_661del5
B. c.1089C > A
C. c.2407dupT
D. c.2207_2212delinsTAGATTC
E. All of the above
F. None of the above

131. A 6-year-old Ashkenazi Jewish girl was brought to a genetics clinic for short status, developmental delay, and intellectual disability. She was born to nonconsanguineous parents after a normal delivery with a good Apgar score and low birth weight. She appeared normal at birth but started to lose weight by 3 months of age. She was able to sit by 3 years and still cannot walk. Her family history was unremarkable. The physical examination revealed that her height was 70.5 cm and her weight 4.94 kg, far below the 5th percentile in each category. She had severe global delay, bilateral cataracts, and severe sensorineural hearing loss. A CT scan revealed bilateral basal ganglia calcification and diffuse cerebral and cerebellar atrophy with mild ventricular dilatation. The medical geneticist suspected that

the patient had Cockayne syndrome and ordered a genetic test to confirm the diagnosis. Which one of the following assays would the medical geneticist most likely have ordered to confirm the diagnosis in this patient?

A. Chromosome breakage study
B. Chromosome karyotype
C. Methylation study
D. Multiplex ligation-dependent probe amplification (MLPA)
E. Sequencing analysis
F. Targeted-mutation analysis
G. None of the above

132. A 6-year-old girl was brought to a genetics clinic for short status, developmental delay, and intellectual disability. She was born to nonconsanguineous parents after a normal delivery with a good Apgar score and low birth weight. She appeared normal at birth but started to lose weight by 3 months of age. She was able to sit by 3 years and still cannot walk. Her family history was unremarkable. The physical examination revealed her height was 70.5 cm and weight 4.94 kg, far below the 5th percentile in each category. She had severe global delay, bilateral cataracts, and severe sensorineural deafness. A CT scan revealed bilateral basal ganglia calcification and diffuse cerebral and cerebellar atrophy with mild ventricular dilatation. The medical geneticist suspected that the patient had Cockayne syndrome and ordered a genetic test to confirm the diagnosis. Which one of the following genes would most likely be included in the molecular genetic test to confirm the diagnosis in this patient?

A. *ERCC3*
B. *ERCC4*
C. *ERCC5*
D. *ERCC6*
E. All of the above
F. None of the above

133. A 6-year-old girl was brought to a genetics clinic for short status, developmental delay, and intellectual disability. She was born to nonconsanguineous parents after a normal delivery with a good Apgar score and low birth weight. She appeared normal at birth but started to lose weight by 3 months of age. She was able to sit by 3 years and still cannot walk. Her family history was unremarkable. The physical examination revealed that her height was 70.5 cm and her weight 4.94 kg, far below the 5th percentile in each category. She had severe global delay, bilateral cataracts, and severe sensorineural deafness. A CT scan revealed bilateral basal

ganglia calcification, diffuse cerebral and cerebellar atrophy with mild ventricular dilatation. The medical geneticist suspected that the patient had Cockayne syndrome and ordered a genetic test to confirm the diagnosis. Which one of the following genes would most likely be included in the molecular genetic test to confirm the diagnosis in this patient?[8]

A. *ERCC1*
B. *ERCC2*
C. *ERCC7*
D. *ERCC8*
E. All of the above
F. None of the above

134. A 6-year-old girl was brought to a genetics clinic for short status, developmental delay, and intellectual disability. She was born to nonconsanguineous parents after a normal delivery with a good Apgar score and low birth weight. She appeared normal at birth but started to lose weight by 3 months of age. She was able to sit by 3 years and still cannot walk. Her family history was unremarkable. The physical examination revealed that her height was 70.5 cm and weight 4.94 kg, far below the 5th percentile in each category. She had severe global delay, bilateral cataracts, and severe sensorineural deafness. A CT scan revealed bilateral basal ganglia calcification and diffuse cerebral and cerebellar atrophy with mild ventricular dilatation. The medical geneticist suspected that the patient had Cockayne syndrome and ordered a genetic test to confirm the diagnosis. A molecular test was ordered and revealed a pathogenic variant in the *ERCC6* gene for Cockayne syndrome. Which one of the following malignancies would the patient have an increased risk of developing in her lifetime?

A. Breast cancer
B. Cervical cancer
C. Colorectal cancer
D. Endometrial carcinoma
E. Leukemia/lymphoma
F. All of the above
G. None of the above

135. Which one of the postnatal growth failure disorders is most likely *NOT* inherited?

A. Bloom syndrome
B. Cockayne syndrome
C. Nijmegen breakage syndrome
D. Progeria
E. Werner syndrome

136. A 7th-grade boy was brought to a dermatology clinic by his parents for abnormally shaped fingernails and toenails, white patches inside the

mouth, and changes in skin coloring around his neck and chest. While talking with the physician, the mother mentioned that her younger brother had similar problems, but not as severe as her son's. Also, her brother did not like exercise and seemed not to be able to tolerate much exercise. One of her uncles on her mother's side, whom she had never met, died of a hematological cancer in another country. The dermatologist suspected that the patient had dyskeratosis congenita and ordered a genetic test for the patient after consulting with a medical geneticist. Which one of the following assays would the dermatologist most likely order to confirm the diagnosis in this patient?

A. Chromosome breakage study
B. Chromosome karyotype
C. Methylation study
D. Multiplex ligation-dependent probe amplification (MLPA)
E. Sequencing analysis
F. Targeted-mutation analysis
G. None of the above

137. A 7th-grade boy was brought to a dermatology clinic by his parents for abnormally shaped fingernails and toenails, white patches inside the mouth, and changes in skin coloring around his neck and chest. While talking with the physician, the mother mentioned that her younger brother had similar problems, but not as severe as her son's. Also, her brother did not like exercise, and seemed not to be able to tolerate much exercise. One of her uncles from her mother's side died of a hematological cancer in another country, whom she had never met. The dermatologist suspected that the patient had dyskeratosis congenita, and ordered a genetic test for the patient after consulting a medical geneticist. Which of the following assays would be the most sensitive one to rule out dyskeratosis congenita in this patient?

A. Chromosome breakage study
B. Chromosome karyotype
C. Methylation study
D. Multicolor flow cytometry FISH (flow-FISH)
E. Sequencing analysis
F. Targeted-mutation analysis
G. None of the above

138. A 7th-grade boy was brought to a dermatology clinic by his parents for abnormally shaped fingernails and toenails, white patches inside the mouth, and changes in skin coloring around his neck and chest. While talking with the physician, the mother mentioned that her younger brother has similar problems, but not as severe as her son's. Also, her brother did not like exercise and

seemed not to be able to tolerate much exercise. One of her uncles from her mother side, whom she had never met, died of a hematological cancer in another country. The dermatologist suspected that the patient had dyskeratosis congenita. Which one of the inherited modes does dyskeratosis congenita have?

A. Autosomal dominant
B. Autosome recessive
C. X-linked
D. All of the above
E. None of the above

139. A 7th-grade boy was brought to a dermatology clinic by his parents for abnormally shaped fingernails and toenails, white patches inside the mouth, and changes in skin coloring around his neck and chest. The family history was significant. The mother's younger brother has similar problem, but not as severe as her son's. Also, her brother did not like exercise and seemed not to be able to tolerate much exercise. One of the mother's uncles from her mother side, whom she'd never met, died of a hematological cancer in another country. The dermatologist suspected that the patient had dyskeratosis congenita and ordered a genetic test for the patient after consulting a medical geneticist. Which one of the genes would most likely harbor a pathogenic variant if the patient had dyskeratosis congenita?

A. *DKC1*
B. *NHP2*
C. *TERC*
D. *TERT*
E. Unknown

140. A 6th-grade boy was brought to a dermatology clinic by his parents for abnormally shaped fingernails and toenails, white patches inside the mouth, and changes in skin coloring around his neck and chest. While talking with the physician, the mother mentioned that her fingernails and toenails do not growth well and that she had some sort of white spots on the back of her neck. She also seemed not to be able to tolerate much exercise any more. Her father died of a hematological cancer right after her family moved to America when she was 5 years old. The dermatologist suspected that the patient had dyskeratosis congenita and ordered a genetic test for the patient after consulting a medical geneticist. Which of the following genes would most likely be included in the genetic test to rule out dyskeratosis congenita in this patient?

A. *DKC1, TERC,* and *TINF2*
B. *TERC, TINF2,* and *TERT*
C. *TERT, NHP2,* and *NOP10*
D. *TINF2, TERT,* and *NHP2*

141. A 6-month-old boy was admitted to a PICU for respiratory difficulties, feeding problems, poor weight gain, recurrent infections, and severe constipation. A medical geneticist was called for consultation. During the physical examination, she noticed that the patient was small for his age. The patient also had developmental delay, broad thumbs and great toes, bilateral undescended testes, and a heart murmur. The medical geneticist suspected that the patient had Rubinstein–Taybi syndrome (RTS). Which one of the following genetic assays would be the most appropriate initial test for this patient?

A. Chromosome breakage study
B. Chromosome microarray
C. Methylation study
D. Multicolor flow cytometry FISH (flow-FISH)
E. Sequencing
F. None of the above

142. A 6-month-old boy was admitted to a PICU for respiratory difficulties, feeding problems, poor weight gain, recurrent infections, and severe constipation. A medical geneticist was called for consultation. During the physical examination, she noticed that the patient was small for his age. The patient also had developmental delay, broad thumbs and great toes, bilateral undescended testes, and a heart murmur. The medical geneticist suspected that the patient had Rubinstein–Taybi syndrome (RTS). In the genetic counseling session, the counselor mentioned that mutations in two genes have been known to cause RTS. How likely would sequencing analyses of both genes detect the pathogenic variant in this patient if he had RTS?

A. 20%
B. 50%
C. 80%
D. 99%
E. Unknown

143. A 6-month-old boy was admitted to a PICU for respiratory difficulties, feeding problems, poor weight gain, recurrent infections, and severe constipation. A medical geneticist was called for consultation. During the physical examination, she noticed that the patient was small for his age. The patient also had developmental delay, broad thumbs and great toes, bilateral undescended testes, and a heart murmur. The medical

geneticist suspected that the patient had Rubinstein–Taybi syndrome (RTS). A molecular sequencing test was ordered, and the results turned out to be negative. The medical geneticist still suspected RTS in this patient, especially since the detection rate of sequencing analysis of the two genes is only approximately 50%. Which one of the following genetic assays would be most appropriate to further rule out RTS in this patient?

A. Chromosome breakage study
B. Chromosome karyotype
C. Chromosome microarray
D. Methylation study
E. Multicolor flow cytometry FISH (flow-FISH)
F. None of the above

144. A 2-year-old boy is brought to a dermatology clinic by his parents for severe sunburn after being on a beach for less than 30 minutes. The parents are immigrants from Turkey. The doctor notices freckling of the skin on the patient's face, arms, and lips in addition to redness and blistering. The boy's development has been normal, and his medical history is unremarkable. The dermatologist suspects that the patient has xeroderma pigmentosum (XP), and a sequencing assay confirms the diagnosis. The mother is pregnant and she wants to find out how likely it will be for her unborn child to have the same condition. What is the estimated recurrent risk of this condition in siblings?

A. <1%
B. 25%
C. 50%
D. 50% in brothers

145. A 2-year-old boy is brought to a dermatology clinic by his parents for severe sunburn after being on a beach for less than 30 minutes. The parents are immigrants from Turkey. The doctor notices freckling of the skin on patient's face, arms, and lips in addition to redness and blistering. The boy's development has been normal, and his medical history is unremarkable. The dermatologist suspects that the patient has xeroderma pigmentosum (XP), and a sequencing assay confirms the diagnosis. Which one of following cancers will have increased incidence in this XP patient?

A. Basal-cell carcinoma
B. Gastric carcinoma
C. Leukemia
D. Lung cancer
E. Melanoma
F. Squamous-cell carcinoma
G. All of the above

146. A 2-year-old boy is brought to a dermatology clinic by his parents for severe sunburn after being on a beach for less than 30 minutes. The parents are immigrants from Turkey. The doctor notices freckling of the skin on patient's face, arms, and lips in addition to redness and blistering. The boy's development has been normal, and his medical history is unremarkable. The dermatologist suspects that the patient has xeroderma pigmentosum (XP), and a sequencing assay confirms the diagnosis. Which one of following cancers will most likely develop in this patient with XP?

A. Brain cancer
B. Gastric carcinoma
C. Leukemia
D. Lung cancer
E. Skin cancer
F. All of the above

147. A 2-year-old boy is brought to a dermatology clinic by his parents for severe sunburn after being on a beach for less than 30 minutes. The parents are immigrants from Turkey. The doctor notices freckling of the skin on patient's face, arms, and lips in addition to redness and blistering. The boy's development has been normal, and his medical history is unremarkable. The dermatologist suspects that the patient has xeroderma pigmentosum (XP), and a sequencing assay confirms the diagnosis. What is expected to be the most characteristic DNA damage after exposure UV light in this patient with XP?

A. AA dimer
B. TT dimer
C. CpG island
D. Double strand breakage
E. Single strand breakage

148. A 4-year-old boy is referred to a surgeon for an abdominal mass found by ultrasound. He is apparently healthy otherwise. After surgical removal of part of the left kidney, the boy is diagnosed with unilateral and unicentric Wilms tumor. The family history is unremarkable. Molecular genetic tests of the *WT1* gene and chromosome microarray analysis are negative. Genetic test for Beckwith–Wiedemann syndrome is negative, too. The parents ask for the estimated recurrent risk for their next child, since the mother is currently pregnant. Which one of the following is the empiric risk of Wilms tumor to the unborn child?

A. 50%
B. 25%
C. 6%–7%
D. <1%
E. None of the above

149. A 1-year-old boy was referred to a genetics clinic by his pediatrician for a history of developmental delay with an inability to move the left limbs and a lump in the left side of the abdomen. The mother's pregnancy and the patient's birth history were unremarkable. His family history was not contributory. The physical examination revealed facial dysmorphic features, aniridia, bilateral undescended testes, and a palpable mass located in the left flank, which was immobile on respiration. An abdominal US detected an echogenic mass lesion measuring $46 \times 48 \times 51$ mm in the inferior pole of the left kidney, a 13-mm lymph node in the left iliac region, and bilateral undescended testes located at the deep inguinal ring; a contrast-enhanced CT suggested Wilms tumor. A contrast-enhanced CT of the brain revealed a large cystic area in the right temporal area with poorly visualized posterior cortical matter and poor separation from the right sylvian fissure; a dilated right frontal horn, temporal horn, trigone and body of right lateral ventricle with regression of right frontal lobe and enlarged CSF space adjacent to it. The gyral enhancement in right parieto-occipital region was suggestive of angiomatosis. Which one of the following genetic assays would most likely be used for the genetic evaluation to confirm/rule out genetic etiologies in this patient?[9]
    A. Chromosome karyotype
    B. Chromosome microarray
    C. Methylation study
    D. Multicolor flow cytometry FISH (flow-FISH)
    E. Sequencing
    F. Targeted-mutation analysis
    G. None of the above

150. A fellow in a clinical molecular genetic laboratory works on a project to develop a next-generation sequencing (NGS) panel for Cowden and Cowden-like syndromes. Which one of the following genes should NOT be included in the panel?
    A. *PTEN*
    B. *SDHB*
    C. *SDHC*
    D. *SDHD*
    E. *VHL*
    F. None of the above

151. An 8-year-old boy was brought to an emergency department by his parents for life-threatening pneumothorax. A CT found multiple cysts with thickening areas in the right lung periphery adjacent to the pleura. The pathological examination of a biopsy of the cysts confirmed the diagnosis of pleuropulmonary blastoma. His family history was remarkable for his father having multinodular goiter and a paternal aunt having ovarian Sertoli—Leydig cell tumor. The physician suspected that the patient had a hereditary cancer syndrome. Which one of the following hereditary cancer predisposition syndromes would this patient most likely have?
    A. *DICER1* syndrome
    B. Gorlin syndrome
    C. Li—Fraumeni syndrome
    D. *PTEN* hamartomatous tumor syndrome
    E. Xeroderma pigmentosum
    F. None of the above

152. An 18-month-old girl was brought to an emergency department by her parents for shortness of breath. An X-ray detected pneumothorax of the left chest. A follow-up CT found multiple cysts with thickening areas in the right lung periphery adjacent to the pleura. The pathological examination of a biopsy of the cysts confirmed the diagnosis of pleuropulmonary blastoma. Her family history revealed that the patient's paternal uncle died from short of breath at 2 years old. The physician suspected that the patient had a hereditary cancer syndrome. After consulting with a medical geneticist, the physician ordered a sequencing test for the patient. Which one of the following genes would most likely be sequenced to rule out genetic etiologies in this patient?
    A. *DICER1*
    B. *ERCC2*
    C. *RET*
    D. *PTEN*
    E. *TP53*
    F. None of the above

153. An 8-year-old boy was brought to an emergency department by his parents for life-threatening pneumothorax. A follow-up CT found multiple cysts with thickening areas in the right lung periphery adjacent to the pleura. The pathological examination of a biopsy of the cysts confirmed the diagnosis of pleuropulmonary blastoma. His family history was remarkable for his father having multinodular goiter and a paternal aunt having ovarian Sertoli—Leydig cell tumor. The physician suspected that the patient had a hereditary cancer syndrome. After consulting a medical geneticist, the physician ordered a

sequencing test for the patient to rule out genetic etiologies. Which one of the following genes would be the most appropriate first-line genetic workup to rule out genetic etiologies in this patient?

A. *DICER1*
B. *ERCC2*
C. *PTCH1*
D. *PTEN*
E. *TP53*
F. *VHL*
G. *XPA*

154. An 8-year-old boy was brought to an emergency department by his parents for life-threatening pneumothorax. CT found multiple cysts with thickening areas in the right lung periphery adjacent to the pleura. Pathological examination of a biopsy of the cysts confirmed the diagnosis of pleuropulmonary blastoma. In his medical record, the physician noticed bilateral cystic nephroma. The family history was remarkable for his father with multinodular goiter. Which one of the following malignancies would other family members have an increased risk of developing?

A. Breast cancer
B. Ovarian Sertoli–Leydig cell tumor
C. Parathyroid tumor
D. Pheochromocytoma
E. Renal-cell carcinoma
F. None of the above

155. An 8-year-old boy was brought to an emergency department for life-threatening pneumothorax. CT found multiple cysts with thickening areas in the right lung periphery adjacent to the pleura. The pathological examination of a biopsy of the cysts confirmed the diagnosis of pleuropulmonary blastoma. The physician noticed bilateral cystic nephroma in his medical record. His family history was remarkable for his father having multinodular goiter and a paternal aunt having ovarian Sertoli–Leydig cell tumor. Which one of the following assays would most likely be used for the genetic evaluation of pleuropulmonary blastoma for this patient?

A. Chromosome karyotype
B. Chromosome microarray
C. Methylation study
D. Multicolor flow cytometry FISH (flow-FISH)
E. Sequencing
F. Targeted-mutation analysis
G. None of the above

156. A 12-year-old Caucasian boy was referred to a genetics clinic for a recent diagnosis of keratocystic odontogenic tumors (KCOTs) in the jaws and bifid ribs. The perinatal history was

uncomplicated. His family history was unremarkable. The physical examination revealed macrocephaly, hypertelorism, pectus excavatum, scoliosis, and polydactyly of both hands. The tumors were removed surgically. Pathological examination of the specimen established a diagnosis of Gorlin syndrome. Which one of the following malignancies would most likely be seen in this patient with Gorlin syndrome?

A. Breast cancer
B. Melanoma
C. Basal-cell carcinoma
D. Pheochromocytoma
E. Renal-cell carcinoma
F. None of the above

157. Which one of the following skin cancers is the most common in Caucasians?

A. Actinic keratosis
B. Basal-cell carcinoma
C. Dysplastic nevi
D. Melanoma
E. Squamous-cell carcinoma
F. None of the above

158. A 28-year-old female patient presented to a clinic for multiple asymptomatic pigmented lesions over her face, chest, and thighs, all of which had presented for more than 10 years. The patient had noticed an increase in the number and size of the lesions in the past 6 months. The physical examination revealed macrocephaly (>2 SD), bossing of the forehead, coarse facial features, and numerous pits over her palms and soles. A biopsy of the skin lesion and pathological examinations revealed basal-cell carcinoma. Her family history was remarkable for his maternal uncle dying of "brain tumor" in his childhood. The physician suspected that the patient had a hereditary cancer syndrome. After consulting with a medical geneticist, the physician ordered a molecular test for the patient to rule out genetic etiologies. Which one of the following genes would most likely harbor a pathogenic variant in this patient if she had a genetic condition?

A. *DICER1*
B. *ERCC2*
C. *PTCH1*
D. *PTEN*
E. *TP53*
F. *VHL*

159. A 28-year-old female patient presented to a clinic for multiple asymptomatic pigmented lesions over her face, chest, and thighs, all of which had presented for more than 10 years. The patient had noticed an increase in the number and size of the lesions in the past 6

months. The physical examination revealed macrocephaly (>2 SD), bossing of the forehead, coarse facial features, and numerous pits over her palms and soles. A biopsy of the skin lesion and pathology examinations revealed basal-cell carcinoma. Her family history was remarkable for the maternal uncle dying of "brain tumor" in his childhood. The physician suspected that the patient had a hereditary cancer syndrome. After consulting with a medical geneticist, the physician ordered a molecular test for the patient to rule out genetic etiologies. The results confirmed the patient had Gorlin syndrome. From which one of the following brain tumors did the patient's maternal uncle most likely die in his childhood?[10]

A. Astrocytoma
B. Ependymoma
C. Glioblastoma
D. Medulloblastoma
E. Meningioma
F. Oligodendroglioma

160. An 11-year-old female patient was brought to a clinic by her parents for a white patch on the tongue with burning sensation for 6 months. The patient did not have a history of tobacco use. Her family history was remarkable for the maternal uncle dying of "pulmonary fibrosis" in early adulthood. The physical examination revealed a bald tongue with a 3×5 cm^2 leukoplakic patch. There was dryness of skin and reticular pigmentation on the sun-exposed areas, especially the back and the neck, as well as the palms and soles. She also had brittle and cracked nails, which were painful and had been present for the same amount of time. Occasionally, there was pus discharge from the nails, which had been treated with antibiotics. The patient also had mild photophobia and epiphora. Laboratory examinations revealed pancytopenia. The physician suspected that the patient had a hereditary syndrome. After consulting a medical geneticist, the physician ordered a sequencing test for the patient. Which one of the following genes would most likely be included in the test ordered for the patient?[11]

A. *DICER1*
B. *ERCC2*
C. *FANCA*
D. *PTCH1*
E. *TERT*
F. *VHL*

161. An 11-year-old girl was brought to a clinic by her parents for a white patch on the tongue with burning sensation for 6 months. The patient did not have a history of tobacco use. Her family history was remarkable for the maternal uncle dying of "pulmonary fibrosis" in early adulthood. The physical examination revealed a bald tongue with a leukoplakic a 3×5 cm^2 patch. There was dryness of skin and reticular pigmentation on the sun-exposed areas, especially the back and the neck, as well as the palms and soles. She also had brittle and cracked nails, which were painful and present for the same amount of time. Occasionally, there was pus discharge from the nails, which had been treated with antibiotics. The patient also had mild photophobia and epiphora. Laboratory examinations revealed pancytopenia. The physician suspected that the patient had a hereditary syndrome. After consulting with a medical geneticist, the physician ordered a molecular test for the patient. Which one of the following assays would be the most sensitive to confirm/rule out genetic etiologies in this patient?[11]

A. Chromosome breakage study
B. Chromosome microarray
C. FISH for gene amplification
D. Next-generation sequencing
E. Telomere-length measurement
F. None of the above

162. A 5-year-old boy was referred to a genetics clinic to rule out a hereditary etiology for his newly diagnosed hepatoblastoma. He was otherwise healthy. Which one of the following hereditary syndromes is the most commonly seen in children with hepatoblastoma?[12]

A. Beckwith—Wiedemann syndrome
B. Familial adenomatous polyposis
C. Gorlin syndrome
D. Li—Fraumeni syndrome
E. None of the above

163. A 42-year-old IT specialist has been healthy all her life except for a "lump" she recently noticed in her neck. She has no symptoms, exercises on a regular basis, and has no history of hospitalizations or serious illnesses. The physical examination reveals an asymmetric thyroid with an approximately 1.6 cm nodule on the left. A needle aspiration reveals C-cell hyperplasia and a possible carcinoma. She undergoes a thyroidectomy. Histological examinations confirm medullary carcinoma of the thyroid. There is no

family history of thyroid cancer. Her mother died of complications of pheochromocytoma after a routine hysterectomy. She has two healthy children, 4 and 8 years old. Which one of the following hereditary cancer predisposition syndromes may be considered to rule out genetic etiologies in this patient?

A. Cowden syndrome
B. Familial adenomatous polyposis
C. Gorlin syndrome
D. Multiple endocrine neoplasms, type 1 (MEN1)
E. Multiple endocrine neoplasms, type 2 (MEN2)
F. All of the above
G. None of the above

164. A 42-year-old IT specialty has been healthy all her life except for a "lump" she recently noticed in her neck. She has no symptoms, exercises on a regular basis, and has no history of hospitalizations or serious illnesses. The physical examination reveals an asymmetric thyroid with an approximately 1.6 cm nodule on the left. A needle aspiration reveals C-cell hyperplasia and a possible carcinoma. She undergoes a thyroidectomy. Histological examinations confirm medullary carcinoma of the thyroid. There is no family history of thyroid cancer. Her mother died of complications of pheochromocytoma after a routine hysterectomy. She has two healthy children, 4 and 8 years old. Which one of the following genes may be tested to rule out genetic etiologies?

A. *DICER1*
B. *MEN1*
C. *PTEN*
D. *RET*
E. *TP53*
F. *VHL*

165. A 42-year-old software engineer who has been healthy all her life except for a "lump" she recently noticed in her neck, for which she seeks evaluation. She has no symptoms, exercises on a regular basis, and has no history of hospitalizations or serious illnesses. Her family history is significant for her paternal uncle dying of pheochromocytoma at a young age. And her mother has benign parathyroid adenomas detected on an annual physical exam. This patient's physical examination reveals an asymmetric thyroid with an approximately 1.5-cm nodule on the right. A needle aspiration reveals C-cell hyperplasia and a possible carcinoma. She undergoes a thyroidectomy. Her mother died of complications of pheochromocytoma after a routine hysterectomy. She has two healthy children, 4 and 8 years old. Which one of the

following thyroid cancers does the patient most likely have if she has multiple endocrine neoplasia type 2 (MEN2)?

A. Anaplastic thyroid cancer
B. Follicular thyroid cancer
C. Medullary thyroid cancer
D. Papillary thyroid cancer
E. None of the above

166. A 26-year-old male came to a clinic with symptoms of goiter for 1 year. No notable symptoms in the history were suggestive of hypothyroidism or hyperthyroidism. He had had pain in right lower chest region for 6 months with no history of respiratory tract infections. He also had a history of three episodes of paroxysmal spells during the past 6 months. Each spell was characterized by headache, sweating, and palpitations. Examinations revealed mucosal neuromas of the lips and tongue, a high arched palate, and a grade 2 hard goiter with no marfanoid habitus. He had hypertension. A fine-needle aspiration of the thyroid revealed solitary nodules of the right lobe. Elevated plasma metanephrine and normetanephrine were noticed. An MRI revealed a right suprarenal mass. A laparotomy and right adrenalectomy were done. Histopathological examinations confirmed the diagnosis of pheochromocytoma. Which one of the following hereditary cancer predisposition syndromes would be considered to rule out genetic etiologies in this patient?[13]

A. Cowden syndrome
B. Familial adenomatous polyposis
C. Gorlin syndrome
D. Multiple endocrine neoplasms, type 1 (MEN1)
E. Multiple endocrine neoplasms, type 2 (MEN2)
F. All of the above
G. None of the above

167. A 26-year-old male came to a clinic with symptoms of goiter for 1 year. No notable symptoms without history suggestive of hypothyroidism or hyperthyroidism. He had had pain in the right lower chest region for 6 months with no history of respiratory tract infections. He also had a history of three episodes of paroxysmal spells during past 6 months. Each spell was characterized by headache, sweating, and palpitations. Examinations revealed mucosal neuromas of lips and tongue, a high arched palate, and a grade 2 hard goiter with no marfanoid habitus. He had hypertension. A fine-needle aspiration of the thyroid revealed solitary nodules of the right lobe. Elevated plasma metanephrine and normetanephrine were noticed. An MRI revealed right suprarenal mass.

A laparotomy and right adrenalectomy were done. Histopathological examinations confirmed the diagnosis of pheochromocytoma. Which one of the following genes may be tested to rule out genetic etiologies in this patient?[13]

A. DICER1
B. MEN1
C. PTEN
D. RET
E. TP53
F. VHL

168. A 23-year-old female underwent surgery for a perforated jejunum due to an injury, and enlarged lymph nodes were found in the stomach incidentally. Histopathological examinations revealed metastases of neuroendocrine carcinoma. During esophagogastroduodenoscopy, the tumor in the stomach was found. Gastric resection and follow-up histopathological examinations established a diagnosis of a well-differentiated neuroendocrine tumor-secreting gastrin. A CT scan of the abdomen identified multiple foci in the pancreas. Later she was again sent to surgery for adhesive intestinal obstruction. Her family history was significant for one of her maternal aunts having a parathyroid tumor. The physician suspected that the patient had a hereditary cancer syndrome. After consulting with a medical geneticist, the physician ordered a molecular test for the patient. Which one of the following hereditary cancer predisposition syndromes might be considered to rule out genetic etiologies in this patient?[14]

A. Cowden syndrome
B. Familial adenomatous polyposis
C. Gorlin syndrome
D. Multiple endocrine neoplasms, type 1 (MEN1)
E. Multiple endocrine neoplasms, type 2 (MEN2)
F. All of the above
G. None of the above

169. A 23-year-old female underwent surgery for a perforated jejunum due to an injury, and enlarged lymph nodes were found in the stomach incidentally. Histopathological examinations revealed metastases of neuroendocrine carcinoma. During esophagogastroduodenoscopy, the tumor in the stomach was found. Gastric resection and follow-up histopathological examinations established a diagnosis of well-differentiated neuroendocrine tumor-secreting gastrin. A CT scan of the abdomen identified multiple foci in the pancreas. Later, she was again sent to surgery for adhesive intestinal obstruction. Her family

history was significant for one of her maternal aunts having a parathyroid tumor. The physician suspected that the patient had a hereditary cancer syndrome. After consulting with a medical geneticist, the physician ordered a sequencing-based test for the patient. Which one of the following genes would most likely be sequenced for this patient to rule out genetic etiologies?[14]

A. DICER1
B. MEN1
C. PTEN
D. RET
E. TP53
F. VHL

170. A 23-year-old female underwent surgery for a perforated jejunum due to an injury, and enlarged lymph nodes were found in the stomach incidentally. Histopathological examinations revealed metastases of neuroendocrine carcinoma. During esophagogastroduodenoscopy, the tumor in the stomach was found. Gastric resection and follow-up histopathological examinations established a diagnosis of well-differentiated neuroendocrine tumor-secreting gastrin. A CT scan of the abdomen identified multiple foci in the pancreas. Later, she was again sent to surgery for adhesive intestinal obstruction. The physician suspected that the patient had a hereditary cancer syndrome. After consulting with a medical geneticist, the physician ordered a genetic test for the patient. Which one of the following assays would be most appropriate to confirm/rule out genetic etiologies in this patient?[14]

A. Chromosome breakage study
B. Chromosome microarray
C. Methylation study
D. Next-generation sequencing
E. Sanger sequencing
F. Targeted-mutation analysis
G. Telomere-length measurement
H. None of the above

171. Which one of the following malignancies is NOT characteristic for multiple endocrine neoplasia syndrome type 1 (MEN1)?

A. Adrenocortical tumors
B. Carcinoid tumors
C. Medullary thyroid cancer
D. Pancreatic tumors
E. Parathyroid tumors with endocrinopathy
F. Pituitary tumors
G. All of the above
H. None of the above

172. Which one of the following genes is associated with multiple endocrine neoplasia syndrome type 1 (MEN1)?
    A. *BRAF*
    B. *KRAS*
    C. *MEN1*
    D. *NRAS*
    E. *PTEN*
    F. *RB1*
    G. *RET*
    H. None of the above

173. Which one of the following malignancies is *NOT* one of characteristics of multiple endocrine neoplasia syndrome type 2 (MEN2)?
    A. Medullary thyroid cancer
    B. Mucosal neuroma
    C. Pheochromocytoma
    D. Pancreatic tumors
    E. Parathyroid adenoma
    F. All of the above
    G. None of the above

174. Which one of the following genes is associated with multiple endocrine neoplasia syndrome type 2 (MEN2)?
    A. *BRAF*
    B. *KRAS*
    C. *MEN1*
    D. *NRAS*
    E. *PTEN*
    F. *RET*
    G. *RB1*
    H. None of the above

175. Which one of the following genes is associated with familial medullary thyroid carcinomas?
    A. *BRAF*
    B. *KRAS*
    C. *MEN1*
    D. *NRAS*
    E. *PTEN*
    F. *RET*
    G. *RB1*
    H. None of the above

176. How often are medullary thyroid carcinomas inherited?
    A. <1%
    B. 5%
    C. 25%
    D. 50%
    E. 75%

177. Which one of the following syndromes is NOT associated with an increased risk for Wilms tumor?
    A. Beckwith—Wiedemann (BWS)
    B. Denys—Drash syndrome (DDS)
    C. Neurofibromatosis type 1
    D. Simpson—Golabi—Behmel syndrome (SGBS)
    E. Trisomy 18
    F. WAGR syndrome
    G. None of the above

178. A 12-month-old boy was brought to a genetics clinic for mild developmental delay. His perinatal history was unremarkable. The physical examination revealed eight café au lait spots over 5 mm in diameter. Otherwise he was healthy. His family history was remarkable for one of his two older brothers being seen in the same clinic previously with similar findings. Another brother was healthy. A genetic etiology was not identified in the sick brother previously. The latest information made the medical geneticist suspect that the patient and his affected brother had a hereditary cancer predisposition syndrome (HCPS). Which one of the following HCPSs might be considered to rule out genetic etiologies in this family?
    A. Denys—Drash syndrome
    B. Neurofibromatosis type 1
    C. Neurofibromatosis type 2
    D. Tuberous sclerosis
    E. All of the above
    F. None of the above

179. A 12-month-old boy was brought to a genetics clinic for mild developmental delay. His perinatal history was unremarkable. The physical examination revealed eight café au lait spots over 5 mm in diameter. Otherwise he was healthy. His family history was remarkable for one of his two older brothers being seen in the same clinic previously with similar findings. Another brother was healthy. A genetic etiology was not identified in the sick brother previously. The latest information made the medical geneticist suspect that the patient and his affected brother had a hereditary cancer predisposition syndrome (HCPS). So the medical geneticist ordered a sequencing-based test for the patient. Which one of the genes would most likely be sequenced to rule out genetic etiologies in this patient?
    A. *NF1*
    B. *NF2*
    C. *TSC1*
    D. *TSC2*
    E. *WT1*
    F. None of the above

180. Which one of the following symptoms is *NOT* likely manifested in individuals with neurofibromatosis type 1 (NF1)?
    A. Acoustic schwannoma
    B. Axillary freckling
    C. Cutaneous neurofibromas
    D. Lisch nodules
    E. Malignant peripheral-nerve-sheath tumor
    F. Optic-pathway tumor

181. A 26-year-old male came to a clinic for a history of bilateral tinnitus and progressive hearing loss for 9 months. He also had swaying toward both sides on walking for 4 months. Otherwise his medical history was uneventful. His mother had an intracranial lesion and died at the age of 33. The physical examination revealed bilateral severe sensorineural hearing loss, a mild bilateral lower motor neuron—type of facial palsy, and cerebellar signs. Ophthalmology evaluations revealed loss of corneal reflex on the right side and papilledema. A CT scan revealed bilateral ovoid well-circumscribed masses at both cerebellopontine angles with heterogeneous contrast enhancement. He had no café au lait spots and no axillary or inguinal freckling. The physician suspected that the patient had a genetic condition. After consulting with a medical geneticist, the physician ordered a sequencing-based test for the patient. Which one of the following hereditary cancer predisposition syndromes would be considered to rule out genetic etiologies in this family?[15]
    A. Denys—Drash syndrome
    B. Neurofibromatosis type 1
    C. Neurofibromatosis type 2
    D. Tuberous sclerosis
    E. All of the above
    F. None of the above

182. A 26-year-old male came to a clinic for a history of bilateral tinnitus and progressive hearing loss for 9 months. He also had swaying toward both sides on walking for 4 months. Otherwise his medical history was uneventful. His mother had an intracranial lesion and died at the age of 33. The physical examination revealed bilateral severe sensorineural hearing loss, a mild bilateral lower motor neuron—type of facial palsy, and cerebellar signs. Ophthalmology evaluations revealed loss of corneal reflex on right side and papilledema. A CT scan revealed bilateral ovoid well-circumscribed masses at both cerebellopontine angles with heterogeneous contrast enhancement. He had no café au lait spots and no axillary or inguinal freckling. The physician suspected that the patient had a

genetic condition. After consulting with a medical geneticist, the physician ordered a sequencing-based test for the patient. Which one of the following genes would most likely be sequenced to rule out genetic etiologies in this family?[15]
    A. *NF1*
    B. *NF2*
    C. *TSC1*
    D. *TSC2*
    E. *WT1*
    F. None of the above

183. A 26-year-old male came to a clinic for a history of bilateral tinnitus and progressive hearing loss for 9 months. He also had swaying toward both sides on walking for 4 months. Otherwise his medical history was uneventful. His mother had an intracranial lesion and died at the age of 33. The physical examination revealed bilateral severe sensorineural hearing loss, a mild bilateral lower motor neuron—type of facial palsy, and cerebellar signs. Ophthalmology evaluations revealed loss of corneal reflex on right side and papilledema. A CT scan revealed bilateral ovoid well-circumscribed masses at both cerebellopontine angles with heterogeneous contrast enhancement. He had no café au lait spots and no axillary or inguinal freckling. The physician suspected that the patient had a genetic condition. After consulting with a medical geneticist, the physician ordered a sequencing-based test for the patient. Which one of the following conditions would most likely cause hearing loss in this patient?[15]
    A. Astrocytomas
    B. Ependymoma
    C. Meningioma
    D. Neurofibromas
    E. Schwannoma
    F. All of the above
    G. None of the above

184. A 26-year-old male came to a clinic for a history of bilateral tinnitus and progressive hearing loss for 9 months. He also had swaying toward both sides on walking for 4 months. Otherwise his medical history was uneventful. His mother had an intracranial lesion and died at the age of 33. The physical examination revealed bilateral severe sensorineural hearing loss, a mild bilateral lower motor neuron—type of facial palsy, and cerebellar signs. Ophthalmology evaluations revealed loss of corneal reflex on right side and papilledema. A CT scan revealed bilateral ovoid well-circumscribed masses at both cerebellopontine angles with heterogeneous contrast enhancement. He had no café au lait

spots and no axillary or inguinal freckling. The physician suspected that the patient had a genetic condition. After consulting with a medical geneticist, the physician ordered a genetic test for the patient. Which one of the following assays would most likely be used for the genetic test that the physician ordered for this patient?[15]

A. Chromosome breakage study
B. Chromosome microarray
C. Methylation study
D. Next-generation sequencing
E. Sanger sequencing
F. Targeted-mutation analysis
G. Telomere-length measurement
H. None of the above

185. A 30-year-old Caucasian female was referred to a cardiology clinic with a history of hypertension for 6 years, chronic sweating, episodes of flushing, throbbing headache, pain in the right flank, and 20-kg weight loss in a year. Her family history revealed that one of her cousins had similar symptoms and was seeking medical attention. The examination revealed that the patient's blood pressure was 130/80 mmHg. An ultrasound study of the kidneys was negative. Laboratory tests detected elevated metanephrine and normetanephrine. Thyroid-function tests were normal. Surgery was performed. Histopathological evaluations confirmed the diagnosis of pheochromocytoma. The physician suspected that the patient had hereditary pheochromocytoma. After consulting with a medical geneticist, the physician ordered a genetic test for the patient. Which one of the following assays would most likely be used for the genetic test that the physician ordered for this patient?[16,17]

A. Chromosome breakage study
B. Chromosome microarray
C. Methylation study
D. Next-generation sequencing
E. Sanger sequencing
F. Targeted-mutation analysis
G. Telomere-length measurement
H. None of the above

186. A 30-year-old Caucasian female was referred to a cardiology clinic with a history of hypertension for 6 years, chronic sweating, episodes of flushing, throbbing headache, pain in the right flank, and 20 kg weight loss in a year. Her family history revealed that one of her cousins had similar symptoms and was seeking medical attention. The physical examination revealed the patient's blood pressure was 130/80 mmHg. An ultrasound study of the kidneys was negative.

Laboratory tests detected elevated metanephrine and normetanephrine. Thyroid-function tests were normal. Surgery was performed. Histopathological evaluations confirmed the diagnosis of pheochromocytoma. The physician suspected that the patient had hereditary pheochromocytoma. After consulting with a medical geneticist, the physician ordered a next-generation sequencing (NGS) panel for the patient. Which one of the following genes would most likely be included in the panel for hereditary form of pheochromocytoma to rule out genetic etiologies in this patient?[16,17]

A. *BRAF*
B. *KRAS*
C. *MEN1*
D. *NRAS*
E. *PTEN*
F. *SDHB*
G. None of the above

187. A 30-year-old Caucasian female was referred to a cardiology clinic with a history of hypertension for 6 years, chronic sweating, episodes of flushing, throbbing headache, pain in the right flank, and 20-kg weight loss in a year. Her family history revealed that one of her cousins had similar symptoms and was seeking medical attention. The physical examination revealed that the patient's blood pressure was 130/80 mmHg. An ultrasound study of the kidneys was negative. Laboratory tests detected elevated metanephrine and normetanephrine. Thyroid-function tests were normal. Surgery was performed. Histopathological evaluations confirmed the diagnosis of pheochromocytoma. The physician suspected that the patient had hereditary pheochromocytoma. After consulting with a medical geneticist, the physician ordered a next-generation sequencing (NGS) panel for the patient. Which one of the following genes would most likely *NOT* be included in this panel for the hereditary form of pheochromocytoma to rule out genetic etiologies in this patient?[16,17]

A. *MEN1*
B. *NF1*
C. *RET*
D. *SDHB*
E. *SDHC*
F. *SDHD*
G. *VHL*
H. None of the above

188. A 38-year-old female presented to a clinic with increased frequency and intensity of headache, vertigo, unsteadiness, and left facial numbness, which started as tinnitus along with hearing

impairment 10 years ago. MRI of the head revealed a mass in the left cerebellopontine angle (CPA) and a durally based mass in the anterior aspect of interhemisphere fissure characteristic of meningioma. The patient underwent left CPA tumor excision. The pathological report revealed two schwannomas originating from the fifth cranial nerve and the eighth cranial nerve, respectively. The physician suspected that the patient had hereditary pheochromocytoma. After consulting with a medical geneticist, the physician ordered a next-generation sequencing (NGS) panel for the patient. Which one of the following hereditary cancer predisposition syndromes would most likely this patient have if she had one?

A. Li—Fraumeni syndrome
B. Multiple endocrine neoplasia syndrome, type 1 (MEN1)
C. Neurofibromatosis type 1
D. Neurofibromatosis type 2
E. von Hippel—Lindau syndrome
F. Cowden syndrome

189. When does retinoblastoma(s) usually occur in an individual?

A. Any age
B. Before 3 years of age
C. Before 5 years of age
D. Before 7 years of age
E. 12 years of age
F. 40 years of age

190. A 2-year-old boy is brought to a clinic for bilateral retinoblastomas (Rb). What is the chance that the patient has a germline pathogenic variant in the *RB1* gene?

A. >99%
B. 80%
C. 50%
D. 20%
E. <1%

191. Jonny, a 3-year-old boy, was referred to a pediatric ophthalmologist because his mother noticed that his right pupil changed from black to light brown, and Jonny had blurry vision in his right eye. Fundus examinations of his left eye were difficult because of diffuse vitreous opacities. There was the impression of a possible mass lesion in the posterior and temporal aspect of the globe. After testing, the patient was diagnosed with bilateral retinoblastoma. After consulting with a medical geneticist, the physician ordered a sequencing-based test for the patient. Which one of the following genes would most likely be sequenced to rule out genetic etiologies in this patient?

A. *GPC3*
B. *GPC4*
C. *RB1*
D. *RET*
E. *WT1*
F. None of the above

192. A 14-year-old girl was brought to a clinic by her mother for pain in the region of her right lower back tooth for 10 days. Her medical history revealed that she had been delayed for her milestones. She had undergone cardiac surgery for severe pulmonary stenosis, moderate right ventricular hypertrophy, and large ostium secundum atrial septal defect (ASD). She had also undergone surgery in her anal region for an anovestibular fistula. The physical examination revealed that she was short for her age (<2 SD). She had facial asymmetry, hypertelorism, down-slanting palpebral fissures, depressed nasal bridge, low-set ears with auricular tags, broad philtrum, short neck, and clubbed fingers. Oral manifestations included incompetent lips, high-arched palate, hypoplastic left jaw, retrognathic maxilla, and prognathic mandible. Intraoral examination revealed dental caries in the retained primary teeth. Pain on percussion was elicited. The physician suspected that the patient had Noonan syndrome. After consulting a medical geneticist, the physician ordered a genetic test for the patient. Which one of the following assays would be most likely be used for the genetic test to rule out Noonan syndrome in this patient?[18]

A. Chromosome breakage study
B. Chromosome microarray
C. Methylation study
D. Next-generation sequencing
E. Sanger sequencing
F. Targeted-mutation analysis
G. Telomere-length measurement
H. None of the above

193. A 14-year-old girl was brought to a clinic by her mother for pain in the region of her right lower back tooth for 10 days. Her medical history revealed that she had delayed milestones. She had undergone cardiac surgery for severe pulmonary stenosis, moderate right ventricular hypertrophy, and large ostium secundum atrial septal defect (ASD). She had also undergone surgery in her anal region for an anovestibular fistula. The physical examination revealed that she was short for her age (<2 SD). She had facial asymmetry, hypertelorism, down-slanting palpebral fissures, depressed nasal bridge, low-set ears with auricular tags, broad philtrum, short neck, and clubbed fingers. Oral manifestations

included incompetent lips, high-arched palate, hypoplastic left jaw, retrognathic maxilla, and prognathic mandible. Intraoral examination revealed dental caries in the retained primary teeth. Pain on percussion was elicited. The physician suspected that the patient had Noonan syndrome. After consulting a medical geneticist, the physician ordered a genetic test for the patient. Which one of the following genes would most likely *NOT* be sequenced to rule out Noonan syndrome in this patient?[18]

A. *BRAF*
B. *HRAS*
C. *KRAS*
D. *NRAS*
E. *PTPN11*
F. *RAF1*
G. All of the above
H. None of the above

194. Cardiofaciocutaneous syndrome (CFC), Costello syndrome, multiple lentigines syndrome (also called "LEOPARD syndrome"), and Noonan syndrome are clinically overlapping conditions. Which one of the following pathways seems to be involved in the process of the pathogenesis of these syndromes?

A. Sonic hedgehog pathway
B. PI3K/Akt pathway
C. RAS/RAF pathway
D. Wnt signal pathway
E. All of the above
F. None of the above

195. A 12-year-old girl was brought to a clinic for decreased hearing in both ears. Her medical history was uneventful. The physical examination revealed that she had a distinctive white forelock of hair in the midline, along with striking bilateral blue irises. A white depigmented patch was present on the right forearm. Both eyes had a bright red fundal reflex with choroidal depigmentation. Her family history was remarkable for her younger brother having similar blue eyes, white forelock of hair, depigmented skin patch, and choroidal depigmentation but with normal hearing. Their father had a history of premature graying of hair. The physician suspected that the patient had a genetic condition. Which one of the following hereditary syndromes would the patient most likely have if she had a genetic condition?[19]

A. Cardiofaciocutaneous syndrome (CFC)
B. Costello syndrome
C. Noonan syndrome
D. Waardenburg syndrome
E. None of the above

196. A 12-year-old girl was brought to a clinic for decreased hearing in both ears. Her medical history was uneventful. The physical examination revealed that she had a distinctive white forelock of hair in the midline, along with striking bilateral blue iris. A white depigmented patch was present on the right forearm. Both eyes had bright a red fundal reflex with choroidal depigmentation. Her family history was remarkable for her younger brother having similar blue eyes, white forelock of hair, depigmented skin patch, and choroidal depigmentation but with normal hearing. Their father had a history of premature graying of hair. The physician suspected that the patient had Waardenburg syndrome. After consulting a medical geneticist, the physician ordered a genetic test for the patient. Which one of the following genes would most likely be included in the genetic test for this patient?[19]

A. *PAX2*
B. *PAX3*
C. *PAX5*
D. *PXP6*
E. All of the above
F. None of the above

197. A 12-year-old girl was brought to a clinic for decreased hearing in both ears. Her medical history was uneventful. The physical examination revealed that she had a distinct white forelock of hair in the midline, along with striking bilateral blue irises. A white depigmented patch was present on the right forearm. Both eyes had bright a red fundal reflex with choroidal depigmentation. Her family history was remarkable for her younger brother having similar blue eyes, white forelock of hair, depigmented skin patch, and choroidal depigmentation but with normal hearing. Their father had a history of premature graying of hair. The physician suspected that the patient had Waardenburg syndrome. After consulting a medical geneticist, the physician ordered a genetic test for the patient. Which one of the following assays would most likely be used for the genetic test to rule out Waardenburg syndrome in this patient?[19]

A. Chromosome breakage study
B. Chromosome microarray
C. Methylation study
D. Next-generation sequencing
E. Sanger sequencing
F. Targeted-mutation analysis
G. Telomere-length measurement
H. None of the above

198. An 18-month-old child was brought to a clinic with a history of ambiguous genitalia noted at birth and increasing abdominal distention for 1 month. The perinatal and developmental histories were uneventful. The family history was remarkable for a sister dying at 25 days of age with a history of loose stools since birth. The physical examination revealed that a large lump was palpable in the right lumbar region, which was ballotable and not crossing the midline. There was no ascites. The external genitalia were ambiguous, with a stretched phallus length of 1.5 cm. Labioscrotal folds were present, but no gonads were palpable. The uterus was not palpable by rectal examination. Laboratory tests revealed that the blood urea was 30 mg/dL, creatinine 0.7 mg/dL, sodium 136 mmol/L, and potassium 3.2 mmol/L. The total serum protein was 5.7 g/dL (albumin 2.7 and globulin 3.0). Urinalysis showed 3 + proteinuria, five to eight WBCs per high-power field, and no red blood cells or casts. Histological evaluations biopsy specimen from the abdominal mass confirmed the diagnosis of Wilms tumor. The patient's karyotype was 46,XY. The physician suspected that the patient had a genetic condition. Which one of the following hereditary syndromes would the patient most likely have?[20]
    A. Beckwith–Wiedemann syndrome
    B. Denys–Drash syndrome
    C. Frasier syndrome
    D. Isolated Wilms tumor
    E. WAGR syndrome
    F. None of the above

199. An 18-month-old child was brought to a clinic with a history of ambiguous genitalia noted at birth and increasing abdominal distention for 1 month. The perinatal and developmental histories were uneventful. The family history was remarkable for a sister dying at 25 days of age with a history of loose stools since birth. The physical examination revealed that a large lump was palpable in the right lumbar region, which was ballotable and not crossing the midline. There was no ascites. The external genitalia were ambiguous, with a stretched phallus length of 1.5 cm. Labioscrotal folds were present, but no gonads were palpable. The uterus was not palpable by rectal examination. Laboratory tests revealed that the blood urea was 30 mg/dL, creatinine 0.7 mg/dL, sodium 136 mmol/L, and potassium 3–2 mmol/L. The total serum proteins was 5.7 g/dL (albumin 2.7 and globulin 3.0). Urinalysis showed 3 + proteinuria, five to eight WBCs per high-power field, and no red blood

cells or casts. Histological evaluations of the abdominal mass biopsy specimen confirmed the diagnosis of Wilms tumor. The patient's karyotype was 46,XY. The physician suspected that the patient had a genetic condition. After consulting with a medical geneticist, the physician ordered a genetic test for the patient. Which one of the following genes would most likely provide an appropriate molecular diagnosis for this patient?[20]
    A. ALK
    B. CDKN1A
    C. PAX6
    D. WT1
    E. All of the above
    F. None of the above

200. An 18-month-old child was brought to a clinic with a history of ambiguous genitalia noted at birth and increasing abdominal distention for 1 month. The perinatal and developmental histories were uneventful. The family history was remarkable for a sister dying at 25 days of age with a history of loose stools since birth. The physical examination revealed that a large lump was palpable in the right lumbar region, which was ballotable and not crossing the midline. There was no ascites. The external genitalia were ambiguous, with a stretched phallus length of 1.5 cm. Labioscrotal folds were present, but no gonads were palpable. The uterus was not palpable by rectal examination. Laboratory tests revealed that the blood urea was 30 mg/dL, creatinine 0.7 mg/dL, sodium 136 mmol/L and potassium 3–2 mmol/L. The total serum protein was 5.7 g/dL (albumin 2.7 and globulin 3.0). Urinalysis showed 3 + proteinuria, five to eight WBCs per high-power field, and no red cells or casts. Histological evaluation of the biopsy specimen from the abdominal mass confirmed the diagnosis of Wilms tumor. The patient's karyotype was 46,XY. The physician suspected that the patient had a genetic condition. After consulting a medical geneticist, the physician ordered a genetic test for the patient. Which one of the following assays would most likely be used for the genetic test to rule out genetic etiologies in this patient?[20]
    A. Chromosome breakage study
    B. Chromosome microarray
    C. Methylation study
    D. Next-generation sequencing
    E. Sanger sequencing
    F. Targeted-mutation analysis
    G. Telomere-length measurement
    H. None of the above

201. A 3-month-old boy was brought to a clinic by his parents for feeding difficulty. He had lost 900 g in 1 month. His medical history revealed severe hydramnios, macrosomia with a birth weight of 4700 g, and neonatal hypoglycemia and hypocalcemia. The physical examination revealed macrocephaly, epicanthus, strabismus, flattened nose, low-set ears, macroglossia, short neck, laxity of small joints of the hand, and axial hypotonia. Echocardiographic studies showed an asymmetric nonobstructive hypertrophic cardiomyopathy involving especially the basal part of the ventricular septum measured at 9 mm. The physician suspected that the patient had Costello syndrome. After consulting a medical geneticist, the physician ordered a genetic test for the patient. Which one of the following genes would most likely provide an appropriate molecular diagnosis for this patient?

   A. *BRAF*
   B. *HRAS*
   C. *KRAS*
   D. *NRAS*
   E. *PTPN11*
   F. *RAF1*
   G. All of the above
   H. None of the above

202. A 3-month-old boy was brought to a clinic by his parents for feeding difficulty. He had lost 900 g in 1 month. His medical history revealed severe hydramnios, macrosomia with a birth weight of 4700 g, and neonatal hypoglycemia and hypocalcemia. The physical examination revealed macrocephaly, epicanthus, strabismus, flattened nose, low-set ears, macroglossia, short neck, laxity of small joints of the hand, and axial hypotonia. Echocardiographic studies showed an asymmetric nonobstructive hypertrophic cardiomyopathy involving especially the basal part of the ventricular septum measured at 9 mm. The physician suspected that the patient had Costello syndrome. Sequencing of the *HRAS* gene identified a pathogenic variant in this patient. Which one of the following cancers would this patient have an increased risk of developing in his lifetime?

   A. Breast cancer
   B. Colorectal cancer
   C. Endometrial cancer
   D. Melanoma
   E. Neuroblastoma
   F. Thyroid cancer

203. A 3-month-old boy was brought to a clinic by his parents for feeding difficulty. He had lost 900 g in 1 month. His medical history revealed severe hydramnios, macrosomia with a birth weight of 4700 g, and neonatal hypoglycemia and hypocalcemia. The physical examination revealed macrocephaly, epicanthus, strabismus, flattened nose, low-set ears, macroglossia, short neck, laxity of small joints of the hand, and axial hypotonia. Echocardiographic studies showed an asymmetric nonobstructive hypertrophic cardiomyopathy involving especially the basal part of the ventricular septum measured at 9 mm. The physician suspected that the patient had Costello syndrome. Sequencing of the *HRAS* gene identified a pathogenic variant in this patient. Which one of the following cancers would this patient have an increased risk of developing in his lifetime?

   A. Breast cancer
   B. Colorectal cancer
   C. Endometrial cancer
   D. Melanoma
   E. Thyroid cancer
   F. Transitional-cell carcinoma of the bladder

204. Which one of the following malignancies do patients with Birt–Hogg–Dubé syndrome (BHDS) have an increased risk of developing?

   A. Breast cancer
   B. Colorectal cancer
   C. Endometrial cancer
   D. Melanoma
   E. Renal-cell carcinoma
   F. Thyroid cancer

205. Which one of the following hereditary cancer predisposition syndromes is caused by activating mutations in a proto-oncogene?

   A. Birt–Hogg–Dubé syndrome
   B. Li–Fraumeni syndrome
   C. Multiple endocrine neoplasia type 1 (MEN1)
   D. Multiple endocrine neoplasia type 2 (MEN2)
   E. von Hippel–Lindau syndrome
   F. All of the above
   G. None of the above

206. Which one of the following hereditary cancer predisposition syndromes is caused by activating mutations in a proto-oncogene?

   A. Birt–Hogg–Dubé syndrome
   B. Costello syndrome
   C. Li–Fraumeni syndrome
   D. Multiple endocrine neoplasia type 2 (MEN2)
   E. Neurofibromatosis type 1
   F. von Hippel–Lindau syndrome
   G. All of the above
   H. None of the above

ANSWERS

1. **C.** The diagnosis of Lynch syndrome can be made on the basis of family history in families that meet the Amsterdam criteria and that have tumor microsatellite instability (MSI) or on the basis of molecular genetic testing in an individual or family with a germline pathogenic variant in one of four mismatch repair (MMR) genes (*MLH1, MSH2, MSH6,* and *PMS2*) or in *EPCAM*.

   In 1990 the International Collaborative Group on Hereditary Nonpolyposis Colorectal Cancer (HNPCC) established the first clinical criteria, the Amsterdam criteria, to define hereditary nonpolyposis colorectal cancer (HNPCC, Lynch syndrome) for the purpose of identifying families for research studies. But when used clinically, these criteria identify only *60%* of patients with Lynch syndrome. This lack of sensitivity led to the development of the revised criteria (Amsterdam II criteria), which take into account the presence of extracolonic cancers and have a detection sensitivity of *approximately 80%* (http://www.ncbi.nlm.nih.gov/books/NBK1211/).

   Therefore, the detection sensitivity of the revised Amsterdam criteria (Amsterdam II criteria) is about 80% to the clinical diagnosis of Lynch syndrome.

2. **C.** Familial adenomatous polyposis (FAP) is a colon cancer predisposition syndrome in which hundreds to thousands of precancerous colonic polyps develop, beginning, on average, at age 16 years (range, 7–36). By age 35 years, 95% of individuals with FAP have polyps. Without colectomy, colon cancer is inevitable. The mean age at colon cancer diagnosis in untreated individuals is 39 years (range, 34–43). *APC* is the only gene in which pathogenic variants cause FAP. Molecular genetic testing of *APC* detects pathogenic variants in up to 90% of individuals with typical FAP (http://www.ncbi.nlm.nih.gov/books/NBK1345/).

   The most efficient way for cascade testing for a familial disease is to *test the proband* for the pathogenic variant in the family first, then test the other family member for the targeted mutation. This principle is especially true when the risk has to be estimated prenatally.

   Therefore, the wife's brother should be tested first to estimate the risk in this family.

3. **F.** Familial adenomatous polyposis (FAP) is a colon cancer predisposition syndrome in which hundreds to thousands of precancerous colonic polyps develop, beginning, on average, at age 16 years (range, 7–36). By age 35 years, 95% of individuals with FAP have polyps. Without colectomy, colon cancer is inevitable. The mean age of colon cancer diagnosis in untreated individuals is 39 years (range, 34–43). *APC* is the only gene in which pathogenic variants cause FAP. The diagnosis relies primarily on clinical findings. Molecular genetic testing of *APC* detects pathogenic variants in up to 90% of individuals with typical FAP. *Full sequencing appears to be more sensitive than deletion/duplication analysis. Approximately 90% of pathogenic variants are detected by full sequencing,* and 8%–12% of mutations are detected by deletion/duplication analysis (http://www.ncbi.nlm.nih.gov/books/NBK1345/).

   Therefore, sequencing analysis of the *APC* gene is the first choice to establish/rule out genetic etiologies in this family.

4. **C.** Utilization of clinical criteria and modeling to identify patients with Lynch syndrome (LS) has been criticized for their less-than-optimal sensitivity and efficiency. Studies of molecular testing of all colorectal cancers (CRCs) reveal that up to 28% of LS patients would be missed with the most liberal of clinical criteria—the revised Bethesda guidelines. Evaluation of Genomic Applications in Practice and Prevention (EGAPP), a project sponsored by the Office of Public Health Genomics at the Centers for Disease Control and Prevention (CDC), determined that *sufficient evidence exists to offer genetic testing for LS to all individuals with newly diagnosed CRC.* The rationale was to reduce morbidity and mortality for relatives of patients with LS. Universal testing for LS has also been endorsed by the Healthy People 2020 and the National Comprehensive Cancer Network (NCCN).

   Therefore, Lynch syndrome should be ruled out in this patient even with the negative family history.

5. **C.** This 35-year-old female had Lynch syndrome with a familial pathogenic variant in the *MLH1* gene. The general cancer risks for people with Lynch syndrome are:

• Colorectal cancer	80%
• Stomach cancer	11%–19%
• Hepatobiliary tract cancer (liver/bile duct)	2%–7%
• Urinary tract cancer	4%–5%
• Small bowel cancer (intestines)	1%–4%
• Brain or central nervous system tumor	1%–3%

Cancer risks specific for women with Lynch syndrome are:

•	Endometrial cancer	20%−60%
•	Ovarian cancer	9%−12%

Lung cancer and breast cancer are not associated with Lynch syndrome (http://www.cancer.net/cancer-types/lynch-syndrome).

Therefore, this patient would not have an increased risk of developing lung cancer due to Lynch syndrome.

6. **A.** This 35-year-old female had Lynch syndrome with a familial pathogenic variant in the *MLH1* gene. The general cancer risks for people with Lynch syndrome are:

• Colorectal cancer	80%
• Stomach cancer	11%−19%
• Hepatobiliary tract cancer (liver/bile duct)	2%−7%
• Urinary tract cancer	4%−5%
• Small bowel cancer (intestines)	1%−4%
• Brain or central nervous system tumor	1%−3%

Cancer risks specific for women with Lynch syndrome are:

Endometrial cancer	20%−60%
Ovarian cancer	9%−12%

Lung cancer and breast cancer are not associated with Lynch syndrome (http://www.cancer.net/cancer-types/lynch-syndrome).

Therefore, this patient would not have an increased risk of developing breast cancer due to Lynch syndrome.

7. **D.** Lynch syndrome is the most common form of inherited colorectal cancer (CRC). It is an autosomal dominant disease with a population incidence of 1 in 400−500 and is responsible for about *3% of all CRCs*. Nearly all CRCs associated with Lynch syndrome exhibit microsatellite instability (MSI). *Approximately 10%−15% of sporadic CRCs also exhibit MSI.* The molecular basis for instability in these tumors is most often methylation of the *MLH1* promoter, leading to loss of both mRNA and protein expression. In total, 10%−20% of CRCs exhibit MSI (http://www.ncbi.nlm.nih.gov/books/NBK1345/).

Therefore, it would be most likely the patient had sporadic colon cancer.

8. **D.** Lynch syndrome is the most common form of inherited colorectal cancer (CRC). It is an autosomal dominant disease with a population incidence of 1 in 400−500 and is responsible for about *3% of all CRCs*. Nearly all CRCs associated with Lynch syndrome exhibit microsatellite instability (MSI). *Approximately 10%−15% of sporadic CRCs also exhibit MSI.* The molecular basis for instability in these tumors is most often methylation of the *MLH1* promoter, leading to loss of both mRNA and protein expression. In total, 10%−20% of CRCs exhibit MSI (http://www.ncbi.nlm.nih.gov/books/NBK1345/).

Therefore, it would be most likely the patient had sporadic colon cancer.

9. **C.** Microsatellites are particularly susceptible to acquire errors in patients with Lynch syndrome when the mismatch repair (MMR) gene function is impaired. Therefore, *somatic microsatellite instability testing of tumor tissue is used to identify tumors caused by defective MMR in a panel of microsatellite markers.* The number of nucleotide repeats in normal tissue is compared with the number from tumor tissue in the same individual. Microsatellite stability (MSS) is recorded if the same number of repeats is present in each marker in both the tumor and the normal tissue. Microsatellite instability (MSI) is demonstrated if the number of repeats in the tumor and the normal tissue differs (http://www.ncbi.nlm.nih.gov/books/NBK1345/).

Therefore, resected tumor tissue would be the most appropriate specimen for the MSI test in this patient.

10. **A.** Microsatellite unstable tumors are often unstable in many microsatellite markers, but sometimes not in all of them. Instability can vary depending upon the markers tested. The greater the length of the microsatellite instability (MSI), the greater the mutation rate. *Mononucleotide repeat markers are more likely to be unstable than other microsatellites in mismatch repair (MMR)−deficient tumors.* Additionally, mononucleotide repeat markers are more likely to be homozygous in patients as compared with other microsatellite markers, allowing for easier analysis. The MSI Analysis System, Version 1.2, from Promega is a fluorescent multiplex PCR−based method that detects microsatellite instability (MSI) with five mononucleotide repeats, and two pentanucleotide repeats are the identity controls. The ABI kit is a fluorescent multiplex PCR−based method that detects microsatellite instability (MSI) with five dinucleotide repeats.

Therefore, in this patient, mononucleotide polymorphisms most likely were unstable than single-nucleotide polymorphisms (SNPs), trinucleotide polymorphisms, and pentanucleotide polymorphisms if he had Lynch syndrome.

11. **B.** Microsatellites are particularly susceptible to acquire errors in patients with Lynch syndrome when the mismatch repair (MMR) gene function is impaired. Therefore, microsatellite instability (MSI) testing is used to identify tumors caused by defective MMR in a panel of microsatellite markers. The number of nucleotide repeats in normal tissue is compared with the number from tumor tissue in the same individual. Microsatellite stability (MSS) is recorded if the same number of repeats is present in each marker in both the tumor and the normal tissue. Microsatellite instability (MSI) is demonstrated if the number of repeats in the tumor and the normal tissue differs.

An MSI-high profile is reported if 40% or more of the repeats are unstable. An MSI-stable profile is reported if no repeats are unstable. An MSI-low profile is reported if fewer than 40% of repeats are unstable. Only a high degree of MSI is considered to be indicative of potential Lynch syndrome (http://www.ncbi.nlm.nih.gov/books/NBK1345/).

Therefore, 40% or more of the repeats are unstable if an MSI-high profile was reported.

12. **B.** Approximately *20%—30% of endometrial cancers* exhibit MSI, and as with colon cancers, the majority are the result of somatic *MLH1* promoter methylation (http://www.ncbi.nlm.nih.gov/books/NBK1345/).

Therefore, endometrial carcinoma has high incidence of microsatellite instability (MSI) besides colon cancer.

13. **C.** Approximately *20%—30% of endometrial cancers* exhibit MSI, and as with colon cancers the majority is the result of somatic *MLH1* promoter methylation (http://www.ncbi.nlm.nih.gov/books/NBK1345/).

Therefore, MSI are seen in about 20—30% of patients with endometrial carcinoma.

14. **E.** Lynch syndrome is the most common form of inherited colorectal cancer (CRC). It is an autosomal dominant disease with a population incidence of 1 in 400—500 and is responsible for about 3% of all CRCs. *Nearly all CRCs associated with Lynch syndrome exhibit microsatellite instability (MSI).*

Therefore, the correct answer is E (>99%).

15. **C.** Both *microsatellite instability (MSI) and loss of heterozygosity (LOH)* are relatively common in colorectal cancer and endometrial adenocarcinoma. LOH may be demonstrated by homozygous genotype with control markers through MSI molecular analysis.

Therefore, this patient's MSI molecular results may be explained by high MSI in the tumor sample with loss of heterozygosity (LOH).

16. **C.** It is a good practice to consider *Lynch syndrome* when there are early-onset colon and endometrial cancers in the same individual or close relatives. Lynch syndrome, also known as hereditary nonpolyposis colorectal cancer (HNPCC) syndrome, is an autosomal dominant inherited cancer susceptibility syndrome caused by a germline mutation in one of the DNA mismatch repair (MMR) genes. *Lynch syndrome is associated with early onset of cancer and the development of multiple cancer types, particularly colon and endometrial cancer.* A combination of family and personal medical history and tumor testing provides an efficient combination for diagnosing this syndrome (http://www.ncbi.nlm.nih.gov/books/NBK1345/).

Cowden syndrome is on the list of differential diagnoses. It is associated with an increased risk of developing breast cancers, thyroid cancers, and endometrial cancers. Colorectal cancers (CRCs) have been identified in individuals with Cowden syndrome, too. However, almost everyone with Cowden syndrome develops hamartomas, sometimes macrocephaly. CRCs and endometrial carcinomas are not commonly seen in patients with Li—Fraumeni syndrome, multiple endocrine neoplasia type 1 (MEN1), and von Hippel—Lindau syndrome.

Therefore, it would be most likely that this family had Lynch syndrome comparing the other options in this question.

17. **D.** Lynch syndrome (hereditary nonpolyposis colon cancer [HNPCC]) is the most common form of inherited colorectal cancer (CRC), responsible for about 3% of all CRCs. It is most frequently caused by pathogenic variants in the mismatch repair (MMR) genes (*MLH1, MSH2, MSH6,* and *PMS2*) or in *EpCAM*. Nearly all CRCs associated with Lynch syndrome exhibit microsatellite instability (MSI). However, approximately 10%—15% of sporadic CRCs also exhibit MSI. The molecular basis for instability in these sporadic CRCs is methylation of the *MLH1* promoter, leading to loss of both mRNA and protein expression. *MSI testing is used to identify tumors caused by defective mismatch repair by comparing the number of nucleotide repeats with a panel of microsatellite markers in normal tissue with the number from tumor tissue from the same individual.* It is much cheaper than NGS testing of all the candidate genes at one time. *BRAF* p.V600E mutation analysis is used to rule out sporadic CRCs when the MSI test is positive because *BRAF* p.V600E mutation is associated with *MLH1*

hypermethylation. Therefore, *ACMG recommends MSI testing as the initial screening test in individuals with CRC to rule out sporadic CRC.*

Germline pathogenic variants in the *APC* gene are associated with autosomal dominant familial adenomatous polyposis (FAP). Germline pathogenic variants in the *MUTYH* gene are associated with autosomal recessive adenomatous polyposis. Germline pathogenic variants in the *BMPR1A* and *SMAD4* genes are associated with autosomal dominant juvenile polyposis syndrome. Germline pathogenic variants in the *STK11* gene are associated with autosomal dominant Peutz–Jeghers syndrome. Germline pathogenic variants in the *PTEN* gene are associated with autosomal dominant *PTEN* hamartomatous tumor syndrome. Hamartomatous polyposis is seen in juvenile polyposis syndrome, Peutz–Jeghers syndrome, or *PTEN* hamartomatous tumor syndrome.

Therefore, microsatellite instability testing should be done to rule out Lynch syndrome, according to ACMG Technical Standard and Guidelines for Genetic Testings for Inherited CRC, 2014.

18. **B**. Lynch syndrome (hereditary nonpolyposis colon cancer [HNPCC]) is the most common form of inherited colorectal cancer (CRC), responsible for about 3% of all CRCs. It is most frequently caused by pathogenic variants in the mismatch repair (MMR) genes (*MLH1, MSH2, MSH6,* and *PMS2*). According to the ACMG Technical Standard and Guidelines, microsatellite instability (MSI) should be done first to rule out sporadic CRC, since most sporadic CRCs do not exhibit MSI. Then *BRAF p.V600E mutation analysis may be used to further rule out sporadic CRCs when the MSI test is positive because BRAF p.V600E mutation is associated with MLH1 hypermethylation.*

Germline pathogenic variants in the *APC* gene are associated with autosomal dominant familial adenomatous polyposis (FAP). Germline pathogenic variants in the *MUTYH* gene are associated with autosomal recessive adenomatous polyposis. Germline pathogenic variants in the *BMPR1A* and *SMAD4* genes are associated with autosomal dominant juvenile polyposis syndrome. Germline pathogenic variants in the *STK11* gene are associated with autosomal dominant Peutz–Jeghers syndrome. Germline pathogenic variants in the *PTEN* gene are associated with autosomal dominant *PTEN* hamartomatous tumor syndrome. Hamartomatous polyposis is seen in juvenile polyposis syndrome, Peutz–Jeghers syndrome, and *PTEN* hamartoma tumor syndrome.

Therefore, the *BRAF* p.V600E mutation test should be done to further rule out Lynch syndrome if a high level of MSI was detected in a patient according to ACMG Technical Standard and Guidelines for Genetic Testing for Inherited CRC, 2014.

19. **D**. It is a good practice to consider Lynch syndrome when there are early onset colon and endometrial cancers in the same individual or close relatives. Lynch syndrome, also known as hereditary nonpolyposis colorectal cancer (HNPCC), an autosomal dominant inherited cancer susceptibility syndrome caused mostly by a germline pathogenic variant in one of the DNA mismatch repair (MMR) genes (*MLH1, MSH2, MSH6, and PMS2*) or the *EpCAM* gene. Lynch syndrome is associated with the early onset of cancer and the development of multiple cancer types, particularly colon and endometrial cancer (http://www.ncbi.nlm.nih.gov/books/NBK1345/).

Cowden syndrome is on the list of differential diagnoses. It is associated with an increased risk of developing several types of cancer, particularly breast cancers, thyroid cancers, and endometrial cancers. Colorectal cancers (CRCs) have been identified in people with Cowden syndrome, too. Germline pathogenic variants in the *PTEN* gene are associated with Cowden syndrome. However, almost everyone with Cowden syndrome develops hamartomas and, sometimes, macrocephaly. Germline pathogenic variants in the *BMPR1A* and *SMAD2* genes are associated with juvenile polyposis syndrome (JPS). Individuals with JPS have an increased risk of developing CRCs. However, women with JPS do not have an increased risk of developing endometrial carcinomas. The *STK11* gene (also called *LKB1*) is a tumor suppressor gene. Germline pathogenic variants in the *STK11* gene are associated with Peutz–Jeghers syndrome (PJS). Individuals with PJS have an increased risk of developing cancers of the gastrointestinal tract, pancreas, cervix, ovary, and breast during their lifetimes.

Chromosome microarray analysis (CMA) is a technique to detect copy-number changes in the human genome instead of single-nucleotide variants in genes. Multiplex ligation-dependent probe amplification (MLPA) is a time-efficient technique to detect genomic deletions and insertions bigger than single-nucleotide variants and in/dels, but smaller than what CMA can detect.

Therefore, an NGS panel with *MLH1, MSH2, MSH6, PMS2,* and *PSM6* would be an appropriate test for this family in order to rule out genetic etiologies.

20. C. A pathogenic variant in the *PMS2* gene confirmed the diagnosis of Lynch syndrome. Lynch syndrome, also known as hereditary nonpolyposis colorectal cancer (HNPCC), an autosomal dominant inherited cancer susceptibility syndrome caused mostly by a germline pathogenic variant in one of the DNA mismatch repair (MMR) genes (*MLH1, MSH2, MSH6, and PMS2*) or the *EpCAM* gene. Lynch syndrome is associated with the early onset of cancer and the development of multiple cancer types, particularly colon and endometrial cancer (http://www.ncbi.nlm.nih.gov/books/NBK1345/). Individuals with Lynch syndrome have up to a 20% risk for colorectal cancer and up to a 15% risk for endometrial cancer by age 70. Cancer risks for *PMS2*-associated Lynch syndrome are somewhat lower than those associated with other Lynch-related genes.

Germline pathogenic variants in the *APC* gene are associated with autosomal dominant familial adenomatous polyposis (FAP). FAP is characterized by the development of hundreds to thousands of precancerous colonic polyps, beginning, on average, at age 16 years (range, 7–36). Germline pathogenic variants in the *BMPR1A* and *SMAD2* genes are associated with juvenile polyposis syndrome (JPS). Individuals with JPS have an increased risk of developing CRCs. However, women with JPS do not have an increased risk of developing endometrial carcinomas. The *STK11* gene (also called *LKB1*) is a tumor suppressor gene. Germline pathogenic variants in the *STK11* gene are associated with Peutz–Jeghers syndrome (PJS). Individuals with PJS have an increased risk of developing cancers of the gastrointestinal tract, pancreas, cervix, ovary, and breast during their lifetimes.

Therefore, this female patient had Lynch syndrome as a result of a deleterious pathogenic variant in the *PMS2* gene.

21. A. Lynch syndrome is the most common form of inherited colorectal cancer (CRC). It is an autosomal dominant disease with a population incidence of 1 in 400–500 and is responsible for about 3% of all CRCs. Lynch syndrome occurs in patients and families with a germline pathogenic variant in one of the DNA mismatch repair genes (*MLH1, MSH2, MSH6, PMS2*) or the *EpCAM* gene. Nearly all CRCs associated with Lynch syndrome exhibit microsatellite instability (MSI) (http://www.ncbi.nlm.nih.gov/books/NBK1345/).

Familial adenomatous polyposis (FAP) is caused by germline pathogenic variants in the *APC* gene. The *APC* gene is a tumor suppressor gene that is responsible for regulating the Wnt pathway.

Therefore, the *APC* gene is not a mismatch repair gene, and is not related to Lynch syndrome.

22. A. Lynch syndrome is the most common form of inherited colorectal cancer (CRC). It is an autosomal dominant disease with a population incidence of 1 in 400–500 and is responsible for about 3% of all CRCs. Lynch syndrome is most frequently caused by mutations in the mismatch repair (MMR) genes (*MLH1, MSH2, MSH6, and PMS2*). MSI testing is an effective method for determining which tumors arise from MMR deficiency (http://www.ncbi.nlm.nih.gov/books/NBK1345/).

A small portion of Lynch syndrome–related tumors are caused by certain pathogenic variants in the *EpCAM* gene, such as an *EpCAM deletion* in the 3′ region. These pathogenic variants account for up to 6% of Lynch syndrome cases. On chromosome 2, the *EpCAM* gene lies next to *MSH2*. The *EpCAM* pathogenic variants involved in Lynch syndrome remove a region that signals the end of the gene, which leads to formation of a long mRNA that includes both *EpCAM* and *MSH2*. And these *EpCAM* pathogenic variants cause the *MSH2* gene to be inactivated by promoter hypermethylation (https://ghr.nlm.nih.gov/gene/EPCAM#conditions).

Therefore, pathogenic variants in the *EpCAM* gene may cause Lynch syndrome with an MSI-high profile and loss of *MSH2* and *MSH6* by IHC although it is not a mismatch repair gene.

23. A. Lynch syndrome is the most common form of inherited colorectal cancer (CRC). It is an autosomal dominant disease with a population incidence of 1 in 400–500 and is responsible for about 3% of all CRC. Lynch syndrome is most frequently caused by mutations in the mismatch repair (MMR) genes (*MLH1, MSH2, MSH6, and PMS2*). MSI testing is an effective method for determining which tumors arise from MMR deficiency. And nearly all CRC associated with Lynch syndrome exhibit microsatellite instability (MSI-high profile) (http://www.ncbi.nlm.nih.gov/books/NBK1345/).

A small portion of Lynch syndrome–related tumors are caused by certain pathogenic variants in the *EpCAM* gene, such as an *EpCAM* deletion in the 3′ region. These pathogenic variants account for up to 6% of Lynch syndrome cases. On chromosome 2, the *EpCAM* gene lies next to *MSH2*. The *EpCAM* pathogenic variants involved in Lynch syndrome remove a region that signals the end of the gene, which leads to formation of a long mRNA that includes both *EpCAM* and *MSH2*. And these *EpCAM* pathogenic variants cause the *MSH2* gene to be inactivated by promoter hypermethylation (https://ghr.nlm.nih. gov/gene/EPCAM#conditions).

Therefore, pathogenic variants in the *EpCAM* gene may cause Lynch syndrome with an MSI-high profile and loss of *MSH2* and *MSH6* by IHC, although it is not a mismatch repair gene.

24. **C.** Lynch syndrome is the most common form of inherited colorectal cancer (CRC). It is an autosomal dominant disease with a population incidence of 1 in 400–500 and is responsible for about 3% of all CRC. Lynch syndrome is most frequently caused by mutations in the mismatch repair (MMR) genes (*MLH1, MSH2, MSH6,* and *PMS2*). MSI testing is an effective method for determining which tumors arise from MMR deficiency. The MMR gene products function as dimers. MSH2 protein may complex with MSH6 or MSH3 protein, and MLH1 protein complexes with PMS2 or PMS1 protein. MSH6 and PMS2 proteins are unstable when not paired in a complex. Thus *a germline pathogenic variant in* MSH2 *typically results in loss of expression of the proteins MSH2/MSH6 and a germline pathogenic variant in MLH1 results in loss of expression of* the proteins MLH1/PMS2. However, germline pathogenic variants in *MSH6* and *PMS2* typically do not result in loss of MSH2 or MLH1 expression because these proteins are still present in other pairings (http://www.ncbi.nlm.nih.gov/books/NBK1345/).

A small portion of Lynch syndrome–related tumors are caused by certain pathogenic variants in the *EpCAM* gene, such as an *EpCAM* deletion in the 3′ region. These pathogenic variants account for up to 6% of Lynch syndrome cases. On chromosome 2, the *EpCAM* gene lies next to *MSH2*. The *EpCAM* pathogenic variants involved in Lynch syndrome remove a region that signals the end of the gene, which leads to formation of a long mRNA that includes both *EpCAM* and *MSH2*. And *these EpCAM pathogenic variants cause the MSH2 gene to be inactivated by promoter hypermethylation* (https://ghr.nlm.nih.gov/gene/EPCAM#conditions).

Therefore, pathogenic variants in the *EpCAM* gene may cause Lynch syndrome with an MSI-high profile and loss of *MSH2* and *MSH6* by IHC, although it is not a mismatch repair gene.

25. **C.** It is a good practice to consider Lynch syndrome when there are early-onset colon and endometrial cancers in the same individual or close relatives. Lynch syndrome (hereditary nonpolyposis colon cancer) is caused by pathogenic variants in one the mismatch repair (MMR) genes (*MLH1, MSH2, MSH6,* and *PMS2,* or in *EpCAM*). It is inherited in an autosomal dominant manner. Somatic pathogenic variants in the *MSH3* gene are associated with endometrial carcinoma (http://www.ncbi.nlm.nih.gov/books/NBK1345/). However, *germline pathogenic variants in* MSH3 *have not found to be associated with Lynch syndrome.*

Therefore, a molecular test of the *MSH3* gene would most likely not provide information to confirm or rule out genetic etiologies in this patient.

26. **F.** Lynch syndrome is the most common form of inherited colorectal cancer (CRC). It is an autosomal dominant disease with a population incidence of 1 in 400–500 and is responsible for about 3% of all CRCs. Nearly all CRCs associated with Lynch syndrome exhibit microsatellite instability (MSI). Approximately 10%–15% of sporadic CRCs also exhibit MSI. The molecular basis for instability in these tumors is most often methylation of the *MLH1* promoter, leading to loss of both mRNA and protein expression. Therefore, in total, 10%–20% of CRCs exhibit MSI. The following guidelines were created for determining microsatellite instability (MSI) in a sample:

- MSI-high: >30%–40% of the markers unstable
- MSI-low: <30%–40% of the markers unstable
- Microsatellite stable (MSS): all markers stable

The results showed that three of five mononucleotide polymorphisms were unstable. So this tumor sample is MSI-high. Since immunohistochemistry (IHC) staining for *MLH1, MSH2, PMS2, MSH6* showed no staining for *MHL1* and *PMS2,* but staining for *MSH2* and *MSH6*. This suggested that a molecular defect was present in the *MLH1* gene, or less likely *PMS2.* CRC with a *BRAF* mutation is extremely rare in patients with Lynch syndrome, whereas it appears in about 40%–60% of sporadic MSI-high CRC. *The molecular basis for instability in these sporadic tumors is most often methylation of the* MLH1 *promoter,* leading to loss of both mRNA and protein expression (http://www.ncbi.nlm.nih.gov/books/NBK1345/).

Therefore, the presence of a *BRAF* mutation in this patient with an MSI-high CRC is associated with hypermethylation of *MLH1* promoter. These results rule out Lynch syndrome.

27. **A.** Lynch syndrome is the most common form of inherited colorectal cancer (CRC). It is an autosomal dominant disease with a population

incidence of 1 in 400–500 and is responsible for about 3% of all CRCs. Lynch syndrome occurs in patients and families with a germline mutation in one of the DNA mismatch repair genes (*MLH1*, *MSH2*, *MSH6*, and *PMS2*) or the *EpCAM* gene. Nearly all CRCs associated with Lynch syndrome exhibit microsatellite instability (MSI). However, approximately 10%–15% of sporadic CRCs also exhibit MSI. The molecular basis for instability in these sporadic tumors is most often *methylation of the MLH1 promoter*, leading to loss of both mRNA and protein expression (http://www.ncbi.nlm. nih.gov/books/NBK1345/).

Therefore, the *MLH1* gene is tended to be hypermethylated in individuals with sporadic CRCs.

28. **B.** This female patient had Lynch syndrome because she had a pathogenic variant in one of the mismatch repair genes, *MSH2*. Patients with Lynch syndrome have up to an 80% lifetime risk of developing colon cancer. *Women with Lynch syndrome have up to a 60% lifetime risk of developing endometrial carcinoma.* Affected individuals are also at greater risk for other cancers, such as stomach, ovarian, small bowel, biliary, renal pelvis, and ureteral cancers (http://www.ncbi. nlm.nih.gov/books/NBK1345/).

Therefore, this female patient would have higher lifetime risk of developing endometrial carcinoma than the other malignancies listed in the question.

29. **D.** *Patients with Lynch syndrome have up to an 80% lifetime risk of developing colon cancer* and, in women, up to a 60% lifetime risk of developing endometrial carcinoma. Affected individuals are also at greater risk for other cancers, such as stomach, ovarian, small bowel, biliary, renal pelvis, and ureteral cancers (http://www.ncbi. nlm.nih.gov/books/NBK1345/).

This female patient had Lynch syndrome because she had a pathogenic variant in one of the mismatch repair genes, *MSH2*.

Therefore, she had up to an 80% risk of developing colon cancer in her lifetime.

30. **C.** Patients with Lynch syndrome have up to an 80% lifetime risk of developing colon cancer and, *in women, up to a 60% lifetime risk of developing endometrial carcinoma.* Affected individuals are also at greater risk for other cancers, such as stomach, ovarian, small bowel, biliary, renal pelvis, and ureteral cancers (http://www.ncbi. nlm.nih.gov/books/NBK1345/).

This female patient had Lynch syndrome because she had a pathogenic variant in one of the mismatch repair genes, *MSH2*.

Therefore, she had up to an 60% risk of developing endometrial carcinoma in her lifetime.

31. **E.** It is a good practice to consider Lynch syndrome when there are early-onset colon and endometrial cancers in the patient or close relatives. Lynch syndrome is the most common form of inherited colorectal cancer (CRC). It is an autosomal dominant disease with a population incidence of 1 in 400–500 and is responsible for about 3% of all CRCs. Nearly all CRCs associated with Lynch syndrome exhibit microsatellite instability (MSI). Individuals with Lynch syndrome have a germline mutation in one of the DNA mismatch repair genes (*MLH1*, *MSH2*, *MSH6*, and *PMS2*) or in *EpCAM* (http://www.ncbi.nlm.nih.gov/books/ NBK1345/).

The mismatch repair (MMR) machinery exists as protein dimers, such as MLH1 and PMS2, and MSH2 and MSH6. Loss of one member of the dimer often results in proteolytic degradation of the other half. Because of this, mutations of *MLH1* often lead to the loss of both MLH1 and PMS2 proteins, and mutations of *MSH2* often lead to the loss of MSH2 and MSH6. However, the opposite is often not true. Loss of PMS2 does not necessarily cause loss of MLH1, and mutation in *MSH6* may not cause loss of MSH2 protein expression. And a small portion of Lynch syndrome—related tumors are caused by pathogenic variants in the *EpCAM* gene, such as a common *EpCAM* deletion in the 3′ region. On chromosome 2, the *EpCAM* gene lies next to *MSH2*. The *EpCAM* pathogenic variants involved in Lynch syndrome remove a region that signals the end of the gene, which leads to formation of a long mRNA that includes both *EpCAM* and *MSH2*. And these *EpCAM* pathogenic variants cause the *MSH2* gene to be inactivated by promoter hypermethylation.

Therefore, sequence analysis of *MLH1* and *PMS1* would be appropriate next step workup for the diagnosis in this patient.

32. **C.** It is a good practice to consider Lynch syndrome when there are early-onset colon and endometrial cancers in the patient or close relatives. Lynch syndrome is the most common form of inherited colorectal cancer (CRC). It is an autosomal dominant disease with a population incidence of 1 in 400–500 and is responsible for about 3% of all CRCs. Nearly all CRCs associated with Lynch syndrome exhibit microsatellite instability (MSI). Individuals with Lynch syndrome have a germline mutation in one of the DNA mismatch repair genes (*MLH1*, *MSH2*,

MSH6, and *PMS2*) or in *EpCAM* (http://www.ncbi.nlm.nih.gov/books/NBK1345/).

A small portion of Lynch syndrome—related tumors are caused by certain pathogenic variants in the *EpCAM* gene, such as *a common EpCAM deletion in the 3' region*. These pathogenic variants account for up to 6% of Lynch syndrome cases. On chromosome 2, the *EpCAM* gene lies next to *MSH2*. The *EpCAM* pathogenic variants involved in Lynch syndrome remove a region that signals the end of the gene, which leads to formation of a long mRNA that includes both *EpCAM* and *MSH2*. And these *EpCAM* pathogenic variants cause the *MSH2* gene to be inactivated by promoter hypermethylation. Deletions in the 3' region of the *EpCAM* gene can be detected using Southern blotting, MLPA, or gene-targeted array comparative genomic hybridization (aCGH) and should be analyzed in patients with IHC results showing loss of *MSH2* and/or *MSH6* (https://ghr.nlm.nih.gov/gene/EPCAM#conditions).

Therefore, molecular analysis of the *EpCAM* gene should be considered and offered to this patient to further rule out Lynch syndrome.

33. **A.** It is a good practice to consider Lynch syndrome when there are early-onset colon and endometrial cancers in the patient or close relatives. Lynch syndrome is the most common form of inherited colorectal cancer (CRC). It is an autosomal dominant disease with a population incidence of 1 in 400—500 and is responsible for about 3% of all CRCs. Nearly all CRCs associated with Lynch syndrome exhibit microsatellite instability (MSI). Individuals with Lynch syndrome have a germline mutation in one of the DNA mismatch repair genes (*MLH1*, *MSH2*, *MSH6*, and *PMS2*) or in *EpCAM* (http://www.ncbi.nlm.nih.gov/books/NBK1345/).

A small portion of Lynch syndrome—related tumors are caused by certain pathogenic variants in the *EpCAM* gene, such as *a common EpCAM deletion in the 3' region*. These pathogenic variants account for up to 6% of Lynch syndrome cases. On chromosome 2, the *EpCAM* gene lies next to *MSH2*. The *EpCAM* pathogenic variants involved in Lynch syndrome remove a region that signals the end of the gene, which leads to formation of a long mRNA that includes both *EpCAM* and *MSH2*. And these *EpCAM* pathogenic variants cause the *MSH2* gene to be inactivated by promoter hypermethylation. Deletions in the 3' region of the *EpCAM* gene can be detected using Southern blotting, MLPA, or gene-targeted aCGH and should be analyzed in patients with IHC results showing loss of *MSH2* and/or *MSH6*

(https://ghr.nlm.nih.gov/gene/EPCAM#conditions).

Therefore, it would be most likely the patient had the common deletion in the *EpCAM* gene.

34. **B.** It is a good practice to consider Lynch syndrome when there are early-onset colon and endometrial cancers in the same individual or close relatives. Lynch syndrome is the most common form of inherited colorectal cancer (CRC). It is an autosomal dominant disease with a population incidence of 1 in 400—500 and is responsible for about 3% of all CRCs. Nearly all CRCs associated with Lynch syndrome exhibit microsatellite instability (MSI). Individuals with Lynch syndrome have a germline mutation in one of the DNA mismatch repair genes (*MLH1*, *MSH2*, *MSH6*, and *PMS2*) or in *EpCAM* (http://www.ncbi.nlm.nih.gov/books/NBK1345/).

A small portion of Lynch syndrome—related tumors are caused by certain pathogenic variants in the *EpCAM* gene, such as a common *EpCAM* deletion in the 3' region. These pathogenic variants account for up to 6% of Lynch syndrome cases. On chromosome 2, the *EpCAM* gene lies next to *MSH2*. The *EpCAM* pathogenic variants involved in Lynch syndrome remove a region that signals the end of the gene, which leads to formation of a long mRNA that includes both *EpCAM* and *MSH2*. And *these EpCAM pathogenic variants cause the MSH2 gene to be inactivated by promoter hypermethylation*. Deletions in the 3' region of the *EpCAM* gene can be detected using Southern blotting, MLPA, or gene-targeted aCGH and should be analyzed in patients with IHC results showing loss of *MSH2* and/or *MSH6* (https://ghr.nlm.nih.gov/gene/EPCAM#conditions).

Therefore, in this patient the deletion in the *EpCAM* gene caused somatic hypermethylation of *MSH2*.

35. **C.** Individuals with Lynch syndrome have a germline mutation in one of the DNA mismatch repair genes (*MLH1*, *MSH2*, *MSH6*, and *PMS2*) or in *EpCAM*. The stability of *PMS2* depends on its ability to form a complex with *MHL1* (a similar situation exists with *MSH2* and *MSH6*). Therefore, *loss of expression of MLH1 will lead to functional loss of expression of both MLH1 and PMS2*. However, the converse is usually not true because tumors with defects in *PMS2* or *MSH6* may maintain expression of *MLH1* and *MSH2*, respectively. A tumor with loss of *MLH1* and *PMS2* may be either sporadic or associated with Lynch syndrome because either *MLH1* promoter methylation or a germline mutation in *MHL1* will

lead to this same IHC profile (http://www.ncbi.nlm.nih.gov/books/NBK1345/).

Therefore, it would be likely that the tumor specimen from this patient lost expression of PMS2, in addition to MLH1.

36. **B.** A majority of individuals with Lynch syndrome have a germline mutation in one of the DNA mismatch repair genes (MLH1, MSH2, MSH6, and PMS2). The stability of MSH62 depends on its ability to form a complex with MHS2 (a similar situation exists with MLH1 and PMS2). Therefore, *loss of expression of MHS2 will lead to functional loss of expression of both MHS2 and MSH62.* However, the converse is usually not true because tumors with defects in PMS2 or MSH6 may maintain expression of MLH1 and MSH2, respectively. A tumor with loss of MHS2 and MSH6 is likely from a germline mutation (http://www.ncbi.nlm.nih.gov/books/NBK1345/).

Therefore, it would be likely that the tumor specimen from this patient lost expression of MSH6, in addition to MSH2.

37. **A.** A colon cancer with loss of MLH1 may be either sporadic or associated with Lynch syndrome because either MLH1 promoter methylation or a germline mutation in MHL1 will lead to this same IHC profile. Therefore, most likely the cancer is sporadic when both MSI and IHC on MHL1 are positive. *More than half of sporadic MSI tumors (50%−68%) have the p.V600E mutation in BRAF, which is rarely detected in Lynch syndrome−associated cancers. It makes BRAF p.V600E the next step in the workup.* If an unstable tumor harbors the BRAF p.V600E mutation, it is most likely sporadic, and germline testing is not necessary. If the BRAF p.V600E mutation is not present, then the tumor may be either sporadic or associated with Lynch syndrome.

Therefore, *BRAF p.V600E will be the most appropriate follow-up test to further rule out Lynch syndrome in this patient.*

38. **F.** Lack of expression of MSH2 and/or MSH6 is usually not seen in sporadic unstable tumors. The stability of MSH6 depends on the stability of MSH2. On the other hand, tumors with defects in MSH6 may maintain expression of MSH2. Molecular genetic tests should be done for germline evaluation of both genes.

Therefore, the most appropriated test will be the MSH2 and MSH6 gene-mutation test.

39. **E.** Germline pathogenic variants in the APC gene are associated with autosomal dominant Familial Adenomatous polyposis (FAP). Germline pathogenic variants in the MUTYH gene are associated with autosomal recessive MYH-associated polyposis (MAP). *With the absence of family history in MAP and the high rate of de novo mutations in attenuated FAP and FAP (20%), analysis of both MUTYH and APC gene mutations should be considered for patients with or without adenomatous polyps.* About 10%−15% of APC mutations are gross deletions and duplications. MLH1 and MSH2 are associated with autosomal dominant hereditary nonpolyposis colorectal cancer (HNPCC), Lynch syndrome (http://www.ncbi.nlm.nih.gov/books/NBK1345/).

Therefore, sequencing analyses of the APC and MUTYH genes with reflex to APC and MUTYH del/dup analysis would be the most appropriate molecular tests as the next step in the workup.

40. **B.** *BRAF mutation is associated with sporadic colorectal cancers.* If a colorectal cancers (CRC) or endometrial cancer is microsatellite instability (MSI)-high and MLH1 methylation negative, it is most likely to be from a patient with Lynch syndrome. Any carcinoma with loss of MSH2 and/or MSH6 is likely to be from a patient with Lynch syndrome. The patient in answer E has an MSI-high tumor and meets the Amsterdam criteria for Lynch syndrome.

Therefore, patients with MLH1 immunohistochemistry (IHC)−negative and BRAF mutation−positive colorectal cancer do not have Lynch syndrome.

41. **C.** Germline pathogenic variants in the APC gene are associated with autosomal dominant familial adenomatous polyposis (FAP). Germline pathogenic variants in the MUTYH gene are associated with autosomal recessive MYH-associated adenomatous polyposis (MAP). With the absence of family history in MAP and the high rate of de novo mutations in attenuated FAP and MAP (20%), both FAP and MAP are on the list of differential diagnoses. *A molecular hallmark of carcinomas caused by MUTYH deficiency is the presence of a specific somatic KRAS mutation, c.34G > T in codon 12 in 64% of MAP CRCs, which does not appear in FAP* (http://www.ncbi.nlm.nih.gov/books/NBK1345/).

Hereditary nonpolyposis colorectal cancer (HNPCC; Lynch syndrome), is an autosomal dominant hereditary cancer syndrome with a germline pathogenic variant in one of the DNA mismatch repair genes (MLH1, MSH2, MSH6, and PMS2) or in the EpCAM gene. Peutz−Jeghers syndrome and PTEN hamartomatous syndrome are associated hamartomatous polyposis instead of adenomatous polyposis.

Therefore, it would be most likely that this female patient had *MYH*-associated polyposis if she had one of the hereditary cancer predisposition syndromes.

42. **A.** Germline pathogenic variants in the *APC* gene are associated with autosomal dominant familial adenomatous polyposis (FAP). A majority of them may be detected by sequencing. FAP patients have normal intelligence and normal appearance. *Interstitial deletions of chromosome 5q22 that include APC have been reported in individuals with attenuated adenomatous polyposis and classic adenomatous polyposis.* In all reports, such individuals have had cognitive impairment, usually in the mild-to-moderate range, and the majority had dysmorphic features (http://www.ncbi.nlm.nih.gov/books/NBK1345/).

Germline pathogenic variants in the *MUTYH* gene are associated with autosomal recessive MYH-associated adenomatous polyposis (MAP). MAP is typically associated with 10 to a few hundred colonic adenomatous polyps that are evident at a mean age of about 50 years. However, colonic cancer develops in some individuals with biallelic *MUTYH* pathogenic variants in the absence of polyposis.

It was most likely that this patient had FAP with additional symptoms due to lack of expression of genes on 5q22.

Therefore, chromosome microarray copy-number variation analysis may be pursued in this patient for a deletion on 5q22.

43. **F.** Colon cancers and endometrial carcinomas are common in patients with Lynch syndrome. Individuals with Lynch syndrome have a germline mutation in one of the DNA mismatch repair (MMR) genes (*MLH1*, *MSH2*, *MSH6*, and *PMS2*) or in the *EpCAM* gene. *The PMS2 gene has at least 15 pseudogenes,* which have a significantly high homology with the active gene (http://www.ncbi.nlm.nih.gov/books/NBK1345/).

Therefore, the *PMS2* gene has more pseudogenes than the others listed.

44. **D.** Immunohistochemistry (IHC) tests can be performed on tumor tissue to establish the probability of Lynch syndrome, and to identify which gene is most likely to have a causative germline variant in a candidate. IHC detects the presence or absence of the protein products expressed by mismatch repair (MMR) genes. The MMR gene products function as dimers. MSH2 protein may complex with MSH6 or MSH3 protein, and MLH1 protein complexes with PMS2 or PMS1 protein. MSH6 and PMS2 proteins are unstable when not paired in a complex. So a germline pathogenic variant in *MSH2* typically results in loss of expression of the proteins MSH2 and MSH6. A germline pathogenic variant in *MLH1* results in loss of expression of the proteins MLH1 and PMS2. However, germline pathogenic variants in *MSH6* and *PMS2* typically do not result in loss of MSH2 or MLH1 expression because these proteins are still present in other pairings.

Antibodies for *MSH2*, *MLH1*, *MSH6*, and *PMS2* have demonstrated 92% sensitivity for identifying tumors that arise in individuals with a germline pathogenic variant. However, false positive and false negative immunohistochemistries (IHCs) have seen with certain antibodies and fixation conditions. *Not all MSH6-mutated tumors may show an MSI-high phenotype* (http://www.ncbi.nlm.nih.gov/books/NBK1345/).

Therefore, it was possible that this patient had a germline pathogenic variant in the *MSH6* gene and the IHC was false negative.

45. **E.** Juvenile polyposis syndrome (JPS) is characterized by predisposition to hamartomatous polyps in the gastrointestinal (GI) tract, specifically in the stomach, small intestine, colon, and rectum. Most individuals with JPS have some polyps by age 20 years. Some may have only four or five polyps over their lifetime, whereas others in the same family may have more than a hundred. If the polyps are left untreated, they may cause bleeding and anemia. Approximately 20% of individuals with JPS have pathogenic variants in *BMPR1A*. Approximately 20% have pathogenic variants in *SMAD4* (http://www.ncbi.nlm.nih.gov/books/NBK1469/).

Germline pathogenic variants in the *APC* gene are associated with autosomal dominant familial adenomatous polyposis (FAP). Germline pathogenic variants in the *STK11* also called *LKB1*) gene are associated with autosomal dominant Peutz–Jeghers syndrome, which also has hamartomatous polyps.

Therefore, both *BMPR1A* and *SMAD4* would likely be included in the genetic evaluation for this patient.

46. **E.** Juvenile polyposis syndrome (JPS) is characterized by predisposition to hamartomatous polyps in the gastrointestinal (GI) tract, specifically in the stomach, small intestine, colon, and rectum. Most individuals with JPS have some polyps by age 20 years. Some may have only four or five polyps over their lifetime, whereas others in the same family may have more than a

hundred. If the polyps are left untreated, they may cause bleeding and anemia.

Approximately 20% of individuals with JPS have pathogenic variants in *BMPR1A*. Approximately 20% have pathogenic variants in *SMAD4*. Mucocutaneous telangiectasias and pulmonary arteriovenous malformations could be symptoms of hereditary hemorrhagic telangiectasia (HHT). *A combined syndrome of JPS and HHT (termed JPS/HHT) is present in most individuals with an SMAD4 pathogenic variant. A majority of SMAD4 pathogenic variants are single-nucleotide mutations* (http://www.ncbi. nlm.nih.gov/books/NBK1469/).

Therefore, *SMAD4* gene sequencing would most likely be used for the genetic evaluation to rule out genetic etiologies in this patient.

47. **B.** Juvenile polyposis syndrome (JPS) is characterized by predisposition to hamartomatous polyps in the gastrointestinal (GI) tract, specifically in the stomach, small intestine, colon, and rectum. Most individuals with JPS have some polyps by age 20 years. Some may have only four or five polyps over their lifetime, whereas others in the same family may have more than a hundred. If the polyps are left untreated, they may cause bleeding and anemia. Most juvenile polyps are benign. However, malignant transformation can occur. The genes known to be associated with JPS are *BMPR1A* and *SMAD4*. JPS caused by *BMPR1A* or *SMAD4* does not have associated cognitive impairment or macrocephaly.

A 10q22-q23 microdeletion syndrome that includes both the PTEN and BMPR1A genes has been reported. Germline pathogenic variants in the *PTEN* gene are associated with Cowden syndrome. Individuals with 10q22-q23 deletions may display hamartomatous polyps due to deletion of *BMPR1A*, cognitive impairments, problems with behavior, and macrocephaly due to the deletion of *PTEN* (http://www.ncbi.nlm.nih.gov/books/ NBK1469/). The resolution of chromosome karyotype may not be enough to determine whether microdeletions involving *BMPR1A* and *PTEN* are deleted. And karyotype cannot determine whether *BMPR1A* and *PTEN* are involved in a deletion detected by karyotype.

Therefore, chromosome microarray for copy-number analysis would most likely be used to characterize the gain of loss *BMPR1A* and/or *PTEN* to rule out genetic etiologies in this patient.

48. **D.** Peutz—Jeghers syndrome is autosomal dominant cancer predisposition disorder caused by pathogenic variants in the *STK11* (also called *LKB1*) gene. The hallmark freckling usually is absent at birth and will begin to develop in early childhood, around 5—6 years of age. The freckles tend to be perioral but can also appear on the eyes, hands, and feet. During the teenage years, many of the freckles will tend to fade. One location with preserved freckling is the buccal mucosa (http:// www.ncbi.nlm.nih.gov/books/NBK1266/).

Germline pathogenic variants in the *APC* gene are associated with autosomal dominant familial adenomatous polyposis (FAP). Germline pathogenic variants in the *MUTYH* gene are associated with autosomal recessive MYH-associated polyposis (MAP). Hereditary nonpolyposis colorectal cancer (HNPCC), also called Lynch syndrome, is autosomal dominant and associated with a germline pathogenic variant in one of the DNA mismatch repair (MMR) genes (*MLH1*, *MSH2*, *MSH6*, and *PMS2*) or in the *EpCAM* gene.

Therefore, it is likely that this patient has Peutz—Jeghers syndrome if he has a hereditary cancer syndrome.

49. **F.** Peutz—Jeghers syndrome (PJS) is an autosomal dominant cancer predisposition disorder caused by pathogenic variants in the *STK11* gene (also called *LKB1*) on 19p13.3. PJS is characterized by the occurrence of gastrointestinal hamartomatous polyps in association with mucocutaneous hyperpigmentation. The diagnosis of PJS is based on clinical findings and histopathological patterns of polyps. PJS is associated with considerable predisposition to gastrointestinal and nongastrointestinal malignancies (http://www. ncbi.nlm.nih.gov/books/NBK1266/).

Germline pathogenic variants of *APC* are associated with autosomal dominant familial adenomatous polyposis (FAP). Germline pathogenic variants *BMPR1A* and *SMAD4* are associated with autosomal dominant juvenile polyposis syndrome (JPS).

Therefore, molecular analysis of the *STK11* gene would be most likely included in the genetic test for this patient.

50. **B.** Peutz—Jeghers syndrome (PJS) is an autosomal dominant inherited gastrointestinal condition caused by germline pathogenic variants in the *STK11* gene (also called *LKB1*) on 19p13.3. PJS is characterized by the occurrence of gastrointestinal hamartomatous polyps in association with mucocutaneous hyperpigmentation. The diagnosis of PJS is based on clinical findings and histopathological patterns of polyps. A significant number of patients with PJS have deletion or duplication of *STK11* (45%) (http://www.ncbi.nlm. nih.gov/books/NBK1266/).

Therefore, *the detection rate of sequencing analysis of STK11 is approximately 55%*.

51. **B.** Peutz–Jeghers syndrome (PJS) is an autosomal dominant inherited gastrointestinal condition caused by germline pathogenic variants in the *STK11* gene (also called *LKB1*) on 19p13.3. PJS is characterized by the occurrence of gastrointestinal hamartomatous polyps in association with mucocutaneous hyperpigmentation. Individuals with PJS are at increased risk of developing intestinal and extraintestinal malignancies. *The relative risks (RR) were highest for gastrointestinal cancer and breast cancer.* The breast cancer risk in women with PJS approaches that of women who have a pathogenic variant in *BRCA1* or *BRCA2* (http://www.ncbi.nlm.nih.gov/books/NBK1266/).

Therefore, the female patient in the question was at increased risk of developing breast cancer because of PJS.

52. **A.** Peutz–Jeghers syndrome (PJS) is an autosomal dominant inherited gastrointestinal condition caused by germline pathogenic variants in the *STK11* gene (also called *LKB1*) on 19p13.3. PJS is characterized by the occurrence of gastrointestinal hamartomatous polyps in association with mucocutaneous hyperpigmentation. Individuals with PJS are at increased risk for intestinal and extraintestinal malignancies. The relative risks were highest for gastrointestinal cancer and breast cancer.

The patient has Peutz–Jeghers syndrome (PJS) due to the deletion of the *STK11* gene. Therefore, *this finding would be clinically significant (pathogenic) to the patient even though it was not related to the referral reason, autism.*

53. **E.** All the hereditary cancer syndromes listed are associated with an increased risk for gastrointestinal malignancies. Cowden syndrome (CS) is a type of *PTEN* hamartomatous tumor syndrome. Affected individuals usually have macrocephaly (> 97th percentile head circumference), trichilemmomas, and papillomatous papules. The lifetime risk of developing benign and malignant tumors of the thyroid, breast, and endometrium is increased significantly.

None of the other syndromes listed are associated with intellectual disability and/or macrocephaly. Patients with Peutz–Jeghers syndrome (PJS) have an increased risk for gastrointestinal malignancies and breast cancers in women, but not thyroid cancers. Patients with familial adenomatous polyposis (FAP) have an increased risk of developing gastrointestinal malignancies, but not the other cancers in this

family. *MYH*-associated polyposis is an autosomal recessive hereditary cancer syndrome. Most families with this disorder have a positive family history. Patients with Lynch syndrome (hereditary nonpolyposis colon cancer [HNPCC]) have an increased risk of developing colorectal cancer (CRC) without polyposis and endometrial carcinomas, but not thyroid cancers.

Therefore, it would be most likely that this patient had *PTEN* hamartomatous tumor syndrome.

54. **E.** Cowden syndrome (CS) is a type of *PTEN* hamartomatous tumor syndrome. Affected individuals usually have macrocephaly (> 97th percentile head circumference), trichilemmomas, and papillomatous papules. The lifetime risk of developing benign and malignant tumors of the thyroid, breast, and endometrium is increased significantly. *PTEN* is the only gene in which pathogenic variants are known to cause CS.

Germline pathogenic variants in *BRCA1* and *BRCA2* are associated with hereditary breast and ovarian cancer, but they are not common in patients with thyroid and endometrial cancers. Germline pathogenic variants in *CDH1* are associated with hereditary diffuse gastric cancer, also can be seen in some patients with breast or ovarian cancer but are not common in patients with thyroid and endometrial cancers. Germline pathogenic variants in *STK11* (also called *LKB1*) are associated with Peutz–Jeghers syndrome (PJS). Individuals with PJS are at increased risk for gastrointestinal malignancies and breast cancer in women. Germline pathogenic variants in *VHL* are associated with von Hippel–Lindau syndrome (VHLS). Gastrointestinal malignancies are not common in patients with VHLS.

Therefore, sequencing analysis of the *PTEN* gene would be the most appropriate first-tier genetic evaluation for this patient.

55. **A.** *Familial adenomatous polyposis (FAP) caused by germline pathogenic variants in the APC gene is the only disorder in the question associated with adenomatous polyposis.* The rest are associated with hamartomatous polyposis. Germline pathogenic variants in the *BMPR1A* and *SMAD4* genes are associated with autosomal dominant juvenile polyposis syndrome. Germline pathogenic variants in the *STK11* gene are associated with autosomal dominant Peutz–Jeghers syndrome. Germline pathogenic variants in the *PTEN* gene are associated with autosomal dominant Cowden syndrome.

Therefore, the *APC* gene would most likely *NOT* be sequenced in this patient to rule out genetic etiologies.

56. **B.** *Individuals with juvenile polyposis syndrome (JPS), Peutz–Jeghers syndrome (PJS), or Cowden syndrome have hamartomatous polyposis.* Germline pathogenic variants in the *BMPR1A* and *SMAD4* genes are associated with autosomal dominant Juvenile polyposis syndrome. Germline pathogenic variants in the *STK11* gene are associated with autosomal dominant Peutz–Jeghers syndrome. Germline pathogenic variants in the *PTEN* gene are associated with autosomal dominant *PTEN* hamartomatous tumor syndrome, such as Cowden syndrome.

Individuals with familial adenomatous polyposis (FAP) or *MYH*-associated polyposis have adenomatous polyposis. Germline pathogenic variants in the *APC* gene are associated with autosomal dominant familial adenomatous polyposis (FAP). Germline pathogenic variants in the *MUTYH* gene are associated with autosomal recessive adenomatous polyposis. Patients with Lynch syndrome (hereditary nonpolyposis colon cancer) have an increased risk of developing colorectal cancer without polyposis. Germline pathogenic variants in the *MLH1*, *MSH2*, *MSH6*, *PMS2*, and *EpCAM* genes are associated with autosomal dominant Lynch syndrome.

Therefore, the gene panel for this patient should include at least *BMPR1A*, *SMAD*, *STK11*, and *PTEN*.

57. **A.** *Familial adenomatous polyposis (FAP) is an autosomal dominant hereditary cancer predisposition syndrome that is caused by germline pathogenic variants in the APC gene located on 5q21.* FAP is characterized by multiple adenomatous polyps, typically more than 100. The most common symptoms of FAP are rectal bleeding, anemia, abdominal pain, tenesmus, and diarrhea. Without colectomy, colon cancer is inevitable (http://www.ncbi.nlm.nih.gov/books/NBK1345/).

Germline pathogenic variants in the *MUTYH* gene are associated with autosomal recessive adenomatous polyposis. *MYH*-associated with adenomatous polyposis (MAP) usually does not have family history. Individuals with juvenile polyposis syndrome have hamartomatous polyposis. Germline pathogenic variants in the *BMPR1A* gene are associated with autosomal dominant juvenile polyposis syndrome. Germline pathogenic variants in the *MLH1* gene are associated with autosomal dominant Lynch syndrome (hereditary nonpolyposis colon cancer [HNPCC]).

Therefore, sequence analysis of the *APC* gene would be the most appropriate first-tier genetic evaluation for this patient.

58. **C.** Individuals with familial adenomatous polyposis (FAP) or *MYH*-associated adenomatous polyposis (MAP) have adenomatous polyposis. Familial adenomatous polyposis (FAP) is an autosomal dominant hereditary cancer predisposition syndrome that is caused by germline pathogenic variants in the *APC* gene located on 5q21. Since sequencing analysis of the *APC* gene did not identify a pathogenic variant, MAP should be ruled out, too, especially when the family history was unremarkable.

MAP is an autosomal recessive adenomatous polyposis syndrome. Individuals with MAP usually have less adenomatous polyposis than patients with familial adenomatous polyposis (FAP), and they have an increased risk of colorectal cancer (CRC). The mean age at onset is about 50 years. Family history is usually negative. *The diagnosis is established in individuals with characteristic clinical findings and biallelic germline MUTYH pathogenic variants* (http://www.ncbi.nlm.nih.gov/books/NBK107219/).

None of the rest on the choices are associated with adenomatous polyposis. Germline pathogenic variants in the *BMPR1A* and *SMAD4* genes are associated with autosomal dominant juvenile polyposis syndrome (JPS). Individuals with JPS have hamartomatous polyposis. Germline pathogenic variants in the *MLH1* gene are associated with autosomal dominant Lynch syndrome (hereditary nonpolyposis colon cancer [HNPCC]).

Therefore, the *MUTYH* gene would be the most appropriate next step in the genetic evaluation for this patient.

59. **A.** *Individuals with familial adenomatous polyposis (FAP) or MYH-associated adenomatous polyposis (MAP) have adenomatous polyposis.* Germline pathogenic variants in the *APC* gene are associated with autosomal dominant familial adenomatous polyposis (FAP). Germline pathogenic variants in *MUTYH* are associated with autosomal recessive adenomatous polyposis.

Individuals with Juvenile polyposis syndrome (JPS), Peutz–Jeghers syndrome (PJS), or Cowden syndrome have hamartomatous polyposis. Germline pathogenic variants in the *BMPR1A* and *SMAD4* genes are associated with autosomal dominant JPS. Germline pathogenic variants in the *STK11* gene are associated with autosomal dominant PJS. Germline pathogenic variants in the *PTEN* gene are associated with autosomal dominant *PTEN* hamartomatous tumor syndrome, including Cowden syndrome. Patients with Lynch syndrome (hereditary nonpolyposis colon cancer [HNPCC]) have an increased risk of developing colorectal cancer without polyposis. Germline pathogenic variants in *MLH1*, *MSH2*, *MSH6*, *PMS2*, and *EpCAM* are associated with autosomal dominant Lynch syndrome.

Therefore, a panel including *APC* and *MUTYH* would be the most appropriate first genetic evaluation for this patient.

60. **B.** Germline pathogenic variants in the *BRCA1* and *BRCA2* genes increase the risk of female breast and ovarian cancers and several additional types of cancer. Together, *BRCA1* and *BRCA2* pathogenic variants account for about 20%−25% of hereditary breast cancers and *about 5%−10% of all breast cancers.* In addition, pathogenic variants in *BRCA1* and *BRCA2* account for around 15% of ovarian cancers overall. Breast and ovarian cancers associated with *BRCA1* and *BRCA2* pathogenic variants tend to develop at younger ages than their nonhereditary counterparts (http://www.cancer.gov/about-cancer/causes-prevention/genetics/brca-fact-sheet#q1).

Therefore, about 5%−10% of patients with breast cancer(s) have predisposition mutations in the *BRCA1* or *BRCA2* genes.

61. **D.** Germline pathogenic variants in the *BRCA1* and *BRCA2* genes increase the risk of female breast and ovarian cancers and several additional types of cancer. Together, *BRCA1* and *BRCA2* pathogenic variants account for *about 20%−25% of hereditary breast cancers* and about 5%−10% of all breast cancers. In addition, pathogenic variants in *BRCA1* and *BRCA2* account for around 15% of ovarian cancers overall. Breast and ovarian cancers associated with *BRCA1* and *BRCA2* pathogenic variants tend to develop at younger ages than their nonhereditary counterparts (http://www.cancer.gov/about-cancer/causes-prevention/genetics/brca-fact-sheet#q1).

Therefore, about 20%−25% of patients with hereditary breast cancer(s) have predisposition mutations in the *BRCA1* or *BRCA2* genes.

62. **C.** Triple-negative breast cancers (TNBCs) are those lacking estrogen and progesterone receptors, and *HER2* expression accounts for approximately 15%−20% of all breast cancer diagnoses. *Ten to twenty percent of women with TNBC have a BRCA1 mutation, while a BRCA2 mutation is much less common.* Thus, given this high frequency, *NCCN guidelines recommend that women with TNBC diagnosed at age 60 or younger should be offered BRCA1/2 counseling and testing regardless of ethnicity and family history.*

These cancers tend to occur more often in younger women and in women who are African American or Hispanic/Latina. Triple-negative breast cancers tend to grow and spread more quickly than most other types of breast cancer. Because the tumor cells do not have hormone receptors, hormone therapy is not helpful in treating these cancers. Because they do not have too much *HER2*, drugs that target *HER2* are not helpful, either. Chemotherapy can still be useful, though.

Human epidermal receptor growth factor 2 (*HER2*, *ERBB2*) gene amplification is the primary mechanism for HER2 overexpression and occurs in 18% to 20% of breast cancer. *HER2* gene amplification is predictive for patient outcomes with HER2-targeting agents. Several targeted agents are approved for the treatment of *HER2*-positive breast cancer, such as trastuzumab, ado-trastuzumab emtansine, pertuzumab, and lapatinib.

Therefore, *BRCA1* and *BRCA2* sequencing would be appropriate in this patient.

63. **D.** *The term triple-positive is used to describe cancers that are ER-positive and PR-positive and have too much HER2.* Breast cancers with *HER2* gene amplification or HER2 protein overexpression are called HER2-positive in pathology reports. These cancers can be treated with hormone drugs as well as drugs that target *HER2*.

Therefore, *HER2* FISH would be appropriate in this patient.

64. **H.** *Germline pathogenic variants in the VHL gene for von Hippel−Lindau syndrome are not associated with an increased risk for breast cancer.*

In addition to the *BRCA1* and *BRCA2* genes, a significantly increased risk of breast cancer is a feature of several other genetic syndromes. These include Cowden syndrome, which is caused by germline pathogenic variants in the *PTEN* gene; hereditary diffuse gastric cancer, which results from germline pathogenic variants in the *CDH1* gene; Li−Fraumeni syndrome, which is caused by germline pathogenic variants in the *TP53* gene; and Peutz−Jeghers syndrome, which results from germline pathogenic variants in the *STK11* gene. Pathogenic variants in *ATM*, *CHEK2*, and *PALB2* are also associated with an increased risk for breast cancer.

Therefore, *VHL* usually is not tested in patients with breast cancer.

65. **C.** The family history on both sides was significant for breast cancers. It suggested the possibility of hereditary cancer syndromes. Since germline pathogenic variants in the *BRCA1* and *BRCA2* genes account for 20%−25% of hereditary breast cancers and about 5%−10% of all breast cancers, these two genes are at the top of the list of differential diagnoses in this family. Since male breast cancer is more commonly associated with pathogenic variants in the *BRCA2* gene than in

the *BRCA1* gene, the likelihood of harboring a pathogenic variant in the *BRCA2* gene is high in both the husband and the wife. Ashkenazi Jews have a founder mutation in *BRCA2*, c.5946delT.

BRCA2 is also known as *FANCD1*. If offspring inherit pathogenic variants in *BRCA2* from both parents, they will have *Fanconi anemia subtype D1 (FA-D1)*, an autosomal recessive syndrome that is associated with childhood solid tumors and development of acute myeloid leukemia (http://www.cancer.gov/about-cancer/causes-prevention/genetics/brca-fact-sheet#q1).

Therefore, this couple's children would be at risk of developing Fanconi anemia.

66. **B.** The family history on both sides was significant for breast cancers, indicating the possibility of hereditary cancer syndromes. Since germline pathogenic variants in the *BRCA1* and *BRCA2* genes account for 20%−25% of hereditary breast cancers and about 5%−10% of all breast cancers, these two genes are at the top of the list of differential diagnoses in this family. Since male breast cancer is more commonly associated with pathogenic variants in the *BRCA2* gene than in the *BRCA1* gene, the likelihood of harboring a pathogenic variant in the *BRCA2* gene is high in both the husband and the wife. Ashkenazi Jews have a founder mutation in *BRCA2*, c.5946delT.

The *BRCA2* gene is also known as *FANCD1*. If offspring inherit pathogenic variants in *BRCA2* from both parents, they will have *Fanconi anemia subtype D1 (FA-D1)*, an autosomal recessive syndrome that is associated with childhood solid tumors and development of acute myeloid leukemia (http://www.cancer.gov/about-cancer/causes-prevention/genetics/brca-fact-sheet#q1).

Li−Fraumeni syndrome is caused by germline pathogenic variants in the *TP53* gene; Cowden syndrome is caused by germline pathogenic variants in the *PTEN* gene; von Hippel−Lindau syndrome is caused by germline pathogenic variants in the *VHL* gene. Germline pathogenic variants in the *TP53*, *PTEN*, or *VHL* gene are not associated with an increased risk for Fanconi anemia.

Therefore, if their firstborn child developed Fanconi anemia, it is most likely that both parents had a heterozygous pathogenic variant in the *BRCA2* gene.

67. **C.** The family history on both sides was significant for breast cancers, indicating the possibility of hereditary cancer syndromes. Since germline pathogenic variants in the *BRCA1* and *BRCA2* genes account for 20%−25% of hereditary breast cancers and about 5%−10% of all breast

cancers, these two genes are at the top of list of differential diagnoses in this case.

The *BRCA1* gene is also known as *FANCS*. If offspring inherit pathogenic variants in the *BRCA1* gene from both parents, they will have *Fanconi anemia subtype CS (FA-CS)*, an autosomal recessive syndrome that is associated with childhood solid tumors and development of acute myeloid leukemia (http://www.cancer.gov/about-cancer/causes-prevention/genetics/brca-fact-sheet#q1). Patients with germline pathogenic variants in *BRCA1* are not at risk of developing ataxia telangiectasia, Bloom syndrome, hereditary telangiectasia, or Nijmegen breakage syndrome. Ataxia telangiectasia, Bloom syndrome, and Nijmegen breakage syndrome belong to a family called "chromosome breakage syndromes."

Therefore, this couple's children would be at risk of developing Fanconi anemia.

68. **B.** An increased likelihood of *BRCA1* and *BRCA2* hereditary breast and ovarian cancer is suspected on the basis of a personal and a family history of breast and ovarian cancers. *Male breast cancer is more commonly associated with a BRCA2 mutation than a BRCA1 mutation. And Ashkenazi Jews have a founder mutation in BRCA2, c.5946delT* (http://www.ncbi.nlm.nih.gov/books/NBK1247/).

Germline pathogenic variants in the *STK11* gene are associated with autosomal dominant Peutz−Jeghers syndrome. Germline pathogenic variants in the *PTEN* gene are associated with autosomal dominant *PTEN* hamartomatous tumor syndromes, including Cowden syndrome. Germline pathogenic variants in the *CDH1* gene are associated with autosomal dominant hereditary diffuse gastric cancer (HDGC).

Therefore, in this case the *BRCA2* gene should be tested for, especially the c.5946delT variant in *BRCA2*, since the patient was Ashkenazi Jewish.

69. **D.** Joanne was cancer-free. But her relatives had breast and/or ovarian cancers. If she was tested without knowing whether her relatives carried a familial pathogenic variant, it may be difficult to interpret the finding. *So, usually predictive testing for at risk asymptomatic family members (including children) requires prior identification of the disease-causing variant in the family.* In this family the patient's sister, *Lily*, would be the best person to test in order to identify the disease-causing variant in the family. Once a germline pathogenic variant is identified within the family, the results of testing for the disease-causing variant in Joanne may be done with great accuracy.

Therefore, Lily should be the first in this family to be tested for a potential genetic etiology.

70. **B.** Joanne was cancer-free. The family history on both sides was significant for breast and ovarian cancers, which suggested the possibility of hereditary cancer syndromes. Since germline pathogenic variants in the *BRCA1* and *BRCA2* genes account for 20%–25% of hereditary breast cancers and about 5%–10% of all breast cancers, these two genes are at the top of the list of differential diagnoses in this case. *Male breast cancer is more commonly associated with a BRCA2 mutation than a BRCA1 mutation* (http://www.ncbi.nlm.nih.gov/books/NBK1247/).

Germline pathogenic variants in the *PTEN* gene are associated with autosomal dominant *PTEN* hamartomatous tumor syndromes, including Cowden syndrome. Germline pathogenic variants in the *TP53* gene are associated with autosomal dominant Li–Fraumeni syndrome. Germline pathogenic variants in the *VHL* gene are associated with autosomal dominant von Hippel–Lindau syndrome. Aside from the *BRCA1* and *BRCA2* genes, a significantly increased risk of breast cancer is also a feature of Cowden and Li–Fraumeni syndromes but not von Hippel–Lindau syndrome. But *BRCA2* was still at the top of the list of differential diagnoses, especially since male breast cancer was present in the family.

Therefore, a heterozygous pathogenic variant in the *BRCA2* gene would most likely be detected in this family.

71. **A.** Ashkenazi Jews have a substantially elevated risk for hereditary breast and ovarian cancer secondary to a high frequency of *BRCA1/2* mutations mainly attributable to three well-described founder mutations: *c.68_69delAG in the BRCA1 gene, c.5266dupC in the BRCA1 gene, and c.5946delT in the BRCA2 gene.* The c.68_69delAG in *BRCA1* occurs with a frequency of about 1.1% in Ashkenazi Jews. The c.5266dupC (g.38462606dupC) in *BRCA1* has an estimated prevalence of 0.1%–0.15%. The c.5946delT in *BRCA2* occurs with a frequency of about 1.5%. One of 40 Ashkenazi Jewish carriers have one of these three pathogenic variants in *BRCA1/ BRCA2*, accounting for more than 90% of the mutations identified (http://www.ncbi.nlm.nih.gov/books/NBK1247/).

Therefore, targeted-mutation analysis for the three Ashkenazi Jewish founder mutations in *BRCA1* and *BRCA2* would be an effective and cost-efficient way to assess whether this Ashkenazi Jewish woman had a *BRCA1* or *BRCA2* germline mutation, rather than sequence

analysis, as recommended for all other populations.

72. **A.** Ashkenazi Jews have a substantially elevated risk for hereditary breast and ovarian cancer secondary to a high frequency of *BRCA1/2* mutations mainly attributable to three well-described founder mutations: *c.68_69delAG in the BRCA1 gene*, c.5266dupC in the *BRCA1* gene, and c.5946delT in the *BRCA2* gene. The c.68_69delAG in *BRCA1* occurs with a frequency of about 1.1% in Ashkenazi Jews. The c.5266dupC (g.38462606dupC) in *BRCA1* has an estimated prevalence of 0.1%–0.15%. The c.5946delT in *BRCA2* occurs with a frequency of about 1.5%. One of 40 Ashkenazi Jewish carriers have one of these three pathogenic variants in *BRCA1/ BRCA2*, accounting for more than 90% of the mutations identified. The *BRCA2* mutation 999del5 occurs in 0.6% of the Icelandic population and in 10.4% of women and 38% of men with breast cancer from Iceland (http://www.ncbi.nlm.nih.gov/books/NBK1247/).

Therefore, c.68_69delAG in the *BRCA1* gene would most likely be detected in this patient.

73. **B.** Ashkenazi Jews have a substantially elevated risk for hereditary breast and ovarian cancer secondary to a high frequency of *BRCA1/2* mutations mainly attributable to three well-described founder mutations: c.68_69delAG in the *BRCA1* gene, c.5266dupC in the *BRCA1* gene, and *c.5946delT in the BRCA2 gene*. The c.68_69delAG in *BRCA1* occurs with a frequency of about 1.1% in Ashkenazi Jews. The c.5266dupC (g.38462606dupC) in *BRCA1* has an estimated prevalence of 0.1%–0.15%. The c.5946delT in *BRCA2* occurs with a frequency of about 1.5%. One of 40 Ashkenazi Jewish carriers have one of these three pathogenic variants in *BRCA1/BRCA2*, accounting for more than 90% of the mutations identified. Studies in the Dutch population have identified three large deletions within *BRCA1*. These deletions, detected using Southern blot analysis, accounted for 36% of mutations in a sample of high-risk Dutch families (http://www.ncbi.nlm.nih.gov/books/NBK1247/).

Therefore, c.5946delT in the *BRCA2* gene would most likely be detected in this patient.

74. **A.** Ashkenazi Jews have a substantially elevated risk for hereditary breast and ovarian cancer secondary to a high frequency of *BRCA1/2* mutations mainly attributable to three well-described founder mutations: c.68_69delAG in the *BRCA1* gene, *c.5266dupC in the BRCA1 gene*, and c.5946delT in the *BRCA2* gene. The c.68_69delAG in *BRCA1* occurs with a frequency of about 1.1% in Ashkenazi Jews. The c.5266dupC

(g.38462606dupC) in *BRCA1* has an estimated prevalence of 0.1%−0.15%. The c.5946delT in *BRCA2* occurs with a frequency of about 1.5%. One of 40 Ashkenazi Jewish carriers have one of these three pathogenic variants in *BRCA1/BRCA2*, accounting for more than 90% of the mutations identified (http://www.ncbi.nlm.nih.gov/books/NBK1247/).

Therefore, c.5266dupC in the *BRCA1* gene would most likely be detected in this patient.

75. **A.** One of 40 Ashkenazi Jews carries one of three pathogenic variants in *BRCA1/BRCA2*, c.68_69delAG in the *BRCA1* gene, c.5266dupC in the *BRCA1* gene, and c.5946delT in the *BRCA2* gene, accounting for more than 90% of the mutations identified. This is attributed to *the founder effect*, where a gene mutation is observed with high frequency in a population founded by a small ancestral group that was once geographically or culturally isolated and in which one or more of the founders was a carrier of the mutant gene. The mutation may be rare in the original population (http://www.ncbi.nlm.nih.gov/books/NBK1247/).

Genetic drift, along with natural selection, mutation, and migration, is the basic mechanism of evolution. It is a process in which allele frequencies within a population change by chance alone as a result of sampling error from generation to generation. The term *genetic heterogeneity* is used to describe disorders, or traits caused by genetic factors and nongenetic factors. Another example of genetic heterogeneity is diabetes, which has both genetic and environmental components. The term *variable expressivity* refers to the range of signs and symptoms that can occur in different people with the same genetic condition. For example, the features of Marfan syndrome vary widely—some people have only mild symptoms (such as being tall and thin with long, slender fingers), while others also experience life-threatening complications involving the heart and blood vessels. Although the features are highly variable, most people with this disorder have a mutation in *FBN1* (http://ghr.nlm.nih.gov). *Penetrance* refers to the proportion of people with a particular genetic change who exhibit signs and symptoms of a genetic disorder. If some people with the mutation do not develop features of the disorder, the condition is said to have reduced or incomplete penetrance. For example, many people with a mutation in the *BRCA1* or *BRCA2* gene will develop cancer during their lifetime, but some people will not. Physicians cannot predict which individual with these pathogenic variants will develop cancer or when the tumors will develop (http://ghr.nlm.nih.gov).

Therefore, the high frequency of certain deleterious mutations in those of Ashkenazi Jewish descent is due to the founder effect. It is not only true for *BRCA1*- and *BRCA2*-related hereditary breast/ovarian cancer, but also for other high-frequency diseases in those of Ashkenazi Jewish descent, such as Tay−Sachs disease, Canavan disease, Niemann−Pick disease type 4, Gaucher disease, familial dysautonomia, Bloom syndrome, Fanconi anemia type C, mucolipidosis IV, and cystic fibrosis.

76. **D.** *Penetrance* refers to the proportion of people with a particular genetic change who exhibit signs and symptoms of a genetic disorder. If some people with the mutation do not develop features of the disorder, the condition is said to have *reduced, or incomplete, penetrance*. For example, many people with a mutation in the *BRCA1* or *BRCA2* gene will develop cancer during their lifetime, but some people will not. Physicians cannot predict which individual with these pathogenic variants will develop cancer or when the tumors will develop (http://ghr.nlm.nih.gov).

A founder effect occurs when a new population is started by a few members of the original population and when there is a lack of genetic variation due to a small mating population. Some of the rare pathogenic variants in the original population may become common in this new population. Genetic drift, along with natural selection, mutation, and migration, is the basic mechanisms of evolution. It is a process in which allele frequencies within a population change by chance alone as a result of sampling error from generation to generation. The term *genetic heterogeneity* is used to describe disorders or traits caused by genetic and nongenetic factors. Another example of genetic heterogeneity is diabetes, which has both genetic and environmental components. *Variable expressivity* refers to the range of signs and symptoms that can occur in different people with the same genetic condition. For example, the features of Marfan syndrome vary widely—some people have only mild symptoms (such as being tall and thin with long, slender fingers), while others also experience life-threatening complications involving the heart and blood vessels. Although the features are highly variable, most people with this disorder have a mutation in *FBN1* (http://ghr.nlm.nih.gov).

Therefore, incomplete penetrance is the increased risk and uncertainty of malignances in patients with deleterious mutations for hereditary cancer predisposition syndromes.

77. **F.** Besides the *BRCA1* and *BRCA2* genes, a significantly increased risk of breast cancer is also a feature of several other genetic syndromes. These include Cowden syndrome, which is caused by germline pathogenic variants in the *PTEN* gene; hereditary diffuse gastric cancer, which results from germline pathogenic variants in the *CDH1* gene; Li—Fraumeni syndrome, which is caused by germline pathogenic variants in the *TP53* gene; and Peutz—Jeghers syndrome, which results from germline pathogenic variants in the *STK11* gene. Germline pathogenic variants in the *ATM*, *CHEK2*, and *PALB2* genes are also associated with an increased risk of breast cancer.

However, pathogenic variants *in the VHL gene for Von Hippel—Lindau are not associated with an increased risk for breast cancer.*

78. **C.** Gail and colleagues described a risk-assessment model that focuses primarily *on nongenetic risk factors, with limited information on family history.* The model is an interactive tool designed by scientists at the National Cancer Institute (NCI) and at the National Surgical Adjuvant Breast and Bowel Project to estimate a woman's risk of developing invasive breast cancer. The risk factors used were age at menarche, age at first live birth, number of previous breast biopsies, and number of first-degree relatives with breast cancer. A model of relative risks for various combinations of these factors was developed from case—control data from the Breast Cancer Detection Demonstration Project. The Gail model was originally designed to determine eligibility for the Breast Cancer Prevention Trial and has since been modified (in part to adjust for race) and made available on the NCI website. The model has been validated in a number of settings and probably works best in general assessment clinics, where family history is not the main reason for referral. The major limitation of the Gail model is the inclusion of only first-degree relatives, which results in underestimating risk in the 50% of families with cancer in the paternal lineage and also takes no account of the age at onset of breast cancer.

The Claus model is for familial risk of breast cancer. The BRCAPRO model is about *BRCA1* and *BRCA2* mutation frequencies, cancer penetrance in mutation carriers, cancer status, and age of the consultee's first-degree and second-degree relatives. The Tyrer—Cuzick model integrates family history, surrogate measures of endogenous estrogen exposure, and benign breast disease in a comprehensive fashion.

Therefore, Gail model is suitable to individuals without personal history of breast cancer(s), and limited information on family history.

79. **B.** *Claus and colleagues developed a risk model for familial risk of breast cancer in a large population-based, case—control study conducted by the Centers for Disease Control and Prevention (CDC).* The data were based on 4730 histologically confirmed breast cancer cases in patients 20—54 years of age and on 4688 controls, who were frequency matched to cases on the basis of both geographic region and 5-year categories of age. Family histories with regard to breast cancer in mothers and sisters were obtained through interviews with the cases and controls. The effect of genotype on the risk of breast cancer was shown to be a function of a woman's age. Carriers of the risk allele were at greater risk at all ages, although the ratio of age-specific risks was greatest at young ages and declined steadily thereafter. The cumulative lifetime risk of breast cancer for women who carried the susceptibility allele was predicted to be high, approximately 92%, while the cumulative lifetime risk for noncarriers was estimated to be 10%. An expansion of the original Claus model estimates breast cancer risk in women with a family history of ovarian cancer. The major drawback of the Claus model is that it does not include any of the nonhereditary risk factors. Another potential drawback of the Claus tables is that they reflect risks for women in the 1980s in the United States. These risks are lower than the current incidence in both North America and most of Europe. As such, an upward adjustment of 3%—4% for lifetime risk is necessary for lifetime risks below 20%.

The Gail model focuses primarily on nongenetic risk factors, with limited information on family history. Concordance of the Gail and Claus models has been shown to be relatively poor, with the greatest discrepancies seen with nulliparity, multiple benign breast biopsies, and a strong paternal or first-degree family history. The BRCAPRO model is about *BRCA1* and *BRCA2* mutation frequencies, cancer penetrance in mutation carriers, cancer status, and age of the consultee's first-degree and second-degree relatives. The Tyrer—Cuzick model integrates family history, surrogate measures of endogenous estrogen exposure, and benign breast disease in a comprehensive fashion.

Therefore, the Claus model is suitable to individuals with family history of breast cancer(s) and/or ovarian cancer(s) and not including the unaffected family members.

80. **B.** Parmigiani and colleagues developed a Bayesian model called the "BRCAPRO model." *It incorporated published BRCA1 and BRCA2 mutation frequencies, cancer penetrance in mutation carriers, cancer status, and age of the consultee's first-degree and second-degree relatives.* An advantage of this model is that it includes information on both affected and unaffected relatives. In addition, it provides estimates for the likelihood of finding either a *BRCA1* or a *BRCA2* pathogenic variant in a family. An output that calculates breast cancer risk using the likelihood of *BRCA1/2* can be utilized. None of the nonhereditary risk factors can yet be incorporated into the model.

The major drawback from the aspect of breast cancer risk assessment is that no other "genetic" element is allowed for. As such, this model will underestimate risk only in families with breast cancer. The model predicted only 49% of the breast cancers that actually occurred in the screened group of 1900 women.

The Gail model focuses primarily on nongenetic risk factors, with limited information on family history. The Claus model is for familial risk of breast cancer. The Tyrer–Cuzick model integrates family history, surrogate measures of endogenous estrogen exposure, and benign breast disease in a comprehensive fashion.

Therefore, the BRCAPRO model is suitable for individuals with a family history of breast cancer(s) and/or ovarian cancer(s), including unaffected family members.

81. **F.** The Tyrer–Cuzick model is based partly on a data set acquired from the International Breast Intervention Study and other epidemiological data. *It integrates family history, surrogate measures of endogenous estrogen exposure and benign breast disease in a comprehensive fashion.* The major advantage over the Claus model and the BRCAPRO model is that the Tyrer–Cuzick model allows for the presence of multiple genes of differing penetrance. It does produce a readout of *BRCA1/2*, but also allows for a lower penetrance of *BRCAX*. The Tyrer–Cuzick model addresses many of the pitfalls of the previous models, significantly, the combination of extensive family history, endogenous estrogen exposure and benign breast disease (atypical hyperplasia).

The Gail model focuses primarily on nongenetic risk factors, with limited information on family history. The Claus model is for familial

risk of breast cancer. The BRCAPRO model is about *BRCA1* and *BRCA2* mutation frequencies, cancer penetrance in mutation carriers, cancer status, and age of the consultee's first-degree and second-degree relatives.

Therefore, the Tyrer–Cuzick model is suitable to integrate family history, surrogate measures of endogenous estrogen exposure, and benign breast disease in a comprehensive fashion.

82. **A.** Mutations in all five genes are associated with an increased risk for breast cancer. *BRCA1 and BRCA2 are usually associated with estrogen, progesterone, and Her2/neu negative (triple-negative) breast cancer.* Families who have a predominance of premenopausal breast cancer are more likely to have a *BRCA1* or *BRCA2* mutation than a *TP53* mutation. Germline pathogenic variants in the *TP53* gene are thought to account for fewer than 1% of total breast cancer cases, and Li–Fraumeni syndrome (LFS)–related breast cancers are usually estrogen-, progesterone-, and Her2/neu-positive (triple-positive). Childhood cancers are not increased among people with a single mutated *BRCA1* or *BRCA2* allele. *STK11* and *PALB2* are not associated with early-onset breast cancer.

Therefore, sequencing reflex to del/dup analysis of *BRCA1* and *BRCA2* would be most appropriate for this patient to rule out genetic etiologies.

83. **B.** *Soft-tissue sarcoma, osteosarcoma, and adrenocortical carcinoma (ACC) are common in individuals with Li–Fraumeni syndrome (LFS).* The other common malignancies in individuals with LFS are premenopausal breast cancer, brain tumors, and leukemias. LFS is diagnosed in individuals meeting established clinical criteria or in those who have a germline pathogenic variant in the *TP53* gene regardless of family cancer history. Approximately 80% of individuals diagnosed clinically have an identifiable germline pathogenic variant in *TP53*, the only gene so far identified in which germline pathogenic variants are definitively associated with LFS (http://www.ncbi.nlm.nih.gov/books/NBK1311/).

Lynch syndrome (hereditary nonpolyposis colorectal cancer [HNPCC]) is characterized by an increased risk for colon cancer and cancers of the endometrium, ovary, stomach, small intestine, hepatobiliary tract, urinary tract, brain, and skin. *PTEN* hamartoma tumor syndrome, including Cowden syndrome, is characterized by an increased risk for benign and malignant tumors of the thyroid, breast, and endometrium. Affected individuals usually have macrocephaly, trichilemmomas, and papillomatous papules, and present by the late 20s. von–Hippel–Lindau (VHL) disease is characterized by hemangioblastomas of the brain, spinal cord, and retina; renal cysts and clear-cell renal-cell carcinoma; pheochromocytoma, pancreatic cysts, and neuroendocrine tumors; endolymphatic sac tumors; and epididymal and broad ligament cysts.

This patient had a personal history of adrenocortical carcinoma and rhabdomyosarcoma and a family history of osteosarcoma.

Therefore, it would be most likely this patient had LFS if she had hereditary cancer predisposition syndrome.

84. **F.** Soft-tissue sarcoma, osteosarcoma, and adrenocortical carcinoma (ACC) are common in individuals with Li–Fraumeni syndrome (LFS). The other common malignancies in individuals with LFS are premenopausal breast cancer, brain tumors, and leukemias. LFS is diagnosed in individuals meeting established clinical criteria or in those who have a germline pathogenic variant in the *TP53* gene regardless of family cancer history. *Approximately 80% of individuals diagnosed clinically have an identifiable germline pathogenic in TP53, the only gene so far identified in which germline pathogenic variants are definitively associated with LFS.* The prevalence of LFS in Ashkenazi Jews is not higher than in general population, and no pathogenic variants are more common in Ashkenazi Jews than in other populations (http://www.ncbi.nlm.nih.gov/books/NBK1311/).

Chromosome breakage study is the diagnostic test for Fanconi anemia. Chromosome karyotype is the diagnostic test for cytogenetic abnormalities, such as trisomy 21. Chromosome microarray analysis is the first-line test for individuals with multiple congenital anomalies, developmental delay, intellectual disability, and autism and is used to detect copy-number gain or loss. ACMG-recommended CMA as the first-line test for individuals with multiple congenital anomalies, developmental delay, intellectual disability, and autism. Methylation study is used to identify epigenetic changes in the genome, such as Prader–Willi and Angelman syndromes. Next-generation sequencing (NGS) is a high-throughput test to sequence multiple genes at the same time. *Sanger sequencing* is still the most appropriate molecular test for single-gene disorders when the most pathogenic variants are single-nucleotide variants and in/dels, such as Li–Fraumeni syndrome. Targeted-mutation analysis is used to identify specific mutations, which is a cost-effective test when there is a founder effect in a population, such as sickle cell

disease. Targeted-mutation analysis is also commonly used to diagnose family members after the mutation is identified in the proband. Quantitative measurement of telomere length by flow FISH is the laboratory test are used to aid the diagnosis of dyskeratosis congenita.

Therefore, Sanger sequencing would most likely be used to identify a pathogenic variant in *TP53* to confirm the diagnosis in this patient.

85. **E.** Soft-tissue sarcoma, osteosarcoma, and adrenocortical carcinoma (ACC) are common in individuals with Li–Fraumeni syndrome (LFS). The other common malignancies in individuals with LFS are premenopausal breast cancer, brain tumors, and leukemias. LFS is diagnosed in individuals meeting established clinical criteria or in those who have a germline pathogenic variant in *the TP53 gene* regardless of family cancer history. Approximately 80% of individuals diagnosed clinically have an identifiable germline pathogenic variant in *TP53*, the only gene so far identified in which germline pathogenic variants are definitively associated with LFS (http://www.ncbi.nlm.nih.gov/books/NBK1311/).

Germline pathogenic variants in the *CDH1* gene are associated with hereditary diffuse gastric cancer. Germline pathogenic variants in the *MLH1* gene are associated with Lynch syndrome (hereditary nonpolyposis colon cancer [HNPCC]). Germline pathogenic variants in the *SMAD4* gene are associated with juvenile polyposis syndrome. Germline pathogenic variants in the *PTEN* gene are associated with *PTEN* hamartoma tumor syndrome, including Cowden syndrome.

This patient has a personal history of adrenocortical carcinoma and rhabdomyosarcoma and a family history of osteosarcoma. So most likely this patient had LFS.

Therefore, sequencing analysis of the *TP53* gene would be the most appropriate test for this patient.

86. **D.** Germline pathogenic variants in all five genes are associated with increased risks for breast cancer. The *BRCA1* and *BRCA2* genes are usually associated with estrogen-, progesterone-, and Her2/neu-negative (triple-negative) breast cancer. Families who have a predominance of premenopausal breast cancer are more likely to have a *BRCA1* or *BRCA2* mutation than a *TP53* mutation. However, childhood cancers are not increased among people with a single mutated *BRCA1* or *BRCA2* allele. In this case, the patient had estrogen-, progesterone-, and Her2/neu-positive (triple-positive) breast cancer and childhood rhabdomyosarcoma. The likelihood of

the patient having a *BRCA1* or *BRCA2* mutation is significantly decreased.

The next one on line is germline pathogenic variants in the TP53 gene associated with Li–Fraumeni syndrome (LFS). Germline *TP53* mutations are thought to account for fewer than 1% of total breast cancer cases. LFS-related breast cancers are usually estrogen-, progesterone-, and Her2/neu-positive (*triple-positive*). LFS is a cancer predisposition syndrome associated with the development of the following classic tumors: soft-tissue sarcoma, osteosarcoma, premenopausal breast cancer, brain tumors, adrenocortical carcinoma (ACC), and leukemias. Individuals with LFS are at increased risk of developing cancer at younger than typical ages. Individuals with LFS are also at increased risk of developing multiple primary tumors. The risk to individuals with LFS of developing a second cancer has been estimated at 57% and the risk of a third malignancy 38%. The most commonly occurring sarcomas associated with LFS were rhabdomyosarcomas before age 5 years and osteosarcomas at any age. LFS-related breast cancers are usually estrogen-, progesterone-, and Her2/neu-positive (triple-positive).

Germline pathogenic variants in the *STK11* and *PALB2* genes are associated with an increased risk for breast cancer but not early-onset breast cancer and/or rhabdomyosarcomas.

Therefore, molecular genetic analysis of the *TP53* gene would be most appropriate for this patient to rule out genetic etiologies.

87. **D.** Rhabdomyosarcoma (RMS) is a cancer made up of cells that normally develop into skeletal muscles. *It is one of the most common sarcomas in patients with Li–Fraumeni syndrome.*

von Hippel–Lindau (VHL) disease is characterized by hemangioblastomas of the brain, spinal cord, and retina; renal cysts and clear-cell renal-cell carcinoma; pheochromocytoma, pancreatic cysts, and neuroendocrine tumors; endolymphatic sac tumors; and epididymal and broad ligament cysts. Germline pathogenic variants in the *VHL* gene are associated with VHL (http://www.ncbi.nlm.nih.gov/books/NBK1463/). Wilms tumor, also called "nephroblastoma," is a type of cancer that starts in the kidneys. It is the most common type of kidney cancer in children. Germline pathogenic variants in the *WT1* gene are associated with Wilms tumor. Retinoblastoma is a cancer that starts in the retina. It is the most common type of eye cancer in children. Germline pathogenic variants in the *RB1* gene are associated with retinoblastoma.

Therefore, sequencing reflex to del/dup analysis of *TP53* would be the most appropriate test for this patient to rule out genetic etiologies.

88. **D.** Adrenocortical carcinoma (ACC) is an aggressive cancer originating in the cortex (steroid hormone–producing tissue) of the adrenal gland. *Children with ACC have a 50%–80% chance of having a germline pathogenic variant in the TP53 gene, even in the absence of additional family history.* Individuals with adult-onset ACC may also be at increased risk for a germline *TP53* mutation, especially if diagnosed before age 50 years. In one series, 5.8% of individuals diagnosed with ACC after age 18 years tested positive for a germline *TP53* mutation (http://www.ncbi.nlm.nih.gov/books/NBK1311/).

von Hippel–Lindau (VHL) disease is characterized by hemangioblastomas of the brain, spinal cord, and retina; renal cysts and clear-cell renal-cell carcinoma; pheochromocytoma, pancreatic cysts and neuroendocrine tumors; endolymphatic sac tumors; and epididymal and broad ligament cysts. Germline pathogenic variants in the *VHL* gene are associated with VHL (http://www.ncbi.nlm.nih.gov/books/NBK1463/). Wilms tumor, also called "nephroblastoma," is a type of cancer that starts in the kidneys. It is the most common type of kidney cancer in children. Germline pathogenic variants in the *WT1* gene are associated with Wilms tumor. Retinoblastoma is a cancer that starts in the retina. It is the most common type of eye cancer in children. Germline pathogenic variants in the *RB1* gene are associated with retinoblastoma.

Therefore, sequencing reflex to del/dup analysis of *TP53* would be the most appropriate test for this patient to rule out genetic etiologies.

89. **D.** The choroid plexus papilloma is a rare, benign tumor most common in children under the age of 2. The choroid plexus carcinoma is the malignant form of this tumor. *The likelihood of germline TP53 mutations in children with CPC is high, even in the absence of a family history suggestive of Li–Fraumeni syndrome (LFS).* Individuals with LFS are at increased risk of developing many types of brain tumors, such as astrocytomas, glioblastomas, medulloblastomas, and *choroid plexus carcinomas (CPCs).* LFS-related brain tumors can occur in childhood or adulthood; the median age at onset is 16 years (http://www.ncbi.nlm.nih.gov/books/NBK1311/).

von Hippel–Lindau (VHL) disease is characterized by hemangioblastomas of the brain, spinal cord, and retina; renal cysts and clear-cell renal-cell carcinoma; pheochromocytoma, pancreatic cysts, and neuroendocrine tumors; endolymphatic sac tumors; and epididymal and broad ligament cysts. Germline pathogenic variants in the *VHL* gene are associated with VHL (http://www.ncbi.nlm.nih.gov/books/NBK1463/). Wilms tumor, also called "nephroblastoma," is a type of cancer that starts in the kidneys. It is the most common type of kidney cancer in children. Germline pathogenic variants in the *WT1* gene are associated with Wilms tumor. Retinoblastoma is a cancer that starts in the retina. It is the most common type of eye cancer in children. Germline pathogenic variants in the *RB1* gene are associated with retinoblastoma.

Therefore, sequencing reflex to del/dup analysis of *TP53* would be the most appropriate test for this patient to rule out genetic etiologies.

90. **C.** *Li−Fraumeni syndrome (LFS)* is an autosomal dominant cancer predisposition syndrome associated with the development of soft tissue sarcoma, *osteosarcoma*, premenopausal *breast cancer*, brain tumors, *adrenocortical carcinoma* (ACC), and leukemias. LFS is diagnosed in individuals meeting established clinical criteria or in those who have a germline pathogenic variant in *the TP53 gene,* regardless of family cancer history. At least 70% of individuals diagnosed clinically have an identifiable germline mutation in *TP53. TP53* is the only gene identified to date in which pathogenic variants are definitively associated with LFS (http://www.ncbi.nlm.nih.gov/books/NBK1311/).

Cowden syndrome, caused by a germline pathogenic variant in *PTEN*, is a multiple-hamartoma syndrome with an increased risk for benign and malignant tumors of the thyroid, breast, and endometrium. Hereditary breast and ovarian cancer syndrome (HBOC), caused by a germline pathogenic variant in *BRCA1* or *BRCA2*, is characterized by an increased risk for breast cancer, ovarian cancer, prostate cancer, and pancreatic cancer. Individuals with multiple endocrine neoplasia type 1 (MEN1), caused by germline pathogenic variants in the *MEN1* gene, have an increased risk of developing parathyroid tumors, pituitary tumors, pancreatic tumors, carcinoid tumors, and adrenocortical tumors, but not familial medullary thyroid cancer (FMTC). Individuals with multiple endocrine neoplasia type 2 (MEN2), caused by germline pathogenic variants in the *RET* gene, have an increased risk of developing familial medullary thyroid cancer (FMTC). von Hippel−Lindau (VHL) disease, caused by a germline pathogenic variant in the *VHL* gene, is characterized by hemangioblastomas

of the brain, spinal cord, and retina; renal cysts and clear-cell renal-cell carcinoma, pheochromocytoma, pancreatic cysts and neuroendocrine tumors; endolymphatic sac tumors; and epididymal and broad ligament cysts.

Therefore, LFS would most likely be consistent with the clinical presentations in this family.

91. **D.** Li−Fraumeni syndrome (LFS) is an autosomal dominant cancer predisposition syndrome associated with the development of soft-tissue sarcoma, *osteosarcoma*, premenopausal *breast cancer*, brain tumors, *adrenocortical carcinoma* (ACC), and leukemias. LFS is diagnosed in individuals meeting established clinical criteria or in those who have a germline mutation in *the TP53 gene* regardless of family cancer history. At least 70% of individuals diagnosed clinically have an identifiable germline mutation in *TP53. TP53* is the only gene identified to date in which pathogenic variants are definitively associated with LFS (http://www.ncbi.nlm.nih.gov/books/NBK1311/).

Hereditary breast and ovarian cancer syndrome (HBOC), caused by a germline pathogenic variant in *BRCA1* or *BRCA2*, is characterized by an increased risk for breast cancer, ovarian cancer, prostate cancer, and pancreatic cancer. Cowden syndrome, caused by a germline pathogenic variant in the *PTEN* gene, is a multiple-hamartoma syndrome with an increased risk for benign and malignant tumors of the thyroid, breast, and endometrium. Germline pathogenic variants in the *PTEN* gene are associated Cowden syndrome. von Hippel−Lindau (VHL) disease, caused by a germline pathogenic variant in the *VHL* gene, is characterized by hemangioblastomas of the brain, spinal cord, and retina; renal cysts and clear-cell renal-cell carcinoma, pheochromocytoma, pancreatic cysts and neuroendocrine tumors; endolymphatic sac tumors; and epididymal and broad ligament cysts.

Therefore, *TP53* associated with LFS should be tested first to confirm/rule out for a genetic etiology in this family.

92. **D.** von Hippel−Lindau (VHL) disease is an autosomal dominant hereditary cancer predisposition syndrome characterized by hemangioblastomas of the brain, spinal cord, and retina; renal cysts and *clear-cell renal-cell carcinoma; pheochromocytoma*, pancreatic cysts and neuroendocrine tumors; endolymphatic sac tumors; and epididymal and broad ligament cysts. *Germline pathogenic variants in the VHL gene*

on 3p25.3 is the only gene associated with VLH. Any individual presenting with a pheochromocytoma should be evaluated for VHL (http://www.ncbi.nlm.nih.gov/books/NBK1463/).

Multiple endocrine neoplasia type 2 (MEN2) accounts for more than 12% of individuals with hereditary pheochromocytoma. Approximately 5% of individuals with nonsyndromic pheochromocytoma and no family history of pheochromocytoma demonstrate a pathogenic variant in the *RET* gene for MEN2. However, clear-cell renal-cell carcinoma is not common in patients with MEN2. Approximately 8.5% of individuals with apparently nonfamilial nonsyndromic pheochromocytoma have been shown to have a pathogenic variant in one of the succinate dehydrogenase subunit genes, such as *SDHD* or *SDHB*, that cause the hereditary paraganglioma—pheochromocytoma syndromes.

This patient had pheochromocytoma and a history of multiple focal clear-cell renal-cell carcinomas. It is most likely that he had VHL caused by a pathogenic variant in the *VHL* gene than MEN2 or hereditary paraganglioma—pheochromocytoma syndromes associated with *SDHD* or *SDHB*.

Therefore, sequencing reflex to del/dup analysis of *VHL* would be most appropriate for this patient to rule out genetic etiologies.

93. **D.** The probability that pheochromocytoma is hereditary is estimated to be 84% for multifocal (including bilateral) tumors, and 59% for tumors with onset at or before age 18 years. Approximately 25% of individuals with pheochromocytoma and no known family history of pheochromocytoma may have an inherited disease caused by a mutation in one of four genes: *RET*, *VHL*, *SDHD*, or *SDHB*. The recently discovered pheochromocytoma susceptibility genes *TMEM127*, *MAX*, and *SDHA* further expand the differential diagnosis for nonsyndromic paraganglioma and pheochromocytoma.

Individuals with Li—Fraumeni syndrome (LFS) are at increased risk of developing many types of brain tumors, such as astrocytomas, glioblastomas, medulloblastomas, choroid plexus carcinomas, but not pheochromocytoma. TP53 is the only gene so far identified in which mutations are definitively associated with LFS (http://www.ncbi.nlm.nih.gov/books/NBK1311/).

Therefore, a molecular test of the *TP53* gene would be not an appropriate test for this patient.

94. **F.** *von Hippel—Lindau (VHL) disease*, caused by a germline pathogenic variant in the *VHL* gene, is characterized by *hemangioblastomas of the brain*, spinal cord, and retina; renal cysts and *clear-cell renal-cell carcinoma, pheochromocytoma*, pancreatic cysts, and neuroendocrine tumors; endolymphatic sac tumors; and epididymal and broad ligament cysts.

Cowden syndrome, caused by a germline pathogenic variant in *PTEN*, is a multiple-hamartoma syndrome with an increased risk for benign and malignant tumors of the thyroid, breast, and endometrium. Hereditary breast and ovarian cancer syndrome (HBOC), caused by a germline pathogenic variant in *BRCA1* or *BRCA2*, is characterized by an increased risk for breast cancer, ovarian cancer, prostate cancer, and pancreatic cancer. Li—Fraumeni syndrome (LFS) is an autosomal dominant cancer predisposition syndrome associated with the development of soft-tissue sarcoma, osteosarcoma, premenopausal breast cancer, brain tumors, adrenocortical carcinoma (ACC), and leukemias. LFS is diagnosed in individuals meeting established clinical criteria or in those who have a germline mutation in the *TP53* gene, regardless of family cancer history. Individuals with multiple endocrine neoplasia type 1 (MEN1), caused by germline pathogenic variants in the *MEN1* gene, have an increased risk of developing parathyroid tumors, pituitary tumors, pancreatic tumors, carcinoid tumors, and adrenocortical tumors, but not familial medullary thyroid cancer (FMTC). Individuals with multiple endocrine neoplasia type 2 (MEN2), caused by germline pathogenic variants in the *RET* gene, have an increased risk of developing familial medullary thyroid cancer (FMTC).

Therefore, VHL would most likely be consistent with the clinical presentations in this family.

95. **D.** A pheochromocytoma is a neuroendocrine tumor of the medulla of the adrenal glands originating in the chromaffin cells, or extraadrenal chromaffin tissue that failed to involute after birth and secretes high amounts of catecholamines, mostly norepinephrine, plus epinephrine to a lesser extent. Up to 25% of pheochromocytomas may be familial. Pathogenic variants of the genes *VHL*, *RET*, *NF1*, *SDHB* and *SDHD* are known to be associated with familial pheochromocytoma. Therefore, this disease may be accompanied by von Hippel—Lindau disease, neurofibromatosis, or familial paraganglioma depending on the pathogenic variant.

TP53 is the only gene associated with autosomal dominant Li—Fraumeni syndrome

(LFS), a cancer predisposition syndrome. *Individuals with LFS do not have a significantly increased risk of developing pheochromocytoma.*

Therefore, the *TP53* gene would most likely not be expected in a next-generation sequencing (NGS) panel for pheochromocytoma.

96. **E.** *von Hippel–Lindau (VHL) disease,* caused by a germline pathogenic variant in *the VHL gene,* is characterized by *hemangioblastomas of the brain,* spinal cord, and retina; renal cysts and *clear-cell renal-cell carcinoma, pheochromocytoma,* pancreatic cysts, and neuroendocrine tumors; endolymphatic sac tumors; and epididymal and broad ligament cysts.

Cowden syndrome, caused by a germline pathogenic variant in *PTEN,* is a multiple-hamartoma syndrome with an increased risk for benign and malignant tumors of the thyroid, breast, and endometrium. Germline pathogenic variants in the *PTEN* gene are associated with Cowden syndrome. Hereditary breast and ovarian cancer syndrome (HBOC), caused by a germline pathogenic variant in *BRCA1* or *BRCA2,* is characterized by an increased risk for breast cancer, ovarian cancer, prostate cancer, and pancreatic cancer. Li–Fraumeni syndrome (LFS) is an autosomal dominant cancer predisposition syndrome associated with the development of soft-tissue sarcoma, osteosarcoma, premenopausal breast cancer, brain tumors, adrenocortical carcinoma (ACC), and leukemias. LFS is diagnosed in individuals meeting established clinical criteria or in those who have a germline mutation in the *TP53* gene, regardless of family cancer history. Individuals with multiple endocrine neoplasia type 1 (MEN1), caused by germline pathogenic variants in the *MEN1* gene, have an increased risk of developing parathyroid tumors, pituitary tumors, pancreatic tumors, carcinoid tumors, and adrenocortical tumors but not familial medullary thyroid cancer (FMTC). Individuals with multiple endocrine neoplasia type 2 (MEN2), caused by germline pathogenic variants in the *RET* gene, have an increased risk of developing familial medullary thyroid cancer (FMTC).

Therefore, *VHL,* associated with VHL disease, should be tested first to confirm/rule out for a genetic etiology in this family.

97. **A.** *Cowden syndrome,* caused by a germline pathogenic variant in *PTEN,* is a multiple-hamartoma syndrome with an increased risk for *benign and malignant tumors of the thyroid, breast, and endometrium.*

Hereditary breast and ovarian cancer syndrome (HBOC), caused by a germline

pathogenic variant in *BRCA1* or *BRCA2,* is characterized by an increased risk for breast cancer, ovarian cancer, prostate cancer, and pancreatic cancer. Li–Fraumeni syndrome (LFS) is an autosomal dominant cancer predisposition syndrome associated with the development of soft-tissue sarcoma, osteosarcoma, premenopausal breast cancer, brain tumors, adrenocortical carcinoma (ACC), and leukemias. LFS is diagnosed in individuals meeting established clinical criteria or in those who have a germline mutation in the *TP53* gene, regardless of family cancer history. Individuals with multiple endocrine neoplasia type 1 (MEN1), caused by germline pathogenic variants in the *MEN1* gene, have an increased risk of developing parathyroid tumors, pituitary tumors, pancreatic tumors, carcinoid tumors, and adrenocortical tumors but not familial medullary thyroid cancer (FMTC). Individuals with multiple endocrine neoplasia type 2 (MEN2), caused by germline pathogenic variants in the *RET* gene, have an increased risk of developing familial medullary thyroid cancer (FMTC). von Hippel–Lindau (VHL) disease, caused by a germline pathogenic variant in the *VHL* gene, is characterized by hemangioblastomas of the brain, spinal cord, and retina; renal cysts and clear-cell renal-cell carcinoma, pheochromocytoma, pancreatic cysts, and neuroendocrine tumors; endolymphatic sac tumors; and epididymal and broad ligament cysts.

Therefore, Cowden syndrome would most likely be consistent with the clinical presentations in this family.

98. **C.** *Cowden syndrome, caused by a germline pathogenic variant in PTEN, is a multiple-hamartoma syndrome with an increased risk for benign and malignant tumors of the thyroid, breast, and endometrium.*

Hereditary breast and ovarian cancer syndrome (HBOC), caused by a germline pathogenic variant in *BRCA1* or *BRCA2,* is characterized by an increased risk for breast cancer, ovarian cancer, prostate cancer, and pancreatic cancer. Li–Fraumeni syndrome (LFS) is an autosomal dominant cancer predisposition syndrome associated with the development of soft-tissue sarcoma, osteosarcoma, premenopausal breast cancer, brain tumors, adrenocortical carcinoma (ACC), and leukemias. LFS is diagnosed in individuals meeting established clinical criteria or in those who have a germline mutation in the *TP53* gene, regardless of family cancer history. Individuals with multiple endocrine neoplasia type 1 (MEN1), caused by germline pathogenic variants in the *MEN1* gene, have an increased risk of developing parathyroid tumors, pituitary tumors, pancreatic tumors, carcinoid tumors, and adrenocortical tumors but not familial medullary thyroid cancer (FMTC). Individuals with multiple endocrine neoplasia type 2 (MEN2), caused by germline pathogenic variants in the *RET* gene, have an increased risk of developing familial medullary thyroid cancer (FMTC). von Hippel–Lindau (VHL) disease, caused by a germline pathogenic variant in the *VHL* gene, is characterized by hemangioblastomas of the brain, spinal cord, and retina; renal cysts and clear-cell renal-cell carcinoma, pheochromocytoma, pancreatic cysts, and neuroendocrine tumors; endolymphatic sac tumors; and epididymal and broad ligament cysts.

Therefore, *PTEN* associated with Cowden syndrome should be tested to confirm/rule out a genetic etiology in this family.

99. **B.** The *PTEN* hamartoma tumor syndrome (PHTS), including Cowden syndrome (CS), Bannayan–Riley–Ruvalcaba syndrome (BRRS), *PTEN*-related Proteus syndrome (PS), and Proteus-like syndrome. CS is a multiple-hamartoma syndrome with an increased risk for benign and malignant tumors of the thyroid, breast, and endometrium. Affected individuals usually have macrocephaly, trichilemmomas, and papillomatous papules and present by the late 20s. The lifetime risk of developing breast cancer is 85%, with an average age at diagnosis between 38 and 46 years. The lifetime risk for thyroid cancer is approximately 35%. The risk for endometrial cancer may approach 28%. *PTEN* is the only gene in which pathogenic variants are known to cause PHTS. *The most common type of thyroid cancer in individuals with PHTS is follicular, rarely papillary, but never medullary thyroid cancer* (http://www.ncbi.nlm.nih.gov/books/NBK1116/ ?term = Cowden + syndrome +).

Therefore, it would be most likely the members of this family with PHTS had follicular thyroid cancer.

100. **C.** The *PTEN* hamartoma tumor syndrome (PHTS), including Cowden syndrome (CS), Bannayan–Riley–Ruvalcaba syndrome (BRRS), *PTEN*-related Proteus syndrome (PS), and Proteus-like syndrome. CS is a multiple-hamartoma syndrome with an increased risk for benign and malignant tumors of the thyroid, breast, and endometrium. Affected individuals usually have macrocephaly, trichilemmomas, and papillomatous papules and present by the late

20s. The lifetime risk of developing breast cancer is 85%, with an average age at diagnosis between 38 and 46 years. The lifetime risk for thyroid cancer is approximately 35%. The risk for endometrial cancer may approach 28%. *PTEN* is the only gene in which pathogenic variants are known to cause PHTS. *The most common type of thyroid cancer in individuals with PHTS is follicular, rarely papillary, but never medullary thyroid cancer* (http://www.ncbi.nlm.nih.gov/books/NBK1116/ ?term = Cowden + syndrome +).

Therefore, it would be most likely the members of this family with PHTS did not have medullary thyroid cancer.

101. **A.** *The lifetime risk of developing breast cancer is 85% in patients with Cowden syndrome.* The lifetime risk for thyroid cancer is approximately 35%. The risk for endometrial cancer may approach 28%. Other cancers that have been identified in people with Cowden syndrome include colorectal cancer, kidney cancer, and melanoma (http://www.ncbi.nlm.nih.gov/books/ NBK1116/?term = Cowden + syndrome +).

Therefore, breast cancer is the most common type of malignancy in individuals with Cowden syndrome.

102. **B.** Gastric cancer was the only type of malignancy in this family. And the members had it at an early age. At the top of list of differential diagnoses is *hereditary diffuse gastric cancer (HDGC)*. HDGC confers an autosomal dominant susceptibility for diffuse gastric cancer, a poorly differentiated adenocarcinoma that infiltrates into the stomach wall causing thickening of the wall (linitis plastica) without forming a distinct mass. Diffuse gastric cancer is also referred to as signet-ring carcinoma or isolated cell–type carcinoma. The average age at onset of hereditary diffuse gastric cancer is 38 years (range, 14–69). Germline pathogenic variants in the *CDH1* gene account for an estimated 30%–50% of HDGC. The majority of the cancers in individuals with *CDH1* mutations occur before age 40 years. The estimated cumulative risk for gastric cancer by age 80 years is 67% for men and 83% for women. Women also have a 39%–52% risk for lobular breast cancer (http://www. ncbi.nlm.nih.gov/books/NBK1139/).

Cowden syndrome, caused by a germline pathogenic variant in *PTEN*, is a multiple-hamartoma syndrome with an increased risk for benign and malignant tumors of the thyroid, breast, and endometrium. Germline pathogenic variants in the *PTEN* gene are associated with Cowden syndrome. Li–Fraumeni syndrome (LFS) is an autosomal dominant cancer predisposition syndrome associated with the development of soft-tissue sarcoma, osteosarcoma, premenopausal breast cancer, brain tumors, adrenocortical carcinoma (ACC), and leukemias. LFS is diagnosed in individuals meeting established clinical criteria or in those who have a germline mutation in the *TP53* gene, regardless of family cancer history. Individuals with multiple endocrine neoplasia type 1 (MEN1), caused by germline pathogenic variants in the *MEN1* gene, have an increased risk of developing parathyroid tumors, pituitary tumors, pancreatic tumors, carcinoid tumors, and adrenocortical tumors but not familial medullary thyroid cancer (FMTC). Individuals with multiple endocrine neoplasia type 2 (MEN2), caused by germline pathogenic variants in the *RET* gene, have an increased risk of developing familial medullary thyroid cancer (FMTC). von Hippel–Lindau (VHL) disease, caused by a germline pathogenic variant in the *VHL* gene, is characterized by hemangioblastomas of the brain, spinal cord, and retina; renal cysts and clear-cell renal-cell carcinoma, pheochromocytoma, pancreatic cysts, and neuroendocrine tumors; endolymphatic sac tumors; and epididymal and broad ligament cysts.

Therefore, hereditary diffuse gastric cancer (HDGC) would be consistent with the clinical presentations in this family.

103. **A.** Gastric cancer was the only type of malignancy in this family. And the members had it at an early age. At the top of list of differential diagnoses is *hereditary diffuse gastric cancer (HDGC)*. HDGC confers an autosomal dominant susceptibility for diffuse gastric cancer, a poorly differentiated adenocarcinoma that infiltrates into the stomach wall causing thickening of the wall (linitis plastica) without forming a distinct mass. Diffuse gastric cancer is also referred to as signet-ring carcinoma or isolated cell type carcinoma. The average age at onset of HDGC is 38 years (range, 14–69). *Germline pathogenic variants in the CDH1 gene account for an estimated 30%–50% of HDGC.* The majority of the cancers in individuals with *CDH1* mutations occur before age 40 years. The estimated cumulative risk for gastric cancer by age 80 years is 67% for men and 83% for women. Women also have a 39%–52% risk for lobular breast cancer (http://www.ncbi.nlm.nih. gov/books/NBK1139/).

Gastric cancer has also been recognized as a part of the tumor spectrum in other inherited cancer predisposition syndromes, such as hereditary nonpolyposis colorectal cancer (HNPCC, also called "Lynch syndrome"), and Li–Fraumeni syndrome. HNPCC is caused by germline pathogenic variants in *MLH1, MSH2, MSH6, PMS2,* or *EpCAM.* The most common malignancies in individuals with NHPCC are colorectal cancer (CRC) and endometrial carcinoma in females. Li–Fraumeni syndrome is caused by germline pathogenic variants in *TP53.* The most common malignancies in individuals with Li–Fraumeni syndrome are soft-tissue sarcoma, osteosarcoma, premenopausal breast cancer, brain tumors, adrenocortical carcinoma (ACC), and leukemias. In addition, stomach cancer has been seen in individuals with *BRCA2, RUNX3, HPP1, Caspase-10,* and *SMAD4.*

Cowden syndrome, caused by a germline pathogenic variant in *PTEN,* is a multiple-hamartoma syndrome with an increased risk for benign and malignant tumors of the thyroid, breast, and endometrium. Individuals with multiple endocrine neoplasia type 1 (MEN1), caused by germline pathogenic variants in the *MEN1* gene, have an increased risk of developing parathyroid tumors, pituitary tumors, pancreatic tumors, carcinoid tumors, and adrenocortical tumors, but not familial medullary thyroid cancer (FMTC). Individuals with multiple endocrine neoplasia type 2 (MEN2), caused by germline pathogenic variants in the *RET* gene, have an increased risk of developing familial medullary thyroid cancer (FMTC). von Hippel–Lindau (VHL) disease, caused by a germline pathogenic variant in the *VHL* gene, is characterized by hemangioblastomas of the brain, spinal cord, and retina; renal cysts and clear-cell renal-cell carcinoma, pheochromocytoma, pancreatic cysts, and neuroendocrine tumors; endolymphatic sac tumors; and epididymal and broad ligament cysts.

Therefore, *CDH1* associated with HDGC should be tested first to confirm/rule out a genetic etiology in this family.

104. **A.** Hereditary diffuse gastric cancer (HDGC) confers an autosomal dominant susceptibility for diffuse gastric cancer, a poorly differentiated adenocarcinoma that infiltrates into the stomach wall causing thickening of the wall (linitis plastica) without forming a distinct mass. Diffuse gastric cancer is also referred to as signet-ring carcinoma or isolated cell–type carcinoma. The average age at onset of hereditary diffuse gastric cancer is 38 years (range, 14–69). Mutation of *CDH1* accounts for an estimated 30%–50% of HDGC. The majority of the cancers in individuals with *CDH1* mutations occur before age 40 years.

The estimated cumulative risk for gastric cancer by age 80 years is 67% for men and 83% for women. *Women also have a 39%—52% risk for lobular breast cancer* (http://www.ncbi.nlm.nih.gov/books/NBK1139/).

Therefore, this female patient in the question also has increased risk of developing breast cancer.

105. **B.** Hereditary diffuse gastric cancer (HDGC) confers an autosomal dominant susceptibility for diffuse gastric cancer, a poorly differentiated adenocarcinoma that infiltrates into the stomach wall causing thickening of the wall (linitis plastica) without forming a distinct mass. Diffuse gastric cancer is also referred to as signet-ring carcinoma or isolated cell—type carcinoma. The average age at onset of hereditary diffuse gastric cancer is 38 years (range, 14—69). Mutation of *CDH1* accounts for an estimated 30%—50% of HDGC. The majority of the cancers in individuals with *CDH1* mutations occur before age 40 years. *The estimated cumulative risk for gastric cancer by age 80 years is 67% for men and 83% for women.* Women also have a 39%—52% risk for lobular breast cancer (http://www.ncbi.nlm.nih.gov/books/NBK1139/).

Therefore, women carriers of germline pathogenic variants in the *CDH1* gene have higher risk of developing gastric cancer than male carriers.

106. **C.** Hereditary diffuse gastric cancer (HDGC) is an autosomal dominant susceptibility for diffuse gastric cancer, a poorly differentiated adenocarcinoma that infiltrates into the stomach wall causing thickening of the wall (linitis plastica) without forming a distinct mass. *CDH1* is the only gene in which pathogenic variants are known to cause hereditary HDGC. The average age at onset of HDGC is 38 years (range, 14—69). The majority of the cancers in individuals with a *CDH1* pathogenic variant occur before age 40. The estimated cumulative risk of gastric cancer by age 80 is 80% for both men and women. *Women also have a 39%—52% risk for lobular breast cancer.* At-risk women should undergo regular breast screening as determined by their physicians, including monthly breast self-examinations and a clinical breast examination every 6 months. However, there is no direct evidence that colorectal cancer is part of the spectrum of cancers associated with *CDH1* germline mutations (http://www.ncbi.nlm.nih.gov/books/NBK1139/).

Therefore, this female patient would have an increased risk of developing lobular breast cancer in addition to gastric cancer.

107. **D.** Hereditary diffuse gastric cancer (HDGC) is an autosomal dominant susceptibility for diffuse gastric cancer, a poorly differentiated adenocarcinoma that infiltrates into the stomach wall causing thickening of the wall (linitis plastica) without forming a distinct mass. *CDH1* is the only gene in which pathogenic variants are known to cause hereditary HDGC. The average age at onset of HDGC is 38 years (range, 14—69). The majority of the cancers in individuals with a *CDH1* pathogenic variant occur before age 40. *The estimated cumulative risk of gastric cancer by age 80 is 80% for both men and women* (http://www.ncbi.nlm.nih.gov/books/NBK1139/).

Therefore, this patient would have 80% risk of developing diffused gastric cancer if she did not get gastrectomy.

108. **B.** Fanconi anemia (FA) is characterized by physical abnormalities, bone-marrow failure, and increased risk of malignancy. Physical abnormalities, such as short stature; abnormal skin pigmentation; malformations of the thumbs, forearms, skeletal system, eyes, kidneys, and urinary tract; and developmental delay are present in 60%—75% of affected individuals. Progressive bone-marrow failure with pancytopenia typically presents in the first decade, often initially with thrombocytopenia or leukopenia. Individuals with FA also have an increased risk of developing MDS, AML, or solid tumors (http://www.ncbi.nlm.nih.gov/books/NBK1401/).

The diagnostic test for FA is chromosome breakage study for increased chromosome breakage or rearrangement in the presence of diepoxybutane (DEB) or mitomycin C (MMC). There are at least 15 FA genes identified. Most of abnormalities of Fanconi anemia (FA) genes are inherited in an autosomal recessive manner except for *germline pathogenic variants in FANCB, which are inherited in an X-linked manner.* Therefore, Joseph's only brother, *John,* will be the sibling with an increased risk for Fanconi anemia. The other sisters have a 50% chance to be a carrier, and the mother is an obligate carrier.

109. **D.** Fanconi anemia (FA) is characterized by physical abnormalities, bone-marrow failure, and increased risk of malignancy. There are at least 15 FA genes identified. Most of abnormalities of Fanconi anemia (FA) genes are inherited in an autosomal recessive manner except for germline pathogenic variants in the *FANCB* gene, which are inherited in an X-linked manner. *The FANCD1 gene is also called BRCA2.* Fanconi anemia may be caused by homozygous or compound

heterozygous mutations in the *FANCD1/BRCA2*. *A heterozygous mutation of FANCD1/BRCA2 increases the risk of breast/ovarian cancer in the individual* (http://www.ncbi.nlm.nih.gov/books/NBK1401/).

Therefore, if the mother carried a heterozygous mutation in *FANCD1/BRCA2*, she would be at risk of developing breast and/or ovarian cancer.

110. **D.** Fanconi anemia (FA) is characterized by physical abnormalities, bone-marrow failure, and increased risk of malignancy. There are at least 15 FA genes identified. Most of abnormalities of Fanconi anemia (FA) genes are inherited in an autosomal recessive manner except for germline pathogenic variants in the *FANCB* gene, which are inherited in an X-linked manner.

The FANCN gene is also called PALB2. Fanconi anemia may be caused by homozygous or compound heterozygous mutations in the *FANCN/PALB2. A heterozygous mutation of FANCN/PALB2 increases the risk of breast cancer in females* (http://www.ncbi.nlm.nih.gov/books/NBK1401/).

Therefore, if the mother carried a heterozygous mutation in *FANCN/PALB2*, she would be at risk of developing breast cancer.

111. **D.** Fanconi anemia (FA) is characterized by physical abnormalities, bone-marrow failure, and increased risk of malignancy. There are at least 15 FA genes identified. Most of abnormalities of Fanconi anemia (FA) genes are inherited in an autosomal recessive manner except for germline pathogenic variants in the *FANCB* gene, which are inherited in an X-linked manner.

The FANCJ gene is also called BRIP1. Fanconi anemia may be caused by homozygous or compound heterozygous mutations in the *FANCJ/BRIP1. A heterozygous mutation of FANCJ/BRIP1 increases the risk of breast cancer in females* (http://www.ncbi.nlm.nih.gov/books/NBK1401/).

Therefore, if the mother carried a heterozygous mutation in *FANCJ/BRIP1*, she would be at risk of developing breast cancer.

112. **C.** Fanconi anemia (FA) exhibits extensive genetic heterogeneity. There are at least 15 FA genes identified. *A single pathogenic variant in complementation group FA-C, the c.456 + 4A > C in the FANCC gene, is the most common pathogenic variant to FA patients of Ashkenazi Jewish ancestry,* and has a carrier frequency of greater than 1/89 in this population. In addition, a mutation (c.65G > A) in *FANCA* (FA-A is the most common complementation group in non-Jewish patients) and the mutation c.6174delT in *FANCD1/BRCA2* are relatively common in the Ashkenazi Jewish

population, too, but not as common as the c.456 + 4A > C in the *FANCC* gene (http://www.ncbi.nlm.nih.gov/books/NBK1401/).

Therefore, *FANCC* is more likely mutated in this Ashkenazi Jewish patient than the other genes in the question.

113. **D.** Fanconi anemia (FA) is the most common genetic cause of aplastic anemia and one of the most common genetic causes of hematological malignancy. Management focuses on surveillance and treatment of physical abnormalities, bone-marrow failure, leukemia, and solid tumors. Hematopoietic stem-cell transplantation (HSCT) is the only curative therapy for the hematological manifestations of Fanconi anemia (FA), including aplastic anemia, myelodysplastic syndrome, and acute leukemia. *Individuals whose hematological manifestations have been successfully treated with HSCT appear to be at an increased risk for solid tumors, particularly squamous-cell carcinomas of the tongue* (http://www.ncbi.nlm.nih.gov/books/NBK1401/).

Therefore, this Ashkenazi Jewish FA patient would still have an increased risk for solid tumor after HSCT.

114. **A.** Fanconi anemia (FA) is the most common genetic cause of aplastic anemia and one of the most common genetic causes of hematological malignancy. The diagnostic test for FA is a chromosome breakage study for increased chromosome breakage or rearrangement in the presence of diepoxybutane (DEB) or mitomycin C (MMC). Lymphocyte mosaicism can develop in individuals initially found to be sensitive to DEB/MMC. These individuals may have a falsely normal DEB/MMC test. In individuals with a normal DEB/MMC test in whom a high degree of clinical suspicion of FA remains, *diepoxybutane (DEB)/mitomycin C (MMC) testing to establish the diagnosis could be performed on an alternative cell type, such as skin fibroblasts* (http://www.ncbi.nlm.nih.gov/books/NBK1401/).

The FA complementation group can be identified by identifying which of the cDNA of the 15 Fanconi anemia (FA)—related genes, when expressed in the cells of the affected individual, corrects the DEB/MMC sensitivity phenotype. It helps in the identification of the abnormal gene of FA but not of mosaicisms. Sensitivity of FA next-generation sequencing panel is 80%–99%, depending on genetic subtypes. Large exonic deletions are common in the *FANCA* gene and may not be detected by NGS. So NGS may be used to identify the gene/mutation after the diagnosis is established by chromosome breakage study.

Therefore, chromosome breakage study with fibroblast cells would be most appropriate to establish the diagnosis of mosaicism.

115. **B.** Androgens improve the blood counts in approximately 50% of individuals with Fanconi anemia (FA). Individuals with FA receiving androgen treatment for bone-marrow failure are at *increased risk for liver tumors.* But not every individual with liver tumors had received androgens. Fertility is reduced in males with FA due to hypospermia or azoospermia, which is not related to the androgen therapy. Individuals with FA are prone to MDS/AML and relapse after treatment, but it is not related to androgen therapy (http://www.ncbi.nlm.nih.gov/books/NBK1401/).

Therefore, this patient would have an increased risk of developing liver tumors due to the androgen therapy.

116. **D.** Fanconi anemia (FA) is an autosomal recessive disease except if the pathogenic variants are in the *FANCB* gene on chromosome X. Since the mother of the husband had FA, the pathogenic variants in the family must not be from *FANCB* (http://www.ncbi.nlm.nih.gov/books/NBK1401/). The husband was an obligate carrier of an FA causing pathogenic variant inherited from his mother. The wife's family was negative for FA. So the wife's risk of carrying an FA mutation was 1/89 ($\approx 1/100$), the carrier frequency in the Ashkenazi Jewish population.

Therefore, the risk of FA in their child will be $1 \times 1/100 \times 1/4 = 1/400$.

117. **A.** Fanconi anemia (FA) is the most common genetic cause of aplastic anemia and one of the most common genetic causes of hematological malignancy. The diagnostic test for FA is a chromosome breakage study for increased chromosome breakage or rearrangement in the presence of diepoxybutane (DEB) or mitomycin C (MMC). The increased sensitivity to DEB/MMC is present in patients with FA regardless of phenotype, congenital anomalies, or severity of the disease. A single pathogenic variant in complementation group FA-C, the c.456 + 4A > C in the *FANCC* gene, is the most common pathogenic variant in FA patients of Ashkenazi Jewish ancestry; it has a carrier frequency of greater than 1/89 in this population. In addition, a mutation (c.65G > A) in *FANCA* (FA-A is the most common complementation group in non-Jewish patients) and the mutation c.6174delT in *FANCD1/BRCA2* are relatively common in the Ashkenazi Jewish population, too, but not as common as the c.456 + 4A > C in the *FANCC* gene (http://www.ncbi.nlm.nih.gov/books/NBK1401/).

The FA complementation study can be used to identify the mutated cDNA of the 15 Fanconi anemia (FA)–related genes. When the wild type cDNA is expressed in the cells of the affected individual, it corrects the DEB/MMC sensitivity phenotype. It helps to identify the abnormal gene of FA. Next-generation sequencing (NGS) may be used to identify the gene/mutation after the diagnosis is established by chromosome breakage study.

Therefore, it would be most likely that the physician ordered a chromosome breakage study of the peripheral-blood sample.

118. **A.** A frameshift mutations is more likely to be pathogenic than a variant at upstream (c.-490G > T in *FANCG*), in an intron (c.710-12A > G in *FANCA*), or at splice site. It is also more likely to be pathogenic than a synonymous substitution (p.F713F in *FANCB*) or a missense mutation (p.L717G in *FANCB*).

Therefore, it would be most likely that p. S849Ffs*40 in *FANCA* is the pathogenic variant detected in this patient.

119. **B.** Fanconi anemia (FA) is an autosomal recessive disease, except that the mutation is in the *FANCB* gene, which is on the X chromosome. In this case, the boy had a pathogenic variant in the *FANCB* gene. The mother most likely was a silent carrier of the pathogenic variant. There was 1/2 chance the pathogenic variant in *FANCB* would be passed to the unborn child. And there was 1/2 chance if the unborn child was a boy.

Therefore, the unborn child's risk for FA would be $1/2 \times 1/2 = 1/4$.

120. **A.** *Ataxia telangiectasia (AT)*, Bloom syndrome (BS), Fanconi anemia (FA), and Nijmegen breakage syndrome are so-called chromosomal breakage syndromes. All chromosomal breakage syndromes are autosomal recessive conditions. AT is characterized by progressive cerebellar gait beginning between ages 1 and 4 years, oculomotor apraxia, choreoathetosis, telangiectasias of the conjunctivae, immunodeficiency, frequent infections, and an increased risk for malignancy, particularly leukemia and lymphoma. Other features include premature aging, with strands of gray hair, and endocrine abnormalities, such as insulin-resistant diabetes mellitus. Patients with AT are hypersensitive to ionizing radiation with increased susceptibility to cancer, usually leukemia or lymphoma (http://www.ncbi.nlm.nih.gov/books/NBK26468/).

BS is characterized by marked genetic instability, including a high level of sister chromatid exchanges associated with a greatly increased predisposition to a wide range of cancers that commonly affect the general population. The common clinical features of BS are proportionate prenatal and postnatal growth retardation and caner predisposition. Additional clinical features include dolichocephaly, facial sun-sensitive telangiectatic erythema, patchy areas of hyperpigmentation and hypopigmentation of the skin and moderate to severe immunodeficiency manifested by recurrent respiratory tract and gastrointestinal infections. FA is characterized by physical abnormalities, bone-marrow failure, and increased risk of malignancy. Physical abnormalities, present in 60%−75% of affected individuals, include one or more of the following: short stature; abnormal skin pigmentation; malformations of the thumbs, forearms, skeletal system, eyes, kidneys and urinary tract, ears (and decreased hearing), heart, gastrointestinal system, and central nervous system; hypogonadism; and developmental delay. Nijmegen breakage syndrome is characterized by progressive microcephaly, intrauterine growth retardation and short stature, recurrent sinopulmonary infections, an increased risk for cancer, and premature ovarian failure in females. Developmental milestones are attained at the usual time during the first year; however, borderline delays in development and hyperactivity may be observed in early childhood. Intellectual abilities tend to decline over time, and most children tested after age 7 have mild to moderate intellectual disability. Recurrent pneumonia and bronchitis may result in respiratory failure and early death. Approximately 40% of affected individuals have developed malignancies before age 20, with the risk being highest for T-cell (55%) and B-cell lymphomas (45%).

This patient's medical and family history support the diagnosis of AT.

Therefore, this patient would most likely have AT if she had a genetic condition.

121. **A.** Ataxia telangiectasia (AT), Bloom syndrome (BS), Fanconi anemia (FA), and Nijmegen breakage syndrome are so-called chromosomal breakage syndromes. All chromosomal breakage syndromes are autosomal recessive conditions. AT is characterized by progressive cerebellar gait beginning between ages 1 and 4 years, oculomotor apraxia, choreoathetosis, telangiectasias of the conjunctivae, immunodeficiency, frequent infections, and an increased risk for malignancy, particularly leukemia and lymphoma. Other features include premature aging with strands of gray hair and endocrine abnormalities, such as insulin-resistant diabetes mellitus. Patients with AT are hypersensitive to ionizing radiation with increased susceptibility to cancer, usually leukemia or lymphoma. Germline pathogenic variants in *the ATM gene* are associated with AT (http://www.ncbi.nlm.nih.gov/books/NBK26468/).

Germline pathogenic variants in the *BLM* gene are associated with BS. Germline pathogenic variants in the *BRIP1* gene, also called *FANCJ*, are associated with FA. Germline pathogenic variants in the *NBN* gene are associated with NBS.

This patient's medical and family history supported the diagnosis of AT.

Therefore, the *ATM* gene would most likely be mutated in this girl.

122. **A.** Ataxia telangiectasia (AT) is an autosomal recessive condition, characterized by progressive gait and truncal ataxia, progressively slurred speech, and oculocutaneous telangiectasia. Other features include premature aging, with strands of gray hair, and endocrine abnormalities, such as insulin-resistant diabetes mellitus. Patients with ataxia telangiectasia (AT) are hypersensitive to ionizing radiation and have an increased susceptibility to cancer, usually leukemia or lymphoma. The risk for malignancy in individuals with classic AT is 38%. Leukemia and lymphoma account for about 85% of malignancies. Younger children tend to have acute lymphocytic leukemia (ALL) of T-cell origin and older children an aggressive T-cell leukemia. Lymphomas are usually B-cell types. As individuals with classic AT are living longer, other cancers and tumors, including ovarian cancer, breast cancer, gastric cancer, melanoma, leiomyomas, and sarcomas, have also been observed (http://www.ncbi.nlm.nih.gov/books/NBK26468/).

And AT carriers are heterozygotes for this autosomal recessive disorder. *Carriers are not at increased risk of developing AT neurological manifestations, but are at a fourfold increased risk of developing breast cancer through mechanisms that are not understood.*

Therefore, the mother of the patient, as a carrier of the ATM pathogenic variant, would have an increased risk of developing breast cancer.

123. **B.** Ataxia telangiectasia (AT) is *an autosomal recessive condition* characterized by progressive cerebellar gait beginning between ages 1 and 4

years, oculomotor apraxia, choreoathetosis, telangiectasias of the conjunctivae, immunodeficiency, frequent infections, and an increased risk for malignancy, particularly leukemia and lymphoma. Other features include premature aging, with strands of gray hair, and endocrine abnormalities, such as insulin-resistant diabetes mellitus. Patients with AT are hypersensitivity to ionizing radiation and have an increased susceptibility to cancer, usually leukemia or lymphoma. Germline pathogenic variants in the *ATM* gene are associated with AT (http://www.ncbi.nlm.nih.gov/books/NBK26468/).

The parents were obligate carriers.

Therefore, the unborn sibling of this patient would have 1/4 chance to have same condition.

124. **E.** Bloom syndrome (BS) is one of the chromosomal breakage syndromes caused by homozygous or compound heterozygous pathogenic variants in the *BLM* gene. BS is characterized by marked genetic instability, including a high level of sister chromatid exchanges associated with a greatly increased predisposition to a wide range of cancers that commonly affect the general population. The common clinical features of BS are proportionate prenatal and postnatal growth retardation and caner predisposition. Additional clinical features include dolichocephaly, facial sun-sensitive telangiectatic erythema, patchy areas of hyperpigmentation and hypopigmentation of the skin and moderate to severe immunodeficiency manifested by recurrent respiratory tract and gastrointestinal infections. The diagnosis of BS is established in a proband by identification of biallelic pathogenic variants in *BLM* on molecular genetic testing or, if molecular genetic testing is inconclusive, with *identification of increased frequency of sister chromatid exchanges on specialized cytogenetic studies* (http://www.ncbi.nlm.nih.gov/books/NBK1398/).

Chromosome breakage study is the diagnostic test for Fanconi anemia. Chromosome karyotype is the diagnostic test for cytogenetic abnormalities, such as trisomy 21. Methylation study is used to identify epigenetic changes in the genome, such as Prader—Willi and Angelman syndromes. Multiplex ligation-dependent probe amplification (MLPA) is a time-efficient technique to detect genomic deletions and insertions bigger than single-nucleotide variants and in/dels, but they smaller than what can be detected on CMA. Next-generation sequencing (NGS) is a high-throughput test to sequence multiple genes at the same time. Sanger sequencing is still the most appropriate molecular test for single-gene

disorders when the most pathogenic variants are single-nucleotide variants and in/dels, such as in Li—Fraumeni syndrome.

Therefore, sister chromatid exchange would most likely be used to diagnose Bloom syndrome in this patient.

125. **B.** All the diseases listed in the question are chromosome-instability syndromes. Fanconi anemia causes extensive chromosome breakage with the existence of DEB/MMC. *Bloom syndrome is associate with increased sister chromatic exchange, which can be used to diagnose Bloom syndrome.* Ataxia telangiectasia is associated with increased chromosomal breakage or cell death of white blood cells after exposure to X-rays.

Therefore, it would be most likely that this patient had Bloom syndrome.

126. **B.** *Bloom syndrome (BS) is one of the chromosomal breakage syndromes caused by homozygous or compound heterozygous pathogenic variants in the BLM gene.* BS is characterized by marked genetic instability, including a high level of sister chromatid exchanges associated with a greatly increased predisposition to a wide range of cancers that commonly affect the general population. The common clinical features of BS are proportionate prenatal and postnatal growth retardation and caner predisposition. Additional clinical features include dolichocephaly, facial sun-sensitive telangiectatic erythema, patchy areas of hyperpigmentation and hypopigmentation of the skin and moderate to severe immunodeficiency manifested by recurrent respiratory tract and gastrointestinal infections. The diagnosis of BS is established in a proband with identification of biallelic pathogenic variants in *BLM* on molecular genetic testing or, if molecular genetic testing is inconclusive, with identification of an increased frequency of sister chromatid exchanges on specialized cytogenetic studies (http://www.ncbi.nlm.nih.gov/books/NBK1398/).

Germline pathogenic variants in the *ATM* gene are associated with ataxia telangiectasia (AT). Germline pathogenic variants in the *BRIP1* gene, also called *FANCJ*, are associated with Fanconi anemia (FA). Germline pathogenic variants in the *NBN* gene are associated with Nijmegen breakage syndrome.

This patient's medical and the test results support the diagnosis of BS.

Therefore, the *BLM* gene would most likely be mutated in this girl.

127. **B.** *Bloom syndrome (BS) is one of autosomal recessive chromosomal breakage syndromes caused by homozygous or compound heterozygous pathogenic*

variants in the BLM gene. BS is characterized by marked genetic instability, including a high level of sister chromatid exchanges associated with a greatly increased predisposition to a wide range of cancers that commonly affect the general population. The common clinical features of BS are proportionate prenatal and postnatal growth retardation and caner predisposition. Additional clinical features include dolichocephaly, facial sun-sensitive telangiectatic erythema, patchy areas of hyperpigmentation and hypopigmentation of the skin and moderate to severe immunodeficiency manifested by recurrent respiratory tract and gastrointestinal infections. The diagnosis of BS is established in a proband with identification of biallelic pathogenic variants in *BLM* on molecular genetic testing or, if molecular genetic testing is inconclusive, with identification of increased frequency of sister chromatid exchanges on specialized cytogenetic studies (http://www.ncbi.nlm.nih.gov/books/NBK1398/).

Therefore, this patient's recurrent risk for this autosomal recessive condition was 1/4.

128. **F.** Bloom syndrome (BS) is one of the chromosomal breakage syndromes caused by homozygous or compound heterozygous pathogenic variants in the *BLM* gene. Approximately 1 in 48,000 Ashkenazi Jews are affected by Bloom syndrome, accounting for about one-third of affected individuals worldwide. The predominant pathogenic variant identified in Ashkenazi Jews with Bloom syndrome is c.2207_2212delinsTAGATTC, a 6-bp deletion along with a 7-bp insertion in exon 10 of *BLM*. This mutation is designated blm^{Ash}. The allele frequency of blm^{Ash} in Ashkenazi Jewish individuals with BS is more than 95%. And the carrier frequency of this pathogenic variant is 1% in Ashkenazi Jews. The second most common pathogenic variant is c.2407dupT (http://www.ncbi.nlm.nih.gov/books/NBK1398/). Both sister chromatid exchanges and targeted-mutation analysis can be used to diagnose Bloom syndrome in this Ashkenazi Jewish girl. However, *targeted-mutation analysis is more cost-effective than sister chromatid exchange study.*

Chromosome breakage study is the diagnostic test for Fanconi anemia. Chromosome karyotype is the diagnostic test for cytogenetic abnormalities, such as trisomy 21. Methylation study is used to identify epigenetic changes in the genome, such as Prader–Willi and Angelman syndromes. Multiplex ligation-dependent probe amplification (MLPA) is a time-efficient technique

to detect genomic deletions and insertions bigger than single-nucleotide variants and in/dels, but smaller than what can be detected on CMA. Next-generation sequencing (NGS) is a high-throughput test to sequence multiple genes at the same time. Sanger sequencing is still the most appropriate molecular test for single-gene disorders when the most pathogenic variants are single-nucleotide variants and in/dels, such as in Li–Fraumeni syndrome. Targeted-mutation analysis is used to identify specific mutations, making it a cost-effective test when there is founder effect in a population. Targeted-mutation analysis is also commonly used to diagnose family members after the mutation is identified in the proband.

Therefore, targeted-mutation analysis would be the more cost-effective genetic workup to confirm the diagnosis in this Ashkenazi Jewish girl.

129. **D.** Bloom syndrome (BS) is an autosomal recessive disease caused by germline pathogenic variants in the *BLM* gene. The mother of the wife was an obligate carrier of a BS-causing allelic variant inherited from her mother. The wife has 1/2 of the chance to be a carrier. The husband's family is negative for BS. So his risk of carrying a BS mutation is 1/100 as the carrier frequency in the Ashkenazi Jewish population.

Therefore, the risk of BS in their child will be $1/2 \times 1/100 \times 1/4 = 1/800.$

130. **D.** Bloom syndrome is an autosomal recessive disease caused by pathogenic variants in the *BLM* gene. Approximately 1 in 48,000 Ashkenazi Jews are affected by Bloom syndrome, accounting for about one-third of affected individuals worldwide. *The predominant pathogenic variant identified in Ashkenazi Jews with Bloom syndrome is c.2207_2212delinsTAGATTC, a 6-bp deletion along with a 7-bp insertion in exon 10 of BLM. This* mutation is designated blm^{Ash}, and the carrier frequency of this pathogenic variant is 1% in Ashkenazi Jews. The second most common pathogenic variant is c.2407dupT (http://www.ncbi.nlm.nih.gov/books/NBK1398/).

Nijmegen breakage syndrome is inherited in an autosomal recessive manner, too. The c.657_661del5 pathogenic variant predominates in affected persons from Eastern Europe, accounting for more than 90% of all mutant alleles in the *NBN* gene. In the United States, about 70% of individuals tested to date are homozygous for this common allele, 15% are heterozygous for c.657_661del5 and a second unique pathogenic variant, and 15% are homozygous for a unique pathogenic variant. Individuals homozygous for the *NBN* c.1089C > A pathogenic variant have features of Fanconi anemia (http://www.ncbi.nlm.nih.gov/books/NBK1176/).

Therefore, the c.2207_2212delinsTAGATTC in the *BLM* gene is referred as *blm*^Ash.

131. **E.** Cockayne syndrome is an autosomal recessive disorder characterized by cachectic dwarfism, cutaneous photosensitivity, loss of adipose tissue, mental retardation, skeletal and neurological abnormalities, and retinopathy. The prognosis is poor. Most affected children die by the second decade of life. Unfortunately, there is no treatment other than supportive measures. The diagnosis is basically clinical, though supportive diagnostic tests are available, including computed tomography (CT) of the brain, bone X-ray, and genetic analysis. The two genes in which mutations are known to cause Cockayne syndrome are *ERCC6* (65% of individuals) and *ERCC8* (35% of individuals). *Most variants can be detected by DNA sequence analysis of the coding and flanking intronic regions of the genes.* Deletion/duplication analysis and/or sequencing of the cDNA can detect additional variants in a minority of cases. Because of the founder effect, Ashkenazi Jewish individuals are at high risk for several autosomal recessive diseases, such as Gaucher disease and Bloom syndrome. However, Cockayne syndrome does not show higher prevalence in Ashkenazi Jews than in other populations. So targeted-mutation analysis does not have adequate detection rate for Cockayne syndrome as a diagnostic test (http://www.ncbi.nlm.nih.gov/books/NBK1342/).

Chromosome breakage study is the diagnostic test for Fanconi anemia. Chromosome karyotype is the diagnostic test for cytogenetic abnormalities. Methylation study is used to identify epigenetic changes in the genome. Multiplex ligation-dependent probe amplification (MLPA) is a time-efficient technique to detect genomic deletions and insertions bigger than single-nucleotide variants and in/dels, but smaller than what can be detected on CMA. Next-generation sequencing (NGS) is a high-throughput test to sequence multiple genes at the same time. Sanger sequencing is still the most appropriate molecular test for single-gene disorders when the most pathogenic variants are single-nucleotide variants and in/dels. Targeted-mutation analysis is used to identify specific mutations, which is a cost-effective test when there is founder effect in a population. Targeted-mutation analysis is also commonly used to

diagnose family members after the mutation is identified in the proband.

Therefore, the medical geneticist would most likely have ordered Sanger sequencing of the *ERCC6* and *ERCC8* genes to confirm the diagnosis in this patient.

132. **D.** Cockayne syndrome is an autosomal recessive disorder characterized by cachectic dwarfism, cutaneous photosensitivity, loss of adipose tissue, mental retardation, skeletal and neurological abnormalities, and retinopathy. The prognosis is poor. Most affected children die by the second decade of life. Unfortunately, there is no treatment other than supportive measures. The diagnosis is basically clinical, though supportive diagnostic tests are available, including computed tomography (CT) of the brain, bone X-ray, and genetic analysis. The two genes in which germline pathogenic variants are known to cause Cockayne syndrome are *ERCC6* (65% of individuals) and *ERCC8* (35% of individuals) (http://www.ncbi.nlm.nih.gov/books/NBK1342/).

ERCC3, *ERCC4*, and *ERCC5* are associated with autosomal recessive xeroderma pigmentosum. *ERCC4* is also associated with autosomal recessive Fanconi anemia. Therefore, the *ERCC6* gene would most likely be included in the molecular genetic test to confirm the diagnosis in this patient.

133. **D.** Cockayne syndrome is an autosomal recessive disorder characterized by cachectic dwarfism, cutaneous photosensitivity, loss of adipose tissue, mental retardation, skeletal and neurological abnormalities, and retinopathy. The prognosis is poor. Most affected children die by the second decade of life. Unfortunately, there is no treatment other than supportive measures. The diagnosis is basically clinical, though supportive diagnostic tests are available, including computed tomography (CT) of the brain, bone X-ray, and genetic analysis. The two genes in which mutations are known to cause Cockayne syndrome are *ERCC6* (65% of individuals) and *ERCC8* (35% of individuals) (http://www.ncbi.nlm.nih.gov/books/NBK1342/).

ERCC1 is associated with autosomal recessive cerebro-oculo-facio-skeletal syndrome, which is a syndrome, other than Cockayne syndrome, that is caused by pathogenic variants in one of the excision-repair genes without predisposition to malignancies. *ERCC2* is associated autosomal recessive xeroderma pigmentosum. However, a pathogenic variant in *ERCC2* was reported in one patient with Cockayne syndrome. *ERCC7* is not recognized as a gene entity.

Therefore, the *ERCC8* gene would most likely be included in the molecular genetic test to confirm the diagnosis in this patient.

134. **G.** Cockayne syndrome is an autosomal recessive disorder characterized by cachectic dwarfism, cutaneous photosensitivity, loss of adipose tissue, mental retardation, skeletal and neurological abnormalities, and retinopathy. The prognosis is poor. Most affected children die by the second decade of life. Unfortunately, there is no treatment other than supportive measures. The diagnosis is basically clinical, though supportive diagnostic tests are available, including computed tomography (CT) of the brain, bone X-ray, and genetic analysis. The two genes in which mutations are known to cause Cockayne syndrome are *ERCC6* (65% of individuals) and *ERCC8* (35% of individuals) (http://www.ncbi.nlm.nih.gov/books/NBK1342/). Cockayne syndrome is caused by pathogenic variants in one of the excision-repair genes. However, *individuals with the disease are not predisposed to malignancies.*

Therefore, this patient would have no increased risk of developing any of the malignancies listed.

135. **D.** All five diseases listed in the question have postnatal growth failure. *Progeria* is also called "Hutchinson−Gilford progeria syndrome" (HGPS). It is characterized by clinical features that develop in childhood and resemble some features of accelerated aging. Profound failure to thrive occurs during the first year. Death occurs as a result of complications of severe atherosclerosis, either cardiac disease (myocardial infarction) or cerebrovascular disease (stroke), generally between ages 6 and 20 years. The average lifespan is approximately 13 years. Almost all individuals with HGPS have the disorder as the result of a de novo autosomal dominant mutation. *Because HGPS is typically caused by a de novo mutation, the risk to the sibs of a proband is small.* However, because one instance of apparent somatic and germline mosaicism has been reported, the risk for parents of having another child with HGPS may be on the order of one in 500 (http://www.ncbi.nlm.nih.gov/books/NBK1121/).

Bloom syndrome also has prenatal growth failure, characterized as intrauterine growth retardation (IUGR). Fanconi anemia (FA), ataxia telangiectasia (AT), Bloom syndrome (BS), Nijmegen breakage syndrome, Werner syndrome (WS), xeroderma pigmentosum (XP), and Cockayne syndrome (CS) are a group of inherited conditions associated with chromosomal instability and breakage. They often are referred as chromosome breakage or chromosome-instability syndromes. Patients with AT, are hypersensitive to ionizing radiation, while patients with BS, FA, and XP are sensitive to UV radiation. Nevertheless, they all have an increased tendency to develop certain types of malignancies. All the chromosome breakage syndromes are inherited in autosomal recessive mode.

Therefore, progeria is most likely not inherited because HGPS is typically caused by a de novo mutation.

136. **E.** The patient had the classic triad of dyskeratosis congenita (DC): dysplastic nails, lacy reticular pigmentation of the upper chest and/or neck, and oral leukoplakia. DC is a telomere biology disorder. All individuals with DC have abnormally short telomeres for their age, as determined by multicolor flow cytometry fluorescence in situ hybridization (flow-FISH) on white-blood-cell (WBC) subsets. To date, *CTC1, DKC1, TERC, TERT, TINF2, NHP2, NOP10,* and *WRAP53* are the genes in which germline pathogenic variants are known to cause DC and result in very short telomeres. Germline pathogenic variants in one of these eight genes have been identified in approximately half the individuals who meet clinical diagnostic criteria for DC (http://www.ncbi.nlm.nih.gov/books/NBK22301/).

Chromosome breakage study is the diagnostic test for Fanconi anemia. Chromosome karyotype is the diagnostic test for cytogenetic abnormalities, such as trisomy 21. Chromosome microarray analysis is the ACMG-recommended first-line test for individuals with multiple congenital anomalies, developmental delay, intellectual disability, and autism. It used to detect copy-number gain or loss. Methylation study is used to identify epigenetic changes in the genome, such as Prader−Willi and Angelman syndromes. Next-generation sequencing (NGS) is a high-throughput test to sequence multiple genes at the same time. Sanger sequencing is still the most appropriate molecular test for single-gene disorders when the most pathogenic variants are single-nucleotide variants and in/dels, such as Li−Fraumeni syndrome. Targeted-mutation analysis is used to identify specific mutations, which is a cost-effective test when there is a founder effect in a population, such as sickle cell disease. Targeted-mutation analysis is also commonly used to diagnose family members after the mutation is identified in the proband.

Quantitative measurement of telomere length by flow-FISH is the laboratory test used to aid the diagnosis of dyskeratosis congenita.

Therefore, it would be most likely the dermatologist ordered a next-generation sequencing (NGS) panel for DC to confirm the diagnosis in this patient.

137. **D.** The patient had the classic triad of dyskeratosis congenita (DC): dysplastic nails, lacy reticular pigmentation of the upper chest and/or neck, and oral leukoplakia. DC is a telomere biology disorder. *All individuals with DC have abnormally short telomeres for their age, as determined by multicolor flow cytometry fluorescence in situ hybridization (flow-FISH) on white-blood-cell (WBC) subsets.* Telomere length less than the 1st percentile for age in lymphocytes is 97% sensitive and is 91% specific for DC. To date, *CTC1, DKC1, TERC, TERT, TINF2, NHP2, NOP10,* and *WRAP53* are the genes in which germline pathogenic variants are known to cause DC and result in very short telomeres. Germline pathogenic variants in one of these eight genes have been identified in approximately half the individuals who meet clinical diagnostic criteria for DC (http://www.ncbi.nlm.nih.gov/books/NBK22301/).

Chromosome breakage study is the diagnostic test for Fanconi anemia. Chromosome karyotype is the diagnostic test for cytogenetic abnormalities, such as trisomy 21. Chromosome microarray analysis is the first-line test for individuals with multiple congenital anomalies, developmental delay, intellectual disability, and autism. Chromosome microarray analysis is the ACMG-recommended first-line test for individuals with multiple congenital anomalies, developmental delay, intellectual disability, and autism. It used to detect copy-number gain or loss. Methylation study is used to identify epigenetic changes in the genome, such as Prader–Willi and Angelman syndromes. Next-generation sequencing (NGS) is a high-throughput test to sequence multiple genes at the same time. Sanger sequencing is still the most appropriate molecular test for single-gene disorders when the most pathogenic variants are single-nucleotide variants and in/dels, such as Li–Fraumeni syndrome. Targeted-mutation analysis is used to identify specific mutations, which is a cost-effective test when there is founder effect in a population, such as sickle cell disease. Targeted-mutation analysis is also commonly used to diagnose family members after the mutation is identified in the proband.

Quantitative measurement of telomere length by flow-FISH is the laboratory test used to aid the diagnosis of dyskeratosis congenita.

Therefore, flow-FISH would be the most sensitive test to rule out dyskeratosis congenita in this patient.

138. **D.** The patient had the classic triad of dyskeratosis congenita (DC): dysplastic nails, lacy reticular pigmentation of the upper chest and/or neck, and oral leukoplakia. DC is a telomere biology disorder. All individuals with DC have abnormally short telomeres for their age, as determined by multicolor flow cytometry fluorescence in situ hybridization (flow-FISH) on white-blood-cell (WBC) subsets. To date, *CTC1, DKC1, TERC, TERT, TINF2, NHP2, NOP10,* and *WRAP53* are the genes in which germline pathogenic variants are known to cause DC and result in very short telomeres. Germline pathogenic variants in one of these eight genes have been identified in approximately half the individuals who meet clinical diagnostic criteria for DC (http://www.ncbi.nlm.nih.gov/books/NBK22301/).

The mode of inheritance of DC varies by gene. Germline pathogenic variants in *DKC1* cause X-linked DC. Germline pathogenic variants in *TERC* and *TINF2* cause *autosomal dominant* DC. Germline pathogenic variants in *ACD, RTEL1,* and *TERT* cause *autosomal dominant or autosomal recessive* DC. Germline pathogenic variants in *CTC1, NHP2, NOP10, PARN,* and *WRAP53* cause *autosomal recessive* DC.

Therefore, DC could be autosomal dominant, autosomal recessive, or X-linked although in this family DC seemed to be X-linked.

139. **A.** The patient had the classic triad of dyskeratosis congenita (DC): dysplastic nails, lacy reticular pigmentation of the upper chest and/or neck, and oral leukoplakia. DC is a telomere biology disorder. All individuals with DC have abnormally short telomeres for their age, as determined by multicolor flow cytometry fluorescence in situ hybridization (flow-FISH) on white-blood-cell (WBC) subsets. To date, *CTC1, DKC1, TERC, TERT, TINF2, NHP2, NOP10,* and *WRAP53* are the genes in which germline pathogenic variants are known to cause DC and result in very short telomeres. Germline pathogenic variants in one of these eight genes have been identified in approximately half the individuals who meet clinical diagnostic criteria for DC.

The mode of inheritance of DC varies by gene. *DKC1* is located on the X chromosome.

Pathogenic variants *in the DKC1 gene cause X-linked DC*. Pathogenic variants in *TERC* and *TINF2* cause autosomal dominant DC. Pathogenic variants in *ACD, RTEL1,* and *TERT* cause autosomal dominant or autosomal recessive DC. Pathogenic variants in *CTC1, NHP2, NOP10, PARN,* and *WRAP53* cause autosomal recessive DC (http://www.ncbi.nlm.nih.gov/books/NBK22301/).

The family history of this patient indicated that he had an X-linked DC because his mother was a silent carrier and all the affected members in the family were males. Therefore, it would be most likely that this patient had a pathogenic variant in *DKC1* if he had an X-linked DC.

140. **B.** The patient had the classic triad of dyskeratosis congenita (DC): dysplastic nails, lacy reticular pigmentation of the upper chest and/or neck, and oral leukoplakia. DC is a telomere biology disorder. All individuals with DC have abnormally short telomeres for their age, as determined by multicolor flow cytometry fluorescence in situ hybridization (flow-FISH) on white-blood-cell (WBC) subsets. To date, *CTC1, DKC1, TERC, TERT, TINF2, NHP2, NOP10,* and *WRAP53* are the genes in which germline pathogenic variants are known to cause DC and result in very short telomeres. Germline pathogenic variants in one of these eight genes have been identified in approximately half the individuals who meet clinical diagnostic criteria for DC.

The mode of inheritance of DC varies by gene. *DKC1* is located on X chromosome. Pathogenic variants in *DKC1* cause X-linked DC. Pathogenic variants *in TERC and TINF2 cause autosomal dominant DC. Pathogenic variants in ACD, RTEL1, and TERT cause autosomal dominant or autosomal recessive DC. Pathogenic variants in CTC1, NHP2, NOP10, PARN, and WRAP53 cause autosomal recessive DC* (http://www.ncbi.nlm.nih.gov/books/NBK22301/).

The family history of this patient indicated he had an autosomal dominant DC because there were no skipping of generations and both males and females were affected. Therefore, *TERC, TINF2, ACD, RTEL1,* and *TERT* would most likely be included in the genetic test to rule out dyskeratosis congenita in this patient.

141. **E.** Rubinstein–Taybi syndrome (RTS) is an autosomal dominant cancer predisposition syndrome. RTS typically occurs as the result of a de novo mutation in the family, and most individuals represent the only affected member in a family. The diagnosis is primarily based on clinical features.

CREBBP and *EP300* are the only genes currently known to be associated with RTS. FISH analysis of *CREBBP* detects microdeletions in approximately 10% of individuals with RTS. *Sequence analysis detects CREBBP pathogenic variants in another 40%–50% of affected individuals. Pathogenic variants in EP300 are identified in approximately 3%–8% of individuals with RTS* (http://www.ncbi.nlm.nih.gov/books/NBK1526/).

Chromosome breakage study is the diagnostic test for Fanconi anemia. Chromosome microarray analysis is the ACMG-recommended first-line test for individuals with multiple congenital anomalies, developmental delay, intellectual disability, and autism. It is used to detect copy-number gain or loss. Methylation study is used to identify epigenetic changes in the genome, such as Prader–Willi and Angelman syndromes. Multicolor flow cytometry fluorescence in situ hybridization (flow-FISH) on white-blood-cell (WBC) subsets is a diagnostic test for dyskeratosis congenita (DC). Sequencing may refer to next-generation sequencing (NGS) or Sanger sequencing. NGS is a high-throughput test to sequence multiple genes at the same time. Sanger sequencing is still the most appropriate molecular test for single-gene disorders when the most pathogenic variants are single-nucleotide variants and in/dels.

Therefore, sequencing analysis of *CREBBP* and *EP300* would be the first-line genetic test for this patient.

142. **B.** Rubinstein–Taybi syndrome (RTS) is an autosomal dominant cancer predisposition syndrome. RTS typically occurs as the result of a de novo mutation in the family, and most individuals represent the only affected member in a family. The diagnosis is primarily based on clinical features. *CREBBP* and *EP300* are the only genes currently known to be associated with RTS. FISH analysis of *CREBBP* detects microdeletions in approximately 10% of individuals with RTS. *Sequence analysis detects CREBBP pathogenic variants in another 40%–50% of affected individuals. Pathogenic variants in EP300 are identified in approximately 3%–8% of individuals with RTS* (http://www.ncbi.nlm.nih.gov/books/NBK1526/).

Therefore, sequencing analyses of both genes would have 50% chance to detect the pathogenic variant in this patient if he had RTS.

143. **C.** Rubinstein–Taybi syndrome (RTS) is an autosomal dominant cancer predisposition syndrome. RTS typically occurs as the result of a de novo mutation in the family, and most individuals represent the only affected member in

a family. The diagnosis is primarily based on clinical features. *CREBBP* and *EP300* are the only genes currently known to be associated with RTS. *FISH analysis of CREBBP detects microdeletions in approximately 10% of individuals* with RTS. Sequence analysis detects *CREBBP* pathogenic variants in another 40%−50% of affected individuals. Pathogenic variants in *EP300* are identified in approximately 3%−8% of individuals with RTS (http://www.ncbi.nlm.nih.gov/books/NBK1526/).

Chromosome breakage study is the diagnostic test for Fanconi anemia. Chromosome karyotype is the diagnostic test for cytogenetic abnormalities, such as trisomy 21. Chromosome microarray analysis is the ACMG-recommended first-line test for individuals with multiple congenital anomalies, developmental delay, intellectual disability, and autism. It is used to detect copy-number gain or loss. Methylation study is used to identify epigenetic changes in the genome, such as Prader−Willi and Angelman syndromes. Multicolor flow cytometry fluorescence in situ hybridization (flow-FISH) on white-blood-cell (WBC) subsets is a diagnostic test for dyskeratosis congenita (DC).

Therefore, chromosome microarray study would be an appropriate next step in the genetic workup to rule out microdeletions involving *CREBBP* and/or *EP300* in this patient.

144. **B.** *Xeroderma pigmentosum (XP) is an autosomal recessive disorder*. At conception, each sib of an affected individual has a 25% chance of being affected, a 50% chance of being an asymptomatic carrier, and a 25% chance of being unaffected and not a carrier. Once an at-risk sib is known to be unaffected, the risk of his/her being a carrier is 2/3. Prevalence of XP is estimated at 1:1,000,000 in the United States and in Europe. In certain populations, such as the Middle East (Turkey, Israel, and Syria) the prevalence is increased, especially in communities in which consanguineous marriages are common (http://www.ncbi.nlm.nih.gov/books/NBK1397/).

Therefore, siblings of the patient have a 25% chance to have the condition.

145. **G.** Patients with xeroderma pigmentosum (XP) have greatly increased risk (more than 1000-fold) of cutaneous neoplasms (*basal-cell carcinoma, squamous-cell carcinoma, and melanoma*). Nearly 45% of patients with XP develop basal-cell or squamous-cell carcinoma, or both, and approximately 5% develop melanomas. Patients with XP also have a moderately increased risk (10−50-fold) for internal neoplasms, such as brain

tumors, leukemia, *lung tumors*, and *gastric carcinomas* (http://www.ncbi.nlm.nih.gov/books/NBK1397/).

Therefore, this patient will have an increased risk of developing all the malignancies listed in the question.

146. **E.** Patients with xeroderma pigmentosum (XP) have greatly increased risk (more than 1000-fold) of *cutaneous neoplasms (basal-cell carcinoma, squamous-cell carcinoma, and melanoma)*. Nearly 45% of patients with XP develop basal-cell or squamous-cell carcinoma, or both, and approximately 5% develop melanomas. Patients with XP also have a moderately increased risk (10−50-fold) for internal neoplasms, such as brain tumors, leukemia, lung tumors, and gastric carcinomas (http://www.ncbi.nlm.nih.gov/books/NBK1397/).

Therefore, skin cancers, including basal-cell carcinoma, squamous-cell carcinoma, and melanoma will most likely develop in this patient with XP.

147. **B.** Normally, damage to DNA in epidermal cells occurs during exposure to ultraviolet (UV) light. *The absorption of the high energy light leads to two T's that are next to each other stick together making a TT dimer*. In a healthy human being, the damage is first excised by endonucleases. DNA polymerase then repairs the missing sequence, and ligase "seals" the transaction. This process is known as "nucleotide excision repair." But the cell cannot deal very well with too many TT pairs. Some cells with lots of TT dimers will die. This is the reason why our skin peels after sunburn. Cells that cannot fix themselves and do not die could become cancerous. Melanoma is a common UV-induced skin cancer. Xeroderma pigmentosum (XP) is an autosomal recessive genetic defect in which nucleotide excision repair (NER) enzymes are mutated, leading to a reduction in or elimination of NER. If left unchecked, damage caused by UV light can cause mutations in individual cell's DNA (http://www.ncbi.nlm.nih.gov/books/NBK1397/).

The CpG island is a short stretch of DNA in which the frequency of the CG sequence is higher than in other regions, where "p" simply indicates that "C" and "G" are connected by a phosphodiester bond. CpG islands are often located around the promoters of housekeeping genes or other genes frequently expressed in a cell. At these locations, the CpG sequence is not methylated. By contrast, the CpG sequences in inactive genes are usually methylated to suppress their expression. The methylated cytosine may be converted to thymine by accidental deamination.

Therefore, TT dimers are expected to be the most characteristic DNA damage after exposure to UV light in this patient with XP.

148. **D.** Wilms tumor, also called "nephroblastoma," is an embryonal malignancy of the kidney. It is the most common renal tumor of childhood. Wilms tumor usually presents as an abdominal mass in an otherwise apparently healthy child. It has the potential for both local and distant spread. Approximately 5%–10% of children with Wilms tumor have bilateral or multicentric tumors. A germline pathogenic variant in the *WT1* gene is thought to be the cause of about 10%–15% of Wilms tumors. Individuals with Beckwith–Wiedemann syndrome have an increased risk of developing Wilms tumor and hepatoblastoma. Nonsyndromic Wilms tumor most frequently occurs as a single occurrence in a family. *Empiric risks to the sibs of a proband who represents a simplex case are unknown but likely low (up to 1%)* (http://www.ncbi.nlm.nih.gov/books/NBK1294/).

This patient does not have pathogenic variants in *WT1*. The molecular test for Beckwith–Wiedemann syndrome is negative. He does not have a family history of any malignancies. It is most likely he has sporadic Wilms tumor. Therefore, the empiric recurrent risk in the unborn child is <1%.

149. **B.** WAGR (Wilms tumor, aniridia, genitourinary anomalies, and mental retardation) is a syndrome that affects the development of many organ systems. It is caused by a deletion of 11p13. The size of the deletion varies among affected individuals. The *PAX6* and *WT1* genes on 11p13 are always deleted in people with the typical signs and symptoms of WAGR. Because pathogenic variants in the *PAX6* gene can affect eye development, the loss of *PAX6* may be responsible for the characteristic eye features of WAGR syndrome. *PAX6* may also affect brain development. Wilms tumor and genitourinary abnormalities are often the result of mutations in *WT1*, so deletion of *WT1* is very likely the cause of these features in WAGR syndrome (http://www.ncbi.nlm.nih.gov/books/NBK1294/).

Chromosome karyotype study is used to detect chromosome aneuploidies, and structural abnormalities associated with feeding difficulty, hypotonia, developmental delay, intellectual disability, dysmorphic features, et al. in pediatric populations; and recurrent pregnancy loss, and infertility in adult population. Chromosome microarray analysis (CMA) is the ACMG-recommended first-line test for individuals with multiple congenital anomalies, developmental delay, intellectual disability, and autism. It is used to detect copy-number gain or loss. Methylation study is used to identify epigenetic changes in the genome, such as methylation study for Prader–Willi/Angelman syndromes. Sequencing may refer to next-generation sequencing (NGS) or Sanger sequencing. Next-generation sequencing (NGS) is a high-throughput test to sequence multiple genes at the same time. It is an appropriate test for Fanconi anemia, hearing loss, and other conditions. Sanger sequencing is the most appropriate molecular test for single-gene disorders when the most pathogenic variants are single-nucleotide variants and in/dels. It is an appropriate test for Gaucher disease, Wiskott–Aldrich syndrome (WAS), and other conditions. Targeted-mutation analysis is used to identify specific mutations, which is a cost-effective test when there is founder effect in a population. Targeted-mutation analysis is also commonly used to diagnose family members after the mutation is identified in the proband. It is an appropriate carrier test for cystic fibrosis (CF).

Therefore, chromosome microarray analysis would most likely be used for the genetic evaluation to confirm/rule out genetic etiologies in this patient.

150. **E.** The *PTEN* hamartoma tumor syndrome (PHTS), including Cowden syndrome (CS), Bannayan–Riley_Ruvalcaba syndrome (BRRS), *PTEN*-related Proteus syndrome (PS), and Proteus-like syndrome. CS is a multiple-hamartoma syndrome with an increased risk for benign and malignant tumors of the thyroid, breast, and endometrium. Affected individuals usually have macrocephaly, trichilemmomas, and papillomatous papules, and present by the late 20s. The lifetime risk of developing breast cancer is 85%, with an average age of diagnosis between 38 and 46 years. The lifetime risk for thyroid cancer is approximately 35%. The risk for endometrial cancer may approach 28%. *PTEN* is the only gene in which pathogenic variants are known to cause PHTS.

Some people have some of the characteristic features of Cowden syndrome, particularly the cancers associated with this condition, but do not meet the strict criteria for a diagnosis of Cowden syndrome. These individuals are often described as having Cowden-like syndrome. Cowden-like syndrome may be caused by *KLLN* promoter hypermethylation, pathogenic variants in *SDHB*, *SDHC*, *SDHD*, or in *PIK3CA* and *AKT1* (http://www.ncbi.nlm.nih.gov/books/NBK1116/?term = Cowden + syndrome +).

von Hippel—Lindau (VHL) disease, caused by a germline pathogenic variant in the VHL gene, is characterized by hemangioblastomas of the brain, spinal cord, and retina; renal cysts and clear-cell renal-cell carcinoma, pheochromocytoma, pancreatic cysts, and neuroendocrine tumors; endolymphatic sac tumors; and epididymal and broad ligament cysts.

Therefore, the *VHL* gene should not be included in a next-generation sequencing panel for Cowden and Cowden-like syndrome.

151. **A.** *Pleuropulmonary blastoma (PPB), cystic nephroma, benign multinodular goiter, and ovarian sex-cord stromal tumors (Sertoli—Leydig cell tumor) are parts of a cancer susceptibility syndrome, DICER1 syndrome.* DICER1 syndrome is caused by heterozygous pathogenic variants in the *DICER1* gene, which provides instructions for making a protein that is involved in the production of microRNA (miRNA) (http://www.ncbi.nlm.nih.gov/books/NBK196157/).

Pleuropulmonary blastoma, pneumothorax, multinodular goiter, and ovarian Sertoli—Leydig cell tumor are not commonly seen in individuals with Gorlin syndrome, Li—Fraumeni syndrome (LFS), *PTEN* hamartoma tumor syndrome (PHTS), or xeroderma pigmentosum (XP).

Therefore, it was most likely this patient had DICER1 syndrome if he had a hereditary cancer predisposition syndrome.

152. **A.** *DICER1*-related disorder is a familial tumor susceptibility syndrome that confers increased risk most commonly for pleuropulmonary blastoma (PPB), ovarian sex-cord stromal tumors, cystic nephroma (CN), and thyroid-gland neoplasia (multinodular goiter, MNG). *The diagnosis of a DICER1-related disorder may be confirmed by identification of a heterozygous germline pathogenic variant in the DICER1 gene* (http://www.ncbi.nlm.nih.gov/books/NBK196157/).

Pleuropulmonary blastoma and pneumothorax are not commonly seen in individuals with Li—Fraumeni syndrome (LFS), *PTEN* hamartoma tumor syndrome (PHTS), or xeroderma pigmentosum (XP). Germline pathogenic variants in the *TP53* gene are associated with Li—Fraumeni syndrome (LFS). Germline pathogenic variants in the *PTEN* gene are associated with *PTEN* hamartoma tumor syndrome (PHTS), such as Cowden syndrome. Germline pathogenic variants in the *XPA, ERCC1, ERCC3, XPC, ERCC2, DDB2, ERCC4,* and *ERCC5* genes are associated with xeroderma pigmentosum (XP).

This patient had pleuropulmonary blastoma and a family history of pneumothorax in his

uncle, which raises possibility of familial *DICER1*-related disorder. Therefore, the *DICER1* gene would most likely be sequenced to rule out genetic etiologies in this patient.

153. **A.** Pleuropulmonary blastoma (PPB), cystic nephroma, benign multinodular goiter, and ovarian sex-cord stromal tumors (Sertoli—Leydig cell tumor) are parts of a cancer susceptibility syndrome, *DICER1* syndrome. *DICER1 syndrome is caused by heterozygous mutations in the DICER1 gene,* which provides instructions for making a protein that is involved in the production of microRNA (miRNA) (http://www.ncbi.nlm.nih.gov/books/NBK196157/).

Pleuropulmonary blastoma, pneumothorax, multinodular goiter, and ovarian Sertoli—Leydig cell tumor are not commonly seen in individuals with Gorlin syndrome, Li—Fraumeni syndrome (LFS), *PTEN* hamartoma tumor syndrome (PHTS), von Hippel—Lindau syndrome (VHL), or xeroderma pigmentosum (XP). Germline pathogenic variants in the *ERCC2* and *XPA* genes are associated with xeroderma pigmentosum (XP). Germline pathogenic variants in the *PTCH1* gene are associated with Gorlin syndrome. Germline pathogenic variants in the *TP53* gene are associated with Li—Fraumeni syndrome (LFS). Germline pathogenic variants in the *PTEN* gene are associated with *PTEN* hamartoma tumor syndrome (PHTS), such as Cowden syndrome. Germline pathogenic variants in the *VHL* gene are associated with von Hippel—Lindau syndrome (VHL).

Therefore, the *DICER1* gene would the most appropriate first-line genetic workup to rule out genetic etiologies in this patient.

154. **B.** Pleuropulmonary blastoma (PPB), cystic nephroma, benign multinodular goiter, and *ovarian sex-cord stromal tumors (Sertoli—Leydig cell tumor)* are parts of a cancer susceptibility syndrome, *DICER1* syndrome. DICER1 syndrome is caused by heterozygous pathogenic variants in the *DICER1* gene, which provides instructions for making a protein that is involved in the production of microRNA (miRNA).

Patients with PPB most commonly have an increased risk for pleuropulmonary blastoma (PPB), ovarian sex-cord stromal tumors (Sertoli—Leydig cell tumor [SLCT], juvenile granulosa-cell tumor [JGCT], and gynandroblastoma), cystic nephroma (CN), and thyroid-gland neoplasia (multinodular goiter [MNG], adenomas, or differentiated thyroid cancer). Less commonly observed tumors are ciliary body medulloepithelioma (CBME), botryoid-type embryonal rhabdomyosarcoma

(ERMS) of the cervix or other sites, nasal chondromesenchymal hamartoma (NCMH), renal sarcoma, pituitary blastoma, and pineoblastoma (http://www.ncbi.nlm.nih.gov/books/ NBK196157/).

The patient in the question had *DICER1* syndrome. Therefore, his female family members with the familial pathogenic variant in the *DICER1* gene would have an increased risk of developing ovarian sex-cord stromal tumors (Sertoli—Leydig cell tumor).

155. **E.** Pleuropulmonary blastoma (PPB), cystic nephroma, benign multinodular goiter, and ovarian sex-cord stromal tumors (Sertoli—Leydig cell tumor) are parts of a cancer susceptibility syndrome, *DICER1* syndrome. *DICER1* syndrome is caused by heterozygous mutations in the *DICER1* gene, which provides instructions for making a protein that is involved in the production of microRNA (miRNA). The diagnosis of a *DICER1*-related disorder is confirmed by identification of a heterozygous *DICER1* germline pathogenic variant. Therefore, *Sanger sequencing of DICER1 is the first-line genetic test to diagnosis of PPB* (http://www.ncbi.nlm.nih.gov/books/ NBK196157/).

Chromosome karyotype is the diagnostic test for cytogenetic abnormalities, such as trisomy 21. Chromosome microarray analysis (CMA) is the ACMG-recommended first-line test for individuals with multiple congenital anomalies, developmental delay, intellectual disability, and autism. It is used to detect copy number gain or loss. Methylation study is used to identify epigenetic changes in the genome, such as methylation study for Prader—Willi/Angelman syndromes. Quantitative measurement of telomere length by flow-FISH is the laboratory test used to aid the diagnosis of dyskeratosis congenita. Sequencing may refer to next-generation sequencing (NGS) or Sanger sequencing. Next-generation sequencing (NGS) is a high-throughput test to sequence multiple genes at the same time. It is an appropriate test for Fanconi anemia, hearing loss, and other conditions. Sanger sequencing is the most appropriate molecular test for single-gene disorders when the most pathogenic variants are single-nucleotide variants and in/dels. It is an appropriate test for Gaucher disease, Wiskott—Aldrich syndrome (WAS), and other conditions. Targeted-mutation analysis is used to identify specific mutations, which is a cost-effective test when there is founder effect in a population. Targeted-mutation analysis is also

commonly used to diagnose family members after the mutation is identified in the proband. It is an appropriate carrier test for cystic fibrosis (CF).

Therefore, *Sanger sequencing analysis* would be the most appropriate diagnostic assay for this patient to confirm/rule out genetic etiologies.

156. **C.** The patient had characteristics of Gorlin syndrome. Gorlin syndrome, also known as "nevoid basal-cell carcinoma syndrome" (NBCCS), is one of the autosomal dominant hereditary cancer syndromes. It is characterized by a classic pentad of features comprised of *multiple basal-cell carcinomas*, jaw cysts, calcification of the falx cerebri, pitting of the palmar and plantar surfaces, and rib anomalies. Approximately 60% of individuals with this syndrome have a recognizable appearance, with macrocephaly, frontal bossing, coarse facial features, and facial milia (http://www.ncbi.nlm. nih.gov/books/NBK1151/).

Therefore, basal-cell carcinoma would most likely be seen in this patient with Gorlin syndrome.

157. **B.** *Basal-cell carcinoma* is the most common form of skin cancer diagnosed annually in the United States. BCCs are rarely fatal, but they can be highly disfiguring if allowed to grow. Squamous-cell carcinoma is the second most common form of skin cancer. An estimated 700,000 cases of SCC are diagnosed each year in the United States.

Therefore, basal cell carcinoma is is the most common type of skin cancers in Caucasians.

158. **C.** The patient had characteristics of Gorlin syndrome. Gorlin syndrome is also known as "nevoid basal-cell carcinoma syndrome" (NBCCS). Approximately 60% of individuals have a recognizable appearance, with macrocephaly, bossing of the forehead, coarse facial features, and facial milia. Other features of Gorlin syndrome include small depressions (pits) in the skin of the palms of the hands and soles of the feet. In people with Gorlin syndrome, the type of cancer diagnosed most often is basal-cell carcinoma. And 5% of affected individuals develop medulloblastoma during childhood. *In most individuals, the diagnosis of Gorlin syndrome is established using clinical diagnostic criteria. PTCH1 (formerly PTCH) and SUFU are the only genes in which mutations are known to cause Gorlin syndrome* (http:// www.ncbi.nlm.nih.gov/books/NBK1151/).

Germline pathogenic variants in the *DICER1* gene are associated with *DICER1* syndrome. Germline pathogenic variants in the *ERCC2* gene are associated with xeroderma pigmentosum.

Germline pathogenic variants in the *TP53* gene are associated with Li–Fraumeni syndrome (LFS). Germline pathogenic variants in the *PTEN* gene are associated with *PTEN* hamartoma tumor syndrome (PHTS), such as Cowden syndrome. Germline pathogenic variants in the *VHL* gene are associated with von Hippel–Lindau syndrome (VHL).

Therefore, the *PTCH1* gene would most likely harbor a pathogenic variant in this patient if she had Gorlin syndrome.

159. **D.** The patient had characteristics of Gorlin syndrome. Gorlin syndrome is also known as "nevoid basal-cell carcinoma syndrome." Approximately 60% of individuals have a recognizable appearance, with macrocephaly, bossing of the forehead, coarse facial features, and facial milia. Other features of Gorlin syndrome include small depressions (pits) in the skin of the palms of the hands and soles of the feet. In people with Gorlin syndrome, the type of cancer diagnosed most often is basal-cell carcinoma. *And 5% of affected individuals develop medulloblastoma during childhood.* In most individuals, the diagnosis of Gorlin syndrome is established using clinical diagnostic criteria. *PTCH1* (formerly *PTCH*) is the only gene in which mutation is known to cause Gorlin syndrome (http://www.ncbi.nlm.nih.gov/books/NBK1151/).

Therefore, it would be most likely that the patient's maternal uncle died of medulloblastoma.

160. **E.** Dyskeratosis congenita (DC), a telomere biology disorder, is characterized by a classic triad of dysplastic nails, lacy reticular pigmentation of the upper chest and/or neck, and oral leukoplakia. Individuals with DC have an increased risk of developing several life-threatening conditions, such as bone-marrow failure, and pulmonary fibrosis. Approximately half of people with DC have heterozygous mutations in the *TERT*, *TERC*, *DKC1*, or *TINF2* genes (http://www.ncbi.nlm.nih.gov/books/NBK22301/).

Germline pathogenic variants in the *DICER1* gene are associated with *DICER1* syndrome. Germline pathogenic variants in the *ERCC2* gene are associated with xeroderma pigmentosum (XP). Germline pathogenic variants in the *FANCA* gene are associated with Fanconi anemia. Germline pathogenic variants in the *PTCH1* gene are associated with Gorlin syndrome. Germline pathogenic variants in the *VHL* gene are associated with von Hippel–Lindau syndrome (VHL).

Therefore, the *TERT* gene would most likely be included in the sequencing test for this patient.

161. **E.** Dyskeratosis congenita (DC), a telomere-shortening disorder, is characterized by a classic triad of dysplastic nails, lacy reticular pigmentation of the upper chest and/or neck, and oral leukoplakia. Individuals with DC have an increased risk of developing several life-threatening conditions, such as bone-marrow failure and pulmonary fibrosis. *The most sensitive test for diagnosis is multicolor flow cytometry fluorescence in situ hybridization (flow-FISH) on white-blood-cell (WBC) subsets to find abnormally short telomeres for their age.* The clinical sensitivity of next-generation sequencing panel with all the genes associated with DC so far is about 40%–70% (http://www.ncbi.nlm.nih.gov/books/NBK22301/).

Chromosome breakage study is the diagnostic test for Fanconi anemia. Chromosome microarray analysis (CMA) is the ACMG-recommended first-line test for individuals with multiple congenital anomalies, developmental delay, intellectual disability, and autism. It is used to detect copy-number gain or loss. FISH for gene amplification is a molecular cytogenetic test for some acquired malignancies, such as *HER2* FISH for breast cancer. Next-generation sequencing (NGS) is a high-throughput test to sequence multiple genes at the same time. It is an appropriate test for Fanconi anemia, hearing loss, and other conditions

Therefore, flow-FISH, used o measure telomere-length, would be the most sensitive test to confirm/rule out genetic etiologies in this patient.

162. **A.** Most cases of hepatoblastoma are sporadic, but genetic syndromes are associated with approximately 15% of hepatoblastoma, such as Beckwith–Wiedemann syndrome (BWS) or familial adenomatous polyposis coli (FAP). The occurrence of hepatoblastoma in individuals with FAP is 400-fold higher than in the general population. *Individual with BWS carry higher risk of developing hepatoblastoma than the ones with FAP.* In addition, multiple case reports suggest an increased risk of hepatoblastoma in patients born with trisomy 18.

Therefore, patients with BWS have a higher risk of developing hepatoblastoma than the others listed in this question.

163. **E.** Certain inherited genetic abnormalities have been associated with the development of different types of thyroid cancer. Individuals with *multiple endocrine neoplasia type 2 (MEN2)*, caused by pathogenic variants in the *RET* gene, have an increased risk of developing familial medullary thyroid cancer (FMTC) and pheochromocytoma (http://www.ncbi.nlm.nih.gov/books/NBK1257/).

Other inherited genetic conditions, such as familial adenomatous polyposis (FAP), Gardner syndrome, Cowden disease, and Carney complex type I, are considered risk factors for thyroid cancer, particularly papillary and follicular thyroid cancers. Individuals with multiple endocrine neoplasia type 1 (MEN1), caused by pathogenic variants in the *MEN1* gene, have an increased risk of developing parathyroid tumors, pituitary tumors, pancreatic tumors, carcinoid tumors, and adrenocortical tumors, but not medullary thyroid cancer. And none of the inherited genetic conditions listed in this question are associated with an increased risk for pheochromocytoma except MEN2.

Therefore, MEN2 may be considered in this patient to rule out genetic etiologies in this patient.

164. **D.** Certain inherited genetic abnormalities have been associated with the development of different types of thyroid cancer. Individuals with *multiple endocrine neoplasia type 2 (MEN2), caused by pathogenic variants in the RET gene,* have an increased risk of developing familial medullary thyroid cancer (FMTC). Other inherited genetic conditions, such as familial adenomatous polyposis (FAP), Gardner syndrome, Cowden disease, and Carney complex type I, are considered risk factors for thyroid cancer, particularly papillary and follicular thyroid cancers. So MEN2 may be on the list of differential diagnoses for this patient (http://www.ncbi.nlm.nih.gov/books/NBK1257/).

None of the inherited genetic conditions listed in this question are associated with an increased risk for pheochromocytoma except MEN2. Germline pathogenic variants in the *DICER1* gene are associated with *DICER1* syndrome. Germline pathogenic variants in the *MEN1* gene are associated with multiple endocrine neoplasia type 1 (MEN1). Germline pathogenic variants in the *PTEN* gene are associated with *PTEN* hamartoma tumor syndrome (PHTS), which includes Cowden syndrome (CS). Germline pathogenic variants in the *TP53* gene are associated with Li–Fraumeni syndrome. Germline pathogenic variants in the *VHL* gene are associated with von Hippel–Lindau syndrome (VHL).

Therefore, the *RET* gene may be tested to rule out genetic etiologies in this patient.

165. **C.** Medullary thyroid cancer (MTC) is typically an aggressive cancer, with reduced survival comparing with other thyroid cancers. About 25% of medullary thyroid cancers are due to the inherited condition, multiple endocrine neoplasia

type 2 (MEN2). *This condition is associated with a 95% to 100% lifetime risk of medullary thyroid cancer (MTC).* Other common symptoms in individuals with MEN2 are parathyroid diseases, such as parathyroid adenomas, and pheochromocytoma. Germline pathogenic variants in the *RET* gene are associated with MEN2 (http://www.ncbi.nlm.nih.gov/books/NBK1257/).

Other inherited genetic conditions, such as familial adenomatous polyposis (FAP), Gardner syndrome, Cowden disease, and Carney complex type I, are considered risk factors for thyroid cancer, particularly papillary and follicular thyroid cancers.

Therefore, this female patient most likely has medullary thyroid cancer if she has MEN2.

166. **E.** Certain inherited genetic abnormalities have been associated with the development of different types of thyroid cancer. Individuals with *multiple endocrine neoplasia type 2 (MEN2),* caused by germline pathogenic variants in the *RET* gene, have an increased risk of developing familial medullary thyroid cancer (FMTC). MEN 2A and MEN 2B confer an increased risk for pheochromocytoma; MEN 2A confers an increased risk for parathyroid adenoma or hyperplasia. Additional features in MEN 2B include mucosal neuromas of the lips and tongue, distinctive facies with enlarged lips, ganglioneuromatosis of the gastrointestinal tract, and a "marfanoid" habitus (http://www.ncbi.nlm.nih.gov/books/NBK1257/).

None of the inherited genetic conditions listed in this question are associated with an increased risk for pheochromocytoma except MEN2. But other inherited genetic conditions, such as familial adenomatous polyposis (FAP), Gardner syndrome, Cowden disease, and Carney complex type I, are considered risk factors for thyroid cancer, particularly papillary and follicular thyroid cancers. Individuals with multiple endocrine neoplasia type 1 (MEN1), caused by pathogenic variants in the *MEN1* gene, have an increased risk of developing parathyroid tumors, pituitary tumors, pancreatic tumors, carcinoid tumors, and adrenocortical tumors but not familial medullary thyroid cancer (FMTC) (http://www.ncbi.nlm.nih.gov/books/NBK1538/).

Therefore, MEN2 would be considered in this patient to rule out genetic etiologies in this patient.

167. **D.** Certain inherited genetic abnormalities have been associated with the development of different types of thyroid cancer. Individuals with *multiple endocrine neoplasia type 2 (MEN2),* caused by a

germline pathogenic variant in the *RET* gene, have an increased risk of developing familial medullary thyroid cancer (FMTC). MEN 2A and MEN 2B confer an increased risk for pheochromocytoma; MEN 2A confers an increased risk for parathyroid adenoma or hyperplasia. Additional features in MEN 2B include mucosal neuromas of the lips and tongue, distinctive facies with enlarged lips, ganglioneuromatosis of the gastrointestinal tract, and a "marfanoid" habitus (http://www.ncbi.nlm.nih.gov/books/NBK1257/).

None of the inherited genetic conditions listed in this question are associated with an increased risk for pheochromocytoma except MEN2. But other inherited genetic conditions, such as familial adenomatous polyposis (FAP), Gardner syndrome, Cowden disease, and Carney complex type I, are considered risk factors for thyroid cancer, particularly papillary and follicular thyroid cancers. So MEN2 may be on the list of differential diagnoses for this patient.

Germline pathogenic variants in the *DICER1* gene are associated with *DICER1* syndrome. Germline pathogenic variants in the *MEN1* gene are associated with multiple endocrine neoplasia type 1 (MEN1). Germline pathogenic variants in the *PTEN* gene are associated with *PTEN* hamartoma tumor syndrome (PHTS), including Cowden syndrome (CS). Germline pathogenic variants in the *TP53* gene are associated with Li–Fraumeni syndrome. Germline pathogenic variants in the *VHL* gene are associated with von Hippel–Lindau syndrome (VHL).

Therefore, the *RET* gene might be tested to rule out genetic etiologies in this patient.

168. **D.** Multiple endocrine neoplasia syndrome type 1 (MEN1) is an autosomal dominant hereditary cancer predisposition syndrome, caused by germline pathogenic variants in the *MEN1* gene. *Individuals with MEN1 are predisposed to tumors of the parathyroid glands, anterior pituitary, and enteropancreatic endocrine cells.* Carcinoid tumors, adrenal adenomas, and lipomas are more common in this population than in the general population (http://www.ncbi.nlm.nih.gov/books/NBK1538/).

Cowden syndrome is a multiple-hamartoma syndrome with an increased risk for benign and malignant tumors of the thyroid, breast, and endometrium. Germline pathogenic variants in the *PTEN* gene are associated with PTEN hamartoma tumor syndrome (PHTS), including Cowden syndrome (CS). Familial adenomatous polyposis (FAP) confers an increased risk of

developing colonic polyps and colorectal cancer. And 5% of affected individuals develop medulloblastoma during childhood. Germline pathogenic variants in the *APC* gene are associated with FAP. Gorlin syndrome, also known as "nevoid basal-cell carcinoma syndrome" (NBCCS), is one of the autosomal dominant hereditary cancer syndromes. It is characterized by a classic pentad of features comprised of multiple basal-cell carcinomas, jaw cysts, calcification of the falx cerebri, pitting of the palmar and plantar surfaces, and rib anomalies. Approximately 60% of individuals have a recognizable appearance, with macrocephaly, frontal bossing, coarse facial features, and facial milia. Germline pathogenic variants in the *PTCH1* gene are associated with Gorlin syndrome. Individuals with multiple endocrine neoplasia type 2 (MEN2), caused by a pathogenic variant in the *RET* gene, have an increased risk of developing familial medullary thyroid cancer (FMTC) and pheochromocytoma. MEN 2A also confers an increased risk of developing parathyroid adenoma or hyperplasia. MEN 2B also confers an increased risk of developing mucosal neuromas of the lips and tongue, and ganglioneuromatosis of the gastrointestinal tract. Germline pathogenic variants the *RET* gene are associated with multiple endocrine neoplasia type 2 (MEN2).

Therefore, MEN1 might be considered for this patient to rule out genetic etiologies in this patient.

169. **B.** Multiple endocrine neoplasia syndrome type 1 (MEN1) is an autosomal dominant hereditary cancer predisposition syndrome, caused by germline pathogenic variants in the *MEN1* gene. Individuals with MEN1 are predisposed to tumors of the parathyroid glands, anterior pituitary, and enteropancreatic endocrine cells. Carcinoid tumors, adrenal adenomas, and lipomas are more common in this population than in the general population (http://www.ncbi.nlm.nih.gov/books/NBK1538/).

Individuals with *DICER1* syndrome most commonly have an increased risk for pleuropulmonary blastoma (PPB), ovarian sex-cord stromal tumors (Sertoli–Leydig cell tumor, juvenile granulosa-cell tumor, and gynandroblastoma), cystic nephroma, and thyroid-gland neoplasia (multinodular goiter, adenomas, or differentiated thyroid cancer). Germline pathogenic variants in the *DICER1* gene are associated with *DICER1* syndrome. Individuals with multiple endocrine neoplasia type 2 (MEN 2) most commonly have an increased risk for medullary carcinoma of the thyroid, pheochromocytoma, and parathyroid adenoma or hyperplasia. Germline pathogenic variants the *RET* gene are associated with MEN2. Individuals with *PTEN* hamartoma tumor syndrome (PHTS), including Cowden syndrome (CS), have an increased risk most commonly for benign and malignant tumors of the thyroid, breast, and endometrium. Germline pathogenic variants in the *PTEN* gene are associated with PHTS. Individuals with Li–Fraumeni syndrome (LFS) most commonly have an increased risk for soft-tissue sarcoma, osteosarcoma, premenopausal breast cancer, brain tumors, adrenocortical carcinoma, and leukemias. Germline pathogenic variants in the *TP53* gene are associated with LFS. Individuals with von Hippel–Lindau syndrome (VHL) most commonly have an increased risk for hemangioblastomas of the brain, spinal cord, and retina; renal cysts and clear-cell renal-cell carcinoma; pheochromocytoma; pancreatic cysts; and neuroendocrine tumors, endolymphatic sac tumors, and epididymal and broad ligament cysts. Germline pathogenic variants in the *VHL* gene are associated with VHL.

Therefore, the *MEN1* gene would be most likely sequenced for this patient to rule out genetic etiologies.

170. **E.** Multiple endocrine neoplasia syndrome type 1 (MEN1) is an autosomal dominant hereditary cancer predisposition syndrome, caused by germline pathogenic variants in *the MEN1 gene*. Individuals with MEN1 are predisposed to tumors of the parathyroid glands, anterior pituitary, and enteropancreatic endocrine cells. Carcinoid tumors, adrenal adenomas, and lipomas are more common in this population than in the general population. *Sanger sequencing test may identify 80%–90% of familial cases and 65% of singleton cases* (http://www.ncbi.nlm.nih.gov/books/NBK1538/).

Chromosome breakage study is the diagnostic test for Fanconi anemia. Chromosome microarray analysis (CMA) is the ACMG-recommended first-line test for individuals with multiple congenital anomalies, developmental delay, intellectual disability, and autism. It is used to detect copy number gain or loss. Methylation study is used to identify epigenetic changes in the genome, such as a methylation study for Prader–Willi/Angelman syndromes. Next-generation sequencing (NGS) is a high-throughput test to sequence multiple genes at the same time. It is an appropriate test for Fanconi anemia, hearing loss,

and other conditions. Sanger sequencing is the most appropriate molecular test for single-gene disorders when the most pathogenic variants are single-nucleotide variants and in/dels. It is an appropriate test for Gaucher disease, Wiskott–Aldrich syndrome (WAS), and other conditions. Targeted-mutation analysis is used to identify specific mutations, which is a cost-effective test when there is a founder effect in a population. Targeted-mutation analysis is also commonly used to diagnose family members after the mutation is identified in the proband. It is an appropriate test for carrier test of cystic fibrosis (CF). Quantitative measurement of telomere length by flow-FISH is the laboratory test used to aid the diagnosis of dyskeratosis congenita.

Therefore, Sanger sequencing would be most appropriate to confirm/rule out genetic etiologies in this patient.

171. **C.** Multiple endocrine neoplasia syndrome type 1 (MEN1) is an autosomal dominant hereditary cancer predisposition syndrome, caused by germline pathogenic variants in the *MEN1* gene. Individuals with MEN1 are predisposed to tumors of the parathyroid glands, anterior pituitary, and enteropancreatic endocrine cells. Carcinoid tumors, adrenal adenomas, and lipomas are more common in this population than in the general population. (http://www. ncbi.nlm.nih.gov/books/NBK1538/).

Medullary thyroid cancer is common in multiple endocrine neoplasia type 2 (MEN2), but not in multiple endocrine neoplasia type 1 (MEN1).

Therefore, medullary thyroid cancer is NOT characteristic for multiple endocrine neoplasia syndrome type 1 (MEN1).

172. **C.** *The MEN1 gene is the only gene in which pathogenic variants are known to cause multiple endocrine neoplasia type 1 (MEN1) syndrome.* Sequencing may detect germline pathogenic variants in the *MEN1* gene in approximately 80%–90% of familial cases and in approximately 65% of singleton cases (http://www.ncbi.nlm.nih. gov/books/NBK1538/).

Pathogenic variants in the *BRAF* gene are associated with cardiofaciocutaneous syndrome or LEOPARD syndrome. Pathogenic variants in the *KRAS* gene are associated with acute myeloid leukemia or *RAS*-associated autoimmune lymphoproliferative disorder. Pathogenic variants in the *NRAS* gene are associated with Noonan syndrome. Pathogenic variants in the *PTEN* gene are associated with acute myeloid leukemia or *RAS*-associated autoimmune lymphoproliferative disorder. Pathogenic variants in the *PTEN* gene are associated with *PTEN* hamartoma tumor syndrome (PHTS), including Cowden syndrome (CS). Pathogenic variants in the *RB1* gene are associated with retinoblastoma. Pathogenic variants in the *RET* gene are associated with multiple endocrine neoplasia type 2 (MEN2).

Therefore, heterozygous germline pathogenic variants in the *MEN1* gene are diagnostic for MEN1.

173. **D.** Individuals with multiple endocrine neoplasia type 2 (MEN2), caused by a germline pathogenic variant in the *RET* gene, have an increased risk of developing familial medullary thyroid cancer (FMTC). MEN 2A and MEN confer have an increased risk for pheochromocytoma; MEN 2A confers an increased risk for parathyroid adenoma or hyperplasia. Additional features in MEN 2B include mucosal neuromas of the lips and tongue, distinctive facies with enlarged lips, ganglioneuromatosis of the gastrointestinal tract, and a "marfanoid" habitus (http://www.ncbi.nlm.nih.gov/books/NBK1257/).

Pancreatic tumors are common in multiple endocrine neoplasia type 1 (MEN1), but not in MEN2.

Therefore, pancreatic tumors is NOT one of characteristics of multiple endocrine neoplasia syndrome type 2 (MEN2).

174. **F.** *Individuals with multiple endocrine neoplasia type 2 (MEN2), caused by a germline pathogenic variant in the RET gene,* have an increased risk of developing familial medullary thyroid cancer (FMTC). MEN 2A and MEN 2B confer an increased risk for pheochromocytoma; MEN 2A confers an increased risk for parathyroid adenoma or hyperplasia. Additional features in MEN 2B include mucosal neuromas of the lips and tongue, distinctive facies with enlarged lips, ganglioneuromatosis of the gastrointestinal tract, and a "marfanoid" habitus (http://www.ncbi.nlm.nih.gov/books/NBK1257/).

Pathogenic variants in the *BRAF* gene are associated with cardiofaciocutaneous syndrome or LEOPARD syndrome. Pathogenic variants in the *KRAS* gene are associated with acute myeloid leukemia or *RAS*-associated autoimmune lymphoproliferative disorder. Pathogenic variants in the *MEN1* gene are associated with multiple endocrine neoplasia type 1 (MEN1). Pathogenic variants in the *NRAS* gene are associated with Noonan syndrome. Pathogenic variants in the *PTEN* gene are associated with acute myeloid leukemia or *RAS*-associated autoimmune lymphoproliferative disorder. Pathogenic variants in the *PTEN* gene are associated with *PTEN* hamartoma tumor syndrome (PHTS), including Cowden syndrome (CS). Pathogenic variants in the *RB1* gene are associated with retinoblastoma.

Therefore, heterozygous germline pathogenic variants in the *RET* gene are diagnostic for MEN2.

175. **F.** *Individuals with multiple endocrine neoplasia type 2 (MEN2), caused by a germline pathogenic variant in the RET gene, have an increased risk of developing familial medullary thyroid cancer (FMTC).* MEN 2A and MEN 2B confer an increased risk for pheochromocytoma; MEN 2A confers an increased risk for parathyroid adenoma or hyperplasia. Additional features in MEN 2B include mucosal neuromas of the lips and tongue, distinctive facies with enlarged lips, ganglioneuromatosis of the gastrointestinal tract, and a "marfanoid" habitus (http://www.ncbi.nlm.nih.gov/books/NBK1257/).

Pathogenic variants in the *BRAF* gene are associated with cardiofaciocutaneous syndrome or LEOPARD syndrome. Pathogenic variants in the *KRAS* gene are associated with acute myeloid leukemia or *RAS*-associated autoimmune lymphoproliferative disorder. Pathogenic variants in the *MEN1* gene are associated with multiple endocrine neoplasia type 1 (MEN1). Pathogenic variants in the *NRAS* gene are associated with Noonan syndrome. Pathogenic variants in the *NRAS* gene are associated with acute myeloid leukemia or *RAS*-associated autoimmune lymphoproliferative disorder. Pathogenic variants in the *PTEN* gene are associated with *PTEN* hamartoma tumor syndrome (PHTS), including Cowden syndrome (CS). Pathogenic variants in the *RB1* gene are associated with retinoblastoma.

Therefore, heterozygous germline pathogenic variants in the *RET* gene are diagnostic for FMTC.

176. **C.** Approximately 25% of patients with medullary thyroid carcinoma have familial medullary thyroid carcinoma.

Therefore, about 25% of medullary thyroid carcinomas are inherited.

177. **C.** *Neurofibromatosis type 1*, also called "von Recklinghausen disease," is characterized by multiple café au lait spots, axillary and inguinal freckling, multiple cutaneous neurofibromas, and iris Lisch nodules. Less common but potentially more serious manifestations include plexiform neurofibromas, optic nerve and other central nervous system gliomas, malignant peripheral-nerve-sheath tumors, scoliosis, tibial dysplasia, and vasculopathy. Pathogenic variants in the *NF1* gene are associated with neurofibromatosis type 1 (http://www.ncbi.nlm.nih.gov/books/NBK1109/).

The rest of syndromes listed in the question predisposing to Wilms tumors are WAGR (Wilms tumor, aniridia, genitourinary abnormalities, and mental retardation), Denys–Drash syndrome

(DDS), Beckwith—Wiedemann (BWS), Simpson—Golabi—Behmel syndrome (SGBS), and trisomy 18.

Therefore, individuals with NF1 do not have an increased risk of developing Wilms tumor in their lifetime.

178. **B.** *Neurofibromatosis type 1 (NF1),* also called "von Recklinghausen disease," is characterized by multiple café au lait spots, axillary and inguinal freckling, multiple cutaneous neurofibromas, and iris Lisch nodules. Less common but potentially more serious manifestations include plexiform neurofibromas, optic nerve and other central nervous system gliomas, malignant peripheral-nerve-sheath tumors, scoliosis, tibial dysplasia, and vasculopathy. Pathogenic variants in the *NF1* gene are associated with NF1 (http://www.ncbi. nlm.nih.gov/books/NBK1109/).

Individuals with Denys—Drash syndrome, neurofibromatosis type 2, or tuberous sclerosis do not usually have multiple café au lait spots. Neurofibromatosis 2 (NF2) is characterized by bilateral vestibular schwannomas with associated symptoms of tinnitus, hearing loss, and balance dysfunction. Pathogenic variants in the *NF2* gene are associated with neurofibromatosis type 2. Denys—Drash syndrome is characterized by kidney disease that begins within the first few months of life and abnormal genitalia. Pathogenic variants in the *WT1* gene are associated with autosomal dominant Wilms tumor, Denys—Drash syndrome, Frasier syndrome, and autosomal recessive nephrotic syndrome. Tuberous sclerosis complex is characterized by the growth of numerous benign tumors in many parts of the body. Patients with tuberous sclerosis complex may also have developmental problems. Pathogenic variants in the *TSC1* or *TSC2* gene are associated with tuberous sclerosis.

Therefore, NF1 might be considered to rule out genetic etiologies in this family.

179. **A.** Neurofibromatosis type 1 (NF1), also called "von Recklinghausen disease," is characterized by multiple café au lait spots, axillary and inguinal freckling, multiple cutaneous neurofibromas, and iris Lisch nodules. Less common but potentially more serious manifestations include plexiform neurofibromas, optic nerve and other central nervous system gliomas, malignant peripheral-nerve-sheath tumors, scoliosis, tibial dysplasia, and vasculopathy. Pathogenic variants *in the NF1 gene are associated with NF1* (http://www.ncbi. nlm.nih.gov/books/NBK1109/).

Individuals with Denys—Drash syndrome, neurofibromatosis type 2, or tuberous sclerosis do not usually have multiple café au lait spots.

Neurofibromatosis 2 (NF2) is characterized by bilateral vestibular schwannomas with associated symptoms of tinnitus, hearing loss, and balance dysfunction. Pathogenic variants in the *NF2* gene are associated with neurofibromatosis type 2. Denys—Drash syndrome is characterized by kidney disease that begins within the first few months of life and abnormal genitalia. Pathogenic variants in the *WT1* gene are associated with autosomal dominant Wilms tumor, Denys—Drash syndrome, Frasier syndrome, and autosomal recessive nephrotic syndrome. Tuberous sclerosis complex is characterized by the growth of numerous benign tumors in many parts of the body. Patients with tuberous sclerosis complex may also have developmental problems. Pathogenic variants in the *TSC1* or *TSC2* genes are associated with tuberous sclerosis.

Therefore, the *NF1* gene would most likely be sequenced to rule out genetic etiologies in this patient.

180. **A.** Neurofibromatosis type 1 (NF1), also called "von Recklinghausen disease," is characterized by multiple café au lait spots, axillary and inguinal freckling, multiple cutaneous neurofibromas, and iris Lisch nodules. Less common but potentially more serious manifestations include plexiform neurofibromas, optic nerve and other central nervous system gliomas, malignant peripheral-nerve-sheath tumors, scoliosis, tibial dysplasia, and vasculopathy. Pathogenic variants in the *NF1* gene are associated with NF1 (http://www.ncbi. nlm.nih.gov/books/NBK1109/).

Therefore, *acoustic schwannoma* is a characteristic of neurofibromatosis 2 (NF2) instead of NF1, and the rest are symptoms of NF1.

181. **C.** *Neurofibromatosis 2 (NF2)* is characterized by bilateral vestibular schwannomas with associated symptoms of tinnitus, hearing loss, and balance dysfunction. The average age at onset is 18—24 years. Almost all affected individuals develop bilateral vestibular schwannomas by age 30 years. Affected individuals may also develop schwannomas of other cranial and peripheral nerves, meningiomas, ependymomas, and, very rarely, astrocytomas. *NF2* is the only gene in which pathogenic variants are known to cause NF2. Sequencing analysis is estimated to identify up to 2/3 of the patients with NF2 (http://www. ncbi.nlm.nih.gov/books/NBK1201/).

Denys—Drash syndrome is characterized by kidney disease that begins within the first few months of life and abnormal genitalia. Pathogenic variants in the *WT1* gene are associated with autosomal dominant Wilms tumor, Denys—Drash syndrome, Frasier syndrome, and autosomal recessive nephrotic syndrome. Neurofibromatosis type 1 (NF1), also called "von Recklinghausen disease," is characterized by multiple café au lait spots, axillary and inguinal freckling, multiple cutaneous neurofibromas, and iris Lisch nodules. Pathogenic variants in the *NF1* gene are associated with neurofibromatosis type 1. Tuberous sclerosis complex is characterized by the growth of numerous benign tumors in many parts of the body. Patients with tuberous sclerosis complex may also have developmental problems. Pathogenic variants in the *TSC1* or *TSC2* gene are associated with tuberous sclerosis.

　　Therefore, NF2 would be considered to rule out genetic etiologies in this family.

182. **B.** *Neurofibromatosis 2 (NF2)* is characterized by bilateral vestibular schwannomas with associated symptoms of tinnitus, hearing loss, and balance dysfunction. The average age at onset is 18–24 years. Almost all affected individuals develop bilateral vestibular schwannomas by age 30 years. Affected individuals may also develop schwannomas of other cranial and peripheral nerves, meningiomas, ependymomas, and, very rarely, astrocytomas. *NF2* is the only gene in which pathogenic variants are known to cause NF2. Sequencing analysis is estimated to identify up to 2/3 of the patients with NF2 (http://www.ncbi.nlm.nih.gov/books/NBK1201/).

　　Denys—Drash syndrome is characterized by kidney disease that begins within the first few months of life and abnormal genitalia. Pathogenic variants in the *WT1* gene are associated with autosomal dominant Wilms tumor, Denys—Drash syndrome, Frasier syndrome, and autosomal recessive nephrotic syndrome. Neurofibromatosis type 1 (NF1), also called "von Recklinghausen disease," is characterized by multiple café au lait spots, axillary and inguinal freckling, multiple cutaneous neurofibromas, and iris Lisch nodules. Pathogenic variants in the *NF1* gene are associated with neurofibromatosis type 1. Tuberous sclerosis complex is characterized by the growth of numerous benign tumors in many parts of the body. Patients with tuberous sclerosis complex may also have developmental problems. Pathogenic variants in the *TSC1* or *TSC2* genes are associated with tuberous sclerosis.

　　Therefore, the *NF2* gene would most likely be sequenced to rule out genetic etiologies in this family.

183. **E.** Neurofibromatosis 2 (NF2) is characterized by bilateral vestibular schwannomas with associated symptoms of tinnitus, hearing loss, and balance dysfunction. The average age at onset is 18–24

years. Almost all affected individuals develop bilateral vestibular schwannomas by age 30 years. *Bilateral vestibular schwannomas is a characteristic of NF2 causing patients loss their hearing postnatally.* Affected individuals may also develop schwannomas of other cranial and peripheral nerves, meningiomas, ependymomas, and, very rarely, astrocytomas. *NF2* is the only gene in which pathogenic variants are known to cause NF2 (http://www.ncbi.nlm.nih.gov/books/NBK1201/).

　　Therefore, it would be most likely this patient had bilateral vestibular schwannomas leading to hearing loss.

184. **E.** Neurofibromatosis 2 (NF2) is characterized by bilateral vestibular schwannomas with associated symptoms of tinnitus, hearing loss, and balance dysfunction. The average age at onset is 18–24 years. Almost all affected individuals develop bilateral vestibular schwannomas by age 30 years. Affected individuals may also develop schwannomas of other cranial and peripheral nerves, meningiomas, ependymomas, and, very rarely, astrocytomas. *NF2* is the only gene in which pathogenic variants are known to cause NF2. *Sequencing analysis is estimated to identify up to 2/3 of the patients with NF2. Deletion/duplication analysis may detect approximately 20% of patients. So the total sensitivity of sequencing and deletion/duplication is about 90%* (http://www.ncbi.nlm.nih.gov/books/NBK1201/).

　　Chromosome breakage study is the diagnostic test for Fanconi anemia. Chromosome karyotype is the diagnostic test for cytogenetic abnormalities, such as trisomy 21. Chromosome microarray analysis (CMA) is the ACMG-recommended first-line test for individuals with multiple congenital anomalies, developmental delay, intellectual disability, and autism. It is used to detect copy-number gain or loss. Methylation study is used to identify epigenetic changes in the genome, such as methylation study for Prader—Willi/Angelman syndromes. Next-generation sequencing (NGS) is a high-throughput test to sequence multiple genes at the same time. It is an appropriate test for Fanconi anemia, hearing loss, and other conditions. Sanger sequencing is the most appropriate molecular test for single-gene disorders when the most pathogenic variants are single-nucleotide variants and in/dels. It is an appropriate test for Gaucher disease, Wiskott—Aldrich syndrome (WAS), and other conditions. Targeted-mutation analysis is used to identify specific mutations, which is a cost-effective test when there is founder effect in a population. Targeted-mutation analysis is also commonly used to diagnose family members after the mutation is identified in the proband. It is an appropriate carrier test for cystic fibrosis (CF). Quantitative measurement of telomere length by flow FISH is the laboratory test used to aid the diagnosis of dyskeratosis congenita.

Therefore, Sanger sequencing would most likely be used for the genetic test that the physician ordered for this patient.

185. **D.** Hereditary paraganglioma/ pheochromocytoma syndromes are characterized by paragangliomas (tumors that arise from neuroendocrine tissues symmetrically distributed along the paravertebral axis from the base of the skull to the pelvis) and by pheochromocytomas (paragangliomas that are confined to the adrenal medulla). Sympathetic paraganglioma/ pheochromocytoma hypersecrete catecholamines and are generally confined to the lower mediastinum, abdomen, and pelvis and are typically secretory. Symptoms of paraganglioma/ pheochromocytoma result either from mass effects or from catecholamine hypersecretion, such as sustained or paroxysmal elevations in blood pressure, headache, episodic profuse sweating, forceful palpitations, pallor, and apprehension or anxiety. The risk for malignant transformation is greater for extraadrenal sympathetic paragangliomas than for pheochromocytomas or skull base and neck paragangliomas (http://www.ncbi.nlm.nih.gov/ books/NBK1548/). According to the latest discoveries, already ten genes play an important role in the pathogenesis of pheochromocytomas: *RET, VHL, NF1, SDHA, SDHB, SDHC, SDHD, SDHAF2, SDH5,* and *TMEM127.*

Chromosome breakage study is the diagnostic test for Fanconi anemia. Chromosome microarray analysis (CMA) is the ACMG-recommended first-line test for individuals with multiple congenital anomalies, developmental delay, intellectual disability, and autism. It is used to detect copy-number gain or loss. CMA is the first-line test for individuals with multiple congenital anomalies, developmental delay, intellectual disability, and autism. Methylation study is used to identify epigenetic changes in the genome, such as methylation study for Prader–Willi/Angelman syndromes. Next-generation sequencing (NGS) is a high-throughput test to sequence multiple genes at the same time. It is an appropriate test for Fanconi anemia, hearing loss, and other conditions. Sanger sequencing is the most

appropriate molecular test for single-gene disorders when the most pathogenic variants are single-nucleotide variants and in/dels. It is an appropriate test for Gaucher disease, Wiskott–Aldrich syndrome (WAS), and other conditions. Targeted-mutation analysis is used to identify specific mutations, which is a cost-effective test when there is founder effect in a population. Targeted-mutation analysis is also commonly used to diagnose family members after the mutation is identified in the proband. It is an appropriate carrier test for cystic fibrosis (CF). Quantitative measurement of telomere length by flow FISH is the laboratory test used to aid the diagnosis of dyskeratosis congenita.

Therefore, next-generation sequencing would most likely be used for the genetic test that the physician ordered for this patient.

186. **F.** Hereditary paraganglioma/pheochromocytoma syndromes are characterized by paragangliomas (tumors that arise from neuroendocrine tissues symmetrically distributed along the paravertebral axis from the base of the skull to the pelvis) and by pheochromocytomas (paragangliomas that are confined to the adrenal medulla). Sympathetic paraganglioma/pheochromocytomas hypersecrete catecholamines and are generally confined to the lower mediastinum, abdomen, and pelvis; they are typically secretory. Symptoms of paraganglioma/pheochromocytoma result either from mass effects or catecholamine hypersecretion, such as sustained or paroxysmal elevations in blood pressure, headache, episodic profuse sweating, forceful palpitations, pallor, and apprehension or anxiety. The risk for malignant transformation is greater for extraadrenal sympathetic paragangliomas than for pheochromocytomas or skull base and neck paragangliomas (http://www.ncbi.nlm.nih.gov/ books/NBK1548/). According to the latest discoveries, already ten genes play an important role in the pathogenesis of pheochromocytomas. These genes include: *RET, VHL, NF1, SDHA, SDHB, SDHC, SDHD, SDHAF2, SDH5,* and *TMEM127.*

Pathogenic variants in the *BRAF* gene are associated with cardiofaciocutaneous (CFC) syndrome or LEOPARD syndrome. Pathogenic variants in the *KRAS* gene are associated with acute myeloid leukemia or *RAS*-associated autoimmune lymphoproliferative disorder. Pathogenic variants in the *MEN1* gene are associated with multiple endocrine neoplasia type 1 (MEN1). Pathogenic variants in the *NRAS* gene are associated with Noonan syndrome.

7. ONCOLOGY—CONSTITUTIONAL

Pathogenic variants in the *PTEN* gene are associated with PTEN hamartoma tumor syndrome (PHTS), including Cowden syndrome (CS). None of these cancer predisposition syndromes are associated with an increased risk of developing pheochromocytomas.

Therefore, the *SDHB* gene would most likely be included in the next-generation sequencing (NGS) panel for hereditary form of pheochromocytoma to rule out genetic etiologies in this patient.

187. **A.** Hereditary paraganglioma/pheochromocytoma syndromes are characterized by paragangliomas (tumors that arise from neuroendocrine tissues symmetrically distributed along the paravertebral axis from the base of the skull to the pelvis) and by pheochromocytomas (paragangliomas that are confined to the adrenal medulla). Sympathetic paraganglioma/pheochromocytomas hypersecrete catecholamines and are generally confined to the lower mediastinum, abdomen, and pelvis; they are typically secretory. Symptoms of paraganglioma/pheochromocytoma result either from mass effects or catecholamine hypersecretion, such as sustained or paroxysmal elevations in blood pressure, headache, episodic profuse sweating, forceful palpitations, pallor, and apprehension or anxiety. The risk for malignant transformation is greater for extraadrenal sympathetic paragangliomas than for pheochromocytomas or skull base and neck paragangliomas (http://www.ncbi.nlm.nih.gov/books/NBK1548/). According to the latest discoveries, already ten genes play an important role in the pathogenesis of pheochromocytomas. These genes include: *RET, VHL, NF1, SDHA, SDHB, SDHC, SDHD, SDHAF2, SDH5,* and *TMEM127*.

MEN1 is the only gene associated with multiple endocrine neoplasia type 1 (MEN1). The most common tumors in MEN1 syndrome are parathyroid, pituitary, and pancreatic tumors. But pheochromocytomas are not common in individuals with MEN1 (http://www.ncbi.nlm.nih.gov/books/NBK1538/).

Therefore, the *MEN1* gene would most likely NOT be included in this panel for a hereditary form of pheochromocytoma to rule out genetic etiologies in this patient.

188. **D.** Neurofibromatosis 2 (NF2) is characterized by bilateral vestibular schwannomas with associated symptoms of tinnitus, hearing loss, and balance dysfunction. The average age at onset is 18–24 years. Almost all affected individuals develop bilateral vestibular schwannomas by age 30. Affected individuals may also develop

schwannomas of other cranial and peripheral nerves, meningiomas, ependymomas, and, very rarely, astrocytomas (http://www.ncbi.nlm.nih.gov/books/NBK1201/).

Individuals with Li−Fraumeni syndrome (LFS) are at increased risk of developing many types of brain tumors, such as astrocytomas, glioblastomas, medulloblastomas, choroid plexus carcinomas (CPC), but not pheochromocytoma. Neurofibromatosis type 1 is characterized by multiple café au lait spots, axillary and inguinal freckling, multiple cutaneous neurofibromas, and iris Lisch nodules. Less common but potentially more serious manifestations include plexiform neurofibromas, optic nerve and other central nervous system gliomas, malignant peripheral-nerve-sheath tumors, scoliosis, tibial dysplasia, and vasculopathy. Individuals with multiple endocrine neoplasia syndrome type 1 (MEN1) are predisposed to tumors of the parathyroid glands, anterior pituitary, and enteropancreatic endocrine cells. Carcinoid tumors, adrenal adenomas, and lipomas are more common in this population than in the general population, too.

Therefore, it is most likely that this patient had NF2 if she had a genetic condition.

189. **C.** *Retinoblastoma is a rare type of eye cancer that usually develops in early childhood, typically before the age of 5.* This form of cancer develops in the retina, which is the specialized light-sensitive tissue at the back of the eye that detects light and color. In most children with retinoblastoma, the disease affects only one eye. However, one of three children with retinoblastoma develops cancer in both eyes. The most common first sign of retinoblastoma is a visible whiteness in the pupil called "cat's eye reflex" or leukocoria. This unusual whiteness is particularly noticeable in photographs taken with a flash. Other signs and symptoms of retinoblastoma include crossed eyes or eyes that do not point in the same direction (strabismus); persistent eye pain, redness, or irritation; and blindness or poor vision in the affected eye(s) (https://ghr.nlm.nih.gov/condition/retinoblastoma).

Therefore, retinoblastoma(s) usually happen before 5 years of age in an individual.

190. **A.** *All patients with bilateral disease have germline RB1 mutations.* But not all patients with germline mutations develop bilateral disease.

Therefore, the patient has >99% chance to have a germline pathogenic variant in the *RB1* gene.

191. **C.** Retinoblastoma (Rb) is a malignant tumor of the developing retina that occurs in children, usually before age 5. Rb develops from cells that have cancer-predisposing variants in both copies

SELF-ASSESSMENT QUESTIONS FOR CLINICAL MOLECULAR GENETICS

of *RB1*. Rb may be unifocal or multifocal. Heritable Rb is an autosomal dominant susceptibility disorder caused by a heterozygous pathogenic variant in *the RB1 gene.* Individuals with heritable Rb are also at increased risk of developing nonocular tumors (http://www.ncbi. nlm.nih.gov/books/NBK1452/).

Pathogenic variants in the *GPC3* and *GPC4* genes are associated with Simpson–Golabi–Behmel syndrome type 1 (SGBS1). Pathogenic variants in the *MEN1* gene are associated with multiple endocrine neoplasia type 1 (MEN1). Pathogenic variants in the *NF1* gene are associated with neurofibromatosis type 1 (NF1). Pathogenic variants in the *WT1* gene are associated with Wilms tumor.

Therefore, the *RB1* gene would most likely be sequenced to rule out genetic etiologies in this patient.

192. **D.** Noonan syndrome (NS) is characterized by characteristic facies, short stature, congenital heart defect, and developmental delay of various degrees. Other findings can include broad or webbed neck, unusual chest shape with superior pectus carinatum and inferior pectus excavatum, cryptorchidism, varied coagulation defects, lymphatic dysplasias, and ocular abnormalities. Although birth length is usually normal, final adult height approaches the lower limit of normal (http://www.ncbi.nlm.nih.gov/books/NBK1548/). Germline pathogenic variants in the *PTPN11, SOS1, RAF1, RIT1, KRAS, NRAS, BRAF,* and *MAP2K1* genes are associated with this autosomal dominant condition.

Chromosome breakage study is the diagnostic test for Fanconi anemia. Chromosome microarray analysis (CMA) is the ACMG-recommended first-line test for individuals with multiple congenital anomalies, developmental delay, intellectual disability, and autism. It is used to detect copy-number gain or loss. Methylation study is used to identify epigenetic changes in the genome, such as methylation study for Prader–Willi/Angelman syndromes. Next-generation sequencing (NGS) is a high-throughput test to sequence multiple genes at the same time. It is an appropriate test for Fanconi anemia, hearing loss, and other conditions. Sanger sequencing is the most appropriate molecular test for single-gene disorders when the most pathogenic variants are single-nucleotide variants and in/dels. It is an appropriate test for Gaucher disease, Wiskott–Aldrich syndrome (WAS), and other conditions. Targeted-mutation analysis is used to identify specific mutations, which is a cost-effective test when there is a founder effect in a

population. Targeted-mutation analysis is also commonly used to diagnose family members after the mutation is identified in the proband. It is an appropriate carrier test for cystic fibrosis (CF). Quantitative measurement of telomere length by flow-FISH is the laboratory test used to aid the diagnosis of dyskeratosis congenita.

Therefore, next-generation sequencing (NGS) would be the most appropriate genetic test to rule out Noonan syndrome in this patient.

193. **B.** Noonan syndrome (NS) is characterized by characteristic facies, short stature, congenital heart defect, and developmental delay of various degrees. Other findings can include broad or webbed neck, unusual chest shape with superior pectus carinatum and inferior pectus excavatum, cryptorchidism, varied coagulation defects, lymphatic dysplasias, and ocular abnormalities. Although birth length is usually normal, final adult height approaches the lower limit of normal. Germline pathogenic variants in the *PTPN11, SOS1, RAF1, RIT1, KRAS, NRAS, BRAF,* and *MAP2K1* genes are associated with this autosomal dominant condition (http://www. ncbi.nlm.nih.gov/books/NBK1548/).

Germline pathogenic variants in *the HRAS gene* are associated with Costello syndrome. Therefore, the *HRAS* gene would most likely *NOT* be sequenced to rule out Noonan syndrome in this patient.

194. **C.** Cardiofaciocutaneous syndrome (CFC), Costello syndrome, multiple lentigines syndrome (also called "LEOPARD syndrome"), and Noonan syndrome are clinically overlapping conditions. Pathogenic variants *in the RAS/RAF pathway, genes such as BRAF, HRAS, KRAS, NRAS, and RAF1 are causative for these syndromes.* So most of these syndromes have a mild to moderately increased risk for malignancies, except CFC.

Sonic hedgehog, PI3K/Akt, and Wnt pathways are all relatively well-known signal pathways in cells related to embryonic proliferation.

Therefore, RAS/RAF pathway seems to be involved in the process of the pathogenesis of these syndromes.

195. **D.** *Waardenburg syndrome is a group of genetic conditions that can cause hearing loss and changes in coloring (pigmentation) of the hair, skin, and eyes.* Although most people with Waardenburg syndrome have normal hearing, moderate to profound hearing loss can occur in one or both ears. The hearing loss is present from birth (congenital). People with this condition often have very pale blue eyes or different-colored eyes, such as one blue eye and one brown eye. Sometimes one eye has segments of two different

colors. Distinctive hair coloring (such as a patch of white hair or hair that prematurely turns gray) is another common sign of the condition. Germline pathogenic variants in the *EDN3*, *EDNRB*, *MITF*, *PAX3*, *SNAI2*, and *SOX10* genes are associated with Waardenburg syndrome (https://ghr.nlm.nih.gov/condition/waardenburg-syndrome#genes).

Cardiofaciocutaneous syndrome (CFC), Costello syndrome, and Noonan syndrome are clinically overlapping conditions with congenital cardiac defects. Hearing loss and changes in the coloring of the hair are not common characteristics of these three syndromes. Pathogenic variants in RAS/RAF pathway, such as *BRAF*, *HRAS*, *KRAS*, *NRAS*, and *RAF1* genes, are causative for these syndromes.

Therefore, this patient would most likely have Waardenburg syndrome if she had a genetic condition.

196. **B.** Waardenburg syndrome is a group of genetic conditions that can cause hearing loss and changes in coloring (pigmentation) of the hair, skin, and eyes. Although most people with Waardenburg syndrome have normal hearing, moderate to profound hearing loss can occur in one or both ears. The hearing loss is present from birth (congenital). People with this condition often have very pale blue eyes or different-colored eyes, such as one blue eye and one brown eye. Sometimes one eye has segments of two different colors. Distinctive hair coloring (such as a patch of white hair or hair that prematurely turns gray) is another common sign of the condition. Germline pathogenic variants in the *EDN3*, *EDNRB*, *MITF*, *PAX3*, *SNAI2*, and *SOX10* genes are associated with Waardenburg syndrome (https://ghr.nlm.nih.gov/condition/waardenburg-syndrome#genes).

Germline pathogenic variants in the *PAX2* gene are associated with focal segmental glomerulosclerosis. Germline pathogenic variants in the *PAX6* gene are associated with coloboma.

Therefore, the *PAX3* gene would most likely be included in the genetic test for this patient.

197. **D.** Waardenburg syndrome is a group of genetic conditions that can cause hearing loss and changes in coloring (pigmentation) of the hair, skin, and eyes. Although most people with Waardenburg syndrome have normal hearing, moderate to profound hearing loss can occur in one or both ears. The hearing loss is present from birth (congenital). People with this condition often have very pale blue eyes or different-colored eyes, such as one blue eye and one brown

eye. Sometimes one eye has segments of two different colors. Distinctive hair coloring (such as a patch of white hair or hair that prematurely turns gray) is another common sign of the condition. Germline pathogenic variants in the *EDN3*, *EDNRB*, *MITF*, *PAX3*, *SNAI2*, and *SOX10 genes* are associated with Waardenburg syndrome (https://ghr.nlm.nih.gov/condition/wardenburg-syndrome#genes).

Chromosome breakage study is the diagnostic test for Fanconi anemia. Chromosome microarray analysis (CMA) is the ACMG-recommended first-line test for individuals with multiple congenital anomalies, developmental delay, intellectual disability, and autism. It is used to detect copy number gain or loss. Methylation study is used to identify epigenetic changes in the genome, such as methylation study for Prader—Willi/Angelman syndromes. Next-generation sequencing (NGS) is a high-throughput test to sequence multiple genes at the same time. It is an appropriate test for Fanconi anemia, hearing loss, and other conditions. Sanger sequencing is the most appropriate molecular test for single-gene disorders when the most pathogenic variants are single-nucleotide variants and in/dels. It is an appropriate test for Gaucher disease, Wiskott—Aldrich syndrome (WAS), and other conditions. Targeted-mutation analysis is used to identify specific mutations, which is a cost-effective test when there is a founder effect in a population. Targeted-mutation analysis is also commonly used to diagnose family members after the mutation is identified in the proband. It is an appropriate carrier test for cystic fibrosis (CF). Quantitative measurement of telomere length by flow-FISH is the laboratory test used to aid the diagnosis of dyskeratosis congenita.

Therefore, next-generation sequencing (NGS) is the most appropriate assay for the genes to confirm/rule out Waardenburg syndrome in this patient.

198. **B.** Individuals with WAGR (Wilms tumor, aniridia, genital anomalies, and retardation) syndrome, *Denys—Drash syndrome (DDS)*, and Beckwith—Wiedemann syndrome (BWS) have an increased risk of developing Wilms tumor, but not Frasier syndrome. Germline pathogenic variants in the *WT1* gene are associated with WAGR, DDS and isolated Wilms tumors, and Frasier syndrome. DDS is characterized by diffuse glomerulosclerosis that begins within the first few months of life and abnormal genitalia. Individuals with DDS have an estimated 90% chance of developing Wilms tumor. Males with DDS have gonadal dysgenesis. Females with DDS usually

have normal genitalia (http://www.ncbi.nlm.nih.gov/book/NBK1294/).

WAGR syndrome is also characterized by aniridia, genitourinary anomalies, and intellectual disability. Individuals with BWS usually have hemihyperplasia in addition to an increased risk of Wilms tumor. A deletion on the short arm of chromosome 11, including the *WT1* region, is associated with WAGR syndrome. Frasier syndrome is caused by a germline pathogenic variant in the *WT1* gene, too. Frasier syndrome is characterized by focal segmental glomerulosclerosis in early childhood, but no increased risk for Wilms tumor. Males with Frasier syndrome have gonadal dysgenesis. Females with Frasier syndrome usually have normal genitalia. BWS is associated with epigenetic and genomic alterations of 11p15.

Therefore, this patient would most likely have DDS caused by a germline pathogenic variant in the *WT1* gene.

199. **D.** Denys−Drash syndrome (DDS) is characterized by diffuse glomerulosclerosis that begins within the first few months of life and abnormal genitalia. Individuals with DDS have an estimated 90% chance of developing Wilms tumor. Males with DDS have gonadal dysgenesis. Females with DDS usually have normal genitalia. Germline pathogenic variants in *the WT1 gene* are associated with DDS (http://www.ncbi.nlm.nih.gov/books/NBK1294/).

The *PAX6* and *WT1* genes are on 11p13. Deletion of the both genes is associated with WAGR (Wilms tumor aniridia, genital anomalies, and retardation) syndrome. Somatic mutations in the *ALK* gene are associated with malignancies. But no hereditary cancer predisposition syndromes have been proved to be caused by germline pathogenic variants in *ALK*. Somatic deletion of *CDKN1A* has been seen in leukemias. No hereditary cancer predisposition syndromes have been proved to be caused by germline pathogenic variants in *CDKN1A*.

This patient's symptoms suggested DDS. Therefore, sequencing the *WT1* gene would most likely provide an appropriate molecular diagnosis for this patient.

200. **E.** Denys−Drash syndrome (DDS) is characterized by diffuse glomerulosclerosis that begins within the first few months of life and abnormal genitalia. Individuals with DDS have an estimated 90% chance of developing Wilms tumor. Males with DDS have gonadal dysgenesis. Females with DDS usually have normal genitalia. Germline pathogenic variants in *the WT1 gene* are

associated with DDS (http://www.ncbi.nlm.nih.gov/books/NBK1294/).

Chromosome breakage study is the diagnostic test for Fanconi anemia. Chromosome microarray analysis (CMA) is the ACMG-recommended first-line test for individuals with multiple congenital anomalies, developmental delay, intellectual disability, and autism. It is used to detect copy number gain or loss. Methylation study is used to identify epigenetic changes in the genome, such as methylation study for Prader−Willi/Angelman syndromes. Next-generation sequencing (NGS) is a high-throughput test to sequence multiple genes at the same time. It is an appropriate test for Fanconi anemia, hearing loss, and other conditions. Sanger sequencing is the most appropriate molecular test for single-gene disorders when the most pathogenic variants are single-nucleotide variants and in/dels. It is an appropriate test for Gaucher disease, Wiskott−Aldrich syndrome (WAS), and other conditions. Targeted-mutation analysis is used to identify specific mutations, which is a cost-effective test when there is a founder effect in a population. Targeted-mutation analysis is also commonly used to diagnose family members after the mutation is identified in the proband. It is an appropriate carrier test for cystic fibrosis (CF). Quantitative measurement of telomere length by flow-FISH is the laboratory test used to aid the diagnosis of dyskeratosis congenita.

Therefore, Sanger sequencing would most likely be used for the genetic test to rule out genetic etiologies in this patient.

201. **B.** Costello syndrome is characterized by failure to thrive in infancy as a result of severe postnatal feeding difficulties, short stature, developmental delay or intellectual disability, coarse facial features (full lips, large mouth, and full nasal tip), and other conditions. Individuals with Costello syndrome have an approximately 15% lifetime risk for malignant tumors, including rhabdomyosarcoma and neuroblastoma in young children and transitional-cell carcinoma of the bladder in adolescents and young adults. *Germline pathogenic variants in the HRAS gene are associated with Costello syndrome* (http://www.ncbi.nlm.nih.gov/books/NBK1507/).

Pathogenic variants in the *BRAF* gene are associated with cardiofaciocutaneous (CFC) syndrome or LEOPARD syndrome. Pathogenic variants in the *KRAS* gene are associated with acute myeloid leukemia or *RAS*-associated autoimmune lymphoproliferative disorder. Pathogenic variants in the *NRAS* gene are associated with Noonan syndrome. Pathogenic variants in the Pathogenic variants in the RAF1 gene are associated with LEOPARD syndrome and Noonan syndrome. *RAF1 gene are associated with dilated cardiomyopathy.*

Therefore, sequencing *HRAS* gene would most likely provide an appropriate molecular diagnosis for this patient.

202. **E.** Costello syndrome is characterized by failure to thrive in infancy as a result of severe postnatal feeding difficulties, short stature, developmental delay or intellectual disability, coarse facial features (full lips, large mouth, and full nasal tip), and other conditions. *Individuals with Costello syndrome have an approximately 15% lifetime risk for malignant tumors, including rhabdomyosarcoma and neuroblastoma in young children and transitional-cell carcinoma of the bladder in adolescents and young adults.* Germline pathogenic variants in the *HRAS* gene are associated with Costello syndrome (http://www.ncbi.nlm.nih.gov/books/NBK1507/).

Therefore, this patient would have an increased risk of developing neuroblastoma.

203. **F.** Costello syndrome is characterized by failure to thrive in infancy as a result of severe postnatal feeding difficulties; short stature, developmental delay or intellectual disability, coarse facial features (full lips, large mouth, and full nasal tip), and other conditions. *Individuals with Costello syndrome have an approximately 15% lifetime risk for malignant tumors including rhabdomyosarcoma and neuroblastoma in young children and transitional-cell carcinoma of the bladder in adolescents and young adults.* Germline pathogenic variants in the *HRAS* gene are associated with Costello syndrome (http://www.ncbi.nlm.nih.gov/books/NBK1507/).

Therefore, this patient would have an increased risk of developing transitional-cell carcinoma of the bladder.

204. **E.** Birt—Hogg—Dubé syndrome is characterized by multiple noncancerous (benign) skin tumors, particularly on the face, neck, and upper chest. Skin lesions typically appear during the third and fourth decades of life and typically increase in size and number with age. Lung cysts are mostly bilateral and multifocal; most individuals are asymptomatic but are at high risk for spontaneous pneumothorax. *Individuals with BHDS are at a sevenfold increased risk for renal tumors that are typically bilateral and multifocal and usually slow-growing.* The median age at tumor diagnosis is 48 years. The most common renal tumors are a hybrid of oncocytoma and chromophobe histologic cell types (so-called oncocytic hybrid tumor) and chromophobe histological cell types. Germline pathogenic variants

in the *FLCN* gene are associated with autosomal dominant Birt—Hogg—Dubé syndrome (http://www.ncbi.nlm.nih.gov/books/NBK1522/).

Therefore, individuals with Birt—Hogg—Dubé syndrome have an increased risk of developing renal-cell carcinoma.

205. **C.** *The MEN1 gene for multiple endocrine neoplasia type 1 (MEN1) is a proto-oncogene.* The rest are caused by loss-of-function mutations in tumor suppressor genes.

Germline pathogenic variants in the *FLCN* gene are associated with Birt—Hogg—Dubé syndrome. Germline pathogenic variants in the *TP53* gene are associated with Li—Fraumeni syndrome. Germline pathogenic variants in the *MEN1* gene are associated with multiple endocrine neoplasia syndrome type 1 (MEN1). Germline pathogenic variants in the *RET* gene are associated with multiple endocrine neoplasia syndrome type 2 (MEN2). Germline pathogenic variants in the *VHL* gene are associated with von Hippel—Lindau syndrome.

Therefore, multiple endocrine neoplasia type 1 (MEN1) is caused by activating mutations in a proto-oncogene.

206. **B.** *The HRAS gene for Costello syndrome is a proto-oncogene.* The rest are caused by loss-of-function mutations in tumor suppressor genes.

Germline pathogenic variants in the *FLCN* gene are associated with Birt—Hogg—Dubé syndrome. Germline pathogenic variants in the *HRAS* gene are associated with Costello syndrome. Germline pathogenic variants in the *TP53* gene are associated with Li—Fraumeni syndrome. Germline pathogenic variants in the *RET* gene are associated with multiple endocrine neoplasia syndrome type 2 (MEN2). Germline pathogenic variants in the *NF1* gene are associated with neurofibromatosis type 1 (NF1). Germline pathogenic variants in the *VHL* gene are associated with von Hippel—Lindau syndrome.

Therefore, Costello syndrome is caused by activating mutations in a proto-oncogene.

References

1. Giardiello FM, et al. Guidelines on genetic evaluation and management of Lynch syndrome: a consensus statement by the US Multi-society Task Force on colorectal cancer. *Am J Gastroenterol* 2014;**109**(8):1159–79.
2. Buckingham L. *Molecular diagnostics: fundamentals, methods, and clinical applications.* 2nd ed. Philadelphia: F.A. Davis Co; 2012. xvi, 558 pp.

3. Nussbaum RL, McInnes RR, Willard HF. *Thompson & Thompsongenetics in medicine*. 8th ed. Philadelphia: Elsevier; 2016. xi, 546 pp.

4. Evans DG, Howell A. Breast cancer risk-assessment models. *Breast Cancer Res* 2007;**9**(5):213.

5. Oliveira C, et al. Genetic screening for familial gastric cancer. *Hered Cancer Clin Pract* 2004;**2**(2):51−64.

6. Corso G, et al. CDH1 germline mutations and hereditary lobular breast cancer. *Fam Cancer* 2016;**15**(2):215−19.

7. Seshachalam A, et al. Ataxia telangiectasia: family management. *Indian J Hum Genet* 2010;**16**(1):39−42.

8. Graham Jr JM, et al. Cerebro-oculo-facio-skeletal syndrome with a nucleotide excision-repair defect and a mutated XPD gene, with prenatal diagnosis in a triplet pregnancy. *Am J Hum Genet* 2001;**69**(2):291−300.

9. Mahale A, Poornima V, Shrestha M. WAGR syndrome—a case report. *Nepal Med Coll J* 2007;**9**(2):138−40.

10. Casaroto AR, et al. Early diagnosis of Gorlin-Goltz syndrome: case report. *Head Face Med* 2011;**7**:2.

11. Karunakaran A, Ravindran R, Arshad M, Ram MK, Laxmi MK. Dyskeratosis congenita: a report of two cases. *Case Rep Dent* 2013;845125.

12. Venkatramani R, et al. Congenital abnormalities and hepatoblastoma: a report from the Children's Oncology Group (COG) and the Utah Population Database (UPDB). *Am J Med Genet A* 2014;**164A**(9):2250−5.

13. Manmadha Rao V, Gandhi MVV, Vivekanand B. Multiple endocrine neoplasia type 2b: a rare case report. *Int J Sci Study* 2015;**2**(10):3.

14. Audrius Šileikis EK, Janavičius R, Strupas K. Multiple endocrine neoplasia type 1: a case report and review of the literature. *Central Eur J Med* 2014;**9**(3):7.

15. Zacharia GS. Neurofibromatosis type 2: a case report and brief review of literature. *Indian J Otol* 2013;**19**(4):3.

16. Van Vuuren W, Naude NN, Meyer FSJ, Sathekge BJ, Sathekge MM. Pheochromocytomas/Paragangliomas and two cases. *South Afr Fam Practice* 2007;**49**(5):4.

17. Karasek D, Frysak Z, Pacak K. Genetic testing for pheochromocytoma. *Curr Hypertens Rep* 2010;**12**(6):456−64.

18. Asokan S, Muthu M, Rathna Prabhu V. Noonan syndrome: a case report. *J Indian Soc Pedod Prev Dent* 2007;**25**(3):4.

19. Sharma K, Arora A. Waardenburg syndrome: a case study of two patients. *Indian J Otolaryngol Head Neck Surg* 2015;**67**(3):324−8.

20. Suri M, Kabra M, Kataria A, Singh GR, Sharma S, Gupta AK, et al. Denys-Drash syndrome. *Indian Pediatr* 1995;**32**:4.

21. Evans DG, Howell A. Breast cancer risk-assessment models. *Breast Cancer Res* 2007;**9**(5):213.

SELF-ASSESSMENT QUESTIONS FOR CLINICAL MOLECULAR GENETICS

Oncology—Acquired

Genetic changes in malignancies may be constitutional (see Chapter 7: Oncology—Constitutional) or acquired (this chapter). In addition to identifying germline pathogenic variants for diagnosis, genetic profiling of malignancies helps physicians to determine the origin of the cancer, its risk for metastasis, its specific drug responsiveness, and its recurrent risk.[1] In 2015 President Barack Obama announced the launch of his Precision Medicine Initiative—"the one that delivers the right treatment at the right time." The first step of the initiative is seeking to "focus on oncology for the near-term by coordinating with the National Cancer Institute (NCI) to pinpoint how genetic factors can lead to cancer."

PRIMARY AND SECONDARY GENETIC ABERRATIONS IN ONCOGENESIS/ TUMORIGENESIS/CARCINOGENESIS

Partially or fully transformed cells harbor hundreds to thousands of molecular genetic mutations, chromosomal alterations, and epigenetic aberrations. The great majority are passive changes; a handful are driven forces. Primary genetic alterations are the driven forces of the malignancies caused by interaction between the oncogenic agents and the genetic materials of the host cell. These alterations are mainly somatic (acquired) mutations. For example, mutations in the *RB1* gene are considered to be the initiator of retinoblastoma.

Secondary genetic alterations are passive changes that arise by survival of nondisjunction and structural rearrangements because of the lack of DNA repair mechanisms. These alterations are followed by the selection of cells with changes that amplify the primary change and thus appear to be nonrandom chromosome patterns.[2] For example, the Philadelphia chromosome (Ph+) is diagnostic of and the primary change for chronic myeloid leukemia (CML). When the CML turns from the chronic phase into the accelerated/blast phase(s), secondary genetic changes are usually present, such as additional copies of Ph+, +8, +19, i(17)(q), and/or gene alterations in *TP53*, *RB1*, *MYC*, *CDKN2A*, *RAS*, *RUNX1*, and *EVI1*.

CLONALITY, CLONAL EXPANSION, AND CLONAL EVOLUTION

Primary genetic aberrations provide selective advantages in cell growth, survival, and metabolism, which compete and override normal and premalignant cells for space, energy, and nutrient and lead to clonal emergence. The clonal selection and propagation of dominant clones of malignant cells may be independently sustained by multiple different combinations of primary mutations. During clonal evolution, malignant cells sequentially accumulate genetic and epigenetic mutations in proto-oncogenes and tumor suppressor genes.[3]

TUMOR HETEROGENEITY

Variations between tumors arising at the same site account for intertumoral heterogeneity, while variations in clonal growth, functional properties or expression markers delineate intratumoral heterogeneity. Genetic heterogeneity between different malignant clones and even within the same clones has been seen in many malignancy types. Moreover, cells within a single genetic clone were deemed to display functional variability in tumor propagation potential.

LOSS OF HETEROZYGOSITY

Loss of heterozygosity (LOH) has been seen in the development of many malignancies, suggesting the absence of functional tumor suppressor gene(s) in the lost region. Mitotic nondisjunction, recombination between homologous chromosomes, and chromosomal deletion are among the implicated mechanisms. For example, a deletion of 3p including the *VHL* gene on 3p25.3 is common in clear-cell renal-cell carcinomas (RCCs), and 1p/19q codeletion is common in oligodendrogliomas. SNP chromosome microarray (CMA) studies reveal that acquired copy neutral LOH (also called region of homozygosity (ROH)) is quite common in malignancies, too. It constitutes 20%–80% of the LOH in human malignancies, which may likely represent secondary genetic alterations during clonal evolution.

SAMPLES FOR GENETIC TESTS

The sample of choice for germline pathogenic variants in hereditary malignant predisposition syndromes is a peripheral-blood specimen (see Chapter 7: Oncology—Constitutional). The sample of choice for acquired pathogenic variants in malignancies is the malignant specimen itself (this chapter). A lot of times microdissection/enrichment is necessary to increase the detection of acquired mutations presented in the malignant cells only. Liquid biopsies are newly developed noninvasive tests of cancer cells and/or cell-free DNAs within blood and/or urine.

QUESTIONS

1. A scientist in a clinical molecular laboratory decides to validate a qualitative assay for B-cell clonality (*IGH* and *IGK*) tests by a PCR method based on the BIOMED-2 consensus. For which one of the following malignancies is this assay *NOT* appropriate?[4]
   A. AML with normal karyotype and FISH
   B. CLL with normal FISH
   C. Follicular lymphoma with normal FISH
   D. Plasma-cell myeloma with normal FISH
   E. All of the above
   F. None of the above
2. A scientist in a clinical molecular laboratory decides to validate a qualitative assay for B-cell clonality (*IGH*) tests by a PCR method based on the BIOMED-2 consensus. In which one of the following situations could the results be false negative?[4]
   A. Absent or incomplete IGH rearrangements in immature B-cell neoplasms in pre-B-cell ALL
   B. The presence of extensive somatic mutation in follicular lymphoma
   C. Negative results caused by DNA degradation on the positive control

D. A and B
E. B and C
F. All of the above
G. None of the above

3. A scientist in a clinical molecular laboratory decides to validate a qualitative assay for T-cell clonality (*TCRG* and *TCRB*) tests by a PCR method based on the BIOMED-2 consensus. For which one of the following malignancies is this assay *NOT* appropriate?[4]
   A. AML with normal karyotype and FISH
   B. Follicular lymphoma with normal FISH
   C. Plasma-cell myeloma with normal FISH
   D. All of the above
   E. None of the above
4. A 45-year-old female presented in a clinic for loss of appetite, and weight loss (10 lb) in the past 6 months. Her medical history was significant for chronic gastritis with *Helicobacter pylori* infection. An upper GI endoscopy demonstrated that the entire stomach was thickened and friable, suspicious for linitis plastica. An abdominal CT showed marked thickening of the stomach as well as abnormal soft-tissue stranding extending to the omentum with numerous small abdominal lymph nodes. Histopathological examinations revealed ulcerated mucosa with granulation tissue enriched with polytypic plasma cells, and focally dense lymphoid infiltrate with lamina propria. Immunohistochemistry (IHC) stains demonstrated increased CD20+ B cells. The morphological and immunophenotypic findings were suspicious for extranodal marginal-zone lymphoma (such as MALT lymphoma). The *MALT1* break-apart FISH was negative. Which one of the following assays would help to further establish the diagnosis if the oncologist still suspected that the patient had MALT lymphoma?[4,5]
   A. *ALK* amplification
   B. *BRAF* V600E
   C. *IGH* and *IGK* clonality tests
   D. *TCRG* and *TCRB* clonality test
   E. All of the above
   F. None of the above
5. A 42-year-old male came to a clinic with a 7-month history of nasal obstruction. A CT scan revealed a 3.4 × 2.6 × 2.6 cm lobulated enhancing soft-tissue mass filling the nasopharynx and bulging minimally into the posterior nasal cavity and the oropharynx. There

was no parapharyngeal extension or extension to the skull base. Histopathological examinations revealed CD3+, CD4+, CD8+, TdT+, and EBER+. The karyotype of the tumor specimen was a normal male, or 46,XY. Which one of the following assays would help to further establish the diagnosis of lymphoma?

A. *ALK* amplification
B. *BRAF* V600E
C. *IGH* and *IGK* clonality tests
D. *TCRG* and *TCRB* clonality test
E. All of the above
F. None of the above

6. A 75-year-old male came to a clinic for a left neck mass. He was otherwise healthy and asymptomatic. Biopsies of the mass and bone marrow were obtained. The physician ordered a test to assess clonality in the *IGH* gene. The result of one of the amplicons for the VH frameworks is shown in Fig. 8.1. The top panel was from the bone marrow and the bottom was from the biopsy of the left neck mass. Which one of the following interpretations of the results would be the most appropriate?[4,6]

A. The results of the bone-marrow biopsy indicated a clonal proliferation of B cells.
B. The results of the bone-marrow biopsy indicated a clonal proliferation of T cells.
C. The results of the biopsy from the neck mass indicated a clonal proliferation of B cells.
D. The results of the biopsy from the neck mass indicated a clonal proliferation of T cells.
E. The results of both samples indicated a clonal proliferation of B cells.
F. The results of both samples indicated a clonal proliferation of T cells.

7. A 75-year-old male came to a clinic for a left neck mass. He was otherwise healthy and asymptomatic. Biopsies of the mass and bone marrow were obtained. The physician ordered a test to assess clonality in the *IGH* gene. The result of one of the amplicons for the VH frameworks are shown in Fig. 8.1. The top panel was from the bone marrow and the bottom was from the biopsy of the left neck mass. Which one of the following interpretations of the results would be the most appropriate?[4]

A. The results indicated a clonal proliferation of B cells in the neck mass but not in the bone marrow. Therefore, the patient had B-cell lymphoma that had not metastasized into the bone marrow.
B. The results indicated a clonal proliferation of B cells in the bone marrow but not in the neck mass. Therefore, the patient had B-cell leukemia.
C. The results indicated a clonal proliferation of B cells in the neck mass but not in the bone marrow. These findings supported a diagnosis of B-cell lymphoma, but reactive lymphoproliferations cannot be completely ruled out.
D. The results indicated a clonal proliferation of B cells in the neck mass but not in the bone marrow. Therefore, the patient had B-cell lymphoma that had metastasized into the bone marrow.
E. The results indicated a clonal proliferation of B cells in bone marrow but not in the neck mass. Therefore, the patient had B-cell leukemia that had not metastasized into a remote site, such as the neck.

8. A 7-year-old female with a high white blood cell count was evaluated in an oncology clinic. A bone-marrow biopsy was obtained and revealed 30%

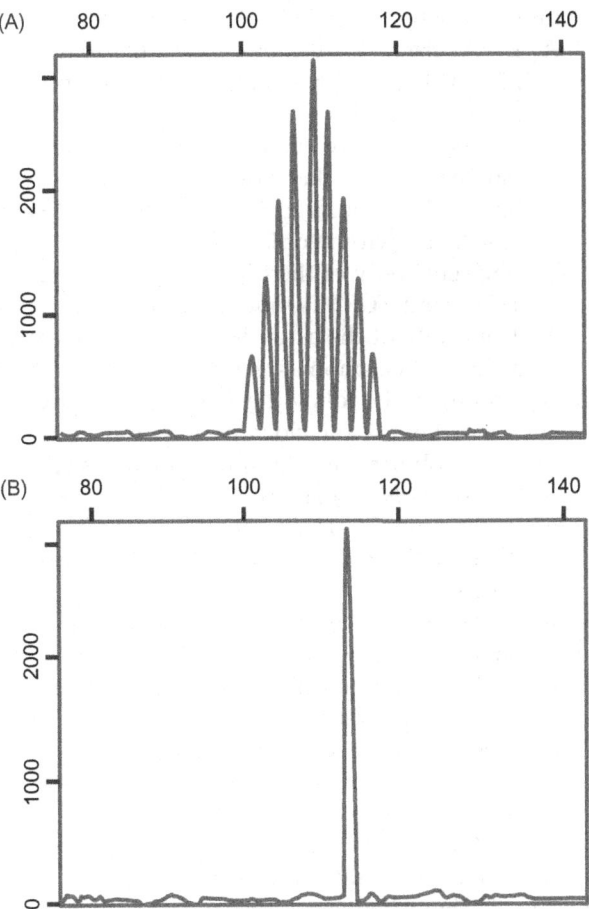

FIGURE 8.1 Electropherograms of (A) bone marrow and (B) left neck mass. The *y*-axis shows relative fluorescence intensity and the *x*-axis the PCR fragment size in base pairs.

lymphoblasts with expression of CD3, CD4, and CD8. A chest CT detected superior mediastinal masses. The physician ordered a test to assess the *TCRG* and *TCRB* gene rearrangement. The result of

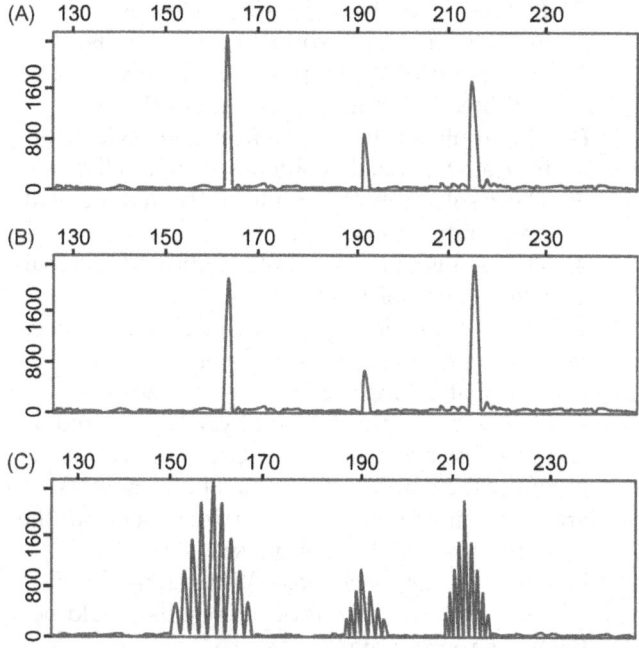

FIGURE 8.2   Electropherograms of (A) bone marrow, (B) mediastinal mass, and (C) normal control. The *y*-axis shows relative fluorescence intensity and the *x*-axis PCR fragment size in base pairs.

one of the amplicons is shown in Fig. 8.2. The top panel was from a normal control, the middle from the bone marrow, and the bottom from the biopsy of the mass.

Which one of the following interpretations of the clonality test is the most appropriate?[4,6]

A. The results of the bone-marrow biopsy indicated a clonal proliferation of B cells.

B. The results of the bone-marrow biopsy indicated a clonal proliferation of T cells.

C. The results of the biopsy from the mass indicated a clonal proliferation of B cells.

D. The results of the biopsy from the mass indicated a clonal proliferation of T cells.

E. The results of both samples indicated a clonal proliferation of B cells.

F. The results of both samples indicated a clonal proliferation of T cells.

9. The EuroClonality (BIOMED-2) consortium has led to standardization and has significantly improved detection of the clonality of malignant B-cell/T-cell lymphomas/leukemias. Which one

of the following is the standard method for the clonal assessment?[4,6]

A. PCR/capillary electrophoresis

B. PCR/Sanger sequencing

C. Next-generation sequencing (NGS)

D. Restriction-fragment—length polymorphism (RFLP)

E. Southern blotting

10. Which one of the following statements regarding molecular T-cell receptor gene rearrangement analysis is CORRECT?[4,6]

A. The *TCRA* gene is the most commonly tested locus.

B. The *TCRB* gene is the most commonly tested locus.

C. The *TCRC* gene is the most commonly tested locus.

D. The *TCRD* gene is the most commonly tested locus.

E. The *TCRG* gene is the most commonly tested locus.

11. Which one of the following statements regarding the assessment of the clonality in the immunoglobulins or TCRs is CORRECT?

A. DNAs from paraffin-embedded tissue have higher detection rate than DNAs from bone-marrow samples.

B. "Pseudoclonality" usually happens when patients have leukocytosis.

C. Single clonal or oligoclonal results are always associated with neoplasms.

D. The sensitivity of the BIOMED-2 assay for *TCRG* and *TCRB* is more than 90%.

E. The utility of the assay is limited in the early stages of lymphomas/leukemias.

12. Which one of the following statements regarding the assessment of the clonality in the immunoglobulins (*IGH* and *IGK*) or TCRs (*TCRG* and *TCRB*) is NOT correct?[4]

A. PCR/capillary electrophoresis works better than Southern blot for paraffin-embedded tissue.

B. PCR/capillary electrophoresis is more sensitive than Southern blot.

C. PCR/capillary electrophoresis is less time consuming than Southern blot.

D. PCR/capillary electrophoresis may detect more possible clonal rearrangements than Southern blot.

E. PCR/capillary electrophoresis has a higher false positive rate than Southern blot.

13. What is the difference between the immunoglobulin (*IGH* and *IGK*) and T-cell receptor (*TCRG* and *TCRB*) clonal rearrangements?[4]

A. A developing T cell has fewer chances to productively rearrange β chains than a developing B cell has for H chains.
B. Somatic hypermutation does not generate diversity in T-cell receptors, while it does in B-cell immunoglobulin.
C. TCR loci are rearranged by the different enzymes from the immunoglobulin loci.
D. TCR has fewer rearrangements than immunoglobulin.
E. TCR rearrangements happen throughout the lifetime, while Ig rearrangements happen only before adolescence.

14. The EuroClonality (BIOMED-2) consortium has led to standardization and has significantly improved detection of the clonality of malignant B-cell/T-cell lymphomas/leukemias. Which immunoglobulin(s) is(are) most commonly used for the clonal assessment?[4]
A. *IGH* D–J and *IGK*
B. *IGH* V–J and *IGK*
C. *IGH* V–J and *IGL*
D. *IGH* D–J and *IGL*
E. *IGH* D–J
F. *IGH* V–J

15. The EuroClonality (BIOMED-2) consortium has led to standardization and has significantly improved detection of the clonality of malignant B-cell/T-cell lymphomas/leukemias. Which T-cell receptor (*TCR*) gene(s) is(are) most commonly used for the clonal assessment?[4]
A. *TCRA*
B. *TCRD*
C. *TCRD* and *TCRA*
D. *TCRB*
E. *TCRG*
F. *TCRG* and *TCRB*

16. An 80-year-old male came to a clinic for a left neck mass. He was otherwise healthy and asymptomatic. A biopsy of the mass was obtained, and it showed a sparse lymphoid infiltration. The physician ordered a test to assess the clonality in the *IGH* gene. The results showed three low-amplitude peaks. The internal control, known polyclonal control, and known clonal control showed the expected results. Which one of the following would be the most appropriate next step in the workup?[4]
A. Repeating the test with the same specimen
B. Requesting second specimen for confirmation
C. Signing the case out as positive for B cell monoclonality
D. Any of the above
E. None of the above

17. An 80-year-old male came to a clinic for a left neck mass. He was otherwise healthy and asymptomatic. A biopsy of the mass was obtained, and it showed a sparse lymphoid infiltration. The physician ordered a test to assess the clonality in the *IGH* gene. The results showed three low amplitude peaks. The internal control, a known polyclonal control, and a known clonal control showed the expected results. The test was repeated with the same sample, and results showed three different low-amplitude peaks. Which one of the following would be the most appropriate interpretation?[4]
A. Presence of oligoclonal *IGH* populations, consistent with diagnosis of a malignancy
B. Presence of oligoclonal *IGH* populations, consistent with reactive clones
C. Presence of oligoclonal *IGH* populations, uncertain significance
D. Pseudoclonality, consistent with a paucity of B cells in the sample
E. Negative, no clonal *IGH* populations
F. Wrong sample in the second test, remedial action form needed

18. A 43-year-old male came to a clinic with high fever and chills for 3 days. He had undergone renal transplantation 6 months ago because of renal-cell carcinoma. He had been on immunosuppressive therapy. A chest X-ray and CT revealed multiple, variably sized nodular lesions at the apical segments of both upper lungs, anterior segment of the left lung, posterobasal segment of the left lower lobe, hilar portion of the right middle lobe, and superior segment of the right lower lobe. Multiple mediastinal lymphadenopathies were also seen in the right paratracheal and subcarinal areas. Minimal pleural effusion was also observed in the right lower thorax. A computed tomogram–guided transthoracic lung biopsy was performed. Irregular thickening of the alveolar septa and the perivascular connective tissue, due to diffuse infiltration of atypical lymphoid cells, were observed. These atypical lymphoid cells were confirmed as B-cell lineage by immunohistochemical staining. Posttransplantation lymphoproliferative disorder (PTLD) was suspected. To establish the cell clonality, which of the following would be the most informative assay?
A. Southern blot analysis of *IGH* and *IGK* gene rearrangement with the biopsy sample
B. Southern blot analysis of *IGH* and *IGK* gene rearrangement with the peripheral-blood sample
C. Southern blot analysis of *IGH* and *IGK* gene rearrangement with the bone-marrow sample

D. PCR/capillary electrophoresis of *IGH* and
IGK gene rearrangement with the biopsy sample

E. PCR/capillary electrophoresis of *IGH* and *IGK* gene rearrangement with the peripheral-blood sample

F. PCR/capillary electrophoresis of *IGH* and *IGK* gene rearrangement with the bone-marrow sample

19. A 43-year-old female was admitted to a local hospital with symptoms of abdominal distention for 6 months, leg swelling for 4 months, and decreased urine output for 4 months. She developed a swelling in the left hypochondrium 6 months ago that progressed to both legs. She had intermittent low-grade fever, loss of appetite, and loss of weight. Otherwise, her medical history was uneventful. Her family history was unremarkable. At admission, her temperature was 98.4°F. Her axillary, cervical, and inguinal lymph nodes were palpable and firm. A mass extending from the left hypochondrium to the hypogastric region was seen, and it moved with respiration. Laboratory tests revealed high WBC (1,400,00/mL; normal range, 4500–11,000/mL) and normocytic hypochromic anemia (Hb, 5.6 g/dL; normal range, 12.0–15.1 g/dL). A bone-marrow biopsy was obtained, and the impression was chronic myeloid leukemia (CML) with lymphoid blast crisis. Which molecular genetic test results would most likely be abnormal with this bone-marrow specimen?[7]

A. *BCR-ABL1*
B. *CEBPA*
C. *FLT3*-ITD
D. *FLT3*-TKD
E. *JAK2*
F. *NPM1*

20. A 32-year-old male was referred to an oncology clinic for leukocytosis (16.6×10^9/L), anemia, and marked thrombocytosis with 2% blasts in the blood. Mild splenomegaly was observed on a physical examination. A bone-marrow aspirate revealed marked myeloid hyperplasia with 1.0% myeloblasts, 2.0% promyelocytes, 3.8% myelocytes, 16.6% metamyelocytes, 29.2% bands, 27.8% segmented neutrophils, 10.2% eosinophils, and 3.0% basophils. The myeloid/erythroid ratio was markedly increased to 26.8:1. A G-banded karyotype demonstrated 46,XY, t(9;22)(q34;q11.2) in 20 of 20 cells analyzed. The oncologist ordered a qualitative *BCR-ABL1* test of this bone-marrow specimen to further characterize this leukemia. Which one of the following statements regarding the qualitative *BCR-ABL1* test is correct?[8,9]

1. It is a DNA-based test.
2. It is a RNA-based test.
3. A single PCR reaction.
4. Multiple PCR reactions.
5. It tests *BCR-ABL1* fusion.
6. It tests *ABL1-BCR* fusion.
   A. 1, 3, and 5
   B. 1, 3, and 6
   C. 1, 4, and 6
   D. 2, 3, and 5
   E. 2, 4, and 5
   F. 2, 4, and 6

21. A 32-year-old male was referred to an oncology clinic for leukocytosis (16.6×10^9/L), anemia, and marked thrombocytosis with 2% blasts in the blood. Mild splenomegaly was observed on a physical examination. A bone marrow aspirate revealed marked myeloid hyperplasia with 1.0% myeloblasts, 2.0% promyelocytes, 3.8% myelocytes, 16.6% metamyelocytes, 29.2% bands, 27.8% segmented neutrophils, 10.2% eosinophils, and 3.0% basophils. The myeloid/erythroid ratio was markedly increased to 26.8:1. A G-banded karyotype demonstrated 46,XY,t(9;22)(q34;q11.2) in 20 of 20 cells analyzed. The oncologist ordered a qualitative *BCR-ABL1* test of this bone-marrow specimen to further characterize this myeloproliferative disorder. Which one of the following statements regarding the quantitative *BCR-ABL1* test is NOT correct?[8,9]

A. It is a DNA-based test.
B. It is a reverse transcriptase (RT-PCR) reaction.
C. There is one amplicon for the p190.
D. There are two amplicons for the p210.
E. There is one amplicon for the p230.

22. How frequently do patients with chronic myelogenous leukemia (CML) have a *BCR-ABL1* fusion gene?[7]

A. 95%
B. 75%
C. 50%
D. 25%
E. <5%

23. How frequently do patients with acute myeloid leukemia (AML) have a *BCR-ABL1* fusion gene?

A. 95%
B. 75%
C. 50%
D. 25%
E. <5%

24. How frequently do adult patients with precursor B ALL have a *BCR-ABL1* fusion gene?[10]

A. 95%
B. 75%
C. 50%

D. 25%

E. <5%

25. How frequently do pediatric patients with precursor B ALL have a *BCR-ABL1* fusion gene?[10]

A. 95%

B. 75%

C. 50%

D. 25%

E. 5%

26. A 46-year-old male presented to an emergency department with severe headaches, dyspnea on exertion, and petechiae on the lower extremities. A complete blood count (CBC) demonstrated a white-blood-cell (WBC) of $56 \times 10^3/\mu L$, hemoglobin (Hb) 9.0 g/dL, hematocrit 23, mean corpuscular volume (MCV) 97 fL, platelets $15 \times 10^9/\mu L$, and absolute neutrophil count (ANC) $0.7 \times 10^3/\mu L$. A bone-marrow biopsy revealed 90% lymphoid blasts with expression of CD19, CD20, CD22, CD10, CD34, TdT, and HLA-DR. The G-banded karyotype result was 46,XY,t (9;22)(q34;q11.2)[20]. The patient was diagnosed with pre-B acute lymphoblastic leukemia (ALL). Which one of the following isoforms of *BCR-ABL1* would the patient most likely have?[9]

A. a19b2

B. b2a2

C. b3a2

D. e1a2

E. e13a2

F. e14a2

27. A 60-year-old male came to a clinic for fatigue, loss of appetite, weight loss, low fever, and night sweats in the past month. Chronic myeloid leukemia (CML) was on the top of the list of differential diagnoses. Cytogenetic and molecular *BCR-ABL1* qualitative tests were ordered. Which one of the following *BCR-ABL1* fusions would most likely be positive if the patient had a t(9;22)?[9]

A. a19b2

B. e1a1

C. e2a2

D. e3a2

E. e14a2

F. e19a2

28. A 66-year-old female came to a clinic for fatigue, loss of appetite, weight loss, low fever, and night sweats in the past month. Chronic myeloid leukemia (CML) was on the top of the list of differential diagnoses. Cytogenetic and molecular *BCR-ABL1* qualitative tests were ordered. Which one of the following *BCR-ABL1* fusions would most likely be positive if the patient had a t(9;22)?[9]

A. a19b2

B. e1a1

C. e2a2

D. e3a2

E. e13a2

F. e19a2

29. A 65-year-old male came to a clinic for fatigue, loss of appetite, weight loss, low fever, and night sweats in the past month. Chronic myeloid leukemia (CML) was on the top of the list of differential diagnoses. Cytogenetic and molecular *BCR-ABL1* qualitative tests were ordered. Which one of the following *BCR-ABL1* fusions would most likely be positive if the patient had a t (9;22)?[9]

A. a19b2

B. b2a2

C. b13a2

D. e1a1

E. e19a2

30. A 66-year-old male came to a clinic for fatigue, loss of appetite, weight loss, low fever, and night sweats in the past month. Chronic myeloid leukemia (CML) was on the top of the list of differential diagnoses. Cytogenetic and molecular *BCR-ABL1* qualitative tests were ordered. Which one of the following fusions of *BCR-ABL1* would most likely be positive if the patient had a t(9;22)?[9]

A. a19b2

B. b3a2

C. b14a2

D. e1a1

E. e19a2

31. Which one of the following *BCR-ABL1* fusions corresponds to the p230 isoform?[9]

A. a19b2

B. b3a2

C. e1a1

D. e13a2

E. e19a2

32. Which one of the following *BCR-ABL1* fusions corresponds to the p230 isoform?[9]

A. a19b2

B. b3a2

C. c3a2

D. e1a1

E. e13a2

33. Which one of the following *BCR-ABL1* fusions corresponds to an isoform with the highest tyrosine kinase activity?[9]

A. a19b2

B. b3a2

C. e1a2

D. e13a2

E. e19a2

34. A 62-year-old male came to a clinic for fatigue, loss of appetite, weight loss, low fever, and night

sweats in the past month. Chronic myeloid leukemia (CML) was on the top of the list of differential diagnoses. Cytogenetic and molecular *BCR-ABL1* quantitative tests were ordered. The results showed that the patient was positive for p210 (b2a2). He was started on imatinib. After 3 months of therapy, he reached remission. However, 6 months after therapy, he relapsed with elevated b2a2. A molecular test was ordered to further assess the resistance. Which one of the following statements regarding the molecular test for imatinib resistance is correct?[11]

A. It is a DNA-based test of the tyrosine kinase domain in the *ABL1* gene.

B. It is a DNA-based test of the tyrosine kinase domain in the *BCR* gene.

C. It is a RNA-based test of the tyrosine kinase domain in the *BCR-ABL1* gene.

D. It is a RNA-based test of the tyrosine kinase domain in the *ABL1* and *BCR-ABL1* genes.

E. It is a RNA-based test of the tyrosine kinase domain in the *ABL1-BCR* gene.

F. It is a RNA based test of the tyrosine kinase domain in the *ABL1* and *ABL1-BCR* genes.

35. Which one of the following malignancies most likely does *NOT* have an acquired *BCR-ABL1* rearrangement?

A. Acute myeloid leukemia (AML)

B. Acute B lymphoblastic leukemia (B ALL)

C. Acute T lymphoblastic leukemia (T ALL)

D. Chronic lymphocytic leukemia (CLL)

E. Myeloid proliferative neoplasm (MPN)

36. A 43-year-old female was admitted to a local hospital with symptoms of abdominal distention for 6 months, leg swelling for 4 months, and decreased urine output for 4 months. She developed a swelling in the left hypochondrium 6 months ago that progressed to both legs. She had intermittent low-grade fever, loss of appetite, and loss of weight. Otherwise, her medical history was uneventful. Her family history was unremarkable. At admission, her temperature was 98.4°F. Her axillary, cervical and inguinal lymph nodes were palpable and firm. A mass extending from the left hypochondrium to the hypogastric region was seen, and it moved with respiration. Laboratory tests revealed a high WBC count (1,400,000/mL; normal range, 4500—11,000/mL) and normocytic hypochromic anemia (Hb, 5.6 g/dL; normal range, 12.0—15.1). A bone-marrow biopsy was obtained and the impression was chronic myeloid leukemia (CML) with lymphoid blast crisis. Chromosome karyotype analyses revealed 46,XX,t(9;22)(q34;q11.2)[6]/48, idem, + 8,der(22)t(9;22)(q34;q11.2)[4]/46,XX[10].

The results of a quantitative *BCR-ABL1* test were positive for p210. Which one of the following targeted therapies would be most appropriate to this patient?

A. Gleevec (imatinib)

B. Herceptin (trastuzumab)

C. Lynparza (olaparib)

D. Zelboraf (vemurafenib)

E. None of the above

37. A 43-year-old female was admitted to a local hospital with symptoms of abdominal distention for 6 months, leg swelling for 4 months, and decreased urine output for 4 months. She developed a swelling in the left hypochondrium 6 months ago that progressed to both legs. She had intermittent low-grade fever, loss of appetite, and loss of and weight. Otherwise, her medical history was uneventful. Her family history was unremarkable. At admission her temperature was 98.4°F. Her axillary, cervical, and inguinal lymph nodes were palpable and firm. A mass extending from the left hypochondrium to the hypogastric region was seen, and it moved with respiration. Laboratory tests revealed a high WBC count (1,400,000/mL; normal range, 4500—11,000/mL) and normocytic hypochromic anemia (Hb, 5.6 g/dL; normal range, 12.0—15.1). A bone-marrow biopsy was obtained and the impression was chronic myeloid leukemia (CML) with lymphoid blast crisis. Which one of the following assays would be the most appropriate for *BCR-ABL1* in order in order to establish the diagnosis of CML in this patient?

A. FISH

B. PCR-capillary electrophoresis

C. Sanger sequencing

D. Targeted-mutation analysis

E. All of the above

F. None of the above

38. A 43-year-old female was admitted to a local hospital with symptoms of abdominal distention for 6 months, leg swelling for 4 months, and decreased urine output for 4 months. She developed a swelling in the left hypochondrium 6 months ago that progressed to both legs. She had intermittent low-grade fever, loss of appetite, and loss of weight. Otherwise, her medical history was uneventful. Her family history was unremarkable. At admission her temperature was 98.4°F. Her axillary, cervical and inguinal lymph nodes were palpable and firm. A mass extending from the left hypochondrium to the hypogastric region was seen, and it moved with respiration. Laboratory tests revealed a high WBC count (1,400,000/mL; normal range, 4500—11,000/mL)

and normocytic hypochromic anemia (Hb, 5.6 g/dL; normal range, 12.0–15.1). A bone-marrow biopsy was obtained and the impression was chronic myeloid leukemia (CML) with lymphoid blast crisis. The results of a chromosome karyotype revealed 46,XX,t(9;22)(q34;q11.2)[6]/48, idem, +8,der(22)t(9;22)(q34;q11.2)[4]/46,XX[10]. The patient responded well to Gleevec (imatinib). One year later the patient had reappearance of BCR-ABL1 p210, even though she had been taking Gleevec (imatinib) as her doctor suggested. The follow-up karyotype results were 46,XX,t(9;22)(q34;q11.2)[12]/46,XX[8]. Which one of the following molecular tests would be appropriate for this patient in order to assistant in the decision about future therapy?

A. Detect amplification of ABL1/BCR rearrangement
B. Detect amplification of BCR/ABL1 rearrangement
C. Detect deletion of BCR/ABL1 rearrangement
D. Identify BCR/ABL1 kinase domain mutation in the ABL1 gene
E. Identify BCR/ABL1 kinase domain mutation in the BCR gene
F. None of the above

39. A 32-year-old male visited a clinic for back pain and lower-extremity paresthesia. At diagnosis, the white-blood-cell count was $5.56 \times 10^4/\mu L$, hemoglobin (Hb) 14.2 g/dL, and platelet count $113 \times 10^4/\mu L$. The blasts were 2% in the peripheral blood and up to 90% in the bone marrow. The immunophenotype of the blasts was CD10+, CD19+, CD13+, cytoplasmic CD22 (cCD22)+, cytoplasmic CD79a (cCD79a)+, HLA-DR+, CD34+, cytoplasmic myeloperoxidase (cMPO)−, and nuclear terminal deoxynucleotidyl transferase (nTdT)+. A morphological diagnosis of acute lymphoblastic leukemia (ALL) was made. The results of a chromosome karyotype revealed 46,XY,t(9;22)(q34;q11.2)[20]. A qualitative reverse-transcriptase polymerase chain reaction (RT-PCR) test for BCR-ABL1 was ordered. For which one of the following BCR-ABL1 fusion types would this patient most likely be positive in this specimen?[9,12]

A. p190
B. p205
C. p210
D. p230
E. All of the above
F. None of the above

40. A 32-year-old male visited a clinic for back pain and low extremity paresthesia. At diagnosis, the white-blood-cell count was $5.56 \times 10^4/\mu L$,

hemoglobin (Hb) 14.2 g/dL, and platelet count $113 \times 10^4/\mu L$. The blasts were 2% in the peripheral blood and up to 90% in the bone marrow. The immunophenotype of the blasts was CD10+, CD19+, CD13+, cytoplasmic CD22 (cCD22)+, cytoplasmic CD79a (cCD79a)+, HLA-DR+, CD34+, cytoplasmic myeloperoxidase (cMPO)−, and nuclear terminal deoxynucleotidyl transferase (TdT)+. A morphological diagnosis of acute lymphoblastic leukemia (ALL) was made. The results of chromosome karyotype revealed 46,XY,t(9;22)(q34;q11.2)[20]. A qualitative reverse-transcriptase polymerase chain reaction (RT-PCR) test for BCR-ABL1 was ordered, and the result was positive for p190. Which one of the following prognoses would this patient most likely have?[9,12]

A. Favorable risk
B. Intermediate risk
C. Unfavorable risk
D. Unclear
E. None of the above

41. A 58-year-old male came to a clinic with symptoms of increasing abdominal discomfort, early satiety, and a weight loss of 20 lb due to poor appetite for approximately 6 months. The white-blood-cell count was 8×10^3 cells/mm^3 with an absolute neutrophil count of 1400 cells/mm^3, hemoglobin 9.3 g/dL, and platelet count 76,000 cells/mm^3. A bone-marrow biopsy resulted in a "dry" aspirate, and the core biopsy was markedly fibrotic. An estimate of the blast count based upon touch preps as well as a CD34+/CD117+ immunostaining of the core biopsy demonstrated only 1.2% blasts. The oncologist suspected that the patient had primary myelofibrosis (PMF). Which one of the following molecular assays would most likely be ordered to confirm the diagnosis in this patient?

A. BCR-ABL1 qualitative test
B. CALR exon 9 mutation
C. JAK2 exon 12 mutation
D. JAK2 V617F mutation
E. MPL exon 10 mutation

42. A 58-year-old male came to a clinic with symptoms of increasing abdominal discomfort, early satiety, and a weight loss of 15 lb due to poor appetite for approximately 6 months. The white-blood-cell count was 8×10^3 cells/mm^3 with an absolute neutrophil count of 1400 cells/mm^3, hemoglobin 9.3 g/dL, and platelet count 76,000 cells/mm^3. A bone marrow biopsy resulted in a "dry" aspirate, and the core biopsy was markedly fibrotic. An estimate of the blast count based upon touch preps as well as a CD34+/CD117+ immunostaining of the core biopsy

demonstrated only 1.2% blasts. A qualitative molecular test demonstrated the *JAK2* V617F mutation. Which one of the following conditions would the patient most likely *NOT* have?

A. Chronic myeloid leukemia (CML)
B. Essential thrombocythemia (ET)
C. Polycythemia vera (PV)
D. Primary myelofibrosis (PMF)
E. None of the above

43. A 68-year-old male came to a clinic with symptoms of exercise intolerance for 2 months. A physical examination was significant for splenomegaly. A complete blood count (CBC) revealed pancytopenia (WBCs, 2×10^3/μL; RBCs, 1.84×10^6/μL; Hgb, 6.6 g/dL, Hct, 19.5%; MCV, 106 fL; and platelet: 22,000/μL). A bone-marrow biopsy showed hypercellularity with no blast clusters. Reticulin staining showed some fibrosis. The oncologist suspected that the patient had primary myelofibrosis (PMF). A qualitative molecular test demonstrated the presence of the *JAK2* V617F mutation. Which one of the following genetic assays would most likely also be positive in this patient?[13]

A. *BCR-ABL1* rearrangement
B. *CALR* exon 9 mutation
C. *JAK2* exon 12 mutation
D. *MPL* exon 10 mutation
E. None of the above

44. A 58-year-old male came to a clinic with symptoms of increasing abdominal discomfort, early satiety, and a weight loss of 20 lb due to poor appetite for approximately 6 months. The white-blood-cell count was 8×10^3 cells/mm^3, with an absolute neutrophil count of 1400 cells/mm^3, hemoglobin 9.3 g/dL, and platelet count 76,000 cells/mm^3. A bone marrow biopsy resulted in a "dry" aspirate, and the core biopsy was markedly fibrotic. An estimate of the blast count based upon touch preps as well as a CD34 + / CD117 + immunostaining of the core biopsy demonstrated only 1.2% blasts. A qualitative molecular test demonstrated the absence of the *JAK2* V617F mutation. Which one of the following conditions would be ruled out in this patient if the *JAK2* V617F molecular test was negative?[13]

A. Chronic myeloid leukemia (CML)
B. Essential thrombocythemia (ET)
C. Polycythemia vera (PV)
D. Primary myelofibrosis (PMF)
E. None of the above

45. A 76-year-old female presented to her primary care physician for a yearly checkup. She reported symptoms of fatigue during the past few months and had been experiencing night sweats, but she explained that the latter were probably due to menopause. The physician learned that the night sweats had become more intense and more frequent in recent months and that the patient had lost about 25 lb in the past year. She had not been dieting, but she said that she could not eat as much as she used to. A physical examination revealed bruising on the extremities, and palpation of the spleen shows slight splenomegaly. A complete blood count revealed WBCs 12.1×10^9/L, RBCs 3200×10^9/L, Hgb 9 g/dL, Hct 34%, platelet count 250×10^9/L, and blasts 0%. A bone-marrow biopsy revealed fibrosis. The karyotype results of the bone marrow showed 46,XX[20]. A qualitative molecular test did not detect the *JAK2* V617F mutation. But the physician still suspected that the patient had primary myelofibrosis (PMF). Which one of the following molecular genetic tests would be helpful in order to further establish/rule out the diagnosis of PMF in this patient?[13]

A. *BCR-ABL1* rearrangement
B. *CALR* exon 9 mutation
C. *JAK2* exon 12 mutation
D. All of the above
E. None of the above

46. A 76-year-old female presented to her primary care physician for a yearly checkup. She reported that she had fatigue during the past few months and had been experiencing night sweats, but she explained that the latter were probably due to menopause. The physician learned that the night sweats had become more intense and more frequent in recent months and that the patient had lost about 25 lb in the past a year. She had not been dieting, but she said that she could not eat as much as she used to. A physical examination revealed bruising on the extremities, and palpation of the spleen showed slight splenomegaly. A complete blood count revealed WBCs 12.1×10^9/L, RBCs 3200×10^9/L, Hgb 9 g/dL, Hct 34%, platelet count 250×10^9/L, and blasts 0%. A bone-marrow biopsy revealed fibrosis. The karyotype results of the bone marrow showed 46,XX[20]. A qualitative molecular test detected the *JAK2* V617F mutation. Which one of the following statements would be most appropriate for this patient?

A. The presence of the *JAK2* V617F mutation rules out the diagnosis of chronic myeloid leukemia (CML).

B. The presence of the *JAK2* V617F mutation establishes the diagnosis of essential thrombocythemia (ET).

C. The presence of the *JAK2* V617F mutation establishes the diagnosis of polycythemia vera (PV).

D. The presence of the *JAK2* V617F mutation establishes the diagnosis of primary myelofibrosis (PMF).

E. None of the above.

47. A 58-year-old male came to a clinic with symptoms of increasing abdominal discomfort, early satiety, and a weight loss of 15 lb due to poor appetite for approximately 6 months. The white-blood-cell count (WBC) was 8×10^3 cells/mm^3, with an absolute neutrophil count of 1400 cells/mm^3, hemoglobin 9.3 g/dL, and platelet count 76,000 cells/mm^3. A bone-marrow biopsy resulted in a "dry" aspirate, and the core biopsy was markedly fibrotic. An estimate of the blast count based upon touch preps as well as a CD34+/CD117+ immunostaining of the core biopsy demonstrated only 1.2% blasts. The oncologist suspected that the patient had primary myelofibrosis (PMF). A qualitative molecular test did not detect the *JAK2* V617F mutation. The oncologist still suspected that the patient had primary myelofibrosis (PMF). Which one of the following molecular genetic tests would be helpful in order to establish the diagnosis in this patient?[13]

A. *BCR-ABL1* rearrangement

B. *JAK2* exon 12 mutation

C. *MPL* exon 10 mutation

D. All of the above

E. None of the above

48. A 76-year-old female presented to her primary care physician for a yearly checkup. She reported that she had fatigue during the past few months and had been experiencing night sweats, but she explained that the latter were probably due to menopause. The physician learned that the night sweats had become more intense and more frequent in recent months that the patient had lost about 25 lb in the past year. She had not been diet, but she said that she could not eat as much as she used to. A physical examination revealed bruising on the extremities, and palpation of the spleen showed slight splenomegaly. A complete blood count revealed WBCs 12.1×10^9/L, RBCs 3200×10^9/L, Hgb 9 g/dL, Hct 34%, platelet count 250×10^9/L, and blasts 0%. A bone-marrow biopsy revealed fibrosis. The karyotype results of the bone marrow showed 46,XX[20]. A qualitative molecular test did not detect the *JAK2* V617F

mutation. A reflex molecular test was ordered in order to further confirm/rule out myeloproliferative neoplasm (MPNs). Which one of the following mutations would *NOT* be part of this reflex test for MPNs in this patient?[13]

A. *FLT3*-ITD mutation

B. *JAK2* T875N mutation

C. *MPL* W515 mutation

D. *MPL* S505N mutation

E. None of the above

49. A 58-year-old male came to a clinic with symptoms of increasing abdominal discomfort, early satiety, and a weight loss of 15 lb due to poor appetite for approximately 6 months. The white-blood-cell count was 0.8×10^3 cells/mm^3 with an absolute neutrophil count of 1400 cells/mm^3, hemoglobin 9.3 g/dL, and platelet count 76,000 cells/mm^3. A bone marrow biopsy resulted in a "dry" aspirate, and the core biopsy was markedly fibrotic. An estimate of the blast count based upon touch preps as well as a CD34+/CD117+ immunostaining of the core biopsy demonstrated only 1.2% blasts. The oncologist suspected that the patient had primary myelofibrosis (PMF). A qualitative molecular test did not detect the *JAK2* V617F mutation. A reflex molecular test was ordered in order to further confirm/rule out myeloproliferative neoplasm (MPNs) in this patient, and a mutation in the *CALR* gene was detected. Which one of the following exons of the *CALR* gene would the detected mutation most likely be located in this patient?[14,15]

A. Exon 9

B. Exon 10

C. Exon 12

D. Exon 18

E. Exon 19

50. A 58-year-old male came to a clinic with symptoms of increasing abdominal discomfort, early satiety, and a weight loss of 15 lb due to poor appetite for approximately 6 months. The white-blood-cell count was $.8 \times 10^3$ cells/mm^3, with an absolute neutrophil count of 1400 cells/mm^3, hemoglobin 9.3 g/dL, and platelet count 76,000 cells/mm^3. A bone marrow biopsy resulted in a "dry" aspirate, and the core biopsy was markedly fibrotic. An estimate of the blast count based upon touch preps as well as a CD34+/CD117+ immunostaining of the core biopsy demonstrated only 1.2% blasts. The oncologist suspected that the patient had primary myelofibrosis (PMF). A qualitative molecular test did not detect the *JAK2* V617F mutation. A reflex molecular test was ordered to further confirm/

rule out myeloproliferative neoplasms (MPNs) in this patient. And a mutation in the exon 9 of the *CALR* gene was detected. Which one of the following types of mutations in *CALR* would most likely be detected in this patient?[13–15]

A. In-frame deletion/insertion
B. Out-of-frame deletion/insertion
C. Single-nucleotide mutation
D. Translocation
E. None of the above

51. A 58-year-old male came to a clinic with symptoms of increasing abdominal discomfort, early satiety, and a weight loss of 15 lb due to poor appetite for approximately 6 months. The white-blood-cell count was $.8 \times 10^3$ cells/mm^3, with an absolute neutrophil count of 1400 cells/mm^3, hemoglobin 9.3 g/dL, and platelet count 76,000 cells/mm^3. A bone marrow biopsy resulted in a "dry" aspirate, and the core biopsy was markedly fibrotic. An estimate of the blast count based upon touch preps as well as a CD34+/CD117+ immunostaining of the core biopsy demonstrated only 1.2% blasts. The oncologist suspected that the patient had primary myelofibrosis (PMF). A qualitative molecular test did not detect the *JAK2* V617F mutation. A reflex molecular test was ordered in order to further confirm/rule out myeloproliferative neoplasm (MPNs) in this patient. And a mutation in the exon 9 of the *CALR* gene was detected. Which one of the following describes the prognostic significance of the mutation detected in the *CALR* gene for this patient?[14,15]

A. Favorable prognosis
B. Intermediate prognosis
C. Unfavorable prognosis
D. Better survival than *JAK2* mutations
E. Worse survival than *JAK2* mutations
F. Unclear
G. None of above

52. A 41-year-old male came to a clinic for an evaluation of his polycythemic status. A physical examination disclosed splenomegaly. His initial complete blood count (CBC) revealed hemoglobin 22.5 g/dL (reference range, 14–17), hematocrit 70.0% (reference range, 39.0–51.0), and platelet count 252,000/μL (reference range, 140,000–400,000) with a white-blood-cell count of 13,400/μL (reference range, 3700–10,000). A subsequent bone-marrow biopsy revealed hypercellular marrow with panmyelosis, large dysmorphic megakaryocytes with clustering, and increased reticulin fibrosis, which was consistent with polycythemia vera (PV) morphology. The serum erythropoietin level was 7.0 μ/mL (reference range, 10.2–25.2). The karyotype of this

bone-marrow specimen was 46,XY[20]. A peripheral-blood specimen was collected for a qualitative *JAK2* V617F mutation analysis, and the results were positive. Which one of the following conditions most likely has *JAK2* V617F?[16]

A. Chronic myeloid leukemia (CML)
B. Essential thrombocythemia (ET)
C. Polycythemia vera (PV)
D. Primary myelofibrosis (PMF)
E. None of the above

53. A 41-year-old male came to a clinic for an evaluation of his polycythemic status. A physical examination disclosed splenomegaly. His initial complete blood count revealed hemoglobin 22.5 g/dL (reference range, 14–17), hematocrit 70.0% (reference range, 39.0–51.0), and platelet count 252,000/μL (reference range, 140,000–400,000), with a white-blood-cell count of 13,400/μL (reference range, 3700–10,000). A subsequent a bone-marrow biopsy revealed a hypercellular marrow with panmyelosis, large dysmorphic megakaryocytes with clustering, and increased reticulin fibrosis, which was consistent with a polycythemia vera (PV) morphology. The serum erythropoietin level was 7.0 μ/mL (reference range, 10.2–25.2). The karyotype results of this bone-marrow specimen was 46,XY [20]. Which one of the following molecular abnormalities would this patient most likely have if he had PV?[13,16]

A. *BCR-ABL1* rearrangement
B. *CALR* mutation
C. *JAK2* V617F mutation
D. *JAK2* mutation in the exon 12
E. *MPL* mutation

54. A 41-year-old male came to a clinic for an evaluation of his polycythemic status. A physical examination disclosed splenomegaly. His initial complete blood count revealed hemoglobin 22.5 g/dL (reference range, 14–17), hematocrit level 70.0% (reference range, 39.0–51.0), and platelet count 252,000/μL (reference range, 140,000–400,000), with a white-blood-cell count of 13,400/μL (reference range, 3700–10,000). A subsequent bone-marrow biopsy revealed a hypercellular marrow with panmyelosis, large dysmorphic megakaryocytes with clustering, and increased reticulin fibrosis, which was consistent with polycythemia vera (PV) morphology. The serum erythropoietin level was 7.0 μ/mL (reference range, 10.2–25.2). The karyotype results of this bone marrow specimen was 46,XY[20]. A peripheral-blood specimen was collected for a qualitative *JAK2* V617F mutation analysis, and the results were

negative. A reflex molecular test was ordered to further confirm/rule out PV in this patient. Which one of the following analyses would most likely be part of this reflex test for this patient with PV?[13,16]

A. *CALR* exon 9 mutation
B. *JAK2* exon 12 mutation
C. *MPL* exon 10 mutation
D. All of the above
E. None of the above

55. A 78-year-old male came to a clinic for severe headache and generalized pruritus. A physical examination disclosed splenomegaly. His initial complete blood count revealed hemoglobin 19.3 g/dL (reference range, 14–17), hematocrit 63.2% (reference range, 39.0–51.0), and platelet count 484,000/μL (reference range, 140,000–400,000/μL), with a white-blood-cell count of 1.84×10^7/μL (reference range, 3,700–10,000/μL). A subsequent a bone-marrow biopsy revealed a hypercellular marrow for age and an increased number of megakaryocytes with normal morphology, which was consistent with polycythemia vera (PV) morphology. The karyotype of this bone-marrow specimen was 46, XY[20]. A peripheral-blood specimen was collected for a qualitative *JAK2* V617F mutation analysis, and the results were positive. Which one of the following targeted therapies would be most appropriate to this patient?[16]

A. Gleevec (imatinib)
B. Herceptin (trastuzumab)
C. Lynparza (olaparib)
D. Zelboraf (vemurafenib)
E. None of the above

56. A 53-year-old female was referred to a hematological clinic for polycythemia vera (PV) 2 years ago. She was treated with phlebotomy alone for the past 2 years. However, she continued to have persistent erythrocytosis. During her last checkup she was found to have an elevated platelet count of 1,020,000/μL (reference range, 150,000–450,000). A quantitative laboratory assay specific for the *JAK2* V617F allele was ordered. The results showed 65% *JAK2* V617F in the peripheral-blood sample. Which one of the following statements would be the most appropriate explanation for this finding?[13]

A. All the cancer cells in the sample are heterozygous for the *JAK2* V617F mutation.
B. All the cancer cells in the sample are homozygous for the *JAK2* V617F mutation.
C. At least some of the cancer cells in the sample are homozygous for the *JAK2* V617F mutation.

D. At least some of the cancer cells in the sample are heterozygous for the *JAK2* V617F mutation.
E. The result is positive, however, it is not possible to predict the zygosity of the sample.

57. A 53-year-old female was referred to a hematological clinic for polycythemia vera (PV) 2 years ago. She was treated with phlebotomy alone for the past 2 years. However, she continued to have persistent erythrocytosis. During her last checkup she was found to have an elevated platelet count of 1,020,000/μL (reference range, 150,000–450,000). A quantitative laboratory assay specific for the *JAK2* V617F allele was ordered. The results were 80% V617F allele, which suggested that the patient was homozygous for the *JAK2* V617K mutation in at least a subset of cells. What would be the most likely explanation for the homozygous *JAK2* mutation in this patient?

A. Both copies of *JAK2* in some cells were mutated to V617F; this fits the two-hit hypotheses.
B. The patient had one inherited copy of the mutation and one somatic mutation.
C. This is a laboratory error.
D. This may be copy neutral loss of heterozygosity (LOH) due to uniparental disomy (UPD).
E. All of the above.
F. None of the above.

58. A 53-year-old female was referred to a hematological clinic for polycythemia vera (PV) 2 years ago. She was treated with phlebotomy alone for the past 2 years. However, she continued to have persistent erythrocytosis. During her last checkup she was found to have an elevated platelet count of 1,020,000/μL (reference range, 150,000–450,000). A quantitative laboratory assay specific for the *JAK2* V617F allele was ordered. The results were 80% V617F allele. Which one of the following statements regarding the quantitative *JAK2* V617F test is correct?[13]

A. It is a DNA-based test.
B. It is a RNA-based test.
C. It is multiple PCR reactions.
D. The recommended test sensitivity is 0.1%.
E. The recommended test sensitivity is 5%.

59. A 78-year-old male came to a clinic for severe headache and generalized pruritus. The physical examination disclosed splenomegaly. His initial complete blood count revealed hemoglobin 19.3 g/dL (reference range, 14–17), hematocrit level 63.2% (reference range, 39.0–51.0), and platelet count 484,000/μL (reference range,

140,000–400,000), with a white-blood-cell count of 18.4×10^9/L (reference range, 3700–10,000). A subsequent a bone-marrow biopsy revealed a hypercellular marrow for age and an increased number of megakaryocytes with normal morphology, which was consistent with polycythemia vera (PV) morphology. The karyotype of this bone-marrow specimen was 46, XY[20]. A peripheral-blood specimen was collected for quantitative *JAK2* V617F mutation analysis, and the result was positive. How frequently is the *JAK2* V617F mutation found in patients with polycythemia vera (PV)?[13]

A. About 3%
B. About 20%
C. About 60%
D. About 80%
E. About 95%

60. How frequently is the *JAK2* V617F mutation found in patients with essential thrombocythemia (ET)?[13]

A. About 3%
B. About 20%
C. About 60%
D. About 80%
E. About 95%

61. How frequently is the *JAK2* V617F mutation found in patients with primary myelofibrosis (PMF)?[13]

A. About 3%
B. About 22%
C. About 60%
D. About 80%
E. About 95%

62. How frequently are the *JAK2* exon 12 mutations found in patients with polycythemia vera (PV)?[13]

A. About 3%
B. About 20%
C. About 60%
D. About 80%
E. About 95%

63. A 78-year-old male came to a clinic for severe headache and generalized pruritus. A physical examination disclosed splenomegaly. His initial complete blood count revealed hemoglobin 19.3 g/dL (reference range, 14–17), hematocrit 63.2% (reference range, 39.0–51.0), and platelet count 484,000/μL (reference range, 140,000–400,000), with a white-blood-cell count of 1.84×10^7/μL (reference range, 3700–10,000/μL). A subsequent bone-marrow biopsy revealed hypercellular marrow for age and increased number of megakaryocytes with normal morphology, which was consistent with polycythemia vera (PV) morphology. The

karyotype results of this bone-marrow specimen was 46,XY[20]. A peripheral-blood specimen was collected for quantitative *JAK2* V617F mutation analysis. The results were 80% V617F allele. What would be the pathogenetic role of *JAK2* V617F in this patient's PV?[13]

A. Activating mutations
B. Dominant negative mutations
C. Gain-of-function mutations
D. Loss-of-function mutations
E. Silent mutations

64. A 13-year-old girl was brought to an emergency department by her parents for severe, global, rapidly worsening headache of 2 days' duration with no history of head trauma, vomiting, fever, seizures, altered sensorium, neck stiffness, or weakness in any part of the body. Her medical and surgical histories were insignificant. A physical examination was unremarkable. Her brain MRI revealed a partial thrombus of the superior sagittal sinus (SSS) with mild engorgement of the venous channels of both cerebral hemispheres. Subsequently, MR venography of the brain confirmed thrombosis of SSS with partial thrombosis of the right transverse sinus. A complete blood count revealed a hemoglobin of 12.5 g/dL, a total leukocyte count of 9×10^9 cells/L, and a differential cell count of polymorphonuclear cells 65%, lymphocytes 30%, eosinophils 5%, and platelets 943×10^9/L. A peripheral-blood smear revealed a high platelet count with mild anisocytosis. Her baseline prothrombin time (PT), activated partial thromboplastin time (aPTT), and fibrinogen levels were normal. The results of antithrombin, protein C, protein S, antiphospholipid antibodies, homocysteine levels, apolipoprotein A/B, lupus anticoagulant, and antinuclear antibodies were all within normal limits. The oncologist suspected that she had essential thrombocythemia (ET). Which one of the following genetic test results would most likely be positive if the patient had ET?[13,17]

A. *BCR-ABL1* FISH
B. *CALR* exon 9 mutation analysis
C. *JAK2* exon 12 mutation analysis
D. *JAK2* V617F mutation analysis
E. *MPL* exon 10 mutation analysis
F. None of the above

65. A 13-year-old girl was brought to an emergency department by her parents for severe, global, rapidly worsening headache of 2 days' duration with no history of head trauma, vomiting, fever, seizures, altered sensorium, neck stiffness, or weakness in any part of the body. Her medical

and surgical histories were insignificant. A physical examination was unremarkable. Her brain MRI revealed a partial thrombus of the superior sagittal sinus (SSS) with mild engorgement of the venous channels of both cerebral hemispheres. Subsequently, MR venography of the brain confirmed thrombosis of SSS with partial thrombosis of the right transverse sinus. A complete blood count revealed a hemoglobin of 12.5 g/dL, a total leukocyte count of 9×10^9 cells/L, and a differential cell count of polymorphonuclear cells 65%, lymphocytes 30%, eosinophils 5%, and platelets 943×10^9/L. A peripheral-blood smear revealed a high platelet count with mild anisocytosis. Her baseline prothrombin time (PT), activated partial thromboplastin time (aPTT), and fibrinogen levels were normal. The antithrombin, protein C, protein S, antiphospholipid antibodies, homocysteine levels, apolipoprotein A/B, lupus anticoagulant, and antinuclear antibodies were all within normal limits. The oncologist suspected that she had essential thrombocythemia (ET). Her JAK2 V617F and BCR-ABL1 test results were negative. A reflex molecular test was ordered to further confirm/rule out ET in this patient. Which one of the following mutations would most likely NOT be part of this reflex test for MPNs?[13,17]

A. CALR exon 9 mutation analysis
B. JAK2 exon 12 mutation analysis
C. MPL exon 10 mutation analysis
D. All of the above
E. None of the above

66. A 13-year-old girl was brought to an emergency department by her parents for severe, global, rapidly worsening headache of 2 days' duration with no history of head trauma, vomiting, fever, seizures, altered sensorium, neck stiffness, or weakness in any part of the body. Her medical and surgical histories were insignificant. A physical examination was unremarkable. Her brain MRI revealed a partial thrombus of the superior sagittal sinus (SSS) with mild engorgement of the venous channels of both cerebral hemispheres. Subsequently, MR venography of the brain confirmed thrombosis of SSS with partial thrombosis of the right transverse sinus. A complete blood count revealed a hemoglobin of 12.5 g/dL, a total leukocyte count of 9×10^9 cells/L, and a differential cell count of polymorphonuclear cell 65%, lymphocytes 30%, eosinophils 5%, and platelets 943×10^9/L. A peripheral-blood smear revealed a high platelet count with mild anisocytosis. Her baseline prothrombin time (PT), activated partial

thromboplastin time (aPTT), and fibrinogen levels were normal. The antithrombin, protein C, protein S, antiphospholipid antibodies, homocysteine levels, apolipoprotein A/B, lupus anticoagulant, and antinuclear antibodies were all in normal limits. The oncologist suspected that she had essential thrombocythemia (ET). Her JAK2 V617F and BCR-ABL1 test results were negative. A reflex molecular test was ordered to further confirm/rule out ET in this patient, and a mutation in the MPL gene was detected. In which one of the following exons of the MPL gene would the mutation most likely be located?[13]

A. Exon 9
B. Exon 10
C. Exon 12
D. Exon 18
E. Exon 19

67. A 36-year-old female presented to a clinic with symptoms of recurrent headache and blackouts. Her medical history was significant for hypertension in the past 6 months. She had been treated for headache without improvement. In the past few days she had experienced numbness in the hands and feet. A physical examination revealed that pain and touch sensation were decreased in the feet but that reflexes and power were normal. Her dorsalis pedis pulse was feeble, but other peripheral pulses were intact. Her spleen was enlarged 6 cm below the subcostal margin, nontender, and firm in consistency. A complete blood count (CBC) demonstrated hemoglobin 12.5 g/dL, hematocrit 48%, platelet count 1517×10^9/L, total leukocyte count 6×10^9/L, polymorphs 62%, lymphocytes 23%, monocytes 3%, and eosinophils 1%. A peripheral-blood smear revealed an abundance of megakaryocytes. Bone marrow revealed hypercellular marrow with giant megakaryocytes and hyperplasia, no fibrosis, and increased platelets. A diagnosis of essential thrombocythemia (ET) was suspected. Karyotype results were 46,XX[20]. JAK2 V617F and BCR-ABL1 test results were negative. A reflex molecular test was ordered to further confirm/rule out ET in this patient, and a mutation in the MPL gene was detected. Which one of the following types of mutation in MPL would most likely be detected in this patient?[13,18]

A. In-frame deletion/insertion
B. Out-of-frame deletion/insertion
C. Single-nucleotide mutation
D. Translocation
E. None of the above

68. A 43-year-old female presented to a clinic with pain and blackish discoloration of the right hand

and weakness of the right half of the body with a left-sided deviation of the face. She had a history of off-and-on headache and pain in the eyes, which were relieved temporarily by taking analgesics. She had not gone to any clinics before for those symptoms because she had been "too busy." A physical examination revealed that reflexes were exaggerated on the right side of body, while right plantar reflex was upgoing. Hand gangrene was present. The tip of her spleen was palpable. A complete blood count (CBC) demonstrated hemoglobin 11.5 g/dL, hematocrit 48%, platelet count 2411×10^9/L, total leukocyte count 11×10^9/L, polymorphs 65%, lymphocytes 21%, monocytes 2%, and eosinophils 3%. A peripheral-blood smear revealed an abundance of megakaryocytes. A bone-marrow sample showed features of thrombocythemia. A brain CT scan showed infarct in the left cerebral hemisphere supplying the middle cerebral artery. Magnetic resonance angiography (MRA) of the right hand showed that the wrist radial artery were completely obliterated and were not visualized in the hand, while the ulnar artery demonstrated a beaded appearance beyond the wrist. The oncologist suspected that she had essential thrombocythemia (ET). Her *JAK2* V617F and *BCR-ABL1* test results were ordered, but both turned out to be negative. What is the required analytic sensitivity of an assay to ensure that 90% of *JAK2* V617F—positive cases are detected?[13]

- A. At least 0.1%
- B. At least 1%
- C. At least 5%
- D. At least 10%
- E. At least 15%

69. Traditionally clinical molecular laboratories have been using Sanger sequencing, restriction-fragment—length polymorphism (RFLP), denaturing high-performance liquid chromatography (dHPLC), high-resolution melting curve analysis, pyrosequencing, and various allele-specific PCR systems with electrophoretic analysis of the products to detect *JAK2* V617F qualitatively. What sensitivity may these methods most likely reach?[13]

- A. 0.1%
- B. 1%
- C. 5%
- D. 10%
- E. 15%

70. A scientist in a clinical molecular pathology laboratory found that the send-out test for *FLT3*-ITD and *FLT3*-TKD had increased significantly in the past 6 months. He decided to validate the test.

With which one of the following malignancies are the *FLT3*-ITD and *FLT3*-TKD mutations associated?

- A. Acute myeloid leukemia (AML)
- B. Essential thrombocytopenia (ET)
- C. Myeloproliferative neoplasm (MPN)
- D. Polycythemia vera (PV)
- E. Primary myelofibrosis (PMF)
- F. None of the above

71. A 49-year-old a marathon runner presented to a clinic with a symptom of unusual fatigue during a 10-km race. A complete blood count (CBC) was notable for a white-blood-cell count of 13×10^9/L, hematocrit of 29%, and platelet count of 116×10^9/L. A bone-marrow biopsy was consistent with poorly differentiated acute myeloid leukemia (AML). The karyotype results on a bone-marrow sample were normal. Which one of the following prognoses would this patient have?

- A. Favorable risk
- B. Intermediate risk
- C. Unfavorable risk
- D. Unclear
- E. None of the above

72. A 43-year-old female presented to a local hospital with fever and cough for 2 days. A physical examination was unremarkable. A complete blood count (CBC) was notable for white blood cells (WBC) 76×10^9/L, neutrophils 33×10^9/L, monocytes 15×10^9/L, hemoglobin 92 g/L, platelet count 296×10^9/L, and 27% blasts. A bone-marrow biopsy revealed that proliferation of nucleated cells was extremely active, whereas myeloid and erythroid proliferation was inhibited. Premonocytes accounted for 49.0% of cells in the bone marrow specimen. Her peroxidase detection was positive, accompanied by periodic acid—Schiff-positive granules. The flow cytometry revealed that CD69(+) and CD14(+) cells accounted for 82.1% of cells, CD33 (+) cells accounted for 68.7%, and CD34(+) cells accounted for 64.2%. The pathological diagnosis was AML-M5b. Karyotype results were normal. A next-generation sequencing (NGS) panel for acute myeloid leukemia (AML) was ordered. Which one of the following genes would most likely *NOT* be included in this NGS panel?[66]

- A. *CEBPA*
- B. *FLT3*
- C. *MPL*
- D. *NPM1*
- E. None of the above

73. A 43-year-old female presented to a local hospital with fever and cough for 2 days. A physical examination was unremarkable. A complete

blood count (CBC) was notable for white blood cells (WBC) 76×10^9/L, neutrophils 33×10^9/L, monocytes 15×10^9/L, hemoglobin 92 g/L, platelet count 296×10^9/L, and 27% blasts. A bone-marrow biopsy revealed that proliferation of nucleated cells was extremely active, whereas myeloid and erythroid proliferation was inhibited. Premonocytes accounted for 49.0%. Her peroxidase detection was positive accompanied by periodic acid—Schiff-positive granules. The flow cytometry revealed that CD69(+) and CD14 (+) cells accounted for 82.1%, CD33(+) cells accounted for 68.7%, and CD34(+) cells accounted for 64.2%. The pathological diagnosis was AML-M5b. Karyotype results were normal. A next-generation sequencing (NGS) panel for acute myeloid leukemia (AML) was ordered, which included the *CEBPA*, c-*KIT*, *DNMT3A*, *FLT3*, *NPM1*, and *RUNX1*, *WT1* genes, and others. Which one of the following genes in the NGS panel is intronless?[19]

A. *CEBPA*
B. c-*KIT*
C. *DNMT3A*
D. *FLT3*
E. *NPM1*
F. *RUNX1*
G. *WT1*
H. None of the above

74. A 49-year-old a marathon runner presented to a clinic with for the symptom of unusual fatigues during a 10-km race. A complete blood count (CBC) was notable for a white-blood-cell count of 13×10^9/L, hematocrit of 29%, and a platelet count of 116×10^9/L. A bone-marrow biopsy was consistent with poorly differentiated acute myeloid leukemia (AML) with normal cytogenetics. A molecular test for *FLT3* and *NPM1* was ordered, and *FLT3*-internal tandem duplication (ITD) was detected. Which one of the following prognoses would this patient have if she had the *FLT3*-ITD mutation?

A. Favorable risk
B. Intermediate risk
C. Unfavorable risk
D. Unclear
E. None of the above

75. A 43-year-old female presented to a local hospital with fever and cough for 2 days. A physical examination was unremarkable. A complete blood count was notable for white blood cells (WBC) 76×10^9/L, neutrophils 33×10^9/L, monocytes 15×10^9/L, hemoglobin 92 g/L, platelet count 296×10^9/L, and 27% blasts. A bone-marrow biopsy revealed that proliferation of

nucleated cells was extremely active, whereas myeloid and erythroid proliferation was inhibited. Premonocytes accounted for 49.0%. Her peroxidase detection was positive accompanied by periodic acid—Schiff-positive granules. The flow cytometry revealed that CD69(+) and CD14 (+) cells accounted for 82.1%, CD33(+) cells accounted for 68.7%, and CD34(+) cells accounted for 64.2%. The pathological diagnosis was AML-M5b. Karyotype results were normal. The oncologist ordered molecular tests on *CEBPA*, *FLT3*-ITD, *FLT3*-TKD, and *NPM1*. Which one of the following assays would most likely be used to detect *FLT3*-ITD in this patient?

A. Fluorescence in situ hybridization (FISH)
B. PCR-capillary electrophoresis
C. Sanger sequencing
D. Targeted-mutation analysis
E. All of the above
F. None of the above

76. A 43-year-old female presented to a local hospital with fever and cough for 2 days. A physical examination was unremarkable. A complete blood count was notable for white blood cells (WBC) 76×10^9/L, neutrophils 33×10^9/L, monocytes 15×10^9/L, hemoglobin 92 g/L, platelet count 296×10^9/L, and 27% blasts. A bone-marrow biopsy revealed that proliferation of nucleated cells was extremely active, whereas myeloid and erythroid proliferation was inhibited. Premonocytes accounted for 49.0%. Her peroxidase detection was positive accompanied by periodic acid—Schiff-positive granules. The flow cytometry revealed that CD69(+) and CD14(+) cells accounted for 82.1%, CD33(+) cells accounted for 68.7%, and CD34(+) cells accounted for 64.2%. The pathological diagnosis was AML-M5b. Karyotype results were normal. The oncologist ordered molecular tests on *CEBPA*, *FLT3*-ITD, *FLT3*-TKD, and *NPM1*. The *FLT3*-ITD mutation was detected. What would be the pathogenetic role of the *FLT3*-ITD mutation in this patient?[20]

A. Activating mutations
B. Dominant negative mutations
C. Gain-of-function mutations
D. Loss-of-function mutations
E. Unclear
F. None of the above

77. A scientist in a clinical molecular pathology laboratory found that the send-out test for the *CEBPA* gene had increased significantly in the past 6 months. He decided to validate the test. With which one of the following malignancies are mutations in the *CEBPA* gene associated?[19]

A. Acute myeloid leukemia (AML)
B. Essential thrombocytopenia (ET)
C. Myeloproliferative neoplasm (MPN)
D. Polycythemia vera (PV)
E. Primary myelofibrosis (PMF)
F. None of the above

78. An 86-year-old female was referred to an oncology clinic for probable acute myeloid leukemia (AML). Her medical history was significant for ovarian and breast cancer. She had had intermittent borderline anemia in the past 6 years and had been prescribed iron in the past, but not recently. Within the past 2 months she had experienced weakness, fatigue, and decreased appetite. Evaluations revealed anemia with increased blasts in a peripheral-blood sample. Flow cytometry results were consistent with AML. Karyotype results were normal. A next-generation sequencing (NGS) panel for myeloid leukemia was ordered, which included the *CEBPA*, c-*KIT*, *DNMT3A*, *FLT3*, *NPM1*, *RUNX1*, *TP53*, *WT1* genes, and others. Which one of the following genes in the NGS panel would be associated with a favorable prognosis if the patient had acquired pathogenic variant(s) of it?[19,21,22]
A. Double *CEBPA* mutations
B. Single *CEBPA* mutation
C. *FLT3*-ITD
D. *FLT3*-TKD
E. *RUNX1*
F. *WT1*
G. *TP53*
H. None of the above

79. A scientist decided to validate a next-generation sequencing (NGS) panel for acute myeloid leukemia (AML). The *CEBPA*, c-*KIT*, *DNMT3A*, *FLT3*, *NPM1*, *RUNX1*, *TP53*, *WT1* genes, and 10 other genes, were included in this NGS panel. Which one of the following genes in the NGS panel is associated with familial acute myeloid leukemia (AML)?[19,22]
A. *CEBPA*
B. c-*KIT*
C. *DNMT3A*
D. *FLT3*
E. *NPM1*
F. *RUNX1*
G. *WT1*
H. None of the above

80. A 15-year-old male presented to a clinic for fatigue, decreased appetite, and general malaise in the past 2 weeks. There had been no fever or night sweats. In the past few weeks he noticed a few "lumps" in his neck, arm pits, and groin. He had lost 10 lb in the past month. Other than these reports, his medical history was uneventful. A physical examination revealed pallor and bilateral nontender cervical adenopathy. A complete blood count (CBC) was notable for white blood cells (WBC) 129×10^9/L, hemoglobin 8.2 g/dL, platelet count 37×10^9/L, and blasts 89%. A peripheral-blood smear demonstrated markedly increased WBCs that were homogeneous in appearance. The majority of WBCs are blasts. Flow cytometry results showed positivity for CD7, CD19, CD34, CD13, CD33, CD65, CD11b, and CD15. Karyotype results were normal. The patient was subsequently diagnosed with acute myeloid leukemia (AML). The oncologist ordered molecular tests on *CEBPA*, *FLT3*-ITD, *FLT3*-TKD, and *NPM1*. Which one of the following assays would most likely be used to detect the *CEBPA* gene in this patient?[19,21,22]
A. FISH
B. PCR-capillary electrophoresis
C. Sanger sequencing
D. Targeted-mutation analysis
E. All of the above
F. None of the above

81. An 18-year-old man came to an emergency department with a 2-week history of fatigue, easy bruising, and acute onset of gross hematuria. The patient had no significant medical or family history. A physical examination revealed a thin-appearing young man with scattered petechiae and ecchymoses of the skin. There were 15% circulating blasts. Karyotype results were normal. Molecular analyses of DNA extracted from the bone-marrow aspirate specimen showed no evidence of *FLT3* or *NPM1* mutations. There were two compound heterozygous mutations in the *CEBPA* gene. Both of them were frameshift mutations, leading to premature termination of amino acids. One was in exon 3, another one was in exon 22. Which one of the following statements regarding these findings would be the most appropriate?[19,22]
A. These two mutations are in *cis*.
B. These two mutations are in *trans*.
C. It is unclear whether these two mutations are in *cis* or *trans*.
D. NGS can help to tell if these two mutations are in *cis* or *trans*.
E. No further tests can help to tell if these two mutations are in *cis* or *trans*.

82. Which one of the following statements regarding *CEBPA* in leukemia is *NOT* correct?
A. Acquired mutations in *CEBPA* are recurrent genetic alterations in AML.

B. Acquired mutations in *CEBPA* are often biallelic in AML.

C. Biallelic *CEBPA* mutations are associated with a favorable prognosis.

D. The *CEBPA* gene is an intronless gene.

E. The prognostic impact of *CEBPA* mutations in the presence of *FLT3* mutations is unfavorable.

83. A scientist in a clinical molecular laboratory decided to validate an assay for the *CEBPA* gene. Which one of the following diseases has indications for *CEBPA* sequence analysis?

A. Acute promyelocytic leukemia (APL)

B. Chronic myelocytic leukemia (CML)

C. Complex karyotype AML raised from myeloid dysplastic syndrome (MDS)

D. Normal karyotype with acute myeloid leukemia (AML)

E. Normal karyotype AML with a *FLT3*-ITD mutation

84. The N-terminal mutations of *CEBPA* lead to overexpress the 30-kD isoform of the CEBPA protein, which typically are which one of the following?

A. Activating mutations

B. Dominant negative mutations

C. Gain-of-function mutations

D. Loss-of-function mutations

E. Silent mutations

85. Which one of the following statements regarding *CEBPA* in leukemia is correct?

A. The most common mutations in *CEBPA* are N-terminal frameshift and C-terminal in-frame mutations.

B. The most common mutations in *CEBPA* are N-terminal in-frame and C-terminal frameshift mutations.

C. Dysregulation of *CEBPA* has been identified only in AML.

D. Patients with monoallelic *CEBPA* mutations have a poor prognosis.

E. Patients with monoallelic *CEBPA* mutations, but not biallelic *CEBPA* mutations, have a favorable prognosis.

86. A 43-year-old female was admitted to a local hospital with fever and cough for 2 days. A physical examination was unremarkable. A complete blood count was notable for white blood cells (WBC) 76×10^9/L, neutrophils 33×10^9/L, monocytes 15×10^9/L, hemoglobin of 92 g/L, platelet count 296×10^9/L, and 27% blasts. A bone-marrow biopsy revealed that proliferation of nucleated cells was extremely active, whereas myeloid and erythroid proliferation was inhibited. Premonocytes accounted for 49.0%. Her peroxidase detection was positive accompanied by periodic acid–Schiff-positive granules. The flow cytometry revealed that CD69(+) and CD14 (+) cells accounted for 82.1%, CD33(+) cells accounted for 68.7%, and CD34(+) cells accounted for 64.2%. The pathological diagnosis was AML-M5b. Karyotype results were normal. The patient was subsequently diagnosed with acute myeloid leukemia (AML). The oncologist ordered a next-generation sequencing (NGS) panel for AML, including *CEBPA*, *FLT3*-ITD, *FLT3*-TKD, *NPM1*, and 10 other genes. An acquired pathogenic mutation in the *NPM1* gene was detected. Which one of the following prognoses would the patient most likely have, according to the genetic findings?[7]

A. Favorable risk

B. Intermediate risk

C. Unfavorable risk

D. Unclear

E. None of the above

87. A 65-year-old male presented to a clinic for fatigue, decreased appetite, and general malaise in the past 2 weeks. There had been no fever or night sweats. In the past few weeks, he noticed a few "lumps" in his neck, armpits, and groin. He had lost 10 lb in the past month. Other than these reports, his medical history was uneventful. A physical examination revealed pallor and bilateral nontender cervical adenopathy. A complete blood count (CBC) was notable for white blood cells (WBC) 129×10^9/L, hemoglobin 8.2 g/dL, platelet count 37×10^9/L, and blasts 89%. A peripheral-blood smear demonstrated markedly increased WBCs that were homogeneous in appearance. The majority of WBC are blasts. Flow cytometry results showed positivity for CD7, CD11b, CD19, CD34, CD13, CD33, and CD65. Karyotype results were normal. The patient was subsequently diagnosed with acute myeloid leukemia (AML). The oncologist ordered molecular tests on *CEBPA*, *FLT3*-ITD, *FLT3*-TKD, and *NPM1*. Which one of the following types of mutation in *NPM1* would most likely be detected in this patient?[7]

A. In-frame deletion/insertion

B. Out-of-frame deletion/insertion

C. Single-nucleotide mutation

D. Translocation

E. None of the above

88. An 86-year-old female was referred to an oncology clinic for probable acute myeloid leukemia (AML). Her medical history was significant for ovarian and breast cancer. She had had intermittent borderline anemia in the past 6 years and had been on prescribed iron in the past,

but not recently. Within the past 2 months she had experienced weakness, fatigue, and decreased appetite. Evaluations revealed anemia with increased blasts in a peripheral-blood sample. Flow cytometry results were consistent with AML. Karyotype results were normal. *FLT3*-ITD and *FLT3*-TKD tests were negative. The oncologist ordered a molecular test for the *NPM1* gene to further assess the prognosis. Which one of the following assays would most likely be used to test the *NPM1* gene in this patient?[7]

- **A.** FISH
- **B.** PCR-capillary electrophoresis
- **C.** Sanger sequencing
- **D.** Targeted-mutation analysis
- **E.** All of the above
- **F.** None of the above

89. Which one of the following statements describes the limitation of the utility of Sanger sequencing in oncology?

- **A.** It is not a sensitive test to detect acquired mutations.
- **B.** It cannot be used to detect large deletions or insertions.
- **C.** It does not help to monitor minimal residue diseases (MRDs).
- **D.** It cannot be used to tell whether compound heterozygous mutations in *CEBPA* are in *cis* or in *trans*.
- **E.** All of the above
- **F.** None of the above

90. Which one of the following genes associated with myeloid neoplasms does *NOT* have a tyrosine kinase domain or domains?

- **A.** *ABL1*
- **B.** *FLT3*
- **C.** *JAK2*
- **D.** *KIT*
- **E.** *NPM1*

91. A 65-year-old male presented to a clinic for fatigue, decreased appetite, and general malaise in the past 2 weeks. There had been no fever or night sweats. In the past few weeks, he noticed a few "lumps" in his neck, armpits, and groin. He had lost 10 lb in the past month. Other than these reports, his medical history was uneventful. A physical examination revealed pallor and bilateral nontender cervical adenopathy. A complete blood count (CBC) was notable for white blood cells (WBC) 129×10^9/L, hemoglobin 8.2 g/dL, platelet count 37×10^9/L, and blasts 89%. A peripheral-blood smear demonstrated markedly increased WBCs that were homogeneous in appearance.

The majority of WBC are blasts. Flow cytometry results showed positivity for CD7, CD11b, CD19, CD34, CD13, CD33, and CD65. Karyotype results were normal. The patient was subsequently diagnosed with acute myeloid leukemia (AML). The oncologist ordered molecular tests on *CEBPA*, *FLT3*-ITD, *FLT3*-TKD, and *NPM1*. Which one of the following genetic alterations would indicate the patient had a favorable prognosis if he had acquired pathogenic variant(s) in this gene?[7]

- **A.** *BAALC*
- **B.** *ERG1*
- **C.** *FLT3-ITD*
- **D.** *MLL-PTD*
- **E.** *MN1*
- **F.** *NPM1*

92. A 76-year-old female was referred to an oncology clinic for abnormal CBC with a significant lymphocytosis. She had had shortness of breath, fatigue, tachycardia/palpitation, and a 10-lb weight loss in the past 2 months. A laboratory evaluation revealed white blood cells (WBCs) 48.4×10^9/L, lymphocytes 82%, hemoglobin 8.0 g/dL, hematocrit 26.5%, mean corpuscular volume (MCV) 107, and platelet count 137×10^9/L. Flow cytometry results on a peripheral-blood smear revealed acute myeloid leukemia (AML), subtype unclear. Karyotype results were normal. A next-generation sequencing (NGS) panel for AML was ordered. Which one of the following genetic alterations would indicate that the patient had an unfavorable prognosis, if he had one?

- **A.** *CEBPA*
- **B.** *FLT3-ITD*
- **C.** *FLT3-TKD*
- **D.** *NPM1*

93. A 70-year-old male came to a clinic for progressive fatigue. A physical examination was unremarkable except for mild pallor of the conjunctiva. A complete blood count (CBC) was notable for white blood cells (WBCs) 2.5×10^3/μL, hemoglobin 9.0 g/dL, and platelet count 2.41×10^5/μL. A bone-marrow biopsy revealed a cellularity of 80%. A bone-marrow aspirate showed moderately dysplastic erythroid precursors with 19% ring sideroblasts and 2% myeloblasts. A diagnosis of myelodysplastic syndrome (MDS) was made. Chromosome karyotype results were normal. A next-generation sequencing (NGS) panel for MDS was ordered to further assess the prognosis. An acquired pathogenic variant in the *SF3B1* gene was

detected. Which one of the following prognoses would this patient most likely have?[23,24]

A. Favorable risk
B. Intermediate risk
C. Unfavorable risk
D. Unclear
E. None of the above

94. The *ASXL1* gene is an epigenetic regulator of gene expression. Acquired pathogenic variants of *ASXL1* are detected in approximately 15% of cases of MDS, 11% of AML, 45% of CMML, 30% of PMF, and 4% of PV/ET and are generally associated with aggressive and poor outcome in these conditions. Which one of the exons in this gene most likely harbors an acquired pathogenic variant in a patient with a myeloid malignancy?[25]

A. Exon 2
B. Exon 9
C. Exon 10
D. Exon 13
E. All of the above
F. None of the above

95. A 3-month-old girl was brought to a clinic for severe respiratory distress, hepatosplenomegaly, anemia, and fever. Her complete blood count was 128.2×10^9/L. Peripheral-blood and bone marrow results revealed 75% and 80% blasts, respectively. Flow cytometry analyses identified atypical cells positive for CD34, CD33, anti-HLA-DR, CD117, CD11b, and myeloperoxidase (MPO) < 3%. Morphologically, the patient was diagnosed with acute myeloid leukemia (AML) M0. Chromosome karyotype results were 47,XX,+ 11[12]/46,XX[8]. Fluorescence in situ hybridization (FISH) analysis for *MLL* rearrangement was ordered, and results revealed three copies of *MLL* but no rearrangement. The oncologist ordered *MLL*-partial tandem duplication (PTD) analysis. Which one of the following assays would most likely be used for the *MLL*-PTD analysis in this patient?[26,27]

A. A DNA-detecting assay
B. An RNA-detecting assay
C. Sequencing
D. Multiple PCR
E. All of the above
F. None of the above

96. A 67-year-old male presented to an emergency department after 36% blasts in the peripheral blood was found during an annual examination. His medical history was significant for prostate cancer diagnosed 6 years ago. A bone-marrow biopsy revealed acute myeloid leukemia (AML) with 30% blasts. Chromosome karyotype results were 47,XX,+ 11[12]/46,XX[8]. Fluorescence in situ hybridization (FISH) analysis for *MLL*

rearrangement revealed three copies of *MLL*, but no rearrangement. The oncologist ordered *MLL*-partial tandem duplication (PTD) analysis, and the results were abnormal. Which one of the following types of changes would this patient most likely have?[26,27]

A. In-frame duplication
B. Out-of-frame duplication
C. Single-nucleotide mutation
D. Translocation
E. None of the above

97. A scientist in a clinical molecular laboratory was developing a next-generation sequencing (NGS) panel for acute myeloid leukemia (AML). Which one of genetic alterations would most likely *NOT* be included in this NGS panel for AML?

A. *CALR*
B. *CEBPA*
C. *FLT3-ITD*
D. *MLL-PTD*
E. *NPM1*
F. None of the above

98. A scientist was developing a next-generation sequencing (NGS) panel for acute myeloid leukemia (AML). Which one of genetic alterations would most like *NOT* be included in this NGS panel for AML?

A. *ASXL1*
B. *CEBPA*
C. *MPL*
D. *RUNX1*
E. *SF3B1*
F. None of the above

99. A 56-year-old male came to a clinic for vertigo, paleness, and fever. Results of a bone-marrow biopsy were consistent with acute myeloid leukemia (AML). Most AML cells were MPO+, CD20 partial+, CD79a partial+, CD3 partial+, some CD138+, CD−, CD5−, Ag+, and Fe+. Cytogenetic karyotype results were 47,XX,+ 8[9]/46,XX[11]. The hematologist ordered a next-generation sequencing (NGS) panel for hematological neoplasms to further assess the prognosis. Which one of the following genes in the NGS panel would most likely be mutated in this patient?[28]

A. *ASXL1*
B. *CEBPA*
C. *GATA1*
D. *GATA2*
E. *SF3B1*
F. All of the above
G. None of the above

100. A 76-year-old female came to a clinic with symptoms of weakness, fatigue, and decreased

appetite. A complete blood count (CBC) revealed hemoglobin 9.9 g/dL, hematocrit 29.5%, white-blood-cell count (WBC) 3200/mm³, platelet count $117 \times 10^3/\mu L$, and blasts 37%. Flow cytometry results was consistent with acute myeloid leukemia (AML). Cytogenetic karyotype results were 47,XX, + 8[9]/46,XX[11]. The hematologist ordered a next-generation sequencing (NGS) panel for hematological neoplasms to further assess the prognosis. An acquired pathogenic variant in the *ASXL1* gene was detected. Which one of the following prognoses would this patient most likely have?[28,29]

A. Favorable risk
B. Intermediate risk
C. Unfavorable risk
D. Unclear
E. None of the above

101. A scientist in a clinical molecular laboratory decided to develop a next-generation sequencing (NGS) panel for acute myeloid leukemia (AML) including the *RUNX1* (*AML1*) gene. Which one of the following aberrations in the *RUNX1* gene is *NOT* a recurrent one in patients with AML?[28,30-34]

A. Amplification
B. Deletion
C. Point mutation
D. Translocation
E. None of the above

102. A 56-year-old male came to a clinic for vertigo, paleness, and fever. Results of bone-marrow examination were consistent with acute myeloid leukemia (AML). Most AML cells were MPO+, CD20 partial+, CD79a partial+, CD3 partial+, some CD138+, CD−, CD5−, Ag+, and Fe+. Cytogenetic karyotype results were 46,XX[20]. The hematologist ordered a next-generation sequencing (NGS) panel for hematological neoplasms to further assess the prognosis. An acquired pathogenic variant in the *KIT* gene was detected. In which one of the exons would the *KIT* mutation most likely be located in this patient?

A. Exon 8
B. Exon 11
C. Exon 13
D. Exon 17
E. None of the above

103. A 2-day-old male was born at 36 weeks' gestation with a prenatal diagnosis of constitutional trisomy 21. Hypoxia developed shortly after birth, followed by respiratory distress requiring mechanical ventilation. A physical examination revealed dysmorphic facial features, hypotonia,

an atrioventricular septal defect, hepatosplenomegaly, ascites, and a diffuse papular skin rash. A complete blood count was notable for white-blood-cell count (WBC) $129 \times 10^3/\mu L$, hematocrit 36.4%, platelet count $119 \times 10^3/\mu L$, and 10%−15% blasts. Flow cytometric analysis confirmed megakaryoblastic differentiation: CD7+, CD23+, CD34+, CD41+, CD42b+, CD56+, CD61+, CD71+, CD2−, CD5−, CD10−, CD13−, CD14−, CD15−, and cytoplasmic MPO−. During the next 3 weeks the WBC count normalized and blasts disappeared from circulation. Which one of the following genetic alterations would most likely be detected in this patient's peripheral-blood sample when his WBC was high?[35]

A. *CALR*
B. *GATA1*
C. *GATA2*
D. *NPM1*
E. *RUNX1*
F. None of the above

104. A 2-day-old male was born at 36 weeks' gestation with a prenatal diagnosis of constitutional trisomy 21. Hypoxia developed shortly after birth, followed by respiratory distress requiring mechanical ventilation. A physical examination revealed dysmorphic facial features, hypotonia, an atrioventricular septal defect, hepatosplenomegaly, ascites, and a diffuse papular skin rash. A complete blood count was notable for white blood cell count (WBC) $129 \times 10^3/\mu L$, hematocrit 36.4%, platelet count $119 \times 10^3/\mu L$, and 10%−15% blasts. Flow cytometric analysis confirmed megakaryoblastic differentiation: CD7+, CD23+, CD34+, CD41+, CD42b+, CD56+, CD61+, CD71+, CD2−, CD5−, CD10−, CD13−, CD14−, CD15−, and cytoplasmic MPO−. Molecular analyses of the *GATA1* gene were ordered. Which one of the following locations in the *GATA1* gene would most likely harbor a pathogenic variant in this patient?[36,37,38]

A. Exon 1
B. Exon 2
C. Exon 3
D. Exon 4
E. Exon 5
F. None of the above

105. A 2-day-old male was born at 36 weeks' gestation with a prenatal diagnosis of constitutional trisomy 21. Hypoxia developed shortly after birth, followed by respiratory distress requiring mechanical ventilation. A physical examination revealed dysmorphic facial features, hypotonia,

an atrioventricular septal defect, hepatosplenomegaly, ascites, and a diffuse papular skin rash. A complete blood count was notable for white blood cell count (WBC) $129 \times 10^3/\mu L$, hematocrit 36.4%, platelet count $119 \times 10^3/\mu L$, and 10%−15% blasts. Flow cytometric analysis confirmed megakaryoblastic differentiation: CD7+, CD23+, CD34+, CD41+, CD42b+, CD56+, CD61+, CD71+, CD2−, CD5−, CD10−, CD13−, CD14−, CD15−, and cytoplasmic MPO−. Molecular analyses of the *GATA1* gene were ordered. Which one of the following assays would most likely be used for the *GATA1* gene in this patient?[36,37,38]

A. FISH
B. PCR-capillary electrophoresis
C. Sanger sequencing
D. Targeted-mutation analysis
E. All of the above
F. None of the above

106. A 46-year-old female was referred to a hematology clinic by her primary care physician for pancytopenia. The patient had a history of fatigue and easy bruising for 2 years and recurrent pneumonia in the past 6 months. Her family history was uneventful. Laboratory studies revealed white blood cells $1.8 \times 10^3/\mu L$, absolute neutrophil count $3.8 \times 10^2/\mu L$, absolute lymphocyte count $3.3 \times 10^2/\mu L$, hemoglobin 7.6 g/dL, and platelets $2.6 \times 10^4/\mu L$. A bone-marrow biopsy demonstrated 20% cellularity with trilineage dysplasia with 10% blasts expressing CD34 (CD34+), but not CD15 (CD15−) or CD33 (CD33−). The cytogenetic karyotype was 46,XX[20]. The hematologist ordered a next-generation sequencing (NGS) panel for hematological neoplasms to further assess the prognosis. An acquired pathogenic variant in the *RUNX1* gene was detected. Which one of the following prognoses would this patient most likely have, based on the NGS results?[39,40,41]

A. Favorable risk
B. Intermediate risk
C. Unfavorable risk
D. Unclear
E. None of the above

107. A 50-year-old female was referred to a hematology clinic by her primary care physician for pancytopenia. The patient had history of fatigue and easy bruising, unexplained lower-extremity swelling, and recurrent herpes infections for 25 years. Her family history was significant for pancytopenia affecting her mother, siblings and their children, and her own children. Both her mother and maternal aunt died from myelodysplastic syndrome (MDS). Laboratory

studies revealed white blood cells 1.8 k/μL, absolute neutrophil count 0.38 k/μL, absolute lymphocyte count 0.33 k/μL, hemoglobin 7.6 g/dL, and platelets 26 k/μL. A bone-marrow biopsy demonstrated 20% cellularity with megakaryocytic atypia, including micromegakaryocytes and erythroid dysplasia without increased CD34+ blasts. The cytogenetic karyotype was 47,XX,+8[9]/46,XX[11]. The hematologist suspected that the patient had a hereditary condition and ordered a molecular test to confirm the suspicion. Which one of the following genes would most likely be tested in this patient for the hereditary condition?

A. *ASXL1*
B. *GATA1*
C. *GATA2*
D. *RUNX1*
E. *RUNX2*
F. *SF3B1*
G. All of the above
H. None of the above

108. A 50-year-old female was referred to a hematology clinic by her primary care physician for pancytopenia. The patient had history of fatigue and easy bruising, unexplained lower-extremity swelling, and recurrent herpes infections for 25 years. Her family history was significant for pancytopenia affecting her mother, siblings and their children, and her own children. Both her mother and maternal aunt died from myelodysplastic syndrome (MDS). Laboratory studies revealed white blood cells 1.8 k/μL, absolute neutrophil count 0.38 k/μL, absolute lymphocyte count 0.33 k/μL, hemoglobin 7.6 g/dL, and platelets 26 k/μL. A bone marrow biopsy demonstrated 20% cellularity with megakaryocytic atypia, including micromegakaryocytes and erythroid dysplasia without increased CD34+ blasts. The cytogenetic karyotype was 47,XX,+8[9]/46,XX[11]. The hematologist suspected that the patient had a hereditary condition and ordered a molecular test to confirm the suspicion. A germline pathogenic variant in the *GATA2* gene was detected. Which one of the following genes would likely be somatically mutated in this patient?[42,43]

A. *ASXL1*
B. *GATA1*
C. *RUNX1*
D. *RUNX2*
E. *SF3B1*
F. All of the above
G. None of the above

109. A 39-year-old female came to an emergency department with severe headaches, dyspnea on exertion, and petechiae on the lower extremities. A complete blood count showed WBCs 56×10^3/µL, hemoglobin 9.0 g/dL, hematocrit 23, mean corpuscular volume 97 fL, platelet count 15×10^9/µL, and absolute neutrophil count 0.7×10^3/µL. A bone marrow biopsy revealed 90% lymphoid blasts. The blast population expressed CD19, CD20, CD22, CD10, CD34, TdT, and HLA-DR. Chromosomal karyotype results were 46,XX[20]. FISH analyses for *BCR-ABL1* were positive. The patient was subsequently diagnosed with pre-B acute lymphoblastic leukemia (ALL). Which one of the following *BCR-ABL1* fusions would the patient most likely have?[44]

   A. p190
   B. p205
   C. p210
   D. p230
   E. All of the above
   F. None of the above

110. A 39-year-old female came to an emergency department with severe headaches, dyspnea on exertion, and petechiae on the lower extremities. A complete blood count showed WBCs 56×10^3/µL, hemoglobin 9.0 g/dL, hematocrit 23, mean corpuscular volume 97 fL, platelet count 15×10^9/µL, and absolute neutrophil count 0.7×10^3/µL. A bone-marrow biopsy was performed and showed 90% lymphoid blasts. The blast population expressed CD19, CD20, CD22, CD10, CD34, TdT, and HLA-DR. The chromosomal karyotype was 46,XX[20]. FISH analyses for *BCR-ABL1* were positive. The patient was subsequently diagnosed with pre-B acute lymphoblastic leukemia (ALL). Which one of the following prognoses would this patient most likely have?[44,45]

   A. Favorable risk
   B. Intermediate risk
   C. Unfavorable risk
   D. Unclear
   E. None of the above

111. A 51-year-old male came to a clinic for generalized weakness and an abdominal lump that had been present for 9 months. On physical examination, mild pallor was noticed. Abdominal examinations revealed enlarged, firm, nontender splenomegaly 10 cm below the costal margin. On ultrasonography, the spleen was measured $18 \times 10 \times 7$ cm with normal echotexture. Laboratory analyses revealed hemoglobin of 9 g/dL, total white-blood-cell count (WBC) of 6.0×10^9/L, red-blood-cell (RBC) count 4.35×10^{12}/L, platelet count

50×10^9/L, and hematocrit 36.2%. A peripheral-blood smear demonstrated 8% atypical cells with light basophilic cytoplasm containing numerous hairy projections on the outer surface, and the nucleus was oval and indented with coarse chromatin. Platelets were reduced in number. Bone marrow aspirations demonstrated a dry tap. A bone-marrow biopsy revealed the typical fried-egg appearance of hairy cells with abnormal areas of fibrosis. Reticulin stains on a marrow biopsy demonstrated increased reticulin fibers. Flow cytometry results revealed positivity for CD19, CD20, CD11c, CD103, FMC-7, and HLA-DR. A diagnosis of hairy-cell leukemia was made. Which one of the following genes would most likely be mutated in this patient?[46–49]

   A. *ASXL1*
   B. *BRAF*
   C. *GATA2*
   D. *RUNX2*
   E. *SF3B1*
   F. None of above

112. A 31-year-old Caucasian male came to a clinic with a 3-week history of breathlessness, fever, diarrhea, and axillary lymphadenopathy. He was diagnosed with infectious mononucleosis 4 years ago. Whole-body CT scanning showed diffuse lymphadenopathy on either side of diaphragm. His white-blood-cell count on presentation rapidly worsened to 8.5×10^4/µL, hemoglobin 11.7 g/dL, and platelets 1.38×10^5/µL. His peripheral-blood smear showed leukocytosis, including neutrophilia and a population of pleomorphic atypical cells, comprising 17% of leukocytes. Flow cytometry on peripheral blood and bone marrow showed an atypical population that expressed bright CD45 and coexpressed CD2, CD56, HLA-DR, CD13, and dim CD4. IHC stains demonstrated that the tumor cells were positive for CD30 and ALK and were distributed in a sinusoidal pattern in the bone marrow. These cells were negative for CD20, CD3, CD8, and EBER (EBV ISH stain). Which one of the following genetic alterations would this patient most likely have?[50]

   A. *ALK* point mutations
   B. *ALK* amplification
   C. inv(2)(p21p23) with *EML4-ALK* fusion
   D. t(2;5)(p23;q35) with *NPM1-ALK* fusion
   E. All of the above
   F. None of the above

113. Which one of the following statements regarding bone-marrow engraftment in molecular analyses is correct?[51]

A. Only the posttransplantation sample is required for the analysis.

B. Chimerism status was usually assessed on bone-marrow samples collected after transplantation.

C. Sanger sequencing is the gold standard method for chimerism status analysis.

D. NGS sequencing has replaced Sanger sequencing as the first-line test for chimerism status analysis.

E. The analytical sensitivity of the chimerism status analysis is about 1%–10%.

114. Which one of the following statements regarding bone-marrow engraftment molecular analyses is *NOT* correct?[51]

A. Choose recipient-specific alleles at least two repeats smaller than the donor alleles if the recipient allele is smaller.

B. It is preferred that both donor and recipient alleles are informative.

C. The chimerism analysis may be used as an indicator for relapse.

D. The chimerism analysis can be used for autologous hematopoietic-cell transplantation.

E. Stutter peaks detected in STR analysis are caused mainly by slippage of *Taq* polymerase during PCR amplification of STR loci.

115. How frequently do patients with Burkitt lymphoma have *c-MYC* translocations?[7]

A. 90%

B. 75%

C. 50%

D. 25%

E. <5%

116. How frequently do patients with diffuse large-B-cell lymphoma (DLBCL) have *c-MYC* translocations?[7]

A. 90%

B. 75%

C. 50%

D. 25%

E. 10%

117. Clinically significant mutations of *EGFR* are typically:

A. Activating mutations

B. Dominant negative mutations

C. Gain-of-function mutations

D. Loss-of-function mutations

E. Silent mutations

118. Genetic alterations in which one of the following is most prevalent in nonsmoking patients with nonsmall-cell lung cancer (NSCLC) in the United States?

A. *ALK*

B. *BRAF*

C. *EGFR*

D. *KRAS*

E. *NRAS*

119. How frequently do patients with nonsmall-cell lung cancer (NSCLC) have *EGFR* mutations in Western populations?

A. <1%

B. 10%

C. 25%

D. 50%

E. 75%

120. How frequently do nonsmokers with nonsmall-cell lung cancer (NSCLC) have *EGFR* mutations in the United States?

A. <1%

B. 10%

C. 25%

D. 50%

E. 75%

121. Which one of the following mutations in *EGFR* most likely is associated with acquired resistance to *EGFR* tyrosine kinase inhibitor (TKI) therapy in patients with nonsmall-cell lung cancer (NSCLC)?

A. G719X in exon 18

B. Deletions in exon 19

C. T790M in exon 20

D. L858R in exon 21

E. None of the above

122. Which one of the following statements regarding acquired genetic alterations in patients with nonsmall-cell lung cancer (NSCLC) is *NOT* correct?

A. Mutations in *EGFR* and *KRAS* are mutually exclusive.

B. Mutations in *EGFR*, *BRAF* and *KRAS* are mutually exclusive.

C. Mutations in *KRAS* and *ALK* are mutually exclusive.

D. Mutations in *BRAF*, *KRAS*, and *ALK* are mutually exclusive.

E. Mutations in *EGFR*, *BRAF*, *KRAS*, and *ALK* are mutually exclusive.

F. None of the above.

123. Which one of the cancers causes the most deaths in the United States?

A. Breast cancer

B. Colorectal cancer

C. Lung cancer

D. Pancreatic cancer

E. Prostate cancer

124. Which one of the following statements regarding erlotinib in therapy for nonsmall-cell lung cancer (NSCLC) is correct?

A. It targets the ligand-binding domain of the *EGFR* gene.

B. It targets the tyrosine kinase domain of the *EGFR* gene.

C. It targets the ligand-binding domain of the *KRAS* gene.

D. It targets the tyrosine kinase domain of the *KRAS* gene.

E. It targets the ligand-binding domain of the *ALK* gene.

F. It targets the tyrosine kinase domain of the *ALK* gene.

125. Which one of the following statements regarding erlotinib in therapy for nonsmall-cell lung cancer (NSCLC) is correct?

A. It is a monoclonal antibody that blocks the ligand-binding domain.

B. It is a small molecule that occupies the ATP-binding groove of the tyrosine kinase.

C. EGFR protein overexpression by immunohistochemistry can predict the response to erlotinib.

D. It can be used for patients with either *EGFR* or *KRAS* mutations, but not those with *ALK* mutations.

E. It can be used effectively to patients with *EGFR* mutations in exons 18 through 21.

126. How frequently do patients with lung adenocarcinoma have acquired *KRAS* mutations?[67]

A. 90%

B. 75%

C. 50%

D. 20%

E. <5%

127. How frequently do patients with nonsmall-cell lung cancer (NSCLC) have acquired an *ALK* rearrangement?

A. 90%

B. 75%

C. 50%

D. 20%

E. 5%

128. Which one of the following techniques is most commonly used to detect *ALK* genetic alterations in patients with nonsmall-cell lung cancer (NSCLC)?

A. FISH

B. OncoScan microarray

C. Quantitative PCR

D. Sanger sequencing

E. TaqMan genotyping assay

129. A patient with nonsmall-cell lung cancer (NSCLC) was found to have a deletion in exon 19 of *EGFR*. She relapsed on erlotinib after a partial remission that lasted 16 months. Which of the following exons of the *EGFR* gene would most likely be tested for resistance?

A. Exon 18

B. Exon 20

C. Exon 21

D. Exon 22

E. All of the above

130. Which one of the following results may be useful to predict whether a patient with nonsmall-cell lung cancer (NSCLC) may *NOT* response well to erlotinib?

A. Amplification of *EGFR*

B. p.G12A mutation in *KRAS*

C. p.L858R in exon 21 of *EGFR*

D. Polysomy of chromosome 7 including *EGFR* on 7p11.2

E. None of the above

131. Which one of the following results may be used to predict whether a patient with nonsmall-cell lung cancer (NSCLC) should *NOT* be treated with erlotinib?

A. Amplification of *EGFR*

B. Asian female nonsmoker

C. *EML4-ALK* translocation detected by FISH

D. p.L858R in exon 21 of *EGFR*

E. Polysomy of chromosome 7 including *EGFR* on 7p11.2

132. A 56-year-old female with a history of stage III melanoma came to an oncology clinic for multiple subcutaneous nodules. A fine-needle aspiration (FNA) of a nodule helped to establish the diagnosis of metastatic melanoma. Which one of the following molecular tests may be useful for prognosis and therapy?

A. *ALK*

B. *BRAF*

C. *EGFR*

D. *KRAS*

E. *NRAS*

133. A 57-year-old female with a history of stage III melanoma came to an oncology clinic for multiple subcutaneous nodules. Fine-needle aspiration (FNA) of a nodule helped to establish the diagnosis of metastatic melanoma. A *BRAF* assay with melting temperature analysis using dual hybridization fluorescence resonance energy transfer (FRET) probes was ordered to detect the V600E mutation. Both the sensor and anchor probes were 100% matched with the wild type *BRAF* sequence. Which one of the following statements regarding this FRET assay is correct?[52]

A. The melting temperature is higher in the wild-type *BRAF* sequence than in the heterozygous mutant.

B. The melting temperature is higher in the heterozygous mutant than in the wild-type *BRAF* sequence.

C. The melting temperature is higher in the heterozygous mutant than in the homozygous *BRAF* mutant.

D. The melting temperature is higher in the homozygous mutant than in the wild-type *BRAF* sequence.

134. A 60-year-old female with a history of stage III melanoma came to an oncology clinic for multiple subcutaneous nodules. Fine-needle aspiration (FNA) of a nodule helped to establish the diagnosis of metastatic melanoma. A *BRAF* assay was ordered. Which one of the following results would be the most likely one for this patient?

A. *BRAF* K581S
B. *BRAF* V600D
C. *BRAF* V600E
D. *BRAF* V600K
E. *BRAF* K601E
F. Wild type

135. A 61-year-old female with a history of stage III melanoma came to an oncology clinic for multiple subcutaneous nodules. Fine-needle aspiration (FNA) of a nodule helped to establish the diagnosis of metastatic melanoma. A *BRAF* assay was ordered. Which one of the following mutations would the patient most likely have?

A. *BRAF* K581S
B. *BRAF* V600D
C. *BRAF* V600E
D. *BRAF* V600K
E. *BRAF* K601E

136. A 59-year-old female with a history of stage III melanoma came to an oncology clinic for multiple subcutaneous nodules. Fine-needle aspiration (FNA) of a nodule helped to establish the diagnosis of metastatic melanoma. A *BRAF* assay with melting-temperature analysis using dual-hybridization fluorescence resonance energy transfer (FRET) probes was ordered to detect the V600E mutation. The melting temperature for the wild type was 64.5°C and for the V600E mutation 59.5°C. A melting temperature of 59.5°C was identified in the tumor sample from this patient. Which one of the following interpretations would be the most appropriate one?

A. A mutation in *BRAF* was identified in this specimen.

B. A V600E mutation was identified in this specimen.

C. Heterozygous V600E mutation was identified in this specimen.

D. Homozygous V600E mutation was identified in this specimen.

E. Sanger sequence is recommended to confirm the finding.

137. A 58-year-old female with a history of stage III melanoma came to an oncology clinic for multiple subcutaneous nodules. Fine-needle aspiration (FNA) of a nodule helped to establish the diagnosis of metastatic melanoma. A *BRAF* assay with melting-temperature analysis using dual-hybridization fluorescence resonance energy transfer (FRET) probes was ordered to detect the V600E mutation. The melting temperature for the wild type was 64.5°C and for the V600E mutation 59.5°C. A melting temperature of 54.5°C was identified besides the 64.5°C for the wild type. Which one of the following actions should be the most appropriate follow-up step?[52]

A. Stating that the V600E mutation is identified and recommending *BRAF* inhibitor therapy.

B. Repeating the test to confirm the finding, then sequencing the region to confirm the mutation.

C. Repeating the test to confirm the finding, then signing it out as a pathogenic variant of V600E.

D. Stating that a variant of V600E mutation is identified and recommending *BRAF* inhibitor therapy.

E. None of above.

138. Acquired *BRAF* mutations are *NOT* common in:
A. Colorectal cancer
B. Ewing sarcoma
C. Metastatic melanoma
D. Nonsmall-cell lung cancer
E. Thyroid carcinoma

139. How frequently do patients with malignant melanomas have somatic mutations in *BRAF*?
A. 90%
B. 75%
C. 45%
D. 20%
E. <5%

140. Which one of the following statements regarding acquired *BRAF* mutations is *NOT* correct?
A. Mutations in *BRAF* are diagnostic for metastatic melanoma.
B. Mutations in *BRAF* are seen in benign melanocytic nevi.

C. Tests for *BRAF* mutations are important in predicting the response of the patient to *BRAF* inhibitors.

D. *BRAF* inhibitors prevent ligands from binding to the receptor.

E. Patients with V600K mutations respond well to *BRAF* inhibitors.

141. Real-time PCR with FRET probes and melting-curve analysis are most useful for detecting which one of the following?
A. Acquired *CEBPA* mutations for AML
B. *BRAF* mutations for melanoma
C. Duchenne muscular dystrophy
D. Fragile X
E. Hemophilia A

142. A *BRAF* V600E mutation can be used in all of the following clinical circumstances EXCEPT:
A. Diagnosing metastatic melanoma
B. Predicting a more aggressive thyroid cancer
C. Predicting response to a *BRAF* inhibitor
D. Predicting response to anti-*EGFR* therapy in colorectal cancer
E. Ruling out Lynch syndrome in patients with colorectal cancer

143. Which one of the following statements regarding erlotinib therapy for nonsmall-cell lung cancer (NSCLC) is correct?
A. It can be used for patients with mutations in *ALK*.
B. It can be used for patients with mutations in *BRAF*.
C. It can be used for patients with mutations in *EGFR*.
D. It can be used for patients with mutations in *KRAS*.
E. It can be used for patients with mutations in *EGFR*, *BRAF*, or *KRAS*.
F. It can be used for patients with mutations in *EGFR*, *BRAF*, *KRAS*, or *ALK*.

144. In which type of thyroid cancers are the *BRAF* mutations most commonly seen?
A. Anaplastic thyroid cancer
B. Follicular thyroid cancer
C. Medullary thyroid cancer
D. Papillary thyroid cancer
E. Poorly differentiated thyroid cancer

145. How frequently do patients with papillary thyroid cancer have acquired mutations in *BRAF*?
A. 90%
B. 75%
C. 45%
D. 20%
E. <5%

146. Which type of thyroid cancers do patients with type 2 multiple endocrine neoplasia (MEN2) most likely have?
A. Anaplastic thyroid cancer
B. Follicular thyroid cancer
C. Medullary thyroid cancer
D. Papillary thyroid cancer
E. Poorly differentiated thyroid cancer

147. Which type of thyroid cancers do patients with Cowden syndrome most likely have?
A. Anaplastic thyroid cancer
B. Follicular thyroid cancer
C. Medullary thyroid cancer
D. Papillary thyroid cancer
E. Poorly differentiated thyroid cancer

148. An 82-year-old male came to an oncology clinic for follow-up. He was diagnosed with papillary thyroid carcinoma (PTC) 25 years ago and treated with a total thyroidectomy. Other history included prostatic carcinoma diagnosed 15 years ago treated with prostatectomy and local radiation. He also had had metastatic thyroid cancer in the lungs treated with partial lung lobectomy 10 years ago. A PET scan demonstrated lesions in the posterior neck. A biopsy of the lesion in his neck revealed a poorly differentiated carcinoma without features of papillary thyroid carcinoma. Which one of the following tests would be most useful in order to confirm or rule out metastatic papillary thyroid carcinoma?
A. *BRAF* V600E mutation
B. *EGFR* mutation analysis
C. *EML4-ALK* translocation
D. *KRAS* mutation analysis
E. *NRAS* mutation analysis

149. A 78-year-old male came to an oncology clinic for follow-up. He was diagnosed with papillary thyroid carcinoma (PTC) 25 years ago and treated with a total thyroidectomy. Other history included prostatic carcinoma diagnosed 15 years ago and treated with prostatectomy and local radiation. He also had had a metastatic thyroid cancer in the lungs treated with partial lung lobectomy 10 years ago. A PET scan demonstrated lesions in the hilum of the left lung. A biopsy of the lesion in his neck revealed a poorly differentiated carcinoma of unknown origin. Which one of the following tests would be most useful in order to confirm or rule out lung carcinoma?
A. *BRAF* V600E mutation
B. *EGFR* mutation analysis
C. *EML4-ALK* translocation FISH
D. *KRAS* mutation analysis

E. *NRAS* mutation analysis

150. Which one of the following genes is most likely mutated in follicular thyroid cancers as a somatic mutation?
   A. *ALK*
   B. *BRAF*
   C. *EGFR*
   D. *KIT*
   E. *RAS*
   F. *RET*

151. A 66-year-old female was diagnosed with gastrointestinal stromal tumor (GIST) 2 months ago, and the tumor was surgically removed 15 days ago. Because the tumor was larger than 10 cm with a high mitotic index, the oncologist wanted to recommend treatment with imatinib. He contacted the pathologist to request a mutation analysis in order to guide treatment and delineate prognosis. Which one of the following genes most likely harbored an acquired pathogenic variant related to the response to imatinib if there was one in this patient?
   A. *BRAF*
   B. *EGFR*
   C. *KIT*
   D. *PDGFRA*
   E. *RAS*

152. How frequently do patients with gastrointestinal stromal tumors (GISTs) have acquired mutations in *KIT*?
   A. 85%
   B. 65%
   C. 45%
   D. 25%
   E. <5%

153. How frequently do patients with gastrointestinal stromal tumors (GISTs) have acquired mutations in *PDGFRA*?
   A. 90%
   B. 70%
   C. 50%
   D. 20%
   E. 10%

154. A 57-year-old male was diagnosed with gastrointestinal stromal tumor (GIST) 1 month ago, and the tumor was surgically removed 10 days ago. Because the tumor was larger than 10 cm with a high mitotic index, the oncologist wanted to recommend treatment with imatinib. He contacted the pathologist to request a *KIT* mutation analysis assay in order to guide treatment and delineate prognosis. Later, a genetic counselor called the oncologist with a positive result. In which one of the following

exons of *KIT* would the acquired pathogenic variant most likely be located in this patient?
   A. Exon 9
   B. Exon 11
   C. Exon 13
   D. Exon 14
   E. Exon 17

155. A 58-year-old male was diagnosed with gastrointestinal stromal tumor (GIST) 1 month ago, and the tumor was surgically removed 10 days ago. Because the tumor was larger than 10 cm with a high mitotic index, the oncologist wanted to recommend treatment with imatinib. After consulting a pathologist, the oncologist ordered a *KIT* mutation analysis assay in order to guide treatment and delineate prognosis. The results of the *KIT* assay turned to be negative. A reflex test was performed according to the note from the oncologist. Which one of the following genes would most likely be analyzed in the reflex test in order to further assess the prognosis, since the mutation analysis of *KIT* was negative?
   A. *ALK*
   B. *BRAF*
   C. *EGFR*
   D. *PDGFRA*
   E. *RAS*

156. A 59-year-old male was diagnosed with gastrointestinal stromal tumor (GIST) 1 month ago, and the tumor was surgically removed 10 days ago. Because the tumor was larger than 10 cm with a high mitotic index, the oncologist wanted to recommend treatment with imatinib. After consulting a pathologist, the oncologist ordered a *KIT* mutation analysis assay in order to guide treatment and further delineate prognosis. The results of the *KIT* assay turned to be negative. A reflex molecular test for *PDGFRA* was performed according to the note from the oncologist, and the result was positive. Which one of the following exons of the *PDGFRA* gene most likely harbored the mutation?
   A. Exon 12
   B. Exon 13
   C. Exon 14
   D. Exon 15
   E. Exon 16
   F. Exon 17
   G. Exon 18

157. A 61-year-old male was diagnosed with gastrointestinal stromal tumor (GIST) 2 months ago, and the tumor was surgically removed 1 month ago. Because the tumor was larger than 10 cm with a high mitotic index, the oncologist wanted to recommend treatment with imatinib.

After consulting a pathologist, the oncologist ordered a *KIT* mutation analysis assay in order to guide treatment and delineate prognosis. The results of the *KIT* assay showed a p.Tyr570del in exon 11. Which one of the following statements is correct with regard to imatinib therapy?[53,54]

A. The patient will respond well to imatinib.

B. The mutation in exon 11 of *KIT* is a positive predictive factor for overall survival.

C. The mutation in exon 11 of *KIT* is a positive predictive factor for progression-free survival.

D. Patients with mutations in exon 11 of *KIT* have a higher risk of secondary mutations.

E. Patients with mutations in exon 11 of *KIT* have improved tumor response with high-dose imatinib.

158. A 64-year-old male was diagnosed with gastrointestinal stromal tumor (GIST) 3 months ago, and the tumor was surgically removed 1 month ago. Because the tumor was larger than 10 cm with a high mitotic index, the oncologist wanted to recommend treatment with imatinib. After consulting a pathologist, the oncologist ordered a *KIT* mutation analysis assay in order to guide treatment and delineate prognosis. The results of the *KIT* assay showed a p. Trp557_Lys558del in exon 11. After 6 months of imatinib therapy, the patient developed resistance. A molecular test was ordered for secondary mutations related to imatinib resistance. In which part of the *KIT* gene would mutations responsible for the imatinib resistance most likely be located in this patient?

A. Exon 9, 13, 14, or 17 of *KIT*

B. Exon 9 or 17 of *KIT*

C. Exon 12−16 of *PDGFRA*

D. Exon 13, 14, or 17 of *KIT*

E. Exon 17 or 18 of *PDGFRA*

159. A 46-year-old female came to a clinic for vague upper abdominal pain and a feeling of an abdominal lump on and off for 2 years. Clinical examinations of the abdomen revealed a well-defined transversely mobile intraabdominal lump in the right hypochondrium of about 8 × 6 cm. The abdomen was explored electively and a 10 × 6 cm tumor was seen arising from the greater curve of the stomach, exophytically, with a sessile base. There was no infiltration of the mass into the surrounding structures, nor any evidence of metastases or lymphadenopathy. Histopathological examinations of the tumor revealed that the gastric submucosa was composed of fusiform and epithelioid cells. Immunohistochemistry stains found that the tumor cells were positive for vimentin, CD34, S-100, SMA, and desmin. The PanCK and LCA were negative. The findings favored the diagnosis of epithelioid gastrointestinal stromal tumor (GIST) of low malignant potential. Which one of the following exons of *KIT* would most likely harbor the mutation in this patient if she has one predicted to respond to a high dose of imatinib therapy?[55]

A. Exon 9

B. Exon 11

C. Exon 13

D. Exon 14

E. Exon 17

160. A 41-year-old female was diagnosed with oligodendroglioma, WHO grade II. A partial resection of the left frontal lobe was done, which removed approximately 80% of the tumor. Which one of the following genetic tests would be appropriate for this patient?[53]

A. *ALK*

B. *BRAF*

C. *EGFR*

D. *RAS*

E. 1p/19q

161. A 41-year-old female was diagnosed with oligodendroglioma, WHO grade II. A partial resection of the left frontal lobe was done, which removed approximately 80% of the tumor. Which one of the following genetic abnormalities would this patient most likely have?

A. 1p/19q amplification

B. 1p/19q deletion

C. 1p/19q duplication

D. Unclear

E. None of above

162. A 45-year-old female was diagnosed with oligodendroglioma, WHO grade II. A partial resection of the left frontal lobe was done, which removed approximately 80% of the tumor. A PCR-based loss-of-heterozygosity (LOH) analysis detected loss of 1p/19q in the tumor. How frequently does the 1p/19 codeletion appear in patients with oligodendroglioma?[53]

A. 100%

B. 80%

C. 60%

D. 40%

E. 20%

163. A 42-year-old male was diagnosed with oligodendroglioma, WHO grade II. A partial resection of the left frontal lobe was done, which removed approximately 80% of the tumor. A PCR-based loss-of-heterozygosity (LOH) analysis

showed loss of 1p/19q in the tumor. Which one of the following statements is *NOT* correct?[53]

A. The 1p/19q codeletion is associated with a favorable response to chemotherapy.

B. The 1p/19q codeletion is associated with significantly better progression-free survival.

C. The 1p/19q codeletion is associated with significantly better overall survival.

D. Loss of 1p alone is associated with a favorable response to chemotherapy.

E. Loss of 19q alone is associated with a favorable response to chemotherapy.

164. A clinical molecular pathology laboratory has been monitoring its send-out test volume to evaluate the need for test validations. In the past 6 months, the volume for 1p/19q tests with a PCR-based loss-of-heterozygosity (LOH) assay with formalin-fixed, paraffin-embedded (FFPE) tissues has increased significantly. The lab director decided to validate an assay for 1p/19q. With which one of the following brain tumors are losses of chromosomes 1p and 19q typically associated?

A. Ependymoma
B. Glioblastoma
C. Meningioma
D. Metastatic prostate cancer
E. Oligodendroglioma

165. A 60-year-old female presented with seizure to an oncology clinic; she had a 3-month history of headaches, nausea, and vomiting. MRI revealed an enhanced mass in the subcortical region of the right frontal lobe. Her family history was unremarkable. A nearly gross total resection was performed. A histological diagnosis of glioblastoma multiforme, WHO grade IV, was made. Which one of the following genetic tests would be most appropriate for diagnosis and estimation of prognosis and therapy in this patient?

A. *BRAF*
B. *MGMT*
C. *PDGFRA*
D. *RAS*
E. 1p/19q FISH

166. A 60-year-old female presented with seizure to an oncology clinic; she had a 3-month history of headaches, nausea, and vomiting. A MRI revealed an enhanced mass in the subcortical region of the right frontal lobe. Her family history was unremarkable. A nearly gross total resection was operated. A histological diagnosis of glioblastoma multiforme, WHO grade IV, was made. Which one of the following genetic tests would be most

appropriate for diagnosis and estimation of prognosis and therapy in this patient?

A. *BRAF*
B. *EGFR*
C. *PDGFRA*
D. *RAS*
E. 1p/19q FISH

167. A 63-year-old male presented with seizure to an oncology clinic; he had a 3-month history of headaches, nausea, and vomiting. MRI revealed an enhanced mass in the subcortical region of the right frontal lobe. His family history was unremarkable. A nearly gross total resection was operated. A histological diagnosis of glioblastoma multiforme, WHO grade IV, was made. *MGMT* and *EGFR* genetic tests were ordered to confirm the diagnosis and estimate prognosis and therapy. Which one of the following *MGMT* regions would most likely be investigated in this patient?

A. Coding region
B. Exon
C. Intron
D. Promoter
E. UTRs
F. Whole gene

168. A 62-year-old female presented with seizure to an oncology clinic; she had a 3-month history of headaches, nausea, and vomiting. MRI revealed an enhanced mass in the subcortical region of the right frontal lobe. Her family history was unremarkable. A nearly gross total resection was operated. A histological diagnosis of glioblastoma multiforme, WHO grade IV, was made. *MGMT* genetic tests were ordered to confirm the diagnosis and estimate prognosis and therapy. Which one of the following techniques would most likely be used for the *MGMT* analysis?

A. Chromosome karyotype
B. Fluorescence in situ hybridization (FISH)
C. Methylation study
D. Sequencing
E. TaqMan SNP genotype

169. A 62-year-old female presented with seizure to an oncology clinic; she had a 3-month history of headaches, nausea, and vomiting. MRI revealed an enhanced mass in the subcortical region of the right frontal lobe. Her family history was unremarkable. A nearly gross total resection was operated. A histological diagnosis of glioblastoma multiforme, WHO grade IV, was made. *MGMT* genetic tests were ordered, and turned out to be negative. The oncologist ordered another genetic test in order to further confirm the diagnosis and estimate prognosis and therapy. Which one of the

following genes would most likely be tested when the *MGMT* genetic test was negative in this patient?

A. *BRAF*
B. *EGFR*
C. *PDGFRA*
D. *RAS*
E. None of the above

170. A 64-year-old female presented with seizure to an oncology clinic; she had a 3-month history of headaches, nausea, and vomiting. MRI revealed an enhanced mass in the subcortical region of the right frontal lobe. Her family history was unremarkable. A nearly gross total resection was operated. A histological diagnosis of glioblastoma multiforme, WHO grade IV, was made. *MGMT* and *EGFR* genetic tests were ordered to confirm the diagnosis and estimate prognosis and therapy. Which one of the following genetic alterations would the *EGFR* assay most likely be designed to detect in this patient?

A. Amplifications
B. Deletions
C. Duplications
D. Microsatellite instability
E. Single-nucleotide mutations
F. Translocation

171. A 62-year-old female presented with seizure to an oncology clinic; she had a 3-month history of headaches, nausea, and vomiting. MRI revealed an enhanced mass in the subcortical region of the right frontal lobe. Her family history was unremarkable. A nearly gross total resection was operated. A histological diagnosis of glioblastoma multiforme, WHO grade IV, was made. *MGMT* and *EGFR* genetic tests were ordered to confirm the diagnosis and estimate prognosis and therapy. Which one of the following techniques would most likely be used for the *EGFR* analysis in order to assist decision making about therapy?

A. Chromosome karyotype
B. Fluorescence in situ hybridization (FISH)
C. Methylation study
D. Sequencing
E. TaqMan SNP genotype

172. A 63-year-old male presented with seizure to an oncology clinic; he had a 3-month history of headaches, nausea, and vomiting. MRI revealed an enhanced mass in the subcortical region of the right frontal lobe. His family history was unremarkable. A nearly gross total resection was operated. A histological diagnosis of glioblastoma multiforme, WHO grade IV, was made. *MGMT* genetic tests were ordered, and the results were positive for

methylation in the promoter region. Which one of the following statements would be the most appropriate interpretation of these results?

A. The patient would be resistant to the alkylating therapy.
B. The patient would respond well to the alkylating therapy.
C. The sample from this patient was bisulfite conversion—positive.
D. The overall survival of this patient would be poor.
E. None of the above.

173. A 61-year-old female presented with seizure to an oncology clinic; she had a 3-month history of headaches, nausea, and vomiting. MRI revealed an enhanced mass in the subcortical region of the right frontal lobe. Her family history was unremarkable. A nearly gross total resection was operated. A histological diagnosis of glioblastoma multiforme, WHO grade IV, was made. *MGMT* and *EGFR* genetic tests were ordered, and results were positive for *EGFR* amplification. Which one of the following statements would be an appropriate interpretation of these results?

A. The patient would respond well to chemotherapy.
B. The patient would respond well to radiation therapy.
C. The patient would respond well to combined chemotherapy and radiation therapy.
D. The patient had oligodendroglioma instead of glioblastoma.
E. The overall survival of this patient would be poor.

174. Which one of the following represents the DNA modification caused by sodium bisulfite treatment for methylation study in the *MGMT* genetic analysis?

A. $A > G$
B. $C > T$
C. $C > U$
D. $T > U$
E. None of above

175. A 61-year-old female presented with seizure to an oncology clinic; she had a 3-month history of headaches, nausea, and vomiting. MRI revealed an enhanced mass in the subcortical region of the right frontal lobe. Her family history was unremarkable. A nearly gross total resection was operated. A histological diagnosis of glioblastoma multiforme, WHO grade IV, was made. *MGMT* genetic tests were ordered, and results showed partial *MGMT* methylation. Which one of the following might result in a pattern of partial methylation in the glioblastoma specimen from this patient?

A. Incomplete conversion
B. Presence of nonneoplastic cells
C. Tumor heterogeneity
D. All of the above
E. None of the above

176. Which one of the following abnormalities is most likely seen in patients with neuroblastoma?
    A. Amplification of *ALK*
    B. c.3520T > A (p.F1174I) in *ALK*
    C. Deletion of the *ALK* gene
    D. inv(2)(p21p23) involving *ALK*
    E. t(2;5)(p23;q35) involving *ALK*

177. Which one of the following abnormalities is most likely seen in patients with anaplastic large-cell lymphoma?
    A. Amplification of *ALK*
    B. c.3520T > A (p.F1174I) in *ALK*
    C. Deletion of the *ALK* gene
    D. inv(2)(p21p23) involving *ALK*
    E. t(2;5)(p23;q35) involving *ALK*

178. With which one of the following malignancies is a *MYCN* amplification most likely associated?
    A. Acute myeloid leukemia
    B. Astrocytoma
    C. B precursor lymphoid neoplasm
    D. Neuroblastoma
    E. Rhabdomyosarcoma

179. A 5-year-old boy was brought to an emergency department (ED) by his parents for symptoms of fever and pain in the lower extremities and refusal to bear weight. A hip X-ray did not have positive findings. He was sent home with pain medications. One month later he was sent to the ED for the same symptoms and significant weight loss (5 lb in the past month). A complete blood count (CBC) revealed normochromic microcytic anemia (RBC, 2.77×10^{12}/L; Hb, 7.5 g/dL; MCV, 78.6 fL). A peripheral-blood smear and a bone-marrow biopsy with immunohistochemical stains led to a diagnosis of metastatic neuroblastoma, poorly differentiated. A genetic test was ordered to assess the prognosis. Which one of the following acquired genetic changes would most likely be detected in this patient?
    A. *C-MYC* amplification
    B. *C-MYC* translocation
    C. *N-MYC* amplification
    D. *N-MYC* translocation
    E. All of the above
    F. None of the above

180. Which one of the following acquired abnormalities is most likely seen in patients with nonsmall-cell lung cancer (NSCLC)?
    A. Amplification of *ALK*
    B. c.3520T > A (p.F1174I) in *ALK*
    C. Deletion of the *ALK* gene

D. inv(2)(p21p23) involving *ALK*
E. t(2;5)(p23;q35) involving *ALK*

181. A 64-year-old male presented to a clinic with an abnormal chest X-ray from an annual physical examination. He had a smoking history of half a pack per day and a history of hypertension. The chest X-ray showed a huge mass on right middle lobe and multiple pulmonary nodules on the right lung. A transcutaneous needle biopsy and pathological examinations confirmed the diagnosis of nonsmall-cell lung carcinoma (NSCLC), adenocarcinoma (ADC) subtype. A molecular battery test was ordered. Which one of the following exons of the *EGFR* gene would most likely be investigated in this molecular battery test?[56]
    A. Exon 9
    B. Exon 11
    C. Exon 13
    D. Exon 14
    E. Exon 19

182. A 64-year-old male presented to a clinic with an abnormal chest X-ray from an annual physical examination. He had a smoking history of half a pack per day and a history of hypertension. The chest X-ray showed a huge mass on right middle lobe and multiple pulmonary nodules on the right lung. A transcutaneous needle biopsy and pathological examinations confirmed the diagnosis of nonsmall-cell lung carcinoma (NSCLC), adenocarcinoma (ADC) subtype. A molecular battery test was ordered. Which one of the following exons of the *EGFR* gene would most likely be investigated in this molecular battery test?[56]
    A. Exon 9
    B. Exon 10
    C. Exon 20
    D. Exon 21
    E. All of the above
    F. None of the above

183. A 64-year-old male presented to a clinic with an abnormal chest X-ray from an annual physical examination. He had a smoking history of half a pack per day and a history of hypertension. The chest X-ray showed a huge mass on right middle lobe and multiple pulmonary nodules on the right lung. A transcutaneous needle biopsy and pathological examinations confirmed the diagnosis of nonsmall-cell lung carcinoma (NSCLC), adenocarcinoma (ADC) subtype. A molecular battery test was ordered, and an acquired pathogenic variant in exon 19 of the *EGFR* gene was detected in the tumor specimen. Which one of the following genetic changes in the *EGFR* gene would this patient most likely have?[56]

A. Amplification
B. In-frame in/dels
C. Out-of-frame in/dels
D. Point mutation
E. All of the above
F. None of the above

184. A 64-year-old male presented to a clinic with an abnormal chest X-ray from an annual physical examination. He had a smoking history of half a pack per day and a history of hypertension. The chest X-ray showed a huge mass on right middle lobe and multiple pulmonary nodules on the right lung. A transcutaneous needle biopsy and pathological examinations confirmed the diagnosis of nonsmall-cell lung carcinoma (NSCLC), adenocarcinoma (ADC) subtype. A molecular battery test was ordered, and an acquired pathogenic variant in exon 21 of the EGFR gene was detected in the tumor specimen. Which one of the following genetic changes in the EGFR gene would this patient most likely have?[56]
A. Amplification
B. In-frame in/dels
C. Out-of-frame in/dels
D. Point mutation
E. All of the above
F. None of the above

185. A 64-year-old male presented to a clinic with an abnormal chest X-ray from an annual physical examination. He had a smoking history of half a pack per day and a history of hypertension. The chest X-ray showed a huge mass on right middle lobe and multiple pulmonary nodules on the right lung. A transcutaneous needle biopsy and pathological examinations confirmed the diagnosis of nonsmall-cell lung carcinoma (NSCLC), adenocarcinoma (ADC) subtype. A molecular battery test was ordered, and an acquired pathogenic variant in exon 21 of the EGFR gene was detected in the tumor specimen. Which kind of clinical significances would this variant in the EGFR gene have for this patient?[57]
A. Diagnostic
B. Prognostic
C. Treatment decisions
D. All of the above
E. None of the above

186. A 64-year-old male presented to a clinic with an abnormal chest X-ray from an annual physical examination. He had a smoking history of half a pack per day and a history of hypertension. The chest X-ray showed a huge mass on right middle lobe and multiple pulmonary nodules on the

right lung. A transcutaneous needle biopsy and pathological examinations confirmed the diagnosis of nonsmall-cell lung carcinoma (NSCLC), adenocarcinoma (ADC) subtype. A molecular battery test was ordered, and an acquired pathogenic variant in exon 21 of the EGFR gene was detected. Gefitinib, a first-generation EGFR tyrosine kinase inhibitor (TKI), was used for treatment. After 6 months, the patient stopped responding to the therapy. The oncologist ordered a molecular test to confirm the resistance. Which one of the following exons of the EGFR gene would most likely be investigated for the resistance?[56]
A. Exon 18
B. Exon 19
C. Exon 20
D. Exon 21
E. All of the above
F. None of the above

187. A 64-year-old male presented to a clinic with an abnormal chest X-ray from an annual physical examination. He had a smoking history of half a pack per day and a history of hypertension. The chest X-ray showed a huge mass on right middle lobe and multiple pulmonary nodules on the right lung. A transcutaneous needle biopsy and pathological examinations confirmed the diagnosis of nonsmall-cell lung carcinoma (NSCLC), adenocarcinoma (ADC) subtype. A molecular battery test was ordered, and an acquired pathogenic variant in exon 21 of the EGFR gene was detected. Gefitinib, a first-generation EGFR tyrosine kinase inhibitor (TKI), was used for treatment. After 6 months, the patient stopped responding to the therapy. The oncologist ordered an EGFR test to confirm the resistance, which turned out to be negative. Which one of the following genetic alterations would most likely be investigated further for the resistance?[56,58]
A. Amplification of ALK
B. Amplification of HER2
C. Amplification of c-MET
D. Amplification of MYCN
E. Amplification of RUNX1
F. None of the above

188. A 64-year-old male presented to a clinic with an abnormal chest X-ray from an annual physical examination. He had a smoking history of half a pack per day and a history of hypertension. The chest X-ray showed a huge mass on right middle lobe and multiple pulmonary nodules on the right lung. A transcutaneous needle biopsy and pathological examinations confirmed the

diagnosis of nonsmall-cell lung carcinoma (NSCLC), adenocarcinoma (ADC) subtype. A molecular battery test was ordered. Which one of the following genetic alterations in the *ALK* gene would most likely be investigated for therapy?[58]

A. Amplification
B. Deletion
C. Duplication
D. Inversion
E. Point mutation
F. All of the above
G. None of the above

189. A 64-year-old male presented to a clinic with an abnormal chest X-ray from an annual physical examination. He had a smoking history of half a pack per day and a history of hypertension. The chest X-ray showed a huge mass on right middle lobe and multiple pulmonary nodules on the right lung. A transcutaneous needle biopsy and pathological examinations confirmed the diagnosis of nonsmall-cell lung carcinoma (NSCLC), adenocarcinoma (ADC) subtype. A molecular battery test was ordered. Which one of the following techniques would most likely be used for the *ALK* analysis in this case?[58]

A. Chromosome karyotype
B. Fluorescence in situ hybridization (FISH)
C. Methylation study
D. Sequencing
E. TaqMan SNP genotype

190. A 64-year-old male presented to a clinic with an abnormal chest X-ray from an annual physical examination. He had a smoking history of half a pack per day and a history of hypertension. The chest X-ray showed a huge mass on right middle lobe and multiple pulmonary nodules on the right lung. A transcutaneous needle biopsy and pathological examinations confirmed the diagnosis of nonsmall-cell lung carcinoma (NSCLC), adenocarcinoma (ADC) subtype. A molecular battery test was ordered. Which one of the following exons of the *KRAS* gene would most likely be investigated in this molecular battery test?[56,58]

A. Exon 2
B. Exon 5
C. Exon 19
D. Exon 21
E. All of the above
F. None of the above

191. A 64-year-old male presented to a clinic with an abnormal chest X-ray from an annual physical examination. He had a smoking history of half a pack per day and a history of hypertension. The chest X-ray showed a huge mass on right middle

lobe and multiple pulmonary nodules on the right lung. A transcutaneous needle biopsy and pathological examinations confirmed the diagnosis of nonsmall-cell lung carcinoma (NSCLC), adenocarcinoma (ADC) subtype. A molecular battery test was ordered. An acquired pathogenic variant in the *KRAS* gene was detected in the tumor specimen. Which one of the following genetic changes in the *KRAS* gene would this patient most likely have?[56,58]

A. Amplification
B. In-frame in/dels
C. Out-of-frame in/dels
D. Point mutation
E. All of the above
F. None of the above

192. A 64-year-old male presented to a clinic with an abnormal chest X-ray from an annual physical examination. He had a smoking history of half a pack per day and a history of hypertension. The chest X-ray showed a huge mass on right middle lobe and multiple pulmonary nodules on the right lung. A transcutaneous needle biopsy and pathological examinations confirmed the diagnosis of nonsmall-cell lung carcinoma (NSCLC), adenocarcinoma (ADC) subtype. A molecular battery test was ordered, which included a sequencing assay for exon 2 of the *KRAS* gene. In addition to exon 2, which one of the following exons of the *KRAS* gene might also harbor acquired pathogenic variants for NSCLC?[56,58]

A. Exon 3
B. Exon 5
C. Exon 19
D. Exon 21
E. All of the above
F. None of the above

193. A 64-year-old male presented to a clinic with an abnormal chest X-ray from an annual physical examination. He had a smoking history of half a pack per day and a history of hypertension. The chest X-ray showed a huge mass on right middle lobe and multiple pulmonary nodules on the right lung. A transcutaneous needle biopsy and pathological examinations confirmed the diagnosis of nonsmall-cell lung carcinoma (NSCLC), adenocarcinoma (ADC) subtype. A molecular battery test was ordered, which included a sequencing assay for exon 2 of the *KRAS* gene. Which kind of clinical significance would a variant in the *KRAS* gene have for this patient?[58]

A. Diagnostic
B. Prognostic
C. Treatment decisions
D. All of the above

E. None of the above

194. A 64-year-old male presented to a clinic with an abnormal chest X-ray from an annual physical examination. He had a smoking history of half a pack per day and a history of hypertension. The chest X-ray showed a huge mass on right middle lobe and multiple pulmonary nodules on the right lung. A transcutaneous needle biopsy and pathological examinations confirmed the diagnosis of nonsmall-cell lung carcinoma (NSCLC), adenocarcinoma (ADC) subtype. A molecular battery test was ordered, and *BRAF* V600E was detected. Which kind of clinical significance would this variant in the *BRAF* gene have in this patient?[56,59,60]

A. Diagnostic
B. Prognostic
C. Treatment decisions
D. All of the above
E. None of the above

195. A 64-year-old male presented to a clinic with an abnormal chest X-ray from an annual physical examination. He had a smoking history of half a pack per day and a history of hypertension. The chest X-ray showed a huge mass on right middle lobe and multiple pulmonary nodules on the right lung. A transcutaneous needle biopsy and pathological examinations confirmed the diagnosis of nonsmall-cell lung carcinoma (NSCLC), adenocarcinoma (ADC) subtype. A molecular battery test was ordered. Which one of the following genetic assays would most likely *NOT* be included in this battery test?[56]

A. *ALK* mutations in the kinase domain
B. *BRAF* mutations
C. *EGFR* in frame deletions of exon 19
D. *EGFR* L858R mutation in exon 21
E. *KRAS* mutations at codon 12 and 13
F. None of the above

196. A 61-year-old female came to a clinic for intermittent bloody stool for 3 weeks. She had had type 2 diabetes for 20 years. A colonoscopy revealed sigmoid colon cancer. A CT of chest, abdomen, and pelvis showed no metastases. A laparoscopy-assisted sigmoid colectomy was done. Histopathological examinations revealed poorly differentiated adenocarcinoma penetrating to the subserosa, and 5 of 16 lymph nodes were positive. A next-generation sequencing (NGS) panel for solid tumor was ordered. Which one of the following genes in this panel is associated with high microsatellite instability (MSI)?[61]

A. *BRAF*
B. *KRAS*
C. *NRAS*
D. *SMAD4*

E. None of the above

197. A 61-year-old female came to a clinic for intermittent bloody stool for 3 weeks. She had had type 2 diabetes for 20 years. A colonoscopy revealed sigmoid colon cancer. A CT of chest, abdomen, and pelvis showed no metastases. A laparoscopy-assisted sigmoid colectomy was done. Histopathological examinations revealed poorly differentiated adenocarcinoma penetrating to the subserosa, and 5 of 16 lymph nodes were positive. A next-generation sequencing panel (NGS) for solid tumor was ordered, and an acquired pathogenic variant in the *KRAS* gene was identified. Which one of the following prognoses would this patient most likely have?[62,63]

A. Favorable risk
B. Intermediate risk
C. Unfavorable risk
D. Unclear
E. None of the above

198. A 72-year-old male was diagnosed with colorectal carcinoma (CRC) by annual endoscopy. He underwent a segmental resection of the sigmoid colon. Histopathological examinations revealed moderately differentiated colorectal adenocarcinoma with gland formation and focal tumor necrosis. A next-generation sequencing (NGS) panel for solid tumor was ordered, and *BRAF* V600E mutation was identified. Which one of the following prognoses would this patient most likely have?[61]

A. Favorable risk
B. Intermediate risk
C. Unfavorable risk
D. Unclear
E. None of the above

199. A 49-year-old female presented to a clinic for vague abdominal pain with progressive constipation and bleeding per rectum. A physical examination revealed right hypochondrial tenderness. A lower GI endoscopy demonstrated a friable, necrotic, and easy-bleeding mass at the rectosigmoid junction. A CT scan revealed dilated bowel loops above the rectosigmoid junction, and multiple hepatic deposits beyond immediate intervention. A final needle biopsy of the mass was done, and confirmed the diagnosis of colorectal carcinoma (CRC). A molecular test of the tumor sample revealed high microsatellite instabilities and *MLH1* hypermethylation. Which one of the following genes would most likely harbor an acquired pathogenic variant with therapeutic significances?[61]

A. *ALK*
B. *BRAF*
C. *EGFR*

D. *KRAS*

E. *NRAS*

F. None of above

200. A 55-year-old Caucasian female presented to a clinic with symptoms of weakness and fatigue. She thought it was because of her irregular menstrual periods. She had lost 10 Ib in the past 6 months. An initial laboratory workup showed that her white-blood-cell (WBC) count was 5200/mm³, hemoglobin 7.5 g/dL, hematocrit 26%, red-blood-cell (RBC) count 3.5×10^6/μL, and platelet count 650,000/μL. Her medical history was significant for chronic constipation and hemorrhoids and hypertension. Her family history was uneventful. While being treated with iron for iron deficiency anemia, she was referred to a GI clinic. A colonoscopy revealed a 6-cm mass located in the ascending colon. A biopsy of the mass was obtained. Histopathological examinations demonstrated adenomatous colorectal carcinoma (CRC). A molecular test of the tumor sample revealed an acquired pathogenic variant in the *KRAS* gene, c.182A > G (p.Q61R). Which one of the following interpretations would most likely be appropriate for this patient?[64]

   A. The patient would respond well to BRAF inhibitor therapy.

   B. The patient would respond well to EGFR inhibitor therapy.

   C. The patient would respond well to KRAS inhibitor therapy.

   D. All of the above.

   E. None of the above.

201. A 55-year-old Caucasian female presented to a clinic with symptoms of weakness and fatigue. She thought it was because of her irregular menstrual periods. She had lost 10 Ib in the past 6 months. An initial laboratory workup showed that her white-blood-cell (WBC) count was 5200/mm³, hemoglobin 7.5 g/dL, hematocrit 26%, red-blood-cell (RBC) count 3.5×10^6/μL, and platelet count 650,000/μL. Her medical history was significant for chronic constipation and hemorrhoids and hypertension. Her family history was uneventful. While being treated with iron for iron deficiency anemia, she was referred to a GI clinic. A colonoscopy revealed a 6-cm mass located in the ascending colon. A biopsy of the mass was obtained. Histopathological examinations demonstrated adenomatous colorectal carcinoma (CRC). A molecular test of the tumor sample for acquired pathogenic variants in the *KRAS* was ordered, and the results were negative. Which one of the following

therapies would most likely be appropriate for this patient?[64]

   A. BRAF inhibitor

   B. EGFR inhibitor

   C. KRAS inhibitor

   D. All of the above

   E. None of the above

202. A 64-year-old Caucasian male presented to a clinic with symptoms of weakness and fatigue. He was evaluated by his primary care physician and diagnosed with iron deficiency anemia. A colonoscopy revealed a 5-cm nonobstructing circumferential mass located in the ascending colon. A biopsy of the mass demonstrated adenomatous colorectal carcinoma (CRC). The patient underwent a right hemicolectomy, revealing a moderately differentiated adenocarcinoma, staged at T4N0 colon cancer. Eight lymph nodes were removed at the time of surgery and all were negative for metastatic cancer. A next-generation sequencing panel (NGS) for DNA analyses of solid tumors was ordered. Which one of the following is a limitation of NGS for DNA analyses of solid tumors?[58]

   A. It needs at least a few micrograms of DNA.

   B. It is not a sensitive test for detecting low-level mosaicism.

   C. It cannot be used on formalin-fixed, paraffin-embedded (FFPE) samples.

   D. It cannot detect inv(2) for *ALK* rearrangement.

   E. All of the above.

   F. None of the above.

203. A 49-year-old marathon runner presented to his primary care physician for his annual physical examination. His family history was significant for his aunt dying of skin cancer in her late 40s. The physician noticed a mole on the back of the patient's left arm proximal to the elbow. The patient told the physician that the mole might have gotten larger over the past 2 years, and he had noticed itchiness in the area of this mole over the past few weeks. The physical examination revealed a hard, enlarged, nontender mass in the left axillary region. The physician removed the mole surgically. Histopathological examination led to a diagnosis of melanoma. A piece of the tumor specimen was sent to a molecular laboratory for a qualitative assay for *BRAF* V600. Which one of the following *BRAF* V600 mutations would the patient most likely have?

   A. V600D

   B. V600E

   C. V600G

   D. V600K

E. V600R

F. None of the above

204. A 49-year-old marathon runner presented to his primary care physician for his annual physical examination. His family history was significant for his aunt dying of skin cancer in her late 40s. The physician noticed a mole on the back of the patient's left arm proximal to the elbow. The patient told the physician that the mole might have gotten larger over the past 2 years, and he had noticed itchiness in the area of this mole over the past few weeks. The physical examination revealed a hard, enlarged, nontender mass in the left axillary region. The physician removed the mole surgically. Histopathological examination led to a diagnosis of melanoma. A piece of the tumor specimen was sent to a molecular laboratory for a qualitative assay for *BRAF* V600. Which one of the following *BRAF* V600 mutations would make the patient suitable for treatment with trametinib (Mekinist tablets, GlaxoSmithKline, LLC) and dabrafenib (Tafinlar capsules, GlaxoSmithKline, LLC) treatment besides V600E, according to the FDA-approval?

A. V600D

B. V600G

C. V600K

D. V600R

E. None of the above

205. A 4-year-old boy was brought to a clinic by his parents for failure to thrive. He was small for his age, cachetic, and mildly lethargic. The parents had noticed progressive weight loss, vomiting, polyuria, and polydipsia for a year. During this time, an extensive cutaneous eruption also became apparent. On physical examination, nearly confluent erythematous macules and papules were present throughout the scalp and extended down the midline of his neck and back. Some of the lesions had an overlying yellow crust, whereas others were petechial or purpuric. In addition, hypopigmented macules were noted in areas of partial resolution. A plain skull X-ray film showed multiple irregular calvarial osteolytic lesions. A complete skeletal survey also revealed osteolytic lesions of the right ileum and the superior aspect of the left iliac wing. On MRI, a thickened pituitary stalk and absent pituitary gland was noted. Histological examinations of a punch biopsy led to a diagnosis of Langerhans-cell histiocytosis (LCH). Which one of the following genes would most likely be somatically mutated in this patient?

A. *ALK*

B. *BRAF*

C. *EGFR*

D. *KRAS*

E. *NRAS*

F. None of the above

206. A scientist in a clinical molecular laboratory decides to validate a qualitative assay for *BRAF* V600E. Which one of the following disorders most likely harbors the *BRAF* V600E mutation?

A. Colorectal carcinoma

B. Langerhans-cell histiocytosis

C. Metastatic melanoma

D. Nonsmall-cell lung cancer

E. Papillary thyroid carcinoma

F. Renal-cell carcinoma

G. None of the above

207. A scientist decides to validate a qualitative assay for *BRAF* V600E in a clinical molecular laboratory. Which one of the following disorders LEAST likely harbors the *BRAF* V600E mutation?

A. Colorectal carcinoma

B. Langerhans-cell histiocytosis

C. Metastatic melanoma

D. Nonsmall-cell lung cancer

E. Papillary thyroid carcinoma

F. Renal-cell carcinoma (RCC)

G. None of the above

208. A scientist in a clinical molecular laboratory decides to validate a targeted solid tumor next-generation sequencing (NGS) panel including *BRAF, EGFR, KRAS, NRAS*, and 13 other genes. For which one of the following malignancies is this assay *NOT* appropriate?[65]

A. Alveolar rhabdomyosarcoma

B. Colorectal carcinoma

C. Embryonal rhabdomyosarcoma

D. Metastatic melanoma

E. Nonsmall-cell lung cancer

F. Papillary thyroid carcinoma

G. None of the above

ANSWERS

1. **A.** Currently, distinguishing between benign and malignant lymphoid proliferations is based on a combination of clinical characteristics, cyto/ histomorphology, immunophenotype, and the identification of well-defined chromosomal aberrations. However, such diagnoses remain challenging in 10%–15% of cases of lymphoproliferative disorders, and clonality assessments often help to confirm diagnostic suspicions. In such cases, molecular gene rearrangement studies have proved useful as an additional diagnostic tool. Molecular clonality

analysis is based on the fact that, in principle, all cells of a malignancy have a common clonal origin and show clonally (identically) rearranged immunoglobulin (Ig) or T-cell receptor (TCR) genes. The diagnosis of malignant B- and T-cell proliferations is therefore supported by the finding of Ig/TCR gene clonality, whereas reactive lymphoproliferations show polyclonally rearranged Ig/TCR genes.

Because this assay is for B cell clonality (IGH and IGK), it will not identify the clonality of myeloid cells. Therefore, it is not an appropriate test for acute myeloid leukemia (AML).

2. **F.** False negative results are seen in the *IGH* or *IGK* PCR assay alone in 5%−20% of B-cell lymphoproliferative neoplasms owing to intrinsic biologic mechanisms. These include *absent or incomplete IGH rearrangements in immature B-cell neoplasms*, such as lymphoblastic leukemia/lymphoma, and *the presence of extensive somatic mutation in some mature B-cell lymphomas*, particularly follicular lymphoma and plasma-cell neoplasms. The combination of *IGH* and *IGK* PCR can overcome these limitations and detect a clonal rearrangement in up to 99% of B-cell neoplasms. Thus, a B-cell clonality panel with both *IGH* and *IGK* is recommended for lymphoblastic neoplasms and in suspected follicular lymphoma.

Technical issues, such as degradation of DNA samples, may also cause false negative results.

Therefore, all of situations listed in the question may cause false negative *IGH* results.

3. **D.** The T-cell clonality tests (*TCRG* and *TCRB*) help to identify a monoclonal population in the right clinical and pathological scenario and suggest the presence of a lymphoid neoplasm (leukemia or lymphoma) even though nonneoplastic lymphocytic proliferations can also present with monoclonal populations. Acute myeloid leukemia (AML) is a myeloid leukemia. Follicular lymphoma (FL), a B-cell lymphoma, is the most common indolent (slow-growing) form of non-Hodgkin lymphoma (NHL), accounting for approximately 20%−30% of all NHLs. Plasma-cell myeloma is a form of tumor in the bone or soft tissue derived from B cells.

Therefore, this T-cell clonality assay is NOT appropriate for all of three disorders.

4. **C.** Mucosa-associated lymphoid tissue (MALT) lymphoma is a type of B-cell non-Hodgkin lymphoma (NHL) that can originate in the gastrointestinal (GI) tract, thyroid, breasts, lungs, and skin. The most common genetic abnormality occurring in MALT lymphomas involves t(11;18)(q21;q21) in the gene *MALT1*. The t(1;14)(p22;q32)

and t(14;18)(q32;q21) are the variants of the t(11;18) translocation in MALT lymphomas. However, not every patient with MALT lymphoma has one of these translocations.

The B-cell clonality test (*IGH* and *IGK*) helps to identify a monoclonal population in the right clinical and pathological scenario, and *suggests the presence of a lymphoid neoplasm* (leukemia or lymphoma), even though nonneoplastic lymphocytic proliferations can also present in monoclonal populations.

ALK amplification is relatively common in patients with nonsmall-cell lung cancer, colorectal carcinoma, and neuroblastoma. *ALK* rearrangement, especially *EML4-ALK*, is common in anaplastic lymphoma (T cell). The *BRAF* V600E mutation is relatively common in solid tumors, such as colorectal cancer (CRC).

Therefore, the B-cell clonality test (*IGH* and *IGK*) would help to further establish the diagnosis if the oncologist still suspected that the patient had MALT lymphoma.

5. **D.** Cancer cells are the progeny of a single malignantly transformed cell, and consequently, these cells are clonally related. So monoclonality is a key feature of populations of malignant tumor cells, which enables discrimination from oligoclonal or polyclonal reactive processes. Clonality assessment is an important tool in the diagnosis of malignant lymphoproliferations, even though clonality does not always imply malignancy because some reactive processes contain large clonal lymphocyte populations.

CD3+, CD4+, CD8+, and TdT+ indicate T-cell involvement. Clonality testing in T lymphoproliferations (*TCRG* and *TCRB*) would help in order to establish the diagnosis in this case.

The B-cell clonality test (*IGH* and *IGK*) helps to identify a monoclonal population in a B lymphoid neoplasm (leukemia or lymphoma), even though nonneoplastic lymphocytic proliferations can also present with monoclonal populations. *ALK* amplification is relatively common in patients with nonsmall-cell lung cancer, colorectal carcinoma, and neuroblastoma. *ALK* rearrangement, especially *EML4-ALK*, is common in anaplastic lymphoma (T cell). The *BRAF* V600E mutation is relatively common in solid tumors, such as colorectal cancer.

Therefore, *TCRG* and *TCRB* clonality test would help to further establish the diagnosis of lymphoma in this case.

6. **C.** In most patients with suspected lymphoproliferative disorders, reactive and malignant cell populations can be discriminated from each other by histomorphology or

cytomorphology supplemented with immunohistochemistry or flow cytometric immunophenotyping. But in 5%–10% of patients, diagnosis is more complicated and less straightforward. Molecular clonality analysis is based on the fact that all cells of a malignancy have a common clonal origin and show clonally rearranged immunoglobulin (Ig) or T-cell receptor (TCR) genes. Therefore, the diagnosis of malignant B- and T-cell proliferations is supported by the finding of Ig/TCR gene clonality, whereas reactive lymphoproliferations show polyclonally rearranged Ig/TCR genes.

Random coupling between one of many V, (D), and J genes results in the formation of an unique V(D)J exon that encodes the actual antigen-binding moiety of the Ig or TCR chain. Because of the huge diversity in Ig/TCR rearrangements, each lymphocyte has a unique antigen-receptor molecule on its membrane, and the chance that two different lymphocytes coincidentally bear the same receptor is almost negligible. Hence, identical rearrangements are not derived from multiple independently generated cells, but rather reflect the clonal nature of the involved cell population. Evaluation of the homogeneous versus the heterogeneous nature of the rearrangements is thus the basis of clonality testing.

In the *IGH* assay of this patient, the amplification products with the bone marrow sample is polyclonal, while the products with the biopsy sample from the left neck mass have only one peak (monoclonal). Therefore, results of the biopsy from the neck mass, but not the bone-marrow sample indicated a clonal proliferation of B cells.

7. **C.** Leukemia and lymphoma of B lymphoid lineage have clonal rearrangements of *IGH* gene derived from the original tumor cell and reproduced in all cells descended from this. In contrast, normal functional cells of B lineage demonstrate patterns of extreme diversity in both antigen specificity and DNA rearrangements. *Monoclonal B cells may be seen in B lymphocytic neoplastic diseases such as multiple myeloma and follicular lymphoma, but also in other illnesses, such as amyloidosis and lupus.*

As a tumor marker, specific DNA rearrangement (monoclonal B cells) identified at diagnosis may be used to identify minimal residual disease after treatment. *IGH* is the first rearranged gene in B-cell development with light-chain genes for kappa (*IGK*) and lambda (*IGL*) occurring only after heavy-chain gene rearrangement has occurred (allelic exclusion). So *IGH* gene rearrangement is an early marker of clonal B lymphoid processes.

Therefore, in this case clonal *IGH* rearrangement in the left neck mass indicated a clonal proliferation of B cells, but not the bone marrow sample. It supported a diagnosis of B-cell lymphoma, whereas reactive lymphoproliferations cannot be completely ruled out. It should be correlated with other clinical and pathological data.

8. **F.** CD3, CD4 and CD8 are T-cell markers. The TCR genes are located on chromosomes 7 and 14. The genes encoding the TCRα (*TCRD*) chain are located within the TCRα (*TCRA*) locus on chromosome 14q11-12, whereas the TCRβ (*TCRB*) and TCRγ (*TCRG*) genes are located at chromosomal positions 7q32-35 and 7p15, respectively. The four genes are composed of C and V regions that are assembled together during thymic ontogeny by somatic recombination. The V domains in the TCRA and TCRG chains are assembled from V and J gene segments, whereas the TCRB and TCRD chains are assembled from V, diversity (D), and J segments. T-cell receptor (TCR) gene rearrangement is an important event in T-cell ontogeny that enables T cells to recognize antigens specifically. Monoclonal T cells may be seen in T-cell lymphocytic neoplastic diseases, but also other illness, such as human immunodeficiency virus (HIV) and Epstein–Barr virus (EBV) infections with specificity for virus, in the elderly, in autoimmunity, in common variable immunodeficiency (CVID), and in severe combined immunodeficiency (SC1D).

As a tumor marker, specific DNA rearrangement (monoclonal B cells) identified at diagnosis may be used to identify minimal residual disease after treatment. *IGH* is the first rearranged gene in B-cell development with light-chain genes for kappa (*IGK*) and lambda (*IGL*) occurring only after heavy-chain gene rearrangement has occurred (allelic exclusion).

In the TCR assay of this patient the amplification products within both the bone marrow and the mediastinal mass samples showed a clonal TCR rearrangement in a polyclonal background. Therefore, the results indicated a clonal proliferation of T cells in both samples.

9. **A.** Gene rearrangement analysis can be performed by Southern blot and by PCR-based techniques. Despite the high reliability of Southern blot analysis, it is increasingly replaced by PCR techniques because of the greater efficiency and sensitivity of PCR. Moreover, PCR is relatively easy, is less labor-intensive, and requires much less high-molecular-weight DNA. Also Southern blot cannot be performed on paraffin-embedded tissue because the DNA is often degraded. *BIOMED-2 consortium multiplex PCR methods*

incorporated with capillary electrophoresis for detecting B- and T-cell clonality have resulted in standardization and significantly improved detection of clonality of malignant B/T-cell lymphomas/leukemias.

To address the challenges of next-generation sequencing (NGS) in Ig/TCR gene analysis, a consortium has been formed for setting standards in Ig/TCR NGS methodology and its applications in hematooncology by EuroClonality (www.euroclonality.org/) in 2013. However, *PCR/capillary electrophoresis is the gold standard for Ig/TCR gene analysis.*

Therefore, PCR/capillary electrophoresis is the standard method for the clonal assessment.

10. E. The TCR genes are located on chromosomes 7 and 14. The genes encoding the TCRα (*TCRD*) chain are located within the TCRα (*TCRA*) loci on chromosome 14q11-12, whereas the TCRβ (*TCRB*) and TCRγ (*TCRG*) genes are located at chromosomal positions 7q32-35 and 7p15, respectively. The four genes are composed of C and V regions that are assembled together during thymic ontogeny by somatic recombination. The V domains in the *TCRA* and *TCRG* chains are assembled from V and J gene segments whereas the *TCRB* and *TCRD* chains are assembled from V, diversity (D), and J segments. T-cell receptor (TCR) gene rearrangement is an important event in T cell ontogeny that enables T cells to recognize antigens specifically.

The rearrangement of *TCRB* and *TCRD* is a two-step process, in which a D gene first recombines with a J gene and then a V gene recombines with the D—J block. Because of the absence of D genes in *TCRA* and *TCRG*, only V—J recombination occurs in these two chains. During these recombination events, diversity at junctional regions is further increased by the incorporation of template-dependent palindromic "P" nucleotides, incorporation of template independent GC-rich "N" nucleotides by TdT, deletion of gene-encoded nucleotides by exonucleolytic activity, and imprecise joining of gene segments.

The TCRG locus is the most commonly tested TCR because the majority of T cells has rearranged TCRG and because the TCRG locus is significantly less complex than TCRB. The TCRG locus has 14 V, 5 J segments, and no D segments. The TCRB locus has 52 V, 2 D, and 13 J segments. Therefore, many labs use TCRG analysis as their first-line clonality assay for T-cell clonality.

To emphasize the importance of testing all the Ig and/or TCR genes, over years research found that false negativity was at least in part caused by the fact that some laboratories only used TCR gamma (TCRG) and complete Ig-heavy chain (IGH) V—J gene rearrangements as PCR targets for reasons of limited primer usage and relatively simple gene structure. The European BIOMED-2 network (now called EuroClonality consortium) initiated the effort, which has resulted in standardized multiplex PCR assays for nearly all Ig/TCR targets, which collectively show an unprecedentedly high rate of detection in the most common B- and T-cell malignancies. This high detection rate was achieved not only by optimized primer design, but also by inclusion of extra Ig/TCR targets (Ig kappa, IGK and TCR beta, TCRB as well as incomplete IGH D—J and TCRB D—J rearrangements).

Therefore, the TCRG gene is the most commonly tested locus for T-cell—receptor gene rearrangement analysis.

11. D. The BIOMED-2 consensus test for TCR clonality includes both the T-cell receptor beta (*TCRB*) locus and the T-cell receptor gamma (*TCRG*) locus, which is useful in patients with suspected T-cell malignancies or to evaluate for residual disease after treatment. *Several published studies have demonstrated that the combination of TCRB and TCRG PCR using the BIOMED-2 method can detect more than 90% of clonal T-cell populations.*

At early stages of lymphomas/leukemias, the ratio of malignant cells to reactive/normal lymphocytes may be below the level of detection, which leads to false negative results. Other reasons for false negative results are:
- Somatic mutations at the primer region may result in the nondetectable single/oligo-clone(s).
- The primers are not located to the V or J segments involved, such as Vγ12 or Jγ12.
- A chromosome translocation is involved in the tested region(s).
- Poor quality of DNA from paraffin-embedded tissue may lead to a false negative result. False positive results may come from:
- Clonal Ig/TCR rearrangement may reactive populations of lymphocytes. The presence of a B/T-cell clone is not always equivalent to the presence of a B/T-cell neoplasm.
- "Pseudoclonality" may happen when only very few B/T cells are in the sample.

Therefore, the sensitivity of the BIOMED-2 assay for *TCRG* and *TCRB* is more than 90%.

12. D. PCR/capillary electrophoresis is less time consuming than Southern blot, and it works well with paraffin-embedded tissue. Southern blot needs a lot of high-quality DNA, which is hard to obtain from paraffin-embedded tissues. On the other side, *PCR/capillary electrophoresis cannot detect all possible rearrangements because of the*

limitation of the primers. Southern blot can theoretically detect all rearrangements. And "pseudoclonality" may happen when only very few B/T cells are in the sample if PCR/capillary electrophoresis is used for the analysis. So PCR/capillary electrophoresis has a higher false positive rate than Southern blot.

Therefore, PCR/capillary electrophoresis may NOT detect more possible clonal rearrangements than Southern blot.

13. **B**. T-cell receptor loci have roughly the same number of V gene segments as do the immunoglobulin loci, but *only B cells diversify rearranged V region genes by somatic hypermutation. Somatic hypermutation does not generate diversity in T-cell receptors.* The T-cell receptor loci comprise sets of gene segments and are rearranged by the same enzymes as the immunoglobulin loci. Most of our T cells are produced when we are less than 12 years old. A developing T cell has more chances to productively rearrange β chains than a developing B cell has for H chains because there are two sets of D, J, and C β loci so that if rearrangement at the first locus fails, rearrangement can still occur at the second.

Therefore, somatic hypermutation does not generate diversity in T cell receptors, while it does in B cell immunoglobulin.

14. **B**. In the EuroClonality network, an algorithm for target selection has been proposed that depends on the suspected cell population. So *in cases of suspected B-cell clonality, generally the three different IGH V-J targets are chosen, in parallel to or followed by the IGK targets.* Although the consecutive use of IGH and IGK PCRs might be the more cost-efficient approach, a parallel approach is more time efficient for both the clinician and the patient. Even though the combination of *IGH* V−J and *IGK* targets should be sufficient in the vast majority of cases (95%), evaluation of the *IGH* D−J and *IGL* targets might occasionally be helpful as a second-line approach. This should be applied to cases with a strong suspicion of B-cell clonality that is not confirmed by *IGH* V−J and *IGK* testing.

Therefore, *IGH* V−J and *IGK* are most commonly used for the clonal assessment.

15. **F**. Analogous to B cells, suspected T-cell clonality can best be addressed by evaluating *two TCR targets (TCRB and TCRG)*, either in parallel or consecutively. Traditionally, *TCRG* is the gold standard target, but the results in the EuroClonality network show that *TCRB* is at least equally informative as the first-line target. Importantly, TCR delta (*TCRD*) (generally together with *TCRG*) should be used as a target only for well-defined clinical requests, that is,

suspected *TCRD* T-cell proliferations or immature (lymphoblastic) T-cell proliferations. Usage of *TCRD* in other situations merely creates difficulties because most *TCRD* rearrangements are removed in *TCRA* lineage T-cells upon rearrangement of the TCR alpha (*TCRA*) locus. So the paucity of *TCRD* templates might easily give rise to preferential amplification and pseudoclonality. Moreover, even authentic clonal *TCRD* rearrangements might not be associated with a malignant lymphoid proliferation.

Therefore, *TCRG* and *TCRB* are most commonly used for the clonal assessment.

16. **A**. For cases with a low percentage of suspected B or T cells, *reproducibility of the profiles is essential.* A low number of lymphocytes in, for example, skin or intestinal lesions can easily result in overinterpretation of coincidental dominant peaks. *To prevent misinterpretation, assessment of the targets in duplicate as well as adjustment of the amount of DNA by increasing the DNA concentration, and hence the number of cells per PCR, are strongly recommended.* When low amplitude peaks are seen, itis most appropriate to repeat the test with the same specimen first in order to rule out pseudoclonality before reaching a conclusion.

Therefore, repeat the test with the same specimen would be the most appropriate next step workup.

17. **D**. *On repeat analysis, different low-amplitude peaks can indicate a paucity of B cells in the sample.* This is called "pseudoclonality," and it is caused by the DNA from only a few cells being amplified in each run. Such results should not be overinterpreted as clonal. The presence of clonal populations is not diagnostic for neoplasm since it may also be reactive.

Therefore, pseudoclonality, consistent with a paucity of B cells in the sample, would be the most appropriate interpretation.

18. **D**. Theoretically, Southern blot can detect all rearrangements and may not cause "pseudoclonality" associated with PCR/capillary electrophoresis when only very few B/T cells are in the sample. However, Southern blot analysis is usually not informative with paraffin-embedded tissue samples owing to insufficient high-molecular-weight DNA.

PCR/capillary electrophoresis is less time consuming than Southern blot and works well with paraffin-embedded tissue. But it cannot detect all possible rearrangements because of the limitation of the primers. And "pseudoclonality" may happen when only very few B/T cells are in the sample if PCR/capillary electrophoresis is used for the analysis.

The lesion is the sample of choice for the IGH and IGK clonality assessment. Therefore, PCR/capillary electrophoresis of *IGH* and *IGK* gene rearrangement with the biopsy sample would be the most informative assay for this patient in order to establish the diagnosis.

19. **A.** Chronic myeloid leukemia (CML) is classified as one of the myeloproliferative neoplasms (MPNs) according to WHO classification, as are polycythemia vera (PV), essential thrombocythemia (ET), and primary myelofibrosis (PMF). The diagnosis of CML is based on the histopathological findings in the peripheral blood and *the BCR-ABL1 rearrangement* in bone marrow. Phases of CML include chronic, accelerated, and blastic. A higher proportion of diseased cells means chronic myelogenous leukemia is at a more advanced stage. The blast phase may be diagnosed when blasts are $\geq 20\%$ of the peripheral-blood WBC or of the nucleated cells of the bone marrow or when there is an extramedullary blast proliferation. In approximately 70% of cases, the blast lineage is myeloid and may include neutrophilic, eosinophilic, basophilic, monocytic, megakaryocytic, or erythroid blasts or any combination thereof, whereas in approximately 20%–30% of cases, the blasts are lymphoblasts.

A somatic point mutation in *JAK2* tyrosine kinase, especially *JAK2* V617F was identifiable in a significant proportion of patients with PV, ET and PMF, but not CML. So *JAK2* mutation analysis may be used to differentiate CML from other MPNs. Somatic mutations in *CEBPA, FLT3-ITD, FLT3-TKD,* and *NPM1* are associated with acute myeloid leukemia (AML).

Therefore, this patient would most likely have the *BCR-ABL1* rearrangement if she had CML.

20. **E.** The Philadelphia (Ph) chromosome is a fusion gene, *BCR-ABL1.* The 5′ part of the *BCR* gene provides strong promoters for the transcription of the fusion gene. And the 3′ part of the *ABL1* gene provides a tyrosine kinase domain to stimulate the cells to divide. The Ph chromosome has been seen in 95% of patients with chronic myeloid leukemia (CML). However, it could be also seen in acute lymphoblastic leukemia (ALL) and occasionally in acute myelogenous leukemia (AML).

Reverse transcriptase polymerase chain reaction (RT-PCR) is the most sensitive method described to date for detecting *BCR-ABL.* Samples from 2% to 3% of patients, which show no cytogenetic evidence of a rearrangement, may be detected to be positive by RT-PCR. And this molecular test can detect the isoforms of this fusion gene owing to the variation of the breakpoints, mainly in the *BCR* gene. The p210

fusion protein is more commonly seen in patients with CML, while p190 is more common in patients with ALL or AML.

Instead of targeting genomic DNA, *the assay targets the chimeric RNA transcripts produced from the fused genes* because the variability in the breakpoints of *BCR* and *ABL1* genes and the large intervening introns complicate direct PCR detection of the *BCR-ABL1* gene rearrangement at the level of genomic DNA. The chimeric RNA is remarkably homogeneous from case to case, which allows reliable detection of nearly all disease-associated translocations. *A couple of pairs of primers usually are used to yield PCR products of different sizes to cover different breakpoint.*

Therefore, a qualitative *BCR-ABL1* test is a RNA-based multiple RT-PCR assay for the *BCR-ABL1* fusion gene.

21. **A.** The Philadelphia (Ph) chromosome is a fusion gene, *BCR-ABL1.* The 5′ part of the *BCR* gene provides strong promoters for the transcription of the fusion gene. And the 3′ part of the *ABL1* gene provides a tyrosine kinase domain to stimulate the cells to divide. The Ph chromosome has been seen in 95% of patients with chronic myeloid leukemia (CML). However, it could be also seen in acute lymphoblastic leukemia (ALL) and occasionally in acute myelogenous leukemia (AML).

Reverse-transcriptase polymerase chain reaction (RT-PCR) is the most sensitive method described to date for detecting *BCR-ABL1.* And this molecular test can identify the isoforms of this fusion gene owing to the variation of the breakpoints, mainly in the *BCR* gene.

The breakpoints on chromosome 9 usually occur in the first two introns of the *ABL1* gene. The breakpoints on chromosome 22 in the *BCR* gene are in one of the three possible breakpoint cluster regions: the major (M) bcr, the minor (m) bcr, or the micro (μ) bcr. In the majority of case of CML, the breakpoints occur in intron 1 or 2 of *ABL1,* which is connected to exon b2 or b3 of the *BCR* gene, giving rise to either the b2a2 or b3a2 variant, both of which are translated into the p210 fusion protein. Less common breakpoints are those in the minor bcr region, leading to an e1a2 fusion gene and an s fusion protein of 190 kDa, which is seen in most cases of Ph-positive ALL patients. The p190 protein has an increased tyrosine kinase activity compared with p210 and is associated with a more aggressive leukemia. Micro bcr breakpoints resulting in the e19a2 (c3a2) fusion gene leading to the p230 protein are also occasionally found. Samples from 2% to 3% of patients, which show no cytogenetic evidence of a rearrangement, may be detected to be positive by RT-PCR. Quantitative assays have been used to estimate the level of residual disease.

Therefore, a quantitative *BCR-ABL1* test is a RNA-based multiple RT-PCR assay for *BCR-ABL1* fusion gene.

22. **A.** At diagnosis, *90%–95%* of cases of chronic myelogenous leukemia (CML) have the characteristic t(9;22)(q34;q11.2) reciprocal translocation that results in the Philadelphia (Ph) chromosome.

Therefore, about 95% of patients with chronic myelogenous leukemia (CML) have a *BCR-ABL1* fusion gene.

23. **E.** The t(9;22)(q34;q11.2) reciprocal translocation appears in 3% of AML and 1% of childhood AML. Therefore, lee than 5% of patients with acute myeloid leukemia (AML) have a *BCR-ABL1* fusion gene.

24. **D.** Among precursor-B ALL cases, t(9;22) translocation occurs in around *20%–30%* of adults and in 5% of children. From the clinical point of view, Ph+ precursor-B ALL is associated with a highly aggressive disease frequently resistant to chemotherapy and with a short survival.

Therefore, about 25% of adult patients with precursor B-ALL have a *BCR-ABL1* fusion gene.

25. **E.** Among precursor-B ALL cases, t(9;22) translocation occurs in around *20%–30%* of adults and in 5% of children. From the clinical point of view, Ph + precursor-B ALL is associated with a highly aggressive disease frequently resistant to chemotherapy and with a short survival.

Therefore, about 5% of pediatric patients with precursor B-ALL have a *BCR-ABL1* fusion gene.

26. **D.** The Philadelphia (Ph) chromosome is a fusion gene, *BCR-ABL1*. The 5′ part of the *BCR* gene provides strong promoters for the transcription of the fusion gene. And the 3′ part of the *ABL1* gene provides a tyrosine kinase domain to stimulate the cells to divide. The Ph chromosome has been seen in 95% of patients with chronic myeloid leukemia (CML). However, it could be also seen in acute lymphoblastic leukemia (ALL) and occasionally in acute myelogenous leukemia (AML).

The breakpoints on chromosome 9 usually occur in the first two introns of the *ABL1* gene. The breakpoints in on chromosome 22 in the *BCR* gene are in one of the three possible breakpoint cluster regions: the major (M) bcr, the minor (m) bcr, or the micro (μ) bcr. In the majority of cases of CML, the breakpoints occur in intron 1 or 2 of ABL1, which is connected to exon b2 or b3 of the *BCR* gene, giving rise to either the b2a2 or b3a2 variant, both of which are translated into the p210 fusion protein. The

b2a2 or b3a2 variants are now called "e13a2" and "e14a2," respectively. *Less common breakpoints are those in the minor bcr region leading to an e1a2 fusion gene and an s fusion protein of 190 kDa, which is seen in most cases of Ph-positive ALL.* The p190 protein has an increased tyrosine kinase activity compared with p210 and is associated with a more aggressive leukemia. Micro bcr breakpoints resulting in the e19a2 (c3a2) fusion gene leading to the p230 protein are also occasionally found. Samples from 2% to 3% of patients, which show no cytogenetic evidence of a rearrangement, may be detected to be positive by RT-PCR.

Therefore, it would be most likely that this patient had *e1a2* of BCR-ABL1 fusion for p190 isoform.

27. **E.** The Philadelphia (Ph) chromosome is a fusion gene, *BCR-ABL1*. The 5′ part of the *BCR* gene provides strong promoters for the transcription of the fusion gene. And the 3′ part of the *ABL1* gene provides a tyrosine kinase domain to stimulate the cells to divide. The Ph chromosome has been seen in 95% of patients with chronic myeloid leukemia (CML). However, it could be also seen in acute lymphoblastic leukemia (ALL) and occasionally in acute myelogenous leukemia (AML).

The breakpoints on chromosome 9 usually occur in the first two introns of the *ABL1* gene. The breakpoints in on chromosome 22 in the *BCR* gene are in one of the three possible breakpoint cluster regions: the major (M) bcr, the minor (m) bcr, or the micro (μ) bcr. In the majority of cases of CML, the breakpoints occur in intron 1 or 2 of ABL1, which is connected to exon b2 or b3 of the *BCR* gene, giving rise to either the b2a2 or b3a2 variant, both of which are translated into the p210 fusion protein. The b2a2 or b3a2 variants are now called "e13a2" and "e14a2," respectively. Less common breakpoints are those in the minor bcr region leading to an e1a2 fusion gene and an s fusion protein of 190 kDa, which is seen in most cases of Ph-positive ALL. The p190 protein has an increased tyrosine kinase activity compared with p210 and is associated with a more aggressive leukemia. Micro bcr breakpoints resulting in the e19a2 (c3a2) fusion gene leading to the p230 protein are also occasionally found. Samples from 2% to 3% of patients, which show no cytogenetic evidence of a rearrangement, may be detected to be positive by RT-PCR.

Therefore, it would be most likely that the patient had an e13a2 (b2a2) or *e14a2 (b3a2)* of *BCR-ABL1* fusion for the p210 isoform.

28. **E.** The Philadelphia (Ph) chromosome is a fusion gene, *BCR-ABL1*. The 5′ part of the *BCR* gene

provides strong promoters for the transcription of the fusion gene. And the 3' part of the *ABL1* gene provides a tyrosine kinase domain to stimulate the cells to divide. The Ph chromosome has been seen in 95% of patients with chronic myeloid leukemia (CML). However, it could be also seen in acute lymphoblastic leukemia (ALL) and occasionally in acute myelogenous leukemia (AML).

The breakpoints on chromosome 9 usually occur in the first two introns of the *ABL1* gene. The breakpoints in on chromosome 22 in the *BCR* gene are in one of three possible breakpoint cluster regions: the major (M) bcr, the minor (m) bcr, or the micro (μ) bcr. *In the majority of case of CML, the breakpoints occur in intron 1 or 2 of ABL1, which is connected to exon b2 or b3 of the BCR gene, giving rise to either the b2a2 or b3a2 variant, both of which are translated into the p210 fusion protein. The b2a2 or b3a2 variants are now called "e13a2" and "e14a2,"* respectively. Less common breakpoints are those in the minor bcr region leading to an e1a2 fusion gene and an s fusion protein of 190 kDa, which is seen in most cases of Ph-positive ALL. The p190 protein has an increased tyrosine kinase activity compared with p210 and is associated with a more aggressive leukemia. Micro bcr breakpoints resulting in the e19a2 (c3a2) fusion gene leading to the p230 protein are also occasionally found. Samples from 2% to 3% of patients, which show no cytogenetic evidence of a rearrangement, may be detected to be positive by RT-PCR.

Therefore, it would be most likely that the patient had an *e13a2 (b2a2)* or e14a2 (b3a2) of *BCR-ABL1* fusion for the p210 isoform.

29. **B.** The Philadelphia (Ph) chromosome is a fusion gene, *BCR-ABL1*. The 5' part of the *BCR* gene provides strong promoters for the transcription of the fusion gene. And the 3' part of the *ABL1* gene provides a tyrosine kinase domain to stimulate the cells to divide. The Ph chromosome has been seen in 95% of patients with chronic myeloid leukemia (CML). However, it could be also seen in acute lymphoblastic leukemia (ALL) and occasionally in acute myelogenous leukemia (AML).

The breakpoints on chromosome 9 usually occur in the first two introns of the *ABL1* gene. The breakpoints in on chromosome 22 in the *BCR* gene are in one of the three possible breakpoint cluster regions: the major (M) bcr, the minor (m) bcr, or the micro (μ) bcr. *In the majority of cases of CML, the breakpoints occur in intron 1 or 2 of ABL1, which is connected to exon b2 or b3 of the BCR gene, giving rise to either the b2a2 or b3a2 variant, both of which are translated into the p210 fusion protein. The b2a2 or b3a2 variants are now called "e13a2" and "e14a2,"*

respectively. Less common breakpoints are those in the minor bcr region leading to an e1a2 fusion gene and an s fusion protein of 190 kDa, which is seen in most cases of Ph-positive ALL. The p190 protein has an increased tyrosine kinase activity compared with p210 and is associated with a more aggressive leukemia. Micro bcr breakpoints resulting in the e19a2 (c3a2) fusion gene leading to the p230 protein are also occasionally found. Samples from 2% to 3% of patients, which show no cytogenetic evidence of a rearrangement, may be detected to be positive by RT-PCR.

Therefore, it would be most likely that the patient had *an e13a2 (b2a2)* or e14a2 (b3a2) of *BCR-ABL1* fusion for the p210 isoform.

30. **B.** The Philadelphia (Ph) chromosome is a fusion gene, *BCR-ABL1*. The 5' part of the *BCR* gene provides strong promoters for the transcription of the fusion gene. And the 3' part of the *ABL1* gene provides a tyrosine kinase domain to stimulate the cells to divide. The Ph chromosome has been seen in 95% of patients with chronic myeloid leukemia (CML). However, it could be also seen in acute lymphoblastic leukemia (ALL) and occasionally in acute myelogenous leukemia (AML).

The breakpoints on chromosome 9 usually occur in the first two introns of the *ABL1* gene. The breakpoints in on chromosome 22 in the *BCR* gene are in one of the three possible breakpoint cluster regions: the major (M) bcr, the minor (m) bcr, or the micro (μ) bcr. *In the majority of cases of CML, the breakpoints occur in intron 1 or 2 of ABL1, which is connected to exon b2 or b3 of the BCR gene, giving rise to either the b2a2 or b3a2 variant, both of which are translated into the p210 fusion protein. The b2a2 or b3a2 variants are now called "e13a2" and "e14a2,"* respectively. Less common breakpoints are those in the minor bcr region leading to an e1a2 fusion gene and an s fusion protein of 190 kDa, which is seen in most cases of Ph-positive ALL. The p190 protein has an increased tyrosine kinase activity compared with p210 and is associated with a more aggressive leukemia. Micro bcr breakpoints resulting in the e19a2 (c3a2) fusion gene leading to the p230 protein are also occasionally found. Samples from 2% to 3% of patients, which show no cytogenetic evidence of a rearrangement, may be detected to be positive by RT-PCR.

Therefore, it would be most likely that the patient had an e13a2 (b2a2) or *e14a2 (b3a2)* of *BCR-ABL1* fusion for the p210 isoform.

31. **E.** The Philadelphia (Ph) chromosome is a fusion gene, *BCR-ABL1*. The 5' part of the *BCR* gene provides strong promoters for the transcription of

the fusion gene. And the 3′ part of the *ABL1* gene provides a tyrosine kinase domain to stimulate the cells to divide. The Ph chromosome has been seen in 95% of patients with chronic myeloid leukemia (CML). However, it could be also seen in acute lymphoblastic leukemia (ALL) and occasionally in acute myelogenous leukemia (AML).

The breakpoints on chromosome 9 usually occur in the first two introns of the *ABL1* gene. The breakpoints in on chromosome 22 in the *BCR* gene is one of the three possible breakpoint cluster regions: the major (M) bcr, the minor (m) bcr, or the micro (μ) bcr. In the majority of cases of CML, the breakpoints occur in intron 1 or 2 of ABL1, which is connected to exon b2 or b3 of the *BCR* gene, giving rise to either the b2a2 or b3a2 variant, both of which are translated into the p210 fusion protein. The b2a2 or b3a2 variants are now called "e13a2" and "e14a2," respectively. Less common breakpoints are those in the minor bcr region leading to an e1a2 fusion gene and an s fusion protein of 190 kDa, which is seen in most cases of Ph-positive ALL. The p190 protein has an increased tyrosine kinase activity compared with p210 and is associated with a more aggressive leukemia. *Micro bcr breakpoints resulting in the e19a2 (c3a2) fusion gene leading to the p230 protein are also occasionally found.* Samples from 2% to 3% of patients, which show no cytogenetic evidence of a rearrangement, may be detected to be positive by RT-PCR.

Therefore, it would be most likely that the patient had an *e19a2 (c3a2)* of *BCR-ABL1* fusion for the p230 isoform.

32. **C.** The Philadelphia (Ph) chromosome is a fusion gene, *BCR-ABL1*. The 5′ part of the *BCR* gene provides strong promoters for the transcription of the fusion gene. And the 3′ part of the *ABL1* gene provides a tyrosine kinase domain to stimulate the cells to divide. The Ph chromosome has been seen in 95% of patients with chronic myeloid leukemia (CML). However, it could be also seen in acute lymphoblastic leukemia (ALL) and occasionally in acute myelogenous leukemia (AML).

The breakpoints on chromosome 9 usually occur in the first two introns of the *ABL1* gene. The breakpoints in on chromosome 22 in the *BCR* gene is one of the three possible breakpoint cluster regions: the major (M) bcr, the minor (m) bcr, or the micro (μ) bcr. In the majority of cases of CML, the breakpoints occur in intron 1 or 2 of ABL1, which is connected to exon b2 or b3 of the *BCR* gene, giving rise to either the b2a2 or b3a2 variant, both of which are translated into the p210 fusion protein. The b2a2 or b3a2 variants are now called "e13a2" and "e14a2," respectively. Less common breakpoints

are those in the minor bcr region leading to an e1a2 fusion gene and an s fusion protein of 190 kDa, which is seen in most cases of Ph-positive ALL. The p190 protein has an increased tyrosine kinase activity compared with p210 and is associated with a more aggressive leukemia. *Micro bcr breakpoints resulting in the e19a2 (c3a2) fusion g leading to the p230 protein are also occasionally found.* Samples from 2% to 3% of patients, which show no cytogenetic evidence of a rearrangement, may be detected to be positive by RT-PCR.

Therefore, it would be most likely that the patient had an *e19a2 (c3a2)* of *BCR-ABL1* fusion for the p230 isoform.

33. **C.** The Philadelphia (Ph) chromosome is a fusion gene, *BCR-ABL1*. The 5′ part of the *BCR* gene provides strong promoters for the transcription of the fusion gene. And the 3′ part of the *ABL1* gene provides a tyrosine kinase domain to stimulate the cells to divide. The Ph chromosome has been seen in 95% of patients with chronic myeloid leukemia (CML). However, it could be also seen in acute lymphoblastic leukemia (ALL) and occasionally in acute myelogenous leukemia (AML).

The breakpoints on chromosome 9 usually occur in the first two introns of the *ABL1* gene. The breakpoints in on chromosome 22 in the *BCR* gene is one of the three possible breakpoint cluster regions: the major (M) bcr, the minor (m) bcr, or the micro (μ) bcr. In the majority of cases of CML, the breakpoints occur in intron 1 or 2 of ABL1, which is connected to exon b2 or b3 of the *BCR* gene, giving rise to either the b2a2 or b3a2 variant, both of which are translated into the p210 fusion protein. The b2a2 or b3a2 variants are now called "e13a2" and "e14a2," respectively. *Less common breakpoints are those in the minor bcr region, leading to an e1a2 fusion gene and the fusion protein of 190 kDa, which is seen in most cases of Ph-positive ALL. The p190 protein has an increased tyrosine kinase activity compared with p210 and is associated with a more aggressive leukemia.* Micro bcr breakpoints resulting in the e19a2 (c3a2) fusion gene leading to the p230 protein are also occasionally found. Samples from 2% to 3% of patients, which show no cytogenetic evidence of a rearrangement, may be detected to be positive by RT-PCR.

Therefore, an *e1a2* of *BCR-ABL1* fusion for p190 isoform has highest tyrosine kinase activity comparing with the p210 and p230 fusion.

34. **C.** The Philadelphia (Ph) chromosome is a fusion gene, *BCR-ABL1*. The 5′ part of the *BCR* gene provides strong promoters for the transcription of the fusion gene. And the 3′ part of the *ABL1* gene provides a tyrosine kinase domain to stimulate

the cells to divide. *Acquired mutations in the BCR-ABL1 tyrosine kinase domain may cause, or contribute to, resistance to tyrosine kinase inhibitors (TKIs) by impairing imatinib's ability to bind to its target in chronic myeloid leukemia patients.* The list of amino acid substitutions detected in imatinib-resistant patients has steadily grown to >90, although some are definitely more frequent than others. Different mutations have been shown to confer variable degrees of resistance to imatinib. Clinical experience with dasatinib and nilotinib, the second-generation TKIs that have thus far received market approval, has demonstrated that definite, much narrower spectra of mutations retain insensitivity to these agents—and these spectra are nonoverlapping, the T315I being the unique exception. The knowledge of the *BCR-ABL1* kinase domain mutation status is a valuable piece of information to be integrated in the decision algorithm aimed at tailoring the best therapeutic strategy for each of these patients: increasing imatinib dose, switching to the second-generation TKI dasatinib or nilotinib, moving to allogeneic stem-cell transplantation, or testing an investigational compound.

Therefore, the molecular test for imatinib resistance is a RNA based test of the tyrosine kinase domain in the *BCR-ABL1* gene.

35. **D.** The Philadelphia (Ph) chromosome is a fusion gene, *BCR-ABL1*. The 5′ part of the *BCR* gene provides strong promoters for the transcription of the fusion gene. And the 3′ part of the *ABL1* gene provides a tyrosine kinase domain to stimulate the cells to divide. The Ph chromosome has been seen in 95% of patients with chronic myeloid leukemia (CML), one of the myeloid proliferative neoplasms (MPNs), according to the WHO classification. However, it could be also seen in patients with acute lymphoblastic leukemia (ALL), occasionally in acute myelogenous leukemia (AML); *it has NOT been seen in chronic lymphocytic leukemia (CLL).*

Therefore, chronic lymphocytic leukemia (CLL) most likely does NOT have an acquired BCR-ABL1 rearrangement.

36. **A.** Chronic myeloid leukemia (CML) is a clonal myeloproliferative disorder resulting from the neoplastic transformation of the primitive hematopoietic stem cell. The disease is monoclonal in origin and affects myeloid cells. CML accounts for 15% of all leukemias in adults. In the United States, approximately 5430 new cases were diagnosed in 2012, with an estimated 610 deaths. *BCR-ABL1* rearrangement has been seen in 95% of patients with CML. BCR-ABL1 fusion protein is a type of tyrosine kinase from

the *ABL1* gene, with a hyperactive promoter from the *BCR* gene causing CML cells to grow and reproduce out of control.

Drugs known as tyrosine kinase inhibitors (TKIs) that targeted BCR-ABL1 fusion protein include *imatinib (Gleevec),* dasatinib (Sprycel), nilotinib (Tasigna), bosutinib (Bosulif), and ponatinib (Iclusig). Imatinib (Gleevec) was the first drug to specifically target the BCR-ABL1 tyrosine kinase protein, and it quickly became the standard treatment for CML. With imatinib (Gleevec) therapy, annual mortality has been reduced significantly.

Olaparib (Lynparza) is known as a PARP [poly (ADP-ribose) polymerase] inhibitor, which blocks the BRCA (the *BRCA1* and *BRCA2* genes) pathway as a treatment for advanced epithelial ovarian cancer. Trastuzumab (Herceptin) and lapatinib (Tykerb) are specifically targeted to amplified *HER*2 in a subset of breast cancer. Vemurafenib (Zelboraf) is a BRAF-enzyme inhibitor for the treatment of *BRAF* V600E-positive metastatic melanoma.

Therefore, imatinib (Gleevec) would be the most appropriate treatment for this patient with CML.

37. **A.** The Philadelphia (Ph) chromosome is a fusion gene, *BCR-ABL1*. The 5′ part of the *BCR* gene provides strong promoters for the transcription of the fusion gene. And the 3′ part of the *ABL1* gene provides a tyrosine kinase domain to stimulate the cells to divide. The Ph chromosome has been seen in 95% of patients with chronic myeloid leukemia (CML). However, it could be also seen in acute lymphoblastic leukemia (ALL) and occasionally in acute myelogenous leukemia (AML) and T lymphoblastic leukemia/lymphoma.

The fusion gene on the derivative chromosome 22q11 produces a chimeric *BCR-ABL1* mRNA transcript and corresponding translated oncoprotein. FISH is the test of choice for aneuploidy, deletion, amplification, inversion, and translocation, such as t(9;22). PCR-capillary electrophoresis is the test of choice for alleles with different sizes, such as *FLT3*-ITD. Sanger sequencing is the test of choice for point mutations and in/dels in all the amplicons, such as *CEBPA*. Targeted-mutation analysis is used to study specific mutations, such as testing of *BRAF* V600E and carrier testing for cystic fibrosis.

Therefore, FISH would be the most appropriate for *BCR-ABL1* in order to establish the diagnosis of CML in this patient.

38. **D.** Chronic myeloid leukemia (CML) is a clonal myeloproliferative disorder resulting from the neoplastic transformation of the primitive

hematopoietic stem cell. The disease is monoclonal in origin and affects myeloid cells. CML accounts for 15% of all leukemias in adults. In the United States. approximately 5430 new cases were diagnosed in 2012, with an estimated 610 deaths. *BCR-ABL1* rearrangement has been seen in 95% of patients with CML and is diagnostic for CML. BCR-ABL1 fusion protein is *a type of tyrosine kinase from the ABL1 gene* with a hyperactive promoter from the *BCR* gene causing CML cells to grow and reproduce out of control.

Drugs known as tyrosine kinase inhibitors (TKIs) that target BCR-ABL1 include imatinib (Gleevec), dasatinib (Sprycel), nilotinib (Tasigna), bosutinib (Bosulif), and ponatinib (Iclusig). Imatinib (Gleevec) was the first drug to specifically target to the BCR-ABL1 tyrosine kinase protein, and it quickly became the standard treatment for CML. With imatinib (Gleevec) therapy, the annual mortality has been reduced significantly.

Acquired mutations in the BCR-ABL1 tyrosine kinase domain may cause, or contribute to, resistance to tyrosine kinase inhibitors (TKIs) by impairing imatinib's ability to bind to its target in chronic myeloid leukemia patients. To date, over 50 distinct mutations have been described, although a smaller subset of these (<20) account for the majority of patients with clinical resistance to TKIs. Recognition of TKI resistance is important in CML, as the effect of some mutations can be overcome by increasing the imatinib dosage, whereas others require switching to either a different (second-generation) TKI or alternative therapy. The common T315I KD mutation is particularly important, given that this alteration confers pan-resistance to all currently employed TKIs except ponatinib.

Therefore, a molecular test for *BCR-ABL1* kinase domain mutation in the *ABL1* part of the fusion gene is appropriate for this patient to confirm/rule out TKIs' resistance in order to make a decision about future therapy.

39. **A**. The Philadelphia (Ph) chromosome is a fusion gene, *BCR-ABL1*. The 5′ part of the *BCR* gene provides strong promoters for the transcription of the fusion gene. And the 3′ part of the *ABL1* gene provides a tyrosine kinase domain to stimulate the cells to divide. The Ph chromosome has been seen in 95% of patients with chronic myeloid leukemia (CML). However, it could be also seen in acute lymphoblastic leukemia (ALL) and occasionally in acute myelogenous leukemia (AML) and T lymphoblastic leukemia/lymphoma.

The breakpoints on chromosome 9 usually occur in the first two introns of the *ABL1* gene. The breakpoints on chromosome 22 in the *BCR* gene are in one of the three possible breakpoint cluster regions: the major (M) bcr, the minor (m) bcr, or the micro (μ) bcr. In the majority of cases of CML, the breakpoints occur in intron 1 or 2 of ABL1, which is connected to exon b2 or b3 of the *BCR* gene, giving rise to either the b2a2 or b3a2 variant, both of which are translated into the p210 fusion protein. The b2a2 or b3a2 variants are now called "e13a2" and "e14a2," respectively. *Less common breakpoints are those in the minor bcr region, leading to an e1a2 fusion gene and an s fusion protein of 190 kDa, which is seen in most cases of Ph positive ALL patients.* The p190 protein has an increased tyrosine kinase activity compared with p210 and is associated with a more aggressive leukemia. Micro bcr breakpoints resulting in the e19a2 (c3a2) fusion gene leading to the p230 protein are also occasionally found. Samples from 2% to 3% of patients, which show no cytogenetic evidence of a rearrangement, may be detected to be positive by RT-PCR.

Therefore, it would be most likely this ALL patient had a p190 isoform of the BCR-ABL1 fusion protein.

40. **C**. The Philadelphia (Ph) chromosome is a fusion gene, *BCR-ABL1*. The 5′ part of the *BCR* gene provides strong promoters for the transcription of the fusion gene. And the 3′ part of the *ABL1* gene provides a tyrosine kinase domain to stimulate the cells to divide. The Ph chromosome has been seen in 95% of patients with chronic myeloid leukemia (CML). However, it could be also seen in acute lymphoblastic leukemia (ALL) and occasionally in acute myelogenous leukemia (AML) and T lymphoblastic leukemia/lymphoma. Ph + ALL is relatively more common in adults than in children, accounting for about 25% of adult ALL but only 2%−4% of childhood ALL.

The breakpoints on chromosome 9 usually occur in the first two introns of the *ABL1* gene. The breakpoints on chromosome 22 in the *BCR* gene are in one of the three possible breakpoint cluster regions: the major (M) bcr, the minor (m) bcr, or the micro (μ) bcr. In the majority of cases of CML, the breakpoints occur in intron 1 or 2 of ABL1, which is connected to exon b2 or b3 of the *BCR* gene giving rise to either the b2a2 or b3a2 variant, both of which are translated into the p210 fusion protein. The b2a2 or b3a2 variants are now called "e13a2" and "e14a2," respectively. Less common breakpoints are those in the minor bcr region, leading to an e1a2 fusion gene and an s fusion protein of 190 kDa, which is seen in most cases of Ph-positive ALL. The p190 protein has an increased tyrosine kinase activity compared with p210 and is associated with a more aggressive leukemia. *In both children and adults, t(9;22) ALL has the worst prognosis among patients with ALL.* Micro bcr breakpoints resulting in the e19a2 (c3a2) fusion gene leading to the p230 protein are also occasionally found. The samples from 2% to 3% of patients, which show no cytogenetic evidence of a rearrangement, may be detected to be positive by RT-PCR.

Therefore, it would be most likely this adult ALL patient had unfavorable risk due to t(9;22).

41. **D.** A somatic point mutation in the *JAK2* tyrosine kinase, especially *JAK2 V617F* was identifiable in a significant proportion of patients with a myeloproliferative neoplasm (MPNs), such as polycythemia vera (PV), essential thrombocythemia (ET), and primary myelofibrosis (PMF) but not chronic myeloid leukemia (CML). So *JAK2* V617 analysis may be used to differentiate CML from other NPMs. The diagnosis of CML is based on the histopathological findings in the peripheral blood and the *BCR-ABL1* rearrangement in bone marrow.

Detection of *JAK2* V617F is helpful in order to establish the diagnosis of MPN. However, a negative *JAK2* V617F result does not exclude the diagnosis of MPN. Other important molecular markers in *BCR-ABL1*–negative MPN include *CALR* exon 9 mutations (20%–30% of PMF and ET) and *MPL* exon 10 mutation (5%–10% of PMF and 3%–5% of ET). Over 50 different mutations have now been reported within exons 12 through 15 of *JAK2*, and essentially all of the non-V617F mutations have been identified in PV. Mutations in *JAK2*, *CALR*, and *MPL* are essentially mutually exclusive.

Therefore, *JAK2* V617F would most likely be ordered first in order to confirm the diagnosis of PMF in this patient.

42. **A.** A somatic point mutation in *JAK2* tyrosine kinase, especially *JAK2* V617F was identifiable in a significant proportion of patients with a myeloproliferative neoplasm (MPN), such as polycythemia vera (PV), essential thrombocythemia (ET), and primary myelofibrosis (PMF) but *not chronic myeloid leukemia (CML)*.

Chronic myeloid leukemia (CML) is a clonal myeloproliferative disorder resulting from the neoplastic transformation of the primitive

hematopoietic stem cell. The diagnosis of CML is based on the histopathological findings in the peripheral blood and the *BCR-ABL1* rearrangement in bone marrow. So *JAK2 mutation analysis may be used to differentiate CML from other NPMs.*

Therefore, it would be most likely that this patient did not have CML since he had the *JAK2* V617F mutation.

43. **E.** DNA sequence mutations in the Janus kinase 2 gene (*JAK2*) are found in the hematopoietic cells of several myeloproliferative neoplasms (MPNs), such as polycythemia vera (PV; close to 100%), essential thrombocythemia (ET; approximately 50%), and primary myelofibrosis (PMF; approximately 50%), but basically never in chronic myelogenous leukemia (CML). Mutations are believed to cause activation of the JAK2 protein, which is an intracellular tyrosine kinase important for signal transduction in many hematopoietic cells. Since it is often difficult to distinguish reactive conditions from the non-CML MPNs, identification of a *JAK2* mutation has a diagnostic value. The potential prognostic significance of *JAK2* mutation detection in MPNs has yet to be clearly established.

The vast majority of *JAK2* mutations occur at base pair 1849 in the gene, resulting in a *JAK2* V617F protein change. In all cases being evaluated for *JAK2* mutation status, *JAK2* V617F mutation detection should be the initial test. However, if no *JAK2* V617F mutation is found, further evaluation of *JAK2* may be clinically indicated. Over 50 different mutations have now been reported within exons 12 through 15 of *JAK2*, and essentially all of the non-V617F mutations have been identified in PV. These mutations include point mutations and small insertions or deletions. Other important molecular markers in *BCR-ABL1*–negative MPNs include *CALR* exon 9 mutations (20%–30% of PMF and ET) and *MPL* exon 10 mutation (5%–10% of PMF and 3%–5% of ET). *Mutations in JAK2, CALR, and MPL are essentially mutually exclusive.*

Therefore, none of assays on the list would be positive, since the patient had the *JAK2* V617F mutation.

44. **E.** DNA sequence mutations in the Janus kinase 2 gene (*JAK2*) are found in the hematopoietic cells of several myeloproliferative neoplasms (MPNs), such as polycythemia vera (PV; close to 100%), essential thrombocythemia (ET; approximately 50%), and primary myelofibrosis (PMF; approximately 50%), but basically never in chronic myelogenous leukemia (CML).

The vast majority of *JAK2* mutations occur at base pair 1849 in the gene, resulting in a *JAK2* V617F protein change. In all cases being evaluated for *JAK2* mutation status, *JAK2* V617F mutation detection should be the initial test. However, if no *JAK2* V617F mutation is found, further evaluation of *JAK2* may be clinically indicated. Over 50 different mutations have now been reported within exons 12 through 15 of *JAK2*, and essentially all of the non-V617F mutations have been identified in PV. These mutations include point mutations and small insertions or deletions. Other important molecular markers in *BCR-ABL1*−negative MPNs include *CALR* exon 9 mutations (20%−30% of PMF and ET) and *MPL* exon 10 mutation (5%−10% of PMF and 3%−5% of ET). Mutations in *JAK2*, *CALR*, and *MPL* are essentially mutually exclusive.

Therefore, a negative *JAK2* V617F mutation analysis could not be used to rule out CML, PV, ET, or PMF in this patient.

45. **B**. DNA sequence mutations in the Janus kinase 2 gene (*JAK2*) are found in the hematopoietic cells of several myeloproliferative neoplasms (MPNs), such as polycythemia vera (PV; close to 100%), essential thrombocythemia (ET; approximately 50%), and primary myelofibrosis (PMF; approximately 50%) but basically never in chronic myelogenous leukemia (CML). Since this patient had a normal karyotype, CML was ruled out owing to a lack of *BCR-ABL1* rearrangement. In a *BCR-ABL1*−negative MPN, *JAK2*, *CALR*, and *MPL* mutations usually help to facilitate a more accurate diagnosis. Mutations in *JAK2*, *CALR*, and *MPL* are essentially mutually exclusive.

In all cases being evaluated for *JAK2* mutation status, *JAK2* V617F mutation detection should be the initial test, since the vast majority of *JAK2* mutations occur as V617F. However, over 50 different mutations have now been reported within exons 12 through 15 of *JAK2*, and essentially all of the non-V617F mutations have been identified in PV. These mutations include point mutations and small insertions or deletions. If no *JAK2* V617F mutation is found, further evaluation of *JAK2* may be clinically indicated if other information suggests PV.

CALR exon 9 mutations were found in 20%−30% of PMF and ET. MPL exon 10 mutations were found in 5%−10% of PMF and 3%−5% of ET.

Therefore, mutation analysis of *CALR* exon 9 mutations would be appropriate in order to further confirm/rule out PMF in this patient.

46. **A**. DNA sequence mutations in the Janus kinase 2 gene (*JAK2*) are found in the hematopoietic cells

of several myeloproliferative neoplasms (MPNs), such as polycythemia vera (PV; close to 100%), essential thrombocythemia (ET; approximately 50%), and primary myelofibrosis (PMF; approximately 50%) but basically never in chronic myelogenous leukemia (CML). Since this patient had a normal karyotype and the *JAK2* V617F mutation, CML was ruled out owing to lack of *BCR-ABL1* rearrangement. In a *BCR-ABL1*−negative MPN, *JAK2*, *CALR*, and *MPL* mutations usually help to facilitate a more accurate diagnosis.

Therefore, a positive *JAK2* V617F mutation analysis ruled out CML in this patient.

47. **C**. DNA sequence mutations in the Janus kinase 2 gene (*JAK2*) are found in the hematopoietic cells of several myeloproliferative neoplasms (MPNs), such as polycythemia vera (PV; close to 100%), essential thrombocythemia (ET; approximately 50%), and primary myelofibrosis (PMF; approximately 50%) but basically never in chronic myelogenous leukemia (CML). Since this patient had a normal karyotype, CML was ruled out owing to lack of *BCR-ABL1* rearrangement. In a *BCR-ABL1*−negative MPN, *JAK2*, *CALR*, and *MPL* mutations usually help to facilitate a more accurate diagnosis. Mutations in *JAK2*, *CALR*, and *MPL* are essentially mutually exclusive.

In all cases being evaluated for *JAK2* mutation status, *JAK2* V617F mutation detection should be the initial test, since the vast majority of *JAK2* mutations occur as V617F. However, over 50 different mutations have now been reported within exons 12 through 15 of *JAK2* and essentially all of the non-V617F mutations have been identified in PV. These mutations include point mutations and small insertions or deletions. If no *JAK2* V617F mutation is found, further evaluation of *JAK2* may be clinically indicated if other information suggests PV.

CALR exon 9 mutations were found in 20%−30% of PMF and ET. *MPL exon 10 mutations were found in 5%−10% of PMF and 3%−5% of ET.*

Therefore, mutation analysis of *MPL* exon 10 mutations would be appropriate to further confirm/rule out PMF in this patient.

48. **A**. DNA sequence mutations in the Janus kinase 2 gene (*JAK2*) are found in the hematopoietic cells of several myeloproliferative neoplasms (MPNs), such as polycythemia vera (PV; close to 100%), essential thrombocythemia (ET; approximately 50%), and primary myelofibrosis (PMF; approximately 50%) but basically never in chronic myelogenous leukemia (CML). Since this patient had a normal karyotype, CML was ruled out

owing to lack of *BCR-ABL1* rearrangement. In a *BCR-ABL1*−negative MPN, *JAK2*, *CALR*, and *MPL* mutations usually help to facilitate a more accurate diagnosis. Mutations in *JAK2*, *CALR*, and *MPL* are essentially mutually exclusive.

In all cases being evaluated for *JAK2* mutation status, *JAK2* V617F mutation detection should be the initial test, since the vast majority of *JAK2* mutations occur as V617F. However, over 50 different mutations have now been reported within exons 12 through 15 of *JAK2* and essentially all of the non-V617F mutations have been identified in PV. These mutations include point mutations and small insertions or deletions. If no *JAK2* V617F mutation is found, further evaluation of *JAK2* may be clinically indicated if other information suggests PV. *CALR* exon 9 mutations were found in 20%−30% of PMF and ET. *MPL* exon 10 mutations were found in 5%−10% of PMF and 3%−5% of ET.

The FLT1-ITD mutation is associated acute myeloid leukemia (AML) instead of MPN. Therefore, *FLT3-ITD* would NOT be part of a reflex test for MPNs in this patient when the *JAK2* V617F test was negative.

49. **A.** The most frequent genetic mutation in *BCR-ABL1*−negative myeloproliferative neoplasms (MPNs) such as polycythemia vera (PV), essential thrombocythemia (ET), and primary myelofibrosis (PMF) is the *JAK2* V617F mutation, which is present in approximately 50%−60% of patients. Detection of the *JAK2* V617F is helpful in order to establish the diagnosis of MPN. However, a negative *JAK2* V617F result does not indicate absence of MPNs. Other important molecular markers in *BCR-ABL1*−negative MPN include *CALR exon 9 mutations* (20%−30% of PMF and ET) and *MPL* exon 10 mutations (5%−10% of PMF and 3%−5% of ET). Mutations in *JAK2*, *CALR*, and *MPL* are essentially mutually exclusive.

The *CALR* gene encodes for calreticulin, a multifunctional protein with a C-terminus rich in acidic amino acids and a KDEL ER-retention motif. All the pathological *CALR* mutations reported to date are *out-of-frame insertions and/or deletions (in/dels) in exon 9*, generating a frame shift and a mutant protein with a novel C-terminus rich in basic amino acids and loss of the KDEL ER-retention signal. The most common mutation types are 52-bp deletion (c.1092_1143del, L367fs*46) and 5-bp insertion (c.1154_1155insTTGCC, K385fs*47), and they comprise approximately 85% of *CALR* mutations in MPN. *CALR* mutations have been found in hematopoietic stem and progenitor cells in MPN patients and may activate the STAT5 signaling pathway. They are associated with a decreased risk of thrombosis in ET, and better survival in PMF compared to *JAK2* mutations.

Therefore, it was most likely that the detected mutation was located in the exon 9 of the *CALR* gene in this patient.

50. **B.** The most frequent genetic mutation in *BCR-ABL1*−negative myeloproliferative neoplasms (MPNs), such as polycythemia vera (PV), essential thrombocythemia (ET), and primary myelofibrosis (PMF) is the *JAK2* V617F mutation, which is present in approximately 50%−60% of patients. Detection of the *JAK2* V617F is helpful in order to establish the diagnosis of MPN. However, a negative *JAK2* V617F result does not indicate absence of MPNs. Other important molecular markers in *BCR-ABL1*−negative MPN include *CALR* exon 9 mutations (20%−30% of PMF and ET) and *MPL* exon 10 mutation (5%−10% of PMF and 3%−5% of ET). Mutations in *JAK2*, *CALR*, and *MPL* are essentially mutually exclusive.

The *CALR* gene encodes for calreticulin, a multifunctional protein with a C-terminus rich in acidic amino acids and a KDEL ER-retention motif. All the pathological *CALR* mutations reported to date are *out-of-frame insertions and/or deletions (in/dels) in exon 9*, generating a frame shift and a mutant protein with a novel C-terminus rich in basic amino acids and loss of the KDEL ER-retention signal. The most common mutation types are 52-bp deletion (c.1092_1143del, L367fs*46) and 5-bp insertion (c.1154_1155insTTGCC, K385fs*47), and they comprise approximately 85% of *CALR* mutations in MPNs. *CALR* mutations have been found in hematopoietic stem and progenitor cells in MPN patients and may activate the STAT5 signaling pathway. They are associated with a decreased risk of thrombosis in ET and better survival in PMF compared to *JAK2* mutations.

Therefore, it was most likely that this patient had an out-of-frame deletion/insertion in the exon 9 of the *CALR* gene.

51. **D.** The *CALR* gene encodes for calreticulin, a multifunctional protein with a C-terminus rich in acidic amino acids and a KDEL ER-retention motif. All the pathological *CALR* mutations reported to date are out-of-frame insertions and/or deletions (in/dels) in exon 9, generating a frame shift and a mutant protein with a novel C-terminus rich in basic amino acids and loss

of the KDEL ER-retention signal. The most common mutation types are 52-bp deletion (c.1092_1143del, L367fs*46) and 5-bp insertion (c.1154_1155insTTGCC, K385fs*47), and they comprise approximately 85% of *CALR* mutations in MPN. *CALR* mutations have been found in hematopoietic stem and progenitor cells in myeloproliferative neoplasms (MPNs) and may activate the STAT5 signaling pathway. *They are associated with a decreased risk of thrombosis in ET, and better survival in PMF compared to JAK2 mutations.*

Therefore, the mutation identified in the *CALR* indicated better survival than *JAK2* mutations.

52. **C.** DNA sequence mutations in the Janus kinase 2 gene (*JAK2*) are found in the hematopoietic cells of several myeloproliferative neoplasms (MPNs), *most frequently polycythemia vera (PV; close to 100%),* essential thrombocythemia (ET' approximately 50%), and primary myelofibrosis (PMF; approximately 50%) but basically never in chronic myelogenous leukemia (CML). Mutations are believed to cause activation of the JAK2 protein, which is an intracellular tyrosine kinase important for signal transduction in many hematopoietic cells. Since it is often difficult to distinguish reactive conditions from the non-CML MPNs, identification of a *JAK2* mutation has diagnostic value. The potential prognostic significance of *JAK2* mutation detection in chronic myeloid disorders has yet to be clearly established. The vast majority of *JAK2* mutations occur at base pair 1849 in the gene, resulting in a *JAK2* V617F protein change. In all cases being evaluated for *JAK2* mutation status, the *JAK2* V617F mutation detection should be the initial test.

Therefore, the *JAK2* V617F mutation is more often detected in patients with PV than ET or PMF, and never in CML.

53. **C.** DNA sequence mutations in the Janus kinase 2 gene (*JAK2*) are found in the hematopoietic cells of several myeloproliferative neoplasms (MPNs), *most frequently polycythemia vera (PV; close to 100%),* essential thrombocythemia (ET; approximately 50%), and primary myelofibrosis (PMF; approximately 50%) but basically never in chronic myelogenous leukemia (CML). Mutations are believed to cause activation of the JAK2 protein, which is an intracellular tyrosine kinase important for signal transduction in many hematopoietic cells.

The vast majority of JAK2 mutations occur at base pair 1849 in the gene, resulting in a JAK2 V617F protein change. In all cases being evaluated for

JAK2 mutation status, *JAK2* V617F mutation detection should be the initial test to help establish the diagnosis of MPN. However, a negative *JAK2* V617F result does not indicate absence of MPNs. Other important molecular markers in *BCR-ABL1*—negative MPNs include *CALR* exon 9 mutations (20%–30% of PMF and ET) and *MPL* exon 10 mutation (5%–10% of PMF and 3%–5% of ET). Mutations in *JAK2, CALR,* and *MPL* are essentially mutually exclusive.

Therefore, this patient would more likely to have the *JAK2* V617F mutation if he had PV.

54. **B.** DNA sequence mutations in the Janus kinase 2 gene (*JAK2*) are found in the hematopoietic cells of several myeloproliferative neoplasms (MPNs), *most frequently polycythemia vera (PV; close to 100%),* essential thrombocythemia (ET; approximately 50%), and primary myelofibrosis (PMF; approximately 50%) but basically never in chronic myelogenous leukemia (CML). The vast majority of *JAK2* mutations occur at base pair 1849 in the gene, resulting in a *JAK2* V617F protein change. However, a negative *JAK2* V617F result does not indicate absence of MPNs. *Over 50 different mutations have now been reported within exons 12 through 15 of JAK2, and essentially all of the non-V617F mutations have been identified in PV.*

Other important molecular markers in *BCR-ABL1*—negative MPN include *CALR* exon 9 mutations (20%–30% of PMF and ET) and *MPL* exon 10 mutation (5%–10% of PMF and 3%–5% of ET). Mutations in *JAK2, CALR,* and *MPL* are essentially mutually exclusive.

Therefore, *JAK2* exon 12 mutation analyses would most likely be part of this reflex test for this patient with PV.

55. **E.** *BCR-ABL1* rearrangement is diagnostic for chronic myeloid leukemia (CML). *Imatinib (Gleevec),* dasatinib (Sprycel), nilotinib (Tasigna), bosutinib (Bosulif), and ponatinib (Iclusig) are known as tyrosine kinase inhibitors (TKIs) and target BCR-ABL1. Imatinib (Gleevec) was the first drug to specifically target the BCR-ABL1 tyrosine kinase protein, and it quickly became the standard treatment for CML. With imatinib (Gleevec) therapy, the annual mortality has been reduced significantly.

Olaparib (Lynparza) is known as a PARP [poly (ADP-ribose) polymerase] inhibitor blocking BRCA (the *BRCA1* and *BRCA2* genes) pathway as a treatment for advanced epithelial ovarian cancer. *Trastuzumab (Herceptin)* and lapatinib (TYKERB) are specifically targeted to amplified *HER2* in a subset of breast cancer. *Vemurafenib*

(Zelboraf) is a BRAF enzyme inhibitor for the treatment of *BRAF* V600E positive metastatic melanoma.

Molecular targeted treatments to *JAK2* V617F are emerging, but they are still very early in their clinical development. Therefore, none of these drugs would be appropriate for this patient with PV.

56. **C.** In the absence of a homozygous population of cells, the greatest percentage of mutant allele would be 50%, which would be the expected result if every cell in the population was heterozygous for the mutation. Therefore, if 65% of the *JAK2* alleles in the sample are positive for the V617F mutation, *it can be concluded that there must be a population of cells present that are homozygous for the mutation.* Although it is possible that a mixture of heterozygous and homozygous cells could produce this finding, the data presented are not sufficient to make this determination.

Therefore, at least some of the cells were homozygous for the *JAK2* V617F mutation in this patient.

57. **D.** The JAK2 kinase is a member of a family of tyrosine kinases involved in cytokine receptor signaling. *JAK2* V617F is *a recurrent acquired mutation* in myeloproliferative neoplasms (MPNs), such as essential thrombocythemia (ET), polycythemia vera (PV), and primary myelofibrosis (PMF). None of these conditions is hereditary. So it is unlikely the patient had an inherited copy of *JKA2* V617F mutation. *JAK2* is a proto-oncogene, rather than a tumor suppressor gene. The *JAK2* V617F mutation activates the tyrosine kinase, which promotes cell proliferation. It is not common to have two copies of this kind of activating mutation in one cell. The chance of two somatic hits of this proto-oncogene in one cell is not entirely impossible, but the possibility is very low.

Acquired uniparental disomy (UPD) due to copy neutral loss of heterozygosity (LOH) is quite common in both hematologic and solid tumors, and was reported to constitute 20%–80% of the LOH in human tumors.

Therefore, this acquired UPD may explain why this patient had homozygous *JAK2* V617F mutation.

58. **A.** The JAK2 kinase is a member of a family of tyrosine kinases involved in cytokine receptor signaling. *JAK2* V617F is a recurrent acquired mutation in myeloproliferative neoplasms (MPNs), such as essential thrombocythemia (ET), polycythemia vera (PV), and primary myelofibrosis (PMF). The vast majority of *JAK2*

mutations occur at base pair 1849 in the gene, resulting in a *JAK2* V617F protein change. *A DNA-based test for single-nucleotide mutation detection is appropriate for JAK2 V617F.*

To ensure that more than 90% of cases are detected, the adequate analytical sensitivity of a clinical *JAK2* assay should be at least 1%. When the *JAK2* V617F level of a particular patient falls below 1%, however, caution must be exercised, because very low levels of *JAK2* V617F mutations (usually <0.1%) have been described in the peripheral blood of unaffected individuals. An assay that detects less than 0.1% of *JAK2* allele, therefore, is more likely to produce false-positive results in the diagnostic setting. On the other hand, low levels (≤1%) of the mutant *JAK2* have been reported in ET patients (as determined by using allele-specific loop-mediated amplification assay). Therefore, if other World Health Organization (WHO) major and minor diagnostic criteria are met, finding such a low positive *JAK2* mutation may still be clinically relevant. If there is doubt, a peripheral-blood or a bone-marrow specimen collected at a later time may be used to confirm the finding.

Therefore, the choice A is correct: the *JAK2* V617F mutation test is a DNA-based assay.

59. **E.** *The JAK2 V617F mutation is found in >95% of patients with polycythemia vera (PV),* approximately 55% of patients with essential thrombocythemia (ET), and 65% of patients with primary myelofibrosis (PMF). The V617F mutation in *JAK2* leads to constitutive activation of the kinase. The active kinase stimulates multiple signal transduction cascades and leads to cellular proliferation in the absence of normal cytokine stimulation, thus leading to expanded cell numbers.

Therefore, the *JAK2* V617F mutation is found in about 95% of patients with polycythemia vera (PV).

60. **C.** The *JAK2* V617F mutation is found in >95% of patients with polycythemia vera (PV), *approximately 55% of patients with essential thrombocythemia (ET),* and 65% of patients with primary myelofibrosis (PMF). The V617F mutation in *JAK2* leads to constitutive activation of the kinase. The active kinase stimulates multiple signal transduction cascades and leads to cellular proliferation in the absence of normal cytokine stimulation, thus leading to expanded cell numbers.

Therefore, the *JAK2* V617F mutation is found in about 60% of patients with essential thrombocythemia (ET).

61. **C.** The *JAK2* V617F mutation is found in >95% of patients with polycythemia vera (PV),

approximately 55% of patients with essential thrombocythemia (ET), and *65% of patients with primary myelofibrosis (PMF)*. The V617F mutation in *JAK2* leads to constitutive activation of the kinase. The active kinase stimulates multiple signal transduction cascades and leads to cellular proliferation in the absence of normal cytokine stimulation, thus leading to expanded cell numbers.

Therefore, the *JAK2* V617F mutation is found in about 60% of patients with primary myelofibrosis (PMF).

62. **A.** The *JAK2* V617F mutation is found in >95% of patients with polycythemia vera (PV). Exon 12 mutations in *JAK2* are far less common, *present in only approximately 3% of PV cases*. In contrast to the V617F mutation, which involves one amino acid codon, exon 12 mutations affect a larger region, spanning codons 533–547. At least 27 clinically verified exon 12 mutations have been identified to date, including amino acid substitutions, deletions, and duplications. Additional exon 12 mutations have been reported, but their clinical significance is unknown.

Therefore, the *JAK2* exon 12 mutations is found in about 3% patients with polycythemia vera (PV).

63. **A.** The *JAK2* V617F mutation is found in >95% of patients with polycythemia vera (PV), approximately 55% of patients with essential thrombocythemia (ET), and 65% of patients with primary myelofibrosis (PMF). *The V617F mutation in JAK2 leads to constitutive activation of the kinase.* The active kinase stimulates multiple signal transduction cascades and leads to cellular proliferation in the absence of normal cytokine stimulation, thus leading to expanded cell numbers.

Therefore, activating mutations would be the pathogenetic role of *JAK2* V617F in this patient's PV.

64. **D.** DNA sequence mutations in the Janus kinase 2 gene (*JAK2*) are found in the hematopoietic cells of several myeloproliferative neoplasms (MPNs), most frequently polycythemia vera (PV; close to 100%), essential thrombocythemia (ET; approximately 50%), and primary myelofibrosis (PMF; approximately 50%) but basically never in chronic myelogenous leukemia (CML). *The vast majority of JAK2 mutations occur at the base pair 1849 in the gene, resulting in a JAK2 V617F protein change.*

Detection of the *JAK2* V617F is useful to help establish the diagnosis of MPN. Other important molecular markers in *BCR-ABL1* negative MPN include *CALR* exon 9 mutations (20%–30% of PMF and ET) and *MPL* exon 10 mutation (5%–10% of PMF and 3%–5% of ET). Over 50 different mutations have now been reported within exons 12 through 15 of *JAK2*, and essentially all of the non-V617F mutations have been identified in PV. Mutations in *JAK2*, *CALR*, and *MPL* are essentially mutually exclusive.

Therefore, *JAK2* V617F mutation analysis would most likely yield a positive result if this patient had ET.

65. **B.** DNA sequence mutations in the Janus kinase 2 gene (*JAK2*) are found in the hematopoietic cells of several myeloproliferative neoplasms (MPNs), most frequently polycythemia vera (PV; close to 100%), essential thrombocythemia (ET; approximately 50%), and primary myelofibrosis (PMF; approximately 50%) but basically never in chronic myelogenous leukemia (CML). The vast majority of *JAK2* mutations occur at base pair 1849 in the gene, resulting in a *JAK2* V617F protein change.

Detection of the *JAK2* V617F is useful to help establish the diagnosis of MPN. Other important molecular markers in *BCR-ABL1* negative MPN include *CALR exon 9 mutations (20%–30% of PMF and ET) and MPL exon 10 mutation (5%–10% of PMF and 3%–5% of ET)*. And over 50 different mutations have now been reported within exons 12 through 15 of *JAK2* and essentially all of the non-V617F mutations have been identified in PV. Mutations in *JAK2*, *CALR*, and *MPL* are essentially mutually exclusive.

Therefore, *JAK2* exon 12 mutation analysis would most likely NOT be part of this reflex test since the patient met all the WHO 2008 diagnostic criteria for ET instead of PV.

66. **B.** *BCR-ABL1* is diagnostic for chronic myeloid leukemia (CML). The most frequent genetic mutation in *BCR-ABL1*−negative myeloproliferative neoplasms (MPNs), such as polycythemia vera (PV), essential thrombocythemia (ET), and primary myelofibrosis (PMF) is the *JAK2* V617F mutation, which is present in approximately 50%–60% of patients. Other important molecular markers in *BCR-ABL1*−negative MPN include *CALR* exon 9 mutations (20%–30% of PMF and ET) and *MPL exon 10 mutation (5%–10% of PMF and 3%–5% of ET)*. Mutations in *JAK2*, *CALR*, and *MPL* are basically mutually exclusive.

MPL codes for a transmembrane tyrosine kinase, and the most common *MPL* mutations are single-base-pair substitutions at codon 515 in exon 10. These mutations have been shown to promote constitutive, cytokine-independent activation of the JAK/STAT signaling pathway and contribute to the oncogenic phenotype. At least eight different *MPL* exon 10 mutations have been identified in PMF and ET to date, and mutations outside of exon 10 have not yet been reported.

Therefore, it was most likely that the detected mutation was located in the exon 10 of the *MPL* gene in this patient.

67. **C.** *BCR-ABL1* is diagnostic for chronic myeloid leukemia (CML). The most frequent genetic mutation in *BCR-ABL1*−negative myeloproliferative neoplasms (MPNs), such as polycythemia vera (PV), essential thrombocythemia (ET), and primary myelofibrosis (PMF), is the *JAK2* V617F mutation, which is present in approximately 50%−60% of patients. Other important molecular markers in *BCR-ABL1*−negative MPNs include *CALR* exon 9 mutations (20%−30% of PMF and ET) and *MPL* exon 10 mutation (5%−10% of PMF and 3%−5% of ET). Mutations in *JAK2*, *CALR*, and *MPL* are essentially mutually exclusive.

DNA sequence mutations in exon 10 of the myeloproliferative leukemia virus oncogene (*MPL*), which are hematopoietic neoplasms classified within the broad category of MPN, have been detected in approximately 5% of patients with PMF and ET. *MPL* codes for a transmembrane tyrosine kinase and *the most common MPL mutations are single base pair substitutions at codon 515*. These mutations have been shown to promote constitutive, cytokine-independent activation of the JAK/STAT signaling pathway and contribute to the oncogenic phenotype. At least eight different *MPL* exon 10 mutations have been identified in PMF and ET to date, and mutations outside of exon 10 have not yet been reported.

Therefore, it was most likely that this patient had a single-nucleotide mutation.

68. **B.** The V617F allele burden in *JAK2* varies greatly (between 1% and 100%) from patient to patient at the time of first diagnosis, and low levels of *JAK2* V617F are not uncommon. With quantitative assessment, it has been reported that approximately 20%−30% of PV patients have less than 25% *JAK2* V617F alleles. Insensitive molecular assays would cause an even bigger problem in ET, in which up to 75% of cases have a *JAK2* V617F level of less than 25% and a considerable number (≤40% of cases) have a *JAK2* V617F level of less than 10%. A quantitative assay or a reasonably sensitive qualitative assay is therefore essential for capturing the cases with low levels of the mutation. An allele burden of greater than 50% suggests homozygosity, which is most likely to occur in PV; it is uncommon in ET. A high allele burden in PV and ET is associated with progression to myelofibrosis.

To ensure that more than 90% of cases are detected, the adequate analytical sensitivity of a clinical JAK2

assay should be at least 1%. When the *JAK2* V617F level of a particular patient falls below 1%, however, caution must be exercised, because very low levels of *JAK2* V617F mutations (usually <0.1%) have been described in the peripheral blood of unaffected individuals. An assay that detects less than 0.1% of *JAK2* allele, therefore, is more likely to produce false positive results in the diagnostic setting. On the other hand, low levels (≤1%) of the mutant *JAK2* have been reported in ET patients (as determined using allele specific loop-mediated amplification assay). Therefore, if other World Health Organization (WHO) major and minor diagnostic criteria are met, finding such a low positive *JAK2* mutation may still be clinically relevant. If there is doubt, a peripheral blood or a bone marrow specimen collected at a later time may be used to confirm the finding.

69. **C.** Although there are no FDA-cleared tests, a number of methods have been developed for detecting *JAK2* V617F mutation. Traditional Sanger sequencing has been used extensively, but it has relatively poor sensitivity. Other methods used to detect V617F include restriction-fragment−length polymorphism, denaturing high-performance liquid chromatography, high-resolution melting curve analysis, pyrosequencing, and various allele-specific PCR systems with electrophoretic analysis of the products. *Most of these methods typically do not achieve sensitivities of less than 5% of alleles.*

Therefore, the sensitivity of these methods most likely may reach to 5%.

70. **A.** *Acute myeloid leukemia (AML)* is an aggressive hematological malignancy that is cured in a minority of patients. An *FLT3*-internal tandem duplication (ITD) mutation, found in approximately a quarter of patients with de novo AML, imparts a particularly poor prognosis. *FTL3*-tyrosine kinase domain (TKD) mutations are reported to occur in approximately 7% of patients, although they seem to be more common in cytogenetically favorable risk AML.

Chronic myeloid leukemia (CML), essential thrombocythemia (ET), polycythemia vera (PV), and primary myelofibrosis (PMF) are all parts of myeloproliferative neoplasms (MPNs). *BCR-ABL1* rearrangement is diagnostic for CML. The most frequent genetic mutation in PV, ET, and PMF is the *JAK2* V617F mutation.

Therefore, the *FLT3*-ITD and *FLT3*-TKD mutations are associated with AML.

71. **B.** Acute myelogenous leukemia (AML) is a heterogeneous group of neoplasms. While cytogenetic aberrations detected at the time of diagnosis are the most commonly used prognostic

features, approximately 20%–40% of AML cases show a normal karyotype, which is considered *an intermediate-risk feature*.

Therefore, this patient would have an intermediate risk, since she had a normal karyotype and no molecular results to further assess the prognosis.

72. **C**. Major insights into the molecular pathogenesis of the cytogenetic standard risk of acute myelogenous leukemia (AML) were provided by discoveries of mutations in the genes encoding CCAAT/enhancer-binding protein α (*CEBPA*) and nucleophosmin (*NPM1*). These entities were recognized in the 2008 WHO Classification and define prognostically relevant subsets of AML. With advanced next-generation sequencing (NGS) technology more and more molecular mutations have been found to carry prognostic significance in patients with AML, such as *CEBPA, c-KIT, DNMT3A, FLT3, NPM1, RUNX1, WT1,* and other conditions. Mutations in the exon 10 of *the MPL gene* are associated with myeloproliferative neoplasm (MPN) instead of AML.

Therefore, the *MPL* gene most likely would not be in an NGS panel for AML.

73. **A**. All the genes listed in this question are associated with acute myelogenous leukemia (AML). *The CEBPA gene is the only intronless gene, though*. The *CEBPA* gene encoded a transcription factor that recognizes the CCAAT motif in the promoters of targeted genes. The encoded protein functions in homodimers and also heterodimers with CCAAT/enhancer-binding proteins beta and gamma. Activity of this protein can modulate the expression of genes involved in cell-cycle regulation as well as in body-weight homeostasis. Mutations of this gene have been identified in approximately 10%–18% of individuals with cytogenetically normal AML.

Therefore, *CEBPA* is the only intronless gene listed in this question.

74. **C**. Acute myeloid leukemia (AML) is an aggressive hematological malignancy that is cured in a minority of patients. An *FLT3*-internal tandem duplication (ITD) mutation, found in approximately a quarter of patients with de novo AML, imparts *a particularly poor prognosis. FTL3*-tyrosine kinase domain (TKD) mutations are reported to occur in approximately 7% of patients, although they seem to be more common in cytogenetically favorable risk AML. Patients with *FLT3*-ITD AML often present with more aggressive disease and have a significantly higher propensity for relapse after remission. The therapeutic approach for these patients has

traditionally included intensive induction chemotherapy, followed by consolidative chemotherapy or hematopoietic-cell transplantation (HCT).

Therefore, this patient would have an unfavorable risk, since she had the *FLT3*-ITD mutation.

75. **B**. Acute myeloid leukemia (AML) is an aggressive hematological malignancy that is cured in a minority of patients. An *FLT3*-internal tandem duplication (ITD) mutation, found in approximately a quarter of patients with de novo AML, imparts a particularly poor prognosis. *FTL3*-tyrosine kinase domain (TKD) mutations are reported to occur in approximately 7% of patients, although they seem to be more common in cytogenetically favorable risk AML. *FLT3*-ITD is located in exon 14 and 15 of the *FLT3* gene, ranging in size from 3 bp to more than hundreds of base pairs. The test of choice for this mutation should be able to distinguish alleles with different sizes.

FISH is a test of choice for aneuploidy, deletion, amplification, inversion, and translocation, such as t(9;22). PCR-capillary electrophoresis is used to tell the size differences between DNA fragments. Sanger sequencing is a test of choice for point mutations and in/dels in all the amplicons, such as *CEBPA*. Targeted-mutation analysis is a test of choice for known point mutations, such as *BRAF* V600E.

Therefore, PCR-capillary electrophoresis would most likely be used to detect the *FLT3*-ITD mutation in this patient.

76. **A**. The *FLT3* gene on 13q12.2 is a proto-oncogene encoded for a growth factor receptor with tyrosine kinase domain(s). *Internal tandem duplication (ITD) mutations cause constitutive activation of the receptor*, the latter being phosphorylated independently of the ligand.

Therefore, the *FLT3*-ITD mutation activates the receptor, which contributes to the leukemia in this patient.

77. **A**. The *CEBPA* gene is an intronless gene encoding a transcription factor that recognizes the CCAAT motif in the promoters of targeted genes. The encoded protein functions in homodimers and also heterodimers with CCAAT/enhancer-binding proteins beta and gamma. Activity of this protein can modulate the expression of genes involved in cell-cycle regulation as well as in body-weight homeostasis. Mutations of this gene have been identified in approximately 10%–18% of individuals with cytogenetically normal *acute myeloid leukemia (AML)*, but not in myeloproliferative neoplasms (MPNs).

Therefore, mutations in the *CEBPA* gene are associated with acute myeloid leukemia (AML).

78. **A**. The *CEBPA* gene is an intronless gene encoding a transcription factor that recognizes the CCAAT motif in the promoters of targeted genes. The encoded protein functions in homodimers and also heterodimers with CCAAT/enhancer-binding proteins beta and gamma. Activity of this protein can modulate the expression of genes involved in cell-cycle regulation as well as in body-weight homeostasis. Mutations of this gene have been identified in approximately 10%−18% of individuals with cytogenetically normal acute myeloid leukemia (AML).

Mutations cluster in both the amino- and carboxy-terminal regions, with the former leading to expression of a truncated isoform of CEBPA (p30) and loss of the full-length protein (p42). Carboxy-terminal mutations affect regions involved in mediating dimerization and DNA binding. In more than half of patients with *CEBPA* mutations, both alleles are involved, combining an upstream mutation in 1 allele with a downstream mutation in the other. *Biallelic CEBPA, but not single CEBPA, mutations are associated with a relatively favorable outcome in individuals with AML.* Acquired mutations in the *RUNX1*, *WT1*, and *TP53*, and *FLT3*-ITD are associated with unfavorable risk in individuals with AML.

Therefore, the patient would have a favorable prognosis if she had acquired biallelic pathogenic variants in the *CEBPA* gene.

79. **A**. Acquired mutations in the *CEPBA* gene have been identified in approximately 10%−18% of individuals with cytogenetically normal acute myeloid leukemia (AML). Mutations cluster in both the amino- and carboxy-terminal regions, with the former leading to expression of a truncated isoform of CEBPA (p30) and loss of the full-length protein (p42). Carboxy-terminal mutations affect regions involved in mediating dimerization and DNA binding. In more than half of patients with *CEBPA* mutations, both alleles are involved, combining an upstream mutation in 1 allele with a downstream mutation in the other. Biallelic *CEBPA* mutations are associated with a relatively favorable outcome in individuals with AML.

Germline pathogenic mutations in the CEPBA gene have been seen in individuals with familial acute myeloid leukemias (AML). If an individual inherits a copy of the variant from one parent, developing AML is associated with acquisition of additional mutation of the other *CEBPA* allele.

Single copy of acquired mutations in the other genes in this question is associated with AML. Germline pathogenic mutations in the *TP53* gene

are associated with Li−Fraumeni syndrome, but not familial AML. Individuals with Li−Fraumeni syndrome are prone to a lot of malignancies, including AML.

Therefore, the *CEPBA* gene in the NGS panel is associated with familial acute myeloid leukemia (AML).

80. **C**. The *CEBPA* gene is an intronless gene encoding a transcription factor that recognizes the CCAAT motif in the promoters of targeted genes. The encoded protein functions in homodimers and also heterodimers with CCAAT/enhancer-binding proteins beta and gamma. Activity of this protein can modulate the expression of genes involved in cell-cycle regulation as well as in body-weight homeostasis. Mutations of this gene have been identified in approximately 10%−18% of individuals with cytogenetically normal acute myeloid leukemia (AML). Biallelic *CEBPA* mutations are associated with a relatively favorable outcome in individuals with AML. *Acquired pathogenic mutations are heterogeneous, and more than 50 mutations have been detected in the full length of the gene. The test of choice for this gene should be able to detect mutations anywhere in the gene.*

FISH is a test of choice for aneuploidy, deletion, amplification, inversion, and translocation, such as t(9;22). PCR-capillary electrophoresis is a test of choice to detect amplicons with different size, such as *FLT3*-ITD. Sanger sequencing is a test of choice for point mutations, in/dels in all the amplicons, such as *CEBPA*. Targeted-mutation analysis is a test of choice for known point mutations, such as *BRAF* V600E.

Therefore, Sanger sequencing would most likely be used to detect the *CEBPA* gene in this patient.

81. **C**. The *CEBPA* gene is an intronless gene encoding a transcription factor that recognizes the CCAAT motif in the promoters of targeted genes. Mutations of this gene have been identified in approximately 10%−18% of individuals with cytogenetically normal acute myeloid leukemia (AML). Biallelic *CEBPA* mutations are associated with a relatively favorable outcome in individuals with AML. Acquired pathogenic mutations are heterogeneous, and more than 50 mutations have been detected in the full length of the gene. Unless two pathogenic mutations are in the same amplicon, it is hard to tell whether they are in *cis* or *trans*. If we are talking about germline pathogenic variants in autosomal recessive disorders, parental testing is helpful to distinguish in *cis* from in *trans* variants.

Therefore, it is unclear whether these two acquired compound heterozygous pathogenic variants in the *CEBPA* gene are in *cis* or in *trans*.

82. **E.** In the current World Health Organization (WHO) classification, acute myeloid leukemia (AML) with mutated *CEBPA* has been designated as a provisional disease entity in the category "AML with recurrent genetic abnormalities."

CEBPA is an intronless gene encoding a transcription factor. Biallelic mutations in the *CEBPA* gene have been described in both adult and pediatric acute myeloid leukemia (AML) patients and are associated with a good prognosis. *The prognostic impact of CEBPA mutations in the presence of FLT3 mutations is unclear.*

The most common mutations in the *CEBPA* gene are N-terminal frameshift mutations and in-frame C-terminal mutations. N-terminal insertions/deletions cause translation of a 30 kDa protein from an internal ATG start site that lacks transactivation domain 1 and has a dominant negative effect over the full-length p42 protein. C-terminal mutations disrupt binding to DNA or dimerization. Patients can have one or two mutations. The latter generally involves N- plus C-terminal alterations that are presumed to be biallelic, although homozygous mutations have also been described. Biallelic *CEBPA* mutations result in a more favorable patient prognosis.

Therefore, the prognostic impact of *CEBPA* mutations in the presence of *FLT3* mutations is unclear, instead of unfavorable.

83. **D.** In the current World Health Organization (WHO) classification, acute myeloid leukemia (AML) with mutated *CEBPA* has been designated as a provisional disease entity in the category "AML with recurrent genetic abnormalities." Acquired biallelic mutations in the *CEBPA* gene have been described in both adult and pediatric AML patients, and are associated with a good prognosis. The prognostic impact of *CEBPA* mutations in the presence of *FLT3* mutations is unclear. However, dysregulation of *CEBPA* is not associated with APL, CML, or MDS.

Therefore, *CEBPA sequence analysis is indicated in patients with normal-karyotype AML.*

84. **B.** The most common mutations in the *CEBPA* gene are N-terminal frameshift mutations and in frame C-terminal mutations. N-terminal insertions/deletions cause translation of a 30 kDa protein. C-terminal mutations disrupt binding to DNA or dimerization in the 42-kDa isoform. Overexpression of the 30-kDa CEBPA protein results in *dominant negative inhibition* of the activity of the 42-kDa isoform of CEBPA protein.

Therefore, the N-terminal mutations of *CEBPA* typically are dominant negative mutations.

85. **A.** In the current World Health Organization (WHO) classification, acute myeloid leukemia (AML) with mutated *CEBPA* has been designated as a provisional disease entity in the category "AML with recurrent genetic abnormalities." Acquired biallelic mutations in the *CEBPA* gene have been described in both adult and pediatric AML patients and are associated with a good prognosis.

The most common mutations in the *CEBPA* gene are *N-terminal frameshift mutations and in frame C-terminal mutations.* N-terminal insertions/deletions cause translation of a 30 kDa protein. C-terminal mutations disrupt binding to DNA or dimerization in the 42-kDa isoform. Overexpression of the 30-kDa CEBPA protein results in dominant negative inhibition of the activity of the 42-kDa isoform of CEBPA protein.

Therefore, the most common mutations in *CEBPA* are N-terminal frameshift and C-terminal in frame mutations.

86. **A.** Acute myeloid leukemia (AML) with mutated *NPM1* usually carries mutations involving exon 12 of the *NPM1* gene. This AML type frequently has myelomonocytic or monocytic features and typically presents de novo in older adults with a normal karyotype. AML with mutated *NPM1* typically shows a good response to induction therapies. *AML with mutated NPM1 and a normal karyotype, in the absence of a FLT3-ITD mutation, has a characteristically favorable prognosis.*[7]

Therefore, this patient would most likely have favorable risk, since she had acquired pathogenic variants in the *NPM1* gene with a normal karyotype.

87. **B.** Acute myeloid leukemia (AML) with mutated *NPM1* usually carries mutations involving exon 12 of the *NPM1* gene. This AML type frequently has myelomonocytic or monocytic features and typically presents de novo in older adults with a normal karyotype. *The majority of mutations in the NPM1 gene are 4-bp insertions.*

Therefore, it would be most likely that an out-of-frame deletion/insertion in *NPM1* was detected in this patient.

88. **B.** Acute myeloid leukemia (AML) with mutated *NPM1* usually carries mutations involving exon 12 of the *NPM1* gene. This AML type frequently has myelomonocytic or monocytic features and typically presents de novo in older adults with a normal karyotype. *The majority of mutations in the NPM1 gene are 4-bp insertions.*

FISH is a test of choice for aneuploidy, deletion, amplification, inversion, and translocation, such as t(9;22). PCR-capillary electrophoresis is a test of choice for amplicons with different sizes, such as *FLT3*-ITD. Sanger sequencing is a test of choice for heterogeneous point mutations, such as *CEBPA*. Targeted-mutation analysis is a test of choice for known point mutations, such as *BRAF* V600E.

Therefore, PCR-capillary electrophoresis would be the most cost-effective way to detect small in/dels, such as a 4-bp insertion, in the *NPM1* gene in this patient.

89. **E.** Automated Sanger sequencing is considered the first generation of sequencing technology. Sanger cancer gene sequencing uses polymerase chain reaction (PCR) amplification of genetic regions of interest followed by sequencing of PCR products using fluorescently labeled terminators, capillary electrophoresis separation of products, and laser-signal detection of nucleotide sequence.

As Sanger-based sequencing efforts moved increasingly into cancer research, it became clear that many tumor specimens and their derivative genomic DNA posed specific challenges that often confounded the detection of specific genomic alterations. The limitations are that it is insensitive to alterations that occur at an allele frequency lower than approximately 20% (a phenomenon that may reflect low tumor content in a specimen), it has limited clinical scalability beyond a few genes, it is unable to detect structural rearrangements or DNA copy-number changes, and it cannot be used to tell whether compound heterozygous mutations are in *cis* or in *trans*.

Therefore, all the statements in the questions describe the limitation of the utility of Sanger sequencing in oncology.

90. **E.** NPM1 is a multifunctional phosphoprotein that encodes for a number of functional domains through which the molecule is able to bind many partners in distinct cellular compartments. NPM displays nucleolar localization and constantly shuttles between the nucleus and the cytoplasm. *NPM1* mutations that relocalize NPM1 from the nucleus into the cytoplasm are associated with the development of acute myeloid leukemia (AML). There is no tyrosine kinase domain in the NPM1 protein. Products of *ABL1*, *FLT3*, *JAK2*, and *c-KIT* have tyrosine kinase domain(s).

Therefore, NPM1, associated with myeloid neoplasms, does **NOT** have tyrosine kinase domain(s).

91. **F.** Acute myeloid leukemia (AML) with mutated *NPM1* usually carries mutations involving exon 12 of the *NPM1* gene. This AML type frequently has myelomonocytic or monocytic features and

typically presents de novo in older adults with a normal karyotype.[7] *AML with mutated NPM1 and a normal karyotype, in the absence of a FLT3-ITD mutation, has a characteristically favorable prognosis.* Mutations in the rest of genes in the question are associated with unfavorable prognoses in patients with AML.

Therefore, the patient would have a favorable prognosis if he had acquired pathogenic variant(s) in *NPM1*.

92. **B.** *Patients with FLT3-ITD tend to have a worse clinical outcome*, whereas the prognostic impact of FLT3-TKD mutation alone is still unclear. Mutations in both *CEBPA* and *NPM1* are associated with favorable prognosis in patients with acute myeloid leukemia (AML).

Therefore, *FLT3-ITD* would indicate the patient had an unfavorable prognosis if he had one.

93. **A.** Recurrent mutations of the *SF3B1* gene can be found in 20% of patients with myelodysplastic syndrome (MDS) and in 65% of patients with MDS with ring sideroblasts. *SF3B1* encodes subunit 1 of the splicing factor 3b protein complex, a core component of the RNA splicing machinery. Patients with MDS who have this mutation have higher platelet counts and higher neutrophil counts. *Acquired SF3B1 mutations were found to be independently associated with better overall survival and lower risk of evolution into AML.*

Therefore, this patient would most likely have a favorable prognosis, since he had a normal karyotype with an acquired pathogenic variant in the *SF3B1* gene.

94. **D.** Somatic mutations in the *ASXL1* gene have been described in all types of myeloid malignancies, including acute myeloid leukemia (AML), myeloproliferative neoplasms (MPNs), myelodysplastic syndromes (MDSs), chronic myelomonocytic leukemia (CMML), and rarely in juvenile myelomonocytic leukemia (JMML). *Most ASXL1 mutations occur in exon 13 (referred to as exon 12 in many publications)* and are frequently frameshift or nonsense mutations that result in C-terminal truncation of the protein upstream of the plant homeodomain finger region. *ASXL1* mutations are associated with poor prognosis typified by aggressive disease and shorter overall survival.

Therefore, exon 13 (referred to as exon 12 in many publications) most likely harbors an acquired pathogenic variant in a patient with a myeloid malignancy.

95. **B.** The mixed lineage leukemia gene (*MLL*), located on 11q23, was initially recognized as a recurrent locus of chromosomal translocation in

acute myeloid leukemia (AML) and acute lymphoid leukemia (ALL). To date, *MLL* has been found in >51 different translocations with distinct fusion partners.

Research showed that in some patients with acute myeloid leukemia (AML), *MLL* is not fused with a partner gene but rather is consistently elongated with a partial tandem duplication (PTD) of exons 11-5 or 12-5 (former exon designations were 6-2 and 8-2). *Leukemia-cell RNA with the MLL-PTD can be detected with RT-PCR using primers that flank the duplication repeat.* This RT-PCR method has a greater sensitivity compared to genomic DNA amplification and Southern blot.

Therefore, a RNA assay would most likely be used to detect *MLL*-PTD in this patient.

96. **A.** The mixed lineage leukemia gene (*MLL*), located on 11q23, was initially recognized as a recurrent locus of chromosomal translocation in acute myeloid leukemia (AML) and acute lymphoid leukemia (ALL). To date, *MLL* has been found in >51 different translocations with distinct fusion partners. Research showed that in some patients with acute myeloid leukemia (AML), *MLL* is not fused with a partner gene but rather is consistently elongated with an *in-frame partial tandem duplication* (PTD) of exons 11-5 or 12-5 (former exon designations were 6-2 and 8-2).

Therefore, this patient would most likely have in frame duplication of *MLL*.

97. **A.** *Acquired pathogenic variants in the exon 9 of the CALR gene are associated with myeloproliferative neoplasms (MPNs), especially essential thrombocythemia (ET) and primary myelofibrosis (PMF) when the patients are JAK2 V617F—negative.* CEBPA, FLT3-internal tandem duplication (ITD), FLT3-tyrosine kinase domain (TKD), MLL-partial tandem duplication (PTD), and NPM1 are associated with acute myeloid leukemia (AML).

Therefore, it would be most likely that the *CALR* gene was not in the NGS panel for AML.

98. **C.** *Acquired pathogenic variants in the exon 10 of the MPL gene are in approximately 5% of patients with primary myelofibrosis (PMF) and essential thrombocythemia (ET), which are hematopoietic neoplasms classified within the broad category of myeloproliferative neoplasms (MPNs). ASXL1, CEBPA, RUNX1,* and *SF3B1* are associated with acute myeloid leukemia (AML).

Therefore, it would be most likely that the *MPL* gene was not in the NGS panel for AML.

99. **A.** Trisomy 8 is one of the most frequent cytogenetically gained aberrations in acute myeloid leukemia (AML). Patients with isolated trisomy 8 (tri 8) are usually older, male, present

with lower WBC counts, and more often harbor acquired pathogenic variants in the *ASXL1*, and *RUNX1* genes but less frequently *FLT3*-ITD, *NPM1* mutations, or double-mutated *CEBPA* than do patients with a normal karyotype.

Therefore, the *ASXL1* gene would most likely be mutated in this patient.

100. **C.** Trisomy 8 is one of the most frequent cytogenetically gained aberrations in acute myeloid leukemia (AML). Patients with isolated trisomy 8 (tri 8) are usually older, male, present with lower WBC counts, and more often harbor acquired pathogenic variants in the *ASXL1* and *RUNX1* genes but less frequently *FLT3*-ITD, *NPM1* mutations, or double-mutated *CEBPA* than do patients with normal karyotype. *ASXL1 exon 12 mutations are frequent in AML with an intermediate-risk karyotype and are independently associated with an adverse outcome.*

Therefore, it would most likely that this patient had an unfavorable risk, since he had an acquired pathogenic variant in the *ASXL1* gene with trisomy 8.

101. **E.** The *RUNX1* gene on 21q22.12 encodes a transcription factor that regulates the differentiation of hematopoietic stem cells into mature blood cells. It is unclear whether *RUNX1* is a proto-oncogene or tumor suppressor gene. In human leukemia, *RUNX1* is involved in various chromosomal translocations that create oncogenic fusion proteins. For example, *RUNX1T1/RUNX1* due to t(8;21)(q21.3;q22.12) is categorized as acute myeloid leukemia (AML) M2. Moreover, structurally intact *RUNX1* is also oncogenic when overexpressed. For example, *RUNX1* duplication/amplification has also been reported in AML. Based on analyses of loss of heterozygosity (LOH) in patients with AML, *RUNX1* was identified as a tumor suppressor gene. AML patients with isolated trisomy 8 (tri 8) more often harbor acquired pathogenic variants in the *ASXL1* and *RUNX1* genes.

Therefore, deletions, duplications/amplifications, point mutations, and translocations of *RUNX1* are all associated with AML.

102. **D.** Several tumors can harbor *KIT* mutations, including gastrointestinal stromal tumors (GIST), mast-cell disease, melanoma, seminoma, acute myeloid leukemia (AML), myeloproliferative neoplasms (MPNs), and lymphomas. The frequency and type of mutations vary among these tumors and have distinct clinical implications.

KIT is mutated in 8.0% of AML. And *KIT* mutations *primarily occur in exon 17* and affect the activation loop of the kinase domain. Some of *KIT* mutations occur in exon 8 (1.8%). These changes result in improved survival and growth of tumor cells. *KIT* mutations fall into class I of the "two-hit" theory of leukemogenesis as a tumor suppressor gene.

Approximately 80% of GISTs harbor a mutation in *KIT* gene, while 2%–5% harbor mutations in *PDGFRA*. In GIST, somatic mutations within the *KIT* gene are located in exons 2, 9, 10, 11, 13, 14, 15, 17, and 18, and somatic mutations within the *PDGFRA* gene are located in exons 12, 14, 15, and 18.

Therefore, it was most likely that the *KIT* mutation in this AML patient was located in exon 17.

103. **B.** Individuals with Down syndrome have an increased risk of leukemia compared to non-Down syndrome individuals. The increased risk is variously estimated at 10- to 100-fold and extends into the adult years. Approximately 10% of Down syndrome neonates manifest transient abnormal myelopoiesis (TAM). In 20%–30% of the affected cases, nonremitting acute megakaryoblastic leukemia subsequently develops in 1–3 years. In addition to myeloid aberrations, Down syndrome individuals also have an increased incidence of acute lymphoblastic leukemia (ALL).

In addition to trisomy 21, acquired GATA1 mutations are present in blast cells of TAM and AML. GATA1 is an erythroid transcription factor expressed by megakaryocytes, erythrocytes, and basophils derived from a specific multipotential progenitor cell (CFU-E/B/Meg).

Therefore, it would be most likely that this neonate had an acquired pathogenic variant in the *GATA1* gene when he had TAM.

104. **B.** In addition to trisomy 21, blast cells in transient abnormal myelopoiesis (TAM) and acute megakaryoblastic leukemia carry acquired mutations in the hematopoietic transcription factor *GATA1*. *Most reported mutations are found in exon 2 of GATA1.* These mutations lead to expression of N-terminally truncated GATA1 protein, and they are detectable in disease but not in remission.

Therefore, most likely this patient would have a pathogenic variant located in exon 2 of the *GATA1* gene.

105. **C.** In addition to trisomy 21, blast cells in transient abnormal myelopoiesis (TAM) and acute megakaryoblastic leukemia carry acquired mutations in *GATA1*. Most reported mutations are found in exon 2 of *GATA1* or, less commonly exon 3, *including insertions, deletions, and point*

mutations. These mutations lead to expression of N-terminally truncated GATA1 protein, and they are detectable in disease but not in remission.

FISH is a test of choice for aneuploidy, deletion, amplification, inversion, and translocation, such as t(9;22). PCR-capillary electrophoresis is a test of choice to detect amplicons with different sizes, such as *FLT3*-ITD. Sanger sequencing is a test of choice for heterogeneous point mutations, such as *CEBPA*. Targeted-mutation analysis is a test of choice for known point mutations, such as *BRAF* V600E.

Therefore, Sanger sequencing would most likely be used for the *GATA1* gene in this patient.

106. **C.** *RUNX1* mutations occur in 8.9% of myelodysplastic syndrome (MDSs). *RUNX1* mutations are most often observed in the refractory cytopenia with multilineage dysplasia (RCMD) and refractory anemia with excess blasts (RAEB) subtypes of high risk. *RUNX1* mutations result in deregulation of the transcription necessary for normal hematopoiesis. *RUNX1 mutations are a prognostic biomarker, associated with shorter overall survival.*

Therefore, it would be likely that this patient had unfavorable risk due to the *RUNX1* mutation and the normal karyotype.

107. **C.** This patient has myelodysplastic syndrome (MDS) associated with *GATA2 deficiency syndrome.* Haploinsufficiency in the *GATA2* gene leads to a wide range of hematologic consequences, including aplastic anemia, chronic neutropenia, and an increased risk of developing MDS or acute myeloid leukemia (AML). Patients are characterized with low or absent B cells, T cells, and natural killer cells. Recurrent herpes infections, lymphedema, and atypical mycobacterial infections are common in *GATA2* deficiency syndromes. AML patients with *GATA2* mutations usually have poor outcomes and require aggressive and early intervention, such as allogeneic stem-cell transplantation. Identification of familial causes of MDS/AML is critical when screening potential sibling donors for stem-cell transplantation as well as identifying additional carriers within a family.

Acquired pathogenic variants in the *ASXL1*, *GATA1*, *RUNX1*, and *SF3B1* genes are associated with myeloid malignancies. Germline pathogenic variants in the *RUNX2* gene are associated with autosomal dominant cleidocranial dysplasia.

Therefore, the *GATA2* gene would most likely be tested in this patient for this hereditary condition.

108. A. This patient has myelodysplastic syndrome (MDS) associated with *GATA2 deficiency syndrome*. Haploinsufficiency in the *GATA2* gene leads to a wide range of hematological consequences, including aplastic anemia, chronic neutropenia, and an increased risk of developing MDS or acute myeloid leukemia (AML). Patients are characterized with low or absent B cells, T cells, and natural killer cells. Recurrent herpes infections, lymphedema, and atypical mycobacterial infections are common in *GATA2* deficiency syndromes. AML patients with *GATA2* mutations usually have poor outcomes and require aggressive and early intervention, such as allogeneic stem-cell transplantation. Approximately 30% of patients with hereditary *GATA2* deficiency syndrome have an acquired heterozygous pathogenic variant in the *ASXL1* gene.

Therefore, it would be likely that *ASXL1* was mutated somatically in this patient.

109. A. *BCR-ABL1*, or Philadelphia (Ph) chromosome, is generated by the der(22) of the t(9;22)(q34;q11) translocation. It is present in over 95% of chronic myelogenous leukemia (CML) cases, 25% of adult ALL cases, and 3%–5% of pediatric ALL cases. The breakpoints on chromosome 9 are scattered over a nearly 200-kb region within the first intron of *ABL1*, whereas the *BCR* breakpoints on chromosome 22 are clustered in two areas: a 5.8-kb major *BCR* (M-bcr) in CML and a minor *BCR* (m-bcr) in most cases of childhood Ph-positive ALL. Nearly all CML patients have a p210 breakpoint. In contrast, *the majority of de novo Ph-positive acute leukemias harbor a p190 breakpoint (m-bcr)*. Patients whose acute leukemia harbors a p210 breakpoint should be evaluated to distinguish de novo acute leukemia from blast crisis of CML.

Therefore, it would be most likely that this patient had a p190 (m-bcr) *BCR-ABL1* fusion.

110. C. *BCR-ABL1*, or Philadelphia (Ph) chromosome, is generated by the der(22) of the t(9;22)(q34;q11) translocation. It is present in over 95% of chronic myelogenous leukemia (CML) cases, 25% of adult ALL cases, and 3%–5% of pediatric ALL cases (29). The breakpoints on chromosome 9 are scattered over a nearly 200-kb region within the first intron of *ABL1*, whereas the *BCR* breakpoints on chromosome 22 are clustered in two areas: a 5.8-kb major *BCR* (M-bcr) in CML and a minor *BCR* (m-bcr) in most cases of childhood Ph-positive ALL. *Presence of any BCR-ABL1 transcript in pre-B ALL predicted a lower chance of initial treatment response and a lower probability of disease-free survival at 3 years.*

Therefore, this patient would have an unfavorable risk due to the *BCR-ABL1*.

111. B. The typical hairy cells of hairy-cell leukemia are so named because of their characteristic cytoplasmic projections, which appear as fine (hairlike) microvilli when seen on light microscopy, phase-contrast microscopy, and electron microscopy. These are mononuclear cells with eccentric or centrally placed nuclei. Hairy cells have a mature-B-cell phenotype and typically express single or multiple immunoglobulin light chains κ/λ and pan–B-cell antigens, such as CD20, CD25, CD11c, and CD103, but not CD21 (late-B-cell marker). These cells have also been distinguished by expression of CD123 and bright annexin A1-positive cells.

In a recent study, *the BRAF V600E mutation was identified in 100% of patients with hairy-cell leukemia*, and not in other lymphoproliferative disorders. Case reports have documented the activity of *BRAF* inhibitors in relapsed/refractory hairy cell leukemia patients harboring *BRAF* V600E.

Therefore, the *BRAF* gene would most likely be mutated in this patient.

112. D. Anaplastic large-cell lymphoma (ALCL) is a relatively rare type of neoplasm, comprising 3% of adult-onset non-Hodgkin lymphoma (NHL) and 10%–15% of pediatric NHL cases. It has unique immunohistochemistry (IHC), staining positive for CD30, a marker for Hodgkin lymphoma, along with coexpression of T-cell markers. A subset (40%–60%) of ALCL cases have translocation t(2;5)(p23;q35), resulting in the formation of nucleophosmin anaplastic lymphoma kinase (NPM1-ALK) protein, a transmembrane tyrosine kinase receptor. Other less common translocations involving the *ALK* gene in cases of ALCL include t(1;2), t(2;3), t(2;17), t(2;19), t(2;22), t(2;X), and inv(2). *ALK*-positive ALCL tends to affect children and young adults, with a higher predilection for males. It carries a good prognosis, with a 5-year survival rate of more than 80% even in advanced stages.

Therefore, this patient would most likely have t(2;5)(p23;q35) with *NPM1-ALK* fusion.

113. E. Chimerism testing (engraftment analysis) by DNA employs methodology commonly used in human identity testing and is accomplished by the analysis of short tandem repeat (STR) loci. The PCR-based STR/CE system can combine the amplification of multiple STR loci in a single tube, permitting analysis of up to 16 loci in one reaction. *STR-based PCR has a moderate analytical sensitivity of 1%–10%.*

Usually, prior to the transplantation, a peripheral-blood sample from the recipient and the donor(s) were analyzed to identify informative markers, which was different between recipient and the donor(s). After transplantation, chimerism status was assessed on peripheral-blood samples collected on days 18, 32, and 51 after transplantation.

Therefore, the analytical sensitivity of the chimerism status analysis is about 1% to 10% using STR-based PCR method.

114. **D**. Major reasons for bone-marrow engraftment (BME)/chimerism testing include:
   - Confirmation of initial engraftment following hematopoietic stem-cell transplantation (HSCT),
   - Monitoring of hematopoietic reconstitution by donor derived cells,
   - Measurement of chimerism in cellular subpopulations to predict graft rejection, GCHD (graft versus host disease) and early relapse,
   - Monitoring effectiveness of posttransplantation therapies,
   - Indicator of relapse.

   BME/chimerism testing cannot be used for autologous HSCT, since there are no informative markers/alleles to distinguish the recipient from the donor.

   Stutter peaks are an artifact of STR PCR amplification that may arise from "slippage" within the repeat sequence during the PCR process. Stutter peaks of tetranucleotide STRs are 4 bp shorter than the main peak, and can have a peak area close to 5% of the main peak area. Therefore, usually laboratories choose recipient-specific alleles at least two repeats smaller than the donor allele(s) if the recipient allele is smaller. Loci at which both of the donor and recipient alleles are informative are preferred because both alleles at each locus can be used for the analysis. Primer sets containing more than one informative locus are preferred because they provide independent confirmation of recipient cells.

   Therefore, the chimerism analysis can be used for autologous hematopoietic cell transplantation.

115. **A**. Most of cases of Burkitt Lymphoma have *c-MYC* translocation at band 8q24 to the IG heavy chain region (*IGH*), 14q32 or, less commonly, at the lambda, 22q11 or kappa (*IGK*), 2p12 light chain loci (*IGL*). *Up to 10% of the cases may lack a demonstrable c-MYC translocation by FISH*, the explanation for which is uncertain.

   Therefore, approximately 90% of patients with Burkitt lymphoma have *c-MYC* rearrangements.

116. **E**. *A c-MYC rearrangement was observed in up to 10% of an unselected series of cases of diffuse large B-cell lymphoma (DLBCL)*, and it is usually associated with a complex pattern of genetic alterations. The *MYC* break partner is an Ig gene in 60% and a non-Ig gene in 40% of cases. Approximately 20% of cases with a *MYC* break have a concurrent *IGH-BCL2* translocation and/or *BCL6* break.

   Therefore, up to 10% of patients with diffuse large B cell lymphoma (DLBCL) have *c-MYC* translocations.

117. **A**. Epidermal growth factor receptor (*EGFR*) is a member of the ErbB family of cell-membrane receptors that are important mediators of cell growth, differentiation, and survival. The EGFR (also known as ErbB1/HER1) is a 170-kDa transmembrane glycoprotein that consists of an extracellular domain that recognizes and binds to specific ligands, a hydrophobic transmembrane domain involved in interactions between receptors within the cell membrane, and an intracellular domain that contains the tyrosine kinase enzymatic activity. Somatic *activating mutations* in exons 18–21 of the *EGFR* gene, corresponding to the cytoplasmic tyrosine kinase domain of the EGFR protein, are the most prevalent and well characterized in nonsmall-cell lung cancer (NSCLC).

   Therefore, clinically significant mutations of *EGFR* are typically activating mutations.

118. **C**. Mutations in *EGFR*, *KRAS*, and *ALK* are mutually exclusive in patients with nonsmall-cell lung cancer (NSCLC). *EGFR mutations are enriched in never-smoking patients and occur in about 50% of never smokers with NSCLC in the United States and in 60%–80% of Asian patients who never smoked with lung cancer.* Approximately 15%–25% of patients with lung adenocarcinoma have tumor-associated *KRAS* mutations. *KRAS* mutations are found in tumors from both former/current smokers and never smokers. They are rarer in never smokers and are less common in East Asian than in U.S. or European patients. Therefore, mutations in *EGFR are* most prevalent in non-smoking patients with non-small cell lung cancer (NSCLC) in USA than in other genes listed in this question.

119. **B**. *EGFR mutations occur in about 10% of nonsmall-cell lung cancer (NSCLC) cancers from Western populations* and, for reasons unknown, are two to three times more common in patients of East Asian descent.

Therefore, about 10% patients with non-small cell lung cancer (NSCLC) have *EGFR* mutations in Western populations.

120. **D**. *EGFR* mutations are enriched in never-smoking patients and *occur in about 50% of never smokers with NSCLC in the United States* and in 60%–80% of Asian patients with lung cancer who never smoked.

Therefore, about 50% non-smokers with non-small cell lung cancer (NSCLC) have *EGFR* mutations in US.

121. **C**. Nonsmall-cell lung cancer (NSCLC) patients with somatic mutations within the EGFR-TK domain, particularly exon 19 deletion, exon 21 L858R, and exon 18 G719X, respond well to the EGFR tyrosine kinase inhibitors (TKIs) gefitinib (Iressa) and erlotinib (Tarceva). By contrast, *the exon 20 T790M mutation is associated with acquired resistance to TKI therapy* (https://www.mycancergenome.org).

Therefore, T790M in exon 20 of *EGFR* is associated with acquired resistance to *EGFR* tyrosine kinase inhibitor (TKI) therapy in patients with non-small cell lung cancer (NSCLC).

122. **F**. *EGFR, KRAS, BRAF*, and *ALK* mutations are all mutually exclusive in patients with nonsmall-cell lung cancer (NSCLC).

123. **C**. *Lung cancer is the most lethal cancer in the United States*, causing more deaths than the next four cancers (colorectal, breast, pancreas, and prostate) combined, according to 2010 American Cancer Society statistics.

Therefore, lung cancer causes most of deaths in the United States.

124. **B**. *Erlotinib targeted to the tyrosine kinase domain in EGFR*. The EGFR-TKIs responsive patients tended to be female nonsmokers with adenocarcinoma, especially the bronchioloalveolar type. Asian ethnicity was also associated with a response. However, these clinical factors alone did not adequately predict outcome, as some men and smokers also responded. EGFR protein overexpression by immunohistochemistry failed to predict response to EGFR-TKIs (https://www.mycancergenome.org).

Therefore, erlotinib targets to the tyrosine kinase domain in the *EGFR* gene in therapy for non-small cell lung cancer (NSCLC).

125. **B**. *Erlotinib is a small molecule that occupies the ATP-binding groove of the tyrosine kinase in EGFR*. Use of the EGFR-TKIs gefitinib (discontinued in the United States), erlotinib, and afatinib is limited to patients with adenocarcinomas who have known activating *EGFR* mutations. *KRAS* mutations in lung cancers occur predominantly in codons 12

(91.7%), 13 (5.7%), and 61 (2.2%). Because of its location downstream of *EGFR*, proliferative signals emanating from a mutated KRAS protein will not be inhibited by EGFR blockade. As a result, and as clinical evidence demonstrates, *KRAS* mutant lung cancers do not respond to EGFR inhibition. *EGFR* and *ALK* mutations are mutually exclusive. Patients with *ALK* rearrangements are not thought to benefit from EGFR-targeting TKIs. Instead, treatment with an ALK inhibitor (crizotinib [Xalkori] or ceritinib [Zykadia]) is indicated (https://www.mycancergenome.org).

Targeted cancer therapies involve drugs designed to interfere with specific molecules necessary for tumor growth and progression and are broadly classified as either monoclonal antibodies or small molecules. Therapeutic monoclonal antibodies target specific antigens found on the cell surface, such as transmembrane receptors or extracellular growth factors. In some cases, monoclonal antibodies are conjugated to radioisotopes or toxins to allow specific delivery of these cytotoxic agents to the intended cancer-cell target. Small molecules can penetrate the cell membrane to interact with targets inside a cell. Small molecules are usually designed to interfere with the enzymatic activity of the target protein.

As with any drug, targeted cancer therapies typically have several different names. One (or more) name is used to designate the chemical compound during development; if successful, the drug receives a generic name and then a brand name used by the pharmaceutical company for marketing. For example, the small molecule STI-571 became known as imatinib (generic name) and is marketed by Novartis under the brand name Gleevec. The name of a targeted agent provides clues to the type of agent and its cellular target.

Monoclonal antibodies end with the stem "-mab" (monoclonal antibody). Small molecules end with the stem "-ib" (indicating that the agent has protein inhibitory properties). Monoclonal antibodies have an additional substem designating the source of the compound—for example, "-ximab" for chimeric human–mouse antibodies, "-zumab" for humanized mouse antibodies, and "-mumab" for fully human antibodies. Both monoclonal antibodies and small molecules contain an additional stem in the middle of the name describing the molecule's target; examples for monoclonal antibodies include "-ci-" for a circulatory system target and "-tu-" for a tumor target, while examples for small molecules include "-tin-" for tyrosine kinase inhibitors and "-zom-" for proteasome inhibitors (https://www.mycancergenome.org).

Therefore, erlotinib is a small molecule that occupies the ATP-binding groove of the tyrosine kinase in therapy for non-small cell lung cancer (NSCLC).

126. **D**. Approximately *15%–25% of patients with lung adenocarcinoma have tumor-associated KRAS mutations. KRAS mutations are uncommon in lung squamous-cell carcinoma.*

Therefore, about 20% of patients with lung adenocarcinoma have acquired KRAS mutations.

127. **E**. Fusion between echinoderm microtubule-associated protein like 4 (*EML4*) and *ALK*, caused by inv(2)(p21p23), is seen in approximately in *2%–7% of patients with nonsmall-cell lung cancer (NSCLC).*

Therefore, about 5% of patients with non-small cell lung cancer (NSCLC) have acquired ALK rearrangement.

128. **A**. Fusion between echinoderm microtubule-associated protein like 4 (EML4) and *ALK*, caused by inv(2)(p21p23), is seen in approximately in 2%–7% of patients with nonsmall-cell lung cancer (NSCLC). This and other ALK rearrangements are more common in nonsmokers or light smokers and in those with adenocarcinomas. *ALK rearrangement may be detected by FISH.* OncoScan microarray analysis can't detect balanced rearrangements, such as inversion. The rest of the methods are used to detect single-nucleotide polymorphisms (SNPs) or small insertions/deletions (in/dels), but not chromosome rearrangements.

Therefore, FISH is most commonly used to detect ALK genetic alterations in patients with non-small cell lung cancer (NSCLC).

129. **B**. The highest response rates to EGFR-TKIs were seen in patients with somatic mutations within the EGFR-TK domain, particularly exon 19 deletions, exon 21 L858R, and exon 18 G719X. By contrast, *the exon 20 T790M mutation is associated with acquired resistance to TKI therapy.* Patients with sensitizing EGFR mutations eventually relapse on therapy, usually after an interval of approximately 1 year. On relapse, about 50% will have the c.2369C > T(p.Thr790Met) mutation in exon 20 of the EGFR gene.

Therefore, exon 20 of the EGFR gene would most likely be tested for resistance in this patient.

130. **B**. *Use of the EGFR-TKIs gefitinib (discontinued in the United States), erlotinib, and afatinib is limited to patients with adenocarcinomas who have known activating EGFR mutations.* Mutations in EGFR,

KRAS, and ALK are mutually exclusive in patients with nonsmall-cell lung cancer (NSCLC).

Therefore, a patient with a p.G12A mutation in KRAS would most likely NOT respond well to erlotinib.

131. **C**. Use of the EGFR-TKIs gefitinib (discontinued in the United States), erlotinib, and afatinib is limited to patients with adenocarcinomas who have known activating EGFR mutations. EGFR mutations and ALK rearrangement in nonsmall-cell lung cancer (NSCLC) are mutually exclusive. Therefore, a patient with a ALK rearrangement would most likely NOT response well to erlotinib.

132. **B**. Mutations in BRAF, GNA11, GNAQ, KIT, MEK1, and NRAS can be found in approximately 70% of all melanomas. *Approximately 50% of melanomas harbor activating BRAF mutations. Inhibitors for BRAF have been developed specific to the oncogenic BRAF mutation V600E (c.1799T > A, or p.Val600Glu).*

Therefore, her tumor sample should be tested for this mutation in order to determine whether this patient is eligible for the BRAF inhibitor therapy.

133. **A**. FRET (Förster or fluorescence resonance energy transfer) is the nonradiative transfer of energy from an excited fluorophore (donor) to another fluorophore (acceptor). FRET occurs only when the molecules concerned are in very close proximity. This makes it a valuable technique for studying interactions between molecules, such as proteins, in solution or in cells. Exciting the donor and then monitoring the relative donor and acceptor emissions, either sequentially or simultaneously, makes it possible to determine when FRET has occurred.

In FRET, the fluorescent signal is detected only when the two probes are adjacent to each other. The signal is generated by using a wavelength that excites one probe's fluorophore and by detecting the fluorophore of the other probe. Fluorescence will be detected only if the two probes are adjacent and in the proper orientation for the excitation. And emission of the first probe's fluorophore, which excited the second probe's fluorophore, in turn emitting the light that is detected.

Melting curve analysis is an assessment of the dissociation characteristics of double-stranded DNA during heating. As the temperature is raised, the double strand begins to dissociate, leading to a rise in the absorbance intensity, hyperchromicity. The temperature at which 50% of DNA is denatured is known as the melting point. As the temperature increases, the sensor probe is eventually no longer able to hybridize to the target, and the fluorescence is lost. Since both the sensor and anchor probes were 100% match with the wild-type *BRAF* sequence, *the sensor probe melts off the wild-type sequence at a higher temperature than that for the c.1799T > A(p.V600E) mutation.*

Therefore, the melting temperature is higher in wild type BRAF sequence than heterozygous mutant.

134. **F.** Approximately 50% of melanomas harbor activating *BRAF* mutations. Among the *BRAF* mutations observed in melanoma, over 90% are at codon 600, and among these, over 90% are a single-nucleotide mutation resulting in substitution of glutamic acid for valine (*BRAF* V600E: nucleotide 1799 T > A; codon GTG > GAG). So about 45% of patients have *BRAF* V600E, while 59% have wild type.

Therefore, it would be most likely that this patient does not have a *BRAF* mutation (wild type).

135. **C.** *BRAF* is a serine/threonine protein kinase, encoded on chromosome 7q34, that activates the MAP kinase/ERK-signaling pathway. Approximately 50% of melanomas harbor activating *BRAF* mutations. *Among the BRAF mutations observed in melanoma, over 90% are at codon 600, and among these, over 90% are a single-nucleotide mutation resulting in substitution of glutamic acid for valine (BRAF V600E: nucleotide 1799 T > A; codon GT > GAG).* The second most common mutation is *BRAF* V600K substituting lysine for valine, that represents 5%–6% (GTG > AAG), followed by *BRAF* V600R (GTG > AGG), an infrequent two-nucleotide variation of the predominant mutation, *BRAF* V600 "E2" (GTG > GAA), and *BRAF* V600D (GTG > GAT). The prevalence of *BRAF* V600K has been reported as higher in some populations.

Therefore, the patient most likely have the *BRAF* V600E mutation.

136. **B.** Melting curve analysis is an assessment of the dissociation characteristics of double-stranded DNA during heating. As the temperature is raised, the double strand begins to dissociate, leading to a rise in the absorbance intensity, hyperchromicity. The temperature at which 50% of DNA is denatured is known as the melting point. The absence of the wild-type *BRAF* signal may have been caused by amplification of the mutant *BRAF* sequence or by loss of the wild-type *BRAF* sequence. Both are possibilities in melanoma. Inhibitors for *BRAF* have been developed specific to the oncogenic *BRAF* mutation V600E (c.1799T > A, or p.Val600Glu). The melting temperature indicated the presence of *BRAF* V600E. There is no need for Sanger confirmation.

Therefore, it would be appropriate to interpret the results as "A V600E mutation was identified in this specimen" instead of specifying heterozygous or homozygous states of the mutation.

137. **B.** In FRET, the fluorescent signal is detected only when the two probes are adjacent to each other. The signal is generated by using a wavelength that excites one probe's fluorophore and by detecting the fluorophore of the other probe. Fluorescence will be detected only if the two probes are adjacent and in the proper orientation for the excitation. And emission of the first probe's fluorophore, which excited the second probe's fluorophore, in turn emitting the light that is detected.

Melting-curve analysis is an assessment of the dissociation characteristics of double-stranded DNA during heating. As the temperature is raised, the double strand begins to dissociate, leading to a rise in the absorbance intensity, hyperchromicity. The temperature at which 50% of DNA is denatured is known as the melting point. As the temperature increases, the sensor probe is eventually no longer able to hybridize to the target and the fluorescence is lost. An abnormal melting curve with a wild-type probe may not be 100% specific for the mutation in question. A change in melting temperature from wild type could also represent another change underneath the probe region. In the case, it may detect other variant, such as V600K and V600D, instead of V600E.

Therefore, Sanger sequencing analysis may be used to confirm the mutation, identified by FRET, if the melting temperature is different from the ones for both wild type and the V600E mutation.

138. **B.** Germline mutations in the *BRAF* gene are associated with cardiofaciocutaneous syndrome, a disease characterized by heart defects, mental retardation, and a distinctive facial appearance. Acquired mutations in this gene have also been associated with various malignancies, including non-Hodgkin lymphoma, colorectal cancer, malignant melanoma, thyroid carcinoma, nonsmall-cell lung carcinoma, and adenocarcinoma of the lung. A pseudogene, which is located on chromosome X, has been identified for this gene (http://www.genecards.org/).

The most common mutation that causes Ewing sarcoma involves two genes, the *EWSR1* gene on chromosome 22 and the *FLI1* gene on chromosome 11. A rearrangement (translocation) of genetic material between chromosomes 22 and 11, written as t(11;22), fuses part of the *EWSR1* gene with part of the *FLI1* gene, creating the *EWSR1/FLI1* fusion gene (http://ghr.nlm.nih.gov/).

Therefore, acquired *BRAF* mutations are NOT common in Ewing sarcoma.

139. **C.** Somatic mutations in *BRAF* have been found in 37%−50% of all malignant melanomas. *BRAF* mutations are found in all melanoma subtypes but are most common in melanomas derived from skin without chronic sun-induced damage. In this category of melanoma, *BRAF* mutations are found in about 59% of samples. (http://www.mycancergenome.org/).

Therefore, about 45% of patients with malignant melanomas have somatic mutations in *BRAF*.

140. **A.** *Somatic mutations in BRAF are not specific for melanoma, and cannot be used for melanoma diagnosis,* as it is often seen in benign melanocytic nevi as well. However, testing for *BRAF* mutations had gained importance in predicting the response of melanoma patients to *BRAF* inhibitors. Vemurafenib and dabrafenib are *BRAF* kinase inhibitors available in the United States. Trametinib, a mitogen-activated extracellular signal regulated kinase (MEK) inhibitor, is also FDA-approved. Patients whose tumors harbored V600E and V600K mutations showed better responses to the MEK inhibitor, trametinib, than to chemotherapy. However, preclinical evidence demonstrates an effect against the V600D mutation.

Therefore, mutations in *BRAF* are NOT diagnostic for metastatic melanoma.

141. **B.** Dual-hybridization FRET probes will show a shift in melting temperature if there are small or single-base-pair mutations underneath the probe. So they are useful for screening or identification of point mutations or small insertion/deletions in either one specific base or a narrowly defined area, such as *BRAF* V600 mutations for melanoma. Large changes, such as deletions of a couple of exons in the *DMD* gene for Duchenne muscular dystrophy or the intron 22 inversion in *F8* for hemophilia A, may not hybridize with the probe, so the results would be interpreted as homozygous wild type. If FRET probes are to be used to screen for multiple mutations in different exons, such as *CEPBA*, multiple different probes will need to be created for each possible area that has a mutation. This may not be feasible or practical in a large gene with mutations scattered throughout.

Therefore, real-time PCR with FRET probes and melting-curve analysis are very useful to detect *BRAF* mutations for melanoma.

142. **A.** *BRAF* mutations are seen in melanoma as well as in benign melanocytic nevi. Therefore, *they can't be used to reliably diagnose a melanoma.* However, they do predict a response to *BRAF* inhibitor therapy, and can predict resistance to *EGFR* therapies in colorectal carcinoma, and predict more aggressive disease in papillary thyroid carcinoma. Mutations in *BRAF* can be used to rule out Lynch syndrome if a patient has colorectal cancer.

Therefore, a *BRAF* V600E mutation can NOT be used to diagnose metastatic melanoma.

143. **C.** *Use of the EGFR-TKIs gefitinib (discontinued in the United States), erlotinib, and afatinib is limited to patients with activating EGFR mutations.* Vemurafenib and dabrafenib are targeted drugs for patients with the *BRAF* V600E activating *mutation. EGFR, KRAS, BRAF,* and *ALK* mutations are mutually exclusive in patient with nonsmall-cell lung cancer (NSCLC). Mutations in *ALK, BRAF,* or *KRAS* do not respond to the *EGFR-TKI.* Therefore, erlotinib therapy can be used to patients with mutations in *EGFR* for non-small cell lung cancer (NSCLC).

144. **D.** *BRAF V600E mutation in the kinase domain appears in 40%−45% of papillary thyroid cancers,* followed by 30%−40% in anaplastic thyroid cancer. It also appears in 20%−40% of poorly differentiated thyroid cancer, but not common in follicular or medullary thyroid cancers.

Medullary thyroid cancer is common in multiple endocrine neoplasia type 2 (MEN2) caused by germline pathogenic variants in the *RET* gene. Follicular thyroid cancer is common in Cowden syndrome caused by germline pathogenic variants in the *PTEN* gene.

Therefore, the *BRAF* mutations most commonly seen in papillary thyroid cancer.

145. **C.** *BRAF V600E mutation in the kinase domain appears in 40%−45% of papillary thyroid cancers,* followed by 30%−40% in anaplastic thyroid cancer. It also appears in 20%−40% of poorly differentiated thyroid cancer, but not common in follicular or medullary thyroid cancers.

Therefore, about 45% of patients with papillary thyroid cancer have acquired mutations in *BRAF*.

146. **C.** *Medullary thyroid cancer* is common in multiple endocrine neoplasia type 2 (MEN2) caused by germline pathogenic variants in the *RET* gene.

BRAF V600E mutation in the kinase domain appears in 40%−45% of papillary thyroid cancers, followed by 30%−40% in anaplastic thyroid cancer. Follicular thyroid cancer is common in Cowden syndrome caused by germline pathogenic variants in the *PTEN* gene.

Therefore, patients with type 2 multiple endocrine neoplasia (MEN2) more likely have medullary thyroid cancer than other thyroid cancers listed in the questions.

147. **B.** *Follicular thyroid cancer* is common in Cowden syndrome caused by germline pathogenic variants in the *PTEN* gene.

Medullary thyroid cancer is common in multiple endocrine neoplasia type 2 (MEN2) caused by germline pathogenic variants in the *RET* gene. *BRAF* V600E mutation in the kinase domain appears in 40%—45% of papillary thyroid cancers, followed by 30%—40% in anaplastic thyroid cancer.

Therefore, patients with Cowden syndrome more likely have follicular thyroid cancer than other thyroid cancers listed in the questions.

148. **A.** Papillary thyroid cancer (PTC) is the most common malignancy of the thyroid gland, representing nearly 80% of all malignant thyroid cancers. *The BRAF V600E mutation is the most common genetic mutation detected in patients with papillary thyroid cancer (PTC).* It appears in 40%—45% of the papillary thyroid cancer. It rarely appears in lung cancer (1%—4% of nonsmall-cell lung cancers, especially adenocarcinoma). It is in about 50% of melanomas and 8%—15% of colorectal cancers. However, there is no history or indication of metastatic melanoma or metastatic colorectal cancer in this patient.

Therefore, detecting *BRAF* V600E would most likely confirm the patient had metastatic papillary thyroid cancer.

149. **E.** Mutations in *BRAF*, *EGFR*, and *KRAS*, and the *ML4-ALK* rearrangement are common and mutually exclusive in patients with nonsmall-cell lung cancer (NSCLC). *NRAS* mutations are rare in NSCLC.

Therefore, negative finding on *NRAS* would indicate that the patient most likely did not have lung cancer.

150. **E.** *RAS (HRAS, KRAS, and NRAS) mutations are identified in 40%—50% of follicular thyroid carcinomas, 10%—20% of papillary thyroid carcinomas, and 20%—40% of poorly differentiated and anaplastic thyroid carcinomas.*

Follicular thyroid cancer is also common in patients with Cowden syndrome with *PTEN* mutations. Medullary thyroid cancer is common in multiple endocrine neoplasia type 2 (MEN2) caused by germline pathogenic variants in the *RET* gene. *BRAF* and *EGFR* gene mutations are not common in follicular or medullary thyroid cancers. Mutations in *ALK* or *KIT* are not common in thyroid cancers.

Therefore, *RAS (HRAS, KRAS,* and *NRAS)* is more likely mutated in follicular thyroid cancers as somatic mutations than other genes listed in this question.

151. **C.** Gastrointestinal stromal tumors (GISTs) are the most common mesenchymal neoplasms of the gastrointestinal tract. GISTs arise in the smooth muscle pacemaker interstitial cell of Cajal or similar cells. They are defined as tumors whose behavior is driven by *mutations in the KIT gene* (85%), *PDGFRA* gene (10%), or *BRAF* kinase (<1%). 95% of GISTs stain positively for *KIT* (CD117). Mutations in KIT activate tyrosine kinase activity in the absence of extracellular stimulator.

Imatinib, also called Gleevec, is a tyrosine kinase inhibitor. It has been used in the treatment of multiple cancers, such as Philadelphia chromosome—positive (Ph +) chronic myelogenous leukemia (CML) and GIST. A subset of GISTs contain mutations in the homologous kinase platelet-derived growth factor receptor alpha (*PDGFRA*), and the most common of these mutations is resistant to imatinib in vitro.

Therefore, it was most likely the *KIT* gene harbored an acquired pathogenic variant related to the response to imatinib if there was one in this patient.

152. **A.** Gastrointestinal stromal tumors (GISTs) are the most common mesenchymal neoplasms of the gastrointestinal tract. GISTs arise in the smooth muscle pacemaker interstitial cell of Cajal or similar cells. They are defined as tumors whose behavior is driven by mutations in the *KIT* gene (85%), *PDGFRA* gene (10%), or *BRAF* kinase (rare). 95% of GISTs stain positively for *KIT* (CD117).

Therefore, about 85% of patients with gastrointestinal stromal tumors (GISTs) have acquired mutations in *KIT*.

153. **E.** Gastrointestinal stromal tumors (GISTs) are the most common mesenchymal neoplasms of the gastrointestinal tract. GISTs arise in the smooth muscle pacemaker interstitial cell of Cajal or similar cells. They are defined as tumors whose behavior is driven by mutations in the *KIT* gene (85%), *PDGFRA* gene (10%), or *BRAF* kinase (rare). And 95% of GISTs stain positively for *KIT* (CD117).

Therefore, about 10% of patients with gastrointestinal stromal tumors (GISTs) have acquired mutations in *PDGFRA*.

154. **B.** The vast majority of *KIT* mutations in gastrointestinal stromal tumors (GISTs) are found *in exon 11 (juxtamembrane domain; about 70%)*, exon 9 (extracellular dimerization motif; 10%—15%), exon 13 (tyrosine kinase 1 domain; 1%—3%), and exon 17 (tyrosine kinase 2 domain and activation loop; 1%—3%). Secondary *KIT* mutations in exons 13, 14, 17, and 18 are commonly identified in biopsy specimens after imatinib treatment, after patients have developed acquired resistance (http://www.mycancergenome.org/).

Therefore, the acquired pathogenic variant in this patient would most likely be located in exon 11 of the *KIT* gene.

155. **D**. Gastrointestinal stromal tumors (GISTs) are the most common mesenchymal neoplasms of the gastrointestinal tract. GISTs arise in the smooth muscle pacemaker interstitial cell of Cajal or similar cells. They are defined as tumors whose behavior is driven by mutations in the *KIT* gene (85%), *PDGFRA* gene (5%–10%), or *BRAF* kinase (rare) (http://www.mycancergenome.org).

Therefore, the *PDGFRA* gene would most likely be analyzed in the reflex test in order to further assess the prognosis, since the mutation analysis of *KIT* was negative.

156. **G**. Gastrointestinal stromal tumors (GISTs) are defined as tumors whose behavior is driven by mutations in the *KIT* gene (85%), *PDGFRA* gene (5%–10%), or *BRAF* kinase (<1%). Mutations of *KIT*, *PDGFRA*, and *BRAF* are mutually exclusive of one another. *In GIST PDGFRA mutations are found mostly in exons 18 (the tyrosine kinase 2 [TK2] domain, 5%)*, exon 12 (juxtamembrane domain; 1%) and 14 (tyrosine kinase 1 [TK1] domain; <1%). Mutations except for D842V in exon 18 are sensitive to imatinib (http://www.mycancergenome.org).

Therefore, it was most likely that an acquired pathogenic variant in the *PDGFRA* gene was located in exon 18 in this patient.

157. **A**. Gastrointestinal stromal tumors (GISTs) are defined as tumors whose behavior is driven by mutations in the *KIT* gene (85%), *PDGFRA* gene (5%–10%), or *BRAF* kinase (<1%). Mutations in exon 11 are in 70% of *KIT*-mutated GISTs. As compared to patients with *KIT* exon 9 mutations and wild-type GIST, patients with exon 11 mutations have a worse relapse-free survival and overall survival. However, *their tumors have the highest sensitivity to imatinib, with a median duration of benefit of approximately 23 months.* Patients with exon 11 mutations are less likely to respond to second-line sunitinib (http://www.mycancergenome.org).

Therefore, the patient will respond well to imatinib.

158. **D**. *KIT* mutations in *exon 14* are generally found as secondary mutations in progressing or refractory GIST. *KIT exon 13 or 17* mutations have also been identified as primary mutations in a small percentage of patients with some responses, but the response is not as good as with mutations in exon 11. In vitro studies suggest that *KIT* double mutants in exon 13/17 are resistant to both imatinib and sunitinib (http://www.mycancergenome.org).

Therefore, it would be most likely that an acquired mutation in exon 13, 14, or 17 of the *KIT*

gene was responsible for the imatinib resistance in this patient.

159. **A**. Mutations in exon 11 are in 70% of *KIT*-mutated GISTs. Patients with exon 11 mutations have the highest sensitivity to imatinib. As compared to patients with *KIT* exon 11 mutations, *patients with exon 9 mutations show intermediate sensitivity to imatinib. A high dose of imatinib is usually required.* The median duration of benefit from imatinib is approximately 7–12 months, as compared to 23 months for patients with exon 11 mutations. As compared to patients with *KIT* exon 11 mutations, patients with exon 9 mutations have a better relapse-free survival and overall survival. Patients with exon 9 mutations are more likely to respond to second-line sunitinib than patients with other *KIT*/*PDGFRA* mutations (http://www.mycancergenome.org).

Therefore, exon 9 of the *KIT* gene would most likely harbor the mutation in this patient if she has one predicted to responsive to high-dose imatinib therapy.

160. **E**. *1p and 19q abnormalities are observed in about 80% of oligodendrogliomas,* 50%–60% of anaplastic oligodendrogliomas and 30%–50% of oligoastrocytomas and anaplastic oligoastrocytomas. *EGFR* amplification is associated with glioblastoma. And *EGFR* amplification and loss of 1p/19q are mutually exclusive.

Therefore, 1p/19q status represents a reliable marker of biological behavior, and testing for 1p/19q is now considered the standard of care.

161. **B**. *Loss of 1p and 19q is observed in about 80% of oligodendrogliomas,* 50%–60% of anaplastic oligodendrogliomas, and 30%–50% of oligoastrocytomas and anaplastic oligoastrocytomas. Numerous studies have shown an association between *1p/19q codeletion* and a favorable response to chemotherapy, including to procarbazine, lomustine, vincristine, and temozolomide, as well as to radiotherapy. Oligodendrogliomas with 1p/19q also have significantly better progression-free survival and overall survival (http://www.mycancergenome.org).

Therefore, it would be most likely the patient had 1p/19q codeletion.

162. **B**. *Loss of 1p and 19q is observed in about 80% of oligodendrogliomas,* 50%–60% of anaplastic oligodendrogliomas, and 30%–50% of oligoastrocytomas and anaplastic oligoastrocytomas.

Therefore, the 1p/19 co-deletion appear in about 80% of patients with oligodendroglioma.

163. **E**. Loss of 1p and 19q is observed in about 80% of oligodendrogliomas, 50%–60% of anaplastic

oligodendrogliomas, and 30%–50% of oligoastrocytomas and anaplastic oligoastrocytomas. Numerous studies have shown an association between 1p/19q codeletion and a favorable response to chemotherapy, including to procarbazine, lomustine, vincristine, and temozolomide, as well as to radiotherapy. Oligodendrogliomas with 1p/19q also have significantly *better progression-free survival and overall survival*. So 1p/19q status thus represents a reliable marker of biological behavior, and testing for 1p/19q loss is now considered the standard of care (http://www.mycancergenome.org).

Loss of 1p alone is also associated with good response to adjuvant therapy. *Isolated 19q loss can be seen in astrocytic tumors, where it is not associated with response to therapy.*

Therefore, loss 19q alone is NOT associated with a favorable response to chemotherapy.

164. **E.** Loss of 1p and 19q is observed in about 80% of *oligodendrogliomas*, 50%–60% of anaplastic oligodendrogliomas, and 30%–50% of oligoastrocytoma and anaplastic oligoastrocytomas.

165. **B.** In glioblastoma multiforme (GBM), the frequency of O^6-*methylguanine-DNA methyltransferase (MGMT) promoter methylation was 45%*. Irrespective of treatment, *MGMT* promoter methylation was an independent favorable prognostic factor. Among patients whose tumor contained a methylated *MGMT* promoter, a survival benefit was observed in patients treated with temozolomide and radiotherapy. The median survival was 22 months for patients with both temozolomide and radiotherapy, as compared with 15 months among those who were assigned to only radiotherapy.

EGFR gene amplification and overexpression are particularly striking features of GBM, observed in approximately 40% of tumors. In approximately 50% of tumors with *EGFR* amplification, a specific *EGFR* mutant (EGFRvIII, also known as *EGFR* type III, del2–7, ∆EGFR) can be detected. Multivariate analysis demonstrated that *EGFR* amplification was an independent, significant, unfavorable predictor for overall survival (OS). *BRAF* mutations are not common in brain tumors. Loss of 1p and 19q is observed in about 80% of oligodendrogliomas, 50%–60% of anaplastic oligodendrogliomas, and 30%–50% of oligoastrocytomas and anaplastic oligoastrocytomas. Gastrointestinal stromal tumors (GISTs) are driven by mutations in the *KIT* gene (85%), *PDGFRA* gene (10%), or *BRAF* kinase (rare) (http://www.mycancergenome.org).

Therefore, *MGMT* promoter methylation study would be appropriate for the diagnosis and estimation of prognosis and therapy of GBM in this patient.

166. **B.** In glioblastoma (glioblastoma multiforme; GBM; WHO Grade IV), the frequency of *MGMT* promoter methylation was 45% and the frequency of *EGFR* gene amplification/overexpression was observed in approximately 40% of tumors. In approximately 50% of tumors with *EGFR* amplification, a specific *EGFR* mutant (EGFRvIII, also known as *EGFR* type III, del2–7, ∆EGFR) can be detected. Multivariate analysis demonstrated that *EGFR amplification was an independent, significant, unfavorable predictor for overall survival (OS)* (http://www.mycancergenome.org).

BRAF mutations are not common in brain tumors. Loss of 1p and 19q is observed in about 80% of oligodendrogliomas, 50%–60% of anaplastic oligodendrogliomas, and 30%–50% of oligoastrocytomas and anaplastic oligoastrocytomas. Gastrointestinal stromal tumors (GISTs) are driven by mutations in the *KIT* gene (85%), *PDGFRA* gene (10%), or *BRAF* kinase (rare).

Therefore, *EGFR* gene amplification study would be appropriate for the diagnosis and estimation of prognosis and therapy of GBM in this patient.

167. **D.** In glioblastoma multiforme (GBM), the frequency of *MGMT* promoter methylation was 45%. Irrespective of treatment, *MGMT promoter methylation was an independent favorable prognostic factor*. Among patients whose tumor contained a methylated *MGMT* promoter, a survival benefit was observed in patients treated with temozolomide and radiotherapy. The median survival was 22 months for patients with both temozolomide and radiotherapy, as compared with 15 months among those who were assigned to only radiotherapy (http://www.mycancergenome.org).

Therefore, promoter of the *MGMT* gene would most likely be investigated in this patient.

168. **C.** In glioblastoma multiforme (GBM), the frequency of *MGMT promoter methylation* was 45%. Irrespective of treatment, *MGMT* promoter methylation was an independent favorable prognostic factor. Methylation-specific PCR is the most common technique used to detect *MGMT* promoter methylation.

Fluorescence in situ hybridization (FISH) testing is used widely in genetics laboratories to test for targeted-chromosome copy-number gain or loss, such as 22q11.2 deletion for velocardiofacial (VCF)/DiGeorge syndrome. The deletion for VCF/DiGeorge syndrome usually encompasses approximately 3 Mb. Methylation study is used to identify epigenetic changes in the genome, such as testing the imprinting center for Prader–Willi/Angelman syndromes. Sequencing analysis included Sanger sequencing, so-called first-generation sequencing, and next-generation sequencing (NGS). NGS is a high-throughput test to sequence multiple genes at the same time, such as more than 15 genes for Fanconi anemia. Sanger sequencing is still the most appropriate molecular test for single-gene disorders when the most pathogenic variants are single-nucleotide variants and in/dels, such as mutation analysis in the *CEBPA* gene for acute myeloid leukemia (AML). TaqMan genotyping assay has been used to detect biallelic single-nucleotide polymorphism (SNP) markers, such as C282Y in *HFE* for hereditary hemochromatosis.

Therefore, methylation study is the most appropriate assay for this patient to detect *MGMT* promoter methylation.

169. **B**. In glioblastoma (glioblastoma multiforme; GBM; WHO Grade IV), the frequency of O^6-methylguanine-DNA methyltransferase (MGMT) promoter methylation was 45%, and the frequency of *EGFR* gene amplification/overexpression was observed in approximately 40% of tumors.

BRAF mutations are not common in brain tumors. Loss of 1p and 19q is observed in about 80% of oligodendrogliomas, 50%–60% of anaplastic oligodendrogliomas, and 30%–50% of oligoastrocytomas and anaplastic oligoastrocytomas. Gastrointestinal stromal tumors (GISTs) are driven by mutations in the *KIT* gene (85%), *PDGFRA* gene (10%), or *BRAF* kinase (rare).

Therefore, *EGFR* amplification would most likely be tested when the *MGMT* genetic test was negative in this patient.

170. **A**. In glioblastoma (glioblastoma multiforme; GBM; WHO Grade IV) the frequency of O^6-methylguanine-DNA methyltransferase (MGMT) promoter methylation was 45%, and the frequency of *EGFR* gene amplification/overexpression was observed in approximately 40% of tumors.

Therefore, an *EGFR* assay would most likely be designed to detect *EGFR* gene amplification/overexpression in this patient.

171. **B**. Glioblastoma (glioblastoma multiforme; GBM; WHO Grade IV) accounts for the majority of primary malignant brain tumors in adults. In GBM, the frequency of *MGMT* promoter

methylation was 45%, and *the frequency of EGFR gene amplification/overexpression was observed in approximately 40% of tumors.* In approximately 50% of tumors with *EGFR* amplification, a specific *EGFR* mutant (EGFRvIII, also known as *EGFR* type III, del2–7, ΔEGFR) can be detected. Multivariate analysis demonstrated that *EGFR* amplification was an independent, significant, unfavorable predictor for overall survival (OS) (http://www.mycancergenome.org).

Chromosome karyotype is used to detect chromosome rearrangements and large gains/losses in the genome, such as t(9;22) for chronic myeloid leukemia (CML). Fluorescence in situ hybridization (FISH) testing is used widely in genetics laboratories to test for targeted chromosome copy-number gain or loss, such as 22q11.2 deletion for velocardiofacial (VCF)/DiGeorge syndrome. The deletion for VCF/DiGeorge syndrome usually encompasses approximately 3 Mb. Methylation study is used to identify epigenetic changes in the genome, such as testing the imprinting center for Prader–Willi/Angelman syndromes. Sequencing analysis included Sanger sequencing, so-called first-generation sequencing, and next-generation sequencing (NGS). NGS is a high-throughput test to sequence multiple genes at the same time, such as more than 15 genes for Fanconi anemia. Sanger sequencing is still the most appropriate molecular test for single-gene disorders when the most pathogenic variants are single-nucleotide variants and in/dels, such as mutation analysis in the *CEBPA* gene for acute myeloid leukemia (AML). TaqMan genotyping assay has been used to detect biallelic single-nucleotide polymorphism (SNP) markers, such as C282Y in *HFE* for hereditary hemochromatosis.

Therefore, FISH would the standard testing method for this genetic alteration in this patient.

172. **B**. In glioblastoma multiforme (GBM), the frequency of *MGMT* promoter methylation was 45%. Irrespective of treatment, *MGMT* promoter methylation was an independent favorable prognostic factor. Among patients whose tumor contained a methylated *MGMT* promoter, *a survival benefit was observed in patients treated with temozolomide and radiotherapy.* The median survival was 22 months for patients with both temozolomide and radiotherapy, as compared with 15 months among those who were assigned to only radiotherapy (http://www.mycancergenome.org).

Methylation-specific PCR is the most common technique used to detect *MGMT* promoter

8. ONCOLOGY—ACQUIRED

methylation. Sodium bisulfite is used to treat the DNA sample from the tumor. The net effect is a substitution of uracils in the place of unmethylated cytosines, while methylated cytosines remain. This difference in sequence between methylated and unmethylated DNA can then be detected by downstream applications. So the methylated *MGMT* promoter will be resistant to the bisulfite conversion.

Therefore, this patient would be respond well to the alkylating therapy and radiotherapy.

173. E. *EGFR gene amplification has been related to decrease overall survival and resistance of glioblastoma multiforme (GBM) cells toward radiation and chemotherapy.* Currently, FISH is the standard testing method for this genetic alteration.

Therefore, the overall survival of this patient would be poor because of the *EGFR* gene amplification.

174. C. Bisulfite modification is a principle tool for analyzing DNA methylation. Sodium bisulfite *deaminates cytosine into uracil,* but it does not affect 5-methylcytosine.

Therefore, sodium bisulfite treatment for methylation study leads to C > U changes in the *MGMT* genetic analysis.

175. D. It is not uncommon to see amplification of both methylated and unmethylated *MGMT* promoter sequences in the same specimen, which may represent tumor-cell heterogeneity with mixtures of hypermethylated and unmethylated *MGMT* promoters or the presence of nonneoplastic cells such as lymphocytes, vascular endothelial cells, and macrophages. In addition, incomplete conversion of nonmethylated cytosine may appear as "methylated" DNA.

Therefore, all of the reasons listed in the question may might result in a pattern of partial methylation in the glioblastoma specimen from this patient.

176. B. *ALK* mutations are found in 8%–9% of patients with neuroblastoma. *Point mutations of ALK predominate in neuroblastoma.*

ALK fusions are found in anaplastic large-cell lymphoma [*t(2;5)(p23;q35) NPM1/ALK* in approximately 50% of patients], colorectal cancer, inflammatory myofibroblastic tumor, nonsmall-cell lung cancer [inv(2)(p21p23) *EML4/ALK* in 4%–5% of patients, *ALK* amplification], and ovarian cancer. All *ALK* fusions contain the entire ALK tyrosine kinase domain. To date, those tested biologically possess oncogenic activity in vitro and in vivo. *ALK* fusions and copy number gains have been observed in renal-cell carcinoma. Finally, *ALK* copy number and protein expression aberrations have also been observed in rhabdomyosarcoma (http://www.mycancergenome.org).

Therefore, c.3520T > A (p.F1174I) in *ALK* is more likely seen in patients with neuroblastoma than the others listed in the question.

177. E. *ALK* fusion is seen in 50%–85% of anaplastic large-cell lymphomas (ALCLs). In 72%–85% of these *ALK*-positive ALCLs, a t(2;5)(p23;q35) translocation resulting in *NPM1-ALK* fusion has been found. In the remaining 15%–28% of the partners include *TPM3, TPM4, TFG, ATIC, CLTC, MSN, MYH9,* and *ALO17. ALK*-positive ALCL has a better prognosis than *ALK*-negative ALCL, and it is diagnosed more frequently in younger patients (http://www.mycancergenome.org).

Point mutations of *ALK* predominate in neuroblastoma. Inv(2)(p21p23) *EML4-ALK* in 4%–5% of patients with nonsmall-cell lung cancer (NSCLC), colorectal cancer, inflammatory myofibroblastic tumor, and ovarian cancer. *ALK* amplification is a poor prognostic marker in patients with NSCLC and colon cancer.

Therefore, t(2;5)(p23;q35) involving *ALK* is more likely seen in patients with anaplastic large cell lymphoma than the others listed in the question.

178. D. *MYCN* amplification is present in about 20% of all cases of *neuroblastoma.* Amplification of *MYCN* is associated with advanced stages of disease, unfavorable biological features, and a poor outcome. In addition, ploidy, 11q, 1p, and 17q gain chromosomal statuses are important in assigning risk. Most recently, *ALK* mutations in neuroblastoma have been identified (http://www.mycancergenome.org).

MYCN amplification is less common in medulloblastoma, rhabdomyosarcoma, and Wilms tumor. Therefore, a *MYCN* amplification is most likely associated with neuroblastoma.

179. C. *MYCN amplification* is present in about 20% of all cases of *neuroblastoma,* but not c-*MYC* amplification. *MYCN* is located on 2p24.3, while c-*MYC* is located in 8q24.21. Amplification of *MYCN* is associated with advanced stages of neuroblastoma, unfavorable biological features, and a poor outcome. In addition, deletions of 1p and 11q are highly recurrent and are associated with a poor prognosis. Most recently, *ALK* mutations in neuroblastoma have been identified (approximately 7%). Development of targeted therapeutics has focused on *ALK* (http://www.mycancergenome.org).

Therefore, N-*MYC* amplification would more likely be detected in this patient than the others listed in the question.

180. D. Approximately 3%–7% of lung tumors harbor *ALK* fusions. *ALK* fusions are more commonly found in light smokers (<10 pack-years) and/or never-smokers. Multiple different *ALK* rearrangements have been described in nonsmall-cell lung cancer (NSCLC). The majority of these *ALK* fusion variants are comprised of portions of the echinoderm microtubule associated protein-like 4 (*EML4*) gene with the *ALK* gene, or *inv(2)(p23p21)* (http://www.mycancergenome.org).

Therefore, inv(2)(p21p23) involving *ALK* is more likely seen in patients with non-small cell lung cancer (NSCLC) than others listed in the question.

181. E. Acquired *EGFR* mutations are present in 10%–15% of patients with nonsmall-cell lung carcinoma (NSCLC) in the United States. Tumors with *EGFR* mutations occur at a higher frequency in East Asians than in non-Asians (30% vs. 8%), in women than in men (59% vs. 26%), in never-smokers than in ever-smokers (66% vs. 22%), and in adenocarcinomas (ADCs) than in other NSCLC histologies (49% vs. 2%). The two most common *EGFR* mutations are located in *exon 19* and exon 21. Gefitinib and erlotinib are the first generation of *EGFR* tyrosine kinase inhibitors (TKIs), which selectively target the intracellular tyrosine kinase domain of *EGFR*, blocking the downstream signaling of the receptor (http://www.mycancergenome.org).

Therefore, exon 19 of the *EGFR* gene would most likely be investigated in this molecular battery test for NSCLC.

182. D. Acquired *EGFR* mutations are present in 10%–15% of patients with nonsmall-cell lung carcinoma (NSCLC) in the United States. Gefitinib and erlotinib are the first generation of *EGFR* tyrosine kinase inhibitors (TKIs). The two most common *EGFR* mutations are located in exon 19 and *exon 21*.

Therefore, exon 21 of the *EGFR* gene would most likely be investigated in this molecular battery test for NSCLC in this patient.

183. B. Acquired *EGFR* mutations are present in 10%–15% of patients with nonsmall-cell lung carcinoma (NSCLC) in the United States. The two most common *EGFR* mutations are located in exon 19 and exon 21. *The one in exon 19 is a short in-frame deletion.*

Therefore, it was most likely this patient had a short in-frame in/del in exon 19 of the *EGFR* gene.

184. D. Acquired *EGFR* mutations are present in 10%–15% of patients with nonsmall-cell lung carcinoma (NSCLC) in the United States. The two most common *EGFR* mutations are located in

exon 19 and exon 21. *The one in exon 21 is a point mutation (CTG to CGG) at nucleotide 2573 that results in substitution of leucine by arginine at codon 858 (L858R).*

Therefore, it was most likely that this patient had a point mutation in exon 21 of the *EGFR* gene.

185. C. Acquired *EGFR* mutations are present in 10%–15% of patients with nonsmall-cell lung carcinoma (NSCLC) in the United States. The American Society of Clinical Oncology recommends *EGFR* mutation testing for patients with advanced NSCLC of the lung who are being considered for first-line therapy with an *EGFR* TKI.

Therefore, detection of the acquired change in the *EGFR* gene would have implications for treatment decisions for this patient.

186. C. Gefitinib and erlotinib are the first generation of *EGFR* tyrosine kinase inhibitors (TKIs), which selectively target the intracellular tyrosine kinase domain of *EGFR*, blocking the downstream signaling of the receptor. *The c.2396C > T(p.T790M) mutation in the exon 20 of the EGFR gene* is associated with acquired resistance to erlotinib/gefitinib (*EGFR* TKI) (http://www.mycancergenome.org).

Therefore, exon 20 of the *EGFR* gene would most likely be investigated for the resistance in this patient.

187. C. The c.2396C > T(p.T790M) mutation in exon 20 of the *EGFR* gene or *amplification of c-MET* is associated with acquired resistance to erlotinib/gefitinib (*EGFR* TKI).

The *c-MET* gene encodes a receptor tyrosine kinase—hepatocyte growth factor receptor (HGFR). Like other receptor tyrosine kinases, it is involved in signal transduction and mediates cell growth. A common mechanism of activation of *c-MET* in nonsmall-cell lung carcinoma (NSCLC) is through amplification of *c-MET*. The *c-MET* gene amplification is occasionally observed in specimens before treatment with targeted therapy. However, a significant proportion of patients who develop acquired resistance to *EGFR* TKIs will have evidence of *c-MET* amplification on a resistance rebiopsy. The *c-MET* gene amplification has been shown to result in resistance to *EGFR* TKIs in vitro (http://www.mycancergenome.org).

ALK amplification is associated with colorectal carcinoma, NSCLC, and neuroblastoma. *EGFR* amplification is associated with glioblastoma. *MYCN* amplification is present in about 20% of all cases of neuroblastoma. *RUNX1* duplication/amplification has been reported in AML.

Therefore, amplification of *c-MET* would most likely be investigated for the resistance in this patient.

188. **D.** A rearrangement in the *ALK* gene, most commonly resulting in an *EML4-ALK* fusion gene, is present in approximately 5% of nonsmall-cell lung carcinoma (NSCLC). Identification of patients with this rearrangement is of key importance, owing to the availability of crizotinib, a newly approved targeted therapy with activity against the kinases of the products of *ALK*, *ROS1*, and *MET* genes. The *EML4* gene is located on 2p21, and the *ALK* gene is located on 2p23.

ALK amplification is associated with NSCLC, too, but not as common as the inv(2)(p23p21). *EGFR* amplification is associated with glioblastoma. *MYCN* amplification is present in about 20% of all cases of neuroblastoma. *RUNX1* duplication/amplification has been reported in AML.

Therefore, the *EML4-ALK* fusion gene caused by an inversion would more likely be investigated than the others for therapy.

189. **B.** A rearrangement in the *ALK* gene, most commonly resulting in an *EML4-ALK* fusion gene, is present in approximately 5% of nonsmall-cell lung carcinoma (NSCLC). Identification of patients with this rearrangement is of key importance, owing to the availability of crizotinib, a newly approved targeted therapy with activity against the kinases of the products of *ALK*, *ROS1*, and *MET* genes. The *EML4* gene is located on 2p21, and the *ALK* gene is located on 2p23.

Chromosome karyotype is used to detect chromosome rearrangements, and large gains/losses, such as t(9;22) for chronic myeloid leukemia (CML). Fluorescence in situ hybridization (FISH) testing is used widely in genetics laboratories to test for targeted chromosome regions, such as 22q11.2 deletion for velocardiofacial (VCF)/DiGeorge syndrome, or the *EML4-ALK* rearrangement. Methylation study is used to identify epigenetic changes in the genome, such as detecting *MGMT* promoter methylation for gastrointestinal stromal tumor (GIST). Reverse-transcriptase PCR (RT-PCR) may be used to detect the *EML4-ALK* fusion transcript. But the variation of the breakpoint decreases the detection rate of this method. Sequencing analysis included Sanger sequencing, so-called first-generation sequencing, and next-generation sequencing (NGS). NGS is a high-throughput test to sequence multiple genes at the same time, such as an acute myeloid leukemia panel with *ASXL1*, *CEBPA*, *DNMT3A*, *FLT3*, *NPM1*, *RUNX1*, *SF3B1*, and *WT1*. Sanger sequencing is still the most

appropriate molecular test for single-gene disorders when the most pathogenic variants are single-nucleotide variants and in/dels, such as detecting mutations in the *HBB* gene for beta thalassemia. TaqMan genotyping assay has been used to detect biallelic single-nucleotide polymorphism (SNP) markers, such as detecting the c.1138G > A(p.Gly380Arg) mutation in the *FGFR3* gene for achondroplasia.

Therefore, FISH analyses would most likely be used for the inv(2) involving *ALK* analysis in this case.

190. **A.** Mutations in *KRAS* are present in approximately 30% of pulmonary adenocarcinomas and 5% of pulmonary squamous-cell carcinomas. As with *EGFR* mutations, *KRAS* mutations are detected mainly in lung adenocarcinomas (ADCs) and are less frequently observed in squamous-cell carcinomas of the lung. By contrast, with lung ADCs harboring *EGFR* mutations, tumors with *KRAS* mutations are seen more frequently (20%– 30%) in Caucasian patients than in East Asian patients (5%). Also, compared with *EGFR* mutations, *KRAS* mutations are more common in current or former smokers than in never-smokers.

In lung cancers, *KRAS* mutations occur *primarily at codons 12 and 13 on exon 2*, and mutations at codon 61 in exon 3 are less frequently seen.

Therefore, it was most likely that exon 2 of the *KRAS* gene was investigated in this molecular battery test.

191. **D.** Mutations in *KRAS* are present in approximately 30% of pulmonary adenocarcinomas and 5% of pulmonary squamous-cell carcinomas.

In lung cancers, *KRAS* mutations occur primarily at codons 12 and 13 on exon 2, and mutations at codon 61 in exon 3 are less frequently seen. The most common *KRAS* mutation in smoking patients with NSCLC is *a G > T transition (84%) at codon 12 resulting in substitution of cysteine (47%), valine (24%), aspartate (15%), or alanine (7%) for wild-type glycine* (http://www.mycancergenome.org).

Therefore, it was most likely this patient had a point mutation in exon 2 of the *KRAS* gene.

192. **A.** Mutations in *KRAS* are present in approximately 30% of pulmonary adenocarcinomas and 5% of pulmonary squamous-cell carcinomas. In lung cancers, *KRAS* mutations occur primarily at codons 12 and 13 on

exon 2, and *mutations at codon 61 in exon 3* are less frequently seen.

Therefore, in addition to exon 2, exon 3 of the *KRAS* gene might also harbor acquired pathogenic variants for NSCLC.

193. **C.** Mutations in *KRAS* are present in approximately 30% of pulmonary adenocarcinomas and 5% of pulmonary squamous-cell carcinomas. The clinical implication of *KRAS* mutation detection is not clear, because the literature regarding the prognostic and predictive usefulness of this marker in nonsmall-cell lung carcinoma (NSCLC) is contradictory, and currently no approved therapeutic agents are available that target *KRAS*. However, presence of a *KRAS* mutation is predictive of resistance to anti-EGFR therapies, since the majority of the time the identification of a *KRAS* mutation is a strong negative predictor for identifying an additional aberration in either *EGFR* or *ALK* (http://www.mycancergenome.org).

Therefore, the identification of a *KRAS* mutation would have therapeutic value to this patient.

194. **C.** Missense mutations of the *BRAF* gene were found in approximately 60% of melanomas, 15% of colorectal cancers, and 3% of nonsmall-cell lung carcinoma (NSCLC). Mutations of *BRAF* were found predominantly in lung adenocarcinomas (ADCs) (97.3%), with approximately 57% being V600E and 43% being non-V600E. Researches have demonstrated the efficacy of the BRAF inhibitor in *BRAF* V600E mutant NSCLC (http://www.mycancergenome.org).

Therefore, the identification of a *BRAF* mutation would have therapeutic value to this patient.

195. **A.** *ALK* rearrangement, especially *EML4-ALK*, *BRAF* mutations, *EGFR* in frame deletions of exon 19, *EGFR* L858R mutation in exon 21, and *KRAS* mutations at codon 12 and 13 are all recurrent abnormalities in patients with nonsmall-cell lung carcinoma (NSCLC), and the presence of these changes appear to be mutually exclusive in NSCLC. *Mutations in the kinase domain of the ALK gene are associated with resistance to ALK tyrosine kinase inhibitor (TKI) therapy* (http://www.mycancergenome.org).

Therefore, detection of *ALK* mutations in the kinase domain would most likely NOT be included in this battery test.

196. **A.** *BRAF mutation is strongly associated with microsatellite instability (MSI).* In sporadic colorectal carcinomas (CRCs), *BRAF* mutation is seen in approximately 60% of MSI-high tumors and only 5%−10% of microsatellite-stable (MSS) tumors. *BRAF* V600E mutation results in hypermethylation of the *MLH1* gene promoter, resulting in loss of the tumor suppressor function and leading to diminished DNA mismatch repair. This occurs exclusive of the germline mismatch repair mutations seen in Lynch syndrome.

The other genes, such as *AKT1*, *KRAS*, *NKRAS*, *PIK3CA*, *PTEN*, and *SMAD4* are associated sporadic CRC without MSI-high. Therefore, *BRAF* is associated with high microsatellite instability (MSI) in colon cancer.

197. **C.** Approximately 36%−40% of patients with colorectal cancer (CRC) have tumor-associated *KRAS* mutations. The majority of the mutations occur at codons 12, 13, and 61 of the *KRAS* gene. The result of these mutations is activating *KRAS* signaling pathways. *KRAS mutated CRC was associated with poor disease-specific survival.*

Therefore, this patient would have poor prognosis owing to the acquired pathogenic variant in the *KRAS* gene.

198. **C.** Approximately 8%−15% of colorectal cancer (CRC) tumors harbor *BRAF* mutations. Both *BRAF* and *KRAS/NRAS* are in the Ras−Raf−MAPK pathway, downstream of epidermal growth factor receptor (EGFR). *BRAF* and *KRAS/NRAS* mutations are mutually exclusive in CRC. *Patients with BRAF mutant CRC have low response rates to conventional therapies and poor overall survival.* This is true for patients regardless of the stage at the time of diagnosis.

Therefore, this patient would have poor prognosis owing to the acquired pathogenic variant in the *BRAF* gene.

199. **B.** *BRAF V600E mutation results in hypermethylation of the MLH1 gene promoter*, resulting in loss of the tumor suppressor function and leading to diminished DNA mismatch repair. This occurs exclusive of the germline mismatch repair mutations seen in Lynch syndrome.

Therefore, this patient would most likely have an acquired pathogenic variant in the *BRAF* gene.

200. **E.** Mutations in *EGFR*, *KRAS*, and *BRAF* are mutually exclusive in patients with colorectal carcinomas (CRCs). *KRAS* mutations have been convincingly associated with poor response to cetuximab and panitumumab, anti-EGFR monoclonal antibodies (MoAbs). Activating mutations in *KRAS* serve to isolate this signaling pathway from the effects of *EGFR* and render *EGFR* inhibition ineffective. Advances have

shown that only tumors with wild-type *KRAS* show significant response to these agents. CRC patients with *KRAS* mutations do not respond to BRAF inhibitor either. There are no effective anti-KRAS inhibitors available (http://www.mycancergenome.org).

Therefore, none of the targeted therapies in the question would be appropriate for this patient.

201. **B**. Mutations in *EGFR*, *KRAS*, and *BRAF* are mutually exclusive in patients with colorectal carcinomas (CRCs). There are no effective anti-KRAS monoclonal antibodies available. Advances have shown that *only tumors with wild-type KRAS show significant response to anti-EGFR monoclonal antibodies (MoAbs, such as cetuximab and panitumumab)* (http://www.mycancergenome.org).

Therefore, anti-EGFR monoclonal antibodies (cetuximab and panitumumab) would most likely be appropriate for this patient.

202. **D**. *A rearrangement in the ALK gene, most commonly due to inv(2) resulting in an EML4-ALK fusion gene, is present in approximately 5% of nonsmall-cell lung carcinoma (NSCLC)*. Identification of patients with this rearrangement is of key importance, owing to the availability of crizotinib, a newly approved targeted therapy with activity against the kinases of the products of *ALK*, *ROS1*, and *MET* genes.

Next-generation sequencing (NGS) has recently emerged as an accurate, cost-effective method to identify mutations across numerous genes known to be associated with response or resistance to specific targeted therapies. Solid tumor targeted cancer gene panels by NGS may be used to assess common mutations in more than 50 genes known to be associated with cancer with formalin-fixed paraffin-embedded tissue (FFPE). Only approximately 200 ng of DNA is needed for an NGS. *NGS is a high-throughput method to detect point mutations and in/dels, but it cannot detect large single- or multiple-exon deletions/duplications, inversions, or translocations*. The results of NGS can be useful for assessing prognosis and guiding treatment of individuals with solid tumors; it can also be used to help determine clinical trial eligibility for patients with mutations in genes not amenable to current FDA-approved targeted therapies.

Therefore, an NGS panel for DNA analyses of solid tumor would not be able to detect an inv(2) rearrangement in the *ALK* gene.

203. **B**. Somatic mutations in *BRAF* have been found in 37%–50% of all malignant melanomas. The most prevalent *BRAF* mutations detected in melanoma are missense mutations that introduce an amino acid substitution at valine 600. Approximately 80%–90% of *BRAF* V600 mutations are *V600E*

(valine to glutamic acid) while 5%–12% are V600K (valine to lysine), and 5% or less are V600R (valine to arginine) or V600D (valine to aspartic acid). The result of these mutations is enhanced BRAF kinase activity and increased phosphorylation of downstream targets, particularly MEK. In the vast majority of cases, *BRAF* mutations are nonoverlapping with other oncogenic mutations found in melanoma, such as *NRAS* and *KIT* mutations.

Therefore, it would be most likely this patient had a *BRAF* V600E mutation.

204. **C**. The U.S. Food and Drug Administration (FDA) granted accelerated approval to trametinib (Mekinist tablets, GlaxoSmithKline, LLC) and dabrafenib (Tafinlar capsules, GlaxoSmithKline, LLC) for use in combination in the treatment of patients with unresectable or metastatic melanoma with a *BRAF* V600E or *V600K* mutation as detected by an FDA-approved test.

Therefore, *BRAF* V600K mutation would make the patient suitable for trametinib (Mekinist tablets, GlaxoSmithKline, LLC) and dabrafenib (Tafinlar capsules, GlaxoSmithKline, LLC) treatment besides V600E according to the FDA-approval.

205. **B**. Mutant *BRAF* has been implicated in the pathogenesis of several cancers, including melanoma, nonsmall-cell lung cancer, colorectal cancer, papillary thyroid cancer, hairy-cell leukemia, non-Hodgkin lymphoma, and ovarian cancer. *Mutant BRAF has been also observed in Langerhans-cell histiocytosis (LCH), glioblastoma, and gastrointestinal stromal tumor (GIST)*. Germline pathogenic variants in *BRAF* are associated with cardiofaciocutaneous (CFC) syndrome. *The BRAF V600E mutation has been identified in 25%–64% of cases of LCH*.

Therefore, it would be most likely this patient had a *BRAF* mutation.

206. **C**. The frequency of *BRAF* mutations varies widely in human cancers, from more than *80% in melanomas and nevi*, to 1%–3% in lung cancers and 5% in colorectal cancer. In 90% of the cases, thymine is substituted with adenine at nucleotide 1799 leading to valine (V) being substituted for by glutamate (E) at codon 600 (V600E). *BRAF* V600E is present in 57% of Langerhans-cell histiocytosis patients.

Therefore, patients with metastatic melanoma most likely have the *BRAF* V600E mutation.

207. **F**. Mutant *BRAF* has been implicated in the pathogenesis of several cancers, including melanoma, nonsmall-cell lung cancer, colorectal cancer, papillary thyroid cancer, hairy-cell leukemia, non-Hodgkin lymphoma, and ovarian

cancer. Mutant *BRAF* has been also observed in Langerhans-cell histiocytosis (LCH), glioblastoma, and gastrointestinal stromal tumor (GIST). Germline pathogenic variants in *BRAF* are associated with cardiofaciocutaneous syndrome. The *BRAF* V600E mutation has been identified in 25%−64% of cases of LCH. *Renal-cell carcinomas (RCC) usually have chromosome abnormalities, but NOT BRAF mutations.* For example, clear-cell RCC usually has a deletion of 3p.

Therefore, it is most likely that patients with RCC do not have a *BRAF* V600E mutation.

208. **A.** The genes listed in the NGS panel are in the Ras_Raf_MAPK pathway. Acquired pathogenic variants in the genes are commonly seen in all the diseases listed except for alveolar rhabdomyosarcoma. Rhabdomyosarcoma is a soft-tissue sarcoma arising from skeletal muscle tissue. Rhabdomyosarcoma most often affects children and is the most common soft-tissue sarcoma diagnosed in children. Alveolar and embryonal rhabdomyosarcoma histologies have distinct molecular profiles. *Approximately 80% of alveolar rhabdomyosarcomas harbor a characteristic translocation between chromosome 1 or 2 and chromosome 13, resulting in a PAX7-FOXO1 or a PAX3-FOXO1 fusion protein.* Aberrant genes observed in embryonal rhabdomyosarcoma include *BRAF, CTNNB1, FGFR4, HRAS, KRAS, NRAS, PIK3CA,* and *PTPN11*.

Therefore, this assay is NOT appropriate for alveolar rhabdomyosarcomas, at least not as a first-line test, even though up to 3% of patients may have an acquired pathogenic variant in the *KRAS* gene.

References

1. Cross D, Burmester JK. The promise of molecular profiling for cancer identification and treatment. *Clin Med Res* 2004;**2**(3):147−50.
2. Greaves M, Maley CC. Clonal evolution in cancer. *Nature* 2012;**481**(7381):306−13.
3. Sabaawy HE. Genetic heterogeneity and clonal evolution of tumor cells and their impact on precision cancer medicine. *J Leuk* 2013;**1**(4):1000124.
4. Langerak AW, et al. EuroClonality/BIOMED-2 guidelines for interpretation and reporting of Ig/TCR clonality testing in suspected lymphoproliferations. *Leukemia* 2012;**26**(10):2159−71.
5 S. Heim, F. Mitelman. *Cancer cytogenetics: Chromosomal and molecular genetic aberrations of tumor cells,* 4th Edition. Wiley-Blackwell, John Wiley & Sons.
6. Sandberg Y, et al. BIOMED-2 multiplex immunoglobulin/T-cell receptor polymerase chain reaction protocols can reliably replace Southern blot analysis in routine clonality diagnostics. *J Mol Diagn* 2005;**7**(4):495−503.
7. Swerdlow SH, Campo E, Harris NL, Jaffe ES, Pileri SA, Stein H, Thiele J, Vardiman JW. *WHO classification of tumors of haematopoietic and lymphoid tissues.* WHO. Stylus Publishing; 2008.

8. Chung HJ, et al. Promyelocytic blast crisis of chronic myeloid leukemia during imatinib treatment. *Ann Clin Lab Sci* 2008;**38**(3):283−6.
9. Crocker John, Murray Paul G. *Molecular biology in cellular pathology.* John Wiley & Sons Ltd; 2003.
10. Tabernero MD, et al. Adult precursor B-ALL with BCR/ABL gene rearrangements displays a unique immunophenotype based on the pattern of CD10, CD34, CD13 and CD38 expression. *Leukemia* 2001;**15**(3):406−14.
11. Soverini S, et al. BCR-ABL kinase domain mutation analysis in chronic myeloid leukemia patients treated with tyrosine kinase inhibitors: recommendations from an expert panel on behalf of European LeukemiaNet. *Blood* 2011;**118**(5):1208−15.
12. Shin SY, et al. Two cases of acute lymphoblastic leukemia with an e1a3 BCR-ABL1 fusion transcript. *Ann Lab Med* 2015;**35**(1):159−61.
13. Gong JZ, et al. Laboratory practice guidelines for detecting and reporting JAK2 and MPL mutations in myeloproliferative neoplasms: a report of the Association for Molecular Pathology. *J Mol Diagn* 2013;**15**(6):733−44.
14. Klampfl T, et al. Somatic mutations of calreticulin in myeloproliferative neoplasms. *N Engl J Med* 2013;**369**(25):2379−90.
15. Nangalia J, et al. Somatic CALR mutations in myeloproliferative neoplasms with nonmutated JAK2. *N Engl J Med* 2013;**369**(25):2391−405.
16. Yoo JH, et al. JAK2 V617F/C618R mutation in a patient with polycythemia vera: a case study and review of the literature. *Cancer Genet Cytogenet* 2009;**189**(1):43−7.
17. Khan AA, et al. JAK2 mutation-negative essential thrombocythemia in a child presenting with cerebral venous thrombosis. *Hematol Oncol Stem Cell Ther* 2012;**5**(1):66−8.
18. Bhatti AB, Ali F, Satti AS. Essential thrombocythemia. *Int J Biomed Adv Res* 2013;**4**(08):5.
19. Grimwade D, Ivey A, Huntly BJ. Molecular landscape of acute myeloid leukemia in younger adults and its clinical relevance. *Blood* 2016;**127**(1):29−41.
20. Abu-Duhier FM, et al. FLT3 internal tandem duplication mutations in adult acute myeloid leukaemia define a high-risk group. *Br J Haematol* 2000;**111**(1):190−5.
21. Lu L, Fan Z, Jian H. Acute myeloid leukemia with t(10;17)(p13; q12) chromosome translocation: a case report and literature review. *Am J Blood Res* 2012;**2**(4):4.
22. Dufour A, et al. Acute myeloid leukemia with biallelic CEBPA gene mutations and normal karyotype represents a distinct genetic entity associated with a favorable clinical outcome. *J Clin Oncol* 2010;**28**(4):570−7.
23. Malcovati L, et al. Clinical significance of SF3B1 mutations in myelodysplastic syndromes and myelodysplastic/myeloproliferative neoplasms. *Blood* 2011;**118**(24):6239−46.
24. Cazzola M, et al. Biologic and clinical significance of somatic mutations of SF3B1 in myeloid and lymphoid neoplasms. *Blood* 2013;**121**(2):260−9.
25. Gelsi-Boyer V, et al. Mutations in ASXL1 are associated with poor prognosis across the spectrum of malignant myeloid diseases. *J Hematol Oncol* 2012;**5**:12.
26. Serravalle S, et al. Trisomy 11 with MLL-PTD in a case of infant AML M0. *Br J Haematol* 2007;**138**(6):817−19.
27. Caligiuri MA, et al. Molecular rearrangement of the ALL-1 gene in acute myeloid leukemia without cytogenetic evidence of 11q23 chromosomal translocations. *Cancer Res* 1994;**54**(2):370−3.
28. Alpermann T, et al. AML with gain of chromosome 8 as the sole chromosomal abnormality (+8sole) is associated with a specific molecular mutation pattern including ASXL1 mutations in 46.8% of the patients. *Leuk Res* 2015;**39**(3):265−72.
29. Schnittger S, et al. ASXL1 exon 12 mutations are frequent in AML with intermediate risk karyotype and are independently associated with an adverse outcome. *Leukemia* 2013;**27**(1):82−91.

30. Cameron ER, Neil JC. The Runx genes: lineage-specific onco-genes and tumor suppressors. *Oncogene* 2004;**23**(24):4308–14.

31. Kirschnerova G, Tothova A, Babusikova O. Amplification of AML1 gene in association with karyotype, age and diagnosis in acute leukemia patients. *Neoplasma* 2006;**53**(2):150–4.

32. Burillo-Sanz S, et al. RUNX1 amplification in AML with myelodysplasia-related changes and ring 21 chromosomes. *Hematol Oncol* 2016;**35**(4):894–9.

33. Silva FP, et al. Identification of RUNX1/AML1 as a classical tumor suppressor gene. *Oncogene* 2003;**22**(4):538–47.

34. Osato M. Point mutations in the RUNX1/AML1 gene: another actor in RUNX leukemia. *Oncogene* 2004;**23**(24):4284–96.

35. Rachel B, Flamholz DMV, Jeroudi M, Sakhalkar VS, Nordberg ML, Cotelingam JD. Myeloblastic proliferation in the peripehral blood of a neonate with down syndrome. *Lab Med* 2004;**35**(7):3.

36. Ito E, et al. Expression of erythroid-specific genes in acute mega-karyoblastic leukaemia and transient myeloproliferative disorder in Down's syndrome. *Br J Haematol* 1995;**90**(3):607–14.

37. Mundschau G, et al. Mutagenesis of GATA1 is an initiating event in Down syndrome leukemogenesis. *Blood* 2003;**101**(11):4298–300.

38. Alford KA, et al. Analysis of GATA1 mutations in Down syn-drome transient myeloproliferative disorder and myeloid leuke-mia. *Blood* 2011;**118**(8):2222–38.

39. Cazzola M, Della Porta MG, Malcovati L. The genetic basis of myelodysplasia and its clinical relevance. *Blood* 2013;**122** (25):4021–34.

40. Bravo GM, et al. Integrating genetics and epigenetics in myelo-dysplastic syndromes: advances in pathogenesis and disease evolution. *Br J Haematol* 2014;**166**(5):646–59.

41. Bejar R, et al. Clinical effect of point mutations in myelodysplas-tic syndromes. *N Engl J Med* 2011;**364**(26):2496–506.

42. Gao J, et al. Heritable GATA2 mutations associated with familial AML-MDS: a case report and review of literature. *J Hematol Oncol* 2014;**7**:36.

43. West RR, et al. Acquired ASXL1 mutations are common in patients with inherited GATA2 mutations and correlate with myeloid transformation. *Haematologica* 2014;**99**(2):276–81.

44. Mullighan CG. Molecular genetics of B-precursor acute lympho-blastic leukemia. *J Clin Invest* 2012;**122**(10):3407–15.

45. Gleissner B, et al. Leading prognostic relevance of the BCR-ABL translocation in adult acute B-lineage lymphoblastic leukemia: a prospective study of the German Multicenter Trial Group and confirmed polymerase chain reaction analysis. *Blood* 2002;**99** (5):1536–43.

46. Kataria SP, Kumar S, Sen R, Singh G, Singh U, Inamdar RG. Hairy cell leukemia: a diagnostic dilemma. *Biomed Int* 2011;**2**:3.

47. Arcaini L, et al. The BRAF V600E mutation in hairy cell leuke-mia and other mature B-cell neoplasms. *Blood* 2012;**119** (1):188–91.

48. Dietrich S, et al. BRAF inhibition in refractory hairy-cell leuke-mia. *N Engl J Med* 2012;**366**(21):2038–40.

49. Follows GA, et al. Rapid response of biallelic BRAF V600E mutated hairy cell leukaemia to low dose vemurafenib. *Br J Haematol* 2013;**161**(1):150–3.

50. Ravilla R, Sasapu A, Ramos JM, Arnaoutakis K. A case of ana-plastic large cell lymphoma presenting in leukemic phase. *J Blood Disord Transfus* 2015;**6**:316.

51. Genetics A.C.o.M. *ACMG standards and guidelines for clinical, CF and Section G*. ACMG; 2011.

52. ACMG. *ACMG standards and guidelines for clinical genetics labora-tories, section G*. ACMG; 2010.

53. Schrijver I. *Diagnostic molecular pathologiy in practice—a case-based approach*. Springer; 2011.

54. Wozniak A, et al. Prognostic value of KIT/PDGFRA mutations in gastrointestinal stromal tumours (GIST): Polish Clinical GIST Registry experience. *Ann Oncol* 2012;**23**(2):353–60.

55. Sashidharan P, et al. Gastrointestinal stromal tumors: a case report. *Oman Med J* 2014;**29**(2):138–41.

56. Brandao GD, Brega EF, Spatz A. The role of molecular pathology in non-small-cell lung carcinoma-now and in the future. *Curr Oncol* 2012;**19**(Suppl. 1):S24–32.

57. Keedy VL, et al. American Society of Clinical Oncology provi-sional clinical opinion: epidermal growth factor receptor (EGFR) mutation testing for patients with advanced non-small-cell lung cancer considering first-line EGFR tyrosine kinase inhibitor ther-apy. *J Clin Oncol* 2011;**29**(15):2121–7.

58. Aisner DL, Marshall CB. Molecular pathology of non-small-cell lung cancer: a practical guide. *Am J Clin Pathol* 2012;**138** (3):332–46.

59. Caparica R, et al. BRAF mutations in non-small-cell lung cancer: has finally Janus opened the door? *Crit Rev Oncol Hematol* 2016;**101**:32–9.

60. Planchard D, et al. Dabrafenib plus trametinib in patients with previously treated BRAF(V600E)-mutant metastatic non-small-cell lung cancer: an open-label, multicentre phase 2 trial. *Lancet Oncol* 2016;**17**(7):984–93.

61. Clarke CN, Kopetz ES. BRAF mutant colorectal cancer as a dis-tinct subset of colorectal cancer: clinical characteristics, clinical behavior, and response to targeted therapies. *J Gastrointest Oncol* 2015;**6**(6):660–7.

62. Arrington AK, et al. Prognostic and predictive roles of KRAS mutation in colorectal cancer. *Int J Mol Sci* 2012;**13**(10):12153–68.

63. Phipps AI, et al. KRAS-mutation status in relation to colorectal cancer survival: the joint impact of correlated tumour markers. *Br J Cancer* 2013;**108**(8):1757–64.

64. Shi C, Washington K. Molecular testing in colorectal cancer: diagnosis of Lynch syndrome and personalized cancer medicine. *Am J Clin Pathol* 2012;**137**(6):847–59.

65. Shukla N, et al. Oncogene mutation profiling of pediatric solid tumors reveals significant subsets of embryonal rhabdomyosar-coma and neuroblastoma with mutated genes in growth signal-ing pathways. *Clin Cancer Res* 2012;**18**(3):748–57.

66. Hu J, Hong X, Li Z, Lu Q. Acute monocytic leukaemia with t(11; 12) (p15; q13)chromosomal changes: A case report and liter-ature review. *Oncol Lett*. 2015;**10**(4):2307–10.

67. Brose MS, Volpe P, Feldman M, Kumar M, Rishi I, Gerrero R, et al. BRAF and RAS mutations in human lung cancer and mela-noma. *Cancer Res*. 2002;**62**(23):6997–7000.

SELF-ASSESSMENT QUESTIONS FOR CLINICAL MOLECULAR GENETICS

CHAPTER

9

Lysosomal Storage Disorders

Lysosomes are subcellular organelles bounded by a single-layer membrane within eukaryotic cells. They contain an array of glycoprotein acid hydrolase enzymes for catabolizing all major classes of biological macromolecules such as proteins, nucleic acids, glycosphingolipids, mucopolysaccharides, and glycogen, as well as sequestered bacteria, viruses, and other foreign substances that are taken up by phagocytosis into white blood cells and macrophages. Lysosomes are also responsible for autophagy, the gradual turnover of each cell's own components as they age and become obsolescent.

Lysosomal storage diseases (LSDs) occur secondary to genetic defects that cause total deficiency or reduced activity of specific native enzymes within the lysosomes. This allows macromolecular compounds that are normally enzymatically catabolized to accumulate within these organelles, expanding them and causing progressive damage in connective tissue, skeletal structure, various organs, and, in some cases, the central nervous system. The damage caused by substrate accumulation results in physical deterioration, functional impairment, and potentially death. At least 50 different LSDs have been identified, broadly divided into categories that are defined by accumulation of a specific macromolecule. Although individually each LSD is somewhat rare, as a group they have an incidence of about 1 per 7000–8000 live births, with regional and genetic population variations. For instance, Gaucher and Tay–Sachs diseases are more prevalent among the Ashkenazi Jewish population. A pathogenic variant associated with Hurler syndrome is known to occur more frequently among Scandinavian and Russian peoples.

Most LSDs are inherited in an autosomal recessive manner. The exceptions are Fabry disease and Hunter syndrome, which follow an X-linked inheritance pattern. All individuals in populations carry four or five abnormal genes. Parents who are close relatives (consanguineous) or belong to certain ethnic groups subject to founder effect (bottle-neck effect), have a higher chance than unrelated parents to both carry the same abnormal gene, which increases the risk to have children with a recessive genetic disorder. Prenatal diagnosis is possible for all LSDs. Early detection is important because when therapies are available, either for the disease itself or for associated symptoms, they may significantly limit the long-term course and impact of the disease.

Gaucher disease type 1 was the first LSD with enzyme-replacement therapy (ERT), which was approved by the U.S. Food and Drug Administration (FDA) in April 1991. Currently, six LSDs (Fabry disease, Gaucher disease type I, Pompe disease, Hurler syndrome, Hunter disease, and Maroteaux–Lamy syndrome) have ERT to augment or replace the activity of a specific endogenous catabolic enzyme within cellular lysosomes (https://www.ncbi.nlm.nih.gov/books/NBK117221/). For many others, there is currently no effective treatment; patients are being treated or investigated with supportive care and allogeneic hematopoietic stem-cell transplantation (HSCT).

In clinical molecular genetic practice, there are Sanger sequencing assays for each individual disorder and next-generation panels for LSDs as a whole. Newborn screening (NBS) for LSDs is under investigation because of the development of treatment options for a subset of these disorders and the demonstration that initiation of treatment shortly after birth often leads to a better outcome. As of February 16, 2016, Pompe and mucopolysaccharidosis I (MPS I) have been approved to be recommended for NBS by the Secretary of the US Department of Health and Human Services' Advisory Committee on Heritable Disorders in Newborns and Children (ACHDNC) in addition to the Recommended Uniform Screening Panel (RUSP) (www.aphlblog.org). Some states have gone beyond the RUSP and have added or are planning to add certain LSDs to their NBS panels. On June 1, 2015, Illinois became one of three states to implement testing for LSDs, joining New York and Missouri (Newborn screening for lysosomal storage diseases.[1]).

Self-assessment Questions for Clinical Molecular Genetics.
DOI: https://doi.org/10.1016/B978-0-12-809967-4.00009-0

Statewide testing in Illinois was implemented for five LSDs (Gaucher, Fabry, MPS I, Niemann–Pick A/B, and Pompe). Because the prevalence of LSDs in specific ethnic groups is high, targeted carrier screening test are also available for presymptomatic individuals in high-risk populations, such as Gaucher screening in Ashkenazi Jewish. *The LSDs disorders covered in this chapter are:*

- *Gaucher disease*
- Hexosaminidase A deficiency (Tay–Sachs disease)
- Sandhoff disease
- Niemann–Pick disease
- Krabbe disease
- Hurler syndrome
- Hunter syndrome
- Metachromatic leukodystrophy
- Fabry disease
- Pompe disease (in Chapter 10: Neuromuscular Disorders also)
- I-cell disease
- Sialidosis type

QUESTIONS

1. Which one of the following enzyme deficiencies causes Gaucher disease?
   A. Beta-galactosidase
   B. Beta-glucocerebrosidase
   C. Beta-hexosaminidase A
   D. Beta-hexosaminidase B
   E. Beta-hexosaminidases A and B

2. A couple in their 30s comes to a clinic for preconception counseling. The husband is Ashkenazi Jewish. The wife is of German/Irish descent. They both are apparently healthy. The medical histories are unremarkable. The husband's family history was significant for his brother dying of a congenital condition in his early 40s. For which one of the following disorders does the husband have the highest risk to be a carrier?
   A. Cystic fibrosis
   B. Familial dysautonomia
   C. Gaucher disease
   D. Tay–Sachs disease
   E. None of the above

3. A 10-year-old Ashkenazi Jewish girl was admitted to a hospital for chronic hepatosplenomegaly and shortening of the right leg. Her development was normal until 5 years of age, when it was noted that her abdomen was becoming progressively enlarged. Since 7 years of age she experienced frequent episodes of epistaxis. At 8 years of age, she began to walk with a limp, and some

shortening of the right lower extremity was noted. At the admission, she was thin, but not ill. She had a low-grade fever, mild systolic hypertension, some enlarged lymph nodes, slight anemia, and an enormous abdomen. Laboratory studies showed leukocytosis and an increased erythrocyte sedimentation rate. Radiography and MRI revealed "cold" bone scans with patchy sclerosis in the right femoral head, suggesting a previous episode of avascular necrosis, as well as abnormalities in bone marrow density, suggesting replacement of marrow fat by an infiltrate. The physician suspected that the patient had Gaucher disease. An enzyme assay showed her glucocerebrosidase level to be 2.0 nmol/mg/h (normal range, 12.5–16.9). A next-generation sequencing (NGS) panel for lysosomal storage disorders was ordered to confirm the diagnosis and to determine family management. Which one of the following genes would most likely harbor pathogenic variant(s) for Gaucher disease in this patient?
   A. GBA
   B. GLB1
   C. HEXA
   D. HEXB
   E. SMPD1
   F. None of the above

4. A couple in their 30s comes to a clinic for preconception counseling. The husband is Ashkenazi Jewish. The wife is of German/Irish descent. They both are apparently healthy. The medical histories are unremarkable. The husband's family history was significant for his brother dying of Gaucher disease in his early 40s. A molecular study has not been done for the family. Which one of the following assays is most likely be used to test the husband for carrier status?
   A. Chromosome microarray
   B. Exome sequence analysis
   C. Multiplex ligation-dependent probe amplification (MLPA)
   D. Next-generation sequencing panel
   E. Sanger sequence analysis
   F. Target variant analysis
   G. None of the above

5. A couple in their 30s comes to a clinic for preconception counseling. The husband is Ashkenazi Jewish. The wife is of German/Irish descent. They both are apparently healthy. The medical histories are unremarkable. The husband's family history was significant for his brother dying of Gaucher disease in his early 40s. The husband was tested before and is a carrier of the L444P variant in *GBA*. Which one of the following genetic

studies most likely is the next step in the workup for this couple?[2,3]

A. Testing the husband for glucocerebrosidase enzyme activity

B. Testing the husband with a sequence assay for *GBA* with reflex to deletion/duplication

C. Testing the wife for glucocerebrosidase enzyme activity

D. Testing the wife for the four common *GBA* pathogenic variants in Ashkenazi Jews

E. Testing the wife with a sequencing assay for *GBA*

F. None of the above

6. A couple in their 30s comes to a clinic for preconception counseling. The husband is Ashkenazi Jewish. The wife is of German/Irish descent. They both are apparently healthy. The medical histories are unremarkable. The husband's family history was significant for his brother dying of Gaucher disease in his early 40s. The husband was tested for the four common pathogenic variants in the *GBA* gene in the past, and the results were negative. Which one of the following is the most appropriate estimation of the false negative rate of the targeted variants in this situation?

A. >99%

B. 80%

C. 45%

D. 10%

E. <1%

7. A Caucasian couple in their 30s comes to a clinic for preconception counseling. They both are apparently healthy. The medical histories are unremarkable. The husband's family history was significant for his brother dying of Gaucher disease in his early 40s. The husband was tested for the four common pathogenic variants in the *GBA* gene in the past, and the results were negative. Which one of the following is the most appropriate estimation of the false negative rate of the targeted variants in this situation?

A. >99%

B. 80%

C. 45%

D. 10%

E. <1%

8. A 10-year-old Ashkenazi Jewish girl was admitted to a hospital for chronic hepatosplenomegaly and shortening of the right leg. Her development was normal until 5 years of age, when it was noted that her abdomen was becoming progressively enlarged. Since 7 years of age, she experienced frequent episodes of epistaxis. At 8 years of age, she began to walk with a limp, and some shortening of the right lower extremity was noted.

At the admission, she was thin, but not ill. She had a low-grade fever, mild systolic hypertension, some enlarged lymph nodes, slight anemia, and an enormous abdomen. Laboratory studies showed leukocytosis and an increased erythrocyte sedimentation rate. Radiography and MRI revealed "cold" bone scans with patchy sclerosis in the right femoral head, suggesting a previous episode of avascular necrosis, as well as abnormalities in bone marrow density, suggesting replacement of marrow fat by an infiltrate. The physician suspected that the patient had Gaucher disease. An enzyme assay showed her glucocerebrosidase level to be 2.0 nmol/mg/h (normal range, 12.5–16.9). A molecular study of *GBA* was ordered to confirm the diagnosis and family management. Which one of the following pathogenic variants in the *GBA* gene would this patient most likely have?[2,3]

A. 84GG: c.84dupG(p.Leu29AlafsTer18)

B. IVS2 + 1G > A: c.115 + 1G > A

C. L444P: c.1448T > C(p.Leu483Pro)

D. N370S: c.1226A > G(p.Gly416Ser)

E. None of the above

9. A 39-year-old single male was admitted to a tertiary health care center in England for intractable grand mal seizures and myoclonus for 22 years. He was born in South Africa to Jewish parents who were first cousins and who originated from Lithuania. The patient had two unaffected sisters. The family history was unremarkable for epilepsy and anemia. At age 17, he had a sudden episode of dizziness followed by brief loss of consciousness and generalized clonic movements of his limbs. Since then, seizures reoccurred monthly with progression gradually to his right arm, more frequently in the early morning. He moved to England at 27 years of age. At the time, his physical examination and laboratory test results were in the normal range. His electroencephalogram was grossly abnormal, with very frequent paroxysms of generalized irregular multiple spikes and waves. He was diagnosed with idiopathic epilepsy. Since age 32, his seizures and myoclonic jerking increased in frequency. He started to have slow deliberate speech broken up by jerks and typical brief irregular shock-like movements of his face and upper limbs with mild incoordination. At the time of admission at age 39, he had urinary incontinence. His muscle tone was in the normal range, but he had finger–nose and heel-shin ataxia. More extensive laboratory testing revealed that his sternal marrow was hypocellular, with normal erythropoiesis and granulopoiesis. In addition, numerous large foamy cells resembling Gaucher cells were present in the marrow. Further

biochemical studies showed that his beta-glucosidase activity of fibroblasts was 35 nmol/mg/h (normal range, 100−500). A molecular study was ordered to further confirm the diagnosis. Which one of the following pathogenic variants in the *GBA* gene would this patient most likely have?[4-6]

A. 84GG: c.84dupG(p.Leu29AlafsTer18)

B. IVS2 + 1G > A: c.115 + 1G > A

C. L444P: c.1448T > C(p.Leu483Pro)

D. N370S: c.1226A > G(p.Gly416Ser)

E. None of the above

10. An Ashkenazi Jewish couple came to a clinic for their first prenatal care. The fetus looked 6 weeks old on ultrasound. A molecular carrier screening panel for Ashkenazi Jews was ordered. The results showed that both the husband and the wife carried the N370S variant in *GBA*. Amniocentesis was done at 14 weeks of gestational age. The results showed that the fetus was homozygous for the N370S variant. Which one of the following symptoms would the unborn baby most likely NOT have in postnatal life?

A. Anemia

B. Hepatosplenomegaly

C. Osteopenia

D. Seizure

E. None of the above

11. An Ashkenazi Jewish couple came to a clinic for their first prenatal care. The fetus looked 6 weeks old on ultrasound. A molecular carrier screening panel for Ashkenazi Jews was ordered. The results showed that both the husband and the wife carried the L444P variant in *GBA*. Amniocentesis was done at 14 weeks of gestational age. The results showed that the fetus was homozygous for the L444P variant. Which one of the following symptoms would the unborn baby most likely NOT have in postnatal life?

A. Anemia

B. Arrhythmia

C. Hepatosplenomegaly

D. Osteopenia

E. Seizure

12. An Ashkenazi Jewish couple came to a clinic for their first prenatal care. The fetus looked 6 weeks old on ultrasound. A molecular carrier screening panel for Ashkenazi Jews was ordered. The results showed that both the husband and the wife carried the L444P variant in *GBA*. Amniocentesis was done at 14 weeks of gestational age. The results showed that the fetus was homozygous for the L444P variant. Which one of the following symptoms would the unborn baby most likely have in postnatal life?

A. Arrhythmia

B. Developmental delay

C. Odd-smelling urine

D. Seizures

E. Sudden death

13. An Ashkenazi Jewish couple comes to a clinic for their preconception counseling. Neither of them had had children before. They both are apparently healthy. The medical histories are unremarkable. The husband's family history is significant for his brother dying of Gaucher disease in his early 40s. What is the risk of the couple's firstborn child having Gaucher disease?

A. 1/54

B. 1/108

C. 3/288

D. 1/144

E. None of the above

14. An Ashkenazi Jewish couple comes to a clinic for their prenatal care when the wife is 6 weeks pregnant. They both are apparently healthy. The medical histories are unremarkable. They have two healthy boys ages 5 and 3. But the husband's family history is remarkable for his brother dying of Gaucher disease in his early 40s. What is the risk that their unborn child will develop Gaucher disease in postnatal life?

A. 1/54

B. 1/108

C. 1/216

D. 1/417

E. 1/1668

F. None of the above

15. The state newborn screening (NBS) laboratory at the Illinois Department of Public Health contacted a local hospital about a positive NBS result. The family came to the hospital for follow-up. The acid-β-glucosidase enzyme activity in the peripheral-blood leukocytes was 10% of normal. The molecular results revealed a compound heterozygous genotype, p.N370S/p.L444P, in *GBA*. Which one of the following symptoms would this patient most likely NOT develop in his lifetime due to Gaucher disease?

A. Hepatomegaly

B. Seizure

C. Splenomegaly

D. Thrombocytopenia

E. None of the above

16. A 12-year-old Ashkenazi Jewish boy is brought to a clinic by his parents for aseptic necrosis of the femur. A physical exam reveals he also has hepatosplenomegaly. A bone-marrow biopsy reveals that patient has macrophages in the bone marrow that look like crumpled paper. A molecular

genetic test detects N370S/L444P variants in *GBA*, which confirms the diagnosis of Gaucher disease. For which one of the following diseases does this patient NOT have an increased risk?

- A. Hepatocarcinoma
- B. Melanoma
- C. Multiple myeloma
- D. Non-Hodgkin's lymphoma
- E. Osteosarcoma
- F. Pancreatic cancer
- G. Parkinson disease
- H. None of the above

17. The diagnosis of hexosaminidase A deficiency relies on the demonstration of which one of the following?
- A. Deficiency of alpha-hexosaminidase B (HEX B) enzymatic activity
- B. Deficiency of beta-hexosaminidase A (HEX A) enzymatic activity
- C. Sequence analysis of *HEXA* with reflex to del/dup analysis
- D. Sequence analysis of *HEXB* with reflex to del/dup analysis
- E. Targeted *HEXA* mutation analysis
- F. Targeted *HEXB* mutation analysis

18. Tay—Sachs disease is caused by deficiency of which one of the following?
- A. Beta-hexosaminidase A
- B. Beta-hexosaminidase B
- C. Beta-hexosaminidase A and B
- D. Beta-galactosidase
- E. Beta-glucocerebrosidase

19. In which one of the following populations is the carrier frequency of Tay—Sachs disease relatively lower?
- A. Ashkenazi Jewish
- B. French Canadians
- C. Louisiana Cajuns
- D. Pennsylvania Amish
- E. Mormons in Utah

20. An Ashkenazi Jewish boy was born normal but started flinching at loud noises at the age of 6 months. He initially could sit up, but then he regressed so far that he could neither roll over nor recognize his parents. An ophthalmological examination revealed a cherry red spot. A clinical diagnosis of Tay—Sachs disease was made. Which one of the following does NOT explain why Tay—Sachs disease has increased prevalence in the Ashkenazi Jewish population?[7]
- A. Bottleneck effect
- B. Founder effect
- C. Genetic drift
- D. Heterozygous advantage
- E. None of the above

21. A couple comes to a clinic for their first prenatal care when the wife is 6 weeks pregnant. The husband has Ashkenazi Jewish ancestry. The wife is of Greek descent. A battery study reveals that the husband's beta-hexosaminidase A (HEX A) enzymatic activity is decreased to approximately 50% of the normal range. Which one of the following studies is the most appropriate next step in the workup for this couple as a part of the prenatal care?
- A. Order targeted *HEXA* pathogenic variant analysis for the husband.
- B. Order targeted *HEXA* pathogenic variant analysis for the wife.
- C. Order *HEXA* sequence analysis reflex to del/dup analysis for the husband.
- D. Order *HEXA* sequence analysis reflex to del/dup analysis for the wife.
- E. Test the wife for beta-hexosaminidase A (HEX A) enzymatic activity.
- F. Test the unborn child for beta-hexosaminidase A (HEX A) enzymatic activity.
- G. Wait for the child to be born, then test the child.
- H. No follow-up is necessary.

22. A couple comes to a clinic for their first prenatal care when the wife is 6 weeks pregnant. The husband has Ashkenazi Jewish ancestry. The wife is of Greek descent. A battery study reveals that the husband's beta-hexosaminidase A (HEX A) enzymatic activity is decreased to approximately 50% of the normal range. A targeted *HEXA* pathogenic variant analysis confirms that the husband carries the p.Tyr427IlefsTer5 pathogenic variant. Which one of the following studies is the most appropriate next step in the workup for this couple as a part of prenatal care?
- A. Order targeted *HEXA* pathogenic variant analysis for the unborn child.
- B. Order targeted *HEXA* pathogenic variant analysis for the wife.
- C. Order *HEXA* sequence analysis reflex to del/dup analysis for the unborn child.
- D. Order *HEXA* sequence analysis reflex to del/dup analysis for the wife.
- E. Test the wife for beta-hexosaminidase A (HEX A) enzymatic activity.
- F. Test the unborn child for beta-hexosaminidase A (HEX A) enzymatic activity.
- G. Wait for the child to be born, then test the child.
- H. No follow-up is necessary.

23. A couple comes to a clinic for their first prenatal care when the wife is 6 weeks pregnant. The husband has Ashkenazi Jewish ancestry. The wife

is of Greek descent. A battery study reveals that the husband's beta-hexosaminidase A (HEX A) enzymatic activity is decreased to approximately 50% of the normal range. A targeted *HEXA* pathogenic variant analysis confirms that the husband carries the p.Tyr427IlefsTer5 pathogenic variant. A HEX A enzymatic activity study with leukocytes from the wife reveals that her enzyme activity is also decreased to approximately 50%. Which one of the following studies is the most appropriate next step in the workup for this couple as a part of the prenatal care?

A. Order targeted *HEXA* pathogenic variant analysis for the unborn child.

B. Order targeted *HEXA* pathogenic variant analysis for the wife.

C. Order *HEXA* sequence analysis reflex to del/dup analysis for the unborn child.

D. Order *HEXA* sequence analysis reflex to del/dup analysis for the wife.

E. Test the wife for beta-hexosaminidase A (HEX A) enzymatic activity.

F. Test the unborn child for beta-hexosaminidase A (HEX A) enzymatic activity.

G. Wait for the child to be born, then test the child.

H. No follow-up is necessary.

24. A couple comes to a clinic for their first prenatal care when the wife is 6 weeks pregnant. The husband has Ashkenazi Jewish ancestry. The wife is of Greek descent. A battery study reveals that the husband's beta-hexosaminidase A (HEX A) enzymatic activity is decreased to approximately 50% of the normal range. A targeted *HEXA* pathogenic variant analysis confirms that the husband carries the p.Tyr427IlefsTer5 pathogenic variant. A HEX A enzymatic activity study with leukocytes from the wife reveals that her enzyme activity is also decreased to approximately 50%. What is the chance that the wife is NOT a silent carrier of Tay–Sachs disease?

A. 90%

B. 50%

C. 35%

D. 10%

E. 2%

25. A couple comes to a clinic for their first prenatal care when the wife is 6 weeks pregnant. The husband has Ashkenazi Jewish ancestry. The wife is of Greek descent. A battery study reveals that the husband's beta-hexosaminidase A (HEX A) enzymatic activity is decreased to approximately 50% of the normal range. A targeted *HEXA* pathogenic variant analysis confirms that the husband carries the p.Tyr427IlefsTer5 pathogenic

variant. A HEX A enzymatic activity study with leukocytes from the wife reveals that her enzyme activity is also decreased to approximately 50%. A targeted *HEXA* pathogenic variant analysis detects a variant, p.Arg247Trp, in the wife. Which one of the following most likely is the risk of the unborn child to develop Tay–Sachs disease?

A. <1%

B. 25%

C. 50%

D. 67%

E. >99%

F. Cannot predict

G. None of the above

26. A couple comes to a clinic for preconception counseling. The husband is a recent French Canadian immigrant from Quebec and the wife is of Native American descent. The husband's brother died of Tay–Sachs disease (TSD) in his childhood. A HEX A enzymatic assay identifies the husband as a carrier. The physician wants to order a targeted molecular study for family management. She calls a couple of clinical laboratories to find out the content of their targeted assays for *HEXA*. Which one of the following pathogenic variants in the *HEXA* gene does the physician try to make sure is covered by the ordered test?

A. c.1073 + G > A

B. c.1421 + 1G > C

C. p.Gly269Ser

D. p.Tyr427IlefsTer5

E. 7.6-kb genomic deletion involving *HEXA*

F. None of the above

27. An Ashkenazi Jewish couple was referred to a genetics clinic for preconception counseling. The wife had a sister who died of Tay–Sachs disease (TSD) in her childhood. The husband had a paternal uncle living in a psychiatric home without a clear diagnosis. A targeted molecular analysis confirmed that the wife is a carrier, but not the husband. The carrier frequency of TSD in Ashkenazi Jews is 1 in 30. If the detection rate of the molecular assay is 90% in Ashkenazi Jews, what is the residual risk of their first child having TSD?

A. 1/291

B. 1/582

C. 1/1164

D. 1/2328

E. None of the above

28. A couple comes to a clinic for their first prenatal care when the wife is 6 weeks pregnant. The husband has Ashkenazi Jewish ancestry. The wife is of Greek descent. The husband's brother died of

Tay—Sachs disease (TSD) in his childhood. A HEX A enzymatic assay with reflex to a targeted molecular study is ordered for the husband. The HEX A enzyme study indicates that he is a carrier. However, the targeted molecular study with the six common variants in *HEXA* (p.Tyr427IlefsTer5, c.1421 + 1G > C, c.1274_1277dupTATC, p. Gly269Ser, p.Arg247Trp, and p.Arg249Trp) did not detect a pathogenic variant. What is the false negative rate of the targeted molecular study with the six common variants in *HEXA*?

A. 90%
B. 50%
C. 35%
D. 10%
E. 5%

29. A 14-year-old Ashkenazi Jewish male was brought to an emergency department by an ambulance for a psychotic and catatonic state. The patient's birth was without complications. His early milestones were met except for speech. His speech was reported to be always difficult to understand. At the age of 5, he was noticed to be thinner and weaker than his peers and could not keep up with other children. The neurological evaluation at the time revealed dysarthria, low muscle mass with increased tone, abnormal wide-based gait, and abnormally brisk bilateral deep tendon reflexes. Between the ages of 11 and 13, the patient gradually developed difficulty with chewing and swallowing and had some drooling and he was noticed to clench his teeth when he spoke. At that time, MRI showed mild cerebellar degeneration. He was the youngest of four children. His siblings and other family members had unremarkable medical histories. At the time of admission at the age of 14, he showed lack of emotion, being withdrawn and almost mute. With medication, he became responsive. His speech remained dysarthric and he still displayed facial grimacing. His gait continued to be wide-based. The suspicion of late-onset Tay—Sachs disease was confirmed by laboratory analyses of serum hexosaminidase A and was only 1% of the total (normal range, 56—80) although the total was in the normal range. In the leukocytes, hexosaminidase A was only 7% of the total (normal range, 63—75). A targeted molecular study for *HEXA* was ordered. Which one of the following pathogenic variants in the *HEXA* gene would the patient most likely have?[8]

A. c.1073 + 1G > A
B. c.1274_1277dupTATC(p.Tyr427IlefsTer5)
C. c.1421 + 1G > C
D. c.533G > A(p.Arg178His)
E. c.739C > T(p.Arg247Trp)

F. c.745C > T(p.Arg249Trp)
G. c.805G > A(p.Gly269Ser)
H. 7.6-kb genomic deletion involving *HEXA*
I. Not sure

30. A 19-month-old Portuguese boy was brought to a hospital for seizures. He presented with a history of neuroregression since he was 6 months old and seizures since he was 12 months old. He was born full-term at 37 weeks with no complications. He was developing normally until he was 6 months old, when it was observed that he was listless and lost the ability to move his limbs and roll over. Since then, the loss of motor skills became progressively evident. He is the only child of a healthy nonconsanguineous couple. The family history is unremarkable. A physical examination revealed he had macrocephaly, spastic quadriplegia, decreased eye contact, and hyperacusis. A neuroimaging examination revealed leukodystrophic changes. An ophthalmic assessment confirmed severe visual impairment and bilateral retinal cherry-red spots. The diagnosis of Tay—Sachs disease (TSD) was made by serum lysosomal enzyme assay with analysis of hexosaminidase A activity (0.02 nmol/min/mL; normal range, 0.5—3.1). A molecular analysis further confirmed the diagnosis by detection of two compound heterozygous pathogenic variants. Which one of the following pathogenic variants in the *HEXA* gene would the patient most likely have?[9]

A. c.1073 + 1G > A
B. c.1274_1277dupTATC(p.Tyr427IlefsTer5)
C. c.1421 + 1G > C
D. c.533G > A(p.Arg178His)
E. c.739C > T(p.Arg247Trp)
F. c.745C > T(p.Arg249Trp)
G. c.805G > A(p.Gly269Ser)
H. 7.6-kb genomic deletion involving *HEXA*
I. Not sure

31. A 1-year 7-month-old boy was brought to a hospital for seizures, cough, and fever for approximately 1 week. His father was of Jewish descent. His mother was a French Canadian from Quebec. His perinatal history was uneventful. He was born at term. At the age of 1 month, he was noticed to have hypotonia, with little power to hold his head up or move his limbs. Since then, the weakness had become progressively evident. His mother suspected he had vision problems. His medical history showed that he came to the same clinic twice for otitis and pneumonia. Four of the mother's relatives had passed away at 2 years of postnatal life. In the hospital, the initial examination revealed that the patient had fever,

rhonchi on chest auscultation, and marasmus-like secondary protein-energy malnutrition. The neurological examination revealed psychomotor retardation, horizontal and bilateral nystagmus, muscle weakness, generalized hyperreflexia, clumsiness, and presence of Babinski and Moro signs. The ophthalmic assessment was complicated by nystagmus and showed chalk-white macular areas with a cherry-red spot in the center of both eyes. The diagnosis of Tay–Sachs disease (TSD) was made by serum lysosomal enzyme assay with analysis of hexosaminidase A activity. Further confirmation was made by detection of two compound heterozygous pathogenic variants through molecular analysis. Which one of the following pathogenic variants in the *HEXA* gene would the patient most likely NOT have?[10]

A. c.1073 + 1G > A
B. c.1274_1277dupTATC(p.Tyr427IlefsTer5)
C. c.1421 + 1G > C
D. c.805G > A(p.Gly269Ser)
E. 7.6-kb genomic deletion involving *HEXA*
F. Not sure

32. A 4-year-old Korean girl was brought to a clinic for progressive physical and mental regression for 3 years. She had been treated with anticonvulsants for her chronic tonic–clonic seizures, but here symptoms were prolonged and uncontrollable. She was born by vaginal delivery at full term without complication. Her family history was significant for her older sister dying at the age of 7 years from the same symptoms. An ophthalmological examination revealed that she fixates her eyes on objects and could not follow moving targets. Oculocephalic reflex and optokinetic nystagmus did not exist. A pale optic disk and a cherry-red spot in the macula were seen in both eyes. Low signal intensity at the bilateral thalamus and high signal intensity at the cerebral white matter were noted in a T2-weighted brain MR image. Cerebral cortex and cerebellum showed general atrophic changes. A lysosomal enzyme assay of the peripheral blood revealed that both β-hexosaminidases A and B isoenzyme were absent in the serum. Which one of the lysosomal disorders would the patient most likely have?[11]

A. Gaucher disease
B. Niemann–Pick disease
C. Sandhoff disease
D. Tay–Sachs disease
E. None of the above

33. An 18-month-old boy was hospitalized for psychomotor regression and drug-resistant myoclonic epilepsy. He was born after an uncomplicated full-term pregnancy. The parents were cousins. There was a history of death of a brother at the age of 16 months under unspecified circumstances. The other three siblings (two brothers and one sister) were unaffected. At the age of 6 months, he was brought to medical attention for myoclonus of the face and upper limbs, recurrent fever, and psychomotor developmental delay. A physical examination revealed a macrocephaly of 51 cm with a dysmorphic syndrome consisting of a frontal bossing and a broadening of the nasal bridge. The neurological examination revealed axial hypotonia. An ophthalmological examination showed a cherry-red-spot without optic atrophy. Cerebral CT scanning showed a bilateral thalamic hyperdensity with hypodensity of the white matter. MRI of the thalamus showed hyperintensities on T1-weighted images and hypointensities on T2-weighted images with an increased T2 signal of the white matter. Enzymatic assays were performed and revealed a deficiency of both hexosaminidases A and B, confirming the diagnosis of Sandhoff disease. A molecular study was ordered to further confirm the diagnosis and for family counseling. Which one of the following genes would most likely be tested to detect Sandhoff disease in this patient?[12]

A. *GBA*
B. *GM2A*
C. *HEXA*
D. *HEXB*
E. *SMPD1*

34. A 14-month-old Indian boy was brought to a hospital with symptoms of disproportionately increasing size of the head (≥2 SD) and multiple episodes of seizures. He was the firstborn child of a nonconsanguineous couple and had an uneventful antenatal period. The perinatal transition was uneventful and there was no family history of seizures. He had a delay in attaining age-appropriate milestones. Head control, recognition of mother, and social smile were attained by 6 months of age and sitting with support by 9 months of age. There was no language development. After 10 months of age, there was regression of the above milestones, and by 1 year, all were lost. A physical examination revealed macrocephaly, open anterior fontanel with frontal bossing, no dentition, bilateral undescended testes, and hepatosplenomegaly. The child had no gaze fixation and an occasional startle response to sounds. The neurological examination revealed generalized hypotonia, exaggerated deep tendon reflexes, clonus, and extensor plantar response. A fundus examination revealed a macular cherry-red-spot. Brain MRI showed

hypomyelination with increase in T2 signal intensity in bilateral frontoparietal areas, temporal lobe, subcortical deep white matter, periventricular white matter, and bilaterally in basal ganglia. Enzymatic assays revealed that beta hexosaminidase A and B together was 230 nmol/mg/h (normal range, 905–2878). Beta hexosaminidase A was 101 nmol/mg/h (normal range, 62–310). The patient was diagnosed with Sandhoff disease. A sequence study for the *HEXB* gene was ordered to further confirm the diagnosis and for family counseling. A heterozygous pathogenic variant, c.619A > G (p.Ile207Val), was detected. Which one of following would most likely describe the pathogenesis of Sandhoff disease in this patient?[13]
- A. Dominant negative
- B. Gain of function
- C. Haploinsufficiency
- D. Loss of function
- E. None of the above

35. A couple comes to a clinic for preconception counseling. Both the husband and the wife are of Ashkenazi Jewish descent. The family history is unremarkable on both sides. Genetic counseling is done, and an Ashkenazi Jewish panel is offered. Which one of following is the most appropriate first step in the workup for this couple?
- A. Test the husband immediately.
- B. Test the wife immediately.
- C. Test both the wife and the husband immediately.
- D. Perform a noninvasive prenatal test when the wife is pregnant.
- E. Test the fetus with CVS when the wife is pregnant.
- F. Test the fetus with amniocentesis when the wife is pregnant.
- G. None of the above.

36. A couple comes to a clinic for their first prenatal care when the wife is 6 weeks pregnant. Both the husband and the wife are of Ashkenazi Jewish descent. The family history is unremarkable on both sides. Genetic counseling is done, and an Ashkenazi Jewish panel is offered. Which one of following is the most appropriate first step in the workup for this couple?
- A. Test the husband immediately.
- B. Test the wife immediately.
- C. Test both the wife and the husband immediately.
- D. Perform noninvasive prenatal test when the wife is pregnant.
- E. Test the fetus with CVS when the wife is pregnant.

- F. Test the fetus with amniocentesis when the wife is pregnant.
- G. None of the above.

37. A couple comes to a clinic for preconception counseling. The husband is of Ashkenazi Jewish descent, and the wife is a Caucasian from East Europe. The family history is unremarkable on both sides. Genetic counseling is done, and an Ashkenazi Jewish panel is offered. Which one of following is the most appropriate first step in the workup for this couple?
- A. Test the husband immediately.
- B. Test the wife immediately.
- C. Test both the wife and the husband immediately.
- D. Perform noninvasive prenatal test when the wife is pregnant.
- E. Test the fetus with CVS when the wife is pregnant.
- F. Test the fetus with amniocentesis when the wife is pregnant.
- G. None of the above.

38. An 18-month-old boy was the second child of a second-degree consanguineous marriage with normal delivery. He was brought to a hospital with symptoms of gradually increasing abdominal distention, developmental delay, excessive crying, and low-grade intermittent fever since the age of 2 months. His medical history showed pneumonia at the age of 6 months. His developmental history showed delayed milestones in the form of neck holding at age 7 months and social smiling at age 8 months. On the physical examination, he had mild pallor and was afebrile. He had frontal bossing, depressed nasal bridge, undescended testes, and persistent Mongolian spots all over body, with features of undernutrition. Hepatosplenomegaly, hypotonia, and diminished deep reflexes were also noted. Laboratory evaluations were suggestive of moderately hypochromic anemia. MRI brain showed thalamic involvement. Fundal examination showed cherry-red spots in the macula of both eyes. A bone-marrow examination showed characteristic lipid-laden foamy histiocytes, which were negative on periodic acid–Schiff (PAS) staining. Histopathological examination of a liver biopsy also showed foamy cells with negative PAS staining. A lysosomal enzyme assay of peripheral blood revealed that acid sphingomyelinase (ASM) was absent in the serum. Which one of the lysosomal disorders would the patient most likely have?[14]
- A. Gaucher disease
- B. Niemann–Pick disease
- C. Sandhoff disease

D. Tay–Sachs disease

E. None of the above

39. A 30-month-old Jewish girl was brought to a hospital with symptoms of intermittent fever, bilateral swelling of the feet, and gradually increasing abdominal distention since 4 months of age. She also had developmental delay, excessive crying, milestone regression, progressive hypotension, and deteriorating neurological status. On the physical examination in the hospital, she had mild pallor and icteric features, undernutrition, facial dysmorphism, periorbital swelling, ascites, and hepatosplenomegaly. Her weight was 8 kg. Her liver was measured to be 8 cm, while the spleen was 10 cm below the rib. Her pupils showed sluggish reaction. No responses were seen with respect to the stimuli, and the reflexes were very poor. An abdominal ultrasound revealed hepatosplenomagaly with large mesenteric lymph nodal masses, retroperitoneal lymph nodes, enlarged porta peripancreatic lymph nodes with moderate ascites. Bone-marrow examination showed characteristic lipid-laden foamy histiocytes, which were negative on periodic acid–Schiff (PAS) staining. A lysosomal enzyme assay of peripheral blood revealed that acid sphingomyelinase (ASM) was 5% of normal in the plasma. A molecular study was ordered to further confirm the diagnosis of Niemann–Pick disease and for family counseling. Which one of the following genes would most likely be tested for Niemann–Pick disease in this patient?[15]

A. *GBA*

B. *GM2A*

C. *HEXA*

D. *HEXB*

E. *SMPD1*

40. A 2-year-old girl was admitted to a local hospital in Virginia for recurrent respiratory tract infections from 4 months of age. Her perinatal history was unremarkable. Her parents and a younger brother were healthy and there was no family history of metabolic disorders. Her liver and spleen were palpable 10 cm and 5.5 cm below the costal margin, respectively. The result of laboratory tests (including liver-function tests) were in the normal ranges. Chest X-rays detected a fairly coarse nodular-reticular pattern in both lungs. A pathological examination of the bone marrow revealed foam cells. Liver biopsy detected enlarged and pale hepatocytes, which were vacuolated and scattered throughout the parenchyma in small groups. Since glycolipids and phospholipids were demonstrated by PAS after diastase and Sudan

Black stains, glycolipid storage disease was diagnosed. She came back to the hospital at 3 years of age, and a bone-marrow examination confirmed the presence of foam cells. Since then she has had frequent coughs and bronchitis, but her clinical conditions remained unchanged until she reached 9 years. At the age of 9 years, she began to complain of headaches and abdominal pains, and skin lesions appeared. She returned to the hospital for further investigation at the age of 14 years. On the physical examination she was 131 cm tall, and weighed 31 kg (both under the 3rd percentile). There was no evidence of neurological disorders. A multigene panel for lysosomal storage disorders detected a heterozygous pathogenic variant, c.1829_1831delGCC (p.Arg608Del), in *SMPD1*. Which one of the following would be the most cost-effective next step in the workup for this patient?[16]

A. Diagnose the patient with Niemann–Pick disease and follow with appropriate treatment.

B. Diagnose the patient with acid sphingomyelinase deficiency and follow with appropriate treatment.

C. Perform deletion and duplication analysis of the genes in the multigene panel for lysosomal storage disorders.

D. Perform deletion and duplication analysis of the *SMPD1* gene.

E. None of the above.

41. A 19-month-old Jewish girl was brought to a local hospital in Israel with symptoms of gradual distention of the abdomen and gradual regression of developmental milestones for 14 months. She had a history of apparently normal growth and development up to 5 months of age. The regression of developmental milestones was evidenced as disappearance of social smile, inability to sit, inability to hold neck, and not able to recognize parents. After 5 months of age, she also had an attack of pneumonia. Her birth history was eventful, and she had been fully immunized. On examination, she had mild pallor. Her liver was enlarged and 10 cm below the costal margin. It was firm, smooth, and nontender. The spleen was 12 cm below the costal margin and was nontender. All the deep reflexes were diminished. There was hypotonia in all four limbs. Her blood examination showed reduced hemoglobin. Abdominal ultrasonography revealed hepatosplenomegaly with normal echotexture without ascites. A fundal examination revealed cherry-red spots in the macula of both eyes. A bone-marrow biopsy detected infiltration of numerous foamy cells in the macrophage. There

was also normoblastic erythroid hyperplasia. Her acid sphingomyelinase was approximately 7% of normal. A diagnosis of Niemann—Pick disease type A was made. Which one of the following pathogenic variants in *SMPD1* would the patient most likely have?[17]

A. c.1493G > T(p.Arg498Leu)

B. c.1829_1831delGCC(p.Arg608Del)

C. c.416T > C(p.Leu139Pro)

D. c.592G > C(p.Ala198Pro)

E. c.1426C > T(p.Arg476Trp)

F. None of the above

42. An 8-month-old boy was admitted to a hospital with the symptoms of tremors in the limbs, swallowing difficulty, and excessive salivation for 4 months. The symptoms evolved to vomiting and peaks of fever during the night before admission. His neuropsychomotor development was normal until the age of 1½ months, when he ceased holding up his head and following objects, started losing interest in the environment, and developed irritability. A physical examination showed microcephaly, ogival palate, and diffuse pigmentation of the retina. A neurological examination evidenced flexion and spastic hypertonia of the upper limbs with abduction of thumbs, symmetrical global hyperreflexia with bilateral Babinski sign, rotatory nystagmus, and spontaneous spasms, resulting from sound, tactile, and light stimuli. EEG showed multifocal irritative activity. Cerebrospinal puncture demonstrated clear fluid, at 5 cells/cm^3 (100% leukocytes), and 161 mg/dL of proteins (55.36% albumin and 12.43% gamma globulin). The patient had transitory hyperthermia and vomiting, stertorous respiration with thick bubbles, and died on the 23rd day after admission. Autopsy revealed microcephaly with the encephalon presenting widened and enlarged sulci, and mild venous congestion. Microscopically, numerous globoid cells were identified, mainly in the deep white matter, presenting a voluminous cytoplasm, sometimes binucleated, with nuclei displayed peripherally and slightly colored by the periodic acid—Schiff (PAS) reaction. Moderate astrocyte reaction, demyelination, and a small number of mononuclear cells were also detected. A lysosomal enzyme assay of peripheral blood revealed that galactocerebrosidase (GALC) enzyme activity was 2% of normal in leukocytes. Which one of the lysosomal disorders would the patient most likely have?[18]

A. Gaucher disease

B. Krabbe disease

C. Niemann—Pick disease

D. Sandhoff disease

E. Tay—Sachs disease

F. None of the above

43. A 2-month-old boy was brought to a clinic for feeding problems and irritability. He was the first child of nonconsanguineous parents, born at term with normal birth weight, length, and head circumference. His family history was unremarkable. His Apgar scores were 9 and 10 at 1 minute and 5 minutes after birth, respectively. A neurological examination revealed generalized hypertonia with an opisthotonic posture, hyperreflexia, and spontaneous Babinski sign. At 12 months of age, he demonstrated a dystonic—spastic quadriparesis with episodes of hyperextension of the lower limbs. He had markedly reduced spontaneous movements and could not localize sound. He had microcephaly, with a head circumference of 42.5 cm (<3 SD below the mean). He continued to deteriorate and died at 17 months of age following respiratory arrest. A sleep electroencephalogram showed a diffusely slow and disorganized background with superimposed isolated spikes in the left temporal region. CT scan at 5 months of age demonstrated widespread high density involving the cerebellar cortex, pons, midbrain, thalami, putamen, and anterior limb of the internal capsule, indicating calcification. There was low density in the cerebellar white matter and, to a lesser degree, in the cerebral hemisphere white matter. Urine organic acids were normal. MRI at 5 months of age demonstrated an abnormal signal in the cerebellar white matter and medial globus pallidus. A cerebrospinal fluid (CSF) examination showed a normal glucose level, a cell count of 26, and a protein of 2.90 g/L (normal range, 0.15—0.45). Lysosomal enzyme analysis was performed on skin fibroblasts, with normal activity demonstrated for β-galactosidase, β-hexosaminidase, and α-fucosidase. The physician suspected that the patient had Krabbe disease. This was confirmed by the demonstration of markedly reduced fibroblast activity of β-galactocerebrosidase (0.17 nmoL/mg/h [normal range, 1.50—8.00]). A molecular study was ordered to further confirm the diagnosis of Krabbe disease and for family counseling. Which one of the following genes would most likely be tested for Krabbe disease in this patient?[19]

A. *GALC*

B. *GBA*

C. *GM2A*

D. *HEXA*

E. *HEXB*

F. *SMPD1*

44. A 3-month-old boy was brought to a local hospital in Mexico by his nonconsanguineous parents for seizures, limb stiffness, irritability, fevers, feeding difficulties, and vomiting. He also showed slowing of mental and motor development. The boy had been born in the same hospital uneventfully. At the age of 6 months, he came again for marked hypertonic with extended and crossed legs, flexed arms, and a backward-bent head. Neurological examination revealed hyperactive tendon reflexes. The physician ordered a molecular study for *GALC*, and the result was positive. Which one of the following would most likely be the finding of the molecular study in this patient?

A. Compound heterozygosity for a 30kb deletion and c.857G > A(p.Gly286asp)

B. Heterozygosity for c.857G > A(p.Gly286asp)

C. Homozygosity for a 30-kb deletion

D. Homozygosity for c.857G > A(p.Gly286asp)

E. Negative

F. None of the above

45. A 7-year-old boy was brought to a clinic with the symptoms of dull pain and bilateral facial asymmetry in the lower jaw for 1 month. A physical examination revealed stunted growth and a short neck. The shape of the head was dolichocephalic with marked macrocephaly. Very prominent occipital and frontal bone was present with frontal bossing. A lateral view revealed hypertelorism of the fronto-occipital area. Coarse facial features such as a depressed and broad nasal bridge, flaring of both nostrils, prominent supraorbital rim bilaterally, ptosis of eyeballs with ocular hypertelorism, thick eyelids, and full, thick lips were observed. His facial asymmetry was more marked on the right side owing to diffuse swelling at the angle and body of mandible. Partial trismus was also observed. He also had an enlarged abdomen, a herniated umbilicus, and massive hepatosplenomegaly. Both the hands were short and stubby, with clawed fingers, which he was unable to straighten. Intraoral examination revealed a large tongue, broad arches with interdental spacing, and moderate anterior open bite with thick gingivae. His family history was noncontributory. The medical history revealed frequent episodes of ear and respiratory infections. A very thin lower border of the mandible was left on the right side owing to bone destruction. Hypoplastic mandibular condyles with short neck and rami with flattening of the superior surface of the condyles were observed. The skull radiograph showed features of dysostosis multiplex, which included a large skull with thickened and sclerotic calvarium and base of the skull, frontal and occipital hyperostosis, hypertelorism, and sella turcica with J sign. Urine examination revealed an increased amount of heparan sulfate and dermatan sulfate. Lysosomal enzyme study revealed absence of α-L-iduronidase. Which one of the lysosomal disorders would the patient most likely have?[20]

A. Hunter syndrome

B. Hurler syndrome

C. Krabbe disease

D. Niemann—Pick disease

E. Sanfilippo syndrome

F. None of the above

46. A 17-month-old boy was referred to a genetics clinic for skeletal dysplasia and developmental delay. His prenatal care and birth were uneventful. The APGAR score was 9. The medical history showed umbilical hernia and recurrent upper respiratory infection in the first year of life. A physical examination showed the boy was short for his age (<3 SD), and had hepatosplenomegaly, coarse facial features, and skeletal dysplasia with restricted joint movement. His mother had a brother and a maternal uncle who died from similar symptoms in childhood without a diagnosis. The urinary glycosaminoglycan (GAG) was elevated. A lysosomal enzyme study revealed absence of α-L-iduronidase enzyme activity in leukocytes. A molecular study was ordered to further confirm the diagnosis of Hurler syndrome and for family counseling. Which one of the following genes would most likely be tested for Hurler syndrome in this patient?

A. *GALC*

B. *HEXA*

C. *IDS*

D. *IDUA*

E. None of the above

47. A 2-year 7-month-old boy presented to a clinic with a history of multiple infections of the upper respiratory tract and otitis. He was tall for his age (+3.46 SD) and moderately overweight (+25.97%). He had a short neck, facial dysmorphism, prominent forehead, depressed nasal bridge, small and stubby fingers with the flexion of distal interphalangeal joints, joint stiffness, distended abdomen with umbilical hernia, hepatosplenomegaly, and mild mental retardation. His Mainz plasma iduronate sulfatase was 6.7986 nM/mL/24 h (normal range, 300—800). Rostock plasma iduronate sulfatase had a value of 1.3 mol/L/h (normal range, ≥2). X-ray demonstrated lumbar vertebral bodies with anterior aspect of beak, and chalice-shaped pelvis, with iliac bones bigger than the ischiopubic ones and were horizontal cotyloid, brown, deformed, and bent for bilateral coxofemoral contortion. Ultrasonographic and echocardiographic examinations revealed first-degree aortic insufficiency, first-degree mitral insufficiency, mild ventricular hypertrophy, and mild hepatosplenomegaly. Lysosomal enzyme study revealed absence of iduronate 2-sulfatase (I2S) enzyme activity in leukocytes. Which one of the lysosomal disorders would the patient most likely have?[21]

A. Hunter syndrome
B. Hurler syndrome
C. Krabbe disease
D. Niemann–Pick disease
E. Sanfilippo syndrome
F. None of the above

48. A 17-month-old boy was referred to a genetics clinic for skeletal dysplasia and developmental delay. His prenatal care and birth were uneventful. The Apgar score was 9 at 1 minute and 10 at 5 minutes. The medical history showed umbilical hernia and recurrent upper respiratory infection in the first year of his life. A physical examination showed that the boy was short for his age (<3 SD) and had hepatosplenomegaly, coarse facial features, and skeletal dysplasia with restricted joint movement. His mother had a brother and a maternal uncle who died from similar symptoms in childhood without a diagnosis. The urinary glycosaminoglycan (GAG) was elevated. A lysosomal enzyme study revealed absence of iduronate 2-sulfatase (I2S) enzyme activity in the white blood cells. A molecular study was ordered to further confirm the diagnosis of Hunter syndrome and for family counseling. Which one of the following genes would most likely be tested for Hunter syndrome in this patient?

A. GALC
B. HEXA
C. IDS
D. IDUA
E. None of the above

49. A 38-month-old boy was referred to a genetics clinic for short stature (≤3 SD) and hepatosplenomegaly identified by ultrasound. The parents reported that the patient grew well in the first year, then "slowed down" after the first birthday. The pregnancy was unremarkable. The delivery was natural, with no complications. The immunizations were up to date. The clinical geneticist noticed that the boy had coarse facial features and could not yet speak a full sentence. A skeletal survey showed skeletal anomalies, including joint contractures. His iduronate 2-sulfatase activity was not detectable and the

arylsulfatase A (ARSA) level was normal. This boy was the couple's second child. The family history revealed early death of his mother's two brothers at the age of 13 years with similar symptoms. The patient's older sister was 5 years old and was apparently healthy. The mother was 16 weeks pregnant with another boy while visiting the clinical geneticist. Which one of the following would most likely describe the estimated risk of the unborn boy developing the same condition?

A. >99%
B. 1/2
C. 1/4
D. Up to 1%
E. Not predictable
F. None of the above

50. A 13-year-old boy was brought to a clinic with a symptom of irregularly placed front teeth. His dental history did not reveal delay or early eruption of baby teeth. He had had recurrent seizures since the age of 8 years and growth retardation since the age of 10 years. His medical history revealed surgery for inguinal hernia on the right side at 9 years and on the left side at 12 years of age. The boy is the second of three children. The eldest, a girl, is apparently healthy. His younger brother had similar symptoms of inguinal hernia. Other family history revealed the early death of his mother's two brothers at the age of 13 years. A physical examination revealed that the patient was of short stature (height 116 cm), had an arm span of 109 cm, and weighed 25.2 kg. He had macrocephaly with bilateral temporal and frontal bossing, coarse facial features, depressed nasal bridge with wide nostrils, bilateral periorbital edema, bushy eyebrows, hypertelorism, puffy eyelids, protruding abdomen, and hepatosplenomegaly. He was intellectually normal. He had claw-like hands and stiff joints. The skin of his extremities was thickened and inelastic. A cardiovascular examination revealed systolic murmur that was best heard in the grade 2 mitral area radiating to left auscultatory variable split to the second heart sound. An ophthalmic examination revealed clear corneas with no corneal clouding. An intraoral examination showed incompetent lips, macroglossia, and anterior open bite. X-ray showed a thickened skull vault with parietal protuberance bilaterally and a dolichocephalic shape. The ribs had an oar-shaped configuration, and the clavicles were thickened. Anterior beaking of lumbar vertebral bodies gave a gibbus deformity or focal kyphosis. Urine analysis showed the presence of glycosaminoglycans (GAGs). His serum alkaline phosphatase level was

increased to 539 IU/L. Lysosomal enzyme study revealed absence of iduronate 2-sulfatase (I2S) enzyme activity in the white blood cells. The patient was diagnosed with Hunter syndrome. A Sanger sequencing analysis of *IDS* did not detect pathogenic variants. The reflex deletion/ duplication study also did not detect pathogenic imbalances. Which one of the following would most likely explain the molecular results in this patient?[22,23]

A. A promoter variant missed by Sanger sequencing

B. A translocation involving *IDS*

C. Unequal recombination between *IDS* and *IDSP1*

D. Wrong diagnosis

E. None of the above

51. A 2-year 6-month-old boy came to a clinic with symptoms of progressive developmental delay, generalized tightness, and inability to sit and stand. He had had fairly normal development until 1 year of age. At that time, he was noticed to have weakness in both lower limbs. His family history was unremarkable. Routine investigations detected a low serum calcium level. Supplemental calcium and vitamin D did not improve his weakness. Then bilateral knee reflex was found to be exaggerated, and the Babinski sign was positive. Brain MRI revealed T2 hyperintense signals in the bilateral frontopariental region, parieto-occipital white matter, corona radiata, and posterior capsule, which suggested dysmyelination or demyelination owing to metachromatic leukodystrophy (MLD). A nerve-conduction velocity study indicated bilateral sensory lower limb motor neuropathy. Arylsulfatase A enzyme activity in leukocytes decreased to 5.3% of normal. Which one of the lysosomal disorders would the patient most likely have?[24]

A. Hunter syndrome

B. Hurler syndrome

C. Metachromatic leukodystrophy

D. X-linked adrenoleukodystrophy

E. Zellweger syndrome spectrum disorders

F. None of the above

52. An 18-month-old girl, born to consanguineous parents, presented to a hospital with decreased mental function and generalized rigidity for 12 days and loss of the ability to hold her neck and sit for 15 days. Her medical history showed head nodding with fever at 6 months of age, which was not associated with uprolling of the eyes, twisting of the limbs, frothing from the mouth, or urinary incontinence. She developed a social smile in the 2nd month and had attained neck holding at the

5th month. She was able to sit with support by the 6th month and sitting without support was attained by the end of the 7th month. She showed stranger anxiety by the 11th month. After 1 year of age, her development regressed, with a progressive inability to walk and sit without support. She was not able to crawl and stand on her own by 15 months of age. She could not articulate any real words by 18 months. She was also not able to feed herself with a spoon or drink from a cup. On examination, she was irritable, with high-pitched crying and inflexed postures at the elbows without signs of meningeal irritation. Her anthropometric measurements were within normal ranges. She had frontal and parietal bossing along with presence of oral thrush, prominent rib cage with rachitic rosary, increased muscle tone, decreased bulk of muscle (thin extremities), and brisk deep tendon reflexes. Brain MRI revealed bilateral symmetrical confluent areas of periventricular deep white matter demyelination, in particular around the atria and frontal horns with sparing of subcortical U fibers. There was increased extra-axial CSF space along both cerebral hemispheres with a mildly dilated ventricular system representing mild cerebral atrophy. Arylsulfatase A enzyme activity in leukocytes were decreased to 2.3% of normal. A molecular study was ordered to further confirm the diagnosis of metachromatic leukodystrophy and for family counseling. Which one of the following genes would most likely be tested for metachromatic leukodystrophy in this patient?[25]

A. *ABCD1*

B. *ARSA*

C. *IDS*

D. *IDUA*

E. *PEX1*

F. None of the above

53. Metachromatic leukodystrophy (MLD) is an autosomal recessive disorder caused by deficiency in arylsulfatase A activity, leading to accumulation of sulfatide substrates. Newborn screening (NBS) for MLD has been difficult. Which one of the following explains why development of an NBS test for MLD is a challenge?[26]

A. Instability of the enzyme in dried blood spots

B. Widespread occurrence of pseudodeficiency alleles

C. Lack of available urine samples from NBS programs

D. All of the above

E. None of the above

54. An Ashkenazi Jewish couple came to a clinic for preconception counseling. Neither had a family

history of disorders commonly seen in their ethnic group. The physician ordered a molecular genetic panel to assess whether the wife is a carrier of one of the disorders commonly seen in their ethnic group. Which one of the genes would most likely NOT be included in the carrier panel for Ashkenazi Jews?

A. *CFTR*
B. *GBA*
C. *HEXA*
D. *SMPD1*
E. *SMPD2*

55. An Ashkenazi Jewish couple came to a clinic for preconception counseling. Neither had a family history of disorders commonly seen in their ethnic group. The physician ordered a molecular genetic panel to assess whether the wife is a carrier of one of the disorders commonly seen in their ethnic group. Which one of the following genes would most likely NOT be included in the carrier panel for Ashkenazi Jews?

A. *ASPA*
B. *ELP1 (IKBKAP)*
C. *GLA*
D. *MEFV*
E. None of the above

56. A 22-year-old, nondiabetic man was admitted to a hospital with a history of an acute onset of diplopia, nausea, vomiting, and dizziness for 12 hours. At the age of 12 years, he had undergone surgery for a blocked right femoral artery. At age 21, he had experienced a dysphasic episode associated with gait disturbance and falling to the right; this episode resolved within 5 days. Three months before the present episode, he was admitted to a hospital for right-sided weakness. During this admission, he was found to have chronic renal failure. He was an alcohol abuser and smoked 1 pack of cigarettes per day. At admission, he was drowsy but easily arousable; his blood pressure was 140/90 mmHg, and there was a questionable angiokeratoma on the right buttock. He had right medial rectus paralysis, right internuclear ophthalmoplegia, upbeat nystagmus on upward gaze, and left horizontal-beat nystagmus; tone was increased on the right. And he showed a right pronator drift, with decreased rapid alternating movements over the right upper extremity and difficult tandem walking. Reflexes were brisk all over, with bilateral Babinski signs and clonic ankle jerks. His 26-year-old brother had similar symptoms without a clear diagnosis. Electromyography showed mild peripheral neuropathy of the axonal type; EGG showed increased QRS voltage. Laboratory analyses

showed decreased creatinine clearance and proteinuria (3.5 g/day); leukocyte α-galactosidase was 6.2% of normal. The urine analysis showed cylindroids and amorphous urates. A kidney biopsy revealed prominent small clear vacuoles in cytoplasm with marked enlargement of glomerular and epithelial cells in vascular loops and abundant mononuclear infiltrates in interstitium. Electron microscopy studies showed typical zebra bodies. His serum α-galactosidase A (α-Gal A) enzyme activity was <1% of normal. Which one of the lysosomal disorders would the patient most likely have?[27]

A. Fabry disease
B. Farber disease
C. Hunter syndrome
D. Hurler syndrome
E. Pompe disease
F. None of the above

57. A 12-year-old boy was admitted to a hospital for chronic pain in the palms of his hands and soles of his feet while walking for 4 years. He also had hypohidrosis and a heating sensation. He was given treatment for pes planus in the Physical Medicine and Rehabilitation (PMR) Department for 2 years, but his symptoms did not improve. On examination, angiokeratomas of the penis and scrotum were found. The 24-hour creatinine clearance ratio (Ccr) was 115.5 mL/min (reference range, 75−125) and the 24-hour urine protein was 9.4 mg/day (reference range, 0−100). An ophthalmic examination showed no sign of corneal opacity and the auditory brainstem response test (ABR) and auditory evoked potential (AEP) showed no evidence of hearing loss. Electrocardiography (ECG) was normal and echocardiography showed mitral-valve prolapse. Electromyography (EMG) and nerve-conduction studies showed no abnormalities. Plasma and urine samples, which were taken after admission, showed a significant decrease in GLA level (3.5 AgalU; normal in male, >15.0 AgalU), and a significant increase in the globotriaosylceramide (GL3) level (plasma 9.1 g/mL [reference range, 3.9−9.9]), urine 5.11 g/mgCr (reference range, 0.01−0.9). A molecular study was ordered to confirm the diagnosis of Fabry disease. Which one of the following genes would most likely be tested for Fabry disease in this patient?[28]

A. *ABCD1*
B. *ARSA*
C. *GBA*
D. *GLA*
E. None of the above

58. A 46-year-old Caucasian male was admitted to a hospital for evaluation of proteinuria, nonspecific cardiac symptoms, and a possible vasculopathy. He had reddish macular—papular skin lesions since the age of 13 years. As a youth, he experienced acroparesthesias and joint pain and did not perspire in hot weather. There was no known family history of skin lesions. The patient was referred for a dermatological examination. He had diffused red to blue papules in the gluteal, lower abdominal, and inguinal regions and on the scrotum and penis. In between the papules were reddish macular lesions. He had similar lesions around the navel and the nipples; less numerous lesions were also present in the armpits and on the flexor aspects of the thighs. Lesions were also seen on his buccal mucosa, upper lip, and palms and soles. Renal function was normal except for mild proteinuria, up to 0.46 g/L. Electrocardiography disclosed a sinusoidal rhythm and concentric hypertrophy of the left ventricle. Echography also showed concentric hypertrophy of the left ventricle and normal systolic activity; the intraventricular septum was thickened and had an unusual granular structure. An ophthalmological investigation revealed aneurysmal dilatations of the conjunctival vessels, and diffuse corneal opacities. Biochemical confirmation of the clinical and histological diagnoses of Fabry disease was made by determining the leukocyte α-Gal A activity, which was totally deficient. Subsequently, a molecular assay for the *GLA* gene was ordered to confirm the diagnosis. Which one of the following molecular assays would most likely be used as a first-tier test to detect pathogenic variants for Fabry disease in this patient?[29]

- **A.** Chromosome microarray (CMA)
- **B.** Multiplex ligation-dependent probe amplification (MLPA)
- **C.** Next-generation sequencing (NGS)
- **D.** Sanger sequencing
- **E.** Target variant analysis of the founder pathogenic variants
- **F.** None of the above

59. A 12-hour-old girl, the first child of nonconsanguineous parents, was admitted to a hospital with a hoarse voice after birth. The baby was born at term with a birth weight of 3500 g. Prenatal examinations identified no abnormalities. A physical examination of the baby revealed the liver edge to be ~3 cm below the rib. A cardiac ultrasound was ordered to examine the heart, which indicated the presence of cardiac hypertrophy. Serum muscle enzymes, such as aspartate aminotransferase, lactate dehydrogenase,

and creatine kinase were elevated. The blood acid alpha-glucosidase (GAA) enzyme activity was 0.1 pmol/punch/h (normal range, 2.88—89.02). Which one of the following lysosomal disorders would the patient most likely have?[30]

- **A.** Fabry disease
- **B.** Farber disease
- **C.** Hunter syndrome
- **D.** Hurler syndrome
- **E.** Pompe disease
- **F.** None of the above

60. An boy with a gestational age of 38 weeks and a birth weight of 3.630 kg, was transferred to a tertiary care center with a diagnosis of hypertrophic cardiomyopathy (HCM) at 48 hours of life. He was the third child of nonconsanguineous parents, and his family history was unremarkable. A heart murmur was detected during the first hours of life, and an echocardiogram showed severe biventricular hypertrophy. Upon arrival, the newborn was asymptomatic and had no dysmorphic features or weakness. A cardiac assessment revealed cardiomegaly, and both an ECG and a 2D echocardiogram showed severe biventricular hypertrophy. The 2D echocardiogram also showed a ventricular septal thickness of 11 mm and a left ventricular posterior wall thickness of 8—9 mm, which was more significant at the apical level. Laboratory tests showed that the only abnormal values were increased creatine kinase (4168 IU/L) and glutamic oxaloacetic transaminase (250 IU/L). No acidosis or hypoglycemia was detected. The results of brain and abdominal ultrasonography were normal. Dried blood spots were sent to assess alpha-glucosidase (GAA) activity, and results in the diagnostic range of Pompe disease were obtained at 7 days of life (0.9 μmol/L/h [reference range, 1.35—6.0 at pH 3.8]). A molecular study was ordered to confirm the diagnosis. Which one of the following genes would most likely be tested for Pompe disease in this patient?[31]

- **A.** *ASPA*
- **B.** *ELP1 (IKBKAP)*
- **C.** *GAA*
- **D.** *GLA*
- **E.** *MEFV*
- **F.** None of the above

61. A 22-year-old Caucasian female with a history of limb weakness came to a clinic for chronic morning headaches. She described her headaches as dull, without nausea, vomiting, visual blurring, photophobia, or phonophobia. The headaches had not responded to pain killers and often subsided spontaneously after 3—4 hours after awakening.

Her medical history revealed that she had suffered from gradually progressive limb weakness for 7 years. The weakness was more prominent in the neck, the trunk, and the proximal limbs. She had difficulty in rising from the floor and climbing stairs without using her arms. During the past 7 years, she had not experienced an efficient nocturnal sleep. Four months ago, a respiratory insufficiency attack led to her being admitted to an intensive care unit (ICU), where a tracheostomy was done. She was diagnosed with polymyositis 2 years ago, and a course of prednisone therapy had no therapeutic effect. Then she was diagnosed with limb girdle muscular dystrophy. There was no family history of muscle disease, headaches, or respiratory problems. A neurological examination revealed severe weakness of the sternocleidomastoid muscles, severe wasting and weakness of the arm abductors (score, 2 of 5), proximal leg muscles (the hip flexors, extensors, and adductors: score, 2 of 5), and bilateral mild weakness of dorsal flexors of the foot (score, 4 of 5). Routine laboratory tests revealed moderately elevated serum creatine kinase (582 IU/L [normal range, 10−100]) and lactate dehydrogenase (565 BBU/mL [normal range, 150−500]). Electromyography showed a myopathic pattern. An overnight polysomnography revealed that her sleep efficacy was 27.09%. Severe hypoxemia, severe sleep apnea (AHI = 77.56 per hour of sleep), severe respiratory-related arousal index (76.54 per hour of sleep) were also shown. The activities of alpha-glucosidase at Ph 3.8, with and without specific inhibition, are 1.18, below the reference ranges (1.5−10 nmol/spot × 21 hours). A genetic study was also ordered to confirm the diagnosis of late-onset Pompe disease. Which one of the following molecular assays would most likely be used as a first-tier test to detect pathogenic variants for Fabry disease in this patient?[32]

A. Chromosome microarray (CMA)
B. Multiplex ligation-dependent probe amplification (MLPA)
C. Next-generation sequencing (NGS)
D. Sanger sequencing
E. Target variant analysis of the founder pathogenic variants
F. None of the above

62. A 28-year-old G3 P1 SAB1 female with no prior health concerns was found to have an abnormal integrated maternal serum screen indicating a 1 in 7 risk for trisomy 18. Fetal ultrasound at 19 weeks' gestation revealed short femurs (<2.5% of normal) and an otherwise normal examination. The family history was notable for one nephew with "weak bones." The patient and her husband were of Yemeni ancestry and distantly related. An amniocentesis showed increased α-fetoprotein at 2.26 MoM and absence of an acetylcholinesterase band. A chromosome analysis revealed a normal male karyotype (46,XY). A follow-up ultrasound at 22 weeks' gestation again demonstrated short femurs, measuring 3.5 cm (under 2.5% of the normal curve). The baby was born by C-section at 37 4/7 weeks' gestation owing to fetal deceleration. Upon delivery, the infant was found to have a hoarse cry, weak reflexes, and low muscle tone. Multiple dysmorphic features were discovered, including short humerus and femurs; bowed lower legs; narrow chest; large ear lobes; retrognathia; yellowish hypertrophic gums and a low, flat palate; hypertrichosis of the bilateral temporal region; and light hair color that was atypical for his ethnic background. He exhibited diffuse patchy ecchymoses on the trunk and persistent thrombocytopenia as well as hyperbilirubinemia. An echocardiogram showed a small atrial septal defect and a large patent ductus arteriosus. The infant also experienced respiratory distress, requiring continuous positive airway pressure ventilation. Laboratory studies revealed elevated levels of multiple plasma and leukocyte lysosomal hydrolases in serum. He passed away at 5 weeks of age. Which one of the following lysosomal disorders would the patient most likely have?[33]

A. Canavan disease
B. Fabry disease
C. Farber disease
D. I-cell disease
E. Pompe disease
F. None of the above

63. An 11-month-old Ashkenazi Jewish male child, born as the third offspring of third-degree consanguineous parents, was brought to a hospital for evaluation and management of abnormal skull shape noted since birth. The mother had also had a spontaneous first-trimester abortion before this child. He was delivered by C-section at full term and had normal cry at birth. He was noted to have global developmental delay since early infancy. He could not recognize his mother, had not attained stable head control, and was unable to sit even with support at 11 months of age. On examination, there were microcephaly and craniosynostosis with a head circumference of 40.5 cm (4 SD below the mean for age and sex). The other features, noted on examination, included coarse facial features with bilateral proptosis, upturned tip of nose with depressed nasal bridge, micrognathia, gum hypertrophy, low-set ears, narrow chest, joint

contractures and bent forearms, and thighs and legs with folds of the overlying skin. Hepatomegaly was noted on palpation of the abdomen. Head CT revealed fusion of the anterior sagittal suture, bicoronal sutures, bilateral lambdoid sutures and temporoparietal sutures. There was bilateral temporo-parietal bossing with diffuse thickening of all skull bones. Mild ventriculomegaly was also noted. Skeletal survey showed significant dysostosis with broad oak-shaped ribs, inferior beaking of vertebrae and diaphyseal and epiphyseal dysplasia with periosteal cloaking. The plasma levels of three lysosomal enzymes (iduronate 2-sulfatase, total hexosaminidase and hexosaminidase A) were significantly elevated (more than 10 times above normal range) in the plasma sample. The diagnosis of I-cell disease with craniosynostosis was established in the child. A genetic test study also ordered to confirm the diagnosis. Which one of the following molecular assays would most likely be used as a first-tier test to detect pathogenic variants for I-cell disease in this patient?[34]

A. Chromosomal microarray (CMA)
B. Multiplex ligation-dependent probe amplification (MLPA)
C. Next-generation sequencing (NGS)
D. Sanger sequencing
E. Target variant analysis of the founder pathogenic variants
F. None of the above

64. A 53-year-old man, with nonconsanguineous parents, presented to a hospital with a history of progressive decrease of visual acuity since the age of 26. At 36, he developed generalized myoclonus and ataxic gait. He showed low visual acuity, ataxic gait, dysarthria, and difficulty in writing. No significant medical or pharmacological history was known. An ophthalmological evaluation revealed low visual acuity (best corrected visual acuity: 20/80 on the right eye and 20/40 on the left eye), bilateral horizontal nystagmus, bilateral cortical and posterior subcapsular cataracts and regular intraocular pressure. A funduscopic examination revealed bilateral macular cherry-red spots. Cup-to-disk ratio was 0.3 bilaterally. Optical coherence tomography (OCT) revealed normal results, however, the presence of nystagmus hindered appropriate retinal imaging. OCT of the nerve-fiber layer revealed atrophy of nerve fibers, especially in the upper and lower quadrants. Perimetry tests showed a defective temporal field in the right eye and an arcuate scotoma in the left eye, but these results provided a low level of confidence influenced by the presence of

nystagmus. A multifocal electroretinography was consistent with the presence of maculopathy with cone dysfunction. EEG revealed an epileptic component of myoclonus. Brain MRI revealed cerebellar and cerebral cortical atrophy. The patient refused skin biopsy. A genetic study was also ordered to confirm the diagnosis. Which one of molecular assays would be most likely used as a first-tier test in this patient?[35]

A. Chromosomal microarray (CMA)
B. Multiplex ligation-dependent probe amplification (MLPA)
C. Next-generation sequencing (NGS)
D. Sanger sequencing
E. Target variant analysis of the founder pathogenic variants
F. None of the above

ANSWERS

1. **B**. Deficiencies of the enzymes all cause lysosomal storage disorders. *Gaucher disease is caused by deficiency of beta-glucocerebrosidase (also known as glucosylceramidase), which is a lysosomal membrane—associated glycoprotein.* The mature protein is composed of 497 amino acids, with 4 oligosaccharide chains coupled to specific asparagine residues. The three-dimensional conformation of the enzyme is stabilized by the formation of three disulfide bonds. The enzyme is responsible for hydrolyzing glucosylceramide into glucose and ceramide (https://www.ncbi.nlm.nih.gov/books/NBK1269/).

Sandhoff disease is caused by pathogenic variants in *HEXB*. The *HEXB* gene encodes for a protein that is part of beta-hexosaminidase A (HEX A) and beta-hexosaminidase B (HEX B). Within lysosomes, these enzymes break down fatty substances, complex sugars, and molecules that are linked to sugars. In particular, HEX A helps to break down GM2 ganglioside. The prototype HEX A deficiency is Tay—Sachs disease. The diagnosis of HEX A deficiency relies on the demonstration of absent to near-absent HEX A enzymatic activity in the serum or white blood cells of a symptomatic individual in the presence of normal or elevated activity of the HEX B isoenzyme. HEX B deficiency is not a recognized disease. Absent to near-absent HEX B usually accompanies lack of HEX A in Sandhoff disease. GM1 gangliosidosis is caused by a deficiency of beta-galactosidase, another lysosomal membrane—associated glycoprotein.

Therefore, deficiency of beta-glucocerebrosidase causes Gaucher disease.

2. **C.** There are a number of genetic disorders for which persons of Jewish heritage, defined by having at least one Jewish grandparent, are most likely to be carriers than the general population, such as Gaucher disease, cystic fibrosis, Tay–Sachs disease, Canavan disease, familial dysautonomia, Bloom syndrome, Fanconi anemia, Niemann–Pick disease, and mucolipidosis. Of these, Gaucher disease is the most common in the Ashkenazi Jewish population (see the table below).

Diseases	Carrier frequency
Gaucher disease	1/15
Cystic fibrosis	1/24
Tay–Sachs disease	1/27
Familial dysautonomia	1/31

Gaucher disease occurs in 1 in 50,000 to 1 in 100,000 people in the general population. Type 1 is the most common form of the disorder; it occurs more frequently in people of Ashkenazi (Eastern and Central European) Jewish heritage than in those with other backgrounds. This form of the condition affects 1 in 500 to 1 in 1000 people of Ashkenazi Jewish heritage (https://ghr.nlm.nih.gov).

The husband's brother died of a congenital condition at a young age, indicating that his parents are obligate carriers. The husband has a 2/3 of chance to be a carrier and a 1/3 of chance to have two normal alleles, since he is asymptomatic.

Therefore, the husband has the highest risk to be a carrier of Gaucher disease.

3. **A.** *GBA is the only gene in which pathogenic variants are known to cause Gaucher disease.* It comprises 7 kb with 11 exons; the cDNA is approximately 2.5 kb. Two different upstream ATG codons are utilized as translation initiation sites. A highly homologous (96% identity) pseudogene (5 kb) is located 16 kb downstream (https://www.ncbi.nlm.nih.gov/books/NBK1269/).

Pathogenic variants in *GLB1* cause GM1 gangliosidosis, type I. Pathogenic variants in *HEXA* cause GM2 gangliosidosis, including Tay–Sachs disease. Pathogenic variants in *HEXB* cause Sandhoff disease. Pathogenic variants in *SMPD1* cause Niemann–Pick disease.

Therefore, *GBA* would most likely harbor pathogenic variant(s) for Gaucher disease in this patient.

4. **F.** The carrier frequency for Gaucher disease (GD) is 1:18 in individuals of Ashkenazi Jewish heritage, which is significantly higher than in other populations. Four variants, N370S, L444P, 84GG, and IVS2 + 1, account for approximately 90% of the pathogenic variants in Ashkenazi Jewish individuals with type 1 Gaucher disease. Testing for the four common *GBA* alleles has been included in panels specifically designed for carrier screening in the Ashkenazi Jewish population (https://www.ncbi.nlm.nih.gov/books/NBK1269/).

Therefore, target variant analysis is the most likely be used to test the husband for carrier status, especially since the wife is not of Jewish descent.

5. **E.** Gaucher disease (GD) is an autosomal recessive lysosomal storage disease. The husband is of Ashkenazi Jewish descent and in his 30s. He remains asymptomatic. It is more likely that he is carrier than a patient, especially since he was tested and only one copy of the L444P variant in *GBA* was detected. So testing the husband with a sequencing assay for *GBA* with reflex to deletion/duplication does not help. Measurement of glucocerebrosidase enzyme activity in peripheral-blood leukocytes is unreliable for carrier determination because of significant overlap in residual enzyme activity levels between obligate carriers and the general (noncarrier) population.

Preconception testing of the partner of a known carrier or affected individual may be requested, especially in ethnic groups with a high prevalence. Four pathogenic variants (N370S, L444P, 84GG, and IVS2 + 1) in *GBA* account for approximately 90% of the disease-causing alleles in the Ashkenazi Jewish population. In non-Jewish populations, the same four alleles account for approximately 50%–60% of disease-causing alleles. Non-Jewish individuals with GD tend to be compound heterozygotes with one common and one "rare" variant or a unique variant (https://www.ncbi.nlm.nih.gov/books/NBK1269/).

The wife is not of Ashkenazi Jewish descent. Targeted-mutation analysis has a low detection ability for her. In this instance, targeted analysis for pathogenic variants is insufficient and full-sequence analysis should be undertaken. Therefore, in this instance sequence analysis most likely is the next step in the workup for this couple.

6. **D.** *The four pathogenic variants (N370S, L444P, 84GG, and IVS2 + 1) in* GBA *account for approximately 90% of the Gaucher disease (GD)–causing alleles in the Ashkenazi Jewish population.* In non-Jewish populations, the same four alleles account for approximately 50%–60% of disease-causing alleles. Non-Jewish individuals with GD tend to be compound heterozygotes with one common and one "rare" variant or a unique variant.

Therefore, the most appropriate estimation of the false negative rate of the targeted variants is 10% in this situation, since the husband is of Ashkenazi Jewish descent.

7. **C.** The four pathogenic variants (N370S, L444P, 84GG, and IVS2 + 1) in *GBA* account for approximately 90% of the Gaucher disease (GD)—causing alleles in the Ashkenazi Jewish population. *In non-Jewish populations, the same four alleles account for approximately 50%—60% of disease-causing alleles.* Non-Jewish individuals with GD tend to be compound heterozygotes with one common and one "rare" variant or a unique variant.

Therefore, the most appropriate estimation of the false negative rate of the targeted variants is approximately 45% in this situation, since the husband is Caucasian.

8. **D.** The carrier frequency for Gaucher disease (GD) is 1 in 18 individuals of Ashkenazi Jewish heritage, which is significantly higher than in other populations. The four variants listed in the question account for approximately 90% of the pathogenic variants in Ashkenazi Jewish individuals with type 1 Gaucher disease (GD). In non-Jewish individuals with type 1 GD, the same four alleles account for approximately 50%—60% of pathogenic variants. Non-Jewish individuals with GD tend to be compound heterozygotes with one common and one "rare" pathogenic variant or a unique pathogenic variant. *The c.1226A > G(p. Gly416Ser) variant, historically called "N370S," is the most common deleterious allele of the* GBA *gene in the Ashkenazi Jewish population for Gaucher disease.* The N370S/N370S genotype appears in 41% of Ashkenazi Jewish patients and 9% of non-Jewish patients. Individuals with at least one N370S allele do not develop primary neurological disease. However, the risk for Parkinson disease among individuals with GD is not precluded by the presence of an N370S allele. Individuals who are homozygous for the N370S variant tend to have milder disease than those who are compound heterozygous. Some individuals who undergo carrier testing have been found to be homozygous for N370S (https://www.ncbi.nlm.nih.gov/books/NBK1269/).

Individuals who are homozygous for the c.1448T > C(p.Leu483Pro) variant, historically called "L444P," tend to have severe disease, often with neurological complications (i.e., types 2 and 3), although several individuals (including adults) with this genotype have had no overt neurological problems. Children who are compound heterozygotes for the c.84dupG(p. Leu29AlafsTer18) variant, 84GG (historically called

"N370S"), or c.115 + 1G > A (historically called "IVS2 + 1G > A") tend to have a subacute disease course with progressive pulmonary involvement and death in the first to second decade. No liveborn child homozygous for either variant has been identified. Thus it is presumed that these genotypes are lethal.

Therefore, this Ashkenazi Jewish girl would most likely have N370S in the *GBA* genes. And targeted mutation analysis can be used to detect carriers in Ashkenazi Jewish descendants.

9. **C.** This patient had neurological complications of Gaucher disease (GD; types 2 and 3). *Individuals who are homozygous for the c.1448T > C(p.Leu483Pro) variant, historically called "L444P," tend to have severe disease, often with neurological complications (i.e., types 2 and 3), although several individuals (including adults) with this genotype have had no overt neurological problems.* In a study of 31 individuals with type 2 GD, L444P accounted for 25 alleles (40%). The L444P variant occurred alone (9 alleles), with the E326K polymorphism (1 allele), and as part of a recombinant allele (15 alleles). In another study, homozygosity for the L444P variant was the most common genotype among individuals with type 3 GD (10 of 24 individuals, or 42%). This variant results in an unstable enzyme with little or no residual activity.

The c.1226A > G(p.Gly416Ser) variant was historically called "N370S." Individuals with at least one N370S allele do not develop primary neurological disease. However, the risk for Parkinson disease among individuals with GD is not precluded by the presence of an N370S allele. Individuals who are homozygous for the N370S variant tend to have milder disease than those who are compound heterozygous. Children who are compound heterozygotes for the c.84dupG(p. Leu29AlafsTer18) variant, also 84GG (historically called "N370S"), or c.115 + 1G > A (historically called "IVS2 + 1G > A") tend to have a subacute disease course with progressive pulmonary involvement and death in the first to second decade. No liveborn child homozygous for either variant has been identified. Thus it is presumed that these genotypes are lethal (https://www.ncbi. nlm.nih.gov/books/NBK1269/).

Therefore, this GD patient would most likely have the L444P variant.

10. **D.** Anemia, hepatosplenomegaly, osteopenia, and seizure are all symptoms of Gaucher disease (GD). Anemia, hepatosplenomegaly, and osteopenia are common features in GD type 1. GD types 2 and 3 are characterized by the presence of primary neurological disease. *Individuals with at least one*

N370S allele most likely have type 1 GD and do not develop primary neurological disease. Individuals who are homozygous for the N370S variant tend to have milder disease than those who are compound heterozygous. It is suspected that a significant proportion of Ashkenazi Jewish individuals with this genotype may be asymptomatic and thus do not come to the attention of medical professionals.

Therefore, the unborn baby would most likely NOT have seizures in postnatal life.

11. **B**. *Anemia, hepatosplenomegaly, osteopenia, and seizure, but not arrhythmia, are all symptoms of Gaucher disease (GD).* Anemia, hepatosplenomegaly, and osteopenia are common features in GD type 1. GD types 2 and 3 are characterized by the presence of primary neurological disease. Individuals who are homozygous for the c.1448T > C(p.Leu483Pro) variant, historically called "L444P," tend to have severe disease, often with neurological complications (i.e., types 2 and 3), although several individuals (including adults) with this genotype have had no overt neurological problems (https://www.ncbi.nlm.nih.gov/books/NBK1269/).

Therefore, the unborn baby would most likely NOT have arrhythmia in postnatal life.

12. **D**. Generally, arrhythmia, developmental delay, odd-smelling urine, and sudden death are not common features in patients with Gaucher disease (GD). GD types 2 and 3 are characterized by the presence of primary neurological disease. *Individuals who are homozygous for the c.1448T > C(p.Leu483Pro) variant, historically called "L444P," tend to have severe disease, often with neurological complications (i.e., types 2 and 3), although several individuals (including adults) with this genotype have had no overt neurological problems* (https://www.ncbi.nlm.nih.gov/books/NBK1269/).

Therefore, the unborn baby would most likely have seizures in postnatal life.

13. **B**. Gaucher disease (GD) is an autosomal recessive lysosomal storage disease. The carrier frequency is 1 in 18 in the Ashkenazi Jewish population. The prevalence is only 1 in 57,000 in other populations. Because the husband's brother died of GD, the parents of the husband are obligate carriers. The husband is not an obligate carrier, but he has a 2/3 chance to be a carrier and a 1/3 chance to have two normal alleles, since he does not have GD.

Therefore, the risk of the couple's firstborn child having GD is: $2/3 \times 1/18 \times 1/4 = 1/108$.

14. **C**. Gaucher disease (GD) is an autosomal recessive lysosomal storage disease. The carrier frequency is 1 in 18 in the Ashkenazi Jewish population. The prevalence is only 1 in 57,000 in other populations. Because the husband's brother died from GD, the

parents of the husband are obligate carriers. The husband is not an obligate carrier, but he has a 2/3 chance to be a carrier and a 1/3 chance to have two normal alleles, since he does not have GD. Since the couple has two healthy boys, the risk of the husband being a carrier is 1/3 (see the table below).

Probability	Carrier	Noncarrier
Prior probability	2/3	1/3
Conditional probability	$(1/2)^2$	1
Joint probability	1/6	2/6
Posterior probability	$\dfrac{1/6}{1/6 + 2/6}$	$= 1/3$

Therefore, the risk that their unborn child will develop GD in his postnatal life is $1/3 \times 1/18 \times 1/4 = 1/216$.

15. **B**. Hepatosplenomegaly, seizure, and thrombocytopenia are all symptoms of Gaucher disease (GD). Hepatosplenomegaly and thrombocytopenia are common features in GD type 1. GD types 2 and 3 are characterized by the presence of primary neurological disease. The *GBA* mutation spectrum varies widely according to ethnic group, and homozygosity for the N370S mutation is the most common genotype in the Ashkenazi Jewish population, in which it accounts for 70% of all disease alleles. The most common disease allele of *GBA* worldwide is the L444P mutation. The most frequent genotype of type 1 Gaucher disease in populations of European descent is N370S/L444P. This genotype generally leads to more severe disease compared with N370S homozygosity. However, *patients with the N370S/L444P genotype have GD type 1* (https://www.ncbi.nlm.nih.gov/books/NBK1269/).

Therefore, the newborn baby will most likely NOT develop seizures due to Gaucher disease in his lifetime.

16. **E**. Gaucher disease (GD) type 1 is characterized by the presence of clinical or radiographic evidence of bone disease (osteopenia, focal lytic or sclerotic lesions, and osteonecrosis), hepatosplenomegaly, anemia and thrombocytopenia, lung disease, and the absence of primary central nervous system disease. GD types 2 and 3 are characterized by the presence of primary neurological disease. Individuals with at least one N370S allele most likely have type 1 GD and do not develop primary neurological disease. Patients with the N370S/L444P genotype have GD type 1, and this genotype generally leads to more severe disease as compared with N370S homozygosity. *Patients with*

type 1 Gaucher disease have an increased risk for Parkinson disease, multiple myeloma, hepatocellular carcinoma, non-Hodgkin lymphoma (NHL), malignant melanoma, and pancreatic cancer.

Parkinsonian features have been reported in a few individuals with type 1 GD; although studies suggest a possible cause-and-effect relationship rather than mere coincidence, the underlying basis remains to be established. The precise risk for individuals with Gaucher disease (GD) of developing Parkinson disease (PD) is not known but has been variously estimated as 20- to 30-fold the risk of an individual in the general population. Family studies suggest that the incidence of parkinsonism may be higher in obligate heterozygotes for GD. *GBA* pathogenic variants have been identified in 5%−10% of individuals with PD. PD associated with *GBA* variants (GBA-PD) is clinically, pathologically, and pharmacologically indistinguishable from idiopathic "sporadic" PD, although GBA-PD has a slightly earlier onset (∼5 years earlier) and more frequently results in cognitive dysfunction (https://www.ncbi. nlm.nih.gov/books/NBK1269/).

Therefore, this patient does not have increased risk to develop osteosarcoma, according to the previous reports.

17. **B.** Beta-hexosaminidase is composed of two subunits, alpha and beta, encoding by separate genes. Both beta-hexosaminidase alpha and beta subunits are members of family 20 of glycosyl hydrolases. Pathogenic variants in the alpha or beta subunit genes lead to an accumulation of GM2 ganglioside in neurons and neurodegenerative disorders termed the GM2 gangliosidoses. *The diagnosis of hexosaminidase A deficiency relies on the demonstration of absent to near-absent beta-hexosaminidase A (HEX A) enzymatic activity in the serum or white blood cells of a symptomatic individual* in the presence of normal or elevated activity of the beta-hexosaminidase B (HEX B) isoenzyme. *HEXA* is the only gene in which pathogenic variants cause hexosaminidase A deficiency (https://www.ncbi.nlm.nih.gov/ books/NBK1218/).

Hexosaminidase B is the beta subunit of the lysosomal enzyme beta-hexosaminidase that, together with the cofactor GM2 activator protein, catalyzes the degradation of the ganglioside GM2, and other molecules containing terminal *N*-acetyl hexosamines. Deficiency of beta-hexosaminidase B and pathogenic variants in the *HEXB* gene causes Sandhoff disease.

Therefore, the diagnosis of hexosaminidase A deficiency relies on the demonstration of deficiency of beta-hexosaminidase A (HEX A) enzymatic activity.

18. **A.** Hexosaminidase A deficiency results in a group of neurodegenerative disorders caused by the accumulation of GM2 ganglioside in lysosomes, which is caused by pathogenic variants in *HEXA*. The prototype beta-hexosaminidase A deficiency is Tay−Sachs disease, also known as the "acute infantile variant."

Sandhoff disease is caused by pathogenic variants in *HEXB*, which disrupt the activity of beta-hexosaminidases A and B; in turn, it prevents these enzymes from breaking down GM2 ganglioside and other molecules. Deficiency of beta-glucocerebrosidase is associated with Gaucher disease. Deficiency of beta-galactosidase is associated with GM1 gangliosidosis.

Therefore, Tay−Sachs disease is caused by deficiency of beta-hexosaminidase A.

19. **E.** Tay−Sachs disease (TSD) has been reported in children of virtually all ethnic, racial, and religious groups. It has been well known that TSD has an increased prevalence in the Ashkenazi Jewish population due to a founder effect. Before the advent of population-based carrier screening, education, and counseling programs for the prevention of TSD in Jewish communities, the incidence of TSD was estimated to be approximately 1 in 3600 Ashkenazi Jewish births. At that birth rate, the carrier rate for TSD is approximately 1 in 30 among Jewish Americans of Ashkenazi extraction (i.e., from Central and Eastern Europe). Among Sephardic Jews and all non-Jews, the disease incidence has been observed to be about 100 times lower, corresponding to a 10-fold lower carrier frequency (between 1 in 250 and 1 in 300).

Certain populations that are relatively isolated genetically have been found to carry *HEXA* pathogenic variants with frequencies comparable to or even greater than those observed in Ashkenazi Jews. These include French Canadians of the eastern St. Lawrence River Valley area of Quebec, Cajuns from Louisiana, and the Old Order Amish in Pennsylvania. It is known that TSD is more prevalent in Mormons in Utah than in other populations.

Therefore, the carrier frequency of Tay−Sachs disease is relatively lower in Mormons in Utah as compared with Ashkenazi Jewish, French Canadians of the eastern St. Lawrence River Valley area of Quebec, Cajuns from Louisiana, and the Old Order Amish in Pennsylvania.

20. D. The Ashkenazi Jewish population has been considered as a genetic isolate, having kept itself separate from its European neighbors by religious and cultural practices of endogamy for a long time. Population isolates are frequently used in genetic research, as such groups are presumed to have reduced genetic diversity, along with increased frequencies of recessive disorders, identity-by-descent (IBD), and linkage disequilibrium (LD) as the result of founder events and population bottlenecks. The most compelling genetic evidence of founder effects in the Ashkenazi Jewish population is the elevated frequency of at least 20 rare recessive diseases attributed to genetic drift following bottlenecks. Coalescence times ascribed to founder mutations for some of these diseases correspond well with historical migrations or episodes of extreme persecution, supporting the argument for genetic drift.

Heterozygous advantage is another phenomenon observed in population genetics. The term is used to describe when the heterozygous genotype has a higher relative fitness than either the homozygous dominant or homozygous recessive genotype. A common example is the case where the heterozygote conveys both advantages and disadvantages, while both homozygotes convey a disadvantage. A well-established case of heterozygote advantage is the *HBB* gene involved in sickle cell anemia.

Therefore, heterozygous advantage does NOT explain why Tay–Sachs disease has increased prevalence in the Ashkenazi Jewish population.

21. A. Assay of HEX A enzymatic activity is the primary method of population screening for carrier detection, as it has greater sensitivity than targeted analysis for pathogenic variants.

However, two pseudodeficiency alleles (p.Arg247Trp and p.Arg249Trp) are not associated with neurological disease, but are associated with reduced degradation of the synthetic substrate when HEX A enzymatic activity is determined. The presence of one pseudodeficiency allele reduces HEX A enzymatic activity toward synthetic substrates but does not reduce enzymatic activity with the natural substrate, GM2 ganglioside. All enzymatic assays use the artificial substrate because the naturally occurring GM2 ganglioside is not a stable reagent and is not available. Thus a potential problem exists in distinguishing between a disease-causing allele, which reduces HEX A enzymatic activity to both artificial and natural substrates, and a pseudodeficiency allele, which reduces HEX A enzymatic activity to the artificial substrate only.

The potential problem is avoided by using molecular genetic testing when the enzymatic activity is abnormal in order to determine whether the reduced HEX A enzymatic activity is caused by a pathogenic variant or a pseudodeficiency variant.

About 35% of non-Jewish individuals identified as heterozygotes by HEX A enzyme–based testing are carriers of a pseudodeficiency allele. About 2% of Jewish individuals identified as heterozygotes by HEX A enzyme–based testing in carrier screening programs are actually heterozygous for a pseudodeficiency allele (https://www.ncbi.nlm.nih.gov/books/NBK1218/).

Therefore, the most appropriate next step in the workup for this couple is targeted *HEXA* pathogenic variant analysis for the husband as a part of the prenatal care after a positive finding for beta-hexosaminidase A (HEX A) enzymatic activity.

22. E. Tay–Sachs disease (TSD) is an autosomal recessive lysosomal storage disorder. The p.Tyr427IlefsTer5 variant is one of the three most common null alleles (p.Tyr427IlefsTer5, c.1421 + 1G > C, and c.1073 + G > A), which in the homozygous state or in compound heterozygosity are associated with TSD. The American College of Obstetricians and Gynecologists (ACOG) recommends offering testing of HEX A enzymatic activity to both members of a couple if one member is of Ashkenazi Jewish heritage. If the wife also carries a pathogenic variant, the unborn child has a 1/4 risk to develop TSD. *To test the wife, assay of HEX A enzymatic activity in serum or leukocytes using synthetic substrates may be considered as a simple, inexpensive, and highly accurate method for heterozygote identification to rule out the possibility.* Serum may be used to test all males and those women who are not pregnant and not using oral contraceptives. Leukocytes are used to test: (1) women who are pregnant; (2) women who are using oral contraceptives; and (3) any individual whose serum HEX A enzymatic activity is in an inconclusive range.

Molecular genetic testing of the *HEXA* gene, in which pathogenic variants cause hexosaminidase A deficiency, is used primarily to: (1) distinguish pseudodeficiency alleles from disease-causing variants in healthy individuals with apparent deficiency of HEX A enzymatic activity identified in population screening programs and (2) identify the specific disease-causing variants in an affected individual to allow for genetic counseling of at-risk family members. The detection rate of molecular genetic testing of *HEXA* is about 99% (https://www.ncbi.nlm.nih.gov/books/NBK1218/).

CVS and amniocentesis are invasive prenatal procedures that are associated with the risk of miscarriage. It is preferred to test the wife first for carrier status instead of running prenatal diagnostic tests on the unborn child using invasive methods. Parental study at the prenatal stage is preferred in this situation because it provides better information for patients for early decision making and preparation if it is necessary.

Therefore, assay of HEX A enzymatic activity in leukocytes in this pregnant woman is the most appropriate next step in the workup for this couple as part of the prenatal care after a heterozygous pathogenic variant is found in the husband.

23. **B**. All enzymatic assays use the artificial substrate because the naturally occurring GM2 ganglioside is not a stable reagent and is not available. There are two common pseudodeficiency alleles (p. Arg247Trp and p.Arg249Trp) in HEX A that are not associated with neurological disease but are associated with reduced degradation of the synthetic substrate. The presence of one pseudodeficiency allele reduces HEX A enzymatic activity toward that of synthetic substrates but does not reduce enzymatic activity with the natural substrate, GM2 ganglioside. Thus a potential problem exists in distinguishing between a disease-causing allele, which reduces HEX A enzymatic activity for both artificial and natural substrates, and a pseudodeficiency allele, which reduces HEX A enzymatic activity for the artificial substrate only. The potential problem is avoided by using molecular genetic testing when the enzymatic activity is abnormal, to determine whether the reduced HEX A enzymatic activity is caused by a disease-causing variant or a pseudodeficiency variant (https://www.ncbi.nlm.nih.gov/books/NBK1218/).

Therefore, targeted *HEXA* pathogenic variant analysis with the two common pseudodeficiency alleles for the wife is the most appropriate next step in the workup for this couple as a part of prenatal care after a positive finding for beta-hexosaminidase A (HEX A) enzymatic activity in the wife.

24. **C**. Assay of HEX A enzymatic activity is the primary method of population screening for carrier detection, as it has greater sensitivity than targeted analysis for pathogenic variants. When individuals are identified with an apparent deficiency of HEX A enzymatic activity, targeted analysis for pathogenic variants can then be used to distinguish pseudodeficiency alleles from disease-causing alleles.

About 35% of non-Jewish individuals identified as heterozygotes by HEX A enzyme–based testing are carriers of a pseudodeficiency allele. About 2% of Jewish individuals identified as heterozygotes by HEX A enzyme-based testing in carrier screening programs are actually heterozygous for a pseudodeficiency allele (https://www.ncbi.nlm.nih.gov/books/NBK1218/).

Therefore, the wife has 35% of chance of not being a silent carrier of Tay–Sachs disease.

25. **A**. Tay–Sachs disease (TSD) is an autosomal recessive lysosomal storage disorder. The husband is a silent carrier of TSD. When enzymatic testing is abnormal in any individual, molecular genetic testing of HEX A is performed in order to identify the pathogenic variant, if possible, and/or to rule out the presence of a pseudodeficiency allele. In this case, the p. Arg247Trp variant detected in the wife is a pseudodeficiency allele, which is not associated with neurological disease but is associated with reduced degradation of the synthetic substrate. Another common pseudodeficiency allele is the p. Arg249Trp variant. Individuals who are heterozygotes for a pseudodeficiency allele are not at increased risk of having a child with TSD or any of the other types of hexosaminidase A deficiency because individuals who are compound heterozygotes for a disease-causing allele and a pseudodeficiency allele who have been followed into the seventh decade have not manifested related neurological symptoms. So the wife is not a carrier of TSD (https://www.ncbi.nlm.nih.gov/books/NBK1218/).

Therefore, the risk of the unborn child to develop Tay–Sachs disease is <1%.

26. **E**. The husband's brother died of Tay–Sachs disease (TSD), indicating that the parents of the husband are obligate carriers. The husband has a 2/3 of chance to be a carrier and a 1/3 of chance to have two normal alleles, since he does not have TSD (the lifespan of a patient with classical TSD is usually less than 4 years). Three alleles, p. Tyr427IlefsTer5, c.1421 + 1G > C, and p.Gly269Ser, are the most common pathogenic variants in *HEX A* in the Ashkenazi Jewish population, in addition to the two pseudodeficiency alleles. *In Quebec, a 7.6-kb genomic deletion that involves the HEX A promoter and exon 1 is the most common allele associated with TSD.* The null allele, c.1073 + 1G > A is in about 10%–15% of individuals with Celtic, French Canadian (specifically from the eastern St. Lawrence River Valley of Quebec), Cajun, and Pennsylvania Dutch background. The p.Arg178His pathogenic variant is predominantly found in

individuals of Portuguese background. When testing individuals from the French Canadian population or other populations with founder variants, care should be taken to identify a laboratory that performs analyses for the appropriate pathogenic variants (https://www.ncbi.nlm.nih.gov/books/NBK1218/).

Therefore, the physician tries to make sure the 7.6-kb genomic deletion involving *HEX A* is covered by the ordered test.

27. **C.** Tay–Sachs disease (TSD) is an autosomal recessive lysosomal storage disorder. The wife is a carrier. A targeted molecular analysis did not confirm the husband is a carrier, and the detection rate of the assay is approximately 90%. The detection rate Bayesian analysis of the husband for the carrier probability is 1/291 (see the table below).

	Carrier	Noncarrier
Prior probability	1/30	29/30
Conditional probability	1/10	1
Joint probability	1/300	290/300
Posterior probability	1/291	

The posterior probability is equal to "Joint probability as a carrier/(Joint probability as a carrier + Joint probability as a noncarrier)."

Therefore, the residual risk of their first child with Tay–Sachs disease is $1/291 \times 1/4 = 1/1164$.

28. **E.** The husband's brother died of Tay–Sachs disease (TSD) in his childhood, indicating the parents of the husband are the obligated carriers. The husband is not an obligate carrier. But he has 2/3 of chance to be a carrier, and 1/3 of chance to have two normal alleles since he does not have

TSD (the lifespan of a patient with classical TSD is usually less than 4 years).

Usually, assay of HEX A enzymatic activity is the primary method of population screening for carrier detection. In the Ashkenazi Jewish population, the sensitivity of targeted analysis for pathogenic variants is lower than assay of HEX A enzymatic activity; therefore some carriers are not identified using targeted analysis. *The false negative rate of the targeted molecular study with the six common variants in HEXA is between 1% (1%–99% = 1%) and 6% (1%–94% = 6%) in Ashkenazi Jews (see Table 9.1). In other ethnics, it is supposed to be higher (Table 9.1)* (https://www.ncbi.nlm.nih.gov/books/NBK1218/).

Therefore, the false negative rate of the targeted molecular study with the six common pathogenic variants in *HEXA* is approximately 5%.

29. **G.** The prototype hexosaminidase A deficiency is Tay–Sachs disease (TSD), also known as the "acute infantile variant." Tay–Sachs disease is characterized by progressive weakness, loss of motor skills, decreased attentiveness, and increased startle response beginning between ages 3 and 6 months, with progressive evidence of neurodegeneration, including seizures, blindness, spasticity, eventual total incapacitation, and death, usually before age 4 years. The juvenile (subacute), chronic, and adult-onset variants of hexosaminidase A deficiency have later onset, slower progression, and more variable neurological findings. Targeted analysis of the *HEXA* gene usually includes the six most common pathogenic variants. It comprises:

- Three null alleles (p.Tyr427IlefsTer5, c.1421 + 1G > C, and c.1073 + G > A) which in the homozygous state or in compound heterozygosity are associated with TSD.

TABLE 9.1 Molecular Genetic Testing of *HEXA* Used in Carrier Detection for Hexosaminidase A Deficiency

Mutations	Allele affect	Carrier frequency	
		Jewish	Non-Jewish
p.Tyr427Ilefs[a]	Null	82%	8%–30%
c.1421 + 1G > C	Null	10%–15%	0
c.1073 + 1G > A	Null	0	15%
p.Gly269Ser	Adult onset	2%	5%
p.Arg247Trp and p.Arg249Trp	Pseudodeficiency	2%	4%–32%
All of the above	Not applicable	94%–99%	32%–82%

[a]*This mutation is also called c.1274_1277dupTATC or c.1278insTATC.CH013*

- *The p.Gly269Ser allele, which is associated with the adult-onset form of hexosaminidase A deficiency in the homozygous state or in compound heterozygosity with a null allele.*

- Two pseudodeficiency alleles (p.Arg247Trp and p.Arg249Trp), which are not associated with neurological disease but are associated with reduced degradation of the synthetic substrate when HEX A enzymatic activity is determined.

The detection rate of this panel in Ashkenazi Jewish in approximately 94%−98%. In Quebec, a 7.6-kb genomic deletion that involves the *HEXA* promoter and exon 1 is the most common allele associated with TSD. The null allele, c.1073 + 1G > A is in about 10%−15% of individuals with Celtic, French Canadian (specifically from the eastern St. Lawrence River Valley of Quebec), Cajun, and Pennsylvania Dutch background. The p.Arg178His pathogenic variant is predominantly found in individuals of Portuguese background (https://www.ncbi.nlm. nih.gov/books/NBK1218/).

Therefore, this patient would most likely have the c.805G > A(p.Gly269Ser) allele for late-onset form of hexosaminidase A deficiency.

30. **D**. The c.1073 + G > A, c.1274_1277dupTATC(p. Tyr427IlefsTer5), c.1421 + 1G > C, and c.533G > A (p.Arg178His) pathogenic variants are null alleles, which in the homozygous state or in compound heterozygosity are associated with Tay−Sachs disease (TSD). The c.739C > T(p.Arg247Trp) and c.745C > T(p.Arg249Trp) are pseudodeficiency alleles, which are not associated with neurological disease but are associated with reduced degradation of the synthetic substrate when HEX A enzymatic activity is determined. The c.805G > A(p.Gly269Ser) allele is associated with the adult-onset form of hexosaminidase A deficiency in the homozygous state or in compound heterozygosity with a null allele.

The three null alleles, c.1073 + G > A, c.1274_1277dupTATC(p.Tyr427IlefsTer5), and c.1421 + 1G > C, are increased in Ashkenazi Jews. In Quebec, a 7.6-kb genomic deletion that involves the *HEXA* promoter and exon 1 is the most common allele associated with TSD. The null allele, c.1073 + 1G > A is in about 10%−15% of individuals with Celtic, French Canadian (specifically from the eastern St. Lawrence River Valley of Quebec), Cajun, and Pennsylvania Dutch background. *The p.Arg178His pathogenic variant predominantly found in individuals of Portuguese background* (https://www.ncbi.nlm.nih.gov/ books/NBK1218/).

This Portuguese patient had classical clinical presentation of TSD. Therefore, he would most likely have the c.533G > A(p.Arg178His) variant.

31. **D**. The c.1073 + G > A, c.1274_1277dupTATC(p. Tyr427IlefsTer5), c.1421 + 1G > C, and c.533G > A (p.Arg178His) are null alleles, which in the homozygous state or in compound heterozygosity are associated with Tay−Sachs disease (TSD). The c.739C > T(p.Arg247Trp) and c.745C > T(p. Arg249Trp) are pseudodeficiency alleles, which are not associated with neurological disease but are associated with reduced degradation of the synthetic substrate when HEX A enzymatic activity is determined. *The c.805G > A(p.Gly269Ser) allele, which is associated with the adult-onset form of hexosaminidase A deficiency in the homozygous state or in compound heterozygosity with a null allele.*

The three null alleles, c.1073 + G > A, c.1274_1277dupTATC(p.Tyr427IlefsTer5), c.1421 + 1G > C, are increased in Ashkenazi Jews. In Quebec, a 7.6-kb genomic deletion that involves the *HEXA* promoter and exon 1 is the most common allele associated with TSD. The null allele, c.1073 + 1G > A is in about 10%−15% of individuals with Celtic, French Canadian (specifically from the eastern St. Lawrence River Valley of Quebec), Cajun, and Pennsylvania Dutch background. The p.Arg178His pathogenic variant predominantly found in individuals of Portuguese background (https://www.ncbi.nlm.nih.gov/ books/NBK1218/).

This patient had classical clinical presentation of TSD. Therefore, he would most likely NOT have the c.805G > A(p.Gly269Ser) variant.

32. **C**. *Sandhoff disease is a lysosomal genetic disorder caused by deficiency of beta-hexosaminidases A and B.* It is characterized by progressively destroying nerve cells in the brain and spinal cord, which is not limited to specific ethnic groups.

Tay−Sachs disease is the prototype of beta hexosaminidase A deficiency. It is highly prevalent in those of Eastern European and Ashkenazi Jewish descent. Gaucher disease is associated with a deficiency of beta-glucocerebrosidase. Niemann−Pick disease types A and B are associated with deficiency of acid sphingomyelinase (ASM).

Therefore, this patient would most likely have Sandhoff disease.

33. **D**. Sandhoff disease is a rare but severe lysosomal storage disorder caused by a deficiency of both hexosaminidases A and B, resulting in accumulation of glycosphingolipids and oligosaccharides in the brain. It represents 7% of

cases of GM2 gangliosidosis. *Pathogenic variants in the HEXB gene cause Sandhoff disease.*

Pathogenic variants in the *GBA* gene cause Gaucher disease. Pathogenic variants in the *HEXA* gene cause hexosaminidase A deficiency (the prototype is Tay–Sachs disease). Pathogenic variants in the *GM2A* gene cause GM2-gangliosidosis, AB variant. Pathogenic variants in the *SMPD1* gene cause Niemann–Pick disease, type A.

Therefore, *HEXB* would most likely be tested to detect Sandhoff disease in this patient.

34. **D.** *Sandhoff disease is an autosomal recessive lysosomal storage disorder caused by a deficiency of both hexosaminidases A and B.* This condition appears to be more common in the Creole population of northern Argentina; the Metis Indians in Saskatchewan, Canada; and people from Lebanon. Silent carriers have reduced enzyme activity, and the remaining activity prevents them from having clinical symptoms.

Therefore, loss of function would most likely describe the pathogenesis of Sandhoff disease in this patient, even though only one copy of abnormal alleles was detected by this sequencing assay.

35. **B.** The Jewish community is at increased risk for many autosomal recessive diseases due to a founder effect (bottle-neck), such as Gaucher disease, cystic fibrosis, Tay–Sachs disease, Canavan disease, familial dysautonomia, Bloom syndrome, Fanconi anemia, Niemann–Pick disease, and mucolipidosis. Children with these diseases are often born to families that do not have other affected relatives. There are different genetic concerns for people of Ashkenazi (Eastern European), Sephardi, and Mizrahi backgrounds. It is estimated that nearly 1 in 2 Ashkenazi Jews in the United States is a carrier of at least 1 of 38 Jewish genetic diseases. Regardless of specific Jewish background, all Jewish and interfaith couples should have preconception carrier screening. The American College of Obstetricians and Gynecologists (ACOG) states that ethnicity-specific, pan-ethnic, and expanded carrier screening are all acceptable strategies for prepregnancy and prenatal carrier screening.

The goal of reproductive carrier screening is to provide important information for couples to use when planning their families. If both partners are carriers of a genetic disorder, performing in vitro fertilization (IVF) with preimplantation genetic diagnosis (PGD) and testing the fetus early in the pregnancy using prenatal diagnostic testing such

as chorionic villus sampling (CVS) or amniocentesis are valid options. With PGD, only unaffected embryos are implanted in the womb. In the case of an affected fetus, the couple can decide whether to continue the pregnancy.

In a couple in which both partners are Jewish, the usual practice is to screen the woman first, if she is not pregnant, generally at her Ob/Gyn's office, as there are X-linked conditions on the testing panel for which only females are screened. If she is found to be a carrier of a specific disease(s), her partner must be screened for that disease(s) if they want to know whether they are at risk for having a child with that disease(s).

Therefore, testing the wife is the most appropriate first step in the workup for this couple.

36. **C.** The goal of reproductive carrier screening is to provide important information for couples to use when planning their families. If both partners are carriers of a genetic condition, in vitro fertilization (IVF) with preimplantation genetic diagnosis (PGD) and testing the fetus early in the pregnancy using prenatal diagnostic testing such as chorionic villus sampling (CVS) or amniocentesis are valid options. With PGD, only unaffected embryos are implanted in the womb. In the case of an affected fetus, the couple can decide whether to continue the pregnancy.

Carrier testing for all of the Jewish genetic diseases by DNA analysis can be done using blood or saliva. *If the woman is already pregnant, both partners must be screened simultaneously.* If they are both carriers of the same disease, earlier fetal testing can be planned and there is more time for counseling and decision making.

Therefore, testing of both the wife and the husband is the most appropriate first step in the workup for this couple.

37. **A.** The goal of reproductive carrier screening is to provide important information for couples to use when planning their families. If both partners are carriers of a genetic condition, in vitro fertilization (IVF) with preimplantation genetic diagnosis (PGD) and testing the fetus early in the pregnancy using prenatal diagnostic testing such as chorionic villus sampling (CVS) or amniocentesis are valid options. With PGD, only unaffected embryos are implanted in the womb. In the case of an affected fetus, the couple can decide whether to continue the pregnancy.

If only one partner is of a Jewish background, that partner should be screened first. If he or she is found to be a carrier of a specific disease(s), the other partner must be screened for that disease(s), if they want to know their risk for having a child with that disease(s).

Therefore, testing of the husband is the most appropriate first step in the workup for this couple (https://www.ncbi.nlm.nih.gov/books/NBK1370/).

38. **B**. *Niemann–Pick disease (NPD) types A and B are associated with deficiency of acid sphingomyelinase (ASM).* NPD type A has neuronopathic symptoms. NPD type B is a nonneuronopathic type of acid sphingomyelinase (ASM) deficiency. Both are caused by biallelic pathogenic variants in *SMPD1*. Usually in patients, the residual ASM enzyme activity is less than 10% of controls (in peripheral-blood lymphocytes or cultured skin fibroblasts) (https://www.ncbi.nlm.nih.gov/books/NBK1370/).

Gaucher disease is associated with deficiency of beta-glucocerebrosidase. Sandhoff disease is caused by deficiency of beta-hexosaminidases A and B. Tay–Sachs disease is the prototype of beta hexosaminidase A deficiency.

Therefore, the patient would most likely have Niemann–Pick disease type A.

39. **E**. Niemann–Pick disease (NPD), also called "acid sphingomyelinase deficiency," is an autosomal recessive lysosomal storage disease. NPD type A (NPDA) has neuronopathic symptoms. NPD type B (NPDB) is a nonneuronopathic type of acid sphingomyelinase (ASM) deficiency. The carrier frequency is 1 in 90 in the Ashkenazi Jewish population. The prevalence is estimated to be 1 in 250,000 in the general population. *SMPD1* and *NPD1* are the genes associated with NPD. *SMPD1 is associated with type A and type B NPD and NPC1 and NPC2 with type C NPD.*

Pathogenic variants in the *GBA* gene cause Gaucher disease. Pathogenic variants in the *HEXA* gene cause hexosaminidase A deficiency (the prototype is Tay–Sachs disease). Pathogenic variants in the *HEXB* gene cause Sandhoff disease. Pathogenic variants in the *GM2A* gene cause GM2 gangliosidosis, AB variant. Pathogenic variants in the *SMPD1* gene cause Niemann–Pick disease, type A.

Therefore, *SMPD1* would most likely be tested for NPDA in this patient.

40. **D**. Acid sphingomyelinase (ASM) deficiency is an autosomal recessive lysosomal storage disorder, which has been categorized in the past as either neuronopathic (Niemann–Pick disease type A [NPD-A]), with death in early childhood, or nonneuronopathic (Niemann–Pick disease type B [NPD-B]). The first symptom in NPD-A is hepatosplenomegaly, usually noted by age 3

months; over time, the liver and spleen become massive. Psychomotor development progresses no further than the 12-month level, after which neurological deterioration is relentless. A classic cherry-red spot of the macula of the retina, which may not be present in the first few months, is eventually present in all affected children. Interstitial lung disease caused by storage of sphingomyelin in pulmonary macrophages results in frequent respiratory infections and often respiratory failure. Most children die before the third year. NPD type B is later in onset and milder in manifestations than NPD type A (https://www.ncbi.nlm.nih.gov/books/NBK1370/).

SMPD1 is associated with type A and type B NPD and *NPC1* and *NPC2* with type C NPD. Sequence analysis of the coding region in *SMPD1* may detect pathogenic variants in 95% of individuals with enzymatically confirmed ASM deficiency. In NPD type B, the variant p.Arg610del may account for almost 90% of pathogenic alleles in individuals from the Maghreb region of North Africa (i.e., Tunisia, Algeria, and Morocco), 100% of pathogenic alleles in Gran Canaria Island, and about 20%–30% of pathogenic variants in the United States.

In this case, the patient had NPD type B. But sequence analysis detected only a heterozygous pathogenic variant in *SMPD1*. Gene-targeted deletion/duplication analysis may be considered to further confirm the diagnosis and for family management. Although no deletions or duplications involving *SMPD1* have been reported to cause ASM deficiency, new deletion/duplication testing methods may identify such pathogenic variants in individuals who did not have a pathogenic variant identified by sequence analysis.

Therefore, deletion and duplication analysis of the *SMPD1* gene would be the most cost-effective next step in the workup for this patient.

41. **A**. *SMPD1* is associated with type A and type B Niemann–Pick disease (NPD) and *NPC1* and *NPC2* with type C NPD. *In NPD type A, three variants (p.Arg498Leu, p.Leu304Pro, p.Phe333SerfsTer52) account for approximately 90% of pathogenic alleles in the Ashkenazi Jewish population.* In this population, the combined carrier frequency for the three common *SMPD1* pathogenic variants is between 1 in 80 and 1 in 100. In contrast with the Ashkenazi Jewish population, each individual affected with NPD-A studied in other populations has a unique *SMPD1* pathogenic variant (https://www.ncbi.nlm.nih.gov/books/NBK1370/).

The rest of the variants listed in the question are pathogenic but are associated with NPD type B.

The variant p.Arg608del may account for almost 90% of pathogenic alleles in individuals from the Maghreb region of North Africa (i.e., Tunisia, Algeria, and Morocco), 100% of pathogenic alleles in Gran Canaria Island, and about 20%−30% of pathogenic variants in the United States. In Chile, the carrier frequency of p.Arg608del is approximately 1 in 106. Some evidence suggests that the p.Leu139Pro, p.Ala198Pro, and p.Arg476Trp pathogenic variants result in a less severe form of NPD-B.

Therefore, this Jewish patient would most likely have the c.1493G > T(p.Arg498Leu) variant.

42. **B.** *This patient had Krabbe disease, which is caused by galactocerebrosidase (GALC) enzyme deficiency.* In almost all individuals with Krabbe disease, galactocerebrosidase (GALC) enzyme activity is deficient (0%−5% of normal activity) in leukocytes isolated from whole heparinized blood or in cultured skin fibroblasts.

Gaucher disease is associated with deficiency of beta-glucocerebrosidase. Niemann−Pick disease (NPD) types A and B are associated with deficiency of acid sphingomyelinase (ASM). Sandhoff disease is caused by deficiency of beta-hexosaminidases A and B. Tay−Sachs disease is the prototype of beta hexosaminidase A deficiency.

Therefore, this patient would most likely have Krabbe disease.

43. **A.** *GALC is the only gene known to be associated with classical Krabbe disease due to galactocerebrosidase (GALC) deficiency.* Atypical Krabbe disease may be caused by biallelic pathogenic variants in *PSAP* also due to saposin A deficiency.

Pathogenic variants in the *GBA* gene cause Gaucher disease. Pathogenic variants in the *HEXA* gene cause hexosaminidase A deficiency (the prototype is Tay−Sachs disease). Pathogenic variants in the *HEXB* gene cause Sandhoff disease. Pathogenic variants in the *GM2A* gene cause GM2-gangliosidosis, AB variant. Pathogenic variants in the *SMPD1* gene cause Niemann−Pick disease, type A.

Therefore, *GALC* would most likely be tested for Krabbe disease in this patient.

44. **C.** *GALC is the only gene known to be associated with classical Krabbe disease due to galactocerebrosidase (GALC) deficiency.* Atypical Krabbe disease may be caused by biallelic pathogenic variants in *PSAP* also due to saposin A deficiency. *In infantile Krabbe disease, a 30-kb deletion accounts for approximately 45% of the mutant alleles in individuals of European ancestry and 35% of the mutant alleles in individuals of Mexican heritage.* This large 30-kb deletion results in the classic infantile

phenotype when in the homozygous state or in the compound heterozygous state along with another pathogenic variants known to cause infantile Krabbe disease, but not the c.857G > A variant. Three other pathogenic variants associated with the infantile phenotype, c.1586C > T(p.Thr529Met), c.1700A > C(p.Tyr567Ser), and c.1472delA(p.Lys491ArgfsTer62), make up another 15% of the mutant alleles in individuals of European ancestry (https://www.ncbi.nlm.nih.gov/books/NBK1238/).

In patients with late-onset Krabbe disease, approximately 50% have at least one copy of the c.857G > A variant. One copy of this variant, even in the compound heterozygous state with the 30-kb deletion, always results in late-onset Krabbe disease.

Therefore, homozygosity for the 30-kb deletion would most likely be the finding of the molecular study in this patient.

45. **B.** *Hurler syndrome, also known as "mucopolysaccharidosis type I (MPS I)," is caused by deficiency of α-L-iduronidase, which leads to deficiency in the metabolism of glycosaminoglycans (GAGs) heparan sulfate and dermatan sulfate.* Accumulation of incompletely degraded glycosaminoglycans into various organs of body leads to impairment of organs and bodily functions (https://www.ncbi.nlm.nih.gov/books/NBK1162/).

Hunter syndrome (mucopolysaccharidosis II) is associated with deficiency of iduronate-2-sulfatase (I2S). Krabbe disease is associated with deficiency of galactocerebrosidase (GALC). Niemann−Pick disease (NPD) types A and B are associated with deficiency of acid sphingomyelinase (ASM). Sanfilippo syndrome (mucopolysaccharidosis III) is associated with a deficiency in one of the enzymes needed to break down the glycosaminoglycan heparan sulfate.

Therefore, this patient would most likely have Hurler syndrome.

46. **D.** The patient had Hurler syndrome, also called mucopolysaccharidosis type I (MPS I), which is caused by deficiency of α-L-iduronidase. Alpha-L-iduronidase is a glycosidase that removes nonreducing terminal α-L-iduronide residues during the lysosomal degradation of heparan sulfate and dermatan sulfate, which are glycosaminoglycans in mammalian cells. *The IDUA gene is the only gene, in which biallelic pathogenic variants currently known to cause Hurler syndrome* (https://www.ncbi.nlm.nih.gov/books/NBK1162/).

Pathogenic variants in the *GALC* gene cause Krabbe disease. Pathogenic variants in the *HEXA* gene cause hexosaminidase A deficiency (the prototype is Tay−Sachs disease). Pathogenic variants in the *IDS* gene cause Hunter syndrome (mucopolysaccharidosis II). Pathogenic variants in the *SGSH*, *NAGLU*, *HGSNAT*, and *GNS* genes cause Sanfilippo syndrome (mucopolysaccharidosis III).

Therefore, *IDUA* would most likely be tested for Hurler syndrome in this patient.

47. **A**. *This patient had Hunter syndrome, also known as "mucopolysaccharidosis II," which is caused by deficiency of iduronate 2-sulfatase (I2S), which leads to glycosaminoglycans (GAG) accumulation.*

Hurler syndrome (mucopolysaccharidosis I) is associated with deficiency of α-L-iduronidase. Krabbe disease is associated with deficiency of galactocerebrosidase (GALC). Niemann–Pick disease (NPD) types A and B are associated with deficiency of acid sphingomyelinase (ASM). Sanfilippo syndrome (mucopolysaccharidosis III) is associated with a deficiency in one of the enzymes needed to break down the glycosaminoglycan heparan sulfate.

Therefore, this patient would most likely have Hunter syndrome.

48. **C**. Hunter syndrome, also known as "mucopolysaccharidosis II," is caused by deficiency of iduronate-2-sulfatase (I2S). *The IDS gene is the only gene in which biallelic pathogenic variants are currently known to cause Hurler syndrome.*

Pathogenic variants in the *GALC* gene cause Krabbe disease. Pathogenic variants in the *HEXA* gene cause hexosaminidase A deficiency (the prototype is Tay–Sachs disease). Pathogenic variants in the *IDUA* gene cause Hurler syndrome (mucopolysaccharidosis I). Pathogenic variants in the *SGSH*, *NAGLU*, *HGSNAT*, and *GNS* genes cause Sanfilippo syndrome (mucopolysaccharidosis III).

Therefore, *IDS* would most likely be tested for Hunter syndrome in this patient.

49. **B**. *Mucopolysaccharidosis type II (MPS II), also known as "Hunter syndrome," is an X-linked MPS caused by a deficiency of iduronidate 2-sulfatase (IDS). IDS is the* only gene in which pathogenic variants are known to cause MPS II.

In this family, the mother is an obligate carrier based on the family history (her two brothers died at the age of 13 years with similar symptoms). Therefore, the estimated risk of the unborn boy developing the same condition would be 1/2.

50. **C**. Absence of iduronate 2-sulfatase (I2S) enzyme activity in white blood cells is diagnostic of Hunter syndrome. *IDS* is the only gene in which pathogenic variants cause Hunter syndrome. Lack of enzyme activity causes accumulation of heparan

and dermatan sulfate (two forms of glysosaminoglycans, or GAGs) in lysosomes, disrupting cellular function and causing disease. The *IDS* gene consists of nine exons and spans about 24 kb of genomic DNA. An *IDS* pseudogene, *IDSP1*, is located about 25 kb telomeric to *IDS*. Homologous regions shared by *IDS* and *IDSP1* predispose to unequal recombination events, leading to complex rearrangements and sometimes large deletions (https://www.ncbi.nlm.nih.gov/books/NBK1274/).

Single-nucleotide changes and splicing variants account for 65% of all pathogenic variants; small (i.e., intraexonic) deletions and insertions account for 17% of all pathogenic variants. Sequence analysis may detect 82% of pathogenic variants within *IDS*. Gene-targeted deletion/duplication analysis detects 9% of patients. *Complex rearrangements, resulting from recombination with the IDSP1 pseudogene or from other processes, may be seen in 9% of patients.* Pathogenic variants in the promoter region of *IDS* have been reported occasionally.

Therefore, unequal recombination between *IDS* and *IDSP1* would most likely explain the molecular results in this patient.

51. **C**. *Metachromatic leukodystrophy (MLD), also known as "arylsulfatase A deficiency," is a lysosomal storage disease, which is commonly listed as a leukodystrophy.* Patients usually have progressive neurological dysfunction, leukodystrophy evidenced by MRI, and increased urinary excretion of sulfatides.

Hurler syndrome (mucopolysaccharidosis I) is associated with deficiency of α-L-iduronidase. Hunter syndrome (mucopolysaccharidosis II) is associated with deficiency of iduronate-2-sulfatase (I2S). X-linked adrenoleukodystrophy (X-ALD) is a disorder of peroxisomal fatty acid beta oxidation, which results in the accumulation of very-long-chain fatty acids in tissues throughout the body. Zellweger syndrome spectrum disorders, including infantile Refsum disease, neonatal adrenoleukodystrophy, and Zellweger syndrome, are peroxisome biogenesis disorders (PBDs).

Therefore, this patient would most likely have metachromatic leukodystrophy.

52. **B**. Metachromatic leukodystrophy (MLD) is also known as "arylsulfatase A deficiency." *ARSA is the only gene in which biallelic pathogenic variants cause MLD.*

Pathogenic variants in the *ABCD1* gene cause X-linked adrenoleukodystrophy. Pathogenic variants in the *IDS* gene cause Hunter syndrome (mucopolysaccharidosis II). Pathogenic variants in the *IDUA* gene cause Hurler syndrome (mucopolysaccharidosis I). Pathogenic variants in the *PEX* gene cause Zellweger syndrome.

Therefore, *ARSA* would most likely be tested for MLD in this patient.

53. **D.** Newborn screening (NBS) of metachromatic leukodystrophy (MLD) by direct measurement of arylsulfatase A activity or protein abundance is not likely to be feasible because of a severe pseudodeficiency problem and relative instability of the enzyme in dried blood spots (DBSs). Sulfatides, the natural substrates for arylsulfatase A, have been shown to be highly increased in urine from MLD patients compared with healthy individuals. However, NBS programs typically use DBS, and dried urine samples (DUS) are usually not available.

   ARSA is the only gene in which biallelic pathogenic variants (*ARSA*-MLD) cause MLD. Pseudodeficiency is suggested by ARSA enzyme activity in leukocytes that are 5%–20% of normal controls. Pseudodeficiency is difficult to distinguish from true ARSA enzyme deficiency by biochemical testing alone. The *ARSA* pseudodeficiency alleles (*ARSA*-PD) result in lower-than-average ARSA enzyme activity but do not cause MLD either in the homozygous state or in the compound heterozygous state with an *ARSA*-MLD allele. The homozygous *ARSA*-PD genotype occurs in as many as 0.5%–2% of the European/Euro-American population and may be even more common in Asian and African populations. Thus an *ARSA*-PD homozygous genotype is more than 400-fold more common than the *ARSA*-MLD homozygous genotype, and an *ARSA*-PD/*ARSA*-MLD compound heterozygous genotype is 30- to 50-fold more common than the *ARSA*-MLD homozygous genotype. An *ARSA*-MLD variant is as likely to be found on an *ARSA*-PD allele as on a wild-type allele, implying that 0.5%–1% of *ARSA*-PD alleles are associated with a cis *ARSA*-MLD variant (so-called *ARSA*-MLD-PD alleles) (https://www.ncbi.nlm.nih.gov/books/NBK1130/).

   Therefore, instability of the enzyme in dried blood spots, widespread occurrence of pseudodeficiency alleles, and the lack of available urine samples from NBS programs are all challenges to the development of a newborn screening program for MLD.

54. **E.** There are a number of genetic disease for which persons of Jewish heritage, defined by at least one grandparent, are most likely to be carriers than those in the general population, such as Gaucher disease, Cystic fibrosis, Tay−Sachs disease, Canavan disease, familial dysautonomia, Bloom syndrome, Fanconi anemia, Niemann−Pick disease, and mucolipidosis in Ashkenazi Jews. It is estimated that nearly 1 in 2 Ashkenazi Jews in the United States is a carrier of at least 1 of 38 Jewish genetic diseases. Carrier testing for all of the Jewish genetic diseases by DNA analysis can be done using blood or saliva. In a couple in which both partners are Jewish, the usual practice is to screen the woman first, if she is not pregnant, generally at her Ob/Gyn's office. If she is found to be a carrier of a specific disease(s), her partner must be screened for that disease(s) if they want to know whether they are at risk for having a child with that disease(s).

   Pathogenic variants in *CFTR* cause cystic fibrosis (CF). In the Ashkenazi Jewish population, three founder mutations, p.R496L, p.L302P, and fsP330, account for more than 95% of mutant alleles and are associated with type A NPD. *GBA* is the only gene in which pathogenic variants cause Gaucher disease (GD). *HEXA* is the only gene in which pathogenic variants cause Tay−Sachs disease (TSD). Niemann−Pick disease (NPD) is associated with mutations in *SMPD1*, *NPD1*, *NPD2*, and *SMPD2*. *SMPD1* is associated with type A and type B of Niemann−Pick disease (NPD). *NPD1, NPD2, and SMPD2 are associated with type C of NPD, which is not common in Ashkenazi Jews.* Three founder mutations, p.R496L, p.L302P, and fsP330, in *SMPD1* are common in the Ashkenazi Jewish population.

   Therefore, *SMPD2* associated with type C of NPD would most likely NOT be included in the carrier panel for Ashkenazi Jews.

55. **C.** There are a number of genetic diseases for which persons of Jewish heritage, defined by at least one grandparent, are most likely to be carriers of than the general population, such as Gaucher disease, Cystic fibrosis, Tay−Sachs disease, Canavan disease, familial dysautonomia, Bloom syndrome, Fanconi anemia, Niemann−Pick disease, and mucolipidosis in Ashkenazi Jews. It is estimated that nearly 1 in 2 Ashkenazi Jews in the United States is a carrier of at least 1 of 38 Jewish genetic diseases. Carrier testing for all of the Jewish genetic diseases by DNA analysis can be done using blood or saliva. In a couple in which both partners are Jewish, the usual practice is to screen the woman first, if she is not pregnant, generally at her Ob/Gyn's office. If she is found to be a carrier of a specific disease(s), her partner must be screened for that disease(s) if they want to know whether they are at risk for having a child with that disease(s).

   The carrier frequency of Canavan disease (CD) in Ashkenazi Jewish is approximately 1 in 55. *ASPA* is the only gene in which pathogenic variants cause CD; two founder mutations, c.854A > C(p.Glu285Ala) and c.693C > A(p.Tyr231X), in *ASPA* present in 99% of Ashkenazi Jewish patients. The third one, c.914C > A(p.Ala305 Glu), was detected in 1% of Ashkenazi Jewish patients. The carrier frequency of familial dysautonomia in Ashkenazi Jews is approximately 1 in 31. *ELP1* (*IKBKAP*) is the only gene in which pathogenic variants cause familial dysautonomia; the two founder pathogenic variants, c.2204 + 6T > C and c.2087G > C(p.Arg696Pro), in *ELP1* (*IKBKAP*) present in 99% of Ashkenazi Jewish patients. The carrier frequency of familial Mediterranean fever in Ashkenazi Jews is approximately 1 in 13. *MEFV* is the only gene in which pathogenic variants cause familial Mediterranean fever; more than 15 pathogenic variants are common in Ashkenazi Jewish patients. *Fabry disease (FD) is found among all ethnic, racial, and demographic groups, and is not more prevalent in Ashkenazi Jews.* The incidence of FD is estimated at 1 in 50,000 to 1 in 117,000 males. *GLA is the only gene in which pathogenic variants cause FD.*

Therefore, *GLA* associated with Fabry disease would most likely NOT be included in the carrier panel for Ashkenazi Jews.

56. **A.** The German dermatologist, Johannes Fabry and the English dermatologist, William Anderson, independently described the first patients with Fabry disease in 1898. *Fabry disease is an X-linked recessive inborn error of glycosphingolipid catabolism resulting from the deficient or absent activity of the lysosomal enzyme α-galactosidase A (α-Gal A).*

Farber disease is associated with deficiency of ceramidase, which causes an accumulation of sphingolipids. Hurler syndrome (mucopolysaccharidosis I) is associated with deficiency of α-L-iduronidase. Hunter syndrome (mucopolysaccharidosis II) is associated with deficiency of iduronate-2-sulfatase (I2S). Pompe disease is associated with deficiency of acid alpha-glucosidase.

Therefore, this patient would most likely have Fabry disease.

57. **D.** Fabry disease results from deficient activity of the enzyme alpha-galactosidase A (α-Gal A) and progressive lysosomal deposition of globotriaosylceramide (GL-3) in cells throughout the body. *The GLA gene is the only gene in which pathogenic variants cause Fabry disease.*

Pathogenic variants in the *ABCD1* gene cause X-linked adrenoleukodystrophy. Pathogenic variants in the *ARSA* gene cause metachromatic leukodystrophy (MLD). Pathogenic variants in the *GBA* gene cause Gaucher disease.

Therefore, *GLA* would most likely be tested for Fabry disease in this patient.

58. **D.** *GLA* is the only gene in which pathogenic variants cause Fabry disease. Fabry disease is found among all ethnic, racial, and demographic groups. The incidence of Fabry disease is estimated at 1 in 50,000 to 1 in 117,000 males. In a study of the Taiwan Chinese population, an unexpectedly high prevalence of the cardiac-variant Fabry-causing pathogenic variant c.640−801G > A (also known as IVS4 + 919G > A and c.639 + 919G > A) was found among newborns (~1:1600 males) as well as individuals with idiopathic hypertrophic cardiomyopathy. Targeted analysis for the IVS4 + 919G > A pathogenic variant can be performed first in individuals of Chinese ancestry with atypical presentation. Targeted analysis for the p.Ala143Pro pathogenic variant can be performed first in individuals from Nova Scotia (incidence 1 in 15,000) (https://www.ncbi.nlm.nih.gov/books/NBK1292/).

More than 800 *GLA* pathogenic variants have been identified, and most are family-specific, occurring only in single pedigrees. Therefore, Sanger sequencing would most likely be used as a first-tier test to detect pathogenic variants for Fabry disease in this Caucasian patient.

59. **E.** *Pompe disease is an autosomal recessive disorder caused by deficiency of the lysosomal enzyme acid-α-glucosidase (GAA), leading to generalized accumulation of lysosomal glycogen especially in the heart, skeletal and smooth muscle, and the nervous system.* Rapid and sensitive analysis of GAA enzyme activity can be performed on dried blood spots when using standard conditions. Complete deficiency of GAA enzyme activity (<1% of normal controls) is associated with infantile-onset Pompe disease (IOPD). Partial deficiency of GAA enzyme activity (2%−40% of normal controls) is associated with late-onset Pompe disease (LOPD).

Fabry disease results from the deficient or absent activity of the lysosomal enzyme α-galactosidase A (α-Gal A). Farber disease is associated with deficiency of ceramidase, which causes an accumulation of sphingolipids. Hurler syndrome (mucopolysaccharidosis I) is associated with deficiency of α-L-iduronidase. Hunter syndrome (mucopolysaccharidosis II) is associated with deficiency of iduronate-2-sulfatase (I2S).

Therefore, this patient would most likely have Pompe disease.

60. **C.** Pompe disease (PD) is an autosomal recessive glycogen storage disorder caused by deficient activity of the lysosomal enzyme acid alpha-1,4-glucosidase (GAA), which leads to glycogen

accumulation in lysosomes and the cytoplasm, resulting in tissue destruction. The enzyme is ubiquitous, but the most affected cells are muscle and cardiac tissues. *GAA is the only gene in which pathogenic variants cause PD.*

ASPA is the only gene in which pathogenic variants cause CD. *ELP1* (*IKBKAP*) is the only gene in which pathogenic variants cause familial dysautonomia. *GLA* is the only gene in which pathogenic variants cause FD. *MEFV* is the only gene in which pathogenic variants cause familial Mediterranean fever.

Therefore, *GAA* would most likely be tested for Pompe disease in this patient.

61. **D.** The incidence of Pompe disease (PD) varies, depending on ethnicity and geographic region, from 1 in 14,000 in African Americans to 1 in 100,000 in individuals of European descent. More than 150 pathogenic variants in *GAA* have been identified in individuals with Pompe disease. *Usually sequence analysis of GAA is performed first and followed by gene-targeted deletion/duplication analysis if only one or no pathogenic variant is found.*

Targeted analysis for pathogenic variants can be performed before sequencing analysis in individuals with the following ancestry and clinical findings: (1). African Americans with infantile-onset PD (IOPD). An estimated 50%−60% have the pathogenic variant p.Arg854Ter; (2) Chinese with IOPD. An estimated 40%−80% have the pathogenic variant p.Asp645Glu; and (3) Adults with late-onset PD (LOPD). An estimated 50%−85% have the pathogenic variant c.336−13T > G typically in the compound heterozygous state. None of these apply to this Caucasian female (https://www.ncbi.nlm.nih.gov/books/NBK1261/).

Therefore, Sanger sequencing would most likely be used as a first-tier test to detect pathogenic variants for Fabry disease in this Caucasian adult patient even though targeted-mutations analysis may detect heterozygous c.336−13T > G.

62. **D.** Mucolipidosis II (I-cell disease) is a lysosomal storage disorder caused by deficiency of *N*-acetylglucosamine-1-phosphotransferase. *Nearly all lysosomal hydrolases are elevated in the plasma and bodily fluids of affected individuals because of the failure of targeting lysosomal acid hydrolases to the lysosomes.*

Canavan disease (CD) is a demyelinating disease caused by deficiency of aspartoacyclase, which catalyzes the breakdown of *N*-acetylaspartic acid (NAA). Fabry disease results from the deficient or absent activity of the lysosomal enzyme, α-galactosidase A (α-Gal A). Farber disease is associated with deficiency of ceramidase,

which causes an accumulation of sphingolipids. Pompe disease (PD) is a glycogen storage disorder caused by deficient activity of the lysosomal enzyme acid alpha-1,4-glucosidase (GAA).

Therefore, this patient would most likely have I-cell disease.

63. **D.** Mucolipidosis II (I-cell disease) is a lysosomal storage disorder caused by deficiency of *N*-acetylglucosamine-1-phosphotransferase. Nearly all lysosomal hydrolases are elevated in the plasma and bodily fluids of affected individuals because of the failure of targeting lysosomal acid hydrolases to the lysosomes. *GNPTAB* is the only gene in which pathogenic variants are known to cause I-cell disease. Several dozen pathogenic variants in all 21 exons of the gene are known. Bidirectional sequencing of the entire *GNPTAB* coding region may detect two pathogenic variants in more than 95% of persons with ML II.

The few estimates of the prevalence of I-cell disease confirm that it is rare (approximately 1 in 123,500 live births in Portugal; approximately 1 in 252,500 in Japan; and approximately 1 in 625,500 in the Netherlands). An unusually high prevalence of I-cell disease in 1 in 6184 live births with an estimated carrier rate of 1 in 39 was found in the northeastern region of the province of Quebec, Canada. In this region, I-cell disease in several large pedigrees has been attributed to a founder effect, as only one *GNPTAB* pathogenic variant (c.3503_3504delTC) has been detected in all obligate carriers. The variant was introduced into that part of Canada in the 17th century by immigrants from France and Scotland. However, in Ashkenazi Jews, this disease is not more prevalent than in other populations, and there is no founder effect (https://www.ncbi.nlm.nih.gov/books/NBK1828/).

Therefore, Sanger sequencing of *GNPTAB* would most likely be used as a first-tier test to detect pathogenic variants for I-cell disease in this patient.

64. **C.** Since the patient refused skin biopsy for an enzyme activity test, it is unclear which enzyme deficiency the patient had. The cherry-red spot sign has also been described in Sandhoff disease, galactosialidosis, GM1 gangliosidosis, GM2 gangliosidosis, Goldberg syndrome, metachromatic leukodystrophy, Niemann−Pick disease types A, B, C, and D, Farber lipogranulomatosis, multiple sulfatase deficiency, Gaucher disease, poisoning (dapsone) and Wolman disease, in addition to sialidosis type I.

In the original case report (in 1995), the patient had a skin biopsy with cultured fibroblasts and leukocytes, which showed null neuraminidase activity levels and normal β-galactosidase levels

(354 in cultured fibroblasts [normal range, 166–2037]; 110 in cultured leukocytes 110 [normal range, 73–585]). The chromatographic profile of oligosaccharides was considered compatible with the disease. The molecular study identified presumably causal pathogenic variants (composite heterozygous mutations c.700G > A (p.D234N) exon 4, c.1021C > T(p.R341X) exon 5) in the *NEU1* gene for sialidosis (mucolipidosis I).

Therefore, a next-generation sequencing (NGS) panel would be most likely used as a first-tier test in this patient.

References

1. Gelb MH, Scott CR, Turecek F. Newborn screening for lysosomal storagediseases. *Clin Chem* 2015;**61**(2):335–46.
2. Larsen EC, Connolly SA, Rosenberg AE. Case records of the Massachusetts General Hospital. Weekly clinicopathological exercises. Case 20-2003. A nine-year-old girl with hepatosplenomegaly and pain in the thigh. *N Engl J Med* 2003;**348**(26):2669–77.
3. Herndon CN, Bender JR. Gaucher's disease: cases in 5 related Negro sibships. *Am J Hum Genet* 1950;**2**(1):49–60.
4. King JO. Progressive myoclonic epilepsy due to Gaucher's disease in an adult. *J Neurol Neurosurg Psychiatry* 1975;**38**(9):849–54.
5. Stone DL, et al. Glucocerebrosidase gene mutations in patients with type 2 Gaucher disease. *Hum Mutat* 2000;**15**(2):181–8.
6. Koprivica V, et al. Analysis and classification of 304 mutant alleles in patients with type 1 and type 3 Gaucher disease. *Am J Hum Genet* 2000;**66**(6):1777–86.
7. Bray SM, et al. Signatures of founder effects, admixture, and selection in the Ashkenazi Jewish population. *Proc Natl Acad Sci USA* 2010;**107**(37):16222–7.
8. Saleh O. Late onset Tay-Sachs disease presenting as a brief psychotic disorder with catatonia: a case report and review of literature. *Jefferson J Psychiatry* 2000;**15**:1 Available from: https://doi.org/10.29046/JJP.015.1.006.
9. Chan LY, et al. Tay-Sach disease with "cherry-red spot"–first reported case in Malaysia. *Med J Malaysia* 2011;**66**(5):497–8.
10. Aragao RE, et al. 'Cherry red spot' in a patient with Tay-Sachs disease: case report. *Arq Bras Oftalmol* 2009;**72**(4):537–9.
11. Yun YM, Lee SN. A case refort of Sandhoff disease. *Korean J Ophthalmol* 2005;**19**(1):68–72.
12. Saouab R, et al. A case report of Sandhoff disease. *Clin Neuroradiol* 2011;**21**(2):83–5.
13. Lakshmi S, Fathima Shirly Anitha G, Vinoth S. A rare case of Sandhoff disease: two in the same family. *Int J Contemp Pediatr* 2015;**2**(1):42–5.
14. Tangde A, Pore S, Kulkarni A, Joshi A, Bindu R. Niemann-pick disease type A – a case report. *Int J Res Med Sci* 2018;**6**(1):366–9.
15. Sriram S, Ahmed J, Saminathan S, Annie S, Raj S. Case study on Type A Niemann Pick disease. *IOSR J Pharm Biol Sci (IOSR-JPBS)* 2016;**11**(4):36–8.
16. Pavone L, Fiumara A, LaRosa M. Niemann-Pick disease type B: clinical signs and follow-up of a new case. *J Inherit Metab Dis* 1986;**9**(1):73–8.
17. Iqbal Bari MIH, Siddiqui AB, Asgar Hossain M, Alam T. Niemann-Pick disease: a case report. *J Teach Assoc* 2002;**15**(1):32–4.
18. Noronha LD, et al. Krabbe's disease – case report. *J Pediatr (Rio J)* 2000;**76**(1):79–82.
19. Duffner PK, et al. Developmental and functional outcomes in children with a positive newborn screen for Krabbe disease: a pilot study of a phone-based interview surveillance technique. *J Pediatr* 2012;**161**(2). p. 258–263e1.
20. Sharma S, et al. Clinical manifestation of Hurler syndrome in a 7 year old child. *Contemp Clin Dent* 2012;**3**(1):86–9.
21. Melit LE, Marginean O, Duicu C, Campean C, Marginean MO. A rare case of Hunter syndrome – case report. *Rom J Pediatr* 2015;**64**(1):38–41.
22. Anekar J, et al. A rare case of mucopolysaccharidosis: hunter syndrome. *J Clin Diagn Res* 2015;**9**(4):ZD23–6.
23. Brusius-Facchin AC, et al. Extension of the molecular analysis to the promoter region of the iduronate 2-sulfatase gene reveals genomic alterations in mucopolysaccharidosis type II patients with normal coding sequence. *Gene* 2013;**526**(2):150–4.
24. Lokhande VS, Gaur A. A case of infantile metachromatic leukodystrophy. *J Neurol Res* 2014;**4**(5-6):138–40.
25. Ali Mallick MS, et al. Infantile metachromatic leukodystrophy in an 18 month old girl. *J Pak Med Assoc* 2016;**66**(9):1197–200.
26. Spacil Z, et al. Sulfatide analysis by mass spectrometry for screening of metachromatic leukodystrophy in dried blood and urine samples. *Clin Chem* 2016;**62**(1):279–86.
27. Moumdjian R, et al. Anderson-Fabry disease: a case report with MR, CT, and cerebral angiography. *Am J Neuroradiol* 1989;**10**(5 Suppl.):S69–70.
28. Cho JE, Hong YH, Lee YG, Lee DH, Yoo HW. Two cases of Fabry disease identified in brothers. *Korean J Pediatr* 2010;**53**(2).
29. Kotnik J, Kotnik F, Desnick RJ. Fabry disease. A case report. *Acta Dermatovenerol Alp Pannonica Adriat* 2005;**14**(1):15–19.
30. Liu Y, et al. Infantile Pompe disease: a case report and review of the Chinese literature. *Exp Ther Med* 2016;**11**(1):235–8.
31. Martinez M, et al. Infantile-onset Pompe disease with neonatal debut: a case report and literature review. *Medicine (Baltimore)* 2017;**96**(51):e9186.
32. Rezaeitalab F, Boostani R, Ghabeli-Juibary A, Mali S. Headache: a presentation of Pompe disease; a case report. *Casp J Neurol Sci* 2017;**3**(8):54–9.
33. Capobres T, Sabharwal G, Griffith B. A case of I-cell disease (mucolipidosis II) presenting with short femurs on prenatal ultrasound and profound diaphyseal cloaking. *Br Inst Radiol* 2016;**2**(3):20150420.
34. Chittem L, Bhattacharjee S, Ranganath P. Craniosynostosis in a child with I-cell disease: the need for genetic analysis before contemplating surgery in craniosynostosis. *J Pediatr Neurosci* 2014;**9**(1):33–5.
35. Sobral I, et al. Sialidosis type I: ophthalmological findings. *BMJ Case Rep* 2014;**2014**. Available from: https://doi.org/10.1136/bcr-2014-205871.

Further Reading

- American College of Medical Genetics and Genomics (ACMGG) (www.acmg.net/)
- Children's National Health System (www.childrensnational.org/)
- GeneReviews (www.ncbi.nlm.nih.gov/books/NBK1116/)
- National Gaucher Foundation (www.gaucherdisease.org/)
- National Organization for Rare Disorders (www.rarediseases.org/)
- National Tay–Sachs & Allied Disease Association (www.ntsad.org/)

10

Neuromuscular Disorders

Neuromuscular disorders (NMD) include a wide range of conditions that affect the muscular system or the peripheral nervous system, which consists of all the motor and sensory nerves that connect the brain and spinal cord to the rest of the body. Progressive muscle weakness is the predominant symptoms of these conditions. Some NMD cases are characterized by progressive muscular impairment leading to loss of mobility, being wheelchair-bound, swallowing difficulties, respiratory muscle weakness, death from respiratory failure, and other symptoms. The Cambridge University physicist, Stephen W. Hawking, was diagnosed with amyotrophic lateral sclerosis (ALS), or Lou Gehrig's disease, when he was 21 years old. He died on March 14, 2018, when he was 76 years old. He was regarded as one of the most brilliant theoretical physicists in history. This shows that NMD do not affect intelligence (http://time.com/5199001/stephen-hawking-als/).

NMD can be divided into rapidly progressive and slowly progressive:

- Rapidly progressive disorders are characterized by muscle impairment that worsens over months, and results in death within a few years, such as Pompe disease, amyotrophic lateral sclerosis (ALS), and Duchenne muscular dystrophy (DMD) in teenagers.
- Variable or slowly progressive disorders are characterized by muscle impairment that worsens over years and only mildly reduces life expectancy, such as limb-girdle muscular dystrophy, facioscapulohumeral muscular dystrophy, and myotonic muscular dystrophy.

This chapter is important because a wide variety of genetic conditions have neuromuscular symptoms, and many of these disorders are treatable if the treatment is initiated early and appropriately. In fact, disability can be stopped and potentially reversed. Finding out the exact nature of the disorder will also allow patients and their families to understand all the implications of the condition and, if it is hereditary, what it might mean for the family and offspring.

The chapter is short because some of the neuromuscular conditions are covered in other chapters. Myotonic dystrophy and spinocerebellar ataxia are covered in Chapter 4, "Disorders of Unstable Repeat Sequences," since unstable repeat DNA sequences cause hypotonia and ataxia in these conditions. Patients with mitochondrial diseases usually have neuromuscular symptoms due to mitochondria hypofunction, which are covered in Chapter 12, "Other Common Genetic Syndromes." The disorders covered in this chapter are:

- Duchenne/Becker muscular dystrophy (DMD/BMD)
- Limb-girdle muscular dystrophy
- Barth syndrome
- Spinal muscular atrophy
- Amyotrophic lateral sclerosis
- Facioscapulohumeral muscular dystrophy
- Pompe disease
- Familial dysautonomia

QUESTIONS

1. A 5-year-old boy was referred to a genetics clinic by his pediatrician for an abnormal gait. He was adopted from another country about a year ago and his family history was unknown. He ran on his tiptoes, which had occurred since he was adopted. He had trouble getting up from a sitting position. He had no other symptoms. His medical history was unremarkable in the past year. He had done well academically in kindergarten despite his language difficulty. A physical examination showed he got up to a standing position using a Gowers maneuver. His gait was best described as wide-based waddling. He was unable to jump. He had calf hypertrophy on both sides. Laboratory testing revealed that his serum creatine kinase (CK) concentration was 75 times higher than

normal. Which one of the following molecular genetics studies would most likely be ordered as the next step in the workup for diagnosis?

A. Deletion/duplication analysis of the *DMD* gene
B. Next-generation sequencing all the genes related to muscular dystrophy
C. Sequencing analysis the *DMD* gene
D. Skeletal muscle biopsy for Western blot studies of dystrophin
E. Skeletal muscle biopsy for immunohistochemistry studies of dystrophin
F. None of the above

2. A 5-year-old boy was referred to a genetics clinic by his pediatrician for an abnormal gait. He was adopted from another country about a year ago and his family history was unknown. He ran on his tiptoes, which had occurred since he was adopted. He had trouble getting up from a sitting position. He had no other symptoms. His medical history was unremarkable in the past year. He had done well academically in kindergarten despite his language difficulty. A physical examination showed he got up to a standing position using a Gowers maneuver. His gait was best described as wide-based waddling. He was unable to jump. He had calf hypertrophy on both sides. Laboratory testing revealed that his serum creatine kinase (CK) concentration was 75 times higher than normal. Which one of the following molecular assays would likely provide the most appropriate first-tier molecular workup for this patient?

A. Multiplex ligation-dependent probe amplification
B. Next-generation sequencing analysis
C. Sanger sequencing analysis
D. TaqMan genotype assays
E. None of the above

3. A 5-year-old boy was referred to a genetics clinic by his pediatrician for an abnormal gait. He was adopted from another country about a year ago and his family history was unknown. He ran on his tiptoes, which had occurred since he was adopted. He had trouble getting up from a sitting position. He had no other symptoms. His medical history was unremarkable in the past year. He had done well academically in kindergarten despite his language difficulty. A physical examination showed he got up to a standing position using a Gowers maneuver. His gait was best described as wide-based waddling. He was unable to jump. He had calf hypertrophy on both sides. Laboratory testing revealed that his serum creatine kinase (CK) concentration was 75 times higher than normal. Duchenne muscular dystrophy (DMD) was suspected. The physician ordered a

deletion/duplication study for the *DMD* gene to confirm the diagnosis, and the result was negative. The physician still suspected DMD. Which one of the following molecular assays would most likely be used as the next step in the molecular workup to rule out DMD in this patient?

A. Multiplex ligation-dependent probe amplification
B. Sanger sequencing analysis
C. TaqMan genotype assays
D. Quantitative PCR
E. None of the above

4. James, a 4-year-old male, was brought to a clinic for a long history of progressive weakening of his muscles. In the first year of his life, he reached many gross motor skill milestones, such as holding his head up, rolling over, sitting, and standing, at normal times. However, he did not walk until age 16 months, and by age 2 he had started to assume a lordotic posture while standing but not while sitting. A Gowers sign was noted by age 4, as was a Trendelenburg gait. Duchenne muscular dystrophy (DMD) was suspected. Laboratory testing revealed an elevated serum creatine kinase level (26,000 IU/L; normal range, <160). A muscle biopsy revealed variation in fiber size, foci of necrosis and regeneration, hyalinization, and, later in the disease, deposition of fat and connective tissue. Western blot found abnormal dystrophin protein. The patient was diagnosed with Duchenne muscular dystrophy (DMD) clinically. James has a 2-year-old sister in good health. No other immediate or distant family members have musculoskeletal difficulties. How frequently do patients with Duchenne muscular dystrophy (DMD) have inherited pathogenic variants?[1]

A. <1%
B. 25%
C. 67%
D. 85%
E. >99%
F. None of the above

5. James, a 4-year-old male, was brought to a clinic for a long history of progressive weakening of his muscles. In the first year of his life, he reached many gross motor skill milestones, such as holding his head up, rolling over, sitting, and standing, at normal times. However, he did not walk until age 16 months, and by age 2 he had started to assume a lordotic posture while standing but not while sitting. A Gowers sign was noted by age 4, as was a Trendelenburg gait. Duchenne muscular dystrophy (DMD) was suspected. Laboratory testing revealed an elevated serum creatine kinase level (26,000 IU/L; normal range, <160). A muscle

biopsy revealed variation in fiber size, foci of necrosis and regeneration, hyalinization, and, later in the disease, deposition of fat and connective tissue. Western blot found abnormal dystrophin protein. A molecular study detected a frameshift deletion in the *DMD* gene. The patient was diagnosed with Duchenne muscular dystrophy (DMD). The same molecular study was offered to his mother and 1-month-old brother. The deletion was not detected in his mother, but it was detected in his brother. Which one of the following would most likely be the explanation of this phenomenon?[1]

A. Incomplete penetrance
B. Variable expression
C. De novo mutations
D. Germline mosaicism
E. X inactivation
F. None of the above

6. James, a 4-year-old male, was brought to a clinic for a long history of progressive weakening of his muscles. In the first year of his life, he reached many gross motor skill milestones, such as holding his head up, rolling over, sitting, and standing, at normal times. However, he did not walk until age 16 months, and by age 2 years he had started to assume a lordotic posture while standing but not while sitting. A Gowers sign was noted by age 4, as was a Trendelenburg gait. Duchenne muscular dystrophy (DMD) was suspected. Laboratory testing revealed an elevated serum creatine kinase level (26,000 IU/L; normal range, <160). A muscle biopsy revealed variation in fiber size, foci of necrosis and regeneration, hyalinization, and, later in the disease, deposition of fat and connective tissue. Western blot found abnormal dystrophin protein. A molecular genetics study detected a frameshift deletion in the *DMD* gene. The patient was diagnosed with Duchenne muscular dystrophy (DMD). The same deletion was not detected in his mother. The proband's parents asked about the recurrent risk in future pregnancies. Which one of the following would be the most approximate estimation of the recurrent risk in this family?[1]

A. <1%
B. 5%
C. 25%
D. 36%
E. None of the above

7. An 8-year-old boy presented for difficulty with walking and muscle weakness leading to difficulty in climbing stairs, running, and particularly vigorous physical activities. He also had decreased strength and endurance. He was from

nonconsanguineous parents and had one healthy brother and two healthy sisters. No other family members had similar symptoms. On the physical examination, he had difficulty jumping onto the examination table. A Gowers sign, proximal weakness of pectoral and pelvic girdle muscles, a waddling gait with tight heel cords, and apparently enlarged calf muscles were noted. His serum creatine kinase and aldolase levels were 50-fold higher than normal. Motor-nerve conduction studies revealed low-amplitude compound muscle action potentials with normal conduction velocities. A molecular genetics study was ordered for Duchenne muscular dystrophy (DMD), and an out-of-frame deletion was detected in the *DMD* gene. Which one of the following conditions would this patient most likely have?[2]

A. Becker muscular dystrophy (BMD)
B. Duchenne muscular dystrophy (DMD)
C. *DMD*-associated dilated cardiomyopathy (DCM)
D. Uncertain
E. None of the above

8. An 18-year-old young male was admitted to a hospital for chest discomfort, nausea, and dyspnea at rest. A molecular genetics study was ordered, and an in-frame deletion was detected. The patient did not have a family history of significant muscle disease and was first examined at 3 years of age because of enlarged calves. At the time of the first examination, blood tests revealed elevated serum levels of creatine kinase (6378 U/L). The electromyogram showed myopathic changes, consisting of small polyphasic potentials. The biceps muscle biopsy revealed dystrophic features. Analysis of the dystrophin-encoding gene by multiplex ligation-dependent probe amplification (MLPA) showed an in-frame deletion of exons 45–49 in the *DMD* gene. Which one of the following conditions would this patient most likely have?[3]

A. Becker muscular dystrophy (BMD)
B. Duchenne muscular dystrophy (DMD)
C. *DMD*-associated dilated cardiomyopathy (DCM)
D. Uncertain
E. None of the above

9. An 8-year-old boy presented for difficulty in walking and muscle weakness leading to difficulty in climbing stairs, running, and particularly vigorous physical activities. He also had decreased strength and endurance. He was from nonconsanguineous parents and had one healthy brother and two healthy sisters. No other family members had similar symptoms. On the physical

examination, he had difficulty jumping onto the examination table. A Gowers sign, proximal weakness of pectoral and pelvic girdle muscles, a waddling gait with tight heel cords, and apparently enlarged calf muscles were noted. His serum creatine kinase and aldolase levels were 50-fold higher than normal. Motor-nerve conduction studies revealed low-amplitude compound muscle action potentials with normal conduction velocities. A molecular genetics study was ordered for Duchenne muscular dystrophy (DMD), and an out-of-frame deletion in the *DMD* gene was detected. Which one of the following recommendations would be appropriate in the molecular genetics report?[2]
- **A.** Genetic counseling
- **B.** Maternal testing
- **C.** Paternal testing
- **D.** Prenatal testing for future pregnancies
- **E.** A and B
- **F.** A and C
- **G.** A, B, and C
- **H.** A, B, and D
- **I.** A, C, and D
- **J.** A, B, C, and D

10. An 8-year-old boy presented for difficulty in walking and muscle weakness leading to difficulty in climbing stairs, running, and particularly vigorous physical activities. He also had decreased strength and endurance. He was from nonconsanguineous parents and had one healthy brother and two healthy sisters. No other family members had similar symptoms. On the physical examination, he had difficulty jumping onto the examination table. A Gowers sign, proximal weakness of pectoral and pelvic girdle muscles, a waddling gait with tight heel cords, and apparently enlarged calf muscles were noted. His serum creatine kinase and aldolase levels were 50-fold higher than normal. Motor-nerve conduction studies revealed low-amplitude compound muscle action potentials with normal conduction velocities. A molecular genetics study for the *DMD* gene detected an out-of-frame deletion, which confirmed the diagnosis of Duchenne muscular dystrophy (DMD). Which one of the following mechanisms would most likely contribute to the pathogenesis of DMD in this patient?[2]
- **A.** Dominant negative
- **B.** Gain of function
- **C.** Loss of function
- **D.** None of the above

11. A 7-month-old boy was admitted to a hospital for heart failure. He was born at term with a weight of 2200 g, a length of 44 cm (both <3rd percentile),

and an occipitofrontal circumference (OFC) of 33.5 cm (10th percentile). The medical history was significant for feeding difficulties after birth that subsequently resolved. A 2D echocardiogram revealed a dilated poorly functioning left ventricle and mild mitral regurgitation. Laboratory testing revealed neutropenia. Follow-up monitoring found that the neutropenia had been recurrent, with an absolute neutrophil count as low as zero. Skin and mucous membrane infections were prominent. His early motor development was delayed, but social and language development were preserved. A urine test revealed increased 3-methylglutaconic acid (3-MGC). A clinical diagnosis of Barth syndrome was made. Which one of the following is the inherited mode of this disorder?[4]
- **A.** Autosomal dominant
- **B.** Autosomal recessive
- **C.** X-linked
- **D.** Mitochondrial inherited
- **E.** None of the above

12. A 10-month-old boy was brought to a clinic for respiratory infection. His developmental milestones were normal. The family history was remarkable for two male cousins and uncles dying of heart failure in early childhood. Cardiomegaly, systolic dysfunction, and myopathy were revealed in the follow-up examination. No diagnosis was made at that time. In the following 2 years, he was in and out of hospitals several times. At 3 years of age, a urine organic acid assay, ordered by a medical geneticist, revealed 3-methylglutaconic aciduria. A diagnosis of Barth syndrome was made clinically. The physician ordered a molecular genetics study to confirm the diagnosis, and a pathogenic variant was detected. Which one of the following would most likely describe the risk of any future children with the same condition?[5]
- **A.** <1%
- **B.** 25%
- **C.** 50%
- **D.** 67%
- **E.** 99%
- **F.** Unpredictable

13. A 10-month-old Ashkenazi Jewish boy was brought to a clinic for respiratory infection. His developmental milestones were normal. The family history was remarkable for two male cousins and uncles dying of heart failure in early childhood. Cardiomegaly, systolic dysfunction, and myopathy were revealed in the follow-up examination. No diagnosis was made at that time. In the following 2 years, he had been in and out of hospitals several times. At 3 years of age, a urine organic acid assay, ordered by a medical geneticist, revealed

3-methylglutaconic aciduria. A diagnosis of Barth syndrome was made clinically. Which one of the following molecular assays would most likely be used as the first-line test to confirm the diagnosis in this patient?

A. Deletion/duplication analysis
B. Next-generation sequencing analysis
C. Sanger sequencing analysis
D. Targeted variant analysis
E. None of the above

14. A 10-month-old Ashkenazi Jewish boy was brought to a clinic for respiratory infection. His developmental milestones were normal. The family history was remarkable for two male cousins and uncles dying of heart failure in early childhood. Cardiomegaly, systolic dysfunction, and myopathy were revealed in the follow-up examination. No diagnosis was made at that time. In the following 2 years, he had been in and out of hospitals several times. At 3 years of age, a urine organic acid assay, ordered by a medical geneticist, revealed 3-methylglutaconic aciduria. A diagnosis of Barth syndrome was made clinically. Which one of the following molecular assays would most likely be used to confirm the diagnosis in this patient?[5]

A. Deletion/duplication analysis of mtDNA
B. Sequencing analysis of mtDNA
C. Sequencing analysis of the *TAZ* gene
D. Sequencing analysis of the *TWNK* gene
E. None of the above

15. A 22-year-old female born of nonconsanguineous parents presented with difficulty in raising her arms above her head and difficulty in getting up from the floor and climbing stairs for the past 7 months. She had more weakness in the upper limbs than in the lower limbs. She had fatigue and exercise intolerance. Her condition had remained static for the past 5 years, after an initial 2 years of deterioration. Her intelligence was normal. Her birth history was noncontributory and developmental milestones had been normal. There was no family history of a similar symptoms. She had history of two miscarriages. On examination, the patient had gross atrophy of the shoulder-girdle muscles and mild atrophy of the medial side of the thigh muscles. Pseudohypertrophy of calves was absent. She had a broad-based waddling gait and lumbar lordosis. Which one of the following molecular genetics studies would be the most appropriate first-tier study to establish a diagnosis in this patient?

A. Chromosomal microarray study (CMA)
B. Fluorescent in situ hybridization (FISH)
C. Molecular genetic testing for *DMD*

D. Next-generation sequencing (NGS) for limb-girdle muscular dystrophy
E. Quantitative PCR

16. A 4-month-old girl was referred to a genetics clinic for severe hypotonia. She had intrauterine growth retardation (IUGR). During the visit the geneticist noted that she could not control her head. She could make contact with her mother's eyes, but her posture was severely hypotonic. Her deep tendon reflexes were absent. Tongue fasciculation was observed. A nerve-conduction study showed decreased lower-extremity motor-nerve compound muscle action potential and delayed conduction velocity. Abnormal spontaneous potentials, polyphasic motor-unit action potentials, and reduced recruitment patterns were noted on needle electromyography of her upper and lower extremities. An electrodiagnostic study suggested an anterior horn cell disease, including spinal muscular atrophy (SMA). Molecular testing was ordered for SMA. Which one of the following molecular genetic assays would most likely be used as a first-tier test to confirm/rule out SMA in this patient?[6]

A. Chromosomal microarray
B. Multiplex ligation-dependent probe amplification (MLPA)
C. Next-generation sequencing analysis
D. Sanger sequencing analysis
E. Target variant analysis
F. None of the above

17. A 48-day-old boy was brought to a clinic for inactivity and poor sucking. He was the first child of nonconsanguineous parents and was born with no perinatal problems. His birth weight was 3.01 kg at 40 weeks of gestational age. His family history was unremarkable for NMD. Since the age of 1 month, his motor activity and sucking power had decreased. In the clinic he looked alert. A physical examination revealed that he had normal cranial-nerve function. He showed hypotonic posture. The upper-extremity power was grade 3 and the lower-extremity power grade 2 symmetrically. There were no deep tendon reflexes. Tongue fasciculation was observed. His serum creatine kinase level was 575 IU/L. Electromyography showed abnormal spontaneous activities. In a motor-nerve conduction study, there was no compound muscle-nerve potential in the left median and right common peroneal nerves. Reduced amplitudes and delayed conduction velocities were noted in the right ulnar and both tibial nerves. On the electrodiagnostic study, sensory nerve action potentials were found in the right median, left superficial peroneal, and both

sural nerves. Molecular testing was ordered for SMA. Which one of the following exons of *SMN1* would most likely be the target of this molecular genetics study?[6]

A. Exon 3
B. Exon 6
C. Exon 7
D. Exon 8
E. None of the above

18. A 4-month-old girl was referred to a genetics clinic for severe hypotonia. She had intrauterine growth retardation (IUGR). During the visit the geneticist noted that she could not control her head. She could make contact with her mother's eyes, but her posture was severely hypotonic. Her deep tendon reflexes were absent. Tongue fasciculation was observed. A nerve-conduction study showed decreased lower-extremity motor-nerve compound muscle action potential and delayed conduction velocity. Abnormal spontaneous potentials, polyphasic motor-unit action potentials, and reduced recruitment patterns were noted on needle electromyography of her upper and lower extremities. An electrodiagnostic study suggested an anterior horn cell disease, including spinal muscular atrophy (SMA). A deletion analysis of the *SMN1*/*SMN2* genes revealed the presence of one copy of exon 7. Which one of the following would be the most appropriate next step in the workup to confirm or rule out the diagnosis?[6]

A. Diagnosing the patient with spinal muscular atrophy
B. Ordering exome sequencing analysis
C. Ordering a next-generation panel with 55 genes for neuromuscular disorders
D. Ordering Sanger sequencing analysis of *SMN1*
E. Ordering Sanger sequencing analysis of *SMN2*
F. None of the above

19. An Ashkenazi Jewish newborn boy was the second child of unrelated parents. He was born by spontaneous vaginal delivery at 38 weeks of gestation. His birth weight was 2620 g. His brother had passed away as a newborn from severe hypotonia and respiratory distress. Antenatally, the mother noticed reduced fetal movements in the last 2 weeks of gestation, and there was polyhydramnios on antenatal scans. The baby was born cyanotic; he was floppy and had no respiratory effort and no chest-wall movement. After two cycles of assisted breathing, the patient remained bradycardic, with a heart rate of <20 beats/minute. Chest compressions were initiated, and the conditions was stabilized with intubation. On day 9 of age, a neurological examination revealed a generalized hypotonia with

absent gag and suck reflexes. Contractures of the shoulders, elbows, hips, and knees were also noted. Deep tendon reflexes and jaw jerk were absent. Cranial ultrasound showed a normal appearance of brain and ventricles. Genetics studies for myotonic dystrophy type 1 were negative, but he had a homozygous deletion of exon 7 and a heterozygous deletion of exon 8 of survival motor neuron gene 1 (*SMN1*). The baby died on day 12 after being disconnected from the tubes. Parental testing revealed that the mother had two copies of exon 7 and exon 8 of *SMN1*, but the father had one copy of exon 7 and exon 8 of *SMN1*. Which one of the following would be the most appropriate explanation of this result?[7,8]

A. It is likely both the couple were carriers of a deletion in *SMN1*.
B. It is likely that the mother had a germline mosaicism for a heterozygous deletion of exon 7 in *SMN1*.
C. The proband and his elder brother had a de novo heterozygous deletion of exon 7 in *SMN1*.
D. The mother had a pathogenic variant, which may be detected by Sanger sequencing analysis.
E. All of the above.
F. None of the above.

20. An Ashkenazi Jewish newborn boy was the second child of unrelated parents. He was born by spontaneous vaginal delivery at 38 weeks of gestation. His birth weight was 2620 g. His brother had passed away as a newborn from severe hypotonia and respiratory distress. Antenatally, the mother noticed reduced fetal movements in the last 2 weeks of gestation, and there was polyhydramnios on antenatal scans. The baby was born cyanotic; he was floppy and had no respiratory effort and no chest-wall movement. After two cycles of assisted breathing, the patient remained bradycardic, with a heart rate of <20 beats/minute. Chest compressions were initiated, and the conditions was stabilized with intubation. On day 9 of age, a neurological examination revealed a generalized hypotonia with absent gag and suck reflexes. Contractures of the shoulders, elbows, hips, and knees were also noted. Deep tendon reflexes and jaw jerk were absent. Cranial ultrasound showed a normal appearance of brain and ventricles. Genetics studies for myotonic dystrophy type 1 were negative, but he had a homozygous deletion of exon 7 and a heterozygous deletion of exon 8 of survival motor neuron gene 1 (*SMN1*). The baby died on day 12 after being disconnected from the tubes. Parental testing revealed that the mother had two copies of exon 7 and exon 8 of *SMN1*, but

the father had one copy of exon 7 and exon 8 of *SMN1*. The physician suspected that the mother had a specific haplotype block, [2 + 0], due to a founder effect in Ashkenazi Jews. Which one of the following would be an appropriate way to confirm it?[7,8]

A. Chromosomal microarray

B. Linkage study

C. No need to confirm

D. Southern blot

E. Testing the mother's parents

F. None of the above

21. An Ashkenazi Jewish newborn boy was the second child of unrelated parents. He was born by spontaneous vaginal delivery at 38 weeks of gestation. His birth weight was 2620 g. The family history was unremarkable. Antenatally, the mother noticed reduced fetal movements in the last 2 weeks of gestation, and there was polyhydramnios on antenatal scans. The baby was born cyanotic; he was floppy and had no respiratory effort and no chest-wall movement. After two cycles of assisted breathing, the patient remained bradycardic, with a heart rate of <20 beats/minute. Chest compressions were initiated, and the conditions was stabilized with intubation. On day 9 of age, a neurological examination revealed a generalized hypotonia with absent gag and suck reflexes. Contractures of the shoulders, elbows, hips, and knees were also noted. Deep tendon reflexes and jaw jerk were absent. Cranial ultrasound showed a normal appearance of brain and ventricles. Genetics studies for myotonic dystrophy type 1 were negative, but he had a homozygous deletion of exon 7 and a heterozygous deletion of exon 8 of survival motor neuron gene 1 (*SMN1*). The baby died on day 12 after being disconnected from the tubes. Parental testing revealed that the husband had one copy of exon 7 of the *SMN1* gene, but the wife had none. Which one of the following would be the most appropriate study as the next step in the workup?[9–11]

A. Redesigning the primers and repeat the study with the new primers

B. Requesting another specimen from the mother

C. Testing the maternal grandparents of the proband

D. Testing the copy number changes of *SMN2* in the wife

E. None of the above

22. The carrier frequency of spinal muscular atrophy (SMA) is about 1 in 40 to 1 in 60 in the United States. Population carrier screening has been recommended by the ACMG, but it has not been supported by the American College of Obstetricians and Gynecologists' Committee on Genetics. The detection rate varies by ethnicity, ranging from 71% in African Americans to 95% in Caucasians. What is the major contributor to this ethnicity-based variation in detection rate?[11]

A. The occurrence of two (or more) *SMN1* genes in tandem on a single chromosome 5

B. The occurrence of two (or more) *SMN2* genes in tandem on a single chromosome 5

C. The occurrence of two (or more) *SMN1* and *SMN2* genes in tandem on a single chromosome 5

D. The occurrence of pathogenic point mutations in *SMN1* on chromosome 5

23. Which one of the following statements regarding spinal muscular atrophy (SMA) is true?[11]

A. There are two inverted SMN copies on chromosome 5q, and *SMN1* is at the centromeric side.

B. The *SMN2* is the SMA-determining gene.

C. The *SMN2* gene produces more full-length transcript than *SMN1*.

D. The number of *SMN2* copies has been shown to modulate the clinical phenotype.

E. *SMN2* exon 7 is absent in the majority of patients, independent of the severity of SMA.

F. The coding sequence of *SMN2* differs from that of *SMN1* by a SNP (840C < T), which alters the amino acid sequence.

24. Which one of the following populations has the highest carrier frequency of spinal muscular atrophy (SMA)?[11,12]

A. African American

B. Ashkenazi Jewish

C. Asian

D. Caucasian

E. Hispanic

25. An Ashkenazi Jewish couple comes to a clinic for a preconception consultation. The medical and family histories are negative on both sides. An Ashkenazi Jewish panel is ordered for the wife. The results show that she has three copies in exon 7 of *SMN1* for spinal muscular atrophy (SMA). Which one of the following may be the most appropriate interpretation?[11]

A. The wife is not a carrier of SMA.

B. The wife has reduced risk to be a carrier.

C. The results must be wrong, and need to be repeated.

D. The sample is mixed with other sample(s), and another blood draw is needed.

26. What is the clinical sensitivity of *SMN1* deletion/copy number analysis to diagnose spinal muscular atrophy (SMA) in Caucasians?

A. >99%

B. 95%

C. 80%

D. 60%

E. 40%

F. 20%

27. Which one of the following populations will have the lowest detection rate if an assay for exon 7 of *SMN1* deletion/copy-number analysis is used to identify carriers of spinal muscular atrophy (SMA)?[11,12]

    A. African American

    B. Ashkenazi Jewish

    C. Asian

    D. Caucasian

    E. Hispanic

28. Which one of the following statements regarding spinal muscular atrophy (SMA) is NOT true?[11,12]

    A. The posterior residual risk for a Caucasian with no family history of SMA to be a carrier following the identification of two copies of *SMN1* exon 7 is higher than that of an African American.

    B. The posterior residual risk for a Caucasian with no family history of SMA to be a carrier following the identification of two copies of *SMN1* exon 7 is higher than in a Caucasian with three copies of *SMN1* exon 7.

    C. The posterior residual risk for a Caucasian with no family history of SMA to be a carrier following the identification of two copies of *SMN1* exon 7 is higher than that of an African American with three copies of *SMN1* exon 7.

    D. None of the above.

29. A scientist in a clinical molecular genetic laboratory plans to validate a quantitative polymerase chain reaction (PCR) assay for spinal muscular atrophy (SMA). Which one of the following designs for the assay should NOT be used?[11]

    A. Monitoring the efficiency of PCR amplification of the internal standard reference gene relative to the *SMN1* gene.

    B. Checking the consistency of the copy number of genomic internal standard reference gene within the genome.

    C. Using two independent copy-number internal standard reference genes.

    D. Using sequencing analysis as a reflex study to rule out the presence of subtle intragenic point variants within the *SMN1* gene.

    E. Using exon 8 as the internal control to test the copy number of *SMN1*.

30. A 40-year-old female came to a clinic with progressive weakness and spasticity of the lower limbs of 12 months' duration. First, she noticed weakness of both hands, followed by generalized fasciculations, dysarthria, and dysphagia. Then in 9 months, she had become dependent for most activities. An examination showed normal mental function, mixed dysarthria, sluggish palatal reflex, and wasting of the tongue. Testing of the motor system revealed fasciculations, severe wasting of hand and feet muscles, and spasticity in all limbs. Power was rated as 2–4 in the upper limbs and 3–4 in the lower limbs, according to the Medical Research Council (MRC) muscle scale. Tendon reflexes were exaggerated, and the plantar response was extensor. The jaw jerk was brisk. She could walk independently. Electromyography performed on all limbs revealed active and chronic denervation with reinnervation. Nerve conductions were normal. The patient's mother developed similar symptoms at 42 years of age and passed away at the age of 50. The patient was diagnosed with amyotrophic lateral sclerosis (ALS) clinically. How frequently is ALS familial?[13]

    A. <1%

    B. 5%–10%

    C. 20%–30%

    D. 50%

    E. 70%–80%

    F. 90%

31. A 43-year-old male came to a hospital with progressive spasticity and weakness and atrophy of the right lower limb for 4 months, followed by similar symptoms in the other limbs with fasciculations. One month later, he developed bulbar palsy. He had severe mixed dysarthria, bifacial weakness, sluggish palatal reflex, wasting of the tongue, hypotonia in the upper limbs, spasticity in the lower limbs and severe atrophy of the limb muscles with grade 2–3 power. Tendon reflexes were exaggerated, with extensor plantar response. Serum electrophoresis, bone scan, and MRI of the brain and cervical spinal cord were normal. Electromyography revealed active denervation and chronic reinnervation in all the limbs. Nerve conductions were normal. The patient's father had similar symptoms and passed away at the age of 58. The patient was diagnosed with amyotrophic lateral sclerosis (ALS) clinically. A molecular genetics study was ordered to confirm the diagnosis and to inform genetic counseling. Which one of the following molecular assays would be the most appropriate to confirm the diagnosis in this patient?[13]

    A. Exome sequencing analysis

    B. Multiplex ligation-dependent probe amplification (MLPA)

    C. Next-generation sequencing analysis

    D. Quantitative PCR analysis

E. Restriction-fragment—length polymorphism analysis

F. Sanger sequencing analysis

G. None of the above

32. A 43-year-old male came to a hospital with progressive spasticity and weakness and atrophy of the right lower limb for 4 months, followed by similar symptoms in the other limbs with fasciculations. One month later, he developed bulbar palsy. He had severe mixed dysarthria, bifacial weakness, sluggish palatal reflex, wasting of the tongue, hypotonia in the upper limbs, spasticity in the lower limbs and severe atrophy of the limb muscles with grade 2—3 power. Tendon reflexes were exaggerated, with extensor plantar response. Serum electrophoresis, bone scan, and MRI of the brain and cervical spinal cord were normal. Electromyography revealed active denervation and chronic reinnervation in all the limbs. Nerve conductions were normal. The patient's father had similar symptoms and passed away at the age of 58. The patient was diagnosed with amyotrophic lateral sclerosis (ALS) clinically. A molecular genetics study was ordered to confirm the diagnosis and to inform genetic counseling. A pathogenic variant, c.112G > A(p.Gly37Arg), in the SOD1 gene was detected. The patient asked the physician if his 20-year-old asymptomatic daughter might be tested. Which one of the following would be the most appropriate response to the request from the patient?[13]

A. Referring the patient's daughter to a pediatric clinic

B. Refusing to test the patient's daughter since she did not have symptoms

C. Refusing to test the patient's daughter since insurance would not pay for testing for asymptomatic individuals

D. Testing the patient's daughter for the familial pathogenic variant after obtaining informed consent

E. None of the above

33. A 40-year-old female came to a clinic with progressive weakness and spasticity of the lower limbs of 12 months' duration. First, she noticed weakness of both hands, followed by generalized fasciculations, dysarthria, and dysphagia. Then in 9 months, she had become dependent for most activities. An examination showed normal mental function, mixed dysarthria, sluggish palatal reflex, and wasting of the tongue. Testing of the motor system revealed fasciculations, severe wasting of hand and feet muscles, and spasticity in all limbs. Power was rated as 2—4 in the upper limbs and 3—4 in the lower limbs, according to the Medical

Research Council (MRC) muscle scale. Tendon reflexes were exaggerated, and the plantar response was extensor. The jaw jerk was brisk. She could walk independently. Electromyography performed on all limbs revealed active and chronic denervation with reinnervation. Nerve conductions were normal. The patient's mother developed similar symptoms at 42 years of age and passed away at the age of 50. The patient was diagnosed with amyotrophic lateral sclerosis (ALS) clinically. A pathogenic variant, c.112G > A(p.Gly37Arg), in the SOD1 gene was detected. The patient asked the physician if her 16-year-old asymptomatic daughter might be tested. Which one of the following would be the most appropriate response to the request from the patient?[13,14]

A. Referring the patient's daughter to a pediatric clinic

B. Refusing to test the patient's daughter since she did not have symptoms

C. Refusing to test the patient's daughter since insurance would not pay for testing for asymptomatic individuals

D. Testing the patient's daughter for the familial pathogenic variant after obtaining informed consent

E. None of the above

34. A 51-year-old male presented to his primary care physician with symptoms of persistent lower back pain. He also noted some right-lower-extremity weakness and atrophy, which he thought resulted from an old racquetball injury of the right calf. The weakness made it difficult for him to walk properly at times. He also had difficulty lifting his arms over his head and had a "crooked" smile. A physical examination revealed an asymmetric smile, minimal right lateral scapular winging, and a steppage gait. Atrophy of the right pectoralis major, trapezius, and gastrocnemius muscles were noted. Atrophy of the bilateral tibialis anterior muscles was also noted. Magnetic resonance imaging (MRI) of the lumbar spine showed a broad-based central disk herniation at the L5—S1 level. Routine serologic testing detected an elevated creatine kinase (CK) level of 324 U/L. Electromyography (EMG) demonstrated findings consistent with a myopathic disorder. A needle examination noted abnormal spontaneous activity in the form of fibrillation potentials and positive sharp waves (PSWs) in various muscles, including the right gastrocnemius and bilateral tibialis anterior muscles. Furthermore, short-duration polyphasic potentials were noted in numerous muscles of the right periscapular region as well as of both lower extremities. Facioscapulohumeral

muscular dystrophy (FMD) was suspected and molecular genetic testing confirmed the diagnosis. Which one of the following types of variants would the patient most likely have?[15]

A. Copy-number variants

B. Macrosatellite variants

C. Microsatellite variants

D. Single-nucleotide variants

E. None of the above

35. A 56-year-old right-handed female came to a hospital for hemiatrophy. Since childhood, she had noted right arm weakness and subsequently right foot drop. Her family history was remarkable for her mother dying at breast cancer at 68-year-old. Neurological examinations, including electromyography and imaging, showed predominant right-sided weakness and atrophy. No asymmetry was apparent in systemic organs, including the brain. The patient was diagnosed with muscular dystrophy, probably facioscapulohumeral muscular dystrophy (FMD). A molecular genetic testing confirmed the diagnosis. Which one of the following assays was most likely used for the molecular genetic testing?[16]

A. Exome sequencing analysis

B. Multiplex ligation-dependent probe amplification (MLPA)

C. Next-generation sequencing analysis

D. Quantitative PCR analysis

E. Sanger sequencing analysis

F. Southern blot

G. None of the above

36. A 56-year-old right-handed female came to a hospital for hemiatrophy. Since childhood, she had noted right arm weakness and subsequently right foot drop. Her family history was remarkable for her mother dying at breast cancer at 68-year-old. Neurological examinations, including electromyography and imaging, showed predominant right-sided weakness and atrophy. No asymmetry was apparent in systemic organs, including the brain. The patient was diagnosed with muscular dystrophy, probably facioscapulohumeral muscular dystrophy (FMD). A molecular genetic testing confirmed the diagnosis. Which one of the following pathogenic variants would the patient most likely have?[16,18]

A. c.2068C > T(p.Pro690Ser) in the *SMCHD1* gene

B. 33- and 48-kb alleles for D4Z4 using *Eco*RI and the p13E-11 probe for Southern blot

C. 44- and 52-kb alleles for D4Z4 using *Eco*RI and the p13E-11 probe for Southern blot

D. A t(4;19)(q35;13) involving *DUX4* at 4q35

E. None of the above

37. An 18-year-old male presented to a clinic with progressive weight loss for the past 11 years. He also experienced episodes of feelings of suffocation and palpitations on exertion. His family history was significant for similar symptoms in uncles, aunts, and cousins who died at ages between 20 and 25 years. He also gave a history of consanguineous marriages in the family. On examination his heart rate was regular at 110 beats/minute and the respiratory rate was 22 breaths/minute. His weight was 36.7 kg and the height 165 cm. He was pale and thin-looking, with uniformly decreased muscle mass. A loud second heart sound was heard at the cardiac apex. His serum aminotransferase levels were mildly raised, and the serum aldolase level was elevated to 25.4 U/L (normal range, 0.1−7.6). The, creatine kinase (CK) level was also raised, at 1179 IU/L (reference range for males, 17−176), and the lactate dehydrogenase level (LDH) was 1205 IU/L (reference range for males, 153−548). His electrocardiogram revealed left ventricular hypertrophy by voltage criteria. However, echocardiography revealed normal left ventricular systolic function with no significant left ventricular hypertrophy. A chest X-ray revealed scoliotic deformity of the dorsal spine. An electromyography/nerve-conduction study showed diffuse irritable myopathic process consistent with muscle dystrophy. A muscle biopsy from the left biceps showed findings consistent with glycogen storage disease type II. A molecular genetic testing confirmed the diagnosis. Which one of the following genes most likely harbored the pathogenic variants?[19]

A. *GAA*

B. *GBA*

C. *HEXA*

D. *SMPD1*

E. None of the above

38. A 4-month-old girl was brought to a clinic for difficulty in feeding and sitting and failure to thrive. She was the first child of nonconsanguineous parents and was delivered at 38 weeks' gestational age without complications. Prenatal examinations were in normal ranges. Her family history was unremarkable. A series of consultations with doctors and various tests revealed liver dysfunction. She was admitted to a hospital for pneumonia and cardiomyopathy after aspiration of syrup at 1 year of age. A physical examination revealed the liver edge about 3 cm below the rib. A cardiac ultrasound indicated the presence of cardiac hypertrophy. Laboratory testing revealed that the serum aspartate

aminotransferase, lactate dehydrogenase, and creatine kinase levels were elevated. Her blood acid alpha-glucosidase (GAA) enzyme activity was 0.1 pmol/punch/hour (normal reference range, 2.88–89.02) at pH 3.8. The girl was diagnosed with Pompe disease, and a molecular genetics study confirmed the diagnosis. Which one of the following assays was most likely used for the molecular genetics testing?[20]

A. Exome sequencing analysis
B. Multiplex ligation-dependent probe amplification (MLPA)
C. Next-generation sequencing analysis
D. Quantitative PCR analysis
E. Sanger sequencing analysis
F. Southern blot
G. None of the above

39. A state laboratory contacted a pediatric geneticist for an abnormal newborn screening (NBS) result for Pompe disease in a baby boy. The family was informed, following which repeat testing of enzyme activity of acid alpha-glucosidase (GAA) was done, as was a molecular genetics study for *GAA*. His enzyme activity of GAA was less than 2% of normal in both the NBS and the repeat studies. The sequencing analysis detected a homozygous variant, c.1726G > A(p.Gly576Ser) in the *GAA* gene. Which one of the following would be the most appropriate interpretation of these findings?

A. The patient had infantile-onset Pompe disease.
B. The patient had late-onset Pompe disease.
C. The patient did not have Pompe disease.
D. The patient's results raised concern for a partial or a full deletion of *GAA*.
E. The patient's results raised concern for a variant in the primer region.

40. A 1-year-old Ashkenazi Jewish boy had been seen intermittently in a local hospital for 6 months because of unexplained febrile episodes and deglutition difficulty with weight loss. The perinatal history was uncomplicated. His family history revealed a paternal aunt with mental retardation and muscular weakness, who died at 8 years of age without a diagnosis. The patient presented with growth retardation. On physical examination he was small for his age with a low weight. He had insensitivity to pain, diminished lacrimation with normal corneal reflex, poor muscular tone with abolished deep tendon reflexes, poor coordination, vomiting attacks, and neuropsychomotor retardation. An electroneuromyography revealed a sensory neuropathy. Which one of the following disorders would this patient more likely have than others?[21]

A. Familial dysautonomia
B. Hereditary neuropathy with liability to pressure palsies (HNLPP)
C. Smith–Lemli–Opitz syndrome
D. Smith–Magenis syndrome
E. None of the above

41. A 1-year-old Ashkenazi Jewish boy had been seen intermittently in a local hospital for 6 months because of unexplained febrile episodes and deglutition difficulty with weight loss. He had insensitivity to pain, diminished lacrimation with normal corneal reflex, poor muscular tone with abolished deep tendon reflexes, poor coordination, vomiting attacks, and neuropsychomotor retardation. He also has growth retardation. The pregnancy had been uncomplicated and the delivery normal. The family history was uneventful. On a physical examination, he was small for his age with low weight. Electroneuromyography revealed sensory neuropathy. Which one of the following disorders does the patient most likely have?

A. Canavan disease
B. Familial dysautonomia
C. Gaucher disease
D. Pompe disease
E. None of the above

42. A 1-year-old Ashkenazi Jewish boy had been seen intermittently in a local hospital for 6 months because of unexplained febrile episodes and deglutition difficulty with weight loss. He had insensitivity to pain, diminished lacrimation with normal corneal reflex, poor muscular tone with abolished deep tendon reflexes, poor coordination, vomiting attacks, and neuropsychomotor retardation. He also had growth retardation. The pregnancy had been uncomplicated and the delivery normal. The family history was uneventful. On a physical examination, he was small for his age with low-weight. Electroneuromyography revealed a sensory neuropathy. What will be the recurrent risk in the couple?[21]

A. 3/4
B. 2/3
C. 1/2
D. 1/4
E. Increase to up to 1%
F. Unpredictable

43. A 1-year-old Ashkenazi Jewish boy had been seen intermittently in a local hospital for 6 months because of unexplained febrile episodes and deglutition difficulty with weight loss. The perinatal history was uncomplicated. His family history revealed a paternal aunt with mental retardation and muscular weakness who died at 8

years of age without a diagnosis. The patient presented with growth retardation. On physical examination, he was small for his age with low weight. He had insensitivity to pain, diminished lacrimation with normal corneal reflex, poor muscular tone with abolished deep tendon reflexes, poor coordination, vomiting attacks, and neuropsychomotor retardation. Electroneuromyography revealed a sensory neuropathy. A diagnosis of familial dysautonomia (FD) was made clinically. Molecular testing of the *IKBKAP* gene was ordered to confirm the diagnosis. Which one of the following assays would most likely be used to confirm the diagnosis in this patient?[21]

    A. Chromosomal microarray analysis
    B. Next-generation sequencing
    C. Sanger sequencing
    D. Targeted-mutation analysis
    E. Whole-exome sequencing
    F. None of the above

44. A 4-week-old girl was admitted to a children's hospital for difficult feeding. She was the second child of an Ashkenazi Jewish couple. A maternal uncle died of cerebral hemorrhage at the age of 11 years; otherwise, the family history was unremarkable. Her perinatal history was uneventful. Sometimes she breathed heavily and her face turned gray. At admission, a physical examination revealed opisthotonos, abdominal distention with visible peristalsis, and hypotonia. Her skin was gray but became mottle when she cried. She had dilated pupils and no fungiform or circumvallate papillae on her tongue. Overflow tears were not produced. Corneal reflexes were absent, and there was no response to pinprick. Her blood pressure was extremely labile. A diagnosis of familial dysautonomia (FD) was made clinically. Molecular testing of the *IKBKAP* gene was ordered to confirm the diagnosis. Where would a pathogenic variant most likely be located in the *IKBKAP* gene in this patient?[22]

    A. Promoter
    B. 5′ UTR
    C. Exon
    D. Intron
    E. Splice site
    F. 3′ UTR

ANSWERS

1. **A.** Dystrophinopathies include a spectrum of X-linked muscle diseases caused by pathogenic variants in *DMD* (https://www.hawaii.edu/

medicine/pediatrics/pedtext/s18c14.html). The *DMD* gene encodes the protein dystrophin. The severe end of the spectrum of dystrophinopathies includes progressive muscle diseases that are classified as Duchenne/Becker muscular dystrophy (DMD/BMD) when skeletal muscle is primarily affected and as *DMD*-associated dilated cardiomyopathy (DCM) when the heart is primarily affected. Molecular genetic testing of *DMD* can establish the diagnosis of a dystrophinopathy without muscle biopsy in most individuals with DMD and BMD. Virtually all males with DMD/BMD have identifiable *DMD* pathogenic variants.

Deletions of one or more exons account for approximately 60%−70% of pathogenic variants in individuals with DMD and BMD. Duplications may lead to in-frame or out-of-frame transcripts and account for the pathogenic variants in approximately 5%−10% of males with DMD and BMD. Single-nucleotide variants (SNVs), including small deletions or insertions, single-base changes, and splice-site changes, account for approximately 25%−35% of pathogenic variants in males with DMD and in about 10%−20% of males with BMD (https://www.ncbi.nlm.nih.gov/books/NBK1119/).

To establish the diagnosis in a male proband with DMD or BMD with clinical findings suggesting a dystrophinopathy and an elevated serum CK concentration, the following steps may be followed: (1) *Perform DMD molecular genetic testing using deletion/duplication analysis first.* (2) If a pathogenic variant is not identified, perform sequencing analysis. (3) If no *DMD* pathogenic variant is identified, skeletal muscle biopsy of individuals with suspected DMD or BMD is warranted for Western blot and immunohistochemistry studies of dystrophin. Because of the phenotypic resemblance between DMD/BMD and certain limb-girdle muscular dystrophies (LGMDs) such as LGMD2I, the clinician may choose to order molecular genetic testing for LGMD before performing a muscle biopsy. (4) If a pathogenic variant is identified, the diagnosis of dystrophinopathy is established, but the distinction between DMD and BMD can be difficult in some cases. For example, deletion of exons 3−7, the most extensively investigated deletion associated with both phenotypes, has been found in males with DMD and also in those with BMD.

Therefore, deletion/duplication analysis of the *DMD* gene would most likely be ordered as the next step in the workup for diagnosis of DMD/BMD in this boy.

2. **A.** Duchenne muscular dystrophy (DMD) is the most frequent muscle disorder in childhood; it is

caused by pathogenic variants in the X-linked dystrophin gene (about 65% deletions, about 7% duplications, about 26% point variants, and about 2% unknown variants) (https://www.hawaii.edu/medicine/pediatrics/pedtext/s18c14.html). *Testing that identifies exon or whole-gene deletions/duplications not detectable by sequencing analysis of the coding and flanking intronic regions of genomic DNA may use a variety of methods, such as quantitative PCR, long-range PCR, multiplex ligation-dependent probe amplification (MLPA), and chromosomal microarray (CMA)* (https://www.ncbi.nlm.nih.gov/books/NBK1119/).

Therefore, multiplex ligation-dependent probe amplification (MLPA) would likely provide the most appropriate first-tier molecular workup for this patient.

3. **B.** Duchenne muscular dystrophy (DMD) is the most frequent muscle disorder in childhood; it is caused by pathogenic variants in the X-linked dystrophin gene (about 65% deletions, about 7% duplications, about 26% point variants, and about 2% unknown variants) (https://www.hawaii.edu/medicine/pediatrics/pedtext/s18c14.html). To establish the diagnosis in a male proband with DMD or BMD with clinical findings suggesting a dystrophinopathy and an elevated serum CK concentration, the following steps may be followed: (1) Perform *DMD* molecular genetic testing using deletion/duplication analysis first. (2) *If a pathogenic variant is not identified, perform sequencing analysis.* (3) If no *DMD* pathogenic variant is identified, skeletal muscle biopsy of individuals with suspected DMD or BMD is warranted for Western blot and immunohistochemistry studies of dystrophin. Because of the phenotypic resemblance between DMD/BMD and certain limb-girdle muscular dystrophies (LGMDs) such as LGMD2I, the clinician may choose to order molecular genetic testing for LGMD before performing a muscle biopsy. (4) If a pathogenic variant is identified, the diagnosis of a dystrophinopathy is established, but the distinction between DMD and BMD can be difficult in some cases. For example, deletion of exons 3–7, the most extensively investigated deletion associated with both phenotypes, has been found in males with DMD and also in those with BMD (https://www.ncbi.nlm.nih.gov/books/NBK1119/).

Quantitative PCR and multiplex ligation-dependent probe amplification (MLPA) may be used to detected deletions/duplications. TaqMan genotype assays may be used for targeted mutation analysis. Therefore, Sanger sequencing analysis would most likely be used as the next step in the molecular workup to rule out DMD in this patient.

4. **C.** Duchenne muscular dystrophy (DMD) is the most frequent muscle disorder in childhood; it is caused by pathogenic variants in the X-linked dystrophin gene (about 65% deletions, about 7% duplications, about 26% point variants, and about 2% unknown variants). *Approximately two thirds of mothers of males with DMD and no family history of DMD are carriers.* If the mother does not have the family-specific DMD pathogenic variant detectable in her DNA, it is possible that the proband has a de novo pathogenic variant. However, because the incidence of germline mosaicism in mothers is 15%−20%, the sibs of a proband are at increased risk of inheriting the family-specific DMD pathogenic variant (https://www.ncbi.nlm.nih.gov/books/NBK1119/).

Therefore, 67% of male patients with DMD have inherited pathogenic variants from their mothers.

5. **D.** A woman with more than one affected son and no other family history of a dystrophinopathy has either: (1) A germline pathogenic variant (i.e., present in each of her cells), making her a carrier of the pathogenic variant; or (2) *Germline mosaicism, such as mosaicism for a DMD pathogenic variant that includes her germline.*

In this family, the deletion, detected in the proband and his brother, was not detected in their mother with a peripheral-blood sample. Therefore, it would be likely that the proband's mother had a germline mosaic pathogenic deletion in the *DMD* gene.

6. **B.** When the mother of the proband does not have the family-specific *DMD* pathogenic variant detectable in her DNA, it is possible that the proband has a de novo pathogenic variant. However, *because the incidence of germline mosaicism in mothers is 15%−20%, the sibs of a proband are at increased risk of inheriting the family-specific Duchenne muscular dystrophy (DMD) pathogenic variant* (https://www.ncbi.nlm.nih.gov/books/NBK1119/).

Therefore, the most approximate estimation of the recurrent risk would be approximately $20\% \times 1/2 \times 1/2 = 5\%$ in this family.

7. **B.** Dystrophinopathies include a spectrum of X-linked muscle diseases caused by pathogenic variants in *DMD*. The *DMD* gene encodes the dystrophin protein. The severe end of the spectrum includes progressive muscle diseases that are classified as Duchenne/Becker muscular dystrophy (DMD/BMD) when skeletal muscle is primarily affected and as *DMD*-associated dilated

cardiomyopathy (DCM) when the heart is primarily affected.

The reading frame "rule" states that pathogenic variants that do not alter the reading frame (in-frame deletions/duplications) generally correlate with the milder BMD phenotype, whereas *those that alter the reading frame (out-of-frame) generally correlate with the more severe DMD phenotype.* Very large deletions may lead to absence of dystrophin expression. Pathogenic variants that disrupt the reading frame include stop variants, some splicing variants, and deletions or duplications. They produce a severely truncated dystrophin protein molecule that is degraded, leading to the more severe DMD phenotype. Exceptions to this "reading-frame rule" include deletions in protein-binding domains that may severely affect function even when in-frame and exon-skipping events in which apparently out-of-frame deletions behave as in-frame deletions or vice versa. Some studies suggest that duplications, which occur more commonly in BMD, may result in exceptions to the reading-frame rule in a higher proportion of cases, perhaps up to 30%. The BMD phenotype occurs when some dystrophin is produced, usually resulting from deletions or duplications that juxtapose in-frame exons, some splicing variants, and most nontruncating single-base changes that result in translation of a protein product with intact N and C termini. The shorter-than-normal dystrophin protein molecule, which retains partial function, produces the milder BMD phenotype (https://www.ncbi.nlm.nih.gov/books/NBK1119/).

The type of deletion/duplication can distinguish between the DMD and BMD phenotypes with 91%–92% accuracy in a proband who represent simplex cases. Exceptions to the reading-frame rule have been documented to occur at a rate below 10%.

DMD-associated DCM is caused by pathogenic variants in *DMD* that affect the muscle promoter (PM) and the first exon (E1), resulting in no dystrophin transcripts being produced in cardiac muscle; however, two alternative promoters that are normally only active in the brain (PB) and Purkinje cells (PP) are active in the skeletal muscle, resulting in dystrophin expression sufficient to prevent manifestation of skeletal muscle symptoms.

Therefore, this patient would most likely have DMD due to an out-of-frame deletion.

8. **A.** Dystrophinopathies include a spectrum of X-linked muscle diseases caused by pathogenic variants in *DMD*. The *DMD* gene encodes the dystrophin protein. The severe end of the spectrum includes progressive muscle diseases that are classified as Duchenne/Becker muscular dystrophy (DMD/BMD) when skeletal muscle is primarily affected and as *DMD*-associated dilated cardiomyopathy (DCM) when the heart is primarily affected.

The reading-frame "rule" states that pathogenic variants that *do not alter the reading frame (in-frame deletions/duplications) generally correlate with the milder BMD phenotype, whereas those that alter the reading frame (out-of-frame) generally correlate with the more severe DMD phenotype.* Very large deletions may lead to absence of dystrophin expression. Pathogenic variants that disrupt the reading frame include stop variants, some splicing variants, and deletions or duplications. They produce a severely truncated dystrophin protein molecule that is degraded, leading to the more severe DMD phenotype. Exceptions to this reading-frame rule include deletions in protein-binding domains that may severely affect function even when in-frame and exon-skipping events in which apparently out-of-frame deletions behave as in-frame deletions or vice versa. Some studies suggest that duplications, which occur more commonly in BMD, may result in exceptions to the reading-frame rule in a higher proportion of cases, perhaps up to 30%. The BMD phenotype occurs when some dystrophin is produced, usually resulting from deletions or duplications that juxtapose in-frame exons, some splicing variants, and most nontruncating single-base changes that result in translation of a protein product with intact N and C termini. The shorter-than-normal dystrophin protein molecule, which retains partial function, produces the milder BMD phenotype (https://www.ncbi.nlm.nih.gov/books/NBK1119/).

The type of deletion/duplication can distinguish between the DMD and BMD phenotypes with 91%–92% accuracy in proband who represent simplex cases. Exceptions to the reading-frame rule have been documented to occur at a rate below 10%.

DMD-associated DCM is caused by pathogenic variants in *DMD* that affect the muscle promoter (PM) and the first exon (E1), resulting in no dystrophin transcripts being produced in cardiac muscle; however, two alternative promoters that are normally active only in the brain (PB) and Purkinje cells (PP) are active in the skeletal muscle, resulting in dystrophin expression sufficient to prevent manifestation of skeletal muscle symptoms.

Therefore, this patient would most likely have BMD due to an in-of-frame deletion.

9. **H.** Duchenne muscular dystrophy (DMD) is a X-linked condition caused by pathogenic variants in *DMD* at Xp21. The father of an affected male would not have the disease, nor would he be a carrier of a DMD pathogenic variant, since this is a X-linked condition. Approximately two-thirds of mothers of males with DMD and no family history of DMD are carriers. If the family-specific *DMD* pathogenic variant cannot be detected in a proband's mother, the sibs of a proband are at increased risk of inheriting the variant because the incidence of germline mosaicism in mothers is 15%−20% (https://www.ncbi.nlm.nih.gov/books/NBK1119/).

The proband in this question was the only family member with DMD. The chance for his mother to be a carrier was 67%. Even if his mother did not have an identifiable deletion on testing of her peripheral-blood specimen, she still had a 15%−20% chance to be have germline mosaicism. Therefore, prenatal genetic testing should be considered regardless of the mother's carrier status. Genetic counseling is the process of providing individuals and families with information on the nature, inheritance, and implications of genetic disorders; it would help the family to understand the disease, cope with the situation, and help the family make informed medical and personal decisions.

Therefore, genetic counseling, maternal testing, and prenatal testing for future pregnancies should all be recommended in the molecular genetics report.

10. **C.** *DMD* is the only gene in which pathogenic variants cause Duchenne muscular dystrophy (DMD). *DMD* is one of the largest genes in the human genome. It spans 2.2 Mb of DNA and comprises 79 exons, and it has at least four promoters. More than 5000 pathogenic variants have been identified in persons with Duchenne muscular dystrophy (DMD) or Becker muscular dystrophy (BMD). Disease-causing alleles are highly variable, including deletion of the entire gene, deletion or duplication of one or more exons, and small deletions, insertions, or single-base changes. In both DMD and BMD, partial deletions and duplications cluster in two recombination hot spots, one proximal at the 5′ end of the gene, comprising exons 2−20 (30%), and one more distal, comprising exons 44−53 (70%). Duplications cluster near the 5′ end of the gene, with duplication of exon 2 being the single most common duplication identified (https://www.ncbi.nlm.nih.gov/books/NBK1119/).

Dystrophin, encoded by *DMD*, is a membrane-associated protein present in muscle cells and some neurons. *Pathogenic variants that lead to lack of dystrophin expression tend to cause DMD*, whereas those that lead to abnormal quality or quantity of dystrophin lead to BMD. In *DMD*-associated dilated cardiomyopathy (DCM), functional dystrophin is absent in the myocardium but may be normal or mildly abnormal in skeletal muscle because *DMD*-associated DCM is associated with specific types of *DMD* pathogenic variants that have a differential response to tissue-specific transcription or alternative splicing in cardiac versus skeletal muscle.

Therefore, the deletion in this patient would most likely be a loss−of-function variant.

11. **C.** *The boy had Barth syndrome, a X-linked condition.* In affected males, Barth syndrome is characterized by cardiomyopathy, neutropenia, skeletal myopathy, prepubertal growth delay, and distinctive facial features. Cardiomyopathy, which is almost always present before age 5 years, is typically dilated cardiomyopathy with or without endocardial fibroelastosis (EFE) or left ventricular noncompaction (LVNC); rarely it is hypertrophic cardiomyopathy (HCM). Female heterozygous do not manifest the disease. It is has been proposed that female carriers are healthy owing to selection against cells with the mutated *TAZ* allele on the active X chromosome, based on the study of the X-chromosome inactivation (https://www.ncbi.nlm.nih.gov/books/NBK247162/).

Therefore, Barth syndrome is an X-linked condition.

12. **A.** Barth syndrome is an X-linked condition characterized in affected males by cardiomyopathy, neutropenia, skeletal myopathy, prepubertal growth delay, and distinctive facial features (most evident in infancy); not all features may be present in each patient. Pathogenic variants in the *TAZ* gene on Xq28 cause Barth syndrome. If a mother has a *TAZ* pathogenic variant, the chance of transmitting it in each pregnancy is 50%. Males who inherit the *TAZ* pathogenic variant will be affected; females who inherit the *TAZ* pathogenic variant will be carriers and will not be affected. *Affected males pass the* TAZ *pathogenic variant to all their daughters and none of their sons* (https://www.ncbi.nlm.nih.gov/books/NBK247162/).

Therefore, this male patient's future children would have <1% risk to have Barth syndrome. But the patient would be at risk of having affected grandchildren through his unaffected daughter(s) who inherit(s) the *TAZ* pathogenic variant from him.

13. **C.** *TAZ* is the only gene in which pathogenic variants are known to cause Barth syndrome. *More*

than 90% of patients have pathogenic variants detected by sequencing; the rest are detected by deletion and duplication analysis. Barth syndrome shows no ethnic or racial predilection, as it has been described throughout the world. Since there is no founder effect in Ashkenazi Jewish, targeted variant analysis has not been used to diagnosis patients unless a pathogenic variant has been identified in the family. Next-generation sequence (NGS) is a cost-effective way to investigate multiple genes, but not a single gene (https://www.ncbi.nlm.nih.gov/books/NBK247162/).

Therefore, Sanger sequencing would most likely be used as the first-line test to confirm the diagnosis in this patient.

14. **C.** Barth syndrome is a rare X-linked condition characterized by dilated cardiomyopathy, muscles weakness, recurrent infections due to neutropenia, and short stature. Males with the condition have 5- to 20-fold increases of urine 3-methylglutaconic acid. *Pathogenic variants in the TAZ gene on Xq28 cause Barth syndrome.* Sequencing analysis of *TAZ* identified approximately 93% of pathogenic variants in affected males (https://www.ncbi.nlm.nih.gov/books/NBK247162/).

Pathogenic variants in *TWNK* are associated with autosomal recessive mitochondrial DNA depletion syndrome, hepatocerebral type; autosomal recessive Perrault syndrome; and autosomal dominant progressive external ophthalmoplegia with mitochondrial DNA deletions. Deletions in mtDNA are associated with Kearns–Sayre syndrome. Somatic deletions of mtDNA are associated with Parkinson disease.

Therefore, sequencing analysis of the *TAZ* gene would most likely be used to confirm a diagnosis of Barth syndrome in this patient.

15. **C.** This female patient had a neuromuscular disorder. The most common form of neuromuscular disorder is X-linked dystrophinopathies, caused by pathogenic variants in *DMD* at Xp21. Penetrance of dystrophinopathies is complete in males. Penetrance in carrier females varies and may depend in part on patterns of X-chromosome inactivation. In some instances, female carriers can have classic Duchenne muscular dystrophy (DMD).

Limb-girdle muscular dystrophy (LGMD) is a descriptive term, generally reserved for childhood- or adult-onset muscular dystrophies that are distinct from the X-linked dystrophinopathies. LGMDs are typically nonsyndromic, with clinical involvement usually limited to skeletal muscle. Individuals with LGMD generally show weakness and wasting restricted to the limb musculature,

proximal greater than distal, and muscle degeneration/regeneration on muscle biopsy. Those transmitted by autosomal dominant inheritance are designated as LGMD type 1 and those transmitted by autosomal recessive inheritance are designated as LGMD type 2 (https://www.ncbi.nlm.nih.gov/books/NBK1408/). The limb-girdle muscular dystrophies typically show degeneration/regeneration (dystrophic changes) on muscle biopsy, which is usually associated with elevated serum creatine kinase concentration. *For any male or female suspected of having limb-girdle muscular dystrophy, it is necessary to first rule out an X-linked dystrophinopathy. Especially in female, the incidence of LGMD is nearly as much as that for a DMD carrier.*

Therefore, molecular genetic testing for *DMD* should be done first in this female patient to rule out being a Duchenne muscular dystrophy (DMD) carrier before testing for LGMD.

16. **B.** Spinal muscular atrophy is a common autosomal recessive neuromuscular disorder caused by pathogenic variants in the survival motor neuron (*SMN1*) gene, affecting approximately 1 in 10,000 live births. It is characterized by progressive symmetrical muscle weakness resulting from the degeneration and loss of anterior horn cells in the spinal cord and brain stem nuclei.

Two almost identical *SMN* genes are present on 5q13—*SMN1* and *SMN2*. *SMN2* shares more than 99% nucleotide identity with *SMN1*. Both *SMN1* and *SMN2* are capable of encoding a 294–amino acid RNA-binding protein, SMN, that is required for efficient assembly of small nuclear ribonucleoprotein (snRNP) complexes. The *SMN1* gene is the spinal muscular atrophy—determining gene. *The homozygous absence of the SMN1 exon 7 has been observed in the majority of patients and is being used as a reliable and sensitive spinal muscular atrophy diagnostic test.* Absence of *SMN1* is partially compensated for by *SMN2*, which produces enough SMN protein to allow for relatively normal development in cell types other than motor neurons. However, *SMN2* cannot fully compensate for loss of *SMN1* because, although *SMN2* is transcribed at a level comparable to that of *SMN1*, a large majority of *SMN2* transcripts lack exon 7, resulting in production of a truncated, less stable SMN protein. But the number of *SMN2* copies has been shown to modulate the clinical phenotype. The absence of both copies of the *SMN1* gene is a very reliable and sensitive assay for the molecular diagnosis of SMA (https://www.ncbi.nlm.nih.gov/books/NBK1352/).

Gene-targeted deletion/duplication analysis to determine the dosage of *SMN1* is performed for the exon 7 of *SMN1*. Methods, that may be used, include quantitative PCR and multiplex ligation-dependent probe amplification (MLPA) to detect single-exon deletions or duplications. Note that *SMN1* and *SMN2* are nearly identical; therefore, gene-targeted microarray cannot be used to determine *SMN1* and *SMN2* copy number.

Therefore, multiplex ligation-dependent probe amplification (MLPA) would most likely be used as a first-tier test to confirm/rule out SMA in this patient.

17. **C.** The SMN region on chromosome 5q12.2-q13.3 is unusually complex, with repetitive sequences, pseudogenes, retrotransposable elements, deletions, and inverted duplications. Unaffected individuals have two genes encoding SMN protein that are arranged in tandem on each chromosome: *SMN1* (telomeric copy) and *SMN2* (centromeric copy). *SMN1* produces a full-length survival motor-neuron protein necessary for lower-motor-neuron function. *SMN2* predominantly produces a survival motor-neuron protein that is lacking in exon 7, a less stable protein. SMA is caused by loss of *SMN1* because *SMN2* cannot fully compensate for the loss of *SMN1*-produced protein. However, when the *SMN2* (dosage) copy number is increased, the small amount of full-length transcript generated by *SMN2* is often able to produce a milder type II or type III phenotype.

SMN1 and *SMN2* each comprise nine exons and differ only in eight nucleotides (five intronic; and three exonic, with one each located within exons 6, 7, and 8). Loss of *SMN1* causes SMA. Individuals with SMA are either homozygous for a deletion of at least exon 7 of *SMN1* or are compound heterozygous for such a deletion along with an intragenic *SMN1*-inactivating pathogenic variant. *Exon 7 of SMN1 is undetectable in more than 95% of individuals with SMA irrespective of the clinical subtype,* either as a result of homozygous deletions or gene conversion of *SMN1* sequence into *SMN2* sequences (possible because of their high nucleotide identity) (https://www.ncbi.nlm.nih.gov/books/NBK1352/).

Therefore, exon 7 of *SMN1* is most likely to be the target of the molecular genetics study for SMA.

18. **D.** Spinal muscular atrophy (SMA) is a common autosomal recessive neuromuscular disorder caused by pathogenic variants in the survival motor neuron (*SMN1*) gene, affecting approximately 1 in 10,000 live births. It is characterized by progressive symmetrical muscle weakness resulting from the degeneration and loss of anterior horn cells in the spinal cord and brain stem nuclei.

Two almost identical *SMN* genes are present on 5q13—*SMN1* and *SMN2*. The *SMN1* gene is the spinal muscular atrophy—determining gene. The homozygous absence of the *SMN1* exon 7 has been observed in the majority of patients and is being used as a reliable and sensitive spinal muscular atrophy diagnostic test. The clinical sensitivity (proportion of homozygous Δ7*SMN1* if 5q13-linked SMA is present) of the diagnostic test is approximately 95%. And approximately 5% of affected patients have other types of pathogenic variants in the *SMN1* gene that will not be detected by homozygous deletion testing. *So if exon 7 is deleted from one copy of SMN1 in a symptomatic patient, performance of sequencing analysis of SMN1 may be considered to further rule out SMA* (https://www.ncbi.nlm.nih.gov/books/NBK1352/).

This patient had classic SMA-like clinical presentation, but had one copy of exon 7 of *SMN1*. It is likely that the remaining copy contains a subtler variant, including nonsense variants, missense variants, splice-site variants, insertions, and small deletions. Therefore, a sequencing-based analysis of *SMN1* may identify a variant in another copy of the *SMN1* gene.

19. **A.** Approximately 6% of parents of a child with spinal muscular atrophy (SMA) resulting from a homozygous *SMN1* deletion have normal results of *SMN1* dosage testing in one of the parents for the following two reasons. About 4%–8% of carriers have two copies of *SMN1* on a single chromosome. These carrier individuals with two copies of *SMN1* on one chromosome (a [2 + 0] genotype) are misdiagnosed as noncarriers by the *SMN1* dosage test; this is a false negative test result. *A specific haplotype block is associated with a [2 + 0] genotype in the Ashkenazi Jewish population.* De novo deletion of exon 7 of one *SMN1* allele occurs in 2% of individuals with SMA; thus, only one parent is a carrier. The majority of de novo pathogenic variants are paternal in origin. In the United States' panethnic population, the calculated a priori carrier frequency is 1/54, with a detection rate of 91.2%. Therefore, an individual from this panethnic population with normal *SMN1* dosage testing would have an about 1/500 residual risk of being a carrier. Germline mosaicism for an *SMN1* variant is another possibility, but cases have not been reported, which indicates a low possibility (https://www.ncbi.nlm.nih.gov/books/NBK1352/).

In this case, the proband had a homozygous deletion of exon 7 and a heterozygous deletion of exon 8 of *SMN1*; the likelihood of his mother having a sequenceable pathogenic variant was minimized. Therefore, statistically it would be likely that both parents were carriers of deletions in *SMN1*, and the mother might have a specific haplotype block, [2 + 0], which is more prevalent in Ashkenazi Jews due to a found effect.

20. **E.** Spinal muscular atrophy (SMA) is an autosomal recessive condition. If both parents are carriers, the recurrent risk in the offspring is 25%. So in this case, it was important to confirm whether the mother was a carrier in order to provide genetic counseling and prenatal management. About 4%–8% of carriers have two copies of *SMN1* on a single chromosome. These carrier individuals with two copies of *SMN1* on one chromosome (a [2 + 0] genotype) are misdiagnosed as noncarriers by the *SMN1* dosage test; it is a false negative test result. A specific haplotype block is associated with a [2 + 0] genotype in the Ashkenazi Jewish population. *Testing additional family members of the parent possibly with the [2 + 0] SMN1 genotype may be informative: usually one of the parents has a deletion (1/0 SMN1 genotype) and the other parent has three or more SMN1 copies (2/1 SMN1 genotype)* (https://www.ncbi.nlm.nih.gov/books/NBK1352/).

Since *SMN1* and *SMN2* are nearly identical, microarray analysis cannot be used to determine *SMN1* and *SMN2* copy number. Linkage study needs a large family with multiple affected members. Southern blot is not an appropriate study in this situation because: (1) *SMN1* and *SMN2* differ in only eight nucleotides (five intronic; three exonic, with one each located within exons 6, 7, and 8), and it is hard to find recognition sites for restriction enzymes. (2) Southern blot is usually used to detect large deletions or duplications.

Therefore, in this situation, testing the parents of the mother was a valid option to confirm whether the mother had a specific haplotype block, [2 + 0], due to a founder effect in Ashkenazi Jews.

21. **D.** The SMN region on chromosome 5q12.2-q13.3 is unusually complex, with repetitive sequences, pseudogenes, retrotransposable elements, deletions, and inverted duplications. Two genes encoding SMN protein are arranged in tandem on each chromosome: *SMN1* (telomeric copy) and *SMN2* (centromeric copy). Although *SMN2* produces fewer full-length transcripts than *SMN1*, the number of *SMN2* copies has been shown to modulate the severity of the disease.

The number of copies (dosage) of *SMN2* (arranged in tandem in *cis* configuration on each chromosome) ranges from zero to five. The *SMN2* copy number varies from zero to three copies in the normal population, with approximately 10%–15% of normal individuals having no *SMN2*. The presence of three or more copies of *SMN2* is correlated with a milder phenotype. Three unaffected family members of patients with SMA, with confirmed *SMN1* homozygous deletions, were shown to have five copies of *SMN2*. These cases not only support the role of *SMN2* in modifying the phenotype but they also demonstrate that expression levels consistent with five copies of the *SMN2* genes may be sufficient to compensate for the absence of the *SMN1* gene. Meanwhile, Prior et al. described three unrelated individuals with SMA whose *SMN2* copy numbers did not correlate with the observed mild clinical phenotypes; they were found to have a single-base substitution—c.859G > C (p.Gly287Arg)—in exon 7 of *SMN2* that created a new exonic splicing enhancer (ESE) element. The new ESE increased the amount of exon 7 inclusion and full-length transcripts generated from *SMN2*, thus resulting in the less severe phenotypes. It was also found that in some rare families with unaffected homozygous *SMN1*-deleted females, the expression of plastin 3 (encoded by *PLS3* at chromosome locus Xq23) was higher than in their SMA-affected counterparts (https://www.ncbi.nlm.nih.gov/books/NBK1352/).

Polymorphisms or point mutations under the primer and/or the probe binding regions may influence the analytical and clinical specificity by increasing the false positive rate depending on the technology used. As a measure of additional quality assurance, follow-up sequencing underneath the primer and probe binding regions on all diagnostic (0 or 1 *SMN1* copy number) results is expected to rule out a false positive diagnostic finding attributable to this phenomenon and provide a better understanding of the underlying molecular mechanism of the mutation identified.

Therefore, owing to the complexity of the *SMN* region, it was appropriate to test the copy-number changes of *SMN2* in the asymptomatic mother after finding the homozygous deletion of exon 7 in *SMN1*. If the copy number of *SMN2* could not explain the clinical findings, the other options may be explored, except for testing the maternal grandparents of the proband, which would not help to explain the discrepancy between the molecular results and the clinical presentation in the mother.

22. **A.** The SMN region on chromosome 5q12.2-q13.3 is unusually complex, with repetitive sequences, pseudogenes, retrotransposable elements, deletions, and inverted duplications.

The sensitivity (true positives/true positives and false negatives, or the detection rate) of the carrier test is defined as the proportion of carriers with the heterozygous Δ7*SMN1*, one-copy genotype among all SMA carriers, including point mutation carriers and deletion carriers with two copies of the *SMN1* gene. Detection rate varies by ethnicity, ranging from 71% in African Americans to 95% in Caucasians. *The major contributor to this ethnicity-based variation in detection rate is the occurrence of two (or more)* SMN1 *genes in tandem on a single chromosome 5.* The alleles with two or more copies of *SMN1* is three to eight times more prevalent in African Americans, than in other ethnic groups. This translates to a much higher frequency of individuals with the SMA carrier while having two copies of exon 7 among African Americans as compared with other races. It also has important implications in risk assessment and counseling after carrier screening in individuals of African American ancestry.

Therefore, the occurrence of two (or more) *SMN1* genes in tandem on a single chromosome 5 is the major contributor to this ethnicity-based variation in detection rate.

23. **D.** Spinal muscular atrophy is a common autosomal recessive neuromuscular disorder caused by pathogenic variants in the survival motor neuron (*SMN1*) gene, affecting approximately 1 in 10,000 live births. Two genes encoding SMN protein are arranged in tandem on each chromosome: *SMN1* (telomeric copy) and *SMN2* (centromeric copy). Two inverted SMN copies are present—*SMN1* (telomeric copy), which is the SMA-determining gene, *SMN2* (centromeric copy). The two SMN genes are highly homologous, have equivalent promoters, and they differ at only 5 base pairs. The base-pair differences are used to differentiate *SMN1* from *SMN2*. The coding sequence of *SMN2* differs from that of *SMN1* by a single nucleotide (840C < T), which does not alter the amino acid but has been shown to be important in splicing. SMA results from a reduction in the amount of the SMN protein, and there is a strong correlation between the disease severity and SMN protein levels. *SMN1* exon 7 is absent in the majority of patients independent of the severity of SMA. *Several studies have shown that the SMN2 copy number modifies the severity of the disease although SMN2 produces fewer full-length transcripts than SMN1.*

Therefore, the number of *SMN2* copies has been shown to modulate the clinical phenotype of SMA.

24. **D.** With an incidence of approximately 1 in 10,000 live births and a carrier frequency of 1 in 40–1 in 60, spinal muscular atrophy (SMA) is the leading inherited cause of infant mortality. A recent report provides carrier frequencies in several populations, including white, Ashkenazi Jewish, African American, Asian, and Hispanic; *the observed one-copy genotype frequency was 1 in 37 (2.7%) in Caucasian, 1 in 46 (2.2%) in Ashkenazi Jews, 1 in 56 (1.8%) in Asians, 1 in 91 (1.1%) in African American, and 1 in 125 (0.8%) in Hispanics.* The lower carrier frequencies found in African Americans and Hispanics would suggest a lower prevalence of SMA in these populations.

Therefore, the carrier frequency of spinal muscular atrophy (SMA) is higher in Caucasians than in the other populations listed.

25. **B.** Spinal muscular atrophy is a common autosomal recessive neuromuscular disorder caused by pathogenic variants in the survival motor neuron (*SMN1*) gene, affecting approximately 1 in 10,000 live births. A negative test result is characterized by the presence of detectable amounts of *SMN1* exon 7, with an *SMN1* exon 7 copy number of one, with the presence of subtle intragenic point pathogenic variants within the *SMN1* gene having been ruled out. If the presence of subtle intragenic pathogenic variants has not been ruled out, a negative test result decreases the likelihood but does not exclude the diagnosis of SMA. *Within the context of carrier testing, an SMN1 copy number of 2 is associated with a reduced risk to be a carrier.*

About 4%–8% of carriers have two copies of *SMN1* on a single chromosome. These carrier individuals with two copies of *SMN1* on one chromosome (a [2 + 0] genotype) are misdiagnosed as noncarriers by the *SMN1* dosage test. And a [2 + 0] genotype presents with a higher frequency in the Ashkenazi Jewish population than in other populations owing to a founder effect (https://www.ncbi.nlm.nih.gov/books/NBK1352/). *So it is possible for a healthy Ashkenazi Jew to have three copies of SMN1 (a [2 + 1] genotype).*

Therefore, the wife has reduced risk to be a carrier, and sequencing analysis may further rule out whether the wife carries intragenic point pathogenic variants within the *SMN1* gene.

26. **B.** Spinal muscular atrophy is a common autosomal recessive neuromuscular disorder caused by pathogenic variants in the survival motor neuron (*SMN1*) gene, affecting approximately 1 in 10,000 live births. The analytical sensitivity of *SMN1* deletion/copy-number analysis (proportion of homozygous Δ7 *SMN1* among all pathogenic variants) is >99% (using the dosage assays described in the

guidelines). *The clinical sensitivity (proportion of homozygous Δ7 SMN1 if 5q13-linked SMA is present) of the diagnostic test is approximately 95%.* The remaining 5% of patients may have intragenic point mutations within the *SMN1* gene or two copies of *SMN1* on a single chromosome 5; this is a source of false negative diagnostic test results.

Therefore, the clinical sensitivity of *SMN1* deletion/copy-number analysis is approximately 95% to diagnose spinal muscular atrophy (SMA) in Caucasians.

27. **A.** *Detection rate of deletion/copy number analysis for spinal muscular atrophy (SMA) varies by ethnicity, ranging from 71% in African Americans to 95% in Caucasians.* The major contributor to this ethnicity-based variation in detection rate is the occurrence of two (or more) *SMN1* genes in tandem on a single chromosome 5 (i.e., the [2 + 0] Category 2 carrier genotype). The estimated frequency of alleles with two or more copies of *SMN1* is three to eight times more prevalent in African Americans than in other ethnic groups. This translates to a much higher frequency of individuals with the SMA carrier [2 + 0] genotype among African Americans as compared with other races. It also has important implications in risk assessment and counseling after carrier screening in individuals of African American ancestry.

Therefore, an assay for exon 7 of *SMN1* deletion/copy-number analysis has the lowest detection rate in the African American population.

28. **A.** Spinal muscular atrophy is a common autosomal recessive neuromuscular disorder caused by pathogenic variants in the survival motor neuron (*SMN1*) gene, affecting approximately 1 in 10,000 live births. A negative test result within the context of carrier screening is defined by an *SMN1* exon 7 copy number ≥ 2 with a reduced posterior risk for being a carrier. The posterior risk determination takes into consideration the conditional probability of being either a carrier or a noncarrier after an *SMN1* copy-number analysis result of ≥ 2. *The posterior residual risk for an individual with no family history of SMA to be a carrier following the identification of two copies of SMN1 exon 7 varies by ethnicity, ranging from 1 in 632 for an individual of Caucasian ancestry to 1 in 121 for an individual of African American ancestry.* The residual risk following the identification of three copies of *SMN1* exon 7 is considerably lower and varies from 1 in 3500 for an individual of Caucasian ancestry to 1 in 3000 for an individual of African American ancestry. As with other carrier screening tests, patients need to understand that a negative carrier screening result

reduces but does not eliminate the risk to be a carrier of SMA. Risk assessment calculations using Bayesian analysis are essential for the proper genetic counseling of SMA families.

Therefore, the posterior residual risk for a Caucasian with no family history of SMA to be a carrier following the identification of two copies of *SMN1* exon 7 is lower than that for an African American.

29. **E.** The gene for spinal muscular atrophy (SMA) is within a complex region containing multiple repetitive and inverted sequences. The SMN genes comprise nine exons with a stop codon present near the end of exon 7. Two inverted SMN copies are present: the telomeric or *SMN1* (telomeric copy), which is the SMA-determining gene and *SMN2* (centromeric copy). The two SMN genes are highly homologous, have equivalent promoters, and differ at only five base pairs. The base-pair differences are used to differentiate *SMN1* from *SMN2*. The coding sequence of *SMN2* differs from that of *SMN1* by a single nucleotide (840C < T), which does not alter the amino acid but has been shown to be important in splicing. *Exon 7 appears only in SMN1, while exon 8 appears only in SMN2 mRNA.* *SMN2* predominantly produces a survival motor-neuron protein that is lacking exon 7, a less stable protein. SMA is caused by the loss of *SMN1* because *SMN2* cannot fully compensate for the loss of *SMN1*-produced protein. However, when the *SMN2* (dosage) copy number is increased, patients tend to have a milder clinical presentation. The *SMN2* copy number varies from 0 to 3 in the normal population, with approximately 10%–15% of normal individuals having no *SMN2*. The presence of three or more copies of *SMN2* is correlated with a milder phenotype.

The laboratory must establish validated, nonoverlapping cutoff values that can accurately and reliably distinguish *SMN1* copy numbers of 0, 1, 2, and ≥ 3. The accuracy, precision, and confidence of *SMN1* copy-number measurements around these established cutoff values should be known to the laboratory. Copy-number variations within the genomic internal standard and inefficiency of polymerase-chain-reaction (PCR) amplification of the internal standard reference gene relative to the *SMN1* gene represent additional sources of false positive or incorrect copy-number estimates. Therefore, the copy number of the genomic internal standard reference gene should be constant at two copies within the genome, and the PCR amplification efficiency of the *SMN1* gene relative to the chosen internal reference standard gene should be consistent between analyses. Performing replicate copy-number measurements with two independent copy-number internal standard reference genes can help ensure the accuracy of copy-number analysis.

Therefore, exon 8 cannot be used as the internal control to test the copy number of *SMN1* because the copy number of exon 8 depends on the copy number of *SMN2*.

30. **B.** Amyotrophic lateral sclerosis (ALS) is a group of progressive neurodegenerative disorders, affecting involving both upper motor neurons (UMNs) and lower motor neurons (LMNs) located in the anterior (ventral) horn regions of the spinal cord, the cranial nerve motor nuclei in the pons and medulla, and the frontal cortex. ALS causes muscle weakness, disability, and eventually death. UMN signs include hyperreflexia, extensor plantar response, increased muscle tone, and weakness in a topographic representation. LMN signs include weakness, muscle wasting, hyporeflexia, muscle cramps, and fasciculations. Initial presentation varies. *Familial amyotrophic lateral sclerosis accounts for 5%–10% of all ALS cases* (https://www.ncbi.nlm.nih.gov/books/NBK1450/).

Therefore, the familial type of ALS accounts for 5%–10% of all cases.

31. **C.** An estimated 10% of individuals with amyotrophic lateral sclerosis (ALS) have at least one other affected family member and are said to have familial ALS (FALS). Familial ALS is phenotypically and genetically heterogeneous. Although most familial ALS cases follow an autosomal dominant inheritance pattern, recessive and X-linked forms have been described. *At least 15 different loci are thought to harbor ALS-causing pathogenic variants.* Pathogenic variants in the *SOD1* gene account for approximately 20% of all familial ALS and approximately 3% of sporadic ALS (https://www.ncbi.nlm.nih.gov/books/NBK1450/).

Therefore, next-generation sequencing analysis would be the most appropriate test to confirm the diagnosis in this patient.

32. **D.** Presymptomatic testing for variants associated with amyotrophic lateral sclerosis (ALS) is controversial because of incomplete penetrance, inability to predict the age at onset, and lack of preventive measures. Because of the individualized nature of predictive testing, consultation with a genetic counselor and a psychologist to obtain informed consent is recommended. At this time, no established testing protocol, such as in Huntington disease, exists although establishment of such protocols has been suggested. However, to err on the side of caution, testing centers often

follow a protocol similar to that for Huntington disease (https://www.ncbi.nlm.nih.gov/books/NBK1450/).

Therefore, the patient's daughter may be tested for the familial pathogenic variant after informed consent.

33. **B.** *Testing of asymptomatic individuals younger than age 18 years who are at risk for adult-onset disorders for which no treatment exists is not considered appropriate, primarily because it negates the autonomy of the child with no compelling benefit.* Further, concern exists regarding the potential adverse effects that such information may have on family dynamics, the risk of discrimination and stigmatization in the future, and the anxiety that such information may cause (https://www.ncbi.nlm.nih.gov/books/NBK1450/). There is a position statement from the National Society of Genetic Counselors (NSGC) and a policy statement from American College of Medical Genetics and Genomics (AMGG) on genetic testing of minors for adult-onset conditions (Genetic Testing of Minors for Adult-Onset Conditions: http://www.nsgc.org/p/bl/et/blogaid = 860).

Therefore, the patient's daughter may not be tested for the familial pathogenic variant for amyotrophic lateral sclerosis (ALS).

34. **B.** Although some controversy remains, facioscapulohumeral muscular dystrophy (FSHD) is likely caused by inappropriate expression of the double homeobox–containing gene, *DUX4*, in muscle cells. *DUX4* lies in the macrosatellite repeat D4Z4 on chromosome 4q35, which has a length between 11 and 100 repeat units on normal alleles. Approximately 95% of individuals with FSHD have a D4Z4 allele of between 1 and 10 repeat units. The shortening of the D4Z4 allele causes chromatin relaxation at the D4Z4 locus and *DUX4* promoter and thereby derepression of *DUX4*. This common form of FSHD is designated facioscapulohumeral muscular dystrophy 1 (FSHD1). *Molecular genetic testing measures the length of the D4Z4 allele.* About 5% of individuals with FSHD show chromatin relaxation at D4Z4 without having a D4Z4 contraction. In these individuals with so-called FSHD2, pathogenic variants in the chromatin modifier *SMCHD1* cause the chromatin relaxation at D4Z4 (https://www.ncbi.nlm.nih.gov/books/NBK1443/).

Therefore, this patient would most likely have a short D4Z4 allele, which is a macrosatellite genetic marker.

35. **F.** The shortening of the *D4Z4* allele causes chromatin relaxation at the *D4Z4* locus and *DUX4* promoter and thereby derepression of DUX4. This common form of facioscapulohumeral muscular

dystrophy (FSHD) is designated facioscapulohumeral muscular dystrophy 1 (FSHD1). Molecular genetic testing measures the length of the D4Z4 allele. About 5% of individuals with FSHD show chromatin relaxation at D4Z4 without having a D4Z4 contraction. In these individuals with so-called FSHD2, pathogenic variants in the chromatin modifier *SMCHD1* cause the chromatin relaxation at D4Z4 (https://www.ncbi.nlm.nih.gov/books/NBK1443/).

Molecular genetic testing to determine the length or number of repeat units of the D4Z4 locus relies on Southern blot analysis, typically with a probe, such as the p13E-11 probe, that is localized immediately proximal to D4Z4. Standard DNA diagnostic testing (defined here as linear gel electrophoresis and Southern blot analysis) uses the restriction enzyme *EcoRI,* which recognizes the D4Z4 locus on chromosomes 4 and 10. Pulsed-field gel electrophoresis and Southern blot analysis requires *EcoRI/HindIII* double digestion for a better resolution of DNA fragments between 20 and 50 kb. An *EcoRI/BlnI* double digestion further fragments the chromosome 10 array, allowing one to distinguish D4Z4 arrays located on chromosome 4 from the similar benign arrays on chromosome 10.

Therefore, Southern blot was most likely used to detect the copy-number losses of the macrosatellite, D4Z4, for the molecular genetic testing of facioscapulohumeral muscular dystrophy (FSHD).

36. **B.** There are two different variants of D4Z4 on chromosome 4: 4A and 4B. Only the D4Z4A variant (haplotype) has an extra *DUX4* exon distal to the D4Z4 region that carries the polyadenylation signal of the gene required for stable expression of *DUX4.* The D4Z4B variant (haplotype) is nonpathogenic (benign) because D4Z4 alleles with D4Z4B variant lack the extra *DUX4* exon distal to D4Z4 to stabilize the *DUX4* transcript. In general, *contractions of the D4Z4 allele in the 4A haplotype causes facioscapulohumeral muscular dystrophy 1 (FSHD1) because it is permissive to DUX4 expression.* The normal D4Z4A allele has between 11 and 100 units of the 3.3-kb repeat sequence (fragments of 43 kb or greater using *EcoRI* and the p13E-11 probe). Borderline alleles are defined by a D4Z4 locus with 10 or 11 repeat units (35–40 kb). Individuals with FSHD1 have one D4Z4A allele contracted to between 1 and 10 repeats units and a D4Z4A allele with the normal 11–100 repeat units. About 95% of FSHD patients have FSHD1. About 5% of individuals with FSHD show chromatin relaxation at D4Z4 without having a D4Z4

contraction. In these individuals with so-called FSHD2, pathogenic variants in the chromatin modifier *SMCHD1* cause the chromatin relaxation at D4Z4 (https://www.ncbi.nlm.nih.gov/books/NBK1443/).

A heterozygous c.2068C > T(p.Pro690Ser) variant in the *SMCHD1* gene was reported in a patient with FSHD2. This patient with FSHD2 was also heterozygous for a permissive D4Z4 haplotype; D4Z4 methylation was decreased to 7%. The variant in *SMCHD1* was inherited from her unaffected mother, while the D4Z4 permissive haplotype was inherited from the unaffected father. The t(4;19)(q35;13) involving DUX4 at 4q35 and CIC at 19q13 were detected in two individuals with Ewing-like sarcomas; the patients did not have FSHD symptoms.

Therefore, this patient would most likely have the 33- and 48-kb alleles for D4Z4 using *EcoRI* and the p13E-11 probe for Southern blot.

37. **A.** Pompe disease, also called "glycogen storage disease type II," is a rare, progressive, and often fatal muscular disease. The underlying pathology is a deficiency of the enzyme acid alpha-glucosidase (GAA) that hydrolyzes lysosomal glycogen. *Biallelic pathogenic variants in GAA cause deficiency of acid alpha-glucosidase (GAA) enzyme activity, leading to Pompe disease* (https://www.ncbi.nlm.nih.gov/books/NBK1261/).

Pathogenic variants in *GBA* cause Gaucher disease. Pathogenic variants in *HEXA* cause Tay–Sachs disease. Pathogenic variants in *SMPD1* cause Niemann–Pick disease.

Therefore, the *GAA* gene most likely harbored the pathogenic variants for Pompe disease in this patient.

38. **E.** Pompe disease, also called "glycogen storage disease type II," is a rare, progressive, and often fatal muscular disease (http://pompeindia.org). The underlying pathology is a deficiency of the enzyme acid alpha-glucosidase (GAA) that hydrolyzes lysosomal glycogen. It was the first recognized lysosomal storage disease and is the only glycogen storage disease that is also a lysosomal storage disease. In Pompe disease, lysosomal glycogen accumulates in many tissues, with skeletal, cardiac, and smooth muscle most prominently involved. Biallelic pathogenic variants in *GAA* cause deficiency of acid alpha-glucosidase (GAA) enzyme activity, leading to Pompe disease. More than 150 pathogenic variants in *GAA* have been identified in individuals with Pompe disease. *Sequencing analysis detects 83%–93% of pathogenic variants in probands.* Gene-targeted deletion/

duplication analysis detects 5%−13% of pathogenic variants in probands. An estimated 50%−60% of African American patients have the pathogenic variant p.Arg854Ter. An estimated 40%−80% of Chinese patients have the pathogenic variant p. Asp645Glu. An estimated 50%−85% of adult patients have the pathogenic variant c.336-13T > G, typically in the compound heterozygous state (https://www.ncbi.nlm.nih.gov/books/NBK1261/).

This pediatric patient's ethnic background was not provided in the question. Therefore, Sanger sequencing analysis was most likely used for the molecular genetic testing to test for Pompe disease in this patient.

39. **C.** Caution must be exercised in correlating results from molecular genetic testing and enzyme analysis in the absence of clinical features of Pompe disease, as the pseudodeficiency allele c.1726G > A (p.Gly576Ser), which is relatively common in Asian populations, interferes with interpretation of enzyme testing in NBS programs (confirmed by screening programs in Missouri and New York) (https://www.ncbi.nlm.nih.gov/books/NBK1261/).

Homozygous pathogenic variants are not common in the general population, but may be seen owing to a founder effect or consanguinity. A partial or a full deletion of *GAA* or a variant in the primer region, which may cause homozygous pathogenic variants, was detected by sequencing analysis; this needs to be further investigated if ethnic background and family history does not support it.

Sequencing analysis detects 83%−93% of pathogenic variants in probands. Gene-targeted deletion/duplication analysis detect 5%−13% of pathogenic variants in probands. It was unlikely there were two copies of uncommon pathogenic variants, missed by Sanger sequencing analysis. As a pseudodeficiency allele, c.1726G > A (p.Gly576Ser) may explain the reduced GAA enzyme activity in this patient. Therefore, it would most likely that this newborn boy did not have Pompe disease.

40. **A.** Familial dysautonomia (FD), also known as Riley−Day syndrome, is an autosomal recessive neuropathy that occurs almost exclusively in the Ashkenazi Jewish population. Affected individuals have gastrointestinal dysfunction, vomiting crises, recurrent pneumonia, altered sensitivity to pain and temperature perception, and cardiovascular instability. Age at onset is usually during infancy. About 40% of individuals have autonomic crises, which is life-threatening. Hypotonia contributes to a delay in acquisition of motor milestones. The carrier frequency is approximately 1 in 31 in the Ashkenazi Jewish population (https://www.ncbi.nlm.nih.gov/books/NBK1180/).

Hereditary neuropathy with liability to pressure palsies (HNLPP) is characterized by repeated focal-pressure neuropathies such as carpal tunnel syndrome and peroneal palsy with foot drop. The first attack usually occurs in the second or third decade. Recovery from acute neuropathy is often complete; when recovery is not complete, the resulting disability is usually mild. Smith−Lemli−Opitz syndrome (SLOS) is a congenital multiple anomaly syndrome caused by an abnormality in cholesterol metabolism resulting from deficiency of the enzyme 7-dehydrocholesterol (7-DHC) reductase. It is characterized by prenatal and postnatal growth retardation, microcephaly, moderate-to-severe intellectual disability, and multiple major and minor malformations. Smith−Magenis syndrome (SMS) is characterized by distinctive physical features (particularly facial features that progress with age), developmental delay, cognitive impairment, and behavioral abnormalities. Infants have feeding difficulties, failure to thrive, hypotonia, hyporeflexia, prolonged napping or need to be awakened for feeding, and generalized lethargy. The majority of individuals function in the mild-to-moderate range of intellectual disability. The behavioral phenotype, including significant sleep disturbance, stereotypies, and maladaptive and self-injurious behaviors, is generally not recognized until age 18 months or older and continues to change until adulthood.

Therefore, this Ashkenazi Jewish boy would more likely have familial dysautonomia than other disorders listed in the question.

41. **B.** This patient has classical presentation of familial dysautonomia (FD). FD, also known as Riley−Day syndrome, is almost exclusively occurs in the Ashkenazi Jewish population. The carrier frequency is approximately 1 in 31 Ashkenazi Jewish population. It affects the development and survival of sensory, sympathetic, and parasympathetic neurons. It is a debilitating disease present from birth. Neuronal degeneration progresses throughout life. Affected individuals have gastrointestinal dysfunction, vomiting crises, recurrent pneumonia, altered sensitivity to pain and temperature perception, and cardiovascular instability (https://www.ncbi.nlm.nih.gov/books/NBK1180/).

Canavan disease and Gaucher disease are also relatively high prevalent in Ashkenazi Jewish. But they are also in other populations, especially Caucasian. The clinical symptoms for Canavan disease and Gaucher disease are different from familial dysautonomia.

Therefore, the patient most likely has familial dysautonomia.

42. **D.** Familial dysautonomia (FD), also known as Riley–Day syndrome, is an autosomal recessive neuropathy that occurs almost exclusively in the Ashkenazi Jewish population. The carrier frequency is approximately 1 in 31 Ashkenazi Jews. A single pathogenic variant in intron 20 of the IKBKAP gene ($2507 + 6T \rightarrow C$) accounts for >99% of the mutations in the Ashkenazi Jewish population. A second pathogenic variant, R696P, is included in most carrier screening panels and accounts for the remainder of Ashkenazi Jewish mutations. In a carrier screening program with this detection rate, at least 99% of affected fetuses would be detected if a prenatal procedure was performed (https://www.ncbi.nlm.nih.gov/books/NBK1180/).

Therefore, the recurrent risk in the couple may be estimated to be 1/4.

43. **D.** The carrier frequency of familial dysautonomia is approximately 1 in 31. *A single variant in intron 20 of the IKBKAP gene (c.2507 + 6T > C) accounts for >99% of the pathogenic variants in the Ashkenazi Jewish population.* A second variant, c.2087G > C(p. Arg696Pro), is included in most carrier screening panels and accounts for the remainder of Ashkenazi Jewish pathogenic variants. In a carrier screening program with these two variants, at least 99% of affected fetuses would be detected if a prenatal procedure was performed. In 2003 a third variant, c.2741C > T(p.Pro914Leu), was detected in a patient with familial dysautonomia (https://www.ncbi.nlm.nih.gov/books/NBK1180/).

Therefore, targeted-mutation analysis would be the most cost-effective way to confirm the diagnosis in this Ashkenazi Jewish patient.

44. **D.** The carrier frequency of familial dysautonomia is approximately 1 in 31 in the Ashkenazi Jewish population. *A single pathogenic variant in intron 20 of the IKBKAP gene (c.2507 + 6T > C) accounts for >99% of the mutations in the Ashkenazi Jewish population.* A second variant, c.2087G > C (p.Arg696Pro), is included in most carrier screening panels and accounts for the remainder of Ashkenazi Jewish pathogenic variants. In a carrier screening program with these two variants, at least 99% of affected fetuses would be detected if a

prenatal procedure was performed. In 2003, a third variant, c.2741C > T(p.Pro914Leu), was detected in a patient with familial dysautonomia (https://www.ncbi.nlm.nih.gov/books/NBK1180/).

Therefore, as an Ashkenazi Jewish descendant, it would be most likely that this boy had the c.2507 + 6T > C variant in intron 20 of the IKBKAP gene.

References

1. Grimm T, et al. Risk assessment and genetic counseling in families with Duchenne muscular dystrophy. *Acta Myol* 2012;**31**(3):179–83.
2. Sohail A, Imtiaz F. *A classical case of duchenne muscular dystrophy.* Hereditary Genet; 2015. 4, p. 139.
3. Doo KH, et al. A case of Becker muscular dystrophy with early manifestation of cardiomyopathy. *Korean J Pediatr* 2012;**55**(9):350–3.
4. Christodoulou J, et al. Barth syndrome: clinical observations and genetic linkage studies. *Am J Med Genet* 1994;**50**(3):255–64.
5. Sabater-Molina M, et al. Barth syndrome in adulthood: a clinical case. *Rev Esp Cardiol (Engl Ed)* 2013;**66**(1):68–70.
6. Ran Lee SC, Koh S-E, Lee IK, Lee J. Two cases of spinal muscular atrophy type 1 with extensive involvement of sensory nerves. *Korean J Pediatr* 2008;**51**(12):1350–4.
7. Al Dakhoul S. Very severe spinal muscular atrophy (Type 0). *Avicenna J Med* 2017;**7**(1):32–3.
8. Luo M, et al. An Ashkenazi Jewish SMN1 haplotype specific to duplication alleles improves pan-ethnic carrier screening for spinal muscular atrophy. *Genet Med* 2014;**16**(2):149–56.
9. Nishimura AL, et al. A mutation in the vesicle-trafficking protein VAPB causes late-onset spinal muscular atrophy and amyotrophic lateral sclerosis. *Am J Hum Genet* 2004;**75**(5):822–31.
10. Prior TW, et al. A positive modifier of spinal muscular atrophy in the SMN2 gene. *Am J Hum Genet* 2009;**85**(3):408–13.
11. Prior TW, et al. Technical standards and guidelines for spinal muscular atrophy testing. *Genet Med* 2011;**13**(7):686–94.
12. Hendrickson BC, et al. Differences in SMN1 allele frequencies among ethnic groups within North America. *J Med Genet* 2009;**46**(9):641–4.
13. Nalini A, Yeshraj G, Veerendrakumar M. Familial amyotrophic lateral sclerosis: first report from India. *Neurol India* 2006;**54**(3):304–5.
14. Committee on Bioethics; Committee on Genetics, and; American College of Medical Genetics and; Genomics Social; Ethical; Legal Issues Committee. Ethical and Policy Issues in Genetic Testing and Screening of Children. Pediatrics. 2013;**131**(3):620-2. http://dx.doi.org/10.1542/peds.2012-3680. Epub 2013 Feb 21. PubMed PMID: 23428972.
15. Castellano V, Feinberg J, Michaels J. Facioscapulohumeral dystrophy: case report and discussion. *HSS J* 2008;**4**(2):175–9.
16. Sugie K, et al. Teaching NeuroImages: hemiatrophy as a clinical presentation in facioscapulohumeral muscular dystrophy. *Neurology* 2009;**73**(5):e24.
17. Lemmers RJ, et al. Digenic inheritance of an SMCHD1 mutation and an FSHD-permissive D4Z4 allele causes facioscapulohumeral muscular dystrophy type 2. *Nat Genet* 2012;**44**(12):1370–4.
18. Kawamura-Saito M, et al. Fusion between CIC and DUX4 up-regulates PEA3 family genes in Ewing-like sarcomas with t(4;19)(q35; q13) translocation. *Hum Mol Genet* 2006;**15**(13):2125–37.

19. Jamil S, Ahmed S, Tariq M. Acid maltase deficiency--Pompe's disease. *J Pak Med Assoc* 2011;**61**(8):821−3.
20. Liu Y, et al. Infantile Pompe disease: a case report and review of the Chinese literature. *Exp Ther Med* 2016;**11**(1):235−8.
21. Tonholo-Silva ER, Takahashi SI, Yoshinaga L. Familial dysautonomia (Riley-Day syndrome). *Arq Neuropsiquiatr* 1994;**52**(1):103−5.
22. Goodall J, Shinebourne E, Lake BD. Early diagnosis of familial dysautonomia. Case report with special reference to primary patho-physiological findings. *Arch Dis Child* 1968;**43**(230):455−8.

Further Reading

- American College of Medical Genetics and Genomics (ACMGG) (www.acmg.net/)
- GeneReviews (www.ncbi.nlm.nih.gov/books/NBK1116/)
- Muscular Dystrophy Association (www.mda.org)
- Muscular Dystrophy Canada (www.muscle.ca/)
- Neurology Advisor (www.neurologyadvisor.com/)

SELF-ASSESSMENT QUESTIONS FOR CLINICAL MOLECULAR GENETICS

11

Prenatal, Newborn Screen, and Metabolic Disorders

For more than 30 years, identifying women at increased risk for pregnancies with trisomies 21, 18, and 13 has been the focus of prenatal screening programs that combine maternal age, levels of specific analytes in maternal serum, and ultrasound findings in the first or second trimester to derive a risk estimate for these trisomies. Depending on whether screening is performed in the first or second trimester of pregnancy or both, these programs now reach a detection rate of up to 88%–96% for Down syndrome and up to 85%–95% for trisomy 18.

In parallel, programs for universal parental carrier screening for autosomal recessive disorders, such as cystic fibrosis (CF), as well as ethnicity-based carrier screening, such as for conditions that are more prevalent in the Ashkenazi Jewish population, were developed to identify parents at 25% risk of having an affected child with these disorders. Identified carrier couples can then choose preimplantation genetic diagnosis to avoid affected pregnancies or prenatal diagnosis, which allows them to consider termination of an affected pregnancy or be prepared for the birth of an affected child.

With recent technological advances in methods to identify numerical and structural chromosome abnormalities and point pathogenic variants, such as chromosomal microarray analysis (CMA) and next-generation sequencing (NGS), the screening for and diagnosis of genetic abnormalities in the fetus is undergoing an unprecedented rapid evolution. At the same time, CMA and NGS have also accelerated the discovery of causes of intellectual disability, birth defects, and many rare genetic and genomic disorders. This has, in turn, motivated the development of expansive carrier screenings for hundreds of genetic disorders at once as well as the development of noninvasive fetal cell-free DNA (cfDNA)–based screens for fetal chromosomal aneuploidy, structural chromosomal abnormalities, and single-gene disorders, so-called noninvasive prenatal testing (NIPT)/noninvasive prenatal screening (NIPS). The availability of CMA- and NGS-based methods, such as targeted gene-panel sequencing and, recently, whole-exome sequencing (WES), has also resulted in the ability to diagnose more fetal genetic disorders from specimens obtained through amniocentesis or chorionic villus sampling (CVS) (Recent advances in prenatal genetic screening and testing. F1000Research 2016, 5(F1000 Faculty Rev):2591 Last updated: October 28, 2016).

The Recommended Uniform Screening Panel (RUSP) is a standardized list of disorders that have been supported by the Advisory Committee on Heritable Disorders in Newborns and Children and recommended by the Secretary of the Department of Health and Human Services (HHS) for states to screen as part of their state universal newborn screening (NBS) programs. Disorders on the RUSP are chosen based on evidence that supports the potential net benefit of screening, the ability of states to screen for the disorder, and the availability of effective treatments. Currently there are 34 core disorders specified by the Health Resources and Services Administration (HRSA) in the RUSP (http://ghr.nlm.nih.gov/). These conditions include phenylketonuria (PKU), cystic fibrosis, sickle cell disease, critical congenital heart disease, hearing loss, and others. It is recommended that every newborn be screened for all disorders on the RUSP. Most states screen for the majority of disorders on the RUSP; newer conditions are still in the process of adoption. Some states also screen for additional disorders (http://www.hrsa.gov).

NBS is performed on every infant regardless of the parents' health insurance status or ability to pay. The fees for NBS vary by state, from less than $15 to about $150. Some states do not charge a fee for this testing. When there is a fee, it is often covered by private health insurance plans. This testing is also covered under the Children's Health Insurance Program (CHIP) and Medicaid for those who are eligible (http://ghr.nlm.nih.gov/). Supplemental screening can be done through a private laboratory, which is not covered under the fees charged by each state for NBS. Within 2–3 weeks after NBS tests are performed, results are sent to the pediatrician's office or clinic. The healthcare provider will notify parents of a positive test result and arrange for further testing to determine a diagnosis. Often when there is a positive screening test result, follow-up diagnostic testing shows that the baby does not have the disease.

Congenital metabolic disorders constitute majority of the RUSP, such as propionic acidemia, methylmalonic acidemia (methylmalonyl-CoA mutase), methylmalonic acidemia (cobalamin disorders), isovaleric acidemia, 3-methylcrotonyl-CoA carboxylase deficiency, 3-hydroxy-3-methyglutaric aciduria, holocarboxylase synthase deficiency, ß-ketothiolase deficiency, glutaric acidemia type I, carnitine uptake defect/carnitine transport defect, medium-chain acyl-CoA dehydrogenase deficiency, very-long-chain acyl-CoA dehydrogenase deficiency, long-chain L-3 hydroxyacyl-CoA dehydrogenase deficiency, trifunctional protein deficiency, argininosuccinic aciduria, citrullinemia type I, maple sirup urine disease, homocystinuria, classic phenylketonuria, tyrosinemia type I, biotinidase deficiency, classic galactosemia, Pompe disease, and other conditions. The traditional classification system for inborn errors of metabolism (IEM) groups the disorders according to the general type of metabolism involved, such as urea-cycle defects, organic acidemias, fatty acid oxidation defects, primary lactic acidosis, aminoacidopathies, disorders of carbohydrate metabolism, lysosomal storage disorders, and peroxisomal disorders. Some of the disorders fit into more than one category. Lysosomal storage disorders (LSDs) are covered in Chapter 9, Lysosomal Storage Disorders.

In this chapter, we put prenatal care, NBS, and IEM together because they are related and become an important part of preventive medicine. Even though NBS is not done in private clinical molecular laboratories, it is important to understand it and to provide follow-up diagnostic testing after abnormal NBS in a timely manner. While it is not possible to cover all the disorders that fall into this category, we used the following relatively common disorders as examples to illustrate the study points for the chapter:

- Hemolytic disease of the fetus and newborn (HDFN)
- Ornithine transcarbamoylase (OTC) deficiency
- Glucose-6-phosphate dehydrogenase deficiency (G6PD)

- Phenylalanine hydroxylase (PAH) deficiency (PKU)
- Long-chain L-3-hydroxyacyl-coenzyme A dehydrogenase deficiency (LCHAD)
- Trifunctional protein deficiency
- Medium-chain acyl-coenzyme A dehydrogenase (MCAD) deficiency
- Short-chain acyl-coenzyme A dehydrogenase (SCAD) deficiency
- Very-long-chain acyl-coenzyme A dehydrogenase (VLCAD) deficiency
- X-linked adrenoleukodystrophy
- Rhizomelic chondrodysplasia punctata type 1 (RCDP1) classic type
- Zellweger syndrome
- *HFE*-associated hereditary hemochromatosis
- Menkes disease
- Wilson disease
- Alagille syndrome
- Canavan disease

QUESTIONS

1. Ultrasonographic scanning revealed a 28-week-old fetus whose anterior neural tube had failed to close; this ultimately resulted in degeneration of the forebrain. Which one of the following is the most appropriate genetic term to describe this defect?[1]
   A. Deformation
   B. Disruption
   C. Dysplasia
   D. Malformation
   E. None of the above

2. Ultrasonographic scanning revealed a 32-week-old fetus with multiple symmetrical joint contractures due to abnormal muscle development. It was caused by severe fetal constraint in a pregnancy complicated by oligohydramnios. The physician reassured the couple that intelligence would most likely not be affected and that orthopedic rehabilitation is often successful. Which one of the following is the most appropriate genetic term to describe this defect?[1]
   A. Deformation
   B. Disruption
   C. Dysplasia
   D. Malformation
   E. None of the above

3. Ultrasonographic scanning revealed a 32-week-old fetus had amniotic band sequence with constriction rings around the left hand, and amputation of the thumb. Which one of the

following is the most appropriate genetic term to describe this defect?[1]

A. Deformation
B. Disruption
C. Dysplasia
D. Malformation
E. None of the above

4. A 37-year-old female came to a clinic for a positive pregnancy test at home. She had a 12-year-old daughter and a 10-year-old son. Laboratory testing confirmed the pregnancy. Ultrasonography revealed an approximately 6-week pregnancy. A maternal first-trimester screen was ordered at 11 weeks' gestation. The results indicated a 1 in 90 likelihood of Down syndrome in the fetus, which was higher than the mother's age-related risk of 1 in 287. What is the clinical sensitivity of the first-trimester screen for Down syndrome?[2]

A. 50%
B. 65%
C. 80%
D. 99%
E. None of the above

5. A 37-year-old female came to a clinic for positive pregnancy test at home. She had a 12-year-old daughter and a 10-year-old son. Laboratory testing confirmed the pregnancy. Ultrasonography revealed an approximately 6-week pregnancy. A maternal first-trimester screen was ordered at 11 weeks' gestation. The results indicated a 1 in 90 likelihood of Down syndrome in the fetus, which was higher than the mother's age-related risk of 1 in 287. What is the clinical specificity of the first-trimester screen for Down syndrome?[2]

A. 42%
B. 65%
C. 80%
D. 92%
E. None of the above

6. A 37-year-old female came to a clinic for positive pregnancy test at home. She had a 12-year-old daughter and a 10-year-old son. Laboratory testing confirmed the pregnancy. Ultrasonography revealed an approximately 6-week pregnancy. A maternal first-trimester screen was ordered at 11 weeks' gestation. The results indicated a 1 in 90 likelihood of Down syndrome in the fetus, which was higher than the mother's age-related risk of 1 in 287. She was informed that prenatal diagnosis would involve obtaining chorionic villus samples (CVSs) (usually at approximately 10–12 weeks' gestation) or amniotic fluid by amniocentesis (usually performed between 15 and 18 weeks' gestation). Both procedures involve a small risk of pregnancy loss, estimated at 1 in 100 to 1 in 200 for

CVS and 1 in 200 to 1 in 400 for amniocentesis. She was uncomfortable with any invasive procedure and declined both. The second-trimester screen revealed that the risk had increased to 1 in 45. What is the clinical sensitivity of the second-trimester screen for Down syndrome?[3]

A. 48%
B. 74%
C. 81%
D. 93%
E. None of the above

7. A 37-year-old female came to a clinic for positive pregnancy test at home. She had a 12-year-old daughter and a 10-year-old son. Laboratory testing confirmed the pregnancy. Ultrasonography revealed an approximately 6-week pregnancy. A maternal first-trimester screen was ordered at 11 weeks' gestation. The results indicated a 1 in 90 likelihood of Down syndrome in the fetus, which was higher than the mother's age-related risk of 1 in 287. She was informed that prenatal diagnosis would involve obtaining chorionic villus sampling (CVSs) (usually at approximately 10–12 weeks' gestation) or amniotic fluid by amniocentesis (usually performed between 15 and 18 weeks' gestation). Both procedures involve a small risk of pregnancy loss, estimated at 1 in 100 to 1 in 200 for CVS and 1 in 200 to 1 in 400 for amniocentesis. She was uncomfortable with any invasive procedure and declined both. The second-trimester screen revealed that the risk had increased to 1 in 45. What is the clinical specificity of the second-trimester screen for Down syndrome?

A. 50%
B. 75%
C. 85%
D. 95%
E. None of the above

8. A 28-year-old female came to a Ob/Gyn clinic with her husband for a second-trimester screen. A blood specimen was collected for laboratory testing. Ultrasonographic scanning revealed a 16-weeks fetus whose anterior neural tube had failed to close (anencephaly). Which one of the following would most likely NOT be the results of the second-trimester maternal serum screening?[3]

A. High maternal serum alpha-fetoprotein (AFP)
B. Low hCG
C. Normal μE3 (estriol)
D. All of the above
E. None of the above

9. Which one of the following studies provides the most accurate result for fetal aneuploidy carrier status at 12 weeks' gestational age with a minimum risk of miscarriage?[4]

A. First-trimester screen
B. Second-trimester screen
C. Amniocentesis
D. Chorionic villus sampling
E. Noninvasive prenatal test (NIPT)

10. A 44-year-old pregnant female underwent obstetric ultrasound at 19 weeks of gestation, which revealed increased fetal nuchal translucency. A noninvasive prenatal test (NIPT) suggested Down syndrome. Which one of the following would likely NOT be the results of second-trimester maternal serum screening if the fetus had trisomy 21?
A. High hCG
B. Low inhibin A
C. Low maternal serum alpha-fetoprotein (MS-AFP)
D. Low μE3 (estriol)
E. None of the above

11. A 21-year-old G2P1 female underwent obstetric ultrasound at 19 5/7 weeks of gestation, which revealed multiple fetal anomalies, including hypoplastic left heart, bilateral cleft lip, bilateral echogenic kidneys with hydronephrosis, echogenic bowel, and bowed right femur. Genetic consultation was provided and risks, benefits, and alternatives of further genetic evaluation, including amniocentesis and cfDNA screening, were discussed. The patient expressed concerns regarding the risks of invasive testing and opted to proceed with cfDNA screening. The cfDNA screening was performed at 20 weeks of gestational age. The result indicated that the fetus might have trisomy 13. Which one of the following would likely NOT be the results of second-trimester maternal serum screening if the fetus had trisomy 13?[5]
A. High hCG
B. Low maternal serum alpha-fetoprotein (MS-AFP)
C. Low μE3 (estriol)
D. Normal inhibin A
E. None of the above

12. A 34-year-old female (G2P1) conceived naturally and presented to an Ob/Gyn clinic for prenatal care at 10 weeks 3 days after her last menstrual period. The pregnancy had been uncomplicated. A noninvasive prenatal test (NIPT) with cell-free DNA (cfDNA) was offered due to the advanced maternal age. Which one of the following studies would likely also be offered?[6]
A. First-trimester screen
B. Amniocentesis
C. Chorionic villus sampling (CVS)
D. Ultrasound evaluation
E. None of the above

13. A 34-year-old female (G2P1) conceived naturally and presented to an Ob/Gyn clinic for prenatal care at 10 weeks 3 days after her last menstrual period. The pregnancy had been uncomplicated. A noninvasive prenatal test (NIPT) with cell-free DNA was offered due to the advanced maternal age. The results were indeterminate. Which one of the following studies would likely be offered for follow-up?[6]
A. First-trimester screen
B. Second-trimester screen
C. Amniocentesis
D. Chorionic villus sampling (CVS)
E. Repeat the NIPT
F. Ultrasound evaluation
G. None of the above

14. A 33-year-old female and her 32-year-old husband came to a clinic for a follow-up prenatal checkup at 20 weeks of gestational age. The pregnancy had been uncomplicated. An ultrasound revealed a complete atrioventricular canal defect (CAVCD). The couple was offered an amniocentesis but declined the invasive diagnostic test in favor of a noninvasive prenatal test (NIPT). The NIPT test did not detect aneuploidy. Which one of the following would be the most appropriate next step in the workup?[6,7]
A. Amniocentesis is recommended to further rule out aneuploidy.
B. Chorionic villus sampling (CVS) is recommended to further rule out aneuploidy.
C. NIPT cannot be used to detect an open neural-tube defect; ultrasound is recommended for follow-up.
D. NIPT is a diagnostic study; there is no need for follow-up.
E. None of the above.

15. A 33-year-old female and her 32-year-old husband came to a clinic for a follow-up prenatal checkup at 20 weeks of gestational age. The pregnancy had been uncomplicated. An ultrasound revealed a complete atrioventricular canal defect (CAVCD). The couple was offered an amniocentesis but declined the invasive diagnostic testing in favor of a noninvasive prenatal test (NIPT). The NIPT did not detect aneuploidy. At 37 weeks of gestational age, the wife gave birth to a 7-lb 3-oz (3.26 kg) baby girl by elective cesarean section. Down syndrome was suspected, since baby had hypotonia, a flattened nasal bridge, and upslanting palpebral fissures. A chromosome analysis confirmed the diagnosis of 47,XX, + 21. Complications seen in the neonatal period included respiratory distress with transient tachypnea that required supplemental oxygen.

A CAVCD was confirmed by a newborn echocardiogram. The couple had two healthy children. In general, which one of the following factors most likely affects the analytical sensitivity of NIPT than others?[6,7]

A. Advanced maternal age

B. Robertsonian translocation, 45,XY,der(13;21)(q10;q10), in the father

C. Fetus with increased risk for trisomy 21 by first-trimester screen

D. High maternal body-mass index (BMI)

E. Previous pregnancy with trisomy 21

F. None of the above

16. Which one of the following most likely meets rejection criteria for noninvasive prenatal testing (NIPT)?[6]

A. Gestational age of 32 weeks

B. Robertsonian translocation, 45,XY,der(13;21)(q10;q10) in the father

C. Fetus with decreased risk for trisomy 21 by first-trimester screen

D. Karyotype of 45,XY,der(13;21)(q10;q10) in the mother

E. Multiple gestations

17. Which one of the following does not meet rejection criteria for noninvasive prenatal testing (NIPT)?[6,8]

A. 6 weeks' gestation

B. Maternal BMI >40

C. Karyotype of 45,XY,der(13;21)(q10;q10) in the mother

D. Multiple gestations

E. None of the above

18. Which one of the following prenatal studies is recommended as the most appropriate choice for first-line screening for the low-risk obstetric population by American College of Obstetricians and Gynecologists (ACOG)?[6]

A. First-trimester screen followed by second-trimester screen

B. Amniocentesis

C. Chorionic villus sampling (CVS)

D. Noninvasive prenatal test (NIPT)

E. None of the above

19. Newborn screening (NBS) began in the United States in the[9]:

A. 1950s

B. 1960s

C. 1970s

D. 1980s

E. 1990s

20. Which one of the following factors increases the potential of false positive newborn screening (NBS) results in premature infants?[10]

A. Preterm newborn in NICU with total parenteral nutrition (TPN)

B. Newborn with PKU

C. Newborn with Beckwith−Wiedemann syndrome

D. Newborn from a cesarean section

E. None of the above

21. Which one of the following prenatal studies gives the most accurate information on fetal aneuploidy at 12 weeks' gestational age without the risk of miscarriage?[3,4]

A. First-trimester screen

B. Second-trimester screen

C. Amniocentesis

D. CVS

E. Noninvasive prenatal test (NIPT)

22. Which one of the following prenatal studies has the highest rate for miscarriage if it is done at 12 weeks' gestational age?[11]

A. First-trimester screen

B. Second-trimester screen

C. Amniocentesis

D. CVS

E. Noninvasive prenatal test (NIPT)

23. A full-term, Caucasian baby boy was born to a 30-year-old woman at 38 weeks of gestation. The baby weighed 2.8 kg, with an Apgar score of 9 and 10 at 1 and 5 minutes, respectively. The baby was noted to have mild jaundice with normal vital signs on day 1 of life; there was no evidence to suggest other causes of neonatal jaundice such as intrauterine infections. His glucose-6-phosphate dehydrogenase (G6PD) screen was normal. Laboratory investigations showed that his total bilirubin was 198 μmol/L and hemoglobin 19 g/dL. The mother was G3P1. Her first pregnancy spontaneously aborted 5 years ago and unfortunately no investigation was performed to find out the cause of abortion. Subsequent pregnancies were uneventful, with no history of hemolytic disease of the fetus and newborn (HDFN) in the past 3 years. She reported no previous history of blood transfusion. Which one of the following conditions would most likely account for the HDFN in this newborn?[12]

A. ABO incompatibility

B. Rhc incompatibility

C. RhD incompatibility

D. RhE incompatibility

E. RhK incompatibility

24. A full-term boy, born to a 32-year-old G2P2 Malaysian mother was noticed to have jaundice on day 1 after birth. His birth weight was 2.96 kg. The mother and the baby were grouped AB and B, respectively, both being positive for RhD antigen. The baby was admitted to the neonatal intensive care unit (NICU) on the following day with hepatomegaly 3 cm and splenomegaly 5 cm below

the costal margin. Direct antiglobulin testing (DAT) of the neonate's red blood cells was strongly positive (4+). Hemoglobin was 6.2 g/dL. A sudden rise of total serum bilirubin (TSB) level from 102 μmol/L on day 1 to 401 μmol/L within 24 h prompted doubling of volume for exchange transfusion. The hyperbilirubinemia was mainly of conjugated bilirubin 1 day post-exchange transfusion. Investigations for infectious causes such as blood culture, urine microscopy, and culture were negative. Liver enzymes such as alkaline phosphatase, alanine aminotransferase, and aspartate aminotransferase were also within the normal ranges. G6PD screening was negative. No evidence of biliary atresia was found. Rh genotyping was performed for the mother, father, and the neonate. The mother was typed as R1R1 (DCe/DCe) and the father R1R2 (DCe/ DcE). The baby was typed as R1R2 (DCe/DcE). Which one of the following conditions would this newborn baby most likely have?[12,13]

A. ABO incompatibility
B. Rhc incompatibility
C. RhD incompatibility
D. RhE incompatibility
E. RhK incompatibility

25. Newborn screening (NBS) is the practice of testing every newborn for harmful or potentially fatal conditions, such as hearing loss and certain genetic, endocrine, and metabolic disorders that typically are not otherwise apparent at birth. Newborn screening in the United States began in the 1960s. Universal newborn screening has become a well-established, state-based, public health system involving education, screening, diagnostic follow-up, treatment and management, and system monitoring and evaluation. Each year, >98% of approximately 4 million newborns in the United States are screened. Through early identification, newborn screening provides an opportunity for treatment and significant reductions in morbidity and mortality. In 2006, the American College of Medical Genetics and Genomics (ACMG), under the aegis of the Health Resources and Services Administration (HRSA), convened a group of experts to address the substantial variation in the number of disorders screened for in each state. The experts evaluated scientific and medical information related to screened conditions and recommended a uniform screening panel. How many conditions are in this recommended uniformed screen program?[9,14]

A. 3
B. 29
C. 31

D. 38
E. 43

26. A 3-day-old boy was brought to an emergency department for lethargy, hypotonia, and shallow breathing, which eventually led to apnea and required a mechanical respirator. Laboratory results showed a plasma ammonium concentration of 3044 mmol/L (normal range, 18–54). Plasma amino acid analysis revealed elevated glutamine and undetectable citrulline levels. Urinary orotic acid was extremely elevated. Which one of the following genes would most likely harbor pathogenic variant(s) in this patient?

A. ASS1
B. ASL
C. CPS1
D. NAGS
E. OTC

27. A 2-year-old girl was brought to an emergency room for vomiting and tremors. The plasma ammonium level was 221 μM/L (normal range, 11–40). Laboratory testing revealed an elevated arginine in serum. Which one of the following enzymes would be the least likely to be deficient before further workup in this patient?

A. Carbamoyl phosphate synthetase I
B. Carbamoyl phosphate synthetase II
C. Ornithine transcarbamoylase
D. Arginase
E. Argininosuccinate lyase
F. None of the above

28. A 2-year-old girl was brought to an emergency room for vomiting and tremors. The plasma ammonium level was 221 μM/L (normal range, 11–40). Laboratory testing revealed an elevated serum arginine. Which one of the following enzymes would most likely cause an elevation of the plasma arginine levels?

A. Arginase
B. Argininosuccinate lyase
C. Carbamoyl phosphate synthetase I
D. Carbamoyl phosphate synthetase II
E. Ornithine transcarbamoylase
F. None of the above

29. A 26-year-old primiparous woman was referred to a neurological clinic for intractable seizures on the fifth postpartum day. She was hospitalized on the second postpartum day because of nausea and vomiting after natural delivery of a healthy baby. Altered mental status, disorientation, and seizure activities were added to the clinical condition of the patient. She was transferred to the neurological clinic with the early diagnosis of eclampsia. Her vital signs were normal. Her medical history was uneventful, and she had no signs of preeclampsia.

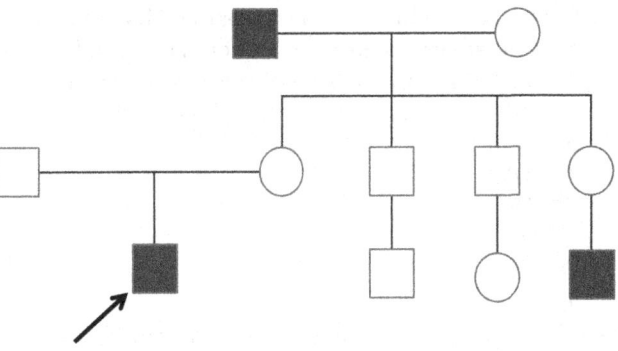

Her lumbar puncture, cerebral CT, and MRI were all normal. An abdominal ultrasonogram was unremarkable. But her arterial ammonia level was 452 μmol/L. Hyperammonemia (550 mmol/L; normal range, 14–38) and respiratory alkalosis led to suspicion for a urea-cycle disorder. There was no sign or finding of acute or chronic hepatic failure or cirrhosis. Which one of the following enzymes would most likely be deficient in this patient?[15]

A. Arginase
B. Argininosuccinate lyase
C. Carbamoyl phosphate synthetase I
D. Carbamoyl phosphate synthetase II
E. Ornithine transcarbamoylase
F. None of the above

30. A 43-year-old man of Mediterranean descent presented to his primary care provider for a routine visit. During the examination, the physician noted some mild splenomegaly and tenderness. Upon further examination, some scleral icterus was noted. Subsequent laboratory studies revealed marginally elevated lactate dehydrogenase (LDH) and bilirubin and slight anemia. This patient was questioned regarding recent food intake and other stressors and was found to have been drinking "several cans of beer" every night. The physician suspected that the patient had glucose-6-phosphate dehydrogenase deficiency (G6PD). Which one of the following statements regarding G6PD is correct?

A. It appears more often in females than in males.
B. It is an autosomal recessive disease.
C. Haploinsufficiency causes the disease.
D. Newborn screening for G6PD deficiency is not performed routinely in the United States.
E. Patients with G6PD have a selection advantage.

31. A 3-year-old boy was admitted to a hospital for severe anemia. His erythrocyte count was 1.25×10^{12}/L, hemoglobin concentration 45 g/L, and total bilirubin level 24.3 μmol/L. He had had jaundice since birth, which was still present at the time of admission. He was first diagnosed with hemolytic anemia, then glucose-6-phosphate dehydrogenase (G6PD) deficiency because his glucose-6-phosphate dehydrogenase activity was less than 1% of normal. After the patient was diagnosed, his family members were tested for G6PD. See the figure below for the pedigree. Why did the proband's mother NOT have any symptoms of this disorder?

A. A de novo pathogenic variant in the proband
B. Clinical heterogeneity
C. Nonpenetrance
D. Variable expression
E. X inactivation

32. In which of the following populations is glucose-6-phosphate dehydrogenase (G6PD) deficiency relatively uncommon?

A. African American
B. Arabic
C. Asian
D. Hispanic
E. None of the above

33. A 21-year-old African American marine was about to be sent overseas. In preparation for his tour of duty, he was given a prophylactic dose of primaquine to prevent malaria. Several days after he began taking the drug, he developed fatigue and hemolytic anemia. Which one of the following pathogenic variants is this patient most likely to have?[35]

A. Hemizygous p.Asn156Asp in G6PD
B. Homozygous p.Asn156Asp in G6PD
C. Hemizygous p.Val32Met in GALK1
D. Homozygous p.Val32Met in GALK1
E. None of the above

34. A 6-year-old Malaysian boy was brought to a hospital for aggressive behavior and developmental delay. He was born in Mecca, Saudi Arabia, after an uneventful pregnancy. His mother noticed that the boy was quiet and could not hold his head up when he was 3 months old. He was able to roll over at 8 months of age, sat without support at 20 months, walked at 2 years, and talked with meaning at 3 years of age. At about 1 year of age, his mother noticed that his normally black hair gradually changed to light brown. There was no history of light hair on either side of the family. The boy had no history of skin rashes. The parents were first cousins and one of the maternal grandfathers was mentally retarded. A physical examination revealed that his height and weight were below the third percentile. He could not follow simple instructions and was not able to read or write. Using the Seguin form board test, his mental age was assessed to be below that of a 3.5-year-old. Laboratory studies revealed increased

phenylalanine in urine and plasma. His family members were negative for phenylalanine. Which one of the following would most likely harbor pathogenic variant(s) for phenylketonuria in this patient?[16]

A. *APC*
B. *PAH*
C. *PC*
D. *PROC*
E. None of the above

35. The newborn screening (NBS) program in Illinois referred a newborn boy, John Doe, to a local hospital for further evaluation for phenylketonuria (PKU). Which one of the following assays has been used in the NBS for phenylketonuria?

A. Tandem mass spectrometry (MS/MS)
B. High-performance liquid chromatography (HPLC)
C. Molecular genetics test
D. Sweat sodium chloride test
E. None of the above

36. Which one of the following assays is most commonly used in newborn screening (NBS) for fatty acid oxidation disorders in United States?

A. Tandem mass spectrometry (MS/MS)
B. Targeted genotyping
C. Sanger sequencing
D. Immunohistochemistry (IHC)
E. Chromosome karyotyping

37. A newborn screening (NBS) sample showed "unsatisfactory" results. A second sample was collected when the infant was 6 days old. Which one of the following disorders would most likely be missed by the repeat NBS in this patient?

A. Amino acid disorders
B. Congenital heart defects
C. Fatty acid oxidation disorders
D. Hearing loss
E. Organic acidemia

38. A 32-year-old mother delivered an infant with intrauterine growth-restricted (IUGR) at 31 weeks of gestational age by cesarean section. The mother had been monitored for HELLP syndrome. The newborn screening (NBS) results were abnormal for elevated C16:0, C18:0, C18:1$_{w}$9, and C18:2$_{w}$6 acylcarnitine. Which one of the following disorders would the infant most likely have?

A. Short-chain acyl CoA dehydrogenase (SCAD) deficiency
B. Medium/short chain hydroxyacyl CoA dehydrogenase (M/SCHAD) deficiency
C. Medium-chain acyl CoA dehydrogenase (MCAD) deficiency
D. Long-chain hydroxyacyl CoA dehydrogenase (LCHAD) deficiency

E. Very-long-chain acyl CoA dehydrogenase (VLCAD) deficiency
F. Trifunctional protein deficiency
G. None of the above

39. A 6-month-old infant girl was brought to the emergency department of a local hospital by her mother for vomiting and lethargy. While in the hospital, the girl had a seizure. A physical examination showed hepatomegaly. A laboratory study revealed that her blood glucose was 26 mg/dL and ketone bodies were absent. MS/MS showed elevated C10:1, C8, and C10 acylcarnitine. Which one of the following disorders would the infant girl most likely have?

A. Short-chain acyl CoA dehydrogenase (SCAD) deficiency
B. Medium/short chain hydroxyacyl CoA dehydrogenase (M/SCHAD) deficiency
C. Medium-chain acyl CoA dehydrogenase (MCAD) deficiency
D. Long-chain hydroxyacyl CoA dehydrogenase (LCHAD) deficiency
E. Very-long-chain acyl CoA dehydrogenase (VLCAD) deficiency
F. Trifunctional protein deficiency
G. None of the above

40. A 2-year-old boy was brought to an emergency department of a local hospital for vomiting and seizures. The medical history revealed that the patient had developmental delay and growth retardation. The blood glucose was 26 mg/dL and ketone bodies were absent. Organic acids analysis revealed elevated C4-carnitine. Which one of the following disorders would the infant girl most likely have?

A. Short-chain acyl CoA dehydrogenase (SCAD) deficiency
B. Medium/short chain hydroxyacyl CoA dehydrogenase (M/SCHAD) deficiency
C. Medium-chain acyl CoA dehydrogenase (MCAD) deficiency
D. Long-chain hydroxyacyl CoA dehydrogenase (LCHAD) deficiency
E. Very-long-chain acyl CoA dehydrogenase (VLCAD) deficiency
F. Trifunctional protein deficiency
G. None of the above

41. A newborn screening (NBS) laboratory detected a mean C16OH concentration significantly higher (0.14 μmol/L) than the population mean, but not above the clinical cut-off of 0.15 μmol/L in a day 5 blood spot sample. A follow-up acylcarnitine testing on the screening sample was performed, and results were considered to be consistent with long-chain hydroxyacyl-CoA dehydrogenase (LCHAD).

The primary pediatrician was notified. The parents brought the baby to the clinic for confirmatory testing, which did not support the diagnosis. The patient was thriving and well and was discharged. At the age of 4 months, the patient presented with lethargy, poor feeding, and vomiting. There was evidence of liver and renal failure, dilated cardiomyopathy, and lactic acidosis. The patient further deteriorated and died after 6 days in the hospital. During the last admission, multiple samples for urine organic acids and blood spot acylcarnitine were analyzed. The results showed biochemical changes consistent with a fatty acid oxidation defect such as LCHADD, mitochondrial trifunctional protein (MTP) deficiency, or *ACAD9* deficiency. Further genetic testing revealed compound heterozygous variants in the *HADHB* gene, c.182G > A(p.Arg61His) and c.788A > G(p. Asp263Gly). One of each of the mutations was identified in each parent. Which one of the following disorders would the patient most likely have had?[17]

A. Long-chain hydroxyacyl CoA dehydrogenase (LCHAD) deficiency
B. Mitochondrial complex I deficiency
C. Trifunctional protein deficiency
D. Not clear
E. None of the above

42. An apparently healthy 18-year-old female was admitted for generalized muscle pain and weakness for a duration of 1 day. The day before admission, she ate dinner at 4:00 p.m. and had not eaten since then. The next morning, the patient woke up with generalized muscle pain and weakness, which worsened throughout the day. She had a history of similar episodes of muscle pain and weakness and passing dark urine since she was 10 years old. The episodes were usually brought on by moderate exercise. She did not have a family history of similar conditions. On examination, she was fully conscious, but appeared weak. Her vital signs were in normal ranges. Laboratory testing revealed elevated lactate and pyruvate. Urinary ketones were absent. Muscle biopsy revealed nonspecific myositis changes. The serum acylcarnitine profile found increased C14:2 (0.26 μmol/L; normal range, <0.08 μmol/L), C14:1 (0.53 μmol/L; normal range, <0.18 μmol/L), and C16:1 (0.16 μmol/L; normal range, <0.08 μmol/L). Which one of the following disorders would the patient most likely have?[18]

A. Short-chain acyl CoA dehydrogenase (SCAD) deficiency
B. Medium/short chain hydroxyacyl CoA dehydrogenase (M/SCHAD) deficiency

C. Medium-chain acyl CoA dehydrogenase (MCAD) deficiency
D. Long-chain hydroxyacyl CoA dehydrogenase (LCHAD) deficiency
E. Very long-chain acyl CoA dehydrogenase (VLCAD) deficiency
F. Trifunctional protein deficiency
G. None of the above

43. A boy was born to unrelated parents at the term by cesarean section due to breech position and oligohydramnios. His birth weight was 2720 g (third percentile) and the head circumference 33 cm (fifth percentile). At birth, he had large anterior and posterior fontanels; widely open sutures; low-set, narrow external auditory canals; antimongoloid slanting of the eyes; nystagmus; subcapsular cataracts; a webbed neck; widely spaced nipples; right undescended testis; extreme laxity of the hips; and bilateral forefoot adduction. At age 4 months, he displayed sensorineural deafness, retinitis pigmentosa (RP), marked axial hypotonicity with dystonic limb hypertonicity, and hepatomegaly. At age 7 months, a urine organic acid study revealed a distinctive dicarboxylic aciduria with reversal of the normal (C6 > C8) ratio and prominence of odd-chain-length dicarboxylic acids, 3-hydroxydicarboxylic acids, 3,6-epoxydicarboxylic acids, and 2-hydroxysebacic acid. The follow-up measurement of very-long-chain fatty acids (VLCFAs) in plasma revealed a marked elevation of both C26:0 and C26:0/C22:0; in addition, there was a significant elevation of the branched-chain fatty acids (BCFAs)—phytanic acid and, particularly, pristanic acid. A diagnosis of peroxisomal biogenesis disorder was made. Which one of the following disorders would the patient least likely have?[19]

A. Infantile Refsum disease
B. Neonatal adrenoleukodystrophy
C. Rhizomelic chondrodysplasia punctata
D. X-linked adrenoleukodystrophy
E. Zellweger syndrome
F. None of the above

44. Which one of the following laboratory results usually is seen in patients with X-linked adrenoleukodystrophy?
A. Increased VLCFA
B. Increased phytanic acids
C. Decreased plasmalogen
D. All of the above
E. None of the above

45. A 7-year-old boy was admitted to an endocrinology clinic in a tertiary hospital for balance and vision disturbances, spastic paraparesis, muscle weakness, and slight

cutaneous hyperpigmentation. He also had gait and coordination disturbances and history of partial left hemibody seizures. His parents and an 18-year-old sister were apparently healthy. A brother had died at the age of 6 with similar signs and symptoms. One of his maternal uncles had died at the age of 6 for unknown reason. His medical history was significant for admission to an emergency department $1\frac{1}{2}$ years ago for nausea, vomiting, severe general health status, and right hemibody tonic–clonic convulsions without fever. The laboratory studies at the time of the previous admission revealed hyponatremia, decreased urinary potassium, hyperglycemia followed by a tendency to hypoglycemia, and extremely low plasma cortisol; he was diagnosed with acute adrenal insufficiency. After symptomatic hormone treatment, he was discharged. Three months after discharge, he developed asthenia, lack of appetite, and altered general status. During the current admission, his plasma cortisol levels were still low ($10 \mu g/dL$). A neurological examination revealed the presence of gait disturbances from a bipyramidal syndrome, coordination disturbances, visual disturbances with decreased visual acuity, narrowed visual field, and convergent strabismus. Concentration and attention disturbances with worsening of school performance were also present. Brain MRI revealed an area of high signal intensity on T2, low signal intensity on T1, and high signal intensity on fluid-attenuated inversion recovery (FLAIR) with a discrete peripheral fixation of the contrast medium and hypofixation inside the lesion in the periventricular cerebral white matter in the parietal and occipital lobes bilaterally and in the splenium of corpus callosum. The physician suspected that the patient had adrenoleukodystrophy and ordered a molecular study for it. Which one of the following genes would most likely harbor pathogenic variant(s) in this patient if he had adrenoleukodystrophy?[20]

A. *ABCD1*
B. *ARX*
C. *FMR2*
D. *SLC6A8*
E. *TNFRSF13B*
F. None of the above

46. A 7-year-old boy was admitted to an endocrinology clinic in a tertiary hospital for balance and vision disturbances, spastic paraparesis, muscle weakness, and slight cutaneous hyperpigmentation. He also had gait and coordination disturbances and history of partial left hemibody seizures. His parents and an 18-year-old sister were apparently healthy.

A brother had died at the age of 6 with similar signs and symptoms. One of his maternal uncles had died at the age of 6 for unknown reason. His medical history was significant for admission to an emergency department $1\frac{1}{2}$ years ago for nausea, vomiting, severe general health status, and right hemibody tonic–clonic convulsions without fever. The laboratory studies at the time of the previous admission revealed hyponatremia, decreased urinary potassium, hyperglycemia followed by a tendency to hypoglycemia, and extremely low plasma cortisol; he was diagnosed with acute adrenal insufficiency. After symptomatic hormone treatment, he was discharged. Three months after discharge, he developed asthenia, lack of appetite, and altered general status. During the current admission, his plasma cortisol levels were still low ($10 \mu g/dL$). A neurological examination revealed the presence of gait disturbances from a bipyramidal syndrome, coordination disturbances, visual disturbances with decreased visual acuity, narrowed visual field, and convergent strabismus. Concentration and attention disturbances with worsening of school performance were also present. Brain MRI revealed an area of high signal intensity on T2, low signal intensity on T1, and high signal intensity on fluid-attenuated inversion recovery (FLAIR) with a discrete peripheral fixation of the contrast medium and hypofixation inside the lesion in the periventricular cerebral white matter in the parietal and occipital lobes bilaterally and in the splenium of corpus callosum. The physician suspected that the patient had adrenoleukodystrophy and ordered a molecular study for it. Which one of the following assays would most likely be used to confirm/rule out the adrenoleukodystrophy in this patient?[20]

A. Chromosomal microarray
B. Exome-sequence analysis
C. Multiplex ligation-dependent probe amplification (MLPA)
D. Next-generation sequencing panel
E. Sanger sequencing analysis
F. Target variant analysis of the founder pathogenic variants
G. None of the above

47. A 6-year-old boy was brought to an emergency department for nausea, vomiting, poor general health status, and right hemibody tonic–clonic convulsions without fever. His parents and an 18-year-old sister are apparently healthy. A brother had died at the age of 6 with similar signs and symptoms. One of his maternal uncles had died at the age of 6 for unknown reason. The laboratory studies at the time of the previous admission

revealed hyponatremia, decreased urinary potassium, hyperglycemia followed by a tendency to hypoglycemia, and extremely low plasma cortisol; he was diagnosed with acute adrenal insufficiency. He was treated with hormones. After his symptom stabilized, the physician ordered exome sequencing analysis to rule out genetic etiology. A pathogenic variant, c.548T > G(p. V183G), in the *ABCD1* gene was detected. His mother and sister carry the same variant. His father does not have the variant. Which one of the following would be the most appropriate next step in the workup for this patient?[20]

A. Confirming the results with deletion and duplication analysis

B. Confirming the results with Sanger sequencing analysis using an alternative pair of primers

C. Reporting it out supporting a clinical diagnosis of adrenoleukodystrophy (ALD)

D. Requesting a second specimen from the patient and his family members for confirmation

E. Not sure

F. None of the above

48. Which one of the following statements regarding rhizomelic chondrodysplasia punctata is correct?

A. It is one of the connective-tissue disorders.

B. It is one of the fatty acid oxidation disorders.

C. It is one of the lysosomal disorders.

D. It is one of the mitochondrial disorders.

E. It is one of the peroxisomal disorders.

F. None of the above.

49. Which one of the following laboratory results usually is seen in patients with rhizomelic chondrodysplasia punctata?

A. Decreased VLCFA

B. Decreased phytanic acids

C. Decreased plasmalogen

D. All of the above

E. None of the above

50. A full-term infant girl was born of third-degree consanguineous parents by spontaneous vaginal delivery to a 25-year-old G3P1 mother. The baby was admitted at birth for respiratory distress and abnormal extremities. The mother had had a spontaneous abortion 3 years ago in the first trimester and an ectopic pregnancy 2 years ago. Prenatal ultrasonographic assessments showed proximal limb shortening. On the clinical examination, the baby had proximal symmetrical shortening of the humerus and to a lesser degree the femur, with flexion contractures in all extremities, midfacial hypoplasia with depressed nasal bridge, anteverted nares with a short neck with nuchal fullness, and ichthyotic skin changes. Radiographic studies showed symmetrical,

bilateral, proximal shortening of upper and lower limbs with multiple punctate calcifications in the epiphyseal cartilage in shoulder, elbow, hip, and knee joints. The physician suspected that the patient had rhizomelic chondrodysplasia punctata (RCDP) and ordered molecular testing for it. Which one of the following genes would most likely harbor pathogenic variant(s) in this patient if she had RCDP?[21]

A. *ABCD1*

B. *COL1A1*

C. *FGFR2*

D. *FGFR3*

E. *PAX3*

F. *PEX7*

G. None of the above

51. A term baby girl was admitted to a neurology department in a local hospital for atypical facial appearance and extremity anomalies at the second hour of her life. Her perinatal history was uneventful except that the prenatal ultrasonographic assessments reported proximal limb shortening. Her parents were unrelated. Her mother had had two miscarriages, as well as a fetus with skeletal abnormalities who was aborted at 22 weeks of gestation, and also had a healthy male child. On physical examination, the patient had a depressed nasal bridge and a highly arched palate. There was shortness of the upper extremities and flexion contractures in all extremities. On a skeletal survey, there was proximal shortness, thick and short diaphyses, and large and irregular metaphyses in the long bones and normal fingers. The radiological findings for the patient were compatible with chondrodysplasia punctata (CDP) with punctate calcifications in the epiphyses and coronal clefts in the vertebral bodies. Further biochemical studies showed high phytanic acid (9.2; normal, <5.28 μmol/L) and low plasmalogen (3.2; normal, >6.6). A Sanger sequencing study detected a homozygous pathogenic variant, c.875T > A(p.Leu292Ter), in the *PEX7* gene. Her mother had the same variant in the heterozygous state. Her father did not have the variant. Which one of the following would be the most appropriate next step in the workup for this patient?[22]

A. Confirming the results with alternative pairs of primers

B. Performing reflex deletion and duplication analysis

C. Reporting it as supporting a clinical diagnosis of rhizomelic chondrodysplasia punctata type 1 (RCDP1)

D. Requesting a second specimen from the patient for confirmation

E. Not sure

F. None of the above

52. A term baby girl was admitted to a neurology department in a local hospital for atypical facial appearance and extremity anomalies at the second hour of her life. Her perinatal history was uneventful except that the prenatal ultrasonographic assessments reported proximal limb shortening. Her parents were unrelated. Her mother had had two miscarriages, as well as a fetus with skeletal abnormalities who was aborted at 22 weeks of gestation, and also had a healthy male child. On physical examination, the patient had a depressed nasal bridge and a highly arched palate. There was shortness of the upper extremities and flexion contractures in all extremities. On a skeletal survey, there was proximal shortness, thick and short diaphyses, and large and irregular metaphyses in the long bones and normal fingers. The radiological findings for the patient were compatible with chondrodysplasia punctata (CDP) with punctate calcifications in the epiphyses and coronal clefts in the vertebral bodies. Further biochemical studies showed high phytanic acid (9.2; normal, $<5.28 \mu mol/L$) and low plasmalogen (3.2; normal, >6.6). A Sanger sequencing study detected a homozygous pathogenic variant, c.875T > A(p.Leu292Ter), in the *PEX7* gene. Her mother had the same variant in the heterozygous state. Her father did not have the variant. Which one of the following would be a more appropriate next step in the workup than others for this patient and her family?[22]

A. Confirming the results with deletion and duplication analysis

B. Confirming the results with Sanger sequencing analysis using an alternative pair of primers

C. Reporting that the patient had an inherited variant from the mother and a de novo variant

D. Requesting a second specimen from the patient and the family members for confirmation

E. Not sure

F. None of the above

53. Which one of the following laboratory results usually is seen in patients with Zellweger syndrome?

A. Overaccumulation of VLCFAs

B. Overaccumulation of phytanic acids

C. Deficiency of plasmalogens

D. All of the above

E. None of the above

54. A boy was delivered by emergency cesarean section at term owing to fetal distress and breech presentation. He received active resuscitation at birth and was admitted to the neonatal intensive care unit. Further clinical examination revealed dysmorphic features and hypotonia, with a wide anterior fontanel, long philtrum, high-arched palate, and broad nasal bridge. This was the first baby for a couple who were first-degree relatives. There was no antenatal care. The initial arterial blood gases showed severe metabolic acidosis. Subsequently, he developed convulsions, which were was managed with phenobarbitone. The baby remained hypotonic with no suck reflex and nasogastric feeding was started. A laboratory study found elevated liver enzymes (raised aspartate aminotransferase [AST], 304 IU/L; raised alanine aminotransferase [ALT], 121 IU/L). Echocardiography revealed a small atrial septal defect (ASD II: secundum-type). One week later, he developed obstructive jaundice. Abdominal ultrasound showed multiple renal cysts. Zellweger syndrome was suspected. STAT laboratory testing revealed elevated C26:0 and C26:1 and the ratios of C24/C22 and C26/C22. His phytanic acid was also elevated, and plasmalogens was reduced. Although he was under intensive care, the baby died when he was 6 months old. A molecular genetic study was ordered to confirm the diagnosis and for family management. Which one of the following molecular assays would be the most cost-effective and most sensitive for this patient?[23]

A. Exome sequencing

B. Multiplex ligation-dependent probe amplification (MLPA)

C. Next-generation sequencing (NGS) panel

D. Sequencing analysis of the *PEX1* gene

E. TaqMan genotype assay

F. None of the above

55. A boy was delivered by emergency cesarean section at term owing to fetal distress and breech presentation. He received active resuscitation at birth and was admitted to the neonatal intensive care unit. Further clinical examination revealed dysmorphic features and hypotonia, with a wide anterior fontanel, long philtrum, high-arched palate, and broad nasal bridge. This was the first baby for a couple who were first-degree relatives. There was no antenatal care. The initial arterial blood gases showed severe metabolic acidosis. Subsequently, he developed convulsions, which were was managed with phenobarbitone. The baby remained hypotonic with no suck reflex and nasogastric feeding was started. A laboratory study found elevated liver enzymes (raised aspartate aminotransferase [AST], 304 IU/L; raised alanine aminotransferase [ALT], 121 IU/L). Echocardiography revealed a small atrial septal defect (ASD II: secundum-type). One week later,

he developed obstructive jaundice. Abdominal ultrasound showed multiple renal cysts. Zellweger syndrome was suspected. STAT laboratory testing revealed elevated C26:0 and C26:1 and the ratios of C24/C22 and C26/C22. His phytanic acid was also elevated, and plasmalogens was reduced. Although he was under intensive care, the baby died when he was 6 months old. A next-generation sequencing panel for peroxisomal biogenesis disorder (PBD) was ordered to confirm the diagnosis and for family management. A homozygous pathogenic variant, c.2097dupT(p. Ile700TyrfsTer42), in *PEX1* was detected in a skin specimen from this patient. Which one of the following would be the most appropriate next step in the workup for this patient and his family?[23]

A. Confirming the results with deletion and duplication analysis

B. Confirming the results with Sanger sequencing analysis using an alternative pair of primers

C. Reporting that the patient had Zellweger syndrome and recommending studies for the parents

D. Requesting a second specimen from the patient and his family members for confirmation

E. Not sure

F. None of the above

56. A 60-year-old male was referred by his family doctor to a hematological outpatient clinic for hyperserotonemia (2.245 ng/L) and a raised level of transferrin saturation (80%−90%). His family history was positive for hereditary hemochromatosis (HH) and Crohn's disease (in his son); two siblings were affected by HH, one with homozygous C282Y variant and the other with heterozygous C282Y variant. A genetic study detected homozygous C282Y variant in *HFE* in this patient. Blood chemistry examinations showed impaired glucose tolerance. Hepatic ultrasonography suggested steatosis and splenomegaly. Liver biopsy showed signs of mild fibrosis, with initial formation of incomplete septa, periportal parenchymal iron accumulation, and biliary siderosis. The patient also had radiographic signs of metacarpophalangeal joint disease of both hands, which is highly suggestive of hemochromatosis. Color Doppler echocardiographic findings revealed concentric left ventricular hypertrophy, left axial shift, and mild mitral and tricuspid failure. A clinical examination of the patient revealed cutaneous hyperpigmentation, mild lack of facial expression, and a fine tremor in both upper limbs, in particular of the fingers of the left hand. The tremor presented at rest but was exacerbated by

emotional stress. The patient was diagnosed with HH clinically. Which one of the following malignancies would the patient be at increased risk to develop?[24]

A. Hepatocarcinoma

B. Colorectal cancer

C. Lung cancer

D. Leukemia

E. Melanoma

F. Rhabdomyosarcoma

57. A couple come to an Ob/Gyn clinic for premarriage counseling. They both are carriers of the C282Y variant in *HFE*. Which one of the following symptoms would their future children NOT be at increased risk to develop due to hereditary hemochromatosis?

A. Arthropathy

B. Diabetes mellitus

C. Dilated cardiomyopathy

D. Hypogonadism

E. Liver cirrhosis

F. Rhabdomyolysis

58. Which one of the following statements regarding *HFE*-associated hereditary hemochromatosis (HH) is appropriate?

A. HH predominantly affects boys of Asian descent.

B. Prenatal diagnosis is recommended to decrease mortality.

C. Linkage analysis is cheaper and more accurate than other molecular diagnostic testing.

D. In order for HH to be symptomatic, both copies of the *HFE* gene must be mutated.

E. None of the above.

59. Which one of the following genes is NOT associated with iron overload?

A. *HFE*

B. *HJV*

C. *HFE2B*

D. *HAMP*

E. *ATP7A*

60. A 47-year-old Caucasian male was brought to an emergency department by his wife for new-onset hyperglycemia after eating Thanksgiving dinner. The family history was unremarkable. A review of systems identified weakness and lethargy, abdominal pain, occasional chest tightness, and pigmentation of the skin and mucosa. A physical examination revealed skin and mucosal pigmentation, hepatomegaly and splenomegaly, and loss of body hair. Hereditary hemochromatosis was suspected. Which one of following molecular tests would be the most appropriate?

A. Chromosomal microarray

B. FISH

C. Sanger sequencing
D. Targeted mutation analysis
E. None of the above

61. A 47-year-old Caucasian male was brought to an emergency department by his wife for new-onset hyperglycemia after eating Thanksgiving dinner. The family history was unremarkable. A review of systems identified weakness and lethargy, abdominal pain, occasional chest tightness, and pigmentation of the skin and mucosa. A physical examination revealed skin and mucosal pigmentation, hepatomegaly and splenomegaly, and loss of body hair. Hereditary hemochromatosis was suspected. A molecular genetics study was ordered. Which one of the following genotypes would this patient be most likely to have if he had hereditary hemochromatosis?
A. p.Cys282Tyr/p.Cys282Tyr
B. p.Cys282Tyr/p.His63Asp
C. p.His63Asp/p.His63Asp
D. p.Cys282Tyr/p.Ser65Cys
E. p.His63Asp/p.Ser65Cys

62. Which one of the following statements regarding hereditary hemochromatosis (HH) is NOT correct?
A. Patients with p.Cys282Tyr/p.Cys282Tyr are at increased risk for hemochromatosis.
B. Patients with p.Cys282Tyr/p.His63Asp are at increased risk for clinical hemochromatosis.
C. Patients with p.His63Asp/p.His63Asp are at increased risk for clinical hemochromatosis.
D. Females have a lower risk for hemochromatosis than males.
E. Population screening for HH is a cost-effective method of proactive management.

63. A 7-month-old white boy from a nonconsanguineous family was admitted to a hospital with a history of clonic seizures of the left upper limb, hypoactivity, and absence of visual contact for 5 months. At 3 months of age, his seizures spread to right upper and lower limbs, along with blinking movements. His perinatal history was uneventful. Prior to his admission, he had had five episodes of pneumonia. At 5 months of age, MRI revealed diffuse brain atrophy, dural thickening, and large subdural and epidural fluid collections, suggesting chronic blood clots at different stages. A physical examination revealed that he was pale and inactive and had little reaction to examination. He had bilateral inguinal hernias. His facial features included epicanthus and thin and brittle hair with a metallic gray tone. He also had a generalized increase in subcutaneous fat with loose and thin skin. A neurological examination revealed that he could

not maintain visual contact, could not follow objects and had a compromised sucking reflex. He was hypotonic in the axial muscles and unable to hold his head up. But his extremities had increased muscle tone. Muscle strength was slightly diminished. His deep tendon reflexes were increased, with extension plantar reflex response. Laboratory studies revealed that his serum ceruloplasmin level (82 mg/L; normal range, >200) and serum copper level (<0.1 µg/L; normal range, 0.7−1.3) were decreased. An X-ray of the long bones revealed epiphyseal fragmentation in the distal extremities of the humerus and femurs. Optic microscopy of a hair sample disclosed pili torti with nodular thickening at the fracture points. The physician diagnosed the patient with Menkes disease clinically. Which one of following genes would most likely harbor pathogenic variant(s) for Menkes disease in this patient?[25]
A. *ATP7A*
B. *ATP7B*
C. *HAMP*
D. *HFE*
E. *HFE2B*
F. *HJV*

64. A 7-month-old white boy from a nonconsanguineous family was admitted to a hospital with a history of clonic seizures of the left upper limb, hypoactivity, and absence of visual contact for 5 months. At 3 months of age, his seizures spread to right upper and lower limbs, along with blinking movements. His perinatal history was uneventful. Prior to his admission, he had had five episodes of pneumonia. At 5 months of age, MRI revealed diffuse brain atrophy, dural thickening, and large subdural and epidural fluid collections, suggesting chronic blood clots at different stages. A physical examination revealed that he was pale and inactive and had little reaction to examination. He had bilateral inguinal hernias. His facial features included epicanthus and thin and brittle hair with a metallic gray tone. He also had a generalized increase in subcutaneous fat with loose and thin skin. A neurological examination revealed that he could not maintain visual contact, could not follow objects and had a compromised sucking reflex. He was hypotonic in the axial muscles and unable to hold his head up. But his extremities had increased muscle tone. Muscle strength was slightly diminished. His deep tendon reflexes were increased, with extension plantar reflex response. Laboratory studies revealed that his serum ceruloplasmin level (82 mg/L; normal range, >200) and serum copper level

(<0.1 μg/L; normal range, 0.7−1.3) were decreased. An X-ray of the long bones revealed epiphyseal fragmentation in the distal extremities of the humerus and femurs. Optic microscopy of a hair sample disclosed pili torti with nodular thickening at the fracture points. The physician diagnosed the patient with Menkes disease clinically. A molecular study detected a homozygous pathogenic variant, c.2938C > T (p.Arg980Ter), in *ATP7A*. Parental testing revealed that his mother carried the same variant in heterozygous state, and remained asymptomatic. His father did not carry the variant. Which one of following would be the most appropriate interpretation of the findings in the family?[25]

A. Menkes disease has incomplete penetrance and variable expression.

B. Reflex deletion/duplication testing was indicated.

C. The patient inherited the variant from the mother and had Menkes disease.

D. The patient had a de novo variant from the paternal side.

E. Not sure.

F. None of the above.

65. A 7-month-old boy was brought to a clinic for gradual-onset hypotonia and seizures. He was born at 34 weeks of gestation to healthy, nonconsanguineous parents. As the first child of the parents, his early development was age-appropriate for 3 months, then regressed. At 5 months of age, he developed myoclonic jerks. A physical examination at 7 months of age revealed a cherubic appearance, with a depressed nasal bridge and brittle, scattered, and hypopigmented scalp hairs. He had no eye contact and no head control. Light microscopic examination of scalp hair showed pili torti. His serum copper level was 15 μg/dL (normal range, 70−150) and his serum ceruloplasmin 58 mg/L (normal range, 187−322). The patient was diagnosed with Menkes disease clinically. A Sanger sequence study was ordered, and no PCR product was detected. The repetitive test did not show PCR products again. Which one of following would be the most appropriate next step in the workup for this patient?[26]

A. Reflex deletion/duplication testing

B. Requesting another specimen from the family

C. Sending the sample to another laboratory for confirmation

D. Using a new lot of all reagents

E. Not sure

F. None of the above

66. A 5-month-old baby boy was brought to a hospital for regression of developmental milestones and seizures. He was born at term to healthy, nonconsanguineous parents. The pregnancy was uneventful. The family history was remarkable for the death of two brothers at the age of 1 month and 18 months; they had severe neurodevelopmental delay without a definite diagnosis. The patient had a history of and 8-day hospital admission on the third day of life for poor feeding, hypothermia, and hyperbilirubinemia (total bilirubin, 16 mg/dL). His early development was age appropriate for 4 months, then he developed tonic and myoclonic seizures. A physical examination at 5 months of age revealed colorless, thin, brittle, and kinky hair. Although eye contact was noted, he had poor head control and no rollover response. Brain CT scan showed cerebral atrophy and subdural effusion. An electroencephalography revealed frequent multifocal epileptiform discharges with disorganized background. His serum copper level was 3 μg/dL (normal range, 70−150), and serum ceruloplasmin 15 mg/L (normal range, 187−322). Light microscopic examination of scalp hair showed pili torti (twisted hair shafts) and trichorrhexis nodosa. No metaphyseal changes of long bones were seen on X-rays. A diagnosis of Menkes disease was made clinically, and a hemizygous pathogenic variant, c.3056G > A (p.Gly1019Asp), was detected in *ATP7A*. Which one of following would most likely describe the pathogenesis of this variant?[26]

A. Dominant negative

B. Gain of function

C. Haploinsufficiency

D. Loss of function

E. None of the above

67. An 8-year-old African boy was brought to an emergency department with symptoms of ascites, facial swelling, and reduced urinary output for 2 weeks. His medical history was unremarkable. There was no previous or current history of similar illness in his four siblings and close contacts. His parents were not known to be related. The initial diagnosis was nephrotic syndrome due to proteinuria and a spot urine protein to creatinine ratio of 1. On day 3 of hospitalization, he became deeply jaundiced, with worsening of the generalized edema. On day 4, he had three brief episodes of generalized clonic seizures over a 2-hour period. After the seizures were managed with anticonvulsant medications, a physical examination revealed ascites and nontender hepatomegaly. On day 8, he developed tremors of his hands while at rest and when reaching for objects. Subsequently, he was observed to be stiff

globally, with his trunk arched forward and fisting of the hands. His gait was noted to be shuffling, with a tendency to fall forward when trying to walk. At the same time, his face retained a wry smile and his speech became slurred and dysarthric. He frequently had generalized body pain and derived some relief when someone helped him to open his clenched fist. He was also noted to be emotionally labile; he cried inconsolably when asking for food. A neurological examination revealed the possible presence of Kayser—Fleischer (KF) rings on both eyes. A slit-lamp examination by an ophthalmologist revealed the presence of both KF rings and sunflower cataracts. A diagnosis of Wilson disease was made clinically. Which one of following genes would most likely harbor pathogenic variant(s) for Wilson disease in this patient?[27]

A. *ATP7A*
B. *ATP7B*
C. *HAMP*
D. *HFE*
E. *HFE2B*
F. *HJV*

68. A 23-year-old female presented to a clinic with symptoms of abdominal pain and intermittent low-grade fever for 5 days. The patient had vomited 500 mL of black-colored vomitus the times and was bleeding from her vagina on the first day of admission. A physical examination revealed she had pallor, icterus, periorbital puffiness, pedal edema, and anasarca. She had distention of the abdomen, with shifting dullness, and the spleen was palpable. Kayser—Fleischer (KF) rings were present in both eyes. The initial diagnosis was cirrhosis with esophageal varices. Her family history was remarkable for the consanguineous marriage of her parents. Her youngest sister had died with similar symptoms at 5 years of age. A liver biopsy and biochemical investigations confirmed a diagnosis of Wilson disease. A Sanger sequencing analysis of *ATP7B* detected a homozygous pathogenic variant, c.2333G > T(p.Arg778Leu). Which one of following would be the most appropriate interpretation of the molecular findings?[28]

A. A new lot of all reagents should be used to confirm the findings.
B. Another set of primers should be used to confirm the findings.
C. Another type of specimen from the patient should be used to confirm the findings.
D. Reflex testing is recommended to confirm/rule out deletions/duplications.
E. The findings confirm the diagnosis of Wilson disease.

F. The findings should be confirmed by another laboratory.
G. None of the above.

69. A 20-year-old male was admitted to a neurological clinic with tremors for 18 months. Initially, he noticed tremor in his right arm when holding a cup. After 2 months, the tremor became continuous and extended to the left arm, head and legs. He also noticed speech changes with the disease progression. Then the tremor occurred even at rest, leaving him bedridden. An ophthalmological examination revealed Kayser—Fleischer rings. A physical examination found jaundice, hepatosplenomegaly, and the presence of abdominal collateral circulation. A neurological examination revealed an intense tremor involving the four limbs, specially the right side, and the head, which presented at rest, and would get worse during voluntary movements. Hypotonia of the upper limbs was also noticed. The orthostatic position was possible only with a wide base, a feature maintained during gait. He also had dysarthria with scanning speech. Pneumoencephalographic scanning revealed ex vacuo enlargement of the third ventricle and lateral ventricles. During the course of the disease, he presented with aggressive behavior that became progressively more intense and required his transfer to a psychiatric hospital, where he died 5 years after the onset of the disease. This was a case of Wilson disease in 1946. Which one of following would most likely describe the pathogenesis of Wilson disease in this patient and others with Wilson disease?[29]

A. Dominant negative
B. Gain of function
C. Haploinsufficiency
D. Loss of function
E. None of the above

70. An 8-year-old boy was brought to a clinic with symptoms of persisting jaundice and itching for 6 years. The parents also reported failure to thrive. In the past 2 years, he has been having difficulty with distant vision. He also had history of one episode of blood-tinged vomitus not associated with melena. He had two healthy older sisters, and his parents were not related. He was developmentally normal for his age with low weight (13 kg; Z score, <−3) and short for his age (99 cm; Z score <−3). On physical examination, he had mild pallor, icterus, clubbing, and scratch marks. His facial features were prominent forehead, deep-set eyes, a pointed chin, and a saddle nose with a bulbous tip. A grade III ejection systolic murmur was audible in the left second intercostal space, with normal S1 and S2.

The liver was palpable 2 cm below costal margin with a span of 8 cm with normal consistency and smooth surface. The spleen was not palpable. There was no ascites. Posterior embryotoxon was found in both eyes, with both also showing Kayser–Fleischer rings. Visual acuity in the right eye was 6/60 and in left eye was 6/FCCF (finger close to face). An upper GI endoscopy revealed mild esophagitis in the lower one-third of the esophagus. A biopsy from the lower esophagus showed mucosal fragments with ulceration and fibrin. A liver biopsy showed paucity of bile ducts with periportal ballooning degeneration and cholestasis. The portal tract showed inflammation and fibrosis. Immunostaining for CK19 did not show bile ducts. His was diagnosed with Alagille syndrome clinically. A molecular genetic study was ordered to confirm the diagnosis. Which one of the following genes would most likely to harbor pathogenic variant(s) in this patient if he had Alagille syndrome?[30]

A. *ATP7A*
B. *ATP7B*
C. *JAG1*
D. *JAG2*
E. *JAG3*
F. None of the above

71. A 4-year-old boy was brought to a clinic for prolonged jaundice since the fifth day of his life. He had history of admission to a hospital at 2 months of age. A physical examination revealed icteric sclera, jaundice, and hepatomegaly. Systolic murmur was audible at the left upper sternal border radiating to left axillary region. An echocardiogram showed mild peripheral left pulmonic arterial stenosis and interatrial left-to-right communication. The serum total bilirubin was 13.9 mg/dL, while the direct bilirubin was 7.35 mg/dL. A liver biopsy was done at 2 months old and revealed paucity of the interlobular bile ducts, but no definite periportal fibrosis could be detected. An eye examination disclosed bilateral posterior embryotoxon. MRI revealed left pulmonary artery stenosis, butterfly vertebrae, and hepatomegaly. He was diagnosed with Alagille syndrome clinically. A molecular genetic study was ordered to confirm the diagnosis. Which one of the following genes most likely harbored pathogenic variant(s) than others in this patient if he had Alagille syndrome?[31]

A. *JAG1*
B. *JAG2*
C. *JAG3*
D. *NOTCH1*
E. *NOTCH2*

F. *NOTCH3*
G. None of the above

72. A 4-year-old boy was brought to a clinic for prolonged jaundice since the fifth day of his life. He had history of admission to a hospital at 2 months of age. A physical examination revealed icteric sclera, jaundice, and hepatomegaly. Systolic murmur was audible at the left upper sternal border radiating to left axillary region. An echocardiogram showed mild peripheral left pulmonic arterial stenosis and interatrial left-to-right communication. The serum total bilirubin was 13.9 mg/dL, while the direct bilirubin was 7.35 mg/dL. A liver biopsy was done at 2 months old and revealed paucity of the interlobular bile ducts, but no definite periportal fibrosis could be detected. An eye examination disclosed bilateral posterior embryotoxon. MRI revealed left pulmonary artery stenosis, butterfly vertebrae, and hepatomegaly. He was diagnosed with Alagille syndrome clinically. A molecular genetic study detected a heterozygous pathogenic variant, c.550C > T(p.Arg184Cys), in *JAG1*. Parental studies detected the same variant in his mother, but not in his father. His mother was apparently healthy. Which one of following would be the most appropriate next step in the workup for this family?[31,32]

A. A new lot of all reagents should be used to confirm the findings.
B. Additional testing of the patient's mother should be considered.
C. Another set of primers should be used to confirm the findings.
D. Another type of specimen from the patient should be used to confirm the findings.
E. Reflex testing to deletion/duplication is recommended in the patient.
F. The findings should be confirmed by another laboratory.
G. None of the above.

73. A 4-year-old boy was brought to a clinic for prolonged jaundice since the fifth day of his life. He had history of admission to a hospital at 2 months of age. A physical examination revealed icteric sclera, jaundice, and hepatomegaly. Systolic murmur was audible at the left upper sternal border radiating to left axillary region. An echocardiogram showed mild peripheral left pulmonic arterial stenosis and interatrial left-to-right communication. The serum total bilirubin was 13.9 mg/dL, while the direct bilirubin was 7.35 mg/dL. A liver biopsy was done at 2 months old and revealed paucity of the interlobular bile ducts, but no definite periportal fibrosis could be

detected. An eye examination disclosed bilateral posterior embryotoxon. MRI revealed left pulmonary artery stenosis, butterfly vertebrae, and hepatomegaly. He was diagnosed with Alagille syndrome clinically. A molecular genetic study detected a heterozygous pathogenic variant, c.550C > T(p.Arg184Cys), in *JAG1*. Which one of following would most appropriately describe the pathogenesis of Alagille syndrome in this patient?[31]

    A. Dominant negative

    B. Gain of function

    C. Haploinsufficiency

    D. Loss of function

    E. None of the above

74. A 4-year-old girl was brought to a tertiary health center for progressive global developmental delay, hypotonia, and ataxia since she was 4 months old. She was born to nonconsanguineous parents, with an uneventful full-term pregnancy. Her parents and two elder brothers are healthy. She appeared normal in the first 3 months of postnatal life. Since the age of 4 months, she has shown delayed developmental milestones, such as poor head control. She could sit up at the age of 33 months but could not roll over. She also presented with severe psychomotor retardation. Since age 3 years, she had had axial hypotonia, peripheral spasticity and ataxia. The physical examination at 4 years of age revealed relative megalencephaly with a head circumference of 51.6 cm (+1.5 SD) and a body height of 93 cm (−2 SD). Bilateral Babinski signs, brisk deep tendon reflexes, and foot clonus with spasticity were demonstrated. No cherry-red spots or pigmentation were evident. She showed almost no voluntary movements. Lysosomal enzyme activities (arylsulfatase, β-galactosidase, and hexosaminidases A and B) were in the normal range. Urinary amino acid analysis revealed an abnormal increased *N*-acetylaspartic acid (NAA). A high level of NAA was also detected in serum and CSF. Assaying for aspartoacylase in fibroblast showed absent activity. A cranial CT scan revealed diffuse symmetrical attenuation in the white matter without ventricular dilatation. An MRI demonstrated marked prolongation of T1 and T2 in the white matter except for the deep part of the frontal area, brain stem, and cerebellum. Which one of the following lysosomal disorders would the patient most likely have?[33]

    A. Canavan disease

    B. Metachromatic leukodystrophy

    C. Pompe disease

    D. X-linked adrenoleukodystrophy

    E. Zellweger syndrome spectrum disorders

    F. None of the above

75. A 4-year-old girl was brought to a tertiary health center for progressive global developmental delay, hypotonia, and ataxia since she was 4 months old. She was born to nonconsanguineous parents, with an uneventful full-term pregnancy. Her parents and two elder brothers are healthy. She appeared normal in the first 3 months of postnatal life. Since the age of 4 months, she has shown delayed developmental milestones, such as poor head control. She could sit up at the age of 33 months but could not roll over. She also presented with severe psychomotor retardation. Since age 3 years, she had had axial hypotonia, peripheral spasticity and ataxia. The physical examination at 4 years of age revealed relative megalencephaly with a head circumference of 51.6 cm (+1.5 SD) and a body height of 93 cm (−2 SD). Bilateral Babinski signs, brisk deep tendon reflexes, and foot clonus with spasticity were demonstrated. No cherry-red spots or pigmentation were evident. She showed almost no voluntary movements. Lysosomal enzyme activities (arylsulfatase, β-galactosidase, and hexosaminidases A and B) were in the normal range. Urinary amino acid analysis revealed an abnormal increased *N*-acetylaspartic acid (NAA). A high level of NAA was also detected in serum and CSF. Assaying for aspartoacylase in fibroblast showed absent activity. A cranial CT scan revealed diffuse symmetrical attenuation in the white matter without ventricular dilatation. An MRI demonstrated marked prolongation of T1 and T2 in the white matter except for the deep part of the frontal area, brain stem, and cerebellum. A molecular study was ordered to confirm the diagnosis of Canavan disease. Which one of the following genes would most likely harbor pathogenic variants for Canavan disease in this patient?[33]

    A. *ASPA*

    B. *ELP1 (IKBKAP)*

    C. *GAA*

    D. *GLA*

    E. *MEFV*

    F. None of the above

76. An Ashkenazi Jewish boy is the fourth child of healthy unrelated parents. The first two children, aged 8 and 7 years are normal. The third child died at the age of 10 months with severe intellectual disability, seizures, and brain CT scan findings compatible with leukodystrophy. Metachromatic and Krabbe leukodystrophies had been excluded by enzyme assays; no autopsy was performed. The proband was born at term after an uneventful pregnancy and normal delivery. At the age of 3 months, he could not support his head.

His eyes were fixed. He had no smile and started having generalized seizures. At the age of 8 months he was admitted to a hospital for status epilepticus. A clinical evaluation revealed that the proband had severe axial hypotonia with peripheral hypertonia. Tendon jerks were brisk, with bilateral ankle clonus. He was almost blind but could react to sound. His head circumference was in the 98th percentile, whereas his height and weight were in the 25th percentile. His brain CT was compatible with leukodystrophy. Urinary amino acid analysis revealed an abnormal increased N-acetylaspartic acid (NAA). A high level of NAA was also detected in serum and CSF. Assaying for aspartoacylase in fibroblast showed absent activity. A molecular study was ordered to confirm the diagnosis of Canavan disease. Which one of molecular assays would most likely be used as a first-tier test to detect pathogenic variants for Canavan disease in this patient?[34]

A. Chromosomal microarray (CMA)
B. Multiplex ligation-dependent probe amplification (MLPA)
C. Next-generation sequencing (NGS)
D. Sanger sequencing
E. Target variant analysis of the founder pathogenic variants
F. None of the above

77. An 8-month-old Caucasian girl was referred to a tertiary health center for investigation of psychomotor retardation, which was evident soon after birth. She was the third child of healthy consanguineous Gypsy parents (second cousins) and was born after an uneventful pregnancy and delivery. Her siblings, a boy and a girl, were phenotypically normal. A clinical examination revealed that she had severe intellectual disability, axial hypotonia, and increased tendon reflexes. She had no head control and was unable to sit unaided. Her head circumference was at the 99th percentile. The brain CT scan was consistent with leukodystrophy. Chromosomal analysis, amino acid analysis, urinary mucopolysaccharides and lysosomal enzymes were all in the normal range. However, an excessive quantity of N-acetylaspartic acid (NAA) was found in urine. Urinary creatinine was 399 μmol/mmol (normal range, <20). Aspartoacylase activity in cultured skin fibroblast was 0.03 μkat/kg of protein. A molecular test was ordered for this patient to confirm the diagnosis of Canavan disease and for family management. Which one of following molecular assays would most likely be used as a first-tier test to detect pathogenic variants for Canavan disease in this patient?[34]

A. Chromosomal microarray (CMA)
B. Multiplex ligation-dependent probe amplification (MLPA)
C. Next-generation sequencing (NGS)
D. Sanger sequencing
E. Target variant analysis of the founder pathogenic variants
F. None of the above

78. An Ashkenazi Jewish couple came to a clinic for preconception counseling. The family history was unremarkable on both sides. An Ashkenazi Jewish carrier screening panel for targeted pathogenic variants was ordered for the wife, which includes the three founder pathogenic variants in the *ASPA* gene. The result revealed that the wife carried a pathogenic variant, c.854A > C(p.Glu285Ala), in the *ASPA* gene for Canavan disease. As a follow-up, the same panel was offered to the husband, and the result was negative. Which one of the following would be the most appropriate estimation of the residual risk of this couple's firstborn child with Canavan disease?

A. 10%
B. 5%
C. 1%
D. 0.25%
E. None of the above

79. An Ashkenazi Jewish couple comes to a clinic in Cincinnati, OH, for their first prenatal counseling when the wife is 8 weeks pregnant. One of the wife's brothers died of Canavan disease when he was 10 years old. The wife's parents live in Israel; they have not been tested for Canavan disease. The husband's family history is unremarkable for the genetic disorders commonly seen in his ethnic group. Which one of the following is the most appropriate first-tier study for this family to estimate the fetus's risk for Canavan disease?

A. Measurement of the concentration of *N*-acetylaspartic acid (NAA) in the urine sample from the wife
B. Measurement of the concentration of *N*-acetylaspartic acid (NAA) in the urine sample from the husband
C. Targeted mutation analysis of *ASPA* in the peripheral-blood sample from the husband
D. Targeted mutation analysis of *ASPA* in the peripheral-blood sample from the wife
E. Testing aspartoacylase enzyme activity with amniocytes
F. Testing aspartoacylase enzyme activity with chorionic villus sampling (CVS)
G. None of the above

ANSWERS

1. D. *Malformations result from intrinsic abnormalities in one or more genetic programs operating in development.* Examples are neural tube defects, cleft lip/palate, extra fingers in the disorder known as Greig cephalopolysyndactyly, and congenital heart defects.

Deformations are caused by extrinsic factors impinging physically on the fetus during development. Most deformations apparent at birth either resolve spontaneously or can be treated by external fixation devices to reverse the effects of the source. Examples include craniofacial asymmetry, arthrogryposis, and talipes (clubfoot). Disruption may be the result of vascular insufficiency, trauma, or teratogens; these can destroy normal tissue, altering the formation of a structure. Examples include some cases of facial clefts and missing digits or limbs. "Amniotic bands" encircling a limb are thought to be one possible mechanism.

Cells go through abnormal changes called "hyperplasia" and "dysplasia" before cancer forms in tissues of the body. In hyperplasia, there is an increase in the number of cells in an organ or tissue that appear normal under a microscope. In dysplasia, the cells look abnormal under a microscope but are not cancerous (https://www.cancer.gov/publications/dictionaries).

Therefore, anencephaly, a neural-tube defect, is an example of malformation, since it results from intrinsic abnormalities during fetal development. Folic acid deficiency may increase the risk for neural-tube defects.

2. A. *Deformations are caused by extrinsic factors impinging physically on the fetus during development.* Most deformations apparent at birth either resolve spontaneously or can be treated by external fixation devices to reverse the effects of the instigating cause. Examples include craniofacial asymmetry, arthrogryposis, and talipes (clubfoot).

Malformations result from intrinsic abnormalities in one or more genetic programs operating in development. Examples are neural-tube defects, cleft lip/palate, extra fingers in the disorder known as Greig cephalopolysyndactyly, and congenital heart defects. Disruption may be the result of vascular insufficiency, trauma, or teratogens; these can destroy normal tissue, altering the formation of a structure. Examples include some cases of facial clefts and missing digits or limbs; "amniotic bands" encircling a limb are thought to be one possible mechanism.

Cells go through abnormal changes called "hyperplasia" and "dysplasia" before cancer forms in tissues of the body. In hyperplasia, there is an increase in the number of cells in an organ or tissue that appear normal under a microscope. In dysplasia, the cells look abnormal under a microscope but are not cancerous (https://www.cancer.gov/publications/dictionaries).

Therefore, deformation is the most appropriate genetic term to describe this defect, since it is caused by extrinsic factors impinging physically on the fetus during development.

3. B. *Disruption may be the result of vascular insufficiency, trauma, or teratogens, which destroys normal tissue altering the formation of a structure.* Examples include some cases of facial clefts and missing digits or limbs. "Amniotic bands" encircling a limb are thought to be one possible mechanism.

Deformations are caused by extrinsic factors impinging physically on the fetus during development. Most deformations apparent at birth either resolve spontaneously or can be treated by external fixation devices to reverse the effects of the instigating cause. Examples include craniofacial asymmetry, arthrogryposis, and talipes. Malformations result from intrinsic abnormalities in one or more genetic programs operating in development. Examples are neural-tube defects, cleft lip/palate, extra fingers in the disorder known as Greig cephalopolysyndactyly, and congenital heart defects.

Cells go through abnormal changes called "hyperplasia" and "dysplasia" before cancer forms in tissues of the body. In hyperplasia, there is an increase in the number of cells in an organ or tissue that appear normal under a microscope. In dysplasia, the cells look abnormal under a microscope but are not cancerous (https://www.cancer.gov/publications/dictionaries).

Therefore, disruption is the most appropriate genetic term to describe amniotic band sequence since it destroys normal tissue, altering the formation of the thumb.

4. C. Down syndrome is the most common chromosome abnormality and constitutes about half of the overall risk at any maternal age. The likelihood of having a child with a chromosome abnormality such as Down syndrome increases with maternal age.

First-trimester screening combines information from a nuchal translucency (NT) measurement (an ultrasound measurement), biochemical analysis of free beta human chorionic gonadotropin (β-hCG) and pregnancy-associated plasma protein A

(PAPP-A), and maternal age to calculate a risk for Down syndrome (trisomy 21), trisomy 18, and trisomy 13. Collection of blood for biochemical analysis is performed between 9 and 13 6/7 weeks' gestation (crown-to-rump length, 24–84 mm). Ultrasound assessment of the NT measurement is performed between 11 and 13 6/7 weeks (crown-to-rump length, 45–84 mm). The combined accuracy rate for the screen to detect the chromosomal abnormalities mentioned above is approximately 85%, with a false positive rate of 5%. It means that approximately 85 of every 100 babies affected by the abnormalities addressed by the screen will be identified, while approximately 5% of all normal pregnancies will receive a positive result or an abnormal level. *The detection rate is 80% for trisomy 21 and 100% for trisomies 13 and 18.* The false positive rate is 7.73% for trisomy 21% and 1.21% for trisomy 18.

Sensitivity, also called the "true positive rate," measures the percentage of sick people who are correctly identified as having the condition. In other words, it answers the question of how often the test is positive if a person has a disease.

Therefore, the clinical sensitivity of the first-trimester screen is approximately 80% for Down syndrome.

5. **D.** Down syndrome is the most common chromosome abnormality and constitutes about half of the overall risk at any maternal age. The likelihood of having a child with a chromosome abnormality such as Down syndrome increases with maternal age. The accuracy rate for the first-trimester screening to detect the chromosomal abnormalities (trisomies 21, 18, and 13) is approximately 85%, with a false positive rate of 5%. It means that approximately 85 of every 100 babies affected by the abnormalities addressed by the screen will be identified, while approximately 5% of all normal pregnancies will receive a positive result or an abnormal level. The detection rate is 80% for trisomy 21 (4 of 5) and 100% for trisomies 13 and 18. The false positive rate is 7.73% for trisomy 21% and 1.21% for trisomy 18.

Specificity, also called the "true negative rate," measures the percentage of healthy people who are correctly identified as not having the condition. In another word, it answers the question how often the test is negative if a person does not have the disease.

$$SPC = \frac{TN}{N} = \frac{TN + FP - FP}{TN + FP} = 1 - \frac{FP}{N} = 1 - FPR$$

FP = false positive; FPR = false positive rate; N = number of negatives; SPC = specificity; TN = number of true positives

The false-positive rate of first-trimester screening is 7.73% for trisomy 21. Therefore, the clinical specificity of the first-trimester screen is approximately 92% for Down syndrome.

6. **C.** Multiple marker screening is used in the second trimester (15–20 weeks) to screen for trisomies 21, 18, and 13, as well as for fetal open neural-tube defects (ONTDs). The most widely used second-trimester screening test is the "quad screen," so named because it uses four biochemical markers: alpha-fetoprotein (AFP), hCG, unconjugated estriol (µE3), and dimeric inhibin A. The quad screen is offered in the second trimester, usually between 15 and 20 weeks of pregnancy. *Using a second-trimester Down syndrome cutoff risk of 1 in 270, screening detects >80% of affected babies in women 35 years and older.* The positive screen rate is 5%. The quad screen detects at least 70% of babies with trisomy 18 and about 85% of those with neural-tube defects.

Therefore, the clinical sensitivity of the second trimester screen is approximately 81% for Down syndrome.

7. **D.** The quad screen is offered in the second trimester, usually between 15 and 20 weeks of pregnancy. It detects at least 70% of babies with trisomy 18 and about 85% of those with-neural tube defects. For Down syndrome, the quad screen detects about 81% of affected babies. *The test also has a 5% false positive rate.*

Specificity, also called the "true negative rate," measures the percentage of healthy people who are correctly identified as not having the condition. In other words, it answers the question of how often the test is negative if a person does not have the disease.

$$SPC = \frac{TN}{N} = \frac{TN + FP - FP}{TN + FP} = 1 - \frac{FP}{N} = 1 - FPR$$

FP = false positive; FPR = false positive rate; N = number of negatives; SPC = specificity; TN = number of true positives.

Therefore, the clinical specificity of the second-trimester screen is approximately 95% for Down syndrome.

8. **C.** In the 1980s, maternal serum screening programs became available to identify pregnancies at risk for open neural-tube defects (ONTDs) and anencephaly; 75%–90% of ONTDs and ≥95% of anencephalies can be detected by elevated maternal serum alpha-fetoprotein (MSAFP) levels with a screen positive rate of 5% or less. The optimal time for ONTDs screening is 16–18 weeks' gestation, but screening can be done between 15 and 20 weeks. In the second trimester, *if the quad*

screen reveals low hCG, low μE3, high AFP, and normal inhibin A, the fetus has increased risk for anencephaly, which is a severe form of neural-tube defect.

Therefore, the μE3 (estriol) should be low instead of normal if the fetus had a neural-tube defect.

9. **E.** Prenatal cell-free DNA (cfDNA) screening, also known as "noninvasive prenatal screening," is a method to screen for certain chromosomal abnormalities, fetal sex, and rhesus (Rh) blood type in a fetus with DNA from the mother and fetus extracted from a maternal blood sample. It is usually offered at or after 10 weeks of gestation. Even though it is not a diagnostic test, having both false positive and false negative rates, *the accuracy (true positive rate) and specificity (true negative rate) of NIPT is greater than 99% for Down syndrome, which is higher than first-trimester screen and second-trimester screen.* Sensitivity and specificity are lower for other aneuploidies like 47, + 18 (97%−99% and >99%, respectively), 47, + 13 (87%−99% and >99%, respectively), and 45,X (92%−95% and 99%, respectively), which are comparatively rare. It may help women make decisions about invasive testing that carries a slight risk of miscarriage, including amniocentesis and chorionic villus sampling (CVS). And it poses no risk of miscarriage or other pregnancy complications.

The first-trimester screen is a noninvasive prenatal evaluation that combines a maternal blood screening test with an ultrasound evaluation of the fetus to identify risk for chromosome aneuploidies. The blood test is used to measure pregnancy-associated plasma protein-A and human chorionic gonadotropin (hCG) in the mother's blood. The ultrasound exam measures the size of the clear space in the tissue at the back of the baby's neck (nuchal translucency). The accuracy rate of the first-trimester screen for chromosome abnormalities is approximately 85%, with a false positive rate of 5%. It poses no risk of miscarriage or other pregnancy complications.

The second-trimester screen, also called the quad screen, is a noninvasive prenatal evaluation for chromosome aneuploidy and neural-tube defects. It tests maternal blood for AFP, hCG, estriol, and inhibin A. The quad screen correctly identifies about 80% of women who are carrying a baby with Down syndrome. About 5% of women have a false positive result. It poses no risk of miscarriage or other pregnancy complications.

Chorionic villus sampling (CVS) is an invasive diagnostic prenatal test for genetic conditions, and is usually done in the first-trimester. It carries various risks, including miscarriage, Rh sensitization, and infection. The risk of miscarriage after CVS is about the same as that associated with transabdominal second-trimester amniocentesis—around 0.7%. The risk of miscarriage might increase if the baby is smaller than normal for gestational age.

Amniocentesis is an invasive diagnostic test, usually done in the second-trimester. It detects chromosome abnormalities, neural-tube defects, and genetic disorders with high level of accuracy (98%−99%). However, it does pose a risk for miscarriage. The risk of miscarriage ranges from 1 in 400 to 1 in 200.

Therefore, noninvasive prenatal test (NIPT) is the most accurate prenatal test for determining fetal aneuploidy carrier status with minimum risk of miscarriage.

10. **B.** In the second trimester, if the quad screen reveals high hCG, low μE3, low AFP, and high inhibin A, the fetus has an increased risk for Down syndrome.

Therefore, the inhibin A level should be high instead of low if the fetus had Down syndrome.

11. **A.** In the second trimester, if the quad screen reveals low hCG, low μE3, low AFP, and normal inhibin A, the fetus has increased risk for trisomy 13.

Therefore, the hCG level should be low instead of high if the fetus had trisomy 13.

12. **D.** Noninvasive prenatal testing (NIPT) does not replace the utility of a first-trimester ultrasound examination, which has been proven to be useful for accurate gestational dating, assessment of the nuchal translucency region to identify a fetus at increased risk for neural-tube defects, a chromosomal abnormality, identification of twins and higher-order pregnancies, placental abnormalities, and congenital anomalies. *Patients who are undergoing cell-free DNA screening should be offered maternal serum alpha-fetoprotein screening or ultrasound evaluation for risk assessment.* Parallel or simultaneous testing with multiple screening methodologies for aneuploidy (first- and/or second-trimester screening) is not cost-effective and should not be performed. Chorionic villus sampling (CVS) and amniocentesis are invasive prenatal diagnostic tests for chromosome abnormalities, which should be offered to a patient who has a positive, indeterminate, or uninterpretable results on screening.

Therefore, in addition to NIPT, ultrasound evaluation should also be offered to assess the risk for fetal anomalies such as neural-tube defects and ventral-wall defects.

13. **D.** First-trimester screen, second-trimester screen, and noninvasive prenatal test (NIPT) with cell-free DNA (cfDNA) are noninvasive prenatal screening tests. Chorionic villus sampling (CVS) and amniocentesis are invasive prenatal diagnostic tests for chromosome abnormalities. Chorionic villus sampling (CVS) usually is done in the first trimester between the 10th and 13th weeks. The second-trimester quad screen is usually offered between 15 and 20 weeks of pregnancy.

"Women whose results are not reported, indeterminate, or uninterpretable (a 'no call' test result) from cell-free DNA screening (cfDNA) should receive further genetic counseling and be offered comprehensive ultrasound evaluation and diagnostic testing because of an increased risk of aneuploidy."

Therefore, a chorionic villus sampling (CVS) would likely be offered for follow-up, since the patient had an indeterminate NIPT result and she was in the first trimester.

14. **A.** Noninvasive prenatal test (NIPT) is a screening test even though its sensitivity and specificity are higher than those reported with traditional first trimester screening or multiple marker screening methods. It cannot replace the high level of accuracy seen by diagnostic testing. Much like traditional screening methods, NIPT test results are categorized into low risk of aneuploidy and high risk of aneuploidy, as well as no-call (undeterminable). Individuals who are determined to be in the low-risk category would not require any further diagnostic evaluation, unless warranted by other clinical findings. *Individuals who are determined to be in the high-risk category should be offered confirmatory diagnostic testing, such as chorionic villus sampling or amniocentesis.*

Chorionic villus sampling (CVS) usually is done in the first trimester between the 10th and 13th weeks. Amniocentesis is usually performed between 14th and 20th weeks. Usually NIPT test is done between 10 and 20 completed weeks gestation age. If the results are positive, uninformative, or test failures, the follow-up test will be amniocentesis between the 15th and 18th weeks.

The cell-free DNA screening test should not be considered in isolation from other clinical findings and test results. Chromosomal abnormalities such as unbalanced translocations, deletions, and duplications will not be detected by NIPT. According to the recommendation from American College of Obstetricians and Gynecologists (ACOG), "If a fetal structural anomaly is identified on ultrasound examination, diagnostic testing

should be offered rather than cell-free DNA screening."

In this case, although the NIPT test was negative, the fetus had a complete atrioventricular canal defect (CAVCD). Therefore, amniocentesis would be the most appropriate next step work up after NIPT testing for this family.

15. **D.** Noninvasive prenatal test (NIPT) is a screening test, though its sensitivity and specificity are higher than those reported with traditional first-trimester screening or multiple-marker screening methods(https://doi.org/10.1155/2014/823504). It cannot replace the high level of accuracy seen by diagnostic testing. Much like traditional screening methods, NIPT results are categorized into low risk of aneuploidy and high risk of aneuploidy, as well as no-call (undeterminable). Individuals who are found to be in the low-risk category would not require any further diagnostic evaluation, unless warranted by other clinical findings. Individuals who are found to be in the high-risk category should be offered confirmatory diagnostic testing, such as chorionic villus sampling or amniocentesis. The no-call category is used to categorize samples that did not generate a result and would require a repeat test sample to be drawn. False positive results can occur in the presence of placental mosaicism, vanishing twin syndrome, or an unidentified maternal condition, such as mosaicism or cancer. False negative results can occur when an insufficient amount of fetal cell-free DNA (cfDNA) is present in the sample, resulting in masking on the fetal phenotype by the maternal cfDNA. When considering NIPT, it is not only important for the patient to receive appropriate pretest counseling on the benefits and limitations of this new technology, but for medical professionals to ensure that testing is offered only when appropriate.

Research showed that for patients weighing more than 250 pounds, 10% or more may have a fetal fraction of less than 4%. According to the CAP Molecular Pathology Checklist, MOL.36330, dated August 21, 2017, *"Maternal weight has a strong impact on fetal fraction (higher weight women have lower fetal fractions). This can reduce analytical sensitivity due to inadequate levels of fetal DNA. This can also result in lower separation between disomic and trisomic fetuses, thereby reducing analytical specificity. BMI may be a suitable replacement for maternal weight, but this has not yet been demonstrated."*

"Maternal age is a useful patient identifier and is used as the primary information to establish the prior risk for common aneuploidies," but not affect analytical sensitivity and/or specificity. "The (NIPT) tests make the assumption that the mother is euploid for each of the autosomal chromosomes examined." Decreased risk of Down syndrome by first-trimester screen does not affect analytical sensitivity and/or analytical specificity of NIPT tests. "If the couple has offspring with Down syndrome, the recurrent risk increases to 1% if both of them have normal karyotypes. If the father has a balanced Robertsonian translocation between chromosomes 13 and 21, the risk of trisomies 13 or 21 in the offspring is increased significantly."

Therefore, in general, high maternal BMI most likely affects the analytical sensitivity.

16. E. According to the CAP Molecular Pathology Checklist, MOL.36350, dated August 21, 2017, *"Insufficient data are currently available to interpret results in triplet or higher number of multiple gestations.* It might be useful to solicit information regarding demise of a co-twin, but data are currently insufficient to provide reliable guideline on the interpretation."

Regardless of the method, the accuracy of screening for aneuploidy is limited in multiple gestations. With any method based on maternal blood (serum analytes or DNA), only a single composite result for the entire gestation is provided, with no ability to distinguish a differential risk between fetuses. The data regarding the performance of cell-free DNA (cfDNA) screening in twin gestations are limited. Although preliminary findings suggest that this screening is accurate, larger prospective studies and published data are needed before this method can be recommended for multiple gestations. Cell-free DNA screening is not recommended for women with multiple gestations. There are no available data on higher-order multiples.

"The [NIPT] tests make the assumption that the mother is euploid for each of the autosomal chromosomes examined." If the mother or father has a balanced Robertsonian translocation between chromosomes 13 and 21, the risk of trisomy 13 or 21 in the offspring is increased significantly. Since the mother is still considered to be euploid, the analysis of the NIPT should not be affected. Decreased risk of Down syndrome by first-trimester screen does not affect analytical sensitivity and/or analytical specificity of NIPTs. The probability of a fetus with aneuploidy is low, but it does not meet exclusion criteria.

Therefore, multiple gestations most likely meet rejection criteria for noninvasive prenatal test (NIPT).

17. C. Noninvasive prenatal screening (NIPS) use cell-free fetal DNA (cfDNA) sequences isolated from a maternal blood sample. Although studies are promising and demonstrate high sensitivity and specificity with low false-positive rates, there are limitations to NIPS.

Uninformative test results due to insufficient isolation of cell-free fetal DNA could lead to a delay in diagnosis or may eliminate the availability of information for risk assessment. Biological factors associated with a reduced availability of cfDNA include a high body-mass index and early gestational age (<10 weeks). Limited data are currently available on the use of NIPS in twins and higher-order pregnancies.

As long as maternal genomic DNA is balanced, the structural variants of the karyotype do not affect the NIPS results. Therefore, a balanced Robertsonian translocation, 45,XY,der(13;21)(q10; q10), in the mother does not meet rejection criteria for NIPS.

18. A. First-trimester screen, second-trimester screen, and noninvasive prenatal test (NIPT) with cell-free DNA (cfDNA) are noninvasive prenatal screening tests. Chorionic villus sampling (CVS) and amniocentesis are invasive prenatal diagnostic tests for chromosome abnormalities.

The American College of Obstetricians and Gynecologists (ACOG) recommendation states, "Given the performance of conventional screening methods, the limitations of cell-free DNA (cfDNA) screening performance, and the limited data on cost-effectiveness in the low-risk obstetric population, conventional screening methods remain the most appropriate choice for first-line screening for most women in the general obstetric population."

Data on the performance of cfDNA testing in the general obstetric population have now become available. The sensitivity and specificity in the general obstetric population are similar to the levels previously published for the aforementioned high-risk population. The positive predictive value, however, is lower in this population, given the lower prevalence of aneuploidy in the general obstetric population (see the table below). That is, fewer women with a positive test result will actually have an affected fetus, and there will be more false positive test results.

Cell-Free DNA Test Performance Characteristics in Patients Who
Receive an Interpretable Result[a]

	Sensitivity (%)	Specificity (%)	Age 25 years	Age 40 years
			PPV (%)	PPV (%)
Trisomy 21	99.3	99.8	33	87
Trisomy 18	97.4	99.8	13	68
Trisomy 13	91.6	99.9	9	57
Sex chromosome aneuploidy	91	99.6	—[b]	—

[a]This table is modeled on 25- and 40-year-old patients based on the presence of
aneuploidy at 16 weeks of gestation. Negative predictive values are not included in the
table, but they are greater than 99% for all patient populations who receive a test
result. Negative predictive values decrease when patients who do not receive a result
are included. Test performance characteristics are derived from a summary of
published reports and are assessed and compiled in published reviews.
[b]The positive and negative predictive values for the sex chromosome aneuploidies
depend on the particular condition identified. In general, however, the PPV ranges
from 20%–40% for most of these conditions.
PPV = positive predictive value.
From the Committee Opinion. Cell-free DNA screening for fetal aneuploidy.
American College of Obstetricians and Gynecologists; 2015, 640.

Another limitation of cfDNA screening in the
general obstetric population is that trisomies 13, 18,
and 21 comprise a smaller proportion of the
chromosome abnormalities found in the general
obstetric population. Traditional serum analyte
screening methods allow for higher detection rates of
these other chromosome abnormalities as well as the
risk of other adverse pregnancy outcomes. For
example, a positive integrated screening test result
may indirectly identify a fetus with an unbalanced
rearrangement of a chromosome other than trisomy
13, 18, or 21. One study of women with abnormal
traditional screening test results who had diagnostic
testing estimated that up to 17% of clinically
significant chromosomal abnormalities would not be
detectable with most of the current cfDNA
techniques. Given the performance of conventional
screening methods and the limitations of cfDNA,
conventional screening methods remain the most
appropriate choice for first-line screening for most
women in the general obstetric population.

However, a recent survey of US obstetrician
opinions indicated that Ob/Gyns "identified NIPT as
clinically superior to traditional screening methods
and indicated that they would like ACOG to formally
recommend NIPT for any pregnant woman."
Insurance coverage, and therefore cost, was noted as
the biggest barrier, and over 81% of surveyed
providers would utilize NIPT as a first-line screening
test if patients' insurance offered full coverage.

Therefore, first-trimester screen followed by
second-trimester screen continues to be the

most appropriate choice of first-line screening for the
low-risk obstetric population, according to ACOG.

19. **B.** *Newborn screening (NBS) testing began in the United
States in the early 1960s, when Robert Guthrie devised a
screening test for phenylketonuria (PKU) using a newborn
blood spot dried onto a filter paper card.* Over the years,
it has evolved into a complex program that tests for
multiple conditions. States and territories mandate
NBS of all infants born within their jurisdiction for
certain treatable disorders that may not otherwise be
detected before developmental disability or death
occurs. Newborns with these disorders typically
appear normal at birth. The testing and follow-up
services of NBS programs are designed to provide
early diagnosis and treatment before significant,
irreversible damage occurs. Appropriate compliance
with the medical management prescribed can allow
most affected newborns to develop normally.

Therefore, newborn screening in the Unites
States began in the 1960s.

20. **A.** An apparent sensitivity of 100% has been reported
by the various states for most of the disorders in the
newborn screen (NBS) panel, and specificity levels are
all above 99%. The positive predictive values (PPVs),
however, range from 0.5%–6.0%. Consequently, for
every infant identified with a true positive screening
result, 12–60 additional infants will receive a false
positive screening result, depending on the disorder
and the specificity of the screening algorithm for that
disorder. The false positive rate was highest in infants
with the lowest of the low birth weights (LBWs).
LBW infants accounted for 3.3% of the total study
population but 89% of the false positive results.

Most infants are born healthy and discharged
within 1–2 days after birth. Infants born ill or
prematurely require longer hospitalization and
often receive intensive medical care in a neonatal
intensive care unit (NICU). *Various medical
therapies, including total parenteral nutrition (TPN),
provided in the NICU, and the liver immaturity of the
preterm infant's metabolic system contribute to higher
rates of presumptive positive NBS results in this group.*

Therefore, preterm newborn in NICU with total
parenteral nutrition (TPN) increases the potential
of false positive newborn screening (NBS) results
in premature infants.

21. **E.** Noninvasive prenatal testing (NIPT), which
analyzes cell-free fetal DNA (cfDNA) circulating in
maternal blood, is a relatively new option in the
prenatal screening and testing paradigm for
trisomy 21 and a few other fetal chromosomal
aneuploidies. Testing can be done any time after 10
weeks; typically it is done between 10 and 22
weeks. Results can take a week or more. The
testing is noninvasive, involving a maternal blood

draw, so the pregnancy is not put at risk for miscarriage or other adverse outcomes associated with invasive testing procedures. *Even though NIPT is not a diagnostic test with both false positive and false negative rate, the accuracy (true positive rate) and specificity (true negative rate) of NIPT is greater than 99% for Down syndrome.*

The accuracy rate for the first-trimester screening to detect the chromosomal abnormalities (trisomies 21, 18, and 13) is approximately 85%, with a false positive rate of 5%. The quad screen is offered in the second trimester, usually between 15 and 20 weeks of pregnancy. It detects at least 70% of fetuses with trisomy 18 and about 85% of those with neural-tube defects. The quad screen detects about 81% of fetuses with Down syndromet.

Chorionic villus sampling (CVS) is an invasive diagnostic prenatal test for genetic conditions, usually done in the first trimester; the miscarriage risk is approximately 1 in 100. Amniocentesis is also an invasive diagnostic test, usually done in the second trimester; the risk of miscarriage ranges from 1 in 400 to 1 in 200.

Therefore, NITP gives the most accurate information on fetal aneuploidy at 12 weeks' gestational age without the risk of miscarriage.

22. **C.** Amniocentesis is usually done between week 15 and 20 of pregnancy; the risk of miscarriage ranges from 1 in 400 to 1 in 200. *Amniocentesis done before week 15 of pregnancy has been associated with a higher rate of complications.* One study of 4334 women found that early amniocentesis was not a safe early alternative compared to second-trimester amniocentesis because of the increased total pregnancy losses (7.6% vs. 5.9%; average relative risk,1.29; 95% confidence interval [CI], 1.03−1.61; high-quality evidence), spontaneous miscarriages (3.6% vs. 2.5%; average RR, 1.41; 95% CI 1.00−1.98; moderate-quality evidence), and a higher incidence of congenital anomalies, including talipes (4.7% vs. 2.7%; average RR, 1.73; 95% CI, 1.26−2.38; high-quality evidence). Chorionic villus sampling (CVS) is an invasive diagnostic prenatal test for genetic conditions, usually done in the first trimester; the miscarriage risk is approximately 1 in 100. More miscarriages were seen after early amniocentesis (AC) compared with transabdominal CVS (2.3% vs. 1.3%; average RR, 1.73; 95% CI, 1.15−2.60).

First-trimester screen, second-trimester screen, and noninvasive prenatal test (NIPT) are noninvasive studies that are not associated with a risk for miscarriage.

Therefore, amniocentesis has highest rate for miscarriage if it is done at 12 weeks' gestational age.

23. **C.** Hemolytic disease of the fetus and newborn (HDFN), also known as "hemolytic disease of the fetus and newborn," is caused by alloimmunization of the mother by exposure to fetal red blood cells, which display a paternally inherited form of an antigen that is different from that in the mother. Maternal alloantibody production is stimulated when fetal red blood cells are positive for an antigen that is absent in the mother's red cells. The maternal IgG antibodies produced will pass through the placenta and attack fetal red cells carrying the corresponding antigen. *Anti-D accounts for the majority of HDFN,* followed by anti-K, anti-c, and anti-E. It can also occur in women of blood type O. Anti-S has been documented as a rare cause of HDFN. The frequency of Rh-negative individuals is more common in Caucasian than in other ethnic groups.

According to the publication, this reported baby's blood group was A RhD-positive with a red-cell phenotype of ccDEe (R2r) and SS. The result of a direct Coombs test (DCT) was positive and red-cell elution studies of the baby's blood identified the presence of anti-D and anti-S antibodies. The mother's transfusion record at the medical center showed that the mother developed anti-S antibodies during her second pregnancy 3 years ago. An antenatal antibody screening test performed at 22 weeks identified only allo-anti-S; no anti-D was detected. She was given RhD Ig prophylaxis at 28 weeks of pregnancy. Her other laboratory results showed that she was categorized as group A RhD-negative with a red-cell phenotype of ccdee (rr), and homozygous ss. At postpartum, the result of her DCT was negative, but the antibody screening test performed using the indirect Coombs test method and antibody investigations showed the presence of anti-D and anti-S, and the anti-D titer was 1:32 (0.25 IU/mL).

Therefore, RhD incompatibility would most likely account for the HDFN in this newborn.

24. **D.** In this case, the mother was e negative. Anti-E most likely would be detected in the mother's serum and eluate from the baby's red cells. Maternal red cell alloimmunization occurs when the fetus is positive for an antigen that is absent on maternal red cells. The mother's body is stimulated to produce immunoglobulin G (IgG) antibodies against the positive fetal red cells; these antibodies pass through the placenta and destroy the antigen-positive fetal red cells. Clinically significant alloantibodies other than anti-D, such as anti-E, anti-K, and anti-c occur in 1 in 300 pregnancies, and the risk of hemolytic disease of the fetus and newborn (HDFN) caused by these antibodies is 1

in 500. Anti-E is the most common clinically significant alloantibody detected in the Malaysian population.

Therefore, this newborn baby would most likely have RhE incompatibility.

25. **B.** States vary widely in their use of newborn screening (NBS) tests, with some mandating screening as few as three conditions and others mandating as many as 43, including varying numbers of the 40 conditions that can be detected by tandem mass spectrometry (MS/MS). In 2006, the American College of Medical Genetics and Genomics (ACMG) convened 292 experts to evaluate 84 conditions. *The experts recommended a uniform screening panel of 29 core (or primary) conditions to be included in state newborn screening (NBS) panels:* 20 inborn errors of metabolism (six amino acidurias, five disorders of fatty oxidation, nine organic acidurias), three hemoglobinopathies, and six other conditions (congenital hypothyroidism (CH), biotinidase deficiency (BTD), congenital adrenal hyperplasia (CAH), classic galactosemia (GALT), hearing loss (HEAR), and cystic fibrosis (CF)).

The Advisory Committee on Heritable Disorders in Newborns and Children (ACHDNC) reviewed nine additional conditions, and recommended the inclusion of two additional conditions—severe combined immunodeficiency and critical congenital heart disease. These were approved by the Secretary in 2010 and 2011, respectively.

Therefore, 29 conditions are included in the uniform screen program recommended by ACMG.

26. **E.** Ornithine transcarbamylase (OTC) deficiency is an X-linked condition of urea biosynthesis characterized by recurrent, often fatal, hyperammonemic encephalopathy in affected males. Males with severe neonatal-onset OTC deficiency are typically normal at birth but become symptomatic from hyperammonemia on day 2–3 of life and are usually catastrophically ill by the time they come to medical attention. After successful treatment of neonatal hyperammonemic coma, these infants can easily become hyperammonemic again despite appropriate treatment; they typically require liver transplantation by age 6 months to improve quality of life. *OTC is the only gene in which pathogenic variants cause OTC deficiency* (https://www.ncbi.nlm.nih.gov/books/NBK154378/).

The *ASS1* gene encodes argininosuccinate synthetase-1, a cytosolic urea cycle enzyme expressed mainly in periportal hepatocytes but also in most other body tissues. Deficiency of argininosuccinate synthetase-1 causes citrullinemia. The *ASL* gene encodes the subunit of argininosuccinate lyase, a urea cycle enzyme that catalyzes the cleavage of argininosuccinate to fumarate and arginine, an essential step in the process of detoxification of ammonia via the urea cycle. Pathogenic variants in *ASL* cause argininosuccinic aciduria. The *CPS1* gene encodes carbamoyl phosphate synthetase I, which is the rate-limiting enzyme that catalyzes the first committed step of the hepatic urea cycle by synthesizing carbamoyl phosphate from ammonia, bicarbonate, and two molecules of ATP. Pathogenic variants in *CPS1* cause carbamoyl phosphate synthetase I deficiency. The *NAGS* gene encodes N-acetylglutamate synthase, a mitochondrial enzyme that catalyzes the formation of N-acetylglutamate (NAG), an essential allosteric activator of carbamoyl phosphate synthase I (CPS1; OMIM# 608307), the first and rate-limiting enzyme in the urea cycle (https://omim.org/). Pathogenic variants in *NAGS* cause N-acetylglutamate synthase deficiency.

Therefore, *OTC* would most likely harbor pathogenic variant(s) in this patient.

27. **C.** The urea cycle is the sole source of endogenous production of arginine and is the principle mechanism for the clearance of waste nitrogen resulting from protein turnover and dietary intake. This extra nitrogen is converted into ammonia (NH_3) and transported to the liver for processing. The urea cycle disorders (UCDs) result from inherited molecular defects that compromise this clearance. *Ornithine transcarbamoylase (OTC) deficiency is the only X-linked condition in UCD, caused by pathogenic variants in OTC at Xp11.4.* OTC deficiency usually affects male, with a severe neonatal onset; females are also somewhat affected, but symptoms are much less severe in females than in males. The other conditions in the urea cycle are autosomal recessive conditions.

Therefore, ornithine transcarbamoylase would the least likely to be the reason for elevated arginine and ammonium in serum before further workup, since the patient was female.

28. **A.** Urea cycle disorders (UCDs) result from inherited deficiencies in any one of the six enzymes or two transporters of the urea cycle pathway. They are carbamoyl phosphate synthetase I (CPS1), ornithine transcarbamylase (OTC), argininosuccinic acid synthetase (ASS1), argininosuccinic acid lyase (ASL), arginase (ARG1), ornithine translocase (ORNT1), and citrin.

Step 1 of the urea cycle is condensation of CO_2, ammonia, and ATP to form carbamoyl phosphate, which is catalyzed by mitochondrial carbamoyl phosphate synthase I (CPS I). Carbamoyl phosphate synthase II (CPS II) uses glutamine rather than ammonia as the nitrogen donor and functions in pyrimidine biosynthesis. Step 2 is L-ornithine transcarbamoylase (OTC) catalyzing transfer of the carbamoyl group of carbamoyl phosphate to ornithine, forming citrulline and orthophosphate, which occurs in the mitochondrial matrix. But both the formation of ornithine and the subsequent metabolism of citrulline take place in cytosol. The entry of ornithine into mitochondria and the exodus of citrulline from mitochondria involve mitochondrial inner-membrane transport systems (ORNT1 and citrin). Step 3 is argininosuccinate synthase (ASS) linking L-aspartate and citrulline via the amino group of aspartates and provides the second nitrogen of urea. Step 4 is cleavage of argininosuccinate, catalyzed by argininosuccinate lyase (ASL), proceeding with retention of nitrogen in arginine and release of aspartate skeleton as fumarate. *Step 5 is hydrolytic cleavage of the guanidine group of arginine, catalyzed by liver arginase (ARG1), releasing urea and ornithine.* Ornithine reenters liver mitochondria for additional rounds of urea synthesis.

A high concentration of arginine indicates a defect in the urea cycle at a level distal to its formation, which may result from arginase deficiency. Therefore, arginase would most likely cause an elevation of the plasma arginine levels.

29. **E.** The patient had postpartum coma due to hyperammonemia related to ornithine transcarbamylase deficiency (OTCD). OTCD is the most common urea-cycle defect, and it can occur as a severe neonatal-onset disease in males (but rarely in females) and as a postneonatal-onset (partial deficiency) disease in males and females. Heterozygous females with postneonatal-onset (partial) OTC deficiency can present from infancy to later childhood, adolescence, or adulthood. No matter how mild the disease, a hyperammonemic crisis can be precipitated by stressors and become a life-threatening event at any age and in any situation, as in this case. Stressors may include crush injury, postoperative events, a high-protein diet, the postpartum period, cancer therapy, prolonged fasting, treatment with high-dose systemic corticosteroids, or febrile illness. Treatment with valproate or haloperidol has been associated with hyperammonemic crises in persons with OTC deficiency.

When children, adolescents, or adults with postneonatal-onset disease become encephalopathic, they may reach stage 2 coma with erratic behavior, combativeness, and delirium

(e.g., not recognizing family members and unintelligible speech). They may come to medical attention if these behavioral abnormalities lead to an emergency medical or psychiatric evaluation. The phenotype of a heterozygous female can range from asymptomatic to significant symptoms with recurrent hyperammonemia and neurological compromise depending on favorable versus nonfavorable X-chromosome inactivation (https://www.ncbi.nlm.nih.gov/books/NBK154378/).

In this case, the patient's ammonia was elevated. She was started on sodium benzoate, and hemodialysis was performed. On the 14th day of hospitalization, she died in the ICU despite all the supportive and specific treatment. Therefore, the patient had ornithine transcarbamoylase deficiency (OTCD).

30. **E.** Glucose-6-phosphate dehydrogenase deficiency (G6PD), the most common enzyme deficiency worldwide, causes a spectrum of diseases, including neonatal hyperbilirubinemia, acute hemolysis, and chronic hemolysis. Persons with this condition may also be asymptomatic. This X-linked condition most commonly affects males of African, Asian, Mediterranean, or Middle Eastern descent. *Like sickle cell disease, G6PD deficiency appears to have reached a substantial frequency in some areas because it confers some resistance to malaria and thus a survival advantage to individuals heterozygous for G6PD deficiency.* Newborn screening (NBS) for G6PD deficiency is not performed routinely in the United States, although it is done in countries with a high prevalence of this disease. The World Health Organization (WHO) recommends screening all newborns in populations with a prevalence of 3%—5% or more in males.

Therefore, patients with G6PD have a selection advantage.

31. **E.** Glucose-6-phosphate dehydrogenase (G6PD) deficiency is an X-linked condition that affects only males and skips generations. The mother of the proband carries one normal copy and one abnormal copy of the gene for the disease. X inactivation is the mechanism by which one of the two chromosome Xs is randomly silenced in each cell of females. Therefore, female carriers of an X-linked condition, such as the mother of the proband in this question, are usually NOT affected or mildly affected except in cases of extremely skewed X inactivation.

Therefore, the proband's mother did NOT have any symptoms of G6PD owing to X inactivation.

32. **D.** *Glucose-6-phosphate dehydrogenase deficiency (G6PD deficiency) is an X-linked recessive disease, which is relatively common in those of African,*

Mediterranean, or Asian descent and less common in Hispanics.

Therefore, glucose-6-phosphate dehydrogenase deficiency (G6PD deficiency) is relatively uncommon in Hispanics as compared with African, Mediterranean, or Asian populations.

33. **A.** Glucose-6-phosphate dehydrogenase (G6PD) deficiency was discovered by Alving and coworkers when they investigated the unusual hemolytic reaction that occurred in ethnic black individuals following the administration of primaquine, an 8-aminoquinoline, for the radical treatment of malaria. Such "primaquine sensitivity" was later observed in other ethnic groups as well. It occurs most often in males. In affected individuals, a defect of G6PD causes red blood cells to break down prematurely, causing hemolysis. Hemolytic anemia is most often triggered by bacterial or viral infections or by certain drugs, such as some antibiotics and medications used to treat malaria. Acute hemolytic anemia can develop as a result of three types of triggers: ingestion of fava beans, infections, and drugs. The drugs that precipitate an attack of hemolytic anemia are antibiotics, antipyretics, and antimalarials. Pathogenic variants in the *G6PD* gene cause G6PD. The gene is located on the chromosome Xq28 region. Affected males have hemizygous variants. The c.466A > G(p.Asn156Asp) in *G6PD* is widely distributed in Africa.

Galactokinase deficiency is caused by homozygous or compound heterozygous pathogenic variants in the *GALK1* gene located on 17q25.1. Galactokinase deficiency is one of the three inborn errors of metabolism that lead to hypergalactosemia. Its major clinical symptom is the development of cataracts during the first weeks or months of life as a result of the accumulation of galactitol, a product of an alternative route of galactose utilization, in the lens. The c94G > A(p.Val32Met) variant in *GALK1* is pathogenic.

Therefore, this male patient would most likely have hemizygous p.Asn126Asp in *G6PD*.

34. **B.** Phenylalanine hydroxylase (PAH) deficiency results in intolerance to the dietary intake of the essential amino acid phenylalanine and produces a spectrum of disorders. The diagnosis of PAH is established in a proband with a plasma phenylalanine concentration persistently above 120 μmol/L (2 mg/dL) and an altered ratio of phenylalanine to tyrosine in the untreated state with normal BH4 cofactor metabolism and/or the finding of biallelic pathogenic variants in *PAH* by molecular genetic testing. *PAH* is the only gene, in which pathogenic variants cause PAH. In the

United States, newborn screening (NBS) can detect 100% of cases (https://www.ncbi.nlm.nih.gov/books/NBK154378/).

Pathogenic variants in *APC* cause autosomal dominant familial adenomatous polyposis (FAP). *PC* encodes pyruvate carboxylase, which is a key enzyme in glucogenesis. Pyruvate carboxylase deficiency is another metabolic disorder. *PROC* encodes protein C. Pathogenic variants in *PROC* cause autosomal dominant or autosomal recessive thrombophilia.

Therefore, *PAH* would most likely harbor pathogenic variant(s) for phenylketonuria in this patient.

35. **A.** All 50 states in the United States require newborns to be screened for phenylketonuria (PKU). Many other countries also routinely screen infants for PKU. Newborn blood testing identifies almost all cases of phenylketonuria. *Measurements with tandem mass spectrometry (MS/MS) determine the concentration of Phe and the ratio of Phe to tyrosine, both of which are elevated in PKU.*

In Illinois, newborn screening (NBS) for sickle cell disease is performed by high-performance liquid chromatography (HPLC) testing. Some states use immunoreactive trypsinogen (IRT) and DNA (molecular genetic) tests for cystic fibrosis (CF) newborn screening, some use IRT-IRT. IRT is secreted in the pancreas. The sweat test is the diagnostic test for CF.

Therefore, tandem mass spectrometry (MS/MS) has been used in newborn screening (NBS) for phenylketonuria.

36. **A.** Newborn screening (NBS) for fatty acid oxidation disorders usually is done before a baby leaves the hospital. The baby's heel is pricked, and a few drops of blood are taken. The blood is sent to the state laboratory to find out if it has more than a normal amount of fatty acids. *The application of tandem mass spectrometry (MS/MS) to newborn screening (NBS) provides an effective means to identify most patients with fatty acid oxidation disorder presymptomatically.* Preventive management is important to decrease the risk for life-threatening hypoglycemia episodes.

Therefore, tandem mass spectrometry (MS/MS) is most commonly used in newborn screening (NBS) for fatty acid oxidation disorders in the United States.

37. **C.** The first specimen for newborn screen (NBS) is usually collected after 24 hours but before 48 hours of age, or prior to the newborn's discharge from the hospital. The second one is collected at 1−2 weeks of age. *Collection of a second sample at 6 days*

could have a large impact because it can lead to false negative results for fatty acid oxidation disorders. Fatty acid markers quickly start to normalize after the first few days of life. Abnormal fatty acid oxidation ranges are higher for first-screen specimens than for second-screen specimens. A specimen collected at 6 days will be analyzed using first-screen reference values. Theoretically, the opposite is also true, collection at 6 days may lead to increased false positives for amino acid and organic acid disorders, since, in general, the reference ranges are lower for first-screen specimens than for second-screen specimens.

Therefore, fatty acid oxidation disorders would most likely be missed by the repeat NBS in this patient.

38. **D.** The short-chain fatty acids contain 2−4 carbon atoms, the medium-chain fatty acids 6−10, the *long-chain fatty acids 12−18*, and the very long-chain fatty acids 20−26. The long-chain fatty acids containing an even number of carbon atoms are important human nutrients, with palmitic acid (16 carbon atoms with 0 double bonds, or 16:0), stearic acid (18:0), oleic acid (18 carbon atoms with 1 double bond at position 9 from the methyl end, or $18:1_{\omega}9$), and linoleic acid ($18:2_{\omega}6$) together account for more than 90% of the fatty acids in the U.S. diet.

Long-chain ʟ-3-hydroxyacyl-coenzyme A dehydrogenase deficiency (LCHAD) is associated with pregnancy-specific disorders, including preeclampsia, HELLP syndrome (hemolysis, elevated liver enzymes, low platelets), hyperemesis gravidarum, acute fatty liver of pregnancy, and maternal floor infarct of the placenta. Since LCHAD is an autosomal recessive disorder, usually both parents are carriers. LCHAD is caused by homozygous or compound heterozygous mutation in *HADHA*.

The mitochondrial trifunctional protein, composed of 4 alpha and 4 beta subunits, catalyzes three steps in mitochondrial beta-oxidation of fatty acids: long-chain 3-hydroxyacyl-CoA dehydrogenase (LCHAD), long-chain enoyl-CoA hydratase, and long-chain thiolase activities. Trifunctional protein deficiency is characterized by decreased activity of all three enzymes. Trifunctional protein deficiency is caused by homozygous or compound heterozygous mutation in the genes encoding either the alpha (*HADHA*) or beta (*HADHB*) subunits of the mitochondrial trifunctional protein.

Therefore, this infant would most likely have long-chain hydroxyacyl CoA dehydrogenase (LCHAD).

39. **C.** The short-chain fatty acids contain 2−4 carbon atoms, the *medium-chain fatty acids 6−10*, the long-chain fatty acids 12−18, and the very-long-chain fatty acids 20−26. Medium-chain acyl-coenzyme A dehydrogenase deficiency (MCAD) is the most common of the fatty acid oxidation disorders. Fatty acids are unable to be metabolized beyond the medium-chain size (8−12 carbons), and gluconeogenesis is effectively inhibited. In response to any fasting or metabolic stress the body is unable to metabolize fat and continues to metabolize glucose. The clinical result is severe hypoglycemia and hypoketonuria, with accumulation of monocarboxylic fatty acids and dicarboxylic organic acids.

Trifunctional protein deficiency is characterized by decreased activity of long-chain 3-hydroxyacyl-CoA dehydrogenase (LCHAD), long-chain enoyl-CoA hydratase, and long-chain thiolase activities.

Therefore, this infant girl would most likely have medium-chain acyl CoA dehydrogenase (MCAD).

40. **A.** *The short-chain fatty acids contain 2−4 carbon atoms,* the medium-chain fatty acids 6−10, the long-chain fatty acids 12−18, and the very-long-chain fatty acids 20−26. Short-chain acyl-CoA dehydrogenase (SCAD) deficiency is characterized by feeding difficulties/failure to thrive, metabolic acidosis, ketotic hypoglycemia, lethargy, developmental delay, seizures, hypotonia, dystonia, and myopathy. It is an autosomal recessive condition leading to elevated 2−4 carbon atoms in plasma.

Therefore, this boy would most likely have short-chain acyl CoA dehydrogenase (SCAD) deficiency.

41. **C.** The mitochondrial trifunctional protein, composed of 4 alpha and 4 beta subunits, catalyzes three steps in mitochondrial beta-oxidation of fatty acids: long-chain 3-hydroxyacyl-CoA dehydrogenase (LCHAD), long-chain enoyl-CoA hydratase, and long-chain thiolase activities. Mitochondrial trifunctional protein deficiency is characterized by decreased activity of all three enzymes. Trifunctional protein deficiency is caused by homozygous or compound heterozygous mutation in the genes encoding either the alpha (*HADHA*) or beta (*HADHB*) subunits of the mitochondrial trifunctional protein. Pathogenic variants in *HADHA* and *HADHB* can affect individual enzymes or the whole MTP complex. Isolated LCHAD deficiency, due to mutation in the *HADHA* gene, is the most common form of MTP deficiency. MTP and LCHAD deficiencies both cause accumulation of long-chain acyl CoA esters and have a similar presentation and phenotype.

Pathogenic variants in *ACAD9* cause mitochondrial complex I deficiency.

Therefore, this patient would most likely have had mitochondrial trifunctional protein deficiency.

42. **E.** Very-long-chain acyl-CoA dehydrogenase (VLCAD) deficiency is a condition that prevents the body from converting very-long-chain fats (C14−C20) to energy, particularly during fasting. Diagnosis relies on: (1) comprehensive acylcarnitine analysis by tandem mass spectrometry (MS/MS) of plasma or a dried blood spot specimen collected during a period of metabolic stress (especially fasting or reduced caloric intake during infectious illness or procedures), followed by (2) molecular genetic testing of *ACADVL*, the only gene in which pathogenic variants are known to cause VLCAD deficiency (VLCADD) (https://www.ncbi.nlm.nih.gov/books/NBK6816/).

Therefore, the patient would most likely have very-long-chain acyl CoA dehydrogenase (VLCAD) deficiency.

43. **D.** Peroxisomal biogenesis disorder (PBD) refers to disorders in the Zellweger spectrum, which include infantile Refsum disease (IRD), neonatal adrenoleukodystrophy (NALD), and Zellweger syndrome. There are also two single-enzyme peroxisomal disorders, acyl-CoA oxidase deficiency and D-bifunctional protein deficiency, that are closely related to PBDs. Rhizomelic chondrodysplasia punctata type 1 (RCDP1) classic type is also a peroxisomal biogenesis disorder (PBD), which is characterized by proximal shortening of the humerus and to a lesser degree the femur (rhizomelia), punctate calcifications in cartilage with epiphyseal and metaphyseal abnormalities (chondrodysplasia punctata, or CDP), coronal clefts of the vertebral bodies, and cataracts that are usually present at birth or appear in the first few months of life.

X-linked adrenoleukodystrophy (ALD) is a disorder of peroxisomal fatty acid beta oxidation that results in the accumulation of very-long-chain fatty acids (VLCFA) in tissues throughout the body. ALD is caused by pathogenic variants in *ABCD1* at Xq28. *The gene defect is NOT an enzyme involved in fatty acid metabolism or peroxisome biogenesis.* Rather, it is a peroxisomal membrane protein, which may be involved in transport of the enzyme. The exact mechanism of the pathogenesis of ALD is not known. Biochemically, individuals with ALD show very high levels of unbranched, saturated, very-long-chain fatty acids, particularly cerotic acid (26:0).

Therefore, the patient would least likely have X-linked adrenoleukodystrophy.

44. **A.** *X-linked adrenoleukodystrophy (X-ALD) is a disorder of peroxisomal fatty acid beta oxidation that results in the accumulation of very-long-chain fatty acids (VLCFA) in tissues throughout the body.* The plasma concentration of very-long-chain fatty acids (VLCFAs) is abnormal in 99% of males with X-ALD. Increased concentration of VLCFA in plasma and/or cultured skin fibroblasts is present in approximately 85% of affected females; 20% of known carriers have normal plasma concentration of VLCFAs (https://www.ncbi.nlm.nih.gov/books/NBK1315/).

Zellweger spectrum disorder (ZSD), including Zellweger syndrome, neonatal adrenoleukodystrophy (NALD), and infantile Refsum disease (IRD), is used to describe defects in the creation and proper function of peroxisomes. Patients with ZSD usually have elevated plasma concentrations of VLCFA (C26:0 and C26:1; elevated ratios of C24/C22 and C26/C22; normal in rhizomelic chondrodysplasia punctata), increased concentrations of phytanic acid and/or pristanic acid (normal in NALD), and reduced amounts of C16 and C18 plasmalogens (normal in IRD) (https://www.ncbi.nlm.nih.gov/books/NBK1448/).

Therefore, patients with X-linked adrenoleukodystrophy usually have increased VLCFAs. Patients with Zellweger syndrome usually have increased VLCFA and phytanic acid and decreased plasmalogens.

45. **A.** X-linked adrenoleukodystrophy (X-ALD) is a disorder of peroxisomal fatty acid beta oxidation that results in the accumulation of very-long-chain fatty acids (VLCFAs) in tissues throughout the body. Biochemically, individuals with ALD show very high levels of unbranched, saturated, very-long-chain fatty acids, particularly cerotic acid (26:0). VLCFAs are usually measured for three parameters: concentration of C26:0, ratio of C24:0 to C22:0, and ratio of C26:0 to C22:0. The plasma concentration of very-long-chain fatty acids (VLCFAs) is abnormal in males with X-ALD, irrespective of age. All three parameters are elevated in the majority of males, though some variation is observed. *X-ALD is caused by pathogenic variants in ABCD1 at Xq28, which encodes a peroxisomal membrane transporter protein* (https://www.ncbi.nlm.nih.gov/books/NBK1315/).

Pathogenic variants in *ARX* cause X-linked lissencephaly. Pathogenic variants in *FMR2*, also called *AFF2*, cause X-linked fragile XE syndrome (FRAXE). Pathogenic variants in *SLC6A8* cause X-linked creatine transporter deficiency, which accounts for up to approximately 1% of cases of X-linked mental retardation (MR). Pathogenic variants in *TNFRSF13B* cause X-linked severe combined immunodeficiency with very low-level T and NK cells.

Therefore, *ABCD1* would most likely harbor pathogenic variant(s) than others in this patient if he had adrenoleukodystrophy. In the case report, this boy had a hemizygous pathogenic variant, c.548T > G(p.V183G), in the *ABCD1* gene. His mother and sister were carriers of this same variant. The boy was discharged with the diagnosis of childhood X-ALD. At home, the neurological disturbances worsened relatively quickly, leading to repeated admissions of the child to the pediatric neurology unit; death occurred 8 months after the diagnosis from generalized paralysis and cardiorespiratory arrest.

46. **E.** The prevalence of X-linked adrenoleukodystrophy (X-ALD) is estimated to be between 1 in 20,000 and 1 in 500,000, and the rate appears to be approximately the same in all ethnic groups. *ABCD1 is the only gene in which pathogenic variants cause X-ALD.* The comprehensive X-linked adrenoleukodystrophy database lists 595 nonrecurrent pathogenic and likely pathogenic variants, as well as rare variants of uncertain significance identified in affected males or obligate heterozygotes. *Nonrecurrent pathogenic variants account for approximately half of the disease-causing variants reported,* which include missense pathogenic variants (~62%), frameshifts (~22%), nonsense pathogenic variants (~10%), in-frame deletions/insertions (~3%), and large deletions (~3%). *Sequencing analysis may detect 93% of probands.* Gene-targeted deletion/duplication analysis may detect 6% of probands (https://www.ncbi.nlm.nih.gov/books/NBK1315/).

Therefore, Sanger sequence analysis would most likely be used to confirm/rule out adrenoleukodystrophy in this patient.

47. **C.** *Pathogenic variants in the ABCD1 gene at Xq28 are associated with X-linked adrenoleukodystrophy (X-ALD).* This male patient had a hemizygous variant, which looked the same as homozygous variants on both next-generation sequencing and Sanger sequencing analysis. This explains why his mother and sister have the same variant in heterozygous state, but his father does not.

Deletion and duplication analysis may be used to detect deletions and duplications that cannot be detected by sequencing analysis and make a heterozygous variant looks like a homozygous variant. Sanger sequence analysis using an alternative pair of primers may be used to detect variants at the primer region, which may also

make a heterozygous variant looks like a homozygous variant.

Therefore, reporting the variant as supporting a clinical diagnosis of X-linked adrenoleukodystrophy (X-ALD) would be a more appropriate next step in the workup for this patient.

48. **E.** *Rhizomelic chondrodysplasia punctata type 1 (RCDP1) classic type is an autosomal recessive peroxisome biogenesis disorder (PBD),* which is characterized by proximal shortening of the humerus and to a lesser degree the femur (rhizomelia), punctate calcifications in cartilage with epiphyseal and metaphyseal abnormalities (chondrodysplasia punctata, or CDP), coronal clefts of the vertebral bodies, and cataracts that are usually present at birth or appear in the first few months of life (http://www.ncbi.nlm.nih.gov/books/NBK1270/).

Ehlers—Danlos syndrome (EDS) is an example of a connective-tissue disorder. Long-chain 3-hydroxyacyl-CoA dehydrogenase (LCHAD) is an example of a fatty acid oxidation disorders. Gaucher disease is an example of a lysosomal disorder. Myoclonic epilepsy with ragged red fibers is an example of a mitochondrial disorder.

Therefore, rhizomelic chondrodysplasia punctate is a peroxisomal biogenesis disorder.

49. **C.** *Patients with rhizomelic chondrodysplasia punctata type 1 (RCDP1) have deficient red-blood-cell concentration of plasmalogens, elevated plasma concentration of phytanic acid, and normal plasma concentration of very-long-chain fatty acids (VLCFA)* (http://www.ncbi.nlm.nih.gov/books/NBK1270/).

Patients with X-linked adrenoleukodystrophy (X-ALD) have an increased concentration of VLCFA in plasma, but not a deficient red-blood-cell concentration of plasmalogens or elevated plasma concentration of phytanic acid. Patients with Zellweger spectrum disorder (ZSD), including Zellweger syndrome, neonatal adrenoleukodystrophy (NALD), and infantile Refsum disease (IRD), usually have elevated plasma concentrations of VLCFA (C26:0 and C26:1; elevated ratios of C24/C22 and C26/C22), increased concentrations of phytanic acid and/or pristanic acid (normal in NALD), reduced amounts of C16 and C18 plasmalogens (normal in IRD) (https://www.ncbi.nlm.nih.gov/books/NBK1448/).

Therefore, patients with rhizomelic chondrodysplasia punctate have a deficient red-blood-cell concentration of plasmalogens.

50. **F.** Rhizomelic chondrodysplasia punctata type 1 (RCDP1) classic type is an autosomal recessive peroxisomal biogenesis disorder (PBD), which is

characterized by proximal shortening of the humerus and to a lesser degree the femur (rhizomelia), punctate calcifications in cartilage with epiphyseal and metaphyseal abnormalities (chondrodysplasia punctata, or CDP), coronal clefts of the vertebral bodies, and cataracts that are usually present at birth or appear in the first few months of life *PEX7 is the only gene in which pathogenic variants cause RCDP1* (http://www.ncbi.nlm.nih.gov/books/NBK1270/).

Pathogenic variants in *ABCD1* cause X-linked adrenoleukodystrophy (X-ALD). Pathogenic variants in *COL1A1* cause autosomal dominant osteogenesis imperfecta. Pathogenic variants in *FGFR2* cause autosomal dominant craniosynostosis, such as Crouzon syndrome, Pfeiffer syndrome, and Saethre–Chotzen syndrome. Pathogenic variants in *PAX3* cause autosomal dominant Waardenburg syndrome.

Therefore, *PEX7* would most likely harbor pathogenic variant(s) in this patient if she had RCDP.

51. **B.** *Rhizomelic chondrodysplasia punctata type 1 (RCDP1) classic type is an autosomal recessive peroxisomal biogenesis disorder (PBD) caused by pathogenic variants in PEX7.* Biochemical tests of peroxisomal function include red-blood-cell concentration of plasmalogens (deficient), plasma concentration of phytanic acid (elevated), and plasma concentration of very long chain fatty acids (VLCFA) (normal) (http://www.ncbi.nlm.nih.gov/books/NBK1270/).

Approximately 39 unique *PEX7* pathogenic variants have been identified thus far (www.dbpex.org). The majority are nonsense, missense, or splice-site variants; small insertions; or deletions. *Sequencing analysis may detect small intragenic deletions/insertions and missense, nonsense, and splice-site variants; typically, exon or whole-gene deletions/duplications are not detected.* Sequence analysis of *PEX7* coding and flanking intronic regions in 133 individuals with RCDP1 from the United States and the Netherlands identified 97% of pathogenic alleles. In all individuals with biochemically confirmed RCDP1, at least one pathogenic *PEX7* allele was identified.

In this case, Sanger sequencing analysis detected a homozygous pathogenic variant for the autosomal recessive condition in the proband, whereas the parents were not related, which raised the suspicion of a large deletion/duplication or pathogenic variant at the primer region. Therefore, reflex deletion and duplication analysis of *PEX7* would be a more appropriate next step in the workup than others listed in the question for this patient. If the results were negative, Sanger sequence analysis using an alternative pair of primers should be considered.

52. **A.** The patient's clinical presentation and biochemical findings supported a clinical diagnosis of rhizomelic chondrodysplasia punctata type 1 (RCDP1), which is an autosomal recessive peroxisome biogenesis disorder (PBD), caused by pathogenic variants in *PEX7*. It is possible that the patient had an inherited variant from the mother and a de novo variant at the paternal derivative allele. However, gross deletion/duplications and variants at the primer regions limitations of Sanger sequencing, and these should be ruled out before interpreting the result as an inherited variant from the mother and a de novo variant at the paternal derivative allele.

Therefore, deletion and duplication analysis would be the most appropriate next step in the workup for this patient and her family. If the results were negative, Sanger sequencing analysis using an alternative pair of primers should be considered.

53. **D.** *Patients with Zellweger syndrome usually have overaccumulation of very-long-chain fatty acids and branched chain fatty acids, such as phytanic acid, and deficient levels of plasmalogens.*

Patients with neonatal adrenoleukodystrophy (NALD) have elevated plasma concentrations of VLCFA (C26:0 and C26:1; elevated ratios of C24/C22 and C26/C22), normal concentrations of phytanic acid and/or pristanic acid, and reduced amounts of C16 and C18 plasmalogens. Patients with infantile Refsum disease (IRD) usually have elevated plasma concentrations of VLCFA (C26:0 and C26:1; elevated ratios of C24/C22 and C26/C22), increased concentrations of phytanic acid and/or pristanic acid, and normal amounts of C16 and C18 plasmalogens. Patients with rhizomelic chondrodysplasia punctata type 1 (RCDP1) have deficient red-blood-cell concentration of plasmalogens, elevated plasma concentration of phytanic acid, and normal plasma concentration of very-long-chain fatty acids (VLCFA). Patients with X-linked adrenoleukodystrophy (X-ALD) have increased concentration of VLCFA in plasma, but not deficient red-blood-cell concentration of plasmalogens or elevated plasma concentration of phytanic acid.

Therefore, patients with Zellweger syndrome have overaccumulation of very-long-chain fatty acids and branched-chain fatty acids, such as phytanic acid, and deficient levels of plasmalogens.

54. C. Zellweger syndrome is an autosomal recessive disorder, caused by pathogenic variants in 12 different PEX genes (*PEX1*, *PXMP3* [*PEX2*], *PEX3*, *PEX5*, *PEX6*, *PEX10*, *PEX12*, *PEX13*, *PEX14*, *PEX16*, *PEX19*, and *PEX26*). *Therefore, next-generation sequencing (NGS) of all 12 genes at one time is the most cost-effective and sensitive method to confirm or rule out the diagnosis.* Pathogenic variants in *PEX1*, the most common cause of Zellweger syndrome are observed in about 68% of affected individuals. Two common *PEX1* mutations have been identified: c.2097dupT(p.Ile700TyrfsTer42; in exon 13) and c.2528G > A(p.Gly843Asp; in exon 15). About 80% of individuals with a *PEX1* defect have at least one of these two common alleles (https://www.ncbi.nlm.nih.gov/books/NBK1448/).

Exome sequencing has been used for patients with rare disorders without a diagnosis. Multiplex ligation-dependent probe amplification (MLPA) is for deletions and duplications smaller than the resolution of chromosomal microarray, but they cannot be detected by sequencing, such as a deletion including one exon and part of introns. Sanger sequencing is cost-effective for one gene not as big as *DMD* with pathogenic variants all over the gene, TaqMan genotyping assay is a target genotyping method to detect known single-nucleotide variants.

Therefore, an NGS panel would be the most cost-effective and sensitive test to confirm the diagnosis and for family management.

55. C. *Zellweger syndrome is an autosomal recessive disorder*, caused by pathogenic variants in 12 different PEX genes (*PEX1*, *PXMP3* [*PEX2*], *PEX3*, *PEX5*, *PEX6*, *PEX10*, *PEX12*, *PEX13*, *PEX14*, *PEX16*, *PEX19*, and *PEX26*). Patients with Zellweger syndrome usually have over-accumulation of very long chain fatty acids and branched chain fatty acids, such as phytanic acid, and deficient levels of plasmalogens.

The patient's parents were first degree relatives. It is likely the patient had a homozygous pathogenic variant, c.2097dupT(p.Ile700TyrfsTer42), in *PEX1* in comparison with other possibilities, such as one heterozygous variant and one deletion/duplication, which may not be detected by a NGS panel. The possibility of one heterozygous variant with a variant at the primer region was also low in this case. Parent testing may confirm if both of the parents were carriers, which might indirectly confirm the patient had a homozygous variant. There was no need to request second specimen from the patient and his family members for confirmation.

Therefore, the most appropriate next step in the workup for this patient and his family was to report that the patient had Zellweger syndrome and to recommend studies for the parents.

56. A. *HFE*-associated hereditary hemochromatosis (*HFE*-HH) is characterized by excessive storage of iron in the liver, skin, pancreas, heart, joints, and testes. It is more common in men than in women. *Advanced iron overload may cause hepatomegaly, hepatic cirrhosis, and hepatocellular carcinoma* (https://www.ncbi.nlm.nih.gov/books/NBK1440/).

Therefore, this patient would be at increased risk to develop hepatocarcinoma.

57. F. Clinical symptoms of *HFE*-associated hereditary hemochromatosis (*HFE*-HH) are hepatomegaly, hepatic cirrhosis, hepatocellular carcinoma, diabetes mellitus, cardiomyopathy, hypogonadism, arthritis (especially involving the metacarpophalangeal joints), and progressive increase in skin pigmentation. But rhabdomyolysis is not one of the symptoms in patients with *HFE*-HH.

Therefore, the couple's future children would NOT be at increased risk to develop rhabdomyolysis due to *HFE*-HH.

58. D. *HFE*-associated hereditary hemochromatosis (*HFE*-HH) is the most common form of HH associated with the homozygous p.C282Y pathogenic variant of the *HFE* gene. Although the prevalence of end-organ damage secondary to *HFE*-HH is relatively low, the p.Cys282Tyr variant is highly prevalent among populations of northern European ancestry, but rare among Asians. The majority of patients with homozygous p.Cys282Tyr variant have neither clinical manifestations of *HFE*-HH nor iron overload. A substantial number of patients have biochemical *HFE*-HH evidenced by iron overload but have no clinical symptoms. Targeted variant analysis for p.Cys282Tyr and p.His63Asp is used in most clinical laboratories, since they account for the vast majority of disease-causing alleles in the population. Because *HFE*-HH is an adult-onset, treatable disorder with low clinical penetrance, prenatal testing is highly unusual even though it is technically feasible (https://www.ncbi.nlm.nih.gov/books/NBK1440/).

Therefore, in order for *HFE*-HH to be symptomatic, both copies of the *HFE* gene must be mutated.

59. E. Hereditary hemochromatosis (HH) is an inherited disorder characterized by progressive iron deposition and tissue injury in multiple organs secondary to an inherited predisposition to excessive and inappropriately regulated intestinal iron absorption. HH has been demonstrated to result from pathogenic variants in several genes involved in the regulation of iron homeostasis such as *HFE, TfR2, HJV, HAMP,* and *SLC40A1* (ferroportin).

HFE-associated hereditary hemochromatosis (*HFE*-HH) is the most common form of HH associated with the homozygous p.C282Y pathogenic variant of the *HFE* gene. At least four additional iron overload hemochromatoses have been identified. Juvenile hemochromatosis, or hemochromatosis type 2 (HFE2), is divided into two forms: HFE2A, caused by mutation in *HJV,* and HFE2B, caused by mutation in *HAMP.* Hemochromatosis type 3 is caused by mutations in *TFR2.* Hemochromatosis type 4 is caused by heterozygous mutations in *SLC40A1.* Pathogenic variants in *ATP7A* cause Menkes disease; pathogenic variants in *ATP7B* cause Wilson disease; both are associated with abnormal copper metabolism.

Therefore, *ATP7A* is NOT associated with iron overload.

60. **D.** At least 28 distinct pathogenic variants in *HFE* have been reported; most are missense or nonsense. Two missense variants account for the vast majority of disease-causing alleles (https://www.gwumc.edu/edu/obgyn/genetics/casestudies/casestudy05.html). They are p.Cys282Tyr and p.His63Asp. *Approximately 60%—90% of patients with HFE-associated hereditary hemochromatosis (HFE-HH) have homozygous p.Cys282Tyr variants. Approximately 3%—8% of HFE-HH patients have compound heterozygous p.Cys282Tyr and p.His63Asp variants.*

In addition, p.Ser65Cys has been seen in combination with p.Cys282Tyr in individuals with iron overload. Unlike individuals heterozygous for the common pathogenic variants, no p.Ser65Cys/wt heterozygotes had elevation of both serum TS (transferrin saturation) and ferritin. A number of private pathogenic variants have also been described, including p.Glu168Ter and p.Trp169Ter, which were found with an allele frequency of 25% and 8.4%, respectively, in individuals with hemochromatosis in two northern regions of Italy (https://www.ncbi.nlm.nih.gov/books/NBK1440/).

Therefore, targeted mutation analysis would be the most appropriate test for this patient.

61. **A.** Hereditary hemochromatosis (HH) is an inherited disorder characterized by progressive iron deposition and tissue injury in multiple organs secondary to an inherited predisposition to excessive and inappropriately regulated intestinal iron absorption (https://www.gwumc.edu/edu/obgyn/genetics/casestudies/casestudy05.html). HH has been demonstrated to result from pathogenic variants in several genes involved in the regulation of iron homeostasis such as *HFE, TfR2, HJV, HAMP,* and *SLC40A1* (ferroportin). *HFE*-associated hereditary hemochromatosis (*HFE*-HH) is the most common form of HH.

Approximately 60%—90% of patients with HFE-associated hereditary hemochromatosis (HFE-HH) have homozygous p.Cys282Tyr variants. Approximately 3%—8% of *HFE*-HH patients have compound heterozygous p.Cys282Tyr and p.His63Asp variants. Individuals who are compound heterozygous for p.Cys282Tyr and p.Ser65Cys may have a small risk for mild hemochromatosis. This rare variant displays a very low penetrance. The p.Ser65Cys variant has been seen in combination with p.Cys282Tyr in individuals with iron overload. But no p.Ser65Cys/wt heterozygotes had elevation of both serum TS (transferrin saturation) and ferritin (https://www.ncbi.nlm.nih.gov/books/NBK1440/).

Therefore, this patient most likely had homozygous the p.Cys282Tyr variant if he had HH.

62. **E.** Approximately 60%—90% of patients with *HFE*-associated hereditary hemochromatosis (*HFE*-HH) have homozygous p.Cys282Tyr variants. Approximately 3%—8% of *HFE*-HH patients have compound heterozygous p.Cys282Tyr and p.His63Asp variants. Individuals who are homozygous for p.His63Asp may have iron overload, which is the diagnosis for biochemical *HFE*-HH.

Three longitudinal population-based screening studies showed that 38%—50% of p.Cys282Tyr homozygotes may develop iron overload (elevated serum ferritin concentration) and 10%—33% may eventually develop hemochromatosis-related symptoms, including nonspecific symptoms, such as fatigue and arthralgia, or end-organ damage, such as diabetes mellitus, cirrhosis, and/or cardiomyopathy. The vast majority of those who develop end-organ damage are male. Women usually develop symptoms after menopause because of a natural correction of iron overload that occurred during the reproductive age. The penetrance for p.Cys282Tyr/p.His63Asp compound heterozygotes is low: only approximately 0.5%—2.0% of such individuals develop clinical evidence of iron overload. The penetrance for p.His63Asp homozygotes is even lower than the penetrance of the p.Cys282Tyr/p.His63Asp compound heterozygotes; although biochemically defined abnormalities may be present, characteristic clinical manifestations are rare. *Because of the low penetrance and variable expressivity, population screening for HFE-HH is not cost-effective* (https://www.ncbi.nlm.nih.gov/books/NBK1440/).

Therefore, population screening for HH is not a cost-effective method of proactive management.

63. **A.** Menkes disease is caused by homozygous or compound heterozygous pathogenic variants in *ATP7A*. Infants with classic Menkes disease appear healthy until the age of 2–3 months, when loss of developmental milestones, hypotonia, seizures, and failure to thrive occur. The diagnosis is usually suspected when infants exhibit typical neurological changes and concomitant characteristic changes of the hair (short, sparse, coarse, twisted, and often lightly pigmented). Temperature instability and hypoglycemia may be present in the neonatal period. Death usually occurs by age 3 years (https://www.ncbi.nlm.nih.gov/books/NBK1413/).

Pathogenic variants in *ATP7B* are associated with Wilson disease. Pathogenic variants in *HFE*, *HJV*, *HAMP*, *TFR2*, and *SLC40A1* are associated with iron overload.

Therefore, *ATP7A* would most likely harbor pathogenic variant(s) in this patient.

64. **C.** Menkes disease is caused by pathogenic variants in *ATP7A* at Xq21.1. The male patient in this question had a hemizygous pathogenic variant in *ATP7A* instead of a homozygous variant. His mother carried the same variant in the heterozygous state, so she was asymptomatic owing to skewed X-inactivation. In theory, unfavorably skewed X-chromosome inactivation in some heterozygous females could be associated with neurological or other clinical findings related to the disorders. About 50% of females who are obligate heterozygotes for an *ATP7A* pathogenic variant demonstrate regions of pili torti, though (https://www.ncbi.nlm.nih.gov/books/NBK1413/).

Therefore, the patient inherited the pathogenic variant from the mother and had Menkes disease.

65. **A.** Menkes disease is caused by pathogenic variants in *ATP7A* at Xq21.1. Sequence analysis of the gene may detect 80% of probands. Gene-targeted deletion/duplication analysis may detect 20% of probands. *Lack of amplification by PCR prior to sequence analysis can suggest a putative (multi)exon or whole-gene deletion on the X chromosome in affected males; confirmation requires additional testing by gene-targeted deletion/duplication analysis* (https://www.ncbi.nlm.nih.gov/books/NBK1413/).

Therefore, reflex deletion/duplication testing would be the most appropriate next step in the workup for this patient.

66. **D.** *ATP7A* contains 23 exons spanning 150 kb of genomic DNA. The coding sequence is 4.5 kb. Pathogenic variants tend to be family-specific. Variant types include small insertions and deletions (35%); nonsense (20%), splicing (15%), and missense (8%) variants; and large deletions or rearrangements (20%).

The protein encoded by *ATP7A*, a P-type ATPase, transports copper across cellular membranes and is critical for copper homeostasis. *ATP7A pathogenic variants may result in a gene product with no copper transport capability (associated with a severe phenotype) or reduced quantity of normally functioning gene product (associated with a milder phenotype)* (https://www.ncbi.nlm.nih.gov/books/NBK1413/).

Therefore, the pathogenic variant detected in this patient would most likely represent a loss-of-function variant in *ATP7A*.

67. **B.** Wilson disease is an autosomal recessive disorder of copper metabolism that can present with hepatic, neurological, or psychiatric disturbances, or a combination of these, in individuals ranging from age 3 years to older than 50 years; symptoms vary among and within families. Kayser–Fleischer rings, frequently present, result from copper deposition in the Descemet membrane of the cornea and reflect a high degree of copper storage in the body. *ATP7B is the only gene in which pathogenic variants cause Wilson disease* (https://www.ncbi.nlm.nih.gov/books/NBK1512/).

Pathogenic variants in *ATP7A* are associated with Menkes disease. Pathogenic variants in *HFE*, *HJV*, *HAMP*, *TFR2*, and *SLC40A1* are associated with iron overload (hemochromatosis).

Therefore, it would be most likely that *ATP7B* harbored pathogenic variant(s) in this patient.

68. **E.** Wilson disease is an autosomal recessive condition cause by biallelic pathogenic variants in *ATP7B*. In this case, the parents of the patient were related, so it was likely that they carried the same pathogenic variant in *ATP7B*. If so, it explained why the patient had a homozygous pathogenic variant. The c.2333G > T(p.Arg778Leu) variant detected in this patient is the only relatively common pathogenic variant, accounting for approximately 57% of Wilson disease–causing alleles in the Asian population younger than age 18 years (https://www.ncbi.nlm.nih.gov/books/NBK1512/).

A new lot of all reagents may be considered if the positive controls showed negative results and/or negative controls showed positive results. Another set of primers may be considered if the controls are in the normal range and the quality and quantity of the DNA from the patient are in the acceptable range but the patient's results are unexplainable. For example, a patient has a homozygous pathogenic variant for an autosomal recessive disorder; but only one of the parents is a carrier. Another type of specimen from a patient may be considered if tissue-type–specific mosaicism is suspected, such as Pallister–Killian syndrome. Reflex testing for deletions/duplications is recommended in situations in which only a heterozygous pathogenic variant is detected by sequencing analysis for an autosomal recessive condition. Clinical tests in a CAP/CLIA-certified laboratory should be done through standard validation. In normal circumstances, there is no need to send samples to another laboratory for confirmation. But it is a widespread practice to send samples to other CAP/CLIA-certified laboratories for confirmation during validation.

Therefore, this molecular result confirmed the clinical diagnosis of Wilson disease in the patient.

69. **D.** Wilson disease is an autosomal recessive condition, cause by biallelic pathogenic variants in *ATP7B*. *ATP7B* is encoded by 21 exons spanning approximately 78 kb on 13q14.3. *ATP7B* has 57% identity with *ATP7A*, the gene defective in Menkes disease. More than 800 pathogenic variants have been identified (see Wilson Disease Mutation Database at https://databases.lovd.nl/shared/genes/ATP7B), including nonsense, missense, frameshift, and splice-site variants as well as large deletions. The c.3207C > A(p.His1069Gln) variant, in a highly conserved motif close to the ATP-binding region, accounts for 35%–45% of Wilson disease–causing alleles in a mixed European population, and a greater proportion in Eastern Europe. It occurs at a frequency of 26%–70% in various populations and is associated with neurological or hepatic disease and a mean age at onset of about 20 years.

The product of *ATP7B* is copper-transporting ATPase 2, an intracellular transmembrane copper transporter that is key in incorporating copper into ceruloplasmin and in moving copper out of the hepatocyte into bile. The protein is a P-type ATPase, characterized by cation-channel and phosphorylation domains containing a highly conserved Asp-Lys-Thr-Gly-Thr (DKTGT) motif, in which the aspartate residue forms a phosphorylated intermediate during the transport cycle. *Tissue damage occurs after excessive copper*

accumulation resulting from lack of copper transport from the liver. Even when no transporter function is present, accumulation of copper occurs over several years (https://www.ncbi.nlm.nih.gov/books/NBK1512/).

Therefore, loss of function would most likely describe the pathogenesis of Wilson disease in this patient and others with Wilson disease.

70. **C.** Alagille syndrome (ALGS) is recognized by a paucity of bile ducts in the liver, along with involvement of the heart, eyes and skeleton and typical facial features. Kayser–Fleischer (KF) rings are usually seen in patients with Wilson disease, but are not specific for Wilson disease. KF rings may in extremely rare cases be seen in copper accumulation associated with cholestatic liver diseases or autoimmune hepatitis. Cholestasis is one of the major clinical manifestations of ALGS. *The two genes in which pathogenic variants are known to cause ALGS are JAG1 and NOTCH2* (http://www.ncbi.nlm.nih.gov/books/NBK1273/).

Pathogenic variants in *ATP7A* cause Menkes disease. Pathogenic variants in *ATP7B* cause Wilson disease. *JAG2* is in the Notch signal pathway with uncertain clinical impact. *JAG3* is not known to be a gene in human genome.

Therefore, *JAG1* would most likely harbor pathogenic variant(s) for Alagille syndrome in this patient if he had Alagille syndrome.

71. **A.** Pathogenic variants in both *JAG1* and *NOTCH2* cause Alagille syndrome (ALGS). *Sequence analysis of JAG1 detects pathogenic variants in more than 89% of individuals who meet clinical diagnostic criteria; deletion/duplication analysis detects exon and whole-gene deletions, including microdeletion of 20p12, in approximately 7% of affected individuals. Pathogenic variants in NOTCH2 are observed in 1%–2% of individuals with ALGS* (http://www.ncbi.nlm.nih.gov/books/NBK1273/).

JAG2 is in the Notch signal pathway with uncertain clinical impact. *JAG3* is not known to be a gene in the human genome. Pathogenic variants in *NOTCH1* cause autosomal dominant Adams–Oliver syndrome and aortic-valve disease. Pathogenic variants in exon 34 of *NOTCH2* cause Hajdu–Chenney syndrome. Pathogenic variants in *NOTCH3* cause autosomal dominant cerebral arteriopathy with subcortical infarcts and leukoencephalopathy (CADASIL), and lateral meningocele syndrome.

Therefore, *JAG1* would the most likely harbor pathogenic variant(s) in this patient if he had Alagille syndrome.

72. **B.** *Alagille syndrome (ALGS) is an autosomal dominant condition.* ALGS demonstrates highly variable

expressivity with incomplete penetrance. The clinical features range from subclinical to severe. To determine the range and frequency of clinical findings in individuals with a *JAG1* pathogenic variant and hence, the penetrance, Kamath et al. studied 53 *JAG1* variant-confirmed relatives of probands with ALGS. Of their findings, 21% met diagnostic criteria independent of family history; 32% were asymptomatic, but met clinical diagnostic criteria when additional testing was performed (analysis of liver enzymes, cardiac examination, eye examination, or skeletal X-rays); 43% had one or two features of ALGS; 4% had no features of ALGS. Based on these data, penetrance is 96%; however, only 53% meet the clinical diagnostic criteria for ALGS (http://www.ncbi.nlm.nih.gov/books/NBK1273/).

A new lot of all reagents may be considered if the positive controls showed negative results and/or negative controls showed positive results. Another set of primers may be considered if the controls are in the normal range and the quality and quantity of the DNA from the patient are in acceptable range; but the patient's results are unexplainable. For example, a patient has a homozygous pathogenic variant for an autosomal recessive disorder, but only one of the parents is a carrier. Another type of specimen from a patient may be considered if tissue-type–specific mosaicism is suspected, such as Pallister–Killian syndrome. Reflex testing for deletions/duplications is recommended in situations in which only a heterozygous pathogenic variant is detected by sequencing analysis for an autosomal recessive disorder. Clinical tests in a CAP/CLIA-certified laboratory should be done through standard validation. In normal circumstances, there is no need to send samples to another laboratory for confirmation. But it is a widespread practice to send samples to other CAP/CLIA-certified laboratories for confirmation during validation.

Therefore, additional testing of the patient's mother should be considered for ALGS.

73. **C.** Alagille syndrome (ALGS) is an autosomal dominant condition, caused by pathogenic variants in *JAG1* and *NOTCH1*. *JAG1* comprises 26 exons. More than 226 pathogenic variants have been identified in individuals with ALGS. Pathogenic variant types have included deletion of the entire *JAG1* gene (4%), protein-truncating variants (frameshift and nonsense) (69%), pathogenic splice variants (16%), and pathogenic missense variants (11%). Jagged-1 is a cell-surface protein that functions as a ligand for the neurogenic locus notch homolog protein 2 (Notch) transmembrane receptors, key signaling molecules found on the surface of a variety of cells. *Haploinsufficiency of Jagged-1 has been shown to result in ALGS as evidenced by those individuals with ALGS who have a cytogenetically detectable deletion of chromosome 20p12 encompassing the entire JAG1 gene.* Haploinsufficiency is likely the pathogenic mechanism in the majority of cases of ALGS, as most pathogenic variants result in or predict a severely truncated protein product, lacking the transmembrane region necessary for the protein product to embed in the cell membrane and participate in signaling (http://www.ncbi.nlm.nih.gov/books/NBK1273/).

Therefore, haploinsufficiency would most appropriately describe the pathogenesis of Alagille syndrome in this patient, though loss of function is technically also correct.

74. **A.** Canavan disease, also called "spongiform degeneration of cerebral white matter," is an autosomal recessive demyelinating disease caused by deficiency of aspartoacyclase, which catalyzes the breakdown of *N*-acetylaspartic acid (NAA). Excessive accumulation of NAA is responsible for the central nervous system changes in this disease.

Metachromatic leukodystrophy (MLD), also known as "arylsulfatase A deficiency," is a lysosomal storage disease that is commonly listed as one of the leukodystrophies. Pompe disease is an autosomal recessive disorder caused by deficiency of the lysosomal enzyme acid-α-glucosidase (GAA), leading to generalized accumulation of lysosomal glycogen, especially in the heart, skeletal and smooth muscle, and the nervous system. X-linked adrenoleukodystrophy (X-ALD) is a disorder of peroxisomal fatty acid beta-oxidation, which results in the accumulation of very-long-chain fatty acids in tissues throughout the body. Zellweger syndrome spectrum disorders, including infantile Refsum disease, neonatal adrenoleukodystrophy, and Zellweger syndrome, are peroxisomal biogenesis disorders (PBDs).

Therefore, the patient would most likely have Canavan disease.

75. **A.** Canavan disease (CD), also called "spongiform degeneration of cerebral white matter," is an autosomal recessive demyelinating disease caused by deficiency of aspartoacyclase, which catalyzes the breakdown of *N*-acetylaspartic acid (NAA). *ASPA is the only gene in which pathogenic variants cause Canavan disease.*

ELP1 (*IKBKAP*) is the only gene in which pathogenic variants cause familial dysautonomia. *GAA* is the only gene in which pathogenic variants cause Pompe disease, also known as "glycogen storage disease II." *GLA* is the only gene in which pathogenic variants cause FD. *MEFV* is the only gene in which pathogenic variants cause familial Mediterranean fever.

Therefore, *ASPA* would most likely be tested for Canavan disease (CD) in this patient.

76. **E.** While Canavan disease occurs in all ethnic groups, most reported individuals are of Ashkenazi Jewish origin. *ASPA* is the only gene in which pathogenic variants are known to cause with Canavan disease. *Two pathogenic variants, p. Glu285Ala and p.Tyr231Ter, account for 98% of pathogenic variants in the Ashkenazi Jewish population.* One pathogenic variant, p.Ala305Glu, accounts for approximately 1% of pathogenic variants in the Ashkenazi Jewish populations (https://www.ncbi.nlm.nih.gov/books/NBK1234/).

Therefore, target variant analysis of the founder pathogenic variants would most likely be used as a first-tier test to detect pathogenic variants for Canavan disease in this Ashkenazi Jewish patient.

77. **D.** Canavan disease occurs in all ethnic groups. But most reported individuals are of Ashkenazi Jewish origin. Two pathogenic variants, p.Glu285Ala and p.Tyr231Ter, account for 98% of pathogenic variants in the Ashkenazi Jewish population and 3% of pathogenic variants in non−Ashkenazi Jewish populations. One pathogenic variant, p.Ala305Glu, accounts for 30%−60% of pathogenic variants in non-Ashkenazi Jewish populations and approximately 1% of pathogenic variants in Ashkenazi Jewish populations. More than 50 other pathogenic variants have been reported in non-Ashkenazi Jewish populations. *Sequence analysis may detect 87% disease-causing alleles in non-Ashkenazi Jewish* (https://www.ncbi.nlm.nih.gov/books/NBK1234/).

Therefore, Sanger sequencing of *ASPA* would most likely be used as a first-tier test to detect pathogenic variants in this non-Ashkenazi Jewish patient.

78. **D.** Canavan disease (CD) is a progressive autosomal recessive disease of the central nervous system. It occurs in all ethnic backgrounds but is highly prevalent in the Ashkenazi Jewish population owing to the founder effect. *ASPA* is the only gene in which pathogenic variants cause CD; two founder mutations, c.854A > C(p.Glu285Ala) and c.693C > A(p.Tyr231X), in *ASPA* present in 98% Ashkenazi Jewish patients. The third one, c.914C > A(p.Ala305 Glu), was detected in 1% of Ashkenazi Jewish patients (https://www.ncbi.nlm.nih.gov/books/NBK1234/).

The residual carrier risk of the husband was 1% with the negative result on these three pathogenic variants in *ASPA*. The wife was a carrier. Therefore, the most appropriate estimation of the residue risk of this couple's first-born child with Canavan disease would be $1\% \times 1 \times 1/4 = 1/400 \ (0.25\%)$.

79. **D.** *ASPA* is the only gene in which pathogenic variants cause Canavan disease (CD). *ASPA* encodes for aspartoacylase, which is responsible for hydrolyzing *N*-acetylaspartic acid (NAA) into aspartic acid and acetate. The specific buildup of NAA in the brain causes demyelinization and other signs of the disease.

Aspartoacylase enzyme activity is extremely low in normal amniocytes and chorionic villus sampling (CVS). Enzyme activity cannot be relied upon for prenatal testing. Carrier detection using biochemical assay is not routinely possible because it relies on a complex enzyme assay in cultured skin fibroblasts. In neonatal/infantile (severe) Canavan disease, the mean concentration of *N*-acetylaspartic acid (NAA) ($n = 117$) was 1440.5 ± 873.3 μmol/mmol of creatinine. Control values in one series ($n = 48$) were 23.5 ± 16.1 μmol/mmol of creatinine. Prenatal testing can be performed by measuring the level of NAA in amniotic fluid at 15−18 weeks' gestation; but it is an invasive procedure, and the couple has to wait several weeks for it.

Two founder mutations, c.854A > C (p.Glu285Ala) and c.693C > A(p.Tyr231X), in *ASPA* present in 98% of Ashkenazi Jewish patients. The third, c.914C > A(p.Ala305 Glu), was detected in 1% of Ashkenazi Jewish patients. The c.433-2A > G splice-site variant was found in a single Ashkenazi Jewish family. All laboratories use at least a two-variant panel for the Ashkenazi Jewish pathogenic variants; many laboratories use a three-variant panel, and a few use a four-variant panel. The detection rate of targeted variant panel is at least 98% in Ashkenazi Jews (https://www.ncbi.nlm.nih.gov/books/NBK1234/).

Testing for at-risk relatives usually requires prior identification of the pathogenic variants in the family. In this case, the proband, the wife's brother passed away without pathogenic variants being identified. The wife's parents are obligate heterozygous carriers, but they are not available for genetic study.

Therefore, targeted mutation analysis of *ASPA* with the peripheral-blood sample from the wife is the most appropriate first-tier study for this family to estimate the fetus's risk for Canavan disease.

References

1. Nussbaum RL, McInnes RR, Willard HF. *Thompson & Thompson genetics in medicine.* 8th ed. Philadelphia: Elsevier; 2016. xi, 546 pp.

2. Park SY, et al. Screening for chromosomal abnormalities using combined test in the first trimester of pregnancy. *Obstet Gynecol Sci* 2016;**59**(5):357–66.

3. Driscoll DA, Gross SJ, Professional Practice Guidelines Committee. Screenin for fetal aneuploidy and neural tube defects. *Genet Med* 2009;**11**(11):818–21.

4. Allyse M, et al. Non-invasive prenatal testing: a review of international implementation and challenges. *Int J Womens Health* 2015;**7**:113–26.

5. Cao Y, et al. False negative cell-free DNA screening result in a newborn with trisomy 13. *Case Rep Genet* 2016;**2016**:7397405.

6. Committee Opinion No. 640: cell-free DNA screening for fetal aneuploidy. *Obstet Gynecol* 2015;**126**(3):e31–7.

7. Smith M, et al. A case of false negative NIPT for Down syndrome-lessons learned. *Case Rep Genet* 2014;**2014**:823504.

8. Gregg AR, et al. ACMG statement on noninvasive prenatal screening for fetal aneuploidy. *Genet Med* 2013;**15**(5):395–8.

9. Newborn screening: toward a uniform screening panel and system. *Genet Med* 2006;**8**(Suppl. 1):1S–252S.

10. Tim-Aroon T, et al. Stopping parenteral nutrition for 3 hours reduces false positives in newborn screening. *J Pediatr* 2015;**167**(2):312–16.

11. Alfirevic Z, Navaratnam K, Mujezinovic F. Amniocentesis and chorionic villus sampling for prenatal diagnosis. *Cochrane Database Syst Rev* 2017;**9**:CD003252.

12. Yousuf R, et al. Hemolytic disease of the fetus and newborn caused by anti-D and anti-S alloantibodies: a case report. *J Med Case Rep* 2012;**6**:71.

13. Usman AS, et al. Hemolytic disease of the fetus and newborn caused by anti-E. *Asian J Transfus Sci* 2013;**7**(1):84–5.

14. Centers for Disease Control and Prevention. CDC grand rounds: newborn screening and improved outcomes. *MMWR Morb Mortal Wkly Rep* 2012;**61**(21):390–3.

15. Acikalin A, Disel NR. A rare cause of postpartum coma: isolated hyperammonemia due to urea cycle disorder. *Am J Emerg Med* 2016;**34**(9):1894–5.

16. Karnaneedi S, et al. Phenylketonuria in a six year old Malay boy – a case report. *Med J Malaysia* 1989;**44**(3):248–51.

17. Mozley E, John K, Cregeen D, Hutton I, Vara R, Olpin S, et al. *A case study from the LCHADD Newborn Bloodspot Screening pilot in England*; 2010. http://www.viapath.co.uk/sites/default/files/upload/PDFs/SSIEM%20LCHADD.pdf.

18. Tong MK, et al. Very long-chain acyl-CoA dehydrogenase deficiency presenting as acute hypercapnic respiratory failure. *Eur Respir J* 2006;**28**(2):447–50.

19. Raas-Rothschild A, et al. A PEX6-defective peroxisomal biogenesis disorder with severe phenotype in an infant, versus mild phenotype resembling Usher syndrome in the affected parents. *Am J Hum Genet* 2002;**70**(4):1062–8.

20. Galesanu C, Lisnic N, Branisteanu D, Moisii L, Tache C, Diaconu G, et al. Adrenoleukodystrophy – case report. *Acta Endocrinol (Buc)* 2005;**1**(3):359–68.

21. Joshi T, Joshi A, Chikhlonde R, Deshmukh L. Rhizomelic chondrodysplasia punctata: a case report. *J Pediatr Neonatol* 2015;**17**(1).

22. Karabayir N, et al. A case of rhizomelic chondrodysplasia punctata in newborn. *Case Rep Med* 2014;**2014**:879679.

23. Kheir AE. Zellweger syndrome: a cause of neonatal hypotonia and seizures. *Sudan J Paediatr* 2011;**11**(2):54–8.

24. Rosana A, La Rosa L. A case of hereditary haemochromatosis in a patient with extrapyramidal syndrome. *Blood Transfus* 2007;**5**(4):241–3.

25. Agertt F, et al. Menkes' disease: case report. *Arq Neuropsiquiatr* 2007;**65**(1):157–60.

26. Barzegar M, Fayyazie A, Gasemie B, Shoja MAM. Menkes disease: report of two cases. *Iran J Pediatr.* 2007;**17**(3):388–92.

27. Esezobor CI, et al. Wilson disease in a Nigerian child: a case report. *J Med Case Rep* 2012;**6**:200.

28. Raju K, et al. Wilson's disease: a clinical autopsy case report with review of literature. *J Nat Sci Biol Med* 2015;**6**(1):248–52.

29. Barbosa ER, et al. Wilson's disease: a case report and a historical review. *Arq Neuropsiquiatr* 2009;**67**(2B):539–43.

30. Bhatia V, Kumar P. Alagille syndrome with a previously undescribed mutation. *Indian Pediatr* 2014;**51**(4):314–16.

31. Mo-Kiu Lau C-MJ, Lee W-Y, Shen C-T, Wang Y-C, Wu C-Y, Kung C-H. Alagille syndrome: a case report. *Chin J Radiol* 1998;**23**(2):61–3.

32. Kamath BM, et al. Consequences of JAG1 mutations. *J Med Genet* 2003;**40**(12):891–5.

33. Hamaguchi H, et al. A case of Canavan disease: the first biochemically proven case in a Japanese girl. *Brain Dev* 1993;**15**(5):367–71.

34. Michelakakis H, et al. Canavan disease: findings in four new cases. *J Inherit Metab Dis* 1991;**14**(2):267–8.

35. Alving AS, Carson PE, Flanagan CL, Ickes CE. Enzymatic deficiency in primaquine-sensitive erythrocytes. *Science.* 1956;**124**(3220):484–5.

Further Reading

- American College of Medical Genetics (ACMG) (www.acmg.net/)
- American Pregnancy Association (www.americanpregnancy.org/)
- American College of Obstetricians and Gynecologists (ACOG) (www.acog.org/)
- Centers for Disease Control and Prevention (www.cdc.gov/)
- dbPEX, PEX Gene Database (www.dbpex.org)
- GeneReviews (www.ncbi.nlm.nih.gov/books/)
- Genetics Home Reference (www.ghr.nlm.nih.gov/)
- Global Variome shared LOVD *ATP7B* (https://databases.lovd.nl/shared/genes/ATP7B)
- Health Resources & Services Administration (www.hrsa.gov/)
- National Cancer Institute (www.cancer.gov)
- Newborn Screening Portal at Centers for Disease Control and Prevention (www.cdc.gov/newbornscreening/)
- Online Mendelian Inheritance in Man (https://omim.org/)
- The American College of Obstetricians and Gynecologists (http://www.acog.org/)
- UpToDate (http://www.uptodate.com/)

12

Other Common Genetic Syndromes

Nearly all human diseases have a genetic component. There are between 4000 and 6000 diagnosed genetic disorders. In Canada, genetic disorders may account for up to 40% of the work of hospital-based pediatric practice.[1] In the United Kingdom, it is estimated that 1 in 25 children is affected by a genetic disorder each year, meaning that 30,000 babies and children are newly diagnosed per year (http://www.geneticdisordersuk.org/). Some genetic disorders are apparent at birth (such as sickle cell disease and most metabolic disorders), whereas others are diagnosed at different stages throughout childhood (such as hearing loss), and sometimes into adulthood (such as Huntington disease). A genetic disorder is a disease caused in whole or in part by a change in the DNA sequence. Traditionally genetic disorders are classified into three main categories: dominant, recessive, and X-linked. The following are also considered to be genetic disorders: Y and mitochondria, abnormalities; susceptibilities to cancer and complex disease, such as BRCA1 and familial breast—ovarian cancer susceptibility, CFH, and macular degeneration; and certain somatic-cell genetic diseases, such as GNAS and McCune—Albright syndrome, and tetrasomy 12p and Pallister—Killian syndrome. According to Online Mendelian Inheritance in Man (OMIM) entry statistics (updated March 1, 2018), there are 15,846 genes. Of these, 6161 phenotypes have a known molecular basis and 3880 genes have phenotype-causing mutations (www.omim.org). And it is not uncommon for one gene to cause more than one phenotypes (1223 of the 3880 genes [32%] correspond to more than one phenotype).

Beyond these, most genetic disorders are "multifactorial inheritance disorders," with a combination of both inherited mutations in multiple genes and environmental factors. Examples of such diseases include many commonly occurring diseases, such as heart disease and diabetes, which are present in many people in different populations around the world. In this sense, genetic disorders may also be classified into three main categories: monogenetic, multifactorial inheritance, and chromosome disorders (including duplications) (www.genome.gov). In recent years, epigenetic changes have been recognized in genetic disorders. The classical example is the imprinting centers at 15q11.2 for Prader—Willi and Angelman syndromes.

Some somatic pathogenic variants do not cause genetic disorders, but rather are related to diagnosis, prognosis, and treatment, which are also frequently tested in clinical genetic laboratories. For example, acquired BRAF pathogenic variants have been found in malignant melanoma, colorectal carcinoma, papillary thyroid carcinoma, astrocytoma, and other disorders, which are related to the eligibility of using BRAF inhibitors, such as vemurafenib (Zelboraf) and dabrafenib (Tafinlar).

This chapter covers the genetic syndromes that affect multiple organ systems, that are not covered in other chapters. In the chapter, you will see that pathogenic variants in one gene may cause more than one syndrome, such as pathogenic variants in the GLI3 gene for Greig cephalopolysyndactyly syndrome and Pallister—Hall syndrome. Also, one syndrome may be caused by multiple genes—for example, Noonan syndrome may be caused by pathogenic variants in PTPN11, SOS1, RAF1, RIT1, NRAS, BRAF, and MAP2K1. Below is a list of selected genetic diseases covered in this chapter:

- Hereditary polycystic kidney diseases
- Bardet—Biedl syndrome
- Alport syndrome
- Alzheimer disease
- Nonsyndromic congenital hearing loss and deafness
- Usher syndrome
- Pendred syndrome
- Branchio-oto-renal (BOR) syndrome
- Waardenburg syndrome

- Mitochondrial DNA (mtDNA) depletion syndromes
- Leber hereditary optic neuropathy
- Maternally inherited diabetes–deafness syndrome
- Myoclonic epilepsy with ragged-red fibers
- MELAS (mitochondrial encephalomyopathy, lactic acidosis, and stroke-like episodes)
- Jervell and Lange-Nielsen syndrome
- Romano–Ward syndrome
- Hypertrophic cardiomyopathy
- Familial hypercholesterolemia
- Hirschsprung disease
- Neurofibromatosis 1
- Neurofibromatosis 2
- Tuberous sclerosis complex
- Rett syndrome
- *MECP2* duplication syndrome
- Benign familial neonatal seizures
- Pseudohypoparathyroidism
- Pseudopseudohypoparathyroidism
- Complete gonadal dysgenesis (*SRY*)
- Azoospermia and oligospermia (*AZF*)
- Swyer syndrome
- Congenital adrenal hyperplasia (deficiency of 21-hydroxylase)
- Prader–Willi/Angelman syndromes
- Alpha-1 antitrypsin deficiency
- Smith–Lemli–Opitz syndrome
- L1 syndrome
- Alpha-thalassemia X-linked intellectual disability
- Cowden syndrome
- Noonan syndrome
- Sotos syndrome
- Beckwith–Wiedemann syndrome
- Russell–Silver syndrome
- Hutchinson–Gilford progeria syndrome
- Cockayne syndrome
- Rubinstein–Taybi syndrome
- Greig cephalopolysyndactyly
- Apert syndrome
- Crouzon syndrome
- Muenke syndrome
- Pfeiffer syndrome
- Saethre–Chotzen syndrome
- Achondroplasia
- Hypochondroplasia
- Leri–Weill dyschondrosteosis
- Costello syndrome
- Hypohidrotic ectodermal dysplasia
- Incontinentia pigmenti
- Immune dysregulation, polyendocrinopathy, enteropathy, X-linked (IPEX) syndrome
- Wiskott–Aldrich syndrome
- Severe combined immunodeficiency

- Adenosine deaminase (ADA) deficiency
- Hyper-IgM (HIGM) syndromes
- Cerebral autosomal dominant arteriopathy with subcortical infarcts and leukoencephalopathy (CADASIL)
- Alagille syndrome

QUESTIONS

1. A 48-hour old full-term girl was admitted to the NICU shortly after birth for respiratory distress. The mother had been told that a prenatal ultrasound might have identified a kidney abnormality. Postnatal STAT abdominal CT confirmed cystic polyposis of both kidneys. The physician suspected that the newborn had polycystic kidney disease. What would most likely be the recurrent risk for this family if the patient had a hereditary form of polycystic kidney disease?
   A. 1/2
   B. 2/3
   C. 1/4
   D. <1%
   E. None of the above

2. A 38-year-old female came to a clinic for elevated blood pressure (145/95 mmHg) found during an annual physical examination. Her serum creatinine was 2.6 mg/dL (normal range 0.5–1.2). Abdominal ultrasound showed bilateral renal cysts and hepatic and pancreatic cysts. Cranial MRI with contrast revealed a 0.4-cm aneurysm of the circle of Willis. What would most likely be the recurrent risk of this disorder in the family?
   A. <1%
   B. 5%–10%
   C. 25%
   D. 50%
   E. 100%
   F. None of the above

3. A 38-year-old Caucasian female came to a clinic for elevated blood pressure (145/95) detected during an annual physical examination. Her serum creatinine was 2.6 mg/dL (normal range 0.5–1.2). Abdominal ultrasound showed bilateral renal cysts and hepatic and pancreatic cysts. Cranial MRI with contrast revealed a 0.4-cm aneurysm of the circle of Willis. Which one of the following molecular genetics studies would most likely be used as a first-tier test to confirm/rule out genetic etiologies in this patient?

A. Chromosomal microarray

B. Multiplex ligation-dependent probe amplification (MLPA)

C. Sequencing the *PDK1* and *PKD2* genes

D. Sequencing the *PKHD1* gene

E. Target variant analysis of the founder pathogenic variants in the *PDK1* and *PKD2* genes

F. Target variant analysis of the founder pathogenic variants in the *PKHD1* gene

G. None of the above

4. A 39-year-old female has progressively worsening renal failure due to polycystic kidney disease. Multiple bilateral renal cysts and renal failure were diagnosed about 7 years ago, after the first episode of hematuria. She also has several cysts in her liver and mild hypertension. She has no other health problems. Her father died of cerebral hemorrhage at the age of 48. Her mother is 62 years old and in good health and has had a normal renal ultrasound study. Her two younger sisters, a younger brother, and two children 6 and 10 years of age are all apparently healthy. She is told that she is likely to require dialysis soon and is advised to consider renal transplantation. Which one of the following polycystic kidney disease does the patient most likely have if she has a genetic form of the disorder?

A. De novo autosomal dominant polycystic kidney disease

B. Inherited autosomal dominant polycystic kidney disease

C. De novo autosomal recessive polycystic kidney disease

D. Inherited autosomal recessive polycystic kidney disease

E. None of the above

5. A 39-year-old female has progressively worsening renal failure due to autosomal dominant polycystic kidney disease. Multiple bilateral renal cysts and renal failure were diagnosed about 6 years ago after an episode of hematuria. She also has two cysts in her liver and mild hypertension that is controlled with medication. She has no other health problems. Her father died of cerebral hemorrhage at age 46 years. Her mother is 55 years old and in good health and has had a normal renal ultrasound study. Her two younger sisters, a younger brother, and three children ages 3, 6, and 10 years are apparently healthy. A molecular study detected a heterozygous pathogenic variant, c.9829C > T(p.Arg3277Cys), in the *PKD1* gene with the peripheral-blood specimen from this patient. She is told that she is likely to require dialysis soon and is advised to

consider renal transplantation. Of the family members who are potential kidney donors, only her youngest sister, age 25 years, is a good tissue match. This sister is evaluated by ultrasound, CT, and MRI as parts of comprehensive renal image analysis, and the results are negative. Which one of the following is the most appropriate next step in the workup?

A. Considering transplantation with a kidney from an unrelated donor

B. Considering transplantation with a kidney from the brother

C. Considering transplantation with a kidney from the youngest sister

D. Considering transplantation with a kidney from a relative who does not have the pathogenic variant

E. Considering transplantation with a kidney from the youngest sister if she doesn't have the pathogenic variant

F. None of the above

6. A 39-year-old female has progressively worsening renal failure due to autosomal dominant polycystic kidney disease. Multiple bilateral renal cysts and renal failure were diagnosed about 6 years ago after an episode of hematuria. Her father died of cerebral hemorrhage at age 46 years. Her mother is 55 years old and in good health and has had a normal renal ultrasound study. A molecular genetics study does not identify pathogenic variants in this patent. She is told that she is likely to require dialysis soon and is advised to consider renal transplantation. A living relative with a good tissue match as the kidney donor may increase long-term survival. Her two younger sisters, a younger brother, and three children ages 3, 6, and 10 years are apparently healthy. Of the family members who are potential kidney donors, only her youngest sister, age 25 years, is a good tissue match. Her youngest sister is evaluated by ultrasound, CT, and MRI as parts of comprehensive renal image analysis, and results are negative. Which one of the following is the most appropriate next step in the workup?

A. Considering transplantation with a kidney from an unrelated donor

B. Considering transplantation with a kidney from the youngest sister

C. Performing linkage study of the family

D. Performing molecular genetics testing of the youngest sister

E. None of the above

7. A 17-year-old male had been followed up for bilateral cystic kidney disease, hypertension, and

obesity since the age of 13 years. The diagnosis was made owing to an accidental finding during abdominal CT at age 13 to rule out appendicitis. A renal ultrasound scan also demonstrated multiple bilateral liver cysts. Because of a paternal history of bilateral renal cysts, genetic testing was ordered to confirm the diagnosis. Which one of the following genes would most likely harbor a pathogenic variant if the patient had autosomal dominant polycystic kidney disease (ADPKD)?[2]

A. PKD1
B. PKD2
C. PKHD1
D. None of the above

8. A 17-year-old male had been followed up for bilateral cystic kidney disease, hypertension, and obesity since the age of 13 years. The diagnosis was made owing to an accidental finding during abdominal CT at age 13 to rule out appendicitis. A renal ultrasound scan also demonstrated multiple bilateral liver cysts. Because of a paternal history of bilateral renal cysts, genetic testing of PKD1 and PKD2 was ordered, and a 3-bp deletion, c.1602_1604TGT, was detected in the PKD2 coding region. Targeted molecular analysis of the father detected the same deletion. Which one of the following mechanisms would most likely contribute to the pathogenesis of the ADPKD in this patient?[2]

A. Dominant negative
B. Gain of function
C. Loss of function
D. None of the above

9. Dr. Z., who is working in a clinical molecular laboratory, decided to validate clinical exome-sequencing testing. One of the validation samples from another clinical laboratory had a pathogenic variant, c.3817C > T(p.Gln1273*), in the PKD1 gene for autosomal dominant polycystic kidney disease (ADPKD). The exome-sequencing testing for this sample was repeated six times by different technologies in three runs as part of the validation for repeatability and reproducibility. None of the studies detected the pathogenic variant, but a 15-bp deletion in exon 3 was detected this patient. Communication with the laboratory that sent the sample confirmed the presence of the c.3817C > T, but not the 15-bp deletion in exon 3. Dr. Z sent this sample to a third clinical laboratory for Sanger sequencing, and the result confirmed the presence of the c.3817C > T, but not the 15-bp deletion in exon 3. Which one of the following mechanisms would most likely contribute to the discrepancy of the testing results with the same specimen in this case?

A. Interference of pseudogenes
B. Primers in polymorphic regions
C. Sample mess-up
D. Variation of enrichment methods
E. None of the above

10. A 29-year-old gravida 2 para 1 Amish American female came to a clinic for ultrasound to assess fetal anatomy at 20 weeks of gestation. Second-trimester fetal anatomy ultrasound revealed enlarged hyperechoic fetal kidneys and normal amniotic fluid index. Follow-up ultrasound at 24 weeks revealed persistently enlarged hyperechoic fetal kidneys. Progressive oligohydramnios was not evident until 29 weeks of gestation, with amphidromous noted by 35 weeks of gestation. A three-generation pedigree did not reveal a significant history of renal disease. A 3.4-kg female neonate with Apgar scores of 4 and 8 at 1 and 5 minutes, respectively, was delivered vaginally at 36 weeks following induction of labor. The newborn required intubation for respiratory distress at 2 minutes after delivery. She continued to have persistent hypoxemia and hypercarbia despite aggressive mechanical ventilation. Chest X-rays, done after birth, revealed low lung volumes with bilateral pneumothorax. The family elected for palliative care and the newborn was extubated approximately 3 hours after delivery and died soon thereafter. The family declined an autopsy. Which one of the following genes would most likely harbor a pathogenic variant in this patient if the patient had a hereditary form of polycystic kidney diseases?[3]

A. PKD1
B. PKD2
C. PKHD1
D. None of the above

11. A 21-year-old gravida 2 para 1 female came to a clinic at 22 weeks of gestation. Ultrasound examination revealed severe oligohydramnios with bilateral symmetrically enlarged, echogenic kidneys filling the fetal abdomen. The urinary bladder was not visible. There was no history of consanguinity between the patient (the pregnant woman) and her partner. And there was no family history of renal disease on either side of the family. The patient and the family were counseled about the possibility of autosomal recessive polycystic kidney disease (ARPKD) and opted to terminate the pregnancy. A male fetus with no gross enlargement of abdomen was delivered. A molecular study of the fetal tissue was ordered. Compound heterozygous pathogenic variants, c.10444C > T and c.5909−2delA, were detected in the PKHD1 gene. Which one of the following

would be the most appropriate next step in the workup for this family?[3,4]

A. Counseling the family about the 25% recurrent risk
B. Recommending prenatal testing for future pregnancies
C. Testing the couple for the pathogenic variants
D. Testing the husband for the pathogenic variants
E. Testing the wife for the pathogenic variants
F. All of the above
G. None of the above

12. A 5-month-old infant boy was brought to a clinic for heart murmur and multiple cardiac masses. There were two cardiac masses in the right ventricular outflow tract and right ventricular free wall at the leaflet of the tricuspid valve. In addition, bilateral multiple renal cysts were found on renal ultrasonography. At age 12 months, generalized tonic–clonic seizure with fever developed. The seizure persisted over 15 minutes with cyanosis. A physical examination revealed hypopigmented patches on the anterior chest, left shoulder, and left leg. There was no palpable abdominal mass. His complete blood count, serum electrolytes, liver enzymes, and routine urinalysis were all normal. Brain MRI revealed multiple cortical and subcortical tubers in bilateral hemispheres and several tiny subependymal hamartomas along the wall of both lateral ventricles. Multiple retinal tumors were found upon ophthalmological examination. The patient's perinatal history was unremarkable. There was no familial history of tuberous sclerosis or polycystic kidney disease. The physician suspected that the patient had tuberous sclerosis and autosomal dominant polycystic kidney disease (ADPKD). Which one of the following molecular genetics assays would be most appropriate for this patient to confirm the diagnosis?[5,6]

A. Multiplex ligation-dependent probe amplification (MLPA)
B. Next-generation sequence (NGS)
C. Quantitative PCR
D. Restriction-fragment–length polymorphism
E. Sanger sequencing
F. None of the above

13. A 26-year-old Caucasian presented to a genetics clinic for evaluation of polycystic kidney disease due to positive family history in multiple individuals (see the figure below for the pedigree). He did not have symptoms. The blood pressure was normal, and the results of ultrasound scanning were negative. A molecular genetics study was ordered to confirm/rule out genetic etiology, and

pathogenic variant(s) were identified. Which one of the following genes would most likely harbor the pathogenic variant(s) in this patient?

A. *PKD1*
B. *PKD2*
C. *PKD3*
D. *PKHD1*
E. *PKHD1L1*

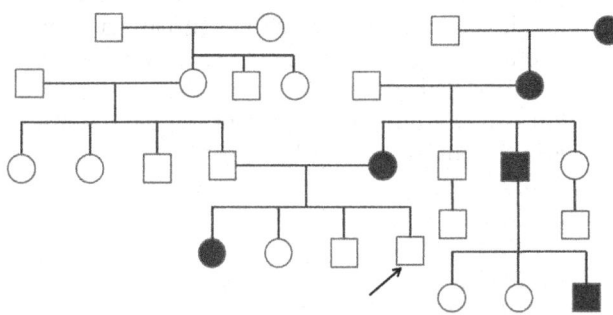

14. A 26-year-old Caucasian presented to a genetics clinic for evaluation of polycystic kidney disease owing to positive family history in multiple individuals (see the figure below for the pedigree). He did not have symptoms. The blood pressure was normal and the results of ultrasound scanning were negative. The *PKD1* and *PKD2* genes were sequenced. The results showed a homozygous pathogenic variant, c.3817C > T(p.Gln1273Ter), in *PKD1*. Which one of the following would be the most appropriate interpretation of the result?

A. The c.3817C > T(p.Gln1273Ter) variant is pathogenic. The patient had polycystic kidney disease.
B. The parents of the proband may be related. The patient needs to be monitored closely for early-onset disease.
C. The result is questionable. The variant needs to be reanalyzed with another pair of primers.
D. The result is questionable. The lab should ask for a redraw of a peripheral-blood sample from the patient.
E. None of the above.

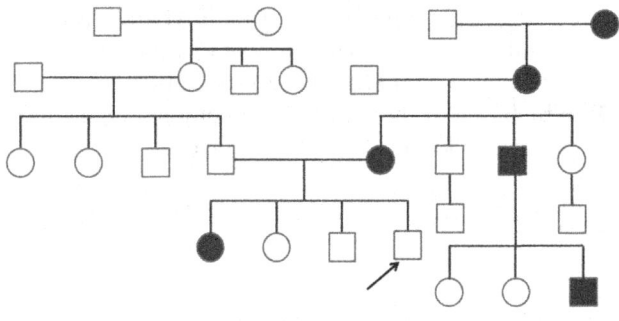

15. A 2-week-old Caucasian infant boy was brought to a genetics clinic for evaluation of polycystic kidney disease owing to positive prenatal ultrasound findings. He did not have symptoms. The blood pressure was normal and the results of ultrasound scanning were negative. His family history was remarkable for a 2-year-old sister with polycystic kidney disease (see the figure below for the pedigree). A molecular genetics study was ordered to confirm/rule out a genetic etiology, and pathogenic variant(s) were identified. Which one of the following genes would most likely harbor the pathogenic variant(s) in this family?
   A. *PKD1*
   B. *PKD2*
   C. *PKD3*
   D. *PKHD1*
   E. *PKHD1L1*

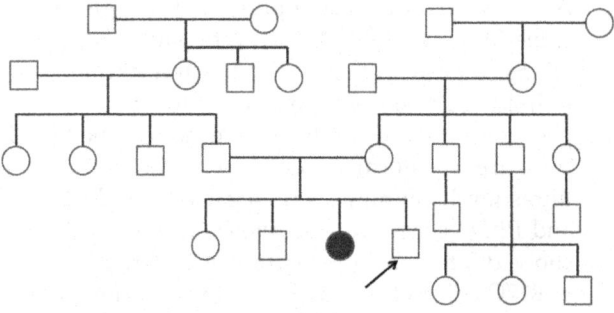

16. Which one of the following statements regarding polycystic kidney diseases is correct?
   A. Autosomal dominant polycystic kidney disease (ADPKD) and autosomal recessive polycystic kidney disease (ARPKD) are caused by same genes.
   B. ADPKD usually causes more significant renal- and liver-related morbidity and mortality than ARPKD.
   C. The onset of ADPKD is usually earlier than that of ARPKD.
   D. The severity of ADPKD disease is attributed primarily to locus heterogeneity.
   E. The contiguous gene deletion syndrome including symptoms for both ADPKD and tuberous sclerosis typically results from a deletion involving both *PKD2* and *TSC1*.

17. Which one of the following statements regarding polycystic kidney diseases is correct?

A. The contiguous gene deletion syndrome including symptoms for both ADPKD and tuberous sclerosis typically results from a deletion involving both *PKD1* and *TSC1*.
B. The contiguous gene deletion syndrome including symptoms for both ADPKD and tuberous sclerosis typically results from a deletion involving both *PKD1* and *TSC2*.
C. The contiguous gene deletion syndrome including symptoms for both in ADPKD and tuberous sclerosis typically results from a deletion involving both *PKD2* and *TSC1*.
D. The contiguous gene deletion syndrome including symptoms for both ADPKD and tuberous sclerosis typically results from a deletion involving both *PKD2* and *TSC2*.
E. None of the above.

18. A 28-year-old Caucasian man has been evaluated as a potential living-relative kidney donor for his mother (see the figure below for the pedigree). He is apparently healthy. Renal ultrasonography results were negative. The *PKD1* and *PKD2* studies for autosomal dominant polycystic kidney disease (ADPKD) did not identify pathogenic variants in the mother. Which one of the following is the most appropriate next step in the workup for this family?

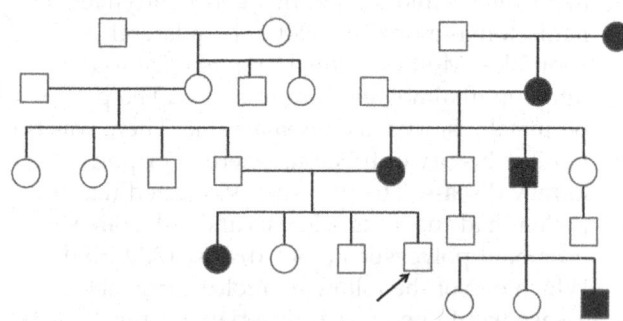

A. Excluding the patient as a renal donor for his mother
B. Performing linkage analysis in the family
C. Sequencing the patient for an ADPKD pathogenic variant
D. Testing *PKHD1* for autosomal recessive polycystic kidney disease (ARPKD)
E. Using a more sensitive renal imaging method, such as MRI or CT
F. None of the above

19. A 4-year-old Caucasian boy was admitted to a local hospital for "febrile seizures." An initial evaluation revealed nystagmus and pigmentary retinopathy, mild central obesity, hypogonadism, mental retardation, behavioral abnormalities, hypothyroidism, hypertension, and severe anemia. He had postaxial polydactyly. Ultrasonography revealed bilateral multiple renal cysts. He was the second offspring of consanguineous parents. His family history was notable for obesity, learning difficulties, six digits on both hands, and visual impairment in his 14-year-old sister; the etiology was unknown. Which one of the following pathogenic variants would this patient most likely have?
    A. c.107C > T(p.T36M) in *PKHD1*
    B. c.12258T > A(p.C4086X) in *PKD1*
    C. c. 547A > G(p.G72S) in *BBS5*
    D. 46,XX,der(16)t(X;16)(q28;p13.2)
    E. None of the above

20. A 14-year-old boy was brought to a clinic with symptoms of underdeveloped genitalia and absence of hair on the pubic and axillary areas. He had developmental delay, intellectual disability, behavioral issues, and diminished vision in both eyes, especially at night. A physical examination revealed severe obesity, postaxial polydactyly with hexadactyly of all four limbs, features of hypogonadism with testicular volume of 2 mL (normal range, 10−12) and micropenis (<2.5 cm), and moderate bilateral conductive deafness. There was proximal lower-limb weakness. The plantar reflex was exaggerated. On eye examination, visual acuity was 6/36 in both eyes, pallor of the optic disks, bilaterally attenuated vessels, and retinal pigmentary changes of retinitis pigmentosa sine pigmento, with mild night blindness and constricted visual field. His parents were first cousins. One of his older brothers died at 18 months of age owing to unknown reasons. One of his maternal cousins, who had similar phenotypic characteristics, died at 11 years of age owing to nephropathy. The medical geneticist suspected that the patient had Bardet−Biedl syndrome and ordered a molecular genetics study to confirm the diagnosis. Which one of the following molecular technologies would provide the most cost-effective testing strategy for this patient?[7]
    A. Next-generation sequencing (NGS)
    B. Quantitative real-time PCR
    C. Restriction-fragment−length polymorphism (RFLP)
    D. Sanger sequencing
    E. None of the above

21. A 22-year-old male was brought to a hospital by his parents with a sudden onset of weakness in all four limbs, both proximal and distal. Initially, he noticed weakness while getting up from a squatting posture and over the next few hours he became bedridden. There was no breathing difficulty. His mother said that he had delayed developmental milestones and was not good at studies in his childhood so he had dropped out of school. Difficulty seeing in the dark had developed over the 3 years, and it was worsening. On physical examination, he was found to have central obesity, a moon-shaped face, acanthosis nigricans, lower-limb polydactyly, a small testicular size, and absence of pubic and axillary hair. His fundus examination revealed retinitis pigmentosa. His central nervous system examination showed hypotonia, grade 0 power, weak neck flexors, and absent reflexes. His urine examination showed trace proteinuria. IQ testing showed a severely impaired social adaptive function. The medical geneticist suspected that the patient had Bardet−Biedl syndrome and ordered a next-generation sequencing (NGS) panel to confirm the diagnosis, which includes 19 genes. Which of the following is this an example of?[6,8]
    A. Allelic heterogeneity
    B. Cellular heterogeneity
    C. Incomplete penetrance
    D. Locus heterogeneity
    E. Variable expression
    F. None of the above

22. Jerry, a 4-year-old boy, was brought to a clinic for an incidental finding of microscopic hematuria and proteinuria on routine screening. The analysis was repeated 2 weeks later with persistent hematuria and proteinuria. Renal ultrasound was normal. Jerry had two healthy sisters. His family history was unremarkable except that one of his cousins had proteinuria found on a dipstick but had been symptom-free (see the figure below for the pedigree). Which one of the following would most likely be the recurrent risk of the same condition in the family if Jerry and his cousin had a hereditary form of renal diseases?
    A. 10%
    B. 25%
    C. 50%
    D. 75%
    E. 99%
    F. Unpredictable

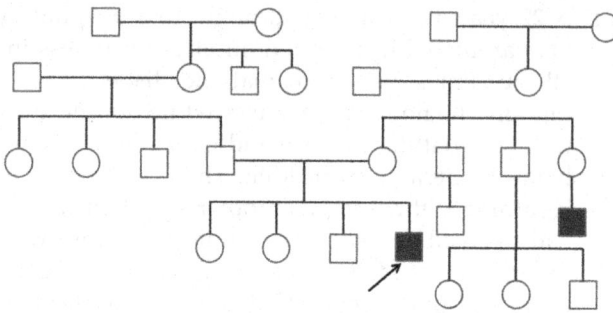

D. Restriction-fragment–length polymorphism (RFLP)

E. Sanger sequencing

F. None of the above

23. Mrs. J., a 52-year-old female, has not been herself lately. She has been misplacing objects more frequently, getting lost in familiar places, having trouble remembering simple words, and not remembering things she recently read or saw. Encouraged by her son, she came to see a neurologist, Dr. Z. After examining her, Dr. Z. suspects that Mrs. J. has early-onset Alzheimer disease. Which one of the following genes is NOT associated with autosomal dominant early-onset Alzheimer disease?

A. *APOE*

B. *APP*

C. *PSEN1*

D. *PSEN2*

E. All of the above

F. None of the above

24. A 52-year-old Caucasian female of Finnish ancestry came to a clinic with symptoms of memory impairment and difficulties in daily life planning and organization since the age of 46. Her family history was notable for progressive cognitive deterioration in her mother and maternal grandfather. Her mother developed memory deficit at the age of 55 and died at 62. Her maternal grandfather developed dementia at 50 years of age and died at 55. A neuropsychological assessment of the proband demonstrated deficit of attention, short- and long-term memory impairment, deficits of executive functions, semantic and phonemic verbal deficits, and abnormalities in praxis and in constructive skills. The physician diagnosed the patient clinically with Alzheimer disease and ordered a molecular genetics study for it. Which one of the following molecular technologies would provide the cost-effective testing strategy for this patient?[9]

A. Multiplex ligation-dependent probe amplification (MLPA)

B. Next-generation sequencing (NGS)

C. Quantitative real-time PCR

25. A 51-year-old Caucasian female of Finnish ancestry came to a clinic with symptoms of memory impairment and difficulties in daily life planning and organization since the age of 46. Her family history was notable for progressive cognitive deterioration in her mother and maternal grandfather. Her mother developed memory deficit at the age of 55 and died at 62. Her maternal grandfather developed dementia at 50 years of age and died at 55. A neuropsychological assessment of the proband demonstrated deficit of attention, short- and long-term memory impairment, deficits of executive functions, semantic and phonemic verbal deficits, and abnormalities in praxis and in constructive skills. The physician diagnosed the patient clinically with Alzheimer disease and ordered a molecular genetics study for it. A 4555-bp deletion spanning exon 9 of *PSEN1* was detected. The patient asked if her 33-year-old asymptomatic daughter may be tested. Which one of the following would be the most appropriate reaction from the physician to this request?[9]

A. A pretesting interview is recommended.

B. Informed consent for such testing is required.

C. Inform the patient that such testing is not useful in predicting age at onset, severity, type of symptoms, and rate of progression.

D. The test should not be offered.

E. A, B, and C.

F. All of the above.

G. None of the above.

26. A 52-year-old Caucasian female of Finnish ancestry came to a clinic with symptoms of memory impairment and difficulties in daily life planning and organization since the age of 46. Her family history was notable for progressive cognitive deterioration in her mother and maternal grandfather. Her mother developed memory deficit at the age of 55 and died at 62. Her maternal grandfather developed dementia at 50 years of age and died at 55. A neuropsychological assessment of the proband demonstrated deficit of attention, short- and long-term memory impairment, deficits of executive functions, semantic and phonemic verbal deficits, and abnormalities in praxis and in constructive skills. The physician diagnosed the patient clinically with Alzheimer disease and ordered a molecular genetics study for it. A 4555-bp deletion spanning exon 9 of *PSEN1* was detected. Her 33-year-old asymptomatic daughter was tested and confirmed to carry the same deletion. Her daughter asked if her 8-year-old son may be tested, too. Which one of the following would be the most appropriate reaction from the physician to this request?[9,10]

A. A pretesting interview is recommended.
B. Informed consent for such testing is required.
C. Inform the patient that such testing is not useful in predicting age at onset, severity, type of symptoms, and rate of progression.
D. The test should not be offered.
E. A, B, and C.
F. All of the above.
G. None of the above.

27. A 52-year-old Caucasian female of Finnish ancestry came to a clinic with symptoms of memory impairment and difficulties in daily life planning and organization since the age of 46. Her family history was notable for progressive cognitive deterioration in her mother and maternal grandfather. Her mother developed memory deficit at the age of 55 and died at 62. Her maternal grandfather developed dementia at 50 years of age and died at 55. A neuropsychological assessment of the proband demonstrated deficit of attention, short- and long-term memory impairment, deficits of executive functions, semantic and phonemic verbal deficits, and abnormalities in praxis and in constructive skills. The physician diagnosed the patient clinically with Alzheimer disease and ordered a molecular genetics study for it. A 4555-bp deletion spanning exon 9 of *PSEN1* was detected. Her 33-year-old asymptomatic daughter was tested and confirmed to carry the same deletion. Her daughter asked if her 8-year-old son may be tested, too. Her daughter was 10 weeks pregnant for her second child, and asked if her unborn child may be tested, too. Which one of the following would be the most appropriate reaction from the physician to this request?[9]

A. The test may be offered.
B. The test should not be offered.
C. Not sure.

28. Mrs. B. is a 41-year-old woman. She works in the fashion industry and is happily married with two sons. Aside from having high cholesterol, she is healthy. Her parents emigrated from Russia before she was born. Her father died from a heart attack at age 68. Her 75-year-old mother currently lives with Mrs. B., and has Alzheimer disease,

which started at 65 years of age. Mrs. B. is concerned about her own risk for Alzheimer disease. Which one of the following genes may be associated with the Alzheimer disease in this family?

A. *APOE*
B. *APP*
C. *PSEN1*
D. *PSEN2*
E. All of the above
F. None of the above

29. Mrs. B. is a 41-year-old woman. She works in the fashion industry and is happily married with two sons. Aside from having high cholesterol, she is healthy. Her parents emigrated from Russia before she was born. Her father died from a heart attack at age 68. Her 75-year-old mother currently lives with Mrs. B., and has Alzheimer disease, which started at 65 years of age. Mrs. B. is concerned about her own risk for Alzheimer disease, and comes to see a doctor. The doctor orders a molecular genetics study for Mrs. B.'s mother. Which one of the following alleles in *APOE* does Mrs. B.'s mother most likely have?

A. e1
B. e2
C. e3
D. e4
E. e5

30. Mrs. B. is a 41-year-old woman. She works in the fashion industry and is happily married with two sons. Aside from having high cholesterol, she is healthy. Her parents emigrated from Russia before she was born. Her father died from a heart attack at age 68. Her 75-year-old mother currently lives with Mrs. B., and has Alzheimer disease, which started at 65 years of age. Mrs. B. is concerned about her own risk for Alzheimer disease, and comes to see a doctor. The doctor orders a molecular genetics study for Mrs. B.'s mother. Which one of the following *APOE* genotypes does Mrs. B.'s mother least likely have?

A. e1/e1
B. e2/e2
C. e3/e3
D. e4/e4
E. e5/e5

31. A 68-year-old female came to a clinic for a family history of dementia. She was in relatively good health and had no symptoms of dementia. However, her two brothers, father, and two other paternal relatives had dementia in their 70s. She wanted to find out whether she would have dementia soon. If so, she would like to find a

lawyer to make a will right away. Which one of the following statements would be the most appropriate?[6]

A. The *APOE* molecular test may be useful as a predictive test.

B. Her risk for Alzheimer is increased threefold to sixfold.

C. She will have Alzheimer disease.

D. She has nothing to worry about.

E. She may consider a next-generation panel for early-onset Alzheimer disease.

32. A 1½-month-old boy was brought to a genetics clinic for congenital bilateral hearing loss. He had abnormal results on a newborn hearing testing and had undergone auditory brain stem response testing. A physical examination did not detect an enlarged thyroid gland. MRI of the inner ear showed bilateral dilation of the vestibular aqueduct with cochlear hypoplasia. Which one of the following genes would most likely be tested for this patient to confirm/rule out genetic etiologies?

A. Connexin 26

B. Connexin 30

C. *GJB2* and *GJB6*

D. *SCL26A4*, *FOXI1*, and *KCNJ10*

E. *MYO7A*, *USH2A*, *CDH23*, *ADGRV1*, *CLRN1*, *PCDH15*, *USH1C*, *USH1G*, and *DFNB31*

33. Which one of the following genes is most likely mutated in patients with hereditary hearing loss?

A. *CDH23*

B. *GJB2*

C. *GJB6*

D. *MYO7A*

E. *SCL26A4*

34. A boy failed a newborn hearing screening in both ears before hospital discharge. However, 4 weeks later, he passed the rescreening in both ears. At 1 year of age, parental concern triggered a referral for a comprehensive audiological evaluation. At this time, the child was diagnosed with severe-to-profound hearing loss in both ears. A physical examination did not detect an enlarged thyroid gland. A CT scan revealed normal temporal-bone anatomy in both ears. An ECG was found to be within normal limits. The family history was unremarkable. Which one of the following molecular sequencing tests would most likely be the next step in the workup to confirm/rule out genetic etiologies in this patient?[11]

A. Connexin 30

B. *GJB2* and *GJB6*

C. *MYO7A*

D. *SCL26A4*, *FOXI1*, and *KCNJ10*

E. Usher syndrome NGS panel

35. A boy failed a newborn hearing screening in both ears before hospital discharge. However, 4 weeks later, he passed the rescreening in both ears. At 1 year of age, parental concern triggered a referral for a comprehensive audiological evaluation. At this time, the child was diagnosed with severe-to-profound hearing loss in both ears. A physical examination did not detect an enlarged thyroid gland. A CT scan revealed normal temporal-bone anatomy in both ears. An ECG was found to be within normal limits. The family history was unremarkable. A molecular study of the *GJB2* and *GJB6* genes was ordered, and the results were negative. Which one of the following molecular sequencing tests would most likely be the next step in the workup to further rule out genetic etiologies in this patient?[11]

A. Connexin 26

B. Connexin 30

C. Mitochondrial panel

D. *SCL26A4*, *FOXI1*, and *KCNJ10*

E. Usher syndrome panel with 11 genes

36. A 36-year-old female came to a genetics clinic for impaired hearing in the past 6 years. A physical examination did not detect an enlarged thyroid gland or dysmorphic facial feature. Her medical history was unremarkable except for the hearing loss. Her family history was not eventful. MRI of inner ear showed normal anatomic structures. A molecular study of the *GJB2* and *GJB6* genes was ordered, and the results were negative. Which one of the following molecular sequencing studies would most likely be the next step in the workup to further rule out genetic etiologies in this patient?

A. Connexin 26

B. Connexin 30

C. Mitochondrial panel

D. *SCL26A4*, *FOXI1*, and *KCNJ10*

E. Usher syndrome panel with 11 genes

37. A 11-year-old girl was seen in a clinic for a cochlear implant evaluation. She was diagnosed with severe to profound hearing loss in both ears. The patient's CT results were equivocal for an enlarged vestibular aqueduct (EVA). Her family history was remarkable for childhood hearing loss; her 4-month-old brother was diagnosed with severe-to-profound hearing loss as well with mild EVAs bilaterally. A molecular study for *SLC26A4* was tested, and the results were negative. Then a molecular study of the *GJB2* and *GJB6* genes detected a homozygous frameshift pathogenic variant, c.35delG, in the *GJB2* gene. The family history was negative

on both sides. Which one of the following recurrent risks would most likely apply to the parents?[11]

A. >99%

B. 50%

C. 25%

D. 5%

E. <1%

F. Unpredictable

38. A 6-month-old Caucasian girl was brought to a genetics clinic for congenital bilateral hearing loss. She had abnormal results on a newborn hearing testing and auditory brain stem response testing. A physical examination did not reveal an enlarged thyroid gland or dysmorphic facial features. The family history was negative on both sides. MRI of the inner ear showed normal anatomic structures. A molecular study of the *GJB2* gene detected a heterozygous frameshift pathogenic variant, c.35delG. Which one of the following molecular genetics studies would most likely be the next step in the workup to further confirm/rule out genetic etiologies in this patient?

A. Connexin 26

B. Connexin 30

C. Mitochondrial panel

D. *SCL26A4*, *FOXI1*, and *KCNJ10*

E. Usher syndrome panel with 11 genes

39. A 1-year old girl with profound congenital bilateral hearing loss was brought to a genetics clinic by her parents. She was born at 40 gestational weeks without complications after an uneventful pregnancy. Her development was normal. There were no identifiable dysmorphic features. An ophthalmologic evaluation was negative. Results of a molecular genetics study revealed that the patient had a heterozygous pathogenic missense variant in the *GJB2* gene and a heterozygous deletion in the *GJB6* gene. Which one of the following statements regarding the pathogenic variants in *GJB2* and *JGB6* would be most appropriate?[12]

A. The variants in *GJB2* and *GJB6* most likely were in *cis*.

B. The variants in *GJB2* and *GJB6* most likely were in *trans*.

C. The deletion in *GJB6* causes hearing loss in this patient, and *GJB2* is a pseudogene.

D. The missense variant in *GJB2* causes hearing loss in this patient, and *GJB6* is a pseudogene.

E. None of the above.

40. A 6-month-old Ashkenazi Jewish girl was brought to a genetics clinic for congenital bilateral hearing loss. She had abnormal results on newborn hearing testing and auditory brain stem response testing. The family history was negative on both sides. A physical examination did not reveal an enlarged thyroid gland or dysmorphic facial features. MRI of the inner ear showed normal anatomic structures. Which one of the following molecular genetics studies would most likely be used to confirm/rule out genetic etiologies in this patient?

A. Chromosomal microarray

B. Exome sequencing

C. Methylation study

D. Next-generation sequencing (NGS)

E. Sanger sequencing

F. Targeted variant assay

G. All of the above

41. A 16-year-old Ashkenazi Jewish girl is brought to a genetics clinic for hearing problem in the past 2 years. Other than it, she has been healthy. Now, she can hear a friend at a close distance but has problems understanding the teachers in the classroom. Her grades have dropped significantly in the past year. She is very frustrated and scared. She was raised by her paternal aunt because her parents died in a car accident when she was 6 years old. The paternal family history is uneventful. The maternal family history is unclear (her mother was an immigrant from Russia). A physical examination is unremarkable. Which one of the following molecular genetics tests is most likely the next step in the workup to confirm/rule out genetic etiologies in this patient?

A. *CLRN1*

B. *GJB2* and *GJB6*

C. *PCDH15*

D. *SCL26A4*, *FOXI1*, and *KCNJ10*

E. Usher syndrome NGS panel

42. An Ashkenazi Jewish couple comes to a clinic for preconception counseling. They are apparently healthy. One of the husband's three siblings has congenital profound bilateral sensorineural hearing loss (SNHL). Otherwise, the family history is uneventful. A molecular genetics study of the husband's affected sibling had a positive finding. Which one of the following most likely describes the risk of the husband being a carrier of the familial pathogenic variant for hearing loss?

A. 1 in 1

B. 1 in 2

C. 1 in 4

D. 2 in 3

E. 1 in 25

43. An Ashkenazi Jewish couple came to a clinic for preconception counseling. They are apparently healthy. One of the husband's three siblings had

congenital profound bilateral sensorineural hearing loss (SNHL). A molecular genetics study of the husband's affected sibling detected a homozygous pathogenic variant in the *GJB2* gene. The couple received genetic counseling. And a targeted genetic testing was ordered for the husband. Which one of the following pathogenic variants would the husband most likely have if he had one?[13,14]

A. c.35delG

B. c.79G > A

C. c.167delT

D. c.235delC

E. c.223C > T

44. A Caucasian couple came to a Ob/Gyn clinic for preconception counseling. They are apparently healthy. One of the husband's three siblings had congenital profound bilateral sensorineural hearing loss (SNHL). A molecular genetics study of the husband's affected sibling detected a homozygous pathogenic variant in the *GJB2* gene. The couple received genetic counseling. And a targeted genetic testing of the husband was ordered. Which one of the following pathogenic variants would the husband most likely have?[13,14]

A. c.35delG

B. c.79G > A

C. c.167delT

D. c.235delC

E. c.223C > T

45. A 13-year-old girl with profound congenital bilateral hearing loss is brought to a genetics clinic for impaired vision in the past 6 months. The patient was born at 40 gestational weeks without complications after an uneventful pregnancy. Her development has been normal except for the hearing loss. There are no identifiable dysmorphic features. An ophthalmologic evaluation confirms retinitis pigmentosa. A molecular genetics study is ordered. Which one of the following molecular genetics assays provides the most cost-effective genetic testing strategy for this patient?

A. Chromosomal microarray

B. Multiplex ligation-dependent probe amplification

C. Next-generation sequencing

D. Quantitative PCR

E. Sanger sequencing

46. A 1-year-old girl was brought to a clinic for bilateral hearing loss. The patient was born at 40 gestational weeks without complications after an uneventful pregnancy. She passed the newborn hearing screen. Her development had been normal. There were no identifiable dysmorphic

features. The mother mentioned that the infant had been given neomycin (aminoglycoside) at 1 month of age for an ear infection. Which one of the following genes would most likely harbor a pathogenic variant in the infant?

A. *GJB2*

B. *GJB6*

C. *MYO7A*

D. 12S rRNA in mtDNA

E. None of the above

47. Hearing loss is one of the most common birth defects; it can affect as many as 3 in 1000 babies born in the United States. How much do genetic factors contribute to congenital hearing loss?

A. 5%

B. 30%

C. 55%

D. 80%

E. > 99%

48. Which one of the following statements regarding hearing loss is NOT correct?

A. Approximately 50% of hearing losses are caused by genetics.

B. Approximately 80% of hearing losses with genetic etiologies have recessive causes.

C. Approximately 70% of hearing losses with genetic etiologies have nonsyndromic causes.

D. Connexin 30 is estimated to be responsible for half of all recessive nonsyndromic hearing losses.

E. None of the above.

49. Which one of the following disorders can NOT cause dominant syndromic hearing loss?

A. Branchio-oto-renal (BOR) syndrome

B. Jervell and Lange-Nielsen syndrome

C. Neurofibromatosis type II (NFII)

D. Stickler syndrome

E. Treacher–Collins syndrome

F. Waardenburg syndrome

50. Which one of the following disorders can NOT cause recessive syndromic hearing loss?

A. Usher syndrome

B. Pendred syndrome

C. Stickler syndrome

D. Branchio-oto-renal (BOR) syndrome

E. Jervell and Lange-Nielsen syndrome

F. Alport syndrome

51. A 12-year-old girl was brought to a clinic for decreased hearing in both ears for years. She had a distinct white forelock of hair in the midline and striking bilateral blue irises. A white depigmented patch was also present on the right forearm. A diffuse swelling was present in the thyroid region of her neck. Her developmental milestones were normal. Her family history was

remarkable for her 8-year-old brother having similar blue eyes and white forelock at birth, and there was spontaneous shedding of this hair by age 2 years. The family history also suggested premature graying of hair in her father since the age of 15 years. But neither her brother nor her father had decreased hearing. Both the patient and her brother had normal IQs and went to regular schools. Their academic performance was normal. A clinical diagnosis of Waardenberg syndrome was made, and a molecular study was ordered to confirm the diagnosis. Which one of the following molecular genetic assays would most likely be used to confirm the diagnosis in this patient?[15]

A. Chromosomal microarray analysis
B. Next-generation sequencing
C. Sanger sequencing
D. Targeted variant assay
E. Whole-exome sequencing
F. None of the above

52. A 32-year-old male came to a clinic for blurry vision since childhood. An eye examination revealed partial heterochromia of the iris. He had congenital hearing loss and a lack of speech development. A physical examination did not reveal abnormal pigmentation of the hair, but hypopigmented patches on his skin were noted. Ptosis of the right upper lid and dystopia canthorum were noted. His firstborn 9-year-old son was mute and deaf since birth, and he had heterochromia, dystopia canthorum, and the same hypopigmented patches on his face as the father. A clinical diagnosis of Waardenberg syndrome was made, and a next-generation sequencing (NGS) panel was ordered for the proband to confirm the diagnosis. Which one of the following genes would most likely be included in this NGS panel for Waardenberg syndrome?[16]

A. *PAX3*
B. *PEX3*
C. *PAX5*
D. *PEX5*
E. *PAX7*
F. *PEX7*

53. A 12-year-old girl was brought to a clinic for decreased hearing in both ears for years. She had a distinct white forelock of hair in the midline and striking bilateral blue irises. A white depigmented patch was also present on the right forearm. A diffuse swelling was present in the thyroid region of her neck. Her developmental milestones were normal. Her family history was remarkable for her

8-year-old brother having similar blue eyes and white forelock at birth, and there was spontaneous shedding of this hair by age 2 years. The family history also suggested premature graying of hair in her father since the age of 15 years. But neither her brother nor her father had decreased hearing. Both the patient and her brother had normal IQs and went to regular schools. Their academic performance was normal. A clinical diagnosis of Waardenberg syndrome was made, and a molecular study was ordered to confirm the diagnosis. A pathogenic variant, p.Asn47His, in *PAX3* was detected; the same variant was detected in her brother and father by a targeted variant analysis. Which one of the following would be the most appropriate estimation of the recurrent risk of the same condition in this family?[15]

A. <1%
B. 5%–7%
C. 14%
D. 25%
E. 50%
F. 100%

54. A 12-year-old girl was brought to a clinic for decreased hearing in both ears for years. She had a distinct white forelock of hair in the midline and striking bilateral blue irises. A white depigmented patch was also present on the right forearm. A diffuse swelling was present in the thyroid region of her neck. Her developmental milestones were normal. Her family history was remarkable for her 8-year-old brother having similar blue eyes and white forelock at birth, and there was spontaneous shedding of this hair by age 2 years. The family history also suggested premature graying of hair in her father since the age of 15 years. But neither her brother nor her father had decreased hearing. Both the patient and her brother had normal IQs and went to regular schools. Their academic performance was normal. A clinical diagnosis of Waardenberg syndrome was made. A next-generation sequencing (NGS) panel detected a pathogenic variant, p.Asn47His, in *PAX3* in the girl. And the same variant was detected in her brother and father by a targeted variant analysis. Which one of the following mechanisms would most likely be the pathogenesis of the variant in this family?[15]

A. Epigenetic change
B. Gain of function
C. Loss of function
D. Unclear
E. None of the above

55. Which one of the following inheritances is most appropriate to describe mitochondrial DNA (mtDNA) depletion syndromes?
   A. Autosomal dominant
   B. Autosomal recessive
   C. Mitochondrial inherited
   D. X-linked
   E. Not clear

56. Which one of the following statements regarding Leber hereditary optic neuropathy (LHON) is NOT correct?
   A. It is caused by pathogenic variants in nuclear DNA encoded for mitochondria proteins.
   B. More than 50% of males with pathogenic variant(s) never experience vision loss or related health problems.
   C. More than 85% of females with pathogenic variant(s) never experience vision loss or related health problems.
   D. LHON is a young-adult-onset disorder.
   E. None of the above.

57. A 20-year-old apparently healthy male was referred to an ophthalmological clinic for unexplained loss of vision. Initial examination revealed a best corrected acuity of 20/20 in the right eye and 20/50 in the left eye with a stable myopic correction. An ophthalmological examination did not reveal abnormal findings. Slit-lamp evaluation revealed healthy anterior segments. The intraocular pressure was 14 mmHg in each eye. Fundus evaluation showed healthy optic disks and maculae. Color vision was 10/14 in the right eye and 6/14 in the left eye by Ishihara plates. Visual fields were unreliable. A retrobulbar optic neuritis was suspected. The MRI was unremarkable. One month later, vision had dropped to 20/30 in the right eye, and to barely count fingers in the left eye. Faint inferior disk swelling was noted in the left eye. Visual fields now demonstrated dense central scotomas in both eyes. Differential diagnosis included drug toxicity, metabolic disease, syphilis, hereditary optic atrophy or neuropathy (LHON), and compressive lesion. A molecular genetics study was ordered for LHON. Which one of the following molecular genetics assays would provide the most cost-effective genetic testing strategy for this patient?[17]
   A. Chromosomal microarray
   B. Multiplex ligation-dependent probe amplification
   C. Next-generation sequencing
   D. Quantitative PCR
   E. Sanger sequencing
   F. Targeted variants analysis

58. A 17-year-old male was referred to a neurological clinic for progressive bilateral visual loss for 6 months. He had first lost sight in his left eye; in a few days, he could see only shadows. One week later, the same symptom occurred in his right eye. At the time of examination, he was able to see only shadows in his right eye. This patient had had generalized tonic–clonic seizures from the age of 7 months until he was 2 years old, with good control using phenobarbital. His two maternal uncles had had similar patterns of visual loss; they died of nonrelated diseases in their 50s without a definite diagnosis. The patient had been smoking about 30 cigarettes/day and drinking heavily every day for 1 year before having vision symptoms. Neuroophthalmological examination revealed visual acuity of 20/800 in both eyes. The direct and consensual pupillary light reflexes were decreased, whereas the extrinsic ocular motility was normal. A campimetric study showed complete visual loss in all fields of both eyes. Fundus examination demonstrated pale optic disks. Visual campimetry showed a marked decrease of retina sensitivity in both eyes. Initial visual evoked potential during the first days of the condition showed discrete signs of conduction disturbances in the optic nerves. Retina fluorescein angiography showed signs of pale optic disks bilaterally, associated with tortuous retinal vessels. Pulse therapy with methylprednisolone did not result in visual improvement. Muscle biopsy was abnormal but nonspecific, with atrophy of fiber types 1 and 2. Hereditary optic atrophy or neuropathy (LHON) was suspected. A molecular genetic study was ordered and confirmed the diagnosis. Which one of the following pathogenic variants would the patient most likely?[18]
   A. m.3243A > G MTTL1
   B. m.3460G > A in MTND1
   C. m.8993T > C in MTATP6
   D. m.8344A > G in MTTK
   E. All of the above
   F. None of the above

59. A 12-year-old boy was brought to a clinic by his parents for progressively blurred vision in both eyes for more than 1 year and worsened visual acuity of the left eye for 2 months. He first started losing sight in his left eye; after a few days, he could see only shadows. His best-corrected visual acuity was 0.08 in the right eye and 0.1 in the left. His medical records revealed no congenital or systemic illness, no drug or substance abuse, and no family history of poor vision. Ophthalmological examination showed bilateral optic disk hyperemia and margin blurring, peripapillary telangiectasias, and a relative afferent pupil defect in his right eye. Fluorescein angiography showed no stain or leakage around the optic disk in the late phase. Visual-field analysis showed central scotoma in the left eye and a near-total defect in the right. Based on the clinical symptoms and signs, hereditary optic atrophy or neuropathy (LHON) was suspected. A molecular genetics study was ordered and confirmed the diagnosis. Which one of the following pathogenic variants would the patient most likely have?[19]

A. Heteroplasmic m.11778G > A in *MTND1*
B. Homoplasmic m.11778G > A in *MTND1*
C. Heteroplasmic m.11778G > A in *MTND4*
D. Homoplasmic m.11778G > A in *MTND4*
E. None of the above

60. A 17-year-old male came to a clinic with progressive bilateral visual loss. Two maternal uncles had similar patterns of visual loss. The patient had a history of smoking and alcohol abuse. A neuroophthalmological examination revealed a visual acuity of 20/800 in both eyes, with decreased direct and consensual pupillary light reflexes. Fundus examination demonstrated pale optic disks. Visual evoked potential testing showed signs of conduction disturbances in both optic nerves and a campimetric study showed complete visual loss in all fields of both eyes. A diagnosis of bilateral optic neuropathy with a clinical suspicion of Leber hereditary optic neuropathy (LHON) was made. Which one of the following statements regarding Leber hereditary optic neuropathy (LHON) is NOT correct?[18]

A. It happens more frequently in males than in females.
B. It is a mitochondrial disorder caused by mtDNA with heteroplasmy in some patients.
C. It is a mitochondrial disorder caused by nuclear DNAs.
D. Patients with LHON usually lose their vision in young adulthood.
E. None of the above.

61. A 17-year-old male came to a clinic with progressive bilateral visual loss. Two maternal uncles had similar patterns of visual loss. The patient had a history of smoking and alcohol abuse. A neuroophthalmological examination revealed a visual acuity of 20/800 in both eyes, with decreased direct and consensual pupillary light reflexes. Fundus examination demonstrated pale optic disks. Visual evoked potential testing showed signs of conduction disturbances in both optic nerves and a campimetric study showed

complete visual loss in all fields of both eyes. A diagnosis of bilateral optic neuropathy with a clinical suspicion of Leber hereditary optic neuropathy (LHON) was made. A blood sample was submitted for genetic analysis, and a homoplasmic pathogenic variant in m.11778 was detected. Which one of the following would be the risk of his future children having vision loss due to LHON?[18]

A. <1%
B. 10%
C. 25%
D. 50%
E. >99%
F. Unpredictable
G. None of the above

62. A 17-year-old male came to a clinic with progressive bilateral visual loss. Two maternal uncles had similar patterns of visual loss. The patient had a history of smoking and alcohol abuse. A neuroophthalmological examination revealed a visual acuity of 20/800 in both eyes, with decreased direct and consensual pupillary light reflexes. Fundus examination demonstrated pale optic disks. Visual evoked potential testing showed signs of conduction disturbances in both optic nerves and a campimetric study showed complete visual loss in all fields of both eyes. A diagnosis of bilateral optic neuropathy with a clinical suspicion of Leber hereditary optic neuropathy (LHON) was made. A blood sample was submitted for genetic analysis, and a homoplasmic pathogenic variant in m.3460 was detected. Which one of the following would be the recurrent risk of LHON in this family?[18]

A. <1%
B. 10%
C. 25%
D. 50%
E. >99%
F. Unpredictable
G. None of the above

63. A 48-year-old female of thin and short appearance (height, 146 cm; weight, 33 kg) was admitted to a hospital for poor blood glucose control. The medical history was significant for diabetes mellitus with onset at age 32, progressive hearing loss in the past 5 years, and a right cerebral infarction 1 year ago. On evaluation, she had mild limb weakness on the left side. A brain CT scan revealed calcification over the bilateral basal ganglia and cerebellum. Brain MRI study revealed cerebral atrophy. The serum glycated hemoglobin (HbA1c) level was elevated (9.5%; normal, <6.2%), and serum immunoreactive

insulin and C-peptide levels were lower than normal controls. Elevated levels of serum creatinine kinase (270 U/L; control range, 15–130) and lactate dehydrogenase (176 U/L; control range, 47–140), and myopathic changes in electromyography suggested concurrent myopathy. A muscle biopsy on the right vastus lateralis revealed ragged red fibers on modified Gomori trichrome staining. An electron microscopic study also revealed a large proportion of abnormal mitochondria of variable sizes in the subsarcolemmal region. Because mitochondrial encephalomyopathy was suspected, muscle, hair follicles, and blood specimens from this patient were sent for mtDNA analysis. Which one of the following genes would most likely harbor a pathogenic variant?[20]

A. *MTATP6*

B. *MTND1*

C. *MTTH*

D. *MTTL1*

E. None of the above

64. A 44-year-old female of normal body weight (body-mass index, calculated as the weight in kilograms divided by the square of the height in meters [BMI], 22) with an 11-year history of diabetes mellitus (DM) came to a clinic for poor recovery from exercise. At age 19, she had been diagnosed with Wolff–Parkinson–White (WPW) syndrome and had experienced several episodes of tachycardia resulting in loss of consciousness; the last episode occurred at age 36. She had been diagnosed with gestational diabetes mellitus (GDM) requiring insulin during her first pregnancy at the age of 23 and her second pregnancy at age 25. After a period of a normalized glucose-tolerance level, she had been diagnosed with DM at age 33. Meanwhile, medical records documented unexplained stable proteinuria since age 25 and progressive bilateral sensorineural hearing loss since age 37. Her family history was remarkable for five of seven siblings having deafness and four having DM. Her mother did not have DM, but she died of a myocardial infarction at age 56. GDM is suspected in the mother of the proband because the birth weights of her last three children ranged from 9 to 11 lb. The two children of the proband, aged 19 and 21, remain healthy, with documented normal glucose tolerance, hearing, and urinalysis. At the time of consultation, the proband's total daily insulin dosage was 60 U and her hemoglobin A1c (HbA1c) was 8.8% (upper limit of the nondiabetic range, 6.1%). The patient had no diabetic retinopathy; however, she exhibited

retinal pigmentation in keeping with macular pattern dystrophy. Her microalbumin-to-creatinine ratio was 32.9 mg/mmol (normal range, <3.4). She reported mild numbness and tingling in her feet and hands. Maternally inherited diabetes and deafness syndrome (MIDD) was suspected and a molecular study was ordered for it. Which one of the following pathogenic variants would the patient most likely have?[21]

A. Heteroplasmic m.11778G > A in *MTND4*

B. Homoplasmic m.11778G > A in *MTND4*

C. Heteroplasmic m.3243A > G *IN MTTL1*

D. Homoplasmic m.3243A > G *IN MTTL1*

E. None of the above

65. A 13-year-old girl born of consanguineous parents developed repeated myoclonic jerks three to four times a day lasting for about 4 seconds after a systemic infection. While on treatment for epilepsy, she developed progressive difficulty in reading over a year, resulting in only finger counting vision at a 1-m distance. She also had progressive hearing loss of 3 months' duration. In addition, there was decreased scholastic performance, mild unsteadiness, and pulsatile-quality headache. Her mother and maternal aunt had a history of similar illnesses at age 17 and were being treated. Both her mother and maternal aunt had large midline lipomas in the neck, and the latter had recurrence after surgical removal. Her mother had a bad obstetric history, with a triplet spontaneous abortion at 3 months and the twin of the index case died during the neonatal period. On examination, the patient was short for her age, with large ears, bilateral primary optic atrophy, sensorineural deafness and mild unsteadiness of gait. Brain stem auditory evoked responses (BAERs) were absent, and visual evoked responses showed prolonged latencies. MRI of the brain was normal except for mild prominence of the cerebellar folia. A muscle biopsy showed ragged red cytochrome C oxidase (COX)-deficient fibers. A molecular study for mtDNA was ordered to confirm the diagnosis of myoclonic epilepsy with ragged red fibers (MERRF), and a pathogenic variant was detected. Which one of the following genes would most likely harbor a pathogenic variant in this patient?[22]

A. *MTATP6*

B. *MTND1*

C. *MTTK*

D. *MTTL1*

E. None of the above

66. A 25-year-old male presented to a clinic with paroxysmal left-upper-limb tics and weakness for 2 years. The involuntary limb tics had a sudden onset

and lasted for seconds, but were not accompanied by a disturbance in consciousness. The patient had approximately 10 attacks per day, which were accompanied by limb weakness. A neurological examination revealed decreased deep tendon reflexes and a decreased sensation of touch, pain and vibration. The gait of the patient was broad and he was unable to walk in a straight line. An EEG revealed diffuse spikes and slow waves, predominantly in the frontal and temporal lobes. An fMRI scan revealed increased signal density on T2-weighted imaging and decreased signal density on T1-weighted imaging in the right temporal occipital cortical lesions. Local cortical atrophy was also observed in the left temporooccipital cortex. In addition, the lactic acid concentration (5.2 mmol/L) had markedly increased. A biopsy of the biceps muscle demonstrated a variation in fiber size and the presence of ragged red fibers. A muscle biopsy showed ragged red COX-deficient fibers. A molecular study for mtDNA was ordered to confirm the diagnosis of myoclonic epilepsy with ragged red fibers (MERRF), and a pathogenic variant was detected. Which one of the following pathogenic variants would the patient most likely have?[23]

A. Heteroplasmic m.14484T > C in *MTND6*
B. Homoplasmic m.14484T > C in *MTND6*
C. Heteroplasmic m.8344A > G in *MTTK*
D. Homoplasmic m.8344A > G in *MTTK*
E. None of the above

67. A 10-year-old boy presented to a clinic with recurrent episodes of headache, nausea, and vomiting for 5 years and hyperlactic acidemia. These episodes were associated with motor weakness on the right side, difficulties in language and memory, and visual disturbances. The mother reported that her brother suffered from the same clinical picture and died by the age of 19 years, but the cause of death was not clear. Neurological examination revealed generalized muscle weakness with mild right-sided hemiparesis. MRI revealed infarction of the left posterior parietal, left occipital, and left medial temporal regions and no visible vascular abnormality on magnetic resonance angiography (MRA). Laboratory testing revealed hyperlactic acidemia and a discrete increase in hepatic transaminases. A diagnosis of mitochondrial encephalomyopathy, lactic acidosis, and stroke-like episodes (MELAS) syndrome was suspected. A molecular study for mtDNA was ordered to confirm the diagnosis, and a pathogenic variant was detected. Which one of the following genes would most likely harbor a pathogenic variant in this patient?[24]

A. *MTATP6*
B. *MTND1*
C. *MTTK*
D. *MTTL1*
E. None of the above

68. A couple came to a genetics clinic for prenatal counseling. Their 2-year-old firstborn son with profound congenital bilateral hearing loss had arrhythmia related to a long QT interval found recently on ECG. The family history was unremarkable on both sides (see the figure below for the pedigree). Which one of the following disorders would the son most likely have if there was a genetic etiology?

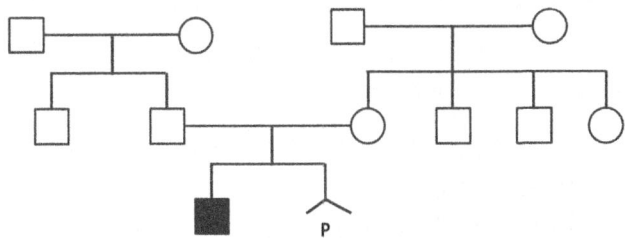

A. Andersen–Tawil syndrome
B. Jervell and Lange-Nielsen syndrome
C. Romano–Ward syndrome
D. Timothy syndrome
E. Usher syndrome

69. A couple came to a genetics clinic for prenatal counseling. Their 2-year-old firstborn son with profound congenital bilateral hearing loss had arrhythmia related to a long QT interval found recently on ECG. The family history was unremarkable on both sides (see below figure for the pedigree). The boy was diagnosed with Jervell and Lange-Nielsen syndrome clinically. A molecular genetics study was pending. What would most likely be the risk that the fetus had the same disorder if the couple's firstborn son had Jervell and Lange-Nielsen syndrome?

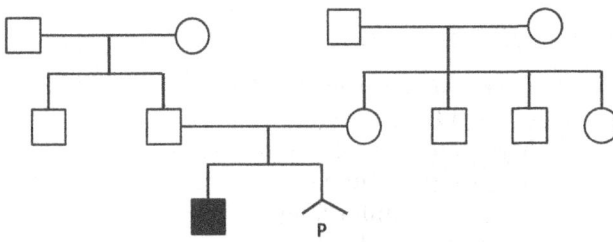

A. <1%
B. 25%
C. 50%
D. 75%
E. >99%

70. A couple came to a genetics clinic for prenatal counseling. Their 2-year-old firstborn son with profound congenital bilateral hearing loss had arrhythmia related to a long QT interval found recently on ECG. The family history was unremarkable on both sides (see the figure below for the pedigree). The boy was diagnosed with Jervell and Lange-Nielsen syndrome clinically. What would most likely be the risk that the fetus had the same long-QT intervals as his brother?

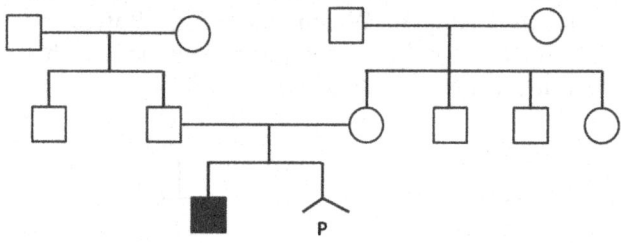

    A. Up to 1%
    B. Up to 25%
    C. Up to 50%
    D. Up to 75%
    E. Up to 100%

71. A couple came to a genetics clinic for prenatal counseling. Their 2-year-old firstborn son had had a couple of fainting episodes and was diagnosed with long-QT syndrome by ECG. The family history was negative on both sides. A molecular test revealed that both the mother and the son has a missense pathogenic variant in the *KCNQ1* gene. Neither the mother nor the son had hearing loss or facial dysmorphic features. The mother had no history of fainting episodes and had been apparently healthy. Subsequent ECG confirmed the diagnosis for the mother. What would most likely be the risk that the fetus had long-QT syndrome?

    A. <1%
    B. 25%
    C. 50%
    D. 75%
    E. 100%

72. What type of genes tend to be mutated in patients with long-QT syndrome?

    A. Myofilament proteins of the sarcomere
    B. Cardiac potassium channels
    C. Cardiac sodium channels
    D. Cardiac chloride channels
    E. Cardiac bicarbonate channels

73. Hypertrophic cardiomyopathy is one of the most common monogenic autosomal dominant cardiovascular diseases, which is caused by pathogenic variants in approximately 20 genes encoding proteins of the cardiac sarcomere. What is the maximum clinical sensitivity of a next-generation sequencing (NGS) panel of all 20 genes for hypertrophic cardiomyopathy?

    A. <1%
    B. 25%
    C. 55%
    D. 85%
    E. >99%

74. A previous healthy 48-year-old Caucasian male came to an emergency department for radiating chest pain, which turned out to be myocardial infarction. His LDL cholesterol level was 249 mg/dL and total cholesterol 465 mg/dL at the time of admission. The family history was remarkable for coronary artery diseases in multiple members (see the figure below for the pedigree). Which one of the following inherited modes would the disorder most likely be in this family if it was genetic?

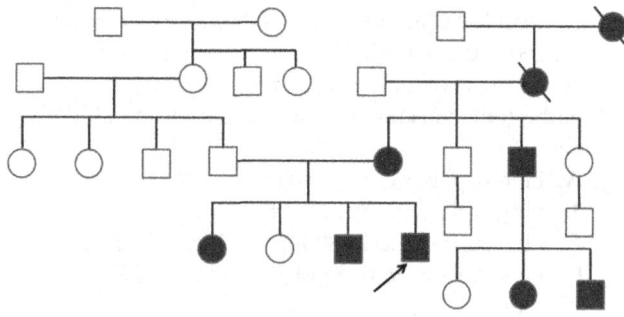

    A. Autosomal dominant
    B. Autosomal recessive
    C. Mitochondrial inherited
    D. X-linked
    E. None of the above

75. A previous healthy 55-year-old Caucasian male came to an emergency department for radiating chest pain, which turned out to be myocardial infarction. His LDL cholesterol level was 189 mg/dL and total cholesterol 218 mg/dL. The family history was remarkable for his father dying of a myocardial infarction at age 61. His brother's untreated LDL cholesterol level was approximately 300 mg/dL at age 58. He was married with a 13-year-old son. A molecular genetics study detected a heterozygous variant c.34C>T(p.Gln12Ter), in *LDLR* in this patient. Which one of the following family members should also be tested for familial hypercholesterolemia?

    A. His wife and son
    B. His brother and son
    C. His wife, brother, and son

D. His brother, son, and all the other first-degree relatives

E. His first-degree relatives older than 18 years

F. None of the above

76. A 21-year-old unmarried female comes to a dermatological clinic with symptoms of multiple soft asymptomatic yellow nodular lesions all over the body that had begun at the age of 2 years. The patient was born to nonconsanguineous parents and her development was normal. There is no history of chest pain, breathlessness, hypertension, diabetes mellitus, hypothyroidism, or any other chronic illness. The patient's parents and two siblings are healthy. However, her paternal uncle and his three sons died at an early age possibly owing to myocardial infarction (younger than 45 years). Dermatological examination reveals extensive and multiple tendinous and tuberous xanthomas of varying sizes, ranging from 1 to 6 cm, distributed mainly over the cubital and popliteal fossae, axillae, shoulders, knees, elbows, hands, and feet. Xanthelasma palpebrarum is noted around the eyelids, and her eyes showed arcus juvenilis. Her total cholesterol is 620 mg/dL, triglyceride 143 mg/dL, LDL 549 mg/dL, HDL 93 mg/dL, and VLDL 27 mg/dL. 2D-electrocardiography reveals posterior annular calcification of the mitral valve, thickened and sclerosed aortic valve with mild aortic regurgitation, and mitral regurgitation. The arteries have extensive atherosclerosis. Familial hypercholesterolemia (FH) is suspected. Which one of the following genes may be tested for pathogenic variant(s) in this patient?[25]

A. *APOB*

B. *LDLR*

C. *PCSK9*

D. All of the above

E. None of the above

77. A 21-year-old unmarried female comes to a dermatological clinic with symptoms of multiple soft asymptomatic yellow nodular lesions all over the body that had begun at the age of 2 years. The patient was born to nonconsanguineous parents and her development was normal. There is no history of chest pain, breathlessness, hypertension, diabetes mellitus, hypothyroidism, or any other chronic illness. The patient's parents and two siblings are healthy. However, her paternal uncle and his three sons died at an early age possibly owing to myocardial infarction (younger than 45 years). Dermatological examination reveals extensive and multiple tendinous and tuberous xanthomas of varying sizes, ranging from 1 to

6 cm, distributed mainly over the cubital and popliteal fossae, axillae, shoulders, knees, elbows, hands, and feet. Xanthelasma palpebrarum is noted around the eyelids, and her eyes showed arcus juvenilis. Her total cholesterol is 620 mg/dL, triglyceride 143 mg/dL, LDL 549 mg/dL, HDL 93 mg/dL, and VLDL 27 mg/dL. 2D-electrocardiography reveals posterior annular calcification of the mitral valve, thickened and sclerosed aortic valve with mild aortic regurgitation, and mitral regurgitation. The arteries have extensive atherosclerosis. Familial hypercholesterolemia (FH) is suspected. Which one of the following pathogenic variants does the patient most likely have?[25]

A. Heterozygous c.3997C > T(p. Arg1306Ter) in *APOB*

B. Homozygous c.3997C > T(p. Arg1306Ter) in *APOB*

C. Heterozygous c.34C > T(p.Gln12Ter) in *LDLR*

D. Homozygous c.34C > T(p.Gln12Ter) in *LDLR*

E. None of the above

78. Which one of the following disorders is associated with age-related penetrance?

A. Familial hypercholesterolemia

B. Hereditary hemochromatosis

C. Huntington disease

D. Hypertrophic cardiomyopathy

E. All of the above

F. None of the above

79. Which one of the following disorders is associated sex-related penetrance?[26]

A. Familial hypercholesterolemia

B. Hereditary hemochromatosis

C. Huntington disease

D. Hypertrophic cardiomyopathy

E. All of the above

F. None of the above

80. A couple brought their 8-year-old daughter to a genetics clinic for Hirschsprung disease 1 month after the surgery to remove the aganglionic segment of colon. The surgeon defined it as "long-segment disease." The child's medical history was negative. Her family history was positive for multiple members on the maternal side having a similar disease. The family was counseled, and a molecular genetics study was ordered for the proband. Which one of the following genes would most likely be tested in this patient?[6]

A. *EDN3*

B. *MEN1*

C. *RAS*

D. *RB1*

E. *RET*

81. A couple brought their 8-year-old son to a genetics clinic for Hirschsprung disease 1 month after the surgery to remove the aganglionic segment of colon. The surgeon defined it as "long-segment disease." The child's medical history was negative. His family history was positive for multiple members on the maternal side having a similar disease. But the mother is phenotypically normal. The molecular genetics test results showed that both the proband and his mother had a pathogenic variant in the *RET* gene. Which one of the following statements explains the discrepancy of clinical presentation in the family?[6]

A. The pathogenic variant from the paternal copy is missed by the molecular test.

B. Low (incomplete) penetrance explains why the mother does not have the disease.

C. The disease affects only males.

D. The test results were wrong. The sample should be sent to another lab to be tested again.

E. Peripheral blood is the wrong sample type. An FFPE sample from resected colon should be sent for the study.

82. A full-term boy was born to a 28-year-old primigravida female with no complications. No meconium was passed in the first 48 hours after birth, then he started to pass nonbilious nonbloody vomitus. He was transferred to the NICU owing to the persistent vomiting and failure of his bowels to open. An upper GI contrast study excluded a malrotation. Hirschsprung disease was then suspected and confirmed on punch rectal biopsies. The genetics of Hirschsprung disease are complex and are not completely understood. How frequently does Hirschsprung disease have an identifiable genetic etiology?

A. 10%
B. 30%
C. 50%
D. 70%
E. 90%
F. >99%

83. An infant boy presents in the second day of life with a large bilious emesis. He had been "spitty" for a day and had yielded 15 mL of greenish gastric aspirate at birth. He had not passed meconium for the first 36 hours of life. He was born at term weighing 3.5 kg. He is an active hungry infant with a moderately distended abdomen. Bowel sounds are very active but not obstructive in nature. No organs or abdominal masses are appreciated, and no

hernias are present. His anus is patent. An abdominal series reveals large dilated loops of bowel but no air in the rectum. A hand-injected contrast enema on the third day of life shows no distinct transition zone. A 24-hour delayed film shows retained contrast and a rectal mucosal suction biopsy reveals an absence of ganglion cells and the presence of hypertrophied nerve fibers consistent with a diagnosis of Hirschsprung disease. If a molecular study is performed to explore the genetic etiology of the Hirschsprung disease in this patient, which one of the following molecular genetic assays is most likely be used to explore the genetic etiology of the Hirschsprung disease in this patient?

A. Chromosomal microarray analysis
B. Next-generation sequencing
C. Sanger sequencing
D. Targeted variant assay
E. Whole-exome sequencing
F. None of the above

84. A full-term male infant was born via an uncomplicated spontaneous vaginal delivery with a birth weight of 3.4 kg in a community hospital. He developed progressive abdominal distention during the first day of life and did not pass meconium. After two bouts of bilious emesis, transfer was arranged for further evaluation and management in a tertiary medical center. On admission, the patient was in mild distress. His abdomen was distended and bowel sounds were present. The anus was patent, with normal sphincter tone, and a small amount of meconium was present on rectal stimulation. No other malformations were apparent on physical exam. Abdominal roentgenography (AXR) showed numerous loops of bowel in a right-sided abdominal distribution and a separate enlarged loop in the left lower quadrant. No free air was appreciated. As well, on the plain film, hemivertebral bodies were seen at the distal thoracic spine with dysplasia of the left ribs. Concern for a distal bowel obstruction was evaluated. Which one of the following disorders is NOT associated with an elevated risk for intestinal obstruction in newborns?[27]

A. Cystic fibrosis
B. Hirschsprung disease
C. Multiple endocrine neoplasia type 1 (MEN1)
D. Multiple endocrine neoplasia type 2 (MEN2)
E. Waardenburg syndrome
F. All of the above
G. None of the above

85. A 26-year-old female came to an emergency department for constipation for many years. She had been evaluated multiple times since the age of 8, and the constipation had been slowly worsening since that time. The results for colonoscopy, barium enema, and anal manometry had been all normal. There was no history of delayed passing of meconium. Her family history was remarkable for similar constipation symptoms in her mother and aunt. A physical examination revealed significant abdominal distention and tympany to palpation. An abdominal CT found severe colonic dilation along with extensive fecal loading and generalized colonic wall thickening. Flexible sigmoidoscopy revealed a markedly distended colon. A gastric emptying study showed severe delay. Rectal biopsy demonstrated a paucity of ganglion cells suggestive of Hirschsprung disease. In which one of the following populations does Hirschsprung disease have the highest incidence?[28]
   A. Female infants
   B. Male infants
   C. Female adults
   D. Male adults
   E. None of the above

86. A Caucasian couple came to a genetics clinic for preconception counseling. The wife had neurofibromatosis 1 (NF1) with a deleterious variant, p.Lys1423Glu, in the *NF1* gene. The husband was apparently healthy. The family history was unremarkable on both sides. Which one of the following would most likely be the risk of their first child having NF1?
   A. <1%
   B. 25%
   C. 50%
   D. >99%
   E. Unclear
   F. None of the above

87. A 16-year-old female came to a genetics clinic with bilateral marked diminution of vision. A physical examination revealed bilateral primary optic atrophy, 12 café au lait spots, and some cutaneous neurofibromatosis. Eight of twelve café au lait spots measured larger than 5 mm in diameter. She was diagnosed with neurofibromatosis 1 (NF1) clinically. A molecular genetics study detected a deleterious variant, p.Lys1423Glu, in the *NF1* gene. Which one of the following would most appropriately describe the pathogenic variant identified in this teenage girl?
   A. Dominant negative variant
   B. Gain-of-function variant
   C. Loss-of-function variant

   D. De novo variant
   E. None of the above

88. A 16-year-old female came to a genetics clinic with bilateral marked diminution of vision. A physical examination revealed bilateral primary optic atrophy, 12 café au lait spots, and some cutaneous neurofibromatosis. Eight of twelve café au lait spots measured larger than 5 mm in diameter. She was diagnosed with neurofibromatosis 1 (NF1) clinically. The family history was unremarkable on both sides. A molecular genetics study detected a deleterious variant, p.Lys1423Glu, in the *NF1* gene. Targeted molecular genetic analysis of the parents did not identify the same variant. Which one of the following descriptions would most likely be appropriate for the genetic etiology of NF1 in this family?[6]
   A. Most likely the teenage girl had a maternally derived de novo pathogenic variant in *NF1*.
   B. Most likely the teenage girl had a paternally derived de novo pathogenic variant in *NF1*.
   C. It is hard to tell the origin of the de novo pathogenic variants in the teenage girl.
   D. Testing of the father may be suggested to further interpret the results in the family.
   E. None of the above.

89. A 6-year-old girl was brought to a genetics clinic by her parents for café au lait spots. A physical examination revealed 12 café au lait spots and some cutaneous neurofibromatosis. Eight of twelve café au lait spots measured larger than 5 mm in diameter. An ophthalmological examination detected Lisch nodules in both eyes. She was diagnosed with neurofibromatosis 1 (NF1) clinically. The family history was remarkable for the girl's 9-year-old brother also being diagnosed with NF1. A molecular genetics study of the girl detected a deleterious variant, p.Lys1423Glu, in the *NF1* gene. Targeted molecular genetic analysis of the parents and the brother found that none of them had the same variant. Subsequently genetics study of the girl's brother identified a deletion involving exons 3, 4, and 5. Which one of the following might explain the discrepancy between clinical diagnoses and genetic testing results in this family?[29,30]
   A. More than one de novo pathogenic variant exists in this family.
   B. Alternative paternity is possible in this family.
   C. Alternative maternity is possible through assisted reproduction in this family.
   D. One or both children in this family was adopted.
   E. All of the above.
   F. None of the above.

90. A 6-year-old girl was brought to a genetics clinic by her parents for café au lait spots. A physical examination revealed 12 café au lait spots and some cutaneous neurofibromatosis. Eight of twelve café au lait spots measured larger than 5 mm in diameter. An ophthalmological examination detected Lisch nodules in both eyes. She was diagnosed with neurofibromatosis 1 (NF1) clinically. The family history was remarkable for the girl's 9-year-old brother also being diagnosed with NF1. A molecular genetics study of the girl detected a deleterious variant, p. Lys1423Glu, in the *NF1* gene. Targeted molecular genetics analysis of the parents and the brother found that the parents did not have the same variant but that the brother did. Which one of the following might explain the genetic findings in this family?[29-32]
  A. More than one de novo pathogenic variant exists in this family.
  B. One of the parents was mosaic for the pathogenic variant.
  C. Alternative paternity is possible in this family.
  D. Alternative maternity is possible through assisted reproduction in this family.
  E. One or both children in this family is adopted.
  F. All of the above.
  G. None of the above.

91. A 6-year-old girl was brought to a genetics clinic by her parents for café au lait spots. A physical examination revealed 12 café au lait spots and some cutaneous neurofibromatosis. Eight of twelve café au lait spots measured larger than 5 mm in diameter. An ophthalmological examination detected Lisch nodules in both eyes. She was diagnosed with neurofibromatosis 1 (NF1) clinically. The family history was remarkable for the girl's 9-year-old brother also being diagnosed with NF1. A molecular genetics study of the girl did not detect pathogenic variant (s) in the *NF1* gene. Which one of the following would be the most appropriate interpretation of the negative genetic results in this patient?
  A. She may still have NF1.
  B. She did not have NF1.
  C. She may have NF2.
  D. She may have NF3.
  E. All of the above.
  F. None of the above.

92. A 16-year-old female came to a genetics clinic with bilateral marked diminution of vision. A physical examination revealed bilateral primary optic atrophy, 12 café au lait spots, and some cutaneous neurofibromatosis. Eight of twelve café au lait spots measured larger than 5 mm in

diameter. She was diagnosed with neurofibromatosis 1 (NF1) clinically. The family history was unremarkable on both sides. Which one of the following benign or malignant tumors would the girl least likely have an increased risk to develop?
  A. Central nervous system tumors
  B. Clear-cell renal-cell carcinoma
  C. Malignant myeloid disorders
  D. Optic-nerve gliomas
  E. Pheochromocytoma

93. In which of the following disorders are Lisch nodules a common feature?
  A. Hereditary hemochromatosis
  B. Neurofibromatosis 1
  C. Neurofibromatosis 2
  D. Tuberous sclerosis
  E. Wilson disease

94. In which of the following disorders is vestibular schwannoma a common feature?
  A. Hereditary hemochromatosis
  B. Neurofibromatosis 1
  C. Neurofibromatosis 2
  D. Tuberous sclerosis
  E. Wilson disease

95. Which one of the following tumors is one of the primary tumor types in patients with neurofibromatosis 2 (NF2)?
  A. Neurofibroma
  B. Optic-nerve glioma
  C. Pheochromocytoma
  D. Schwannoma
  E. None of the above

96. A 28-year-old Caucasian male presented to a clinic with a history of bilateral tinnitus and progressive hearing loss of 9 months' duration. He also had swaying toward either side on walking for 4 months. His family history was unremarkable. A physical examination found that he had a few subcutaneous swellings over the trunk. He had neither café au lait spots nor any axillary or inguinal freckling. He had bilateral severe sensorineural deafness and a mild bilateral lower motor neuron type of facial palsy and cerebellar signs. Ophthalmologic evaluation revealed loss of corneal reflex on right side and papilledema. A brain CT scan revealed bilateral ovoid well-circumscribed masses at both cerebellopontine angles with heterogeneous contrast enhancement. Based on clinical findings, a diagnosis of neurofibromatosis 2 (NF2) was made. Sanger sequencing and deletion/duplication testing of *NF2* did not detect pathogenic variants. Which one of the following would be the most appropriate next step in the workup to identify the genetic etiology of this patient's NF2?[33]

A. Exome sequencing
B. Linkage study
C. Molecular testing for NF1
D. Using fibroblast cells to test *NF2*
E. Whole-genome sequencing
F. None of the above

97. A 28-year-old Ashkenazi Jewish male presented to a clinic with history of bilateral tinnitus and progressive hearing loss of 9 months' duration. He also had swaying toward either side on walking for 4 months. His family history was unremarkable. A physical examination found that he had a few subcutaneous swellings over the trunk. He had neither café au lait spots nor any axillary or inguinal freckling. He had bilateral severe sensorineural deafness and a mild bilateral lower motor neuron type of facial palsy and cerebellar signs. Ophthalmologic evaluation revealed loss of corneal reflex on right side and papilledema. A brain CT scan revealed bilateral ovoid well-circumscribed masses at both cerebellopontine angles with heterogeneous contrast enhancement. Based on clinical findings, a diagnosis of neurofibromatosis 2 (NF2) was made. Sanger sequencing and deletion/duplication testing of *NF2* was pending. The patient's wife was 10 weeks pregnant with their first baby. Which one of the following would be the most appropriate estimation of the fetus's risk for NF2?[33]

A. <1%
B. Up to 25%
C. Up to 50%
D. >99%
E. Not sure
F. None of the above

98. A 23-year-old Caucasian male presented to a clinic with a history of bilateral tinnitus and progressive hearing loss of 9 months' duration. He also had swaying toward either side on walking for 4 months. His mother was documented to have had an intracranial space-occupying lesion and died at the age of 32 years. A physical examination found that he had a few subcutaneous swellings over the trunk. He had neither café au lait spots nor any axillary or inguinal freckling. He had bilateral severe sensorineural deafness and a mild bilateral lower motor neuron type of facial palsy and cerebellar signs. Ophthalmologic evaluation revealed a loss of corneal reflex on the right side and papilledema. A brain CT scan revealed bilateral

ovoid well-circumscribed masses at both cerebellopontine angles with heterogeneous contrast enhancement. Based on clinical findings and family history, a diagnosis of neurofibromatosis 2 (NF2) was made. Sanger sequencing of *NF2* detected a pathogenic variant, c.1604T > C(p.Leu535Pro). The patient had a 14-year-old brother who remained asymptomatic but wanted to find out his risk for NF2. Which one of the following would be the most appropriate response to the request from the proband's younger brother?[33]

A. Referring him to a pediatric clinic
B. Refusing to test him, since NF2 is an adult-onset disease
C. Refusing to test him, since insurance would not pay for testing of asymptomatic individuals
D. Testing him for the familial pathogenic variant
E. None of the above

99. A 13-year-old Caucasian girl was brought to a genetics clinic for epilepsy that began at the age of 6 months. A physical examination revealed hypopigmented skin lesions on the face and abdomen. Radiological studies demonstrated typical cortical tubers, which led to a diagnosis of tuberous sclerosis. Follow-up studies detected a large number of angiomyolipomas in both kidneys. Pathological examination of biopsy specimens demonstrated an unclassified renal-cell carcinoma. A molecular genetics study was ordered to further assist the diagnosis. Which of the following genes would most likely be included in the molecular test for this patient?[34]

A. *TSC1*
B. *TSC2*
C. *TSC3*
D. A and B
E. A and C
F. A, B, and C
G. None of the above

100. A 13-year-old Caucasian girl was brought to a genetics clinic for epilepsy that began at the age of 6 months. Her family history was unremarkable. A physical examination revealed hypopigmented skin lesions on the face and abdomen. Radiological studies demonstrated typical cortical tubers, which led to a diagnosis of tuberous sclerosis. Follow-up studies detected a large number of angiomyolipomas in both kidneys. Pathological examination of biopsy specimens demonstrated an unclassified renal-cell carcinoma. A molecular genetics study was ordered to further assist the diagnosis and was

still pending. Which one of the following would most likely be the recurrent risk of TSC in this family?[34,35]

A. <1%
B. 25%
C. 50%
D. 99%
E. Unpredictable

101. Tuberous sclerosis complex (TSC) is the second most common neurocutaneous disease. It is inherited in an autosomal dominant pattern. What is the de novo mutation rate of TSC?

A. <1%
B. 15%
C. 33%
D. 50%
E. 67%
F. 99%

102. Rett syndrome is a progressive neurodevelopmental disorder. In which one of the following populations is the prevalence of Rett syndrome highest?

A. Ashkenazi Jewish
B. Boys
C. Caucasians
D. Girls
E. Late adulthood
F. Mediterranean

103. A 2-year-old girl was referred to a genetics clinic for decelerating growth and progressive loss of language and motor skills. She had normal development until the age of 18 months. This girl lost her acquired, purposeful hand skills, expressive and receptive language, and reciprocal social interaction. She gradually developed a broad-based gait and typical stereotypic hand movements. No other family members had neurological diseases. Generalized slow waves were observed throughout the EEG recording. MRI showed diffuse cerebral atrophy with T2 hypointensity of the basal ganglia, thalami, and midbrain and a focal T2 hypointense left occipital lobe lesion. Based on these findings, the neurologist suggested a diagnosis of Rett syndrome. Which one of the following genes would most likely be tested to confirm the diagnosis in this patient?[36]

A. CDKL5
B. DCX
C. FMR1
D. FOXG1
E. LIS1
F. MECP2

104. A 3-year-old girl was referred to a clinic for a gradual loss of speech and reciprocal social interaction. She gradually developed a broad-based gait and typical stereotypic hand movements in the past 12 months. She was born to nonconsanguineous parents with an uncomplicated pregnancy. The perinatal history was uneventful. No other family members had neurological diseases. Generalized slow waves were observed throughout the EEG recording. MRI showed diffuse cerebral atrophy with T2 hypointensity of the basal ganglia, thalami, and midbrain and a focal T2 hypointense left occipital lobe lesion. Based on these findings, the neurologist suggested a diagnosis of Rett syndrome. Genetic testing detected a pathogenic variant, c.808C > T(p.Arg270Ter), in the MECP2 gene. Peripheral-blood samples from the parents were collected for a targeted molecular analysis. Which one of the following would most likely be the detection rate in at least one of the parents?[36]

A. <1%
B. 25%
C. 50%
D. >99%
E. Unpredictable

105. A 1-year-old boy was referred to a genetics clinic for decelerating growth and progressive loss of language and motor skills. He had normal development until the age of 3 months. He lost his acquired, purposeful hand skills, expressive and receptive language, and reciprocal social interaction. He gradually developed a broad-based gait and typical stereotypic hand movements. No other family members had neurological diseases. Generalized slow waves were observed throughout the EEG recording. MRI showed diffuse cerebral atrophy with T2 hypointensity of the basal ganglia, thalami, and midbrain and a focal T2 hypointense left occipital lobe lesion. Based on these findings, the neurologist suggested a diagnosis of Rett syndrome. Which one of the following genes would most likely be tested to confirm the diagnosis in this patient?[36]

A. CDKL5
B. DCX
C. FMR1
D. FOXG1
E. LIS1
F. MECP2

106. A 2-year-old girl was referred to a genetics clinic for decelerating growth and progressive loss of

language and motor skills. She had normal development until the age of 18 months. She lost her acquired, purposeful hand skills, expressive and receptive language, and reciprocal social interaction. She gradually developed a broad-based gait and typical stereotypic hand movements. No other family members had any neurological diseases. Generalized slow waves were observed throughout the EEG recording. MRI showed diffuse cerebral atrophy with T2 hypointensity of the basal ganglia, thalami, and midbrain and focal T2 hypointense left occipital lobe lesion. Based on these findings, the neurologist suggested a diagnosis of Rett syndrome. A genetic testing was ordered to confirm the diagnosis. Which one of the following molecular genetic assays would most likely be used for the genetic study offered to this patient as the first-line test?[36]

- **A.** Chromosomal microarray
- **B.** Deletion/duplication array
- **C.** FISH
- **D.** Karyotype
- **E.** Sanger sequencing
- **F.** Targeted variant assays

107. In which one of the following populations does the *MECP2* duplication syndrome most likely occur?

- **A.** Ashkenazi Jewish
- **B.** Boys
- **C.** Caucasians
- **D.** Girls
- **E.** Late adulthood
- **F.** Mediterranean

108. An 8-year-old Indian girl was brought to a clinic for a gradual loss of speech, social interaction, and hand skills; stereotypic movements of the hand and body began at the age of 3. She was born to nonconsanguineous parents with an uncomplicated perinatal history. Her birth weight and height were normal. In the first 3 years of postnatal life, her development reached normal milestones. Then her developmental milestones became gradually delayed. A physical examination revealed gait ataxia, muscle wasting, microcephaly, dental attrition, dental caries, and an absence of meaningful words. Marked cognitive and communication delay suggested severe mental retardation. A brain MRI revealed diffuse cerebral atrophy with T2 hypointensity of basal ganglia, thalami, and midbrain. Her family history suggested mild mental retardation of her older sister. The physician suspected a diagnosis of Rett syndrome. Which one of the following tests

would most likely be ordered than others to confirm or rule out the diagnosis in this patient?[36]

- **A.** Deletion and duplication analysis of the *CDKL5* gene
- **B.** Deletion and duplication analysis of the *FOXG1* gene
- **C.** Deletion and duplication analysis of the *MECP2* gene
- **D.** Sequencing analysis of the *CDKL5* gene
- **E.** Sequencing analysis of the *FOXG1* gene
- **F.** Sequencing analysis of the *MECP2* gene
- **G.** None of the above

109. An 8-year-old Indian girl was brought to a clinic for a gradual loss of speech, social interaction, and hand skills; stereotypic movements of the hand and body began at the age of 3. She was born to nonconsanguineous parents with an uncomplicated perinatal history. Her birth weight and height were normal. In the first 3 years of postnatal life, her development reached normal milestones. Then her developmental milestones became gradually delayed. A physical examination revealed gait ataxia, muscle wasting, microcephaly, dental attrition, dental caries, and an absence of meaningful words. Marked cognitive and communication delay suggested severe mental retardation. A brain MRI revealed diffuse cerebral atrophy with T2 hypointensity of basal ganglia, thalami, and midbrain. Her family history suggested mild mental retardation of her older sister. The physician suspected a diagnosis of Rett syndrome. A molecular genetics study was ordered, and a pathogenic variant, c.806delG (p.V288X) in the *MECP2* gene, was detected. During the evaluation, the mother was pregnant with a boy. Which one of the following would most likely be the risk of this future sibling have Rett syndrome?[36]

- **A.** <1%
- **B.** 25%
- **C.** 50%
- **D.** 67%
- **E.** >99%
- **F.** None of the above

110. A 9-year-old boy, Jason, was brought to a clinic with global developmental delay for 8 years, frequent respiratory infections for 9 years, and seizure for 6 months. He was the second child of unrelated healthy parents and was born after a normal delivery from an uneventful pregnancy. The family history revealed a maternal cousin, Jonathan, with similar symptoms. A physical examination revealed mild dysmorphic facial features and severe mental retardation with poor speech. The EEG studies showed rhythmic theta

activity over the frontal areas and paroxysmal spike and slow waves with frontotemporal predominance. The physician suspected a *MECP2*-related disorder. Which one of the following studies would most likely be ordered to confirm or rule out the diagnosis in this patient?[37]
A. Deletion and duplication analysis of the *ATRX* gene
B. Deletion and duplication analysis of the *L1CAM* gene
C. Deletion and duplication analysis of the *MECP2* gene
D. Sequencing analysis of the *ATRX* gene
E. Sequencing analysis of the *L1CAM* gene
F. Sequencing analysis of the *MECP2* gene
G. None of the above

111. A scientist in a clinical molecular laboratory developed a next-generation sequencing (NGS) panel for epilepsy. Which one of the following genes would least likely be included in this panel?
A. *FOXP3*
B. *KCNQ2*
C. *MECP2*
D. *SCN1A*
E. None of the above

112. A 28-year-old mother gave a birth to a full-term baby girl after an uncomplicated pregnancy. On the third day of life, the baby girl was brought to a clinic for three brief generalized tonic seizures with upward deviation of the eyes and cyanosis of the lips that lasted approximately 1 minute for each. General and neurological examinations were unremarkable. Electrolytes, calcium, glucose, and EEG were all normal. She was administered phenobarbital and discharged in 3 days without seizures. Her phenobarbital was tapered off at 3 months of age. Her seizures recurred at 4 months of age. Her EEG revealed several spike discharges originating from the left and right central-temporal areas. Phenobarbital was restarted and tapered off successfully with no seizures at 7 months of age. She had normal neurodevelopment thereafter. Her family history was remarkable for five affected paternal family members in three generations with uncomplicated neonatal convulsions. Benign familial neonatal seizures were suspected. Which one of the following type of genes would most likely be mutated in this newborn if she had a pathogenic variant for benign familial neonatal seizures?[38]
A. Chloride channels
B. GABA receptor
C. Nicotinic acid receptor
D. Potassium channels
E. Sodium channels

113. A 7-year-old previously healthy boy was brought to an emergency department for a 10-minute tonic–clonic seizure while sleeping. Upon arrival, he was awake and responsive but showed clinical evidence of hypocalcemia and an unremarkable physical exam. His perinatal history and family history were unremarkable. Initial laboratory assessment showed a calcium level of 5.6 mg/dL, phosphate 8.7 mg/dL, and ionized calcium 0.71 mmol/L and 0.64 mmol/L in a 2-hour period. High-dose calcium was infused to prevent further seizure activity. Further assessment showed elevated PTH levels of 321 pg/mL with the concurrent calcium of 5.5 mg/dL, mild 25-hydroxyvitamin D deficiency of 14.1 ng/mL, normal 25-hydroxyvitamin D_1, thyroid-function test, and spot urinary calcium. Pseudohypoparathyroidism type 1B was suspected. A molecular study was ordered to confirm the diagnosis after the patient stabilized. Which one of the following molecular genetic assays would most likely be used as the first-line test to confirm the diagnosis in this patient?[39]
A. Chromosomal microarray
B. FISH
C. Methylation study
D. Multiplex ligation-dependent probe amplification (MLPA)
E. Next-generation sequencing
F. Sanger sequencing

114. A 6-year-old boy was referred to a clinic for absence seizure. There was no family history of endocrine problems or developmental delay. No dysmorphic features or bone deformation were appreciated. Laboratory testing revealed hypocalcemia, hyperphosphatasemia, and an elevated PTH level. A molecular study was ordered. The results showed hypermethylation at the *NESP55* and hypomethylation at *NESPAS*, *GNAS XL* and *GNAS A/B*. Which one of the following genes is exclusively maternally expressed?[40]
A. *GNAS A/B*
B. *GNAS XL*
C. *NESP55*
D. *NESPAS*
E. All of the above
F. None of the above

115. A 6-year-old boy was referred to a clinic for absence seizure. There was no family history of endocrine problems or developmental delay. No dysmorphic features or bone deformation were seen. Laboratory testing revealed hypocalcemia, hyperphosphatasemia, and an elevated PTH level. A molecular study was ordered. The results

showed hypermethylation at the *NESP55* and hypomethylation at the *NESPAS*, *GNAS XL*, and *GNAS A/B*. Which one of the following disorders would this patient most likely have?[40]

A. Pseudohypoparathyroidism type 1A
B. Pseudohypoparathyroidism type 1B
C. Pseudohypoparathyroidism type 2
D. Not sure
E. None of the above

116. A 6-year-old boy was referred to a clinic for absence seizure. There was no family history of endocrine problems or developmental delay. No dysmorphic features or bone deformation were seen. Laboratory testing revealed hypocalcemia, hyperphosphatasemia, and an elevated PTH level. Pseudohypoparathyroidism type 1B (PHP-1B) was suspected. A molecular study was ordered to confirm the diagnosis. Which one of the following testing results would most likely confirm the diagnosis of PHP-1B?[40]

A. Hypermethylation of *GNAS A/B*
B. Hypermethylation of *GNAS XL*
C. Hypermethylation of *NESP55*
D. Hypermethylation of *NESPAS*
E. None of the above

117. Which one of the following pathogenic variants is most likely detected than others in a patient with pseudohypoparathyroidism (PHP)?[41,42]

A. De novo c.725Cdel in *GNAS*
B. Maternally inherited c.725Cdel in *GNAS*
C. Paternally inherited c.725Cdel in *GNAS*
D. All of the above
E. None of the above

118. A 7-year-old previously healthy boy was brought to an emergency department for a 10-minute tonic–clonic seizure while sleeping. Upon arrival, he was awake and responsive but showed clinical evidence of hypocalcemia and an unremarkable physical exam. Initial laboratory assessment showed a calcium level of 5.6 mg/dL, phosphate 8.7 mg/dL, and ionized calcium 0.71 mmol/L and 0.64 mmol/L in a 2-hour period. High-dose calcium was infused to prevent further seizure activity. Further assessment showed elevated PTH levels of 321 pg/mL with the concurrent calcium of 5.5 mg/dL, mild 25-hydroxyvitamin D deficiency of 14.1 ng/mL, normal 25-hydroxyvitamin D_1, thyroid-function test, and spot urinary calcium. The family history was significant for his two older brothers having similar symptoms. Pseudohypoparathyroidism type 1B (PHP-1B) was suspected. A molecular study was ordered to confirm the diagnosis, and a heterozygous 3-bp deletion, p.Ile382del, in the *GNAS* gene was detected in this patient. Targeted

variant studies detected the same pathogenic variant in his two affected brothers, their mother, and the maternal grandfather. At the time, his mother was pregnant with a girl. Which one of the following would most likely be the estimated risk that this unborn girl has the same condition?[39,43]

A. <1%
B. 5%–7%
C. 14%
D. 25%
E. 50%
F. 100%

119. Which one of the following characteristics is NOT common in patients with pseudohypoparathyroidism (PHP)?

A. Increased 1,25-$(OH)_2D_3$
B. Decreased calcitriol
C. Decreased calcium
D. Increased parathyroid hormone (PTH)
E. Increased phosphates

120. A 37-year-old man with a history of having a bicuspid aortic valve surgically replaced at the age of 31 years was admitted to a hospital with symptoms of fever and mild left mandibular pain for 6 weeks. A physical examination revealed short stature (155 cm), and absence of the fourth and fifth metacarpophalangeal knuckles bilaterally. Hands X-ray confirmed shortening of the first and third distal phalanges, and missing fourth and fifth metacarpals bilaterally. His serum calcium and phosphate were normal, and he had intact parathyroid hormone (PTH) levels, confirming the diagnosis of pseudopseudohypoparathyroidism (PPHP). A molecular study detected a pathogenic variant, c.344C > T(p.Pro115Leu), in the *GNAS* gene in his peripheral-blood specimen. Which one of the following would most likely be the estimated risk that this patient's children would have the same condition?[44,45]

A. <1%
B. 5%–7%
C. 14%
D. 25%
E. 50%
F. 100%

121. A 37-year-old woman with a history of having a bicuspid aortic valve surgically replaced at the age of 31 years was admitted to a hospital with symptoms of fever and mild left mandibular pain for 6 weeks. A physical examination revealed short stature (155 cm) and absence of the fourth and fifth metacarpophalangeal knuckles bilaterally. Hands X-ray confirmed shortening of the first and third distal phalanges and missing

fourth and fifth metacarpals bilaterally. Her serum calcium and phosphate were normal, and she had intact parathyroid hormone (PTH) levels, confirming the diagnosis of pseudopseudohypoparathyroidism (PPHP). A molecular study detected a pathogenic variant, c.344C > T(p.Pro115Leu), in the *GNAS* gene in her peripheral-blood specimen. Which one of the following would most likely be the estimated risk that this patient's children would have the same condition?[44,45]

A. <1%

B. 5%–7%

C. 14%

D. 25%

E. 50%

F. 100%

122. Which one of the following characteristics is NOT common in patients with pseudopseudohypoparathyroidism (PPHP)?

A. Decreased calcitriol

B. Decreased calcium

C. Increased parathyroid hormone (PTH)

D. Increased phosphates

E. None of the above

123. A 42-year-old gravid 6 para 4 female of Caucasian descent was evaluated at 20 weeks of gestation for sex discrepancy detected by karyotype and ultrasound. A routine CVS, done at 11 weeks of gestation for advanced maternal age, documented a normal female karyotype (46,XX). An ultrasound evaluation detected normal male external genitalia. Which one of the following analyses would most likely be used as the initial evaluation for the gender discrepancy in this fetus?

A. FISH for the *AZFa*, *AZFb*, and *AZFc* genes

B. FISH for the *SRY* gene

C. Maternal cell contamination testing

D. Sequencing the *AR* gene for androgen insensitivity

E. Sequencing the *CYP21A2* gene for congenital adrenal hyperplasia

F. Waiting until the baby is born

124. A 44-year-old gravid 6 para 4 female of Caucasian descent was evaluated at 20 weeks of gestation for sex discrepancy detected by karyotype and ultrasound. A routine CVS, done at 11 weeks of gestation for advanced maternal age, documented a normal female karyotype (46,XX). An ultrasound evaluation detected normal male external genitalia. Maternal cell contamination testing confirmed the fetal origin of the sample used for the karyotype. Which one of the following analyses would most likely be used as

the next step in the evaluation for the sex discrepancy in this fetus?[6]

A. FISH for the *AZFa*, *AZFb*, and *AZFc* genes

B. FISH for the *SRY* gene

C. Sequencing the *AR* gene for androgen insensitivity

D. Sequencing the *CYP21A2* gene for congenital adrenal hyperplasia

E. None of the above

125. A clinical geneticist is paged by NICU for consultation on a 1-day old girl with ambiguous genitalia. The baby's vital signs are stable, and physical exam is unremarkable except for the genitalia findings. The baby was born at 40 weeks with Apgar scores 9 and 9 at 1 and 5 minutes following an uncomplicated pregnancy. She eats well within normal weight limits. There is no significant family history on either side. A routine amniocentesis, done at 16 weeks' gestation for advanced maternal age, documented a normal female karyotype (46,XX). Which one of the following analyses is most likely used as the initial evaluation for ambiguous genitalia in this fetus?

A. FISH for the *AZFa*, *AZFb*, and *AZFc* genes

B. FISH for the *SRY* gene

C. Sequencing the *AR* gene for androgen insensitivity

D. Sequencing the *CYP21A2* gene for congenital adrenal hyperplasia

E. None of the above

126. A 44-year-old gravid 6 para 4 female of Caucasian descent was evaluated at 20 weeks of gestation for sex discrepancy detected by karyotype and ultrasound. A routine amniocentesis, done at 16 weeks of gestation for advanced maternal age, documented a normal male karyotype (46,XY). An ultrasound evaluation detected normal female external genitalia. Postnatal examinations confirmed the normal female genitalia and normal male karyotype. Which one of the following analyses would least likely be used as the initial evaluation for gonadal dysgenesis in this newborn?[6]

A. Chromosomal microarray analysis

B. Exome sequencing

C. FISH for the *SRY* gene

D. Sequencing the *SRY* gene

E. None of the above

127. A 44-year-old gravid 6 para 4 female of Caucasian descent was evaluated at 20 weeks of gestation for sex discrepancy detected by karyotype and ultrasound. A routine amniocentesis, done at 16 weeks of gestation for advanced maternal age, documented a normal male karyotype (46,XY).

An ultrasound evaluation detected normal female genitalia. Postnatal examinations confirmed the normal female external genitalia and normal male karyotype. A chromosomal microarray analysis identified a microdeletion on chromosome Y including the *SRY* gene. Which one of the following disorders would the newborn NOT be at increased risk to develop?[6]

A. Breast cancer

B. Dysgerminoma

C. Gonadoblastoma

D. Infertility

E. None of the above

128. A 6-month-old infant was brought to a genetics clinic for ambiguous genitalia. A chromosomal analysis revealed a normal female karyotype (46, XX). A physical examination revealed penoscrotal hypospadias and cryptorchidism without identifiable Müllerian structures. Which one of the following would least likely be part of the workup for the diagnosis?[6]

A. Sequencing analysis of *CYO21A2*

B. Sequencing analysis of *SOX9*

C. *SOX3* FISH

D. *SOX9* FISH

E. *SRY* FISH

129. A 3-year-old boy was referred to a genetics clinic for postnatal-onset obesity, hypotonia, and intellectual disability. A physical examination revealed small hands and feet. The physician suspected that the patient had Prader–Willi syndrome. Which one of the following analyses would most likely be used as the initial genetic evaluation for this patient?

A. Chromosomal microarray analysis

B. FISH for the 15q 11.2 deletion

C. Karyotyping

D. Methylation study

E. Sequencing of the *UBE3A* gene

130. A 4-year-old girl was referred to a genetics clinic for absence of speech, severe intellectual disability, and recurrent seizures. Physical exam revealed short stature. The physician suspected that the patient had Angelman syndrome. Which one of the following analyses would most likely be used as the initial genetic evaluation for this patient?

A. FISH for the 15q 11.2 deletion

B. Chromosomal microarray analysis

C. Karyotyping

D. Methylation study

E. Sequencing of the *UBE3A* gene

131. Which one of the following diseases may be detected by Sanger sequencing analysis of *UBE3A* on 15q11.2?

A. Angelman syndrome

B. Charcot–Marie–Tooth syndrome

C. Prader–Willi syndrome

D. Smith–Magenis syndrome

E. None of the above

132. A scientist in a clinical molecular laboratory worked to develop a methylation assay for Prader–Willi and Angelman syndromes. He designed primers for both methylated and unmethylated alleles at the promoter region of the *SNRPN* gene. During the prevalidation studies, one of the specimens showed only one band for methylated allele after sodium bisulfite treatment. What would be the most appropriate interpretation for this specimen if all the controls worked appropriately?

A. The specimen was from a patient with Angelman syndrome.

B. The specimen was from a patient with Prader–Willi syndrome.

C. The specimen was from a patient with Angelman syndrome who has a deletion on 15q11.2.

D. The specimen was from a patient with Prader–Willi syndrome who has a deletion on 15q11.2.

E. None of the above.

133. A scientist in a clinical molecular laboratory worked to develop a methylation assay for Prader–Willi and Angelman syndromes. He designed primers for both methylated and unmethylated alleles at the promoter region of the *SNRPN* gene. During the prevalidation studies, one of the specimens showed only one band for unmethylated allele after sodium bisulfite treatment. What would be the most appropriate interpretation for this specimen if all the controls worked appropriately?

A. The specimen was from a patient with Angelman syndrome.

B. The specimen was from a patient with Prader–Willi syndrome.

C. The specimen was from a patient with Angelman syndrome who has a deletion on 15q11.2.

D. The specimen was from a patient with Prader–Willi syndrome who has a deletion on 15q11.2.

E. None of the above.

134. An 8-year-old boy was referred to a pediatric neurological clinic with symptoms of developmental delay and epilepsy for 6 years. He was the second child of nonconsanguineous parents. The family history was unremarkable. His perinatal history was uneventful. A physical

examination revealed that he had mandibular prognathism, strabismus, and an unusual laughing facial expression. His walking was unsteady, but muscle tone and force and deep tendon reflexes were normal. He had intellectual disability and speech disability with restricted communication abilities. The physician suspected Angelman syndrome and ordered a molecular methylation study to confirm the diagnosis. Which one of the following would be the targeted genomic region for this methylation study?[46]

A. 5′ of *SNRPN*
B. 3′ of *SNRPN*
C. 5′ of *UBE3A*
D. 3′ of *UBE3A*
E. None of the above

135. An 8-year-old boy was referred to a pediatric neurological clinic with symptoms of developmental delay and epilepsy for 6 years. He was the second child of nonconsanguineous parents. The family history was unremarkable. His perinatal history was uneventful. A physical examination revealed that he had mandibular prognathism, strabismus, and an unusual laughing facial expression. His walking was unsteady, but muscle tone and force and deep tendon reflexes were normal. He had intellectual disability and speech disability with restricted communication abilities. The physician suspected Angelman syndrome and ordered a molecular methylation study to confirm the diagnosis. Which one of the following would be the detection rate of the methylation study if the patient had Angelman syndrome?[46]

A. >99%
B. 80%
C. 60%
D. 30%
E. 10%

136. An 8-year-old boy was referred to a pediatric neurological clinic with symptoms of developmental delay and epilepsy for 6 years. He was the second child of nonconsanguineous parents. The family history was unremarkable. His perinatal history was uneventful. A physical examination revealed that he had mandibular prognathism, strabismus, and an unusual laughing facial expression. His walking was unsteady, but muscle tone and force and deep tendon reflexes were normal. He had intellectual disability and speech disability with restricted communication abilities. The physician suspected Angelman syndrome and ordered a molecular methylation study to confirm the diagnosis. The results confirmed the diagnosis of AS. Which one

of the following statements would be the most appropriate interpretation of the positive molecular methylation result?[46]

A. The patient had imprinting center defect.
B. The patient had a deletion involving the imprinting center.
C. The patent had maternal UPD.
D. The patient had paternal UPD.
E. The patient had a duplication involving the imprinting center.
F. None of the above.

137. An 8-year-old boy was referred to a pediatric neurological clinic with symptoms of developmental delay and epilepsy for 6 years. He was the second child of nonconsanguineous parents. The family history was unremarkable. His perinatal history was uneventful. A physical examination revealed that he had mandibular prognathism, strabismus, and an unusual laughing facial expression. His walking was unsteady, but muscle tone and force and deep tendon reflexes were normal. He had intellectual disability and speech disability with restricted communication abilities. The physician suspected Angelman syndrome and ordered a molecular methylation study to confirm the diagnosis. The results confirmed the diagnosis of AS. Which one of the following molecular genetic assays would be the best choice as the next step in the workup to further explore the genetic mechanism of AS in this patient in comparison with the others?[46]

A. Chromosomal karyotyping
B. FISH
C. Oligonucleotide microarray
D. SNP microarray
E. None of the above

138. An 8-year-old boy was referred to a pediatric neurological clinic with symptoms of developmental delay and epilepsy for 6 years. He was the second child of nonconsanguineous parents. The family history was unremarkable. His perinatal history was uneventful. A physical examination revealed that he had mandibular prognathism, strabismus, and an unusual laughing facial expression. His walking was unsteady, but muscle tone and force and deep tendon reflexes were normal. He had intellectual disability and speech disability with restricted communication abilities. The physician suspected Angelman syndrome and ordered a molecular methylation study to confirm the diagnosis. The results confirmed the diagnosis of AS. A follow-up SNP array detected an approximately 5.2-Mb region of copy neutral loss of heterozygosity (ROH) at 15q11.13. Which one of the following

interpretations would be most appropriate for this patient?[46]

A. The patient had a deletion involving the imprinting center.

B. The patent had maternal UPD.

C. The patient had paternal UPD.

D. The ROH region might unmask a homozygous pathogenic variant in the imprinting center.

E. None of the above.

139. An 8-year-old boy was referred to a pediatric neurological clinic with symptoms of developmental delay and epilepsy for 6 years. He was the second child of nonconsanguineous parents. The family history was unremarkable. His perinatal history was uneventful. A physical examination revealed that he had mandibular prognathism, strabismus, and an unusual laughing facial expression. His walking was unsteady, but muscle tone and force and deep tendon reflexes were normal. He had intellectual disability and speech disability with restricted communication abilities. The physician suspected Angelman syndrome and ordered a molecular methylation study to confirm the diagnosis. The results were normal. The physician still suspected that the patient had Angelman syndrome. Which one of the following genetic mechanisms for AS would still be possible in this patient even though results of the methylation study were negative?[46]

A. Deletions of the 15q11.2q13

B. Imprinting defects

C. Maternal uniparental disomy (UPD)

D. Pathogenic variants in the SNRPN gene

E. Pathogenic variants in the UBE3A gene

F. Paternal uniparental disomy (UPD)

140. An 8-year-old boy was referred to a pediatric neurological clinic with symptoms of developmental delay and epilepsy for 6 years. He was the second child of nonconsanguineous parents. The family history was unremarkable. His perinatal history was uneventful. A physical examination revealed that he had mandibular prognathism, strabismus, and an unusual laughing facial expression. His walking was unsteady, but muscle tone and force and deep tendon reflexes were normal. He had intellectual disability and speech disability with restricted communication abilities. The physician suspected Angelman syndrome and ordered a molecular methylation study to confirm the diagnosis. The results were normal. The physician still suspected that the patient had AS. He ordered sequencing analysis of the UBE3A gene, and a pathogenic variant was detected. Parental testing found that his asymptomatic mother carried the same

pathogenic variant. So did his apparently healthy maternal aunt. Which one of the following would most likely be the risk that the patient's maternal aunt would have a child with Angelman syndrome?[46]

A. <1%

B. 25%

C. 50%

D. 75%

E. >99%

141. An 8-year-old boy was referred to a pediatric neurological clinic with symptoms of developmental delay and epilepsy for 6 years. He was the second child of nonconsanguineous parents. The family history was unremarkable. His perinatal history was uneventful. A physical examination revealed that he had mandibular prognathism, strabismus, and an unusual laughing facial expression. His walking was unsteady, but muscle tone and force and deep tendon reflexes were normal. He had intellectual disability and speech disability with restricted communication abilities. The physician suspected Angelman syndrome and ordered a molecular methylation study to confirm the diagnosis. The results were normal. The physician still suspected that the patient had AS. He ordered sequencing analysis of the UBE3A gene, and a pathogenic variant was detected. Parental testing found that his asymptomatic mother carried the same pathogenic variant. So did his apparently healthy maternal uncle. Which one of the following would most likely be the risk that the patient's maternal uncle would have a child with Angelman syndrome?

A. <1%

B. 25%

C. 50%

D. 75%

E. >99%

142. Which one of the following genotypes of the SERPINA1 gene is the most common pathogenic one seen in patients with alpha-1 antitrypsin deficiency?

A. PI*M/M

B. PI*M/Z

C. PI*Null/Null

D. PI*S/Null

E. PI*S/S

F. PI*Z/Z

143. The SERPINA1 gene is the only gene known to cause alpha-1 antitrypsin deficiency (AATD). Which one of the following genotypes of the SERPINA1 gene is the most common one in apparently healthy individuals worldwide?

    A. PI*M/M
    B. PI*M/Z
    C. PI*Null/Null
    D. PI*S/Null
    E. PI*S/S
    F. PI*Z/Z

144. Alpha-1 antitrypsin deficiency (AATD) is an autosomal recessive disease. Which one of the following malignancies has an increased risk in patients with AATD in comparison with individuals from general populations?
    A. Adenocarcinoma of the lung
    B. Hepatocellular carcinoma
    C. Pancreatic cancer
    D. Stomach cancer
    E. None of the above

145. Alpha-1 antitrypsin deficiency (AATD) is an autosomal recessive condition, which is caused by pathogenic variants in the *SERPINA1* gene. Which one of the following is the most important environmental factor for the manifestation of the disease?
    A. Obesity
    B. Sedentary lifestyle
    C. Smoking
    D. Alcohol use
    E. None of the above

146. A 1-year old boy was brought to a clinic for fever, cough, and loose motion that began at the age of 6 days. His parents were related (second cousins) with a history of having four children who died (two stillbirths and two intrauterine deaths). The patient's perinatal history was uneventful. He was blind and had global developmental delay. A physical examination revealed a malnourished child with all three growth parameters below the third percentile. He had broad nasal tip, anteverted nostrils, microphthalmia, roving eye movements, strabismus, epicanthic folds, long philtrum, low-set ears, thin upper lip, and oligodontia. He had an underdeveloped scrotum with microphallus and bilateral undescended testes. Ultrasound revealed a hypoplastic sac of the scrotum, with the left small testis in the inguinal region and the right testis not identifiable in the inguinal region or pelvis. Electrocardiography revealed atrial septal defect with left-to-right shunting and moderate pulmonary stenosis. CT revealed mild brain atrophy. His serum cholesterol was 60 mg/dL and his urine 7-dehydrocholesterol concentration was 165 μg/mL. Chromosomal analysis revealed 46,XY. A molecular test identified a heterozygous nonsense pathogenic variant in the *HDCR7* gene.

Which one of the following interpretations of the results would be most appropriate?[47]
    A. The patient had congenital adrenal hyperplasia.
    B. The patient had Smith−Lemli−Opitz syndrome.
    C. The patient had *SRY* deletion.
    D. It is undetermined, and postnatal evaluation is recommended.
    E. None of the above.

147. A Caucasian nonconsanguineous couple, with one previous healthy child born at term, came for prenatal care. The maternal serum screen showed very low estriol, and the ultrasound scan at 20 weeks of gestation suggested heart defect and ambiguous genitalia. The fetus was significantly small for gestational age, especially the long bones. Amniocentesis revealed that the fetus had 46,XY. The physician suspected that the fetus had Smith−Lemli−Opitz syndrome. Which one of the following would be the most appropriate initial workup to confirm or rule out the diagnosis in this fetus?
    A. Measuring 7-dehydrocholesterol concentration in amniotic fluid
    B. Measuring 7-dehydrocholesterol concentration in the parents
    C. Testing the amniotic fluid for pathogenic variants in the *DHCR7* gene
    D. Testing the parents for pathogenic variants in the *DHCR7* gene
    E. None of the above

148. A Caucasian nonconsanguineous couple, with one previous healthy child born at term, came for prenatal care. The maternal serum screen showed very low estriol, and the ultrasound scan at 20 weeks of gestation suggested a heart defect and ambiguous genitalia. The fetus was significantly small for the gestational age, especially the long bones. Amniocentesis revealed that the fetus had 46,XY. Elevated 7-dehydrocholesterol (7-DHC) reductase was detected in the amniotic fluid. And the follow-up molecular testing detected a heterozygous pathogenic variant, c.356A > T(p. His119Leu), in the *DHCR7* gene. The fetus was diagnosed with Smith−Lemli−Opitz syndrome. What would most likely be the recurrent risk of same condition in this family?[47]
    A. < 1%
    B. 25%
    C. 50%
    D. 75%
    E. 100%
    F. None of the above

149. A 2-year-old boy was referred to a genetics clinic for developmental delay. He was the only child of healthy nonconsanguineous parents. He had no relatives with a hereditary disease or intellectual disability. A prenatal ultrasound in the third trimester had revealed congenital hydrocephalus. A physical examination revealed bilateral flexed adducted thumbs and bilateral clinodactyly of the fifth finger. A brain MRI revealed enlarged lateral ventricles and corpus callosum agenesis. At 4 years of age, he developed spastic paraplegia. The physician suspected L1 syndrome. Which one of the following studies would most likely be ordered to confirm or rule out the diagnosis in this patient?[48]
    A. Deletion and duplication analysis of the *MECP2* gene
    B. HPLC for hemoglobinopathy
    C. Sequencing analysis of the *ATRX* gene
    D. Sequencing analysis of the *L1CAM* gene
    E. Sequencing analysis of the *MECP2* gene
    F. None of the above

150. A 2-year-old boy was referred to a genetics clinic for developmental delay. He was the only child of healthy nonconsanguineous parents. He had no relatives with a hereditary disease or intellectual disability. A prenatal ultrasound in the third trimester had revealed congenital hydrocephalus. A physical examination revealed bilateral flexed adducted thumbs and bilateral clinodactyly of the fifth finger. A brain MRI revealed enlarged lateral ventricles and corpus callosum agenesis. At 4 years of age, he developed spastic paraplegia. The physician suspected L1 syndrome. A molecular study of the *L1CAM* gene was ordered, and a pathogenic variant, c.1754A > C(p.Gln1160*), leading to loss of carboxyl terminal amino acids, was detected. Which one of the following would most likely be the recurrent risk of same condition in the family?[48]
    A. <1%
    B. 6%–10%
    C. 25%
    D. 50%
    E. 67%
    F. >99%
    G. Unpredictable
    H. None of the above

151. A 2-year-old boy was referred to a genetics clinic for developmental delay. He was the only child of healthy nonconsanguineous parents. He had no relatives with a hereditary disease or intellectual disability. A prenatal ultrasound in the third trimester had revealed congenital hydrocephalus. A physical examination revealed bilateral flexed

adducted thumbs and bilateral clinodactyly of the fifth finger. A brain MRI revealed enlarged lateral ventricles and corpus callosum agenesis. At 4 years of age, he developed spastic paraplegia. The physician suspected L1 syndrome. A molecular study of the *L1CAM* gene was ordered, and a pathogenic variant, c.1754A > C(p.Gln1160*), leading to loss of carboxyl terminal amino acids, was detected. Which one of the following would most likely be used as the first step in the workup to estimate the recurrent risk of the same condition in the family?[48]
    A. Targeted variant analysis of the father
    B. Targeted variant analysis of the mother
    C. Targeted variant analysis of the parents
    D. Prenatal testing of future fetuses
    E. Any of above
    F. None of the above

152. A healthy nonconsanguineous couple came to a clinic for preconception counseling because of a family history of intellectual disability. Physical examinations on both husband and wife were negative. The husband had two brothers with intellectual disability. He also had three healthy sisters; all had sons with clinical symptoms of L1 syndrome, such as hydrocephalus, developmental delay, and adducted thumbs. Which one of the following individuals should be tested first to identify a pathogenic variant in the family?[48]
    A. One of the husband's brothers
    B. One of the husband's nephews
    C. One of the husband's sisters
    D. The husband
    E. The husband's parents
    F. The wife
    G. The future fetus
    H. All of the above
    I. None of the above

153. A healthy nonconsanguineous couple came to a clinic for preconception counseling because of a family history of intellectual disability. Physical examinations on both husband and wife were negative. The husband had two brothers with intellectual disability. He also had three healthy sisters; all had sons with clinical symptoms of L1 syndrome, such as hydrocephalus, developmental delay, and adducted thumbs. Sequencing analysis of *L1CAM* with peripheral blood from one of the husband's nephews detected an A > C substitution at nucleotide 1754 (c.1754 A > C) involving the replacement of an aspartic acid at position 585 by an alanine in the extracellular domain of the protein (p.Asp585Ala). Which one of the following individuals in the family would be least likely to be tested due to the minimal possibility?[48]

A. The husband's other nephews
B. The husband's sisters
C. The husband's father
D. The husband's mother
E. All of the above

154. A healthy nonconsanguineous couple came to a clinic for preconception counseling because of a family history of intellectual disability. Physical examinations on both husband and wife were negative. The husband had two brothers with intellectual disability. He also had three healthy sisters; all had sons with clinical symptoms of L1 syndrome, such as hydrocephalus, developmental delay, and adducted thumbs. Sequencing analysis of *L1CAM* with peripheral blood from one of the husband's nephews detected an A > C substitution at the nucleotide 1754 (c.1754 A > C) involving the replacement of an aspartic acid at position 585 by an alanine in the extracellular domain of the protein (p.Asp585Ala). Which one of the following would most likely be the risk that the couple would have a child with L1 syndrome?[48]

A. <1%
B. 6%−10%
C. 25%
D. 50%
E. 67%
F. >99%
G. Unpredictable
H. None of the above

155. A 2½-year-old boy was brought to a clinic by his parents for 2 days of irritability and fever. He was born full term to a healthy 28-year-old gravida 3 para 2 mother and had an uneventful perinatal history except for flexion deformity of both middle fingers. He had had seizures six times since the age of 15 months, which were uncontrollable with antiepilepsy medications. He had severe developmental delay and intellectual disability. His family history was remarkable for a maternal cousin, a 6-year-old boy, with similar symptoms. A physical examination revealed mild hypotonia, a flat and midhypoplastic face with prognathism, narrow and upward slanting palpebral fissures with hypertelorism, low-set ears, a small crashed nose, widely spaced incisors, carp-like mouth, and round back. An X-ray revealed mild scoliosis. Hemoglobin H (HbH) inclusion bodies were detected under microscopy in 1.1% of brilliant cresyl blue−stained RBCs, consistent with a diagnosis of alpha-thalassemia X-linked intellectual disability syndrome. Which one of the following studies would most likely be

ordered to confirm or rule out the diagnosis in this patient?[49]

A. Chromosomal microarray analysis
B. Deletion and duplication analysis of the *MECP2* gene
C. Sequencing analysis of the *ATRX* gene
D. Sequencing analysis of the *MECP2* gene
E. Sequencing analysis of the *RPS6KA3* gene
F. None of the above

156. A 32-month-old boy was brought to a clinic for 2 days of irritability and fever. He was born full term to a healthy 28-year-old gravida 4 para 3 mother and had an uneventful perinatal history except for flexion deformity of both middle fingers. He had had seizures six times since the age of 15 months that were uncontrollable with antiepilepsy medications. He had severe developmental delay and intellectual disability. His family history was unremarkable. A physical examination revealed mild hypotonia, a flat and midhypoplastic face with prognathism, narrow and upward slanting palpebral fissures with hypertelorism, low-set ears, a small crashed nose, widely spaced incisors, carp-like mouth, and round back. An X-ray revealed mild scoliosis. Hemoglobin H (HbH) inclusion bodies were detected under microscopy in 1.1% of brilliant cresyl blue−stained RBCs, consistent with a diagnosis of alpha-thalassemia X-linked intellectual disability syndrome. Sequencing analysis of the *ATRX* gene detected a pathogenic variant, c.109C > T(p.Arg37Ter). Which one of the following individuals should be tested first for the pathogenic variant before cascade testing in the rest of the family?

A. His father
B. His mother
C. His brother
D. His sister
E. All of the above
F. None of the above

157. Constitutional *BRAF* pathogenic variants have NOT been detected in patients with which one of the following?

A. Cardiofaciocutaneous (CFC) syndrome
B. Cowden syndrome
C. LEOPARD syndrome
D. Noonan syndrome
E. None of the above

158. A 10-month-old boy was referred to a genetics clinic for strabismus. His perinatal history was significant for premature delivery (36 weeks gestation, birth weight: 2500 g) with respiratory distress syndrome, first-degree intracranial hemorrhage, dilation of both renal pyelons,

migratory testis, supravalvular pulmonary stenosis, and hypotonia. An ophthalmological examination revealed hypertelorism, down-slanting palpebral fissures, left eye esotropia, and presence of bilateral optic disk pits. A physical examination revealed low-set of ears with irregular shape and posteriorly rotated, high-arched palate, and micrognathia. Cytogenetic results revealed a normal male karyotype, or 46,XY. The physician suspected that the patient had Noonan syndrome. Which one of the following molecular genetic assays would most likely be used to confirm/rule out diagnosis in this patient?[50]

A. Chromosomal microarray analysis
B. Denaturing high-performance liquid chromatography (dHPLC)
C. Exome-sequencing analysis
D. Multiplex ligation-dependent probe amplification (MLPA)
E. Next-generation sequencing analysis
F. Sequencing analysis of the *PTPN11* gene

159. A 10-month-old boy was referred to a genetics clinic for strabismus. His perinatal history was significant for premature delivery (GS 36 weeks, TM 2500 g) with respiratory distress syndrome, first-degree intracranial hemorrhage, dilation of both renal pyelons, migratory testis, supravalvular pulmonary stenosis, and hypotonia. An ophthalmological examination revealed hypertelorism, down-slanting palpebral fissures, left eye esotropia, and presence of bilateral optic disk pits. A physical examination revealed low-set of ears with irregular shape and posteriorly rotated, high-arched palate, and micrognathia. Cytogenetic results revealed a normal male karyotype, or 46,XY. The physician suspected that the patient had Noonan syndrome. Which one of the following genes would least likely harbor a pathogenic variant for Noonan syndrome in this patient?[50]

A. *KIT*
B. *KRAS*
C. *NRAS*
D. *PTPN11*
E. *RAF1*
F. *SOS1*

160. A 10-month-old boy was referred to a genetics clinic for strabismus. His perinatal history was significant for premature delivery (GS 36 weeks, TM 2500 g) with respiratory distress syndrome, first-degree intracranial hemorrhage, dilation of both renal pyelons, migratory testis, supravalvular pulmonary stenosis, and hypotonia. An ophthalmological examination revealed hypertelorism, down-slanting palpebral

fissures, left eye esotropia, and presence of bilateral optic disk pits. A physical examination revealed low-set of ears with irregular shape and posteriorly rotated, high-arched palate, and micrognathia. Cytogenetic results revealed a normal male karyotype, or 46,XY. The physician suspected that the patient had Noonan syndrome. A next-generation sequencing (NGS) panel was ordered, and a pathogenic variant, heterozygous c.214G > T(p.Ala72Ser), in the *PTPN11* gene was detected. Which one of the following malignancies would this patient NOT have an increased risk to develop?[60]

A. Acute lymphoblastic leukemia (ALL)
B. Acute myeloid leukemia (AML)
C. Colorectal cancer
D. Myeloproliferative disorders (MPN)
E. Neuroblastoma
F. Rhabdomyosarcoma

161. A 16-year-old Caucasian boy came to a clinic for seizures of primary generalized tonic–clonic type for 6 years. At the age of 12, he developed insidious onset and progressive bilateral diminution of vision, without field defects. His perinatal history was uneventful except for prolonged labor and being a big baby. Umbilical hernia was noticed at birth and was corrected on the second day of life. Macroglossia and prognathism were also noticed since birth. He had delayed developmental milestones with poor scholastic performance. At 3 years of age, he was noticed to have frontal bossing and acromegaly. At 7, he underwent surgery for cryptorchidism. A physical examination revealed macrocephaly (98th percentile) with a height of 185 cm (> 95th percentile) and a weight of 62 kg. His father, age 62 years, was 165 cm tall and mother, age 50 years, was 155 cm tall. The patient had hypertelorism, megalophthalmos, macroglossia, prognathism, malocclusion of teeth, big nose, prominent superciliary arches, divergent squint, high arched palate and large hands and feet. Fundi revealed bilateral optic atrophy with visual acuity of 2/60 in. right eye and 6/60 in. left eye, with total color blindness. He also had moderate myopia on the right eye and simple myopic astigmatism in the left eye. His brain MRI was normal. The physician suspected that the patient had Sotos syndrome. Which one of the following studies would most likely be ordered first to confirm or rule out the diagnosis in this patient?[51]

A. Chromosomal microarray
B. Karyotype
C. Methylation study of IC1 and IC2 on 11p15
D. Sequencing analysis of the *EZH2* gene

E. Sequencing analysis of the *LMNA* gene

F. Sequencing analysis of the *NSD1* gene

G. None of the above

162. A 16-year-old Japanese boy came to a clinic for seizures of primary generalized tonic–clonic type for 6 years. At the age of 12, he developed insidious onset and progressive bilateral diminution of vision, without field defects. His perinatal history was uneventful except for prolonged labor and being a big baby. Umbilical hernia was noticed at birth and was corrected on the second day of life. Macroglossia and prognathism were also noticed since birth. He had delayed developmental milestones with poor scholastic performance. At 3 years of age, he was noticed to have frontal bossing and acromegaly. At 7, he underwent surgery for cryptorchidism. A physical examination revealed macrocephaly (98th percentile) with a height of 185 cm (>95th percentile) and a weight of 62 kg. His father, age 62 years, was 165 cm tall and mother, age 50 years, was 155 cm tall. The patient had hypertelorism, megalophthalmos, macroglossia, prognathism, malocclusion of teeth, big nose, prominent superciliary arches, divergent squint, high arched palate and large hands and feet. Fundi revealed bilateral optic atrophy with visual acuity of 2/60 in. right eye and 6/60 in. left eye, with total color blindness. He also had moderate myopia on the right eye and simple myopic astigmatism in the left eye. His brain MRI was normal. The physician suspected that the patient had Sotos syndrome. Which one of the following studies would most likely be ordered first to confirm or rule out the diagnosis in this patient?[51]

A. Chromosomal microarray

B. Karyotype

C. Methylation study of IC1 and IC2 on 11p15

D. Sequencing analysis of the *EZH2* gene

E. Sequencing analysis of the *LMNA* gene

F. Sequencing analysis of the *NSD1* gene

G. None of the above

163. A 30-year-old gravida 3 para 2 mother was followed prenatally after a 19-week ultrasound showed a single amniotic band, shortened cervix, and echogenic kidneys and bowel. A female infant was born weighing 1869 g (90th percentile) at 31 weeks gestation via emergency cesarean section for nonreassuring fetal rhythm strip and poor biophysical profile. The baby's Apgar scores were 7 and 1 minutes and 9 at 5 minutes, but her glucose was 22 mg/dL, and persistent profound hypoglycemia continued. Her right leg was bigger than her left. Echocardiography showed PDA, and an abdominal ultrasound showed two nodular soft-tissue foci in the posterior wall of the urinary bladder; the liver was noted to be markedly heterogeneous, with at least two areas of rounded hypodensity. MRI of the abdomen found a pancreatic tail cyst; size discrepancy of the kidneys, with the right kidney measuring larger than the left; numerous tiny medullary cysts; and a right adrenal mass, with numerous enhancing hepatic lesions. Beckwith–Wiedemann syndrome (BWS) was highly suspected. Which one of the following molecular genetic studies would be appropriate for this infant in order to confirm the diagnosis?

A. Chromosomal microarray

B. Methylation study

C. Multiplex ligation-dependent probe amplification (MLPA)

D. Sanger sequencing

E. All of the above

F. None of the above

164. A 30-year-old gravida 3 para 2 mother was followed prenatally after a 19-week ultrasound showed a single amniotic band, shortened cervix, and echogenic kidneys and bowel. A female infant was born weighing 1869 g (90th percentile) at 31 weeks gestation via emergency cesarean section for nonreassuring fetal rhythm strip and poor biophysical profile. The baby's Apgar scores were 7 and 1 minutes and 9 at 5 minutes, but her glucose was 22 mg/dL, and persistent profound hypoglycemia continued. Her right leg was bigger than her left. Echocardiography showed PDA, and an abdominal ultrasound showed two nodular soft-tissue foci in the posterior wall of the urinary bladder; the liver was noted to be markedly heterogeneous, with at least two areas of rounded hypodensity. MRI of the abdomen found a pancreatic tail cyst; size discrepancy of the kidneys, with the right kidney measuring larger than the left; numerous tiny medullary cysts; and a right adrenal mass, with numerous enhancing hepatic lesions. Beckwith–Wiedemann syndrome (BWS) was highly suspected. Paternal uniparental disomy (UPD) 15 was detected. Did this molecular result confirm the diagnosis of BWS in this infant?

A. Yes

B. No

C. Not sure

165. A couple was referred to a genetics clinic because the fetus was large for gestational age and had omphalocele seen on ultrasonography when the wife was 28 weeks pregnant. The family was counseled for the possibility of Beckwith–Wiedemann syndrome (BWS). The

baby boy was delivered by a cesarean section at 37 weeks of gestational age with a birth weight of 9 lb 2 oz and a notably large placenta. Omphalocele and macroglossia were noted at the birth. The family history was negative on both sides. How many imprinting centers are located in the Beckwith–Wiedemann critical region at 11p15?[103]

A. 1
B. 2
C. 3
D. 4
E. 5

166. A boy was born at 33 weeks by cesarean section. He was diagnosed with macroglossia and had omphalocele. He also had congenital hypothyroidism, mild hypotonia, overweight, slight lingual protrusion, and grooves in the earlobes. The family history was negative on both sides. He underwent surgery 12 hours after birth for omphalocele. Beckwith–Wiedemann syndrome (BWS) was at the top of the list of differential diagnoses. An abnormal genetic finding was predicted to cause gain of expression of IGF2 and loss of expression of CDKN1C in the BWS critical region at same time. Which one of the following genetic alterations may result in gain of expression of IGF2 and loss of expression of CDKN1C in the BWS critical region at same time?[52]

A. Gain of methylation of maternal IC1
B. Loss of methylation of maternal IC2
C. Paternal UPD of 11p15
D. Pathogenic variants in the CDKN1C gene
E. Pathogenic variants in the IGF2 gene

167. A 35-year-old pregnant woman was referred to maternal–fetal medicine after her routine 20-week prenatal ultrasound revealed bilaterally enlarged echogenic kidneys with mild pelviectasis. A fetal MRI showed markedly enlarged kidneys bilaterally and a prominent tongue. Beckwith–Wiedemann syndrome was suspected. At birth, a molecular study was ordered to confirm the diagnosis. Which one of the following abnormal findings would NOT confirm the diagnosis of BWS?[53]

A. Gain of methylation on the maternal chromosome at imprinting center 1 (IC1)
B. Loss of methylation on the maternal chromosome at imprinting center 2 (IC2)
C. Paternal uniparental disomy (UPD) of chromosome 11p15
D. Pathogenic variants in the CDKN1C gene
E. Pathogenic variants in the IGF2 gene

168. In the pedigree shown in the figure below, two phenotypically normal sisters have grandchildren with Beckwith–Wiedemann syndrome (BWS). Which one of the following inherited genetic alteration may explain the clinical presentations in this family?

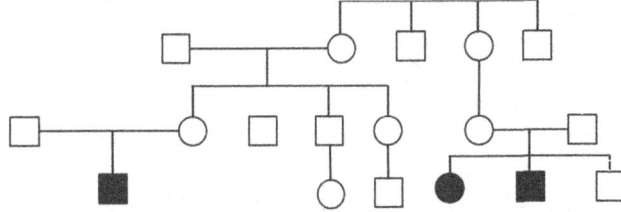

A. A pathogenic variant in the CDKN1C gene
B. A pathogenic variant in the IGF2 gene
C. Gain of methylation on the maternal chromosome at imprinting center 1 (IC1)
D. Loss of methylation on the maternal chromosome at imprinting center 2 (IC2)
E. Paternal uniparental disomy (UPD) of chromosome 11p15

169. Which one of the following genes is overexpressed in patients with Beckwith–Wiedemann syndrome?

A. CDKN1C
B. H19
C. IGF2
D. KCNQ1
E. KCNQOT1

170. Which one of the following genes is underexpressed in patients with Beckwith–Wiedemann syndrome?

A. CDKN1C
B. H19
C. IGF2
D. KCNQ1
E. KCNQOT1

171. A 21-year-old gravida 1 para 0 pregnant woman was referred to maternal–fetal medicine after her 28-week prenatal ultrasound revealed omphalocele. A baby girl was delivered at 39 weeks by cesarean section. The anterior abdominal defect was noted, with bowel in the sac that covered by a transparent membranous and umbilical cord at the top of the sac. Surgery was performed immediately. The girl was 4160 g (75th–90th percentile) in weight and 52 cm (75th–90th percentile) in height and her head circumference was 36 cm (50th–75th percentile). She also had macroglossia. There were no organomegaly or renal anomalies. The family history was unremarkable. Beckwith–Wiedemann syndrome was suspected.

A molecular study was ordered to confirm the diagnosis. Which one of the following would most likely to be the genetic finding if the patient had Beckwith—Wiedemann syndrome?[53,54]

A. *CDKN1C* single nucleotide pathogenic variant
B. Gain of methylation of maternal imprinting center 1 on 11p15.5
C. Loss of methylation of maternal imprinting center 2 on 11p15.5
D. UPD(11p15)mat
E. UPD(11p15)pat

172. In the pedigree illustrated in the figure below, two phenotypically normal sisters have grandchildren with Beckwith—Wiedemann syndrome (BWS). How frequently does BWS demonstrate an autosomal dominant mode of inheritance with incomplete penetrance, as shown in the pedigree?[6,54]

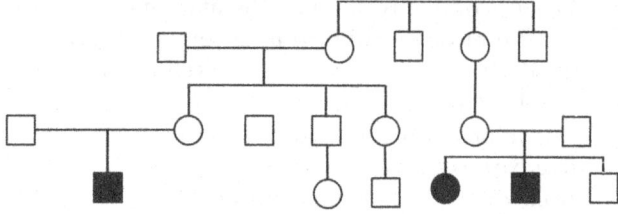

A. <1%
B. 12%
C. 28%
D. 50%
E. 74%

173. A fellow in a clinical molecular laboratory is trained in an assay for Beckwith—Wiedemann syndrome (BWS). This assay includes methylation study, Sanger sequencing of the *CDKN1C* gene, and chromosomal microarray. He was given results from five samples for interpretation. Which one of the following samples is NOT from a patient with Beckwith—Wiedemann syndrome?[6,54]

A. A missense pathogenic variant in *CDKN1C*
B. Gain of methylation of maternal imprinting center 1 on 11p15.5
C. Loss of methylation of maternal imprinting center 2 on 11p15.5
D. UPD(11p15)mat
E. UPD(11p15)pat

174. A fellow in a clinical molecular laboratory is trained in an assay for Beckwith—Wiedemann syndrome (BWS). This assay includes methylation study, Sanger sequencing of the *CDKN1C* gene, and chromosomal microarray. He was given results from 5 samples for interpretation. Which one of the following samples is from a patient with Beckwith—Wiedemann syndrome?[6,54]

A. Duplication of maternal copy of 11p15.5
B. Gain of methylation of maternal imprinting center 2 on 11p15.5
C. Loss of methylation of maternal imprinting center 1 on 11p15.5
D. UPD(11p15)mat
E. UPD(11p15)pat
F. None of the above

175. A 30-year-old gravida 3 para 2 mother was followed prenatally for 19-week ultrasound findings of single amniotic band, shortened cervix, echogenic kidneys and bowel. A female infant was born weighing 1869 g (90th percentile) at 31 weeks' gestation via emergency cesarean section for nonreassuring fetal rhythm strip and poor biophysical profile. The baby's Apgar scores were 7 at 1 minutes and 9 at 5 minutes, but her glucose was 22 mg/dL and persistent profound hypoglycemia continued. Her right leg was bigger than the left. Echocardiography showed PDA, and an abdominal ultrasound showed two nodular soft-tissue foci in the posterior wall of the urinary bladder; the liver was noted to be markedly heterogeneous with at least two areas of rounded hypodensity. MRI of the abdomen revealed a pancreatic tail cyst; a size discrepancy of the kidneys, with the right kidney measuring larger than the left; numerous tiny medullary cysts; and a right adrenal mass, with numerous enhancing hepatic lesions. Beckwith—Wiedemann syndrome (BWS) was highly suspected. A molecular study confirmed that the infant had UPD(15)pat. Which one of the following tumors would this patient have an increased risk to develop in comparison with individuals in general populations?[6]

A. Colon cancer
B. Ewing sarcoma
C. Osteosarcoma
D. Wilms tumor
E. None of the above

176. A couple was referred to a genetics clinic because the fetus was large for gestational age and omphalocele on ultrasonography at 28 weeks' gestation. The family was counseled for the possibility of Beckwith—Wiedemann syndrome (BWS). The boy was delivered by a cesarean section at 37 weeks of gestation, with a birth weight of 9 lb 2 oz and a notably large placenta. Omphalocele and macroglossia were noted at birth. A methylation study confirmed the clinical diagnosis of BWS. Which one of the following tumors would this patient have an increased risk to develop in comparison with individuals in general populations?[6]

A. Acute megakaryoblastic leukemia
B. Ewing sarcoma
C. Hepatoblastoma
D. Retinoblastoma
E. None of the above

177. An 8-year-old girl was referred to a tertiary care center for short stature. She had been diagnosed with intrauterine growth retardation and delivered at a full term. Her birth weight was 1500 g (<3rd percentile), and length 41 cm (<3rd percentile). Her development was delayed; she sat without support at 13 months of age and walked at 2.5 years of age. Her anterior fontanel did not close until 3 years of age. At the time of physical examination, her height was 101 cm and head circumference 54.5 cm. She had a broad forehead with a small triangular face and heavy eyebrows. Her left leg was 2 cm shorter than the right, and the circumference of the left leg was larger than that of the right. The end of her first and fifth fingers was dysplastic, bending interiorly, and the bone age was 3.5 years. Laboratory testing was negative. A diagnosis of Russell–Silver syndrome (RSS) was made clinically. A molecular study was ordered. Which one of the following genetic alterations might be seen in this patient if she had Russell–Silver syndrome (RSS)?[55]
    A. Duplication of maternal copy of 11p15.5
    B. Gain of methylation of maternal imprinting center 1 on 11p15.5
    C. Loss of methylation of maternal imprinting center 2 on 11p15.5
    D. UPD(11p15)pat
    E. None of the above

178. A 15-year-old boy from nonconsanguineous parents was brought to an emergency department for status epilepticus. He had seizure disorder beginning at the age of 1 month. He also had congenital short stature, low birth weight, feeding difficulties, and limb asymmetry. Despite difficulties, he had been attending school regularly. On the physical examination, he was thin and short (97 cm) and had a normal head circumference. He had a broad forehead, triangular facies, low-set prominent ears, and crowed teeth. The third and fourth phalanges of the feet showed clinodactyly. Asymmetry of the hands, phalanges, and lower extremities were noted with hemihypertrophy of the left lower extremity. A diagnosis of Russell–Silver syndrome (RSS) was made clinically. A molecular study was ordered. Which one of the following genetic alterations might be seen in this patient if he had Russell–Silver syndrome (RSS)?[56]

A. Gain of methylation of paternal imprinting center 1 on 11p15.5
B. Gain of methylation of paternal imprinting center 2 on 11p15.5
C. Loss of methylation of paternal imprinting center 1 on 11p15.5
D. Loss of methylation of paternal imprinting center 2 on 11p15.5
E. None of the above

179. An 8-year-old boy was referred to a tertiary care center with symptoms of failure to gain weight and increased size of the left half of the body since birth. He was delivered at 36 weeks of gestation weighing 1000 g. His developmental milestones were delayed (neck control at 1 year, sitting at 2 years, and walking at 3 years). The family history was unremarkable. On examination, he had hemihypertrophy of the left side of the body, frontal bossing with triangular facies, depressed nasal bridge, low-set ears, malocclusion of teeth, and high arched palate. He also had brachydactyly of fingers and toes of both hands and feet and hypoplasia of the fifth finger and little toe and syndactyly of the third and fourth toes. His height was 109 cm (Z score = −3) and his weight 23.5 kg (Z score = −0.7). He had a small penis and absence of the left testis. His IQ was below normal. X-ray of the wrists found delayed bone age (five carpal bones). A diagnosis of Russell–Silver syndrome (RSS) was made clinically. Which one of the following genetic studies would be appropriate for this patient in order to confirm the diagnosis?[57]
    A. Chromosomal microarray
    B. Methylation study
    C. Multiplex ligation-dependent probe amplification (MLPA)
    D. All of the above
    E. None of the above

180. Sam Berns was a patient with progeria, a disease of rapid premature aging that only about 250 children worldwide are known to have. His parents, Drs. Leslie Gordon and Scott Berns, were both pediatricians. Sam Berns was one of 28 children who participated in a research trial conducted by the Progeria Research Foundation (PRF), which his parents founded. In Sam's lifetime, the National Human Genome Research Institute (NHGRI), working with researchers from the PRF, discovered in 2003 that the disease is caused by a pathogenic variant in a single gene, which destabilizes the cell's nuclear membrane in ways that lead to failure of the cardiovascular, skeletal, and muscular systems. Which one of the following is the gene discovered for progeria?[58]

A. *LMNA*
B. *LMNB1*
C. *TERT*
D. *TWINKY*
E. None of the above

181. Hutchinson—Gilford progeria syndrome (progeria) is a premature aging disorder. Cardiovascular problems are the eventual cause of death in most children with progeria. The average life expectancy for a child with progeria is about 13 years. Which one of the following molecular genetic assays would be the most cost-effective, and sensitive one for the diagnosis of progeria?
A. Exome sequencing
B. Multiplex ligation-dependent probe amplification (MLPA)
C. Next-generation sequencing (NGS)
D. Sanger sequencing analysis
E. Targeted variant assay
F. None of the above

182. Sam Berns was a patient with progeria, a disease of rapid premature aging that only about 250 children worldwide are known to have. His parents, Drs. Leslie Gordon and Scott Berns, were both pediatricians. Sam Berns was one of 28 children who participated in a research trial conducted by the Progeria Research Foundation (PRF), which his parents founded. In Sam's lifetime, the National Human Genome Research Institute (NHGRI), working with researchers from the PRF, discovered in 2003 that the disease is caused by a pathogenic variant in a single gene, which destabilizes the cell's nuclear membrane in ways that lead to failure of the cardiovascular, skeletal, and muscular systems. Which one of the following types of pathogenic variants is this variant?[58]
A. Frameshift
B. In/del
C. Missense
D. Nonsense
E. Nonstop
F. Synonymous

183. A 14-year-old girl presented with a progressive history of coarsening of skin, failure to thrive, and inability to squat for the past 3 to 4 years. The girl had also developed global alopecia over the past few years. The perinatal history was uneventful. She was apparently normal until 1 year of age, when the parents started noticing the above features. She had normal intelligence. No family history of similar symptoms could be elicited. General examination revealed the child to be of short stature and malnourished.

The eyes appeared prominent and the chin was hypoplastic chin. Multiple patches of coarse and thickened skin were present, especially over the dorsum of the hands and shoulders. The terminal ends of the fingers appeared broad and stubby. A provisional diagnosis of progeria was made. A targeted variant assay was used to confirm the diagnosis, and the pathogenic variant was detected. The parents asked the genetic counselor for the recurrent risk since the mother was pregnant with their second child. Which one of the following would most likely be the recurrent risks in this family?[59]
A. <1%
B. 6%—10% due to reduced penetrance
C. 25%
D. 50%
E. 67%
F. >99%
G. None of the above

184. Which one of the following DNA repair deficiency disorders does NOT have an increased risk for malignancies?
A. Ataxia telangiectasia
B. Bloom syndrome
C. Cockayne syndrome
D. Werner syndrome
E. Xeroderma pigmentosum

185. A 6-year-old boy was brought to a genetics clinic for intellectual disability, lack of speech development, and dysmorphic facial features. His perinatal history was uneventful. The family history was unremarkable. His general health was good. A physical examination revealed short stature, microbrachycephaly, a characteristic face, broad and angulated thumbs, broad big toes, mild scoliosis, micropenis, and severe intellectual disability. The characteristic craniofacial features were downslanted palpebral fissures, low-hanging columella, high palate, grimacing smile, and talon cusps. Radiographs showed broad ribs and cleft of vertebral body S1. A diagnosis of Rubinstein—Taybi syndrome was made clinically. At the end of the appropriate genetic counseling, the couple asked for the recurrent risk. Which one of the following would most likely be the estimated recurrent risk of the condition in this family?[60]
A. <1%
B. 5%—10%
C. 25%
D. 50%
E. 100%
F. None of the above

186. A 6-year-old boy was brought to a genetics clinic for intellectual disability, lack of speech development, and dysmorphic facial features. His perinatal history was uneventful. The family history was unremarkable. His general health was good. A physical examination revealed short stature, microbrachycephaly, a characteristic face, broad and angulated thumbs, broad big toes, mild scoliosis, micropenis, and severe intellectual disability. The characteristic craniofacial features are downslanted palpebral fissures, low-hanging columella, high palate, grimacing smile, and talon cusps. Radiographs showed broad ribs and cleft of vertebral body S1. A diagnosis of Rubinstein–Taybi syndrome was made clinically. A FISH test detected a microdeletion of 16p13.3 region including *CREBBP* in the patient. Which of the following mechanisms would most likely cause the symptoms of the Rubinstein–Taybi syndrome in this patient?[60,61]
    A. Dominant negative
    B. Epigenetic change
    C. Haploinsufficiency
    D. Unclear
    E. None of the above

187. A 2-year-old girl was referred to a genetics clinic for developmental delay and multiple congenital anomalies. Her perinatal history was uneventful except for macrosomia (>2 SD). Soon after birth, she was noted to have preaxial polydactyly and cutaneous syndactyly of the first to fourth toes on both feet and cutaneous syndactyly of the second to fourth fingers on the left hand. Her developmental milestones were delayed. She gained head control, sitting and crawling at 5, 14, and 20 months, respectively. At age 2 she could not walk independently and lacked speech but could follow simple orders. A physical examination revealed macrocephaly (+2.3 SD) with frontal bossing and hypertelorism. Her brain MRI showed multiple cerebral cavernous malformations, ventricular dilatation, and hypogenesis of corpus callosum. She had no history of febrile seizure and epilepsy. Her family history was unremarkable. A Greig cephalopolysyndactyly contiguous gene deletion syndrome was suspected. Which one of following assays would most likely be used as the first-line test to confirm the diagnosis in this patient?[62]
    A. Chromosome karyotyping
    B. Chromosomal microarray analysis
    C. Exome-sequence analysis
    D. NGS analysis
    E. Sanger sequencing analysis
    F. None of the above

188. A 2-year-old girl was referred to a genetics clinic for developmental delay and multiple congenital anomalies. Her perinatal history was uneventful except for macrosomia (>2 SD). Soon after birth, she was noted to have preaxial polydactyly and cutaneous syndactyly of the first to fourth toes on both feet and cutaneous syndactyly of the second to fourth fingers on the left hand. Her developmental milestones were delayed. She gained head control, sitting and crawling at 5, 14, and 20 months, respectively. At age 2 she could not walk independently and lacked speech but could follow simple orders. A physical examination revealed macrocephaly (+2.3 SD) with frontal bossing and hypertelorism. Her brain MRI showed multiple cerebral cavernous malformations, ventricular dilatation, and hypogenesis of corpus callosum. She had no history of febrile seizure and epilepsy. Her family history was unremarkable. A Greig cephalopolysyndactyly contiguous gene deletion syndrome was suspected. A chromosomal microarray study detected a 7.1-Mb deletion at 17p14, and confirmed the diagnosis. Which one of following genes would most likely be involved in the deletion in this patient?[62]
    A. *GLI1*
    B. *GLI2*
    C. *GLI3*
    D. *GLI4*
    E. None of the above

189. A cytogenetics director worked on a prenatal chromosomal microarray case. The clinical indication for the study was not provided. A terminal deletion of the long arm of chromosome 7, involving the entire *GLI3* gene, was detected. Which one of the following conditions would the fetus most likely have?
    A. Greig cephalopolysyndactyly syndrome (GCPS)
    B. Muenke syndrome
    C. Pallister–Hall syndrome
    D. Pallister–Killian syndrome
    E. All of the above
    F. None of the above

190. A baby girl, the first child of unrelated parents, was born at term weighing 3130 g and with a head circumference of 35 cm. Multiple problems were noted at birth, including choanal atresia, bifid epiglottis, and a cleft upper larynx with a posterior web in the subglottic area. A CT scan of the thorax revealed that the angle of the carina was almost 180 degrees. Facially she had a short nose with depressed nasal bridge and anteverted nares and her ear lobes were anteverted. There

was bilateral hexadactyly with osseous 2/3 syndactyly of the right hand, which may have represented an insertional type of polydactyly. There was mild soft-tissue syndactyly of the left hand. All fingers appeared slightly short and tapering. On X-ray her sacrum appeared hypoplastic. Subsequently, she developed signs of hypopituitarism, recurrent problems with upper airway obstruction, and feeding difficulties. She died at 12 months of age after a respiratory infection. Her chromosomes were normal. Autopsy revealed a tracheal diverticulum and a small right middle lobe of the lung with incomplete separation of the right upper and lower lobes. The pituitary gland was absent, with a rudimentary stalk, and the adrenal glands were markedly fibrotic. The thymus was aplastic histologically. A 2×2 cm soft nodular mass in the brain occupied the position of hypothalamus and replaced it completely, which was diagnosed as hypothalamus hamartoma. Examination of the rest of the brain showed that the frontal, parietal, and occipital lobes appeared disproportionately small with respect to the temporal lobes. The unci were featureless and the olfactory tracts were absent. There was a generalized reduction of bulk of the white matter and the corpus callosum was abnormally thin. A diagnosis of Pallister–Hall syndrome was made. Which one of the following genes would most likely be mutated in this patient?[63]

A. *FGFR2*
B. *FGFR3*
C. *GLI2*
D. *GLI3*
E. *SMAD3*
F. *SMAD4*
G. None of the above

191. Which one of the following disorders causes pathogenic variants in the *GLI3* gene?
    A. Autosomal dominant Greig cephalopolysyndactyly syndrome (GCPS)
    B. Autosomal recessive Greig cephalopolysyndactyly syndrome (GCPS)
    C. Autosomal dominant Pallister–Hall syndrome
    D. Autosomal recessive Pallister–Hall syndrome
    E. A and B
    F. A and C
    G. B and D
    H. C and C
    I. None of the above

192. A 1½-year-old boy was admitted to a hospital with symptoms of cough, cold, and fever. He was born full term of nonconsanguineous parents. He did not have a significant past medical or surgical

history. The child had minimal wheeze. He had broad forehead with frontal bossing, broad nasal root, ocular hypertelorism, macrocephaly (>97th percentile for his age). Postaxial polydactyly in his hands and preaxial polysyndactyly of feet was noted. His anterior fontanel was open. He had attained appropriate motor and mental milestones for his age. Echocardiography and ultrasonography of the cranium and abdomen were normal. The family history revealed polydactyly and syndactyly in sister, mother, and maternal grandfather and delta phalanx in mother and grandfather, suggestive of an autosomal dominant inheritance. There was no family history of neurological abnormalities. His clinical features suggested Greig cephalopolysyndactyly syndrome. Which one of the following molecular genetic assays would most likely be used to detect pathogenic variant (s) in this patient?[64]
    A. Deletion/duplication analysis
    B. Next-generation sequencing analysis
    C. Sanger sequencing analysis
    D. Targeted variant analysis
    E. None of the above

193. A baby girl was born by elective C-section at 31 weeks of gestational age following concerns about intrauterine growth retardation (IUGR) and oligohydramnios. Her birth weight was 1.2 kg (−1.76 SD). Soon after the delivery, she was noted to be pale and to have irregular respirations and desaturations. Endotracheal intubation was extremely difficult, with multiple unsuccessful attempts. The examination of the upper airway showed a bifid epiglottis and uvula and a funnel-shaped trachea. Physical examination revealed oligodactyly, with three fingers and a thumb on the right hand and four fingers and a thumb on the left hand. She had short fingers and a single palmar crease bilaterally. The toes were noted to be overlapping, with slightly rocker-bottom appearances to the feet. She also had a short nose with a depressed nasal bridge and anteverted nares. She had two umbilical vessels, an imperforate anus, and a small urogenital opening. Cardiovascular workups revealed a small patent ductus arteriosus but an otherwise structurally normal heart. A high-resolution CT scan of the chest revealed a trachea of very small diameter— 3.5 mm. Bronchography demonstrated the right upper lobe bronchus arising from the trachea and small airways. MRI of the brain revealed the presence of a large mass in the suprasellar subarachnoid space measuring $25 \times 17 \times 22$ mm, with imaging characteristics of a hypothalamic

hamartoma. The cochlea was noted to be truncated bilaterally with a reduced number of turns. The baby had recurrent hypoglycemia (blood glucose, <2.6 mmol/L) from the first day of life. And her plasma insulin level (65 pmol/L) and C-peptide (775 pmol/L) were inappropriately elevated during hypoglycemia. The plasma free fatty acids (285 μmol/L) and 3-hydroxybutyrate (8 μmol/L) were suppressed during hypoglycemia. Congenital hyperinsulinism due to Pallister−Hall syndrome was suspected. Which one of following genes would most likely be tested to confirm the diagnosis in this patient?[65]

A. *GLI1*
B. *GLI2*
C. *GLI3*
D. *GLI4*
E. None of the above

194. A 3-week-old girl was seen in a clinic for brachycephaly with a flattened occiput and prominent frontal bossing. A physical examination revealed bilateral coronal synostosis by palpation. The metopic and sagittal sutures were wide open, and the metopic suture extended to the nasofrontal junction. The anterior fontanel extended from the nasal to the occipital bone. She had turribrachycephaly because of her craniosynostosis. A slight degree of midface retraction was present, along with downslanting of the palpebral fissures. She also exhibited mild to moderate sensorineural hearing loss and has required use of hearing aids on a full-time basis. At age 4, brachycephaly and mild proptosis were noted. A molecular genetics study did not reveal any sequence changes in *FGFR1*, *FGFR2*, and *FGFR3*. Which one of following genes would most likely be tested as the next step in the workup to further rule out genetic etiology in this patient?[66]

A. *COL1A2*
B. *FBN1*
C. *PEX3*
D. *TWIST1*
E. None of the above

195. A 3-week-old girl was seen in a clinic for brachycephaly with a flattened occiput and prominent frontal bossing. A physical examination revealed bilateral coronal synostosis by palpation. The metopic and sagittal sutures were wide open, and the metopic suture extended to the nasofrontal junction. The anterior fontanel extended from the nasal to the occipital bone. She had turribrachycephaly because of her craniosynostosis. A slight degree of midface retraction was present, along with downslanting

of the palpebral fissures. She also exhibited mild to moderate sensorineural hearing loss and has required use of hearing aids on a full-time basis. At age 4, brachycephaly and mild proptosis were noted. All six of her older siblings had the same characteristics of craniosynostosis. A molecular genetics study was ordered to confirm the diagnosis for syndromic craniosynostosis. Which one of following assays would be the most cost-effective way to confirm the diagnosis in this patient?[66]

A. Chromosome karyotyping
B. Chromosomal microarray analysis
C. Exome-sequence analysis
D. NGS analysis
E. Sanger sequencing analysis
F. None of the above

196. A 3-week-old girl was seen in a clinic for brachycephaly with a flattened occiput and prominent frontal bossing. A physical examination revealed bilateral coronal synostosis by palpation. The metopic and sagittal sutures were wide open, and the metopic suture extended to the nasofrontal junction. The anterior fontanel extended from the nasal to the occipital bone. She had turribrachycephaly because of her craniosynostosis. A slight degree of midface retraction was present, along with downslanting of the palpebral fissures. She also exhibited mild to moderate sensorineural hearing loss and has required use of hearing aids on a full-time basis. At age 4, brachycephaly and mild proptosis were noted. All six of her older siblings had the same characteristics of craniosynostosis. A next-generation sequencing (NGS) test was ordered and revealed a pathogenic variant, p.R191M, in the *TWIST1* gene. At the time of the review of her test results, her mother was 6 weeks pregnant. Which one of following would most likely be the estimated recurrent risk of the same condition in this future child?[66]

A. <1%
B. 5%−10%
C. 25%
D. 50%
E. 100%
F. None of the above

197. A 24-month-old Asian girl was brought to a clinic for plagiocephaly/brachycephaly and dysmorphic facial features. Her perinatal history was uneventful. She had mild neurodevelopmental delay, mild midfacial hypoplasia, hypertelorism, downslanting palpebral fissures, strabismus, and a beak-shaped nose. The family history was significant for her mother, her mother's two

sisters, and her maternal grandfather having similar cephalofacial anomalies, strabismus, and short stature. The severity of the brachycephaly was variable among these family members. The 3D-CT and MRI revealed bilateral coronal craniosynostosis, plagiocephaly/brachycephaly, bilateral lateral ventricle dilation, proptosis, and a small cerebellum. Muenke syndrome was at the top of the differential diagnostic list. Which one of following assays would most likely be used to confirm the diagnosis of Muenke syndrome in this patient?[67]

A. Chromosome karyotyping
B. Chromosomal microarray
C. Exome-sequence analysis
D. NGS analysis
E. Sanger sequencing analysis
F. Targeted variant analysis
G. None of the above

198. A 24-month-old Asian girl was brought to a clinic for plagiocephaly/brachycephaly and dysmorphic facial features. Her perinatal history was uneventful. She had mild neurodevelopmental delay, mild midfacial hypoplasia, hypertelorism, downslanting palpebral fissures, strabismus, and a beak-shaped nose. The family history was significant for her mother, her mother's two sisters, and her maternal grandfather having similar cephalofacial anomalies, strabismus, and short stature. The severity of the brachycephaly was variable among these family members. The 3D-CT and MRI revealed bilateral coronal craniosynostosis, plagiocephaly/brachycephaly, bilateral lateral ventricle dilation, proptosis, and a small cerebellum. A next-generation sequencing (NGS) test was ordered and revealed a pathogenic variant, c.749C > G(p.Pro250Arg), in the *FGFR3* gene. Which one of following conditions would the patient most likely have?[67]

A. Apert syndrome
B. Crouzon syndrome
C. Muenke syndrome
D. Pfeiffer syndrome
E. Saethre–Chotzen syndrome
F. None of the above

199. A full-term baby was born with multiple congenital anomalies, including brachycephaly, maxillary hypoplasia, exophthalmos, proptosis, low-set ears, preauricular skin tags, atresia of the external auditory canal, high arched palate, radially deviated broad thumbs and medially deviated big toes, ankylosed elbows, and a mass on the coccygeal area. 3D-CT revealed closure of

the bilateral coronal sutures and left lambdoidal suture, midface hypoplasia, and shallow orbits. A spinal MRI revealed an outwardly everted coccyx. He was the first child of an apparently healthy nonconsanguineous couple. The family history was unremarkable. A next-generation sequence (NGS) test was ordered and revealed a pathogenic variant, c.755C > G(p.Trp290Cys), in the *FGFR2* gene. Which one of following conditions would the patient least likely have?[68]

A. Apert syndrome
B. Crouzon syndrome
C. Pfeiffer syndrome
D. Saethre–Chotzen syndrome
E. All of the above
F. None of the above

200. During a routine dental checkup, a 9-year-old boy was found to have protruding eyes and enlarged calvarium. A physical examination revealed exophthalmos, strabismus, hypertelorism, irregularly shaped vault with the left side of the head enlarged involving the sagittal and coronal sutures, relatively large mandible, retruded maxilla resulting in midface retrusion, Parrot beak nose, asymmetrical enlargement of the skull, everted lower lip, deep and narrow palate, and reduced vision. An X-ray revealed closure of the sagittal and coronal sutures. A hammered-silver appearance was seen in regions of the skull, due to compression of the developing brain on the fused bone. A CT scan revealed craniosynostosis with premature closure of sutures, shallow orbits with proptosis, hypoplastic maxilla and zygoma, nonpneumatized right middle ear cavity with acellular mastoids, and moderate degree of hydrocephalus with diffuse indentation of inner table of skull and narrowing of diploic space and prominent convolutional margins. A next-generation sequence (NGS) test was ordered and revealed a pathogenic variant, p.Trp290Gly, in the *FGFR2* gene. Which one of following conditions would the patient least likely have?[69]

A. Apert syndrome
B. Crouzon syndrome
C. Muenke syndrome
D. Pfeiffer syndrome
E. Any of the above
F. None of the above

201. During a routine dental checkup, a 9-year-old boy was found to have protruding eyes and enlarged calvarium. A physical examination revealed exophthalmos, strabismus, hypertelorism, irregularly shaped vault with the left side of the

head enlarged involving the sagittal and coronal sutures, relatively large mandible, retruded maxilla resulting in midface retrusion, Parrot beak nose, asymmetrical enlargement of the skull, everted lower lip, deep and narrow palate, and reduced vision. An X-ray revealed closure of the sagittal and coronal sutures. A hammered-silver appearance was seen in regions of the skull, due to compression of the developing brain on the fused bone. A CT scan revealed craniosynostosis with premature closure of sutures, shallow orbits with proptosis, hypoplastic maxilla and zygoma, nonpneumatized right middle ear cavity with acellular mastoids, and moderate degree of hydrocephalus with diffuse indentation of inner table of skull and narrowing of diploic space and prominent convolutional margins. A next-generation sequence (NGS) test was ordered and revealed a pathogenic variant, p.Trp290Gly, in the *FGFR2* gene. Which one of the following would most likely be the pathogenetic mechanism of the variant in this patient?[69–74]

A. Epigenetic change
B. Gain of function
C. Loss of function
D. Unclear
E. None of the above

202. During a routine dental checkup, a 9-year-old boy was found to have protruding eyes and enlarged calvarium. A physical examination revealed exophthalmos, strabismus, hypertelorism, irregularly shaped vault with the left side of the head enlarged involving the sagittal and coronal sutures, relatively large mandible, retruded maxilla resulting in midface retrusion, Parrot beak nose, asymmetrical enlargement of the skull, everted lower lip, deep and narrow palate, and reduced vision. An X-ray revealed closure of the sagittal and coronal sutures. A hammered-silver appearance was seen in regions of the skull, due to compression of the developing brain on the fused bone. A CT scan revealed craniosynostosis with premature closure of sutures, shallow orbits with proptosis, hypoplastic maxilla and zygoma, nonpneumatized right middle ear cavity with acellular mastoids, and moderate degree of hydrocephalus with diffuse indentation of inner table of skull and narrowing of diploic space and prominent convolutional margins. A next-generation sequence (NGS) test was ordered and revealed a pathogenic variant, p.Trp290Gly, in the *FGFR2* gene. Neither of the parents had the same variant. Which one of following is a risk factor for syndromic craniosynostosis?[69,75-77]

A. Increased maternal age
B. Increased paternal age
C. Maternal consumption of alcohol during pregnancy
D. Maternal consumption of tobacco during pregnancy
E. Paternal consumption of alcohol during pregnancy
F. Paternal consumption of tobacco during pregnancy
G. None of the above

203. A 2-month-old boy was admitted to a hospital for recurrent respiratory tract infections and respiratory distress. Pneumonia was diagnosed and treated with antibiotics. After the pneumonia was resolved, the patient was noted to have a large cranium with a prominent forehead. His nasal bridge was moderately flat, and the chest was small in comparison with the abdomen. A diagnosis of achondroplasia was suspected. A skeletal survey further revealed a reduced anteroposterior diameter of the thorax and rhizomelic shortening of the proximal end of the long bones. An X-ray revealed that the bone calvarium was large with a small sella, and there was evidence of a decrease in the interpedicular distance in the lower lumbar spine, suggesting lumbar canal stenosis. A molecular genetics study was ordered to confirm the diagnosis. Which one of following assays would most likely be used to confirm the diagnosis of achondroplasia in this patient?[78]

A. Chromosome karyotyping
B. Chromosomal microarray analysis
C. Exome-sequence analysis
D. NGS analysis
E. Sanger sequencing analysis
F. Targeted variant analysis
G. None of the above

204. A 2-month-old boy was admitted to a hospital for recurrent respiratory tract infections and respiratory distress. Pneumonia was diagnosed and treated with antibiotics. After the pneumonia was resolved, the patient was noted to have a large cranium with a prominent forehead. His nasal bridge was moderately flat, and the chest was small in comparison with the abdomen. A diagnosis of achondroplasia was suspected. A skeletal survey further revealed a reduced anteroposterior diameter of the thorax and rhizomelic shortening of the proximal end of the long bones. An X-ray revealed that the bone calvarium was large with a small sella, and there was evidence of a decrease in the interpedicular distance in the lower lumbar spine, suggesting

lumbar canal stenosis. Which one of following genes would most likely be tested to confirm the diagnosis of achondroplasia in this patient?[78]

A. *FGFR1*
B. *FGFR2*
C. *FGFR3*
D. *FGFR4*
E. None of the above

205. A 2-month-old boy was admitted to a hospital for recurrent respiratory tract infections and respiratory distress. Pneumonia was diagnosed and treated with antibiotics. After the pneumonia was resolved, the patient was noted to have a large cranium with a prominent forehead. His nasal bridge was moderately flat, and the chest was small in comparison with the abdomen. A diagnosis of achondroplasia was suspected. A skeletal survey further revealed a reduced anteroposterior diameter of the thorax and rhizomelic shortening of the proximal end of the long bones. An X-ray revealed that the bone calvarium was large with a small sella, and there was evidence of a decrease in the interpedicular distance in the lower lumbar spine, suggesting lumbar canal stenosis. A molecular study detected a pathogenic variant, c.1138G > A (p.Gly380Arg), in *FGFR3*. Which one of the following would most likely be the pathogenetic mechanism of the variant in this patient?[78,79]

A. Epigenetic change
B. Gain of function
C. Loss of function
D. Unclear
E. None of the above

206. A 2-month-old boy was admitted to a hospital for recurrent respiratory tract infections and respiratory distress. Pneumonia was diagnosed and treated with antibiotics. After the pneumonia was resolved, the patient was noted to have a large cranium with a prominent forehead. His nasal bridge was moderately flat, and the chest was small in comparison with the abdomen. A diagnosis of achondroplasia was suspected. A skeletal survey further revealed a reduced anteroposterior diameter of the thorax and rhizomelic shortening of the proximal end of the long bones. An X-ray revealed that the bone calvarium was large with a small sella, and there was evidence of a decrease in the interpedicular distance in the lower lumbar spine, suggesting lumbar canal stenosis. A molecular study detected a pathogenic variant, c.1138G > A (p. Gly380Arg), in *FGFR3*. Neither of the parents had the variant. Which one of following is a risk factor for achondroplasia?[78]

A. Increased maternal age
B. Increased paternal age
C. Maternal consumption of alcohol during pregnancy
D. Maternal consumption of tobacco during pregnancy
E. Paternal consumption of alcohol during pregnancy
F. Paternal consumption of tobacco during pregnancy
G. None of the above

207. A couple with achondroplasia came to a clinic for premarriage counseling. They both had been tested and had the c.1138G > A (p.Gly380Arg) variant in *FGFR3*. Which one of the following would be expected in this couple in addition to having children with the same condition?

A. Intellectual disability in some of their children
B. No children with normal height
C. Recurrent pregnancy loss
D. Shorter lifespan
E. None of the above

208. A couple with achondroplasia came to a clinic for premarriage counseling. They both had been tested and had the c.1138G > A (p.Gly380Arg) variant in *FGFR3*. Which one of the following would most likely to be the chance of this couple having a child with normal height?

A. < 1%
B. 25%
C. 33%
D. 50%
E. 67%
F. 100%
G. None of the above

209. A 14-year-old girl was brought to a clinic for short stature. She was the second child of a couple in their 20s. Her perinatal history was unremarkable. A physical examination revealed a height of 97 cm (−2.18 SDS), a head circumference of 54 cm (+3.71 SDS); and head circumference standard deviation score (SDS)-height SDS (DHc/Ht) SDS = +5.89. Her skeleton was disproportional, with short limbs and a relatively long trunk (upper-to-lower-segment ratio, 1.21 [> 2 SD]), brachydactyly, metaphyseal flaring, limited elbow extension, short legs, and a short arm span. Her mother's and father's height were 154 cm and 172 cm, respectively. Her developmental milestones were normal, but she showed difficulties in neuropsychological development, especially language skills. Radiographic examination confirmed rhizomelic short stature. Her karyotype was 46,XX. A molecular study for achondroplasia was ordered, and no pathogenic variants were

detected. Reflex testing for hypochondroplasia was initiated. Which one of following genes would most likely be tested for hypochondroplasia in this patient?[80]

A. *FGFR1*

B. *FGFR2*

C. *FGFR3*

D. *FGFR4*

E. None of the above

210. A 14-year-old girl was brought to a clinic for short stature. She was the second child of a couple in their 20s. Her perinatal history was unremarkable. A physical examination revealed a height of 97 cm (−2.18 SD), a head circumference of 54 cm (+3.71 SD); and head circumference SD-height SD = +5.89. Her skeleton was disproportional, with short limbs and a relatively long trunk (upper-to-lower-segment ratio, 1.21 [>2 SD]), brachydactyly, metaphyseal flaring, limited elbow extension, short legs, and a short arm span. Her mother's and father's height were 154 cm and 172 cm, respectively. Her developmental milestones were normal, but she showed difficulties in neuropsychological development, especially language skills. Radiographic examination confirmed rhizomelic short stature. Her karyotype was 46,XX. A molecular study for achondroplasia was ordered, and no pathogenic variants were detected. Reflex testing for hypochondroplasia was initiated. Which one of following assays would most likely be used for the reflex testing for hypochondroplasia in this patient?[80]

A. Chromosome karyotyping

B. Chromosomal microarray analysis

C. Exome-sequence analysis

D. NGS analysis

E. Sanger sequencing analysis

F. Targeted variant analysis

G. None of the above

211. A 7-year-old girl came to an endocrinological clinic for short stature. Her perinatal history was unremarkable, with normal birth weight and height. Her motor and language development were in the normal range. She had always been one of the shortest students in her class. A physical examination revealed that her height was less than the third percentile, her weight approximately in the fifth percentile, and head circumference in the 90th percentile. She had mesomelic limb shortening. An X-ray confirmed bilateral Madelung deformity. A sequencing analysis of *SHOX* with reflex to deletion/duplication was ordered, and a deletion involving the whole gene was detected. Which one of the

following disorders would this patient most likely have?

A. Achondroplasia

B. Hypochondroplasia

C. Leri−Weill dyschondrosteosis

D. Stickler syndrome

E. Turner syndrome

212. A 7-year-old girl came to an endocrinological clinic for short stature. Her perinatal history was unremarkable, with normal birth weight and height. Her motor and language development were in the normal range. She had always been one of the shortest students in her class. A physical examination revealed that her height was less than the third percentile, her weight approximately in the fifth percentile, and head circumference in the 90th percentile. She had mesomelic limb shortening. An X-ray confirmed bilateral Madelung deformity. A sequencing analysis of *SHOX* with reflex to deletion/duplication was ordered, and a deletion involving the whole gene was detected. Which one of the following is the inherited mode of this disease?

A. Autosomal dominant

B. Autosomal recessive

C. X-linked

D. Mitochondrial inherited

E. None of the above

213. A 7-year-old girl came to an endocrinological clinic for short stature. Her perinatal history was unremarkable, with normal birth weight and height. Her motor and language development were in the normal range. She had always been one of the shortest students in her class. A physical examination revealed that her height was less than the third percentile, her weight approximately in the fifth percentile, and head circumference in the 90th percentile. She had mesomelic limb shortening. An X-ray confirmed bilateral Madelung deformity. A sequencing analysis of *SHOX* with reflex to deletion/duplication was ordered, and a deletion involving the whole gene was detected. Which one of the following analyses would most likely be used as the initial genetic evaluation for this patient?

A. Chromosomal microarray analysis

B. Karyotyping

C. Sequencing the *SHOX* gene

D. Targeted variant assay

E. None of the above

214. A 10-month-old girl was admitted to a hospital for heart failure and a history of admission to an intensive care unit for decompensated heart failure and cardiac arrest 1 month before. Her perinatal history was unremarkable. Her parents

were unrelated. She remained asymptomatic until the age of 2 months, when she presented with shortness of breath, poor appetite and weight loss. Electrocardiography revealed dilated cardiac myopathy, especially of the left atrium and left ventricle. There was also hepatomegaly, 4 cm below the right costal margin. No dysmorphic features were observed. The patient evolved with refractory heart failure because of severely deteriorated left ventricular function and became a candidate for heart transplantation. While waiting for the transplantation, a molecular study was ordered for isolated cardiomyopathy. Which one of the following molecular genetic assays would most likely be used to confirm the diagnosis in this patient?[81]

  A. Chromosomal microarray analysis
  B. Next-generation sequencing
  C. Sanger sequencing
  D. Targeted variant assay
  E. Whole-exome sequencing
  F. None of the above

215. A 3-month-old boy was brought to a clinic for feeding difficulty and failure to thrive (loss of 900 g in 1 month). The medical history revealed severe hydramnios, macrosomia with a birth weight of 4700 g, and neonatal hypoglycemia and hypocalcemia. A physical examination revealed macrocephaly (>3 SD), epicanthus, strabismus, flattened nose, low-set ears, macroglossia, and short neck. A follow up electrocardiogram at 6 months of age revealed an asymmetric nonobstructive hypertrophic cardiomyopathy involving especially the basal part of the ventricular septum. A clinical diagnosis of Costello syndrome was made. A molecular study was ordered to confirm the diagnosis. Which one of the following molecular genetic assays would most likely be used to confirm the diagnosis in this patient?[82]

  A. Chromosomal microarray analysis
  B. Next-generation sequencing
  C. Sanger sequencing
  D. Targeted variant assay
  E. Whole-exome sequencing
  F. None of the above

216. An 8-year-old boy was brought to a dental clinic for lack of teeth as well as speech and mastication problems. He was an only child. No others in the family had similar symptoms. Lack of primary and permanent teeth in the oral cavity resulted in dietary problems. A physical examination

revealed saddle nose; soft, dry and light-colored skin; increased pigmentation; as well as thin, linear wrinkles in the perioral region. He had complete absence of primary and permanent teeth, thin alveolar ridges, reduced vertical bone height, and loss of sulcus depth in the posterior regions of the maxillary and mandibular jaws. Complete anodontia was confirmed by panoramic radiography. A clinical diagnosis of anhidrotic ectodermal dysplasia was made. A molecular study was ordered to confirm the diagnosis. Which one of the following molecular genetic assays would most likely be used than others to confirm the diagnosis in this patient?[83]

  A. Chromosomal microarray analysis
  B. Next-generation sequencing
  C. Sanger sequencing
  D. Targeted variant assay
  E. Whole-exome sequencing
  F. None of the above

217. An 8-year-old boy was brought to a dental clinic for lack of teeth as well as speech and mastication problems. He was the only child, and no others in the family had similar symptoms. Lack of primary and permanent teeth in the oral cavity resulted in dietary problems. A physical examination revealed saddle nose; soft, dry and light-colored skin; increased pigmentation; as well as thin, linear wrinkles in the perioral region. He had complete absence of primary and permanent teeth, thin alveolar ridges, reduced vertical bone height, and loss of sulcus depth in the posterior regions of maxillary and mandibular jaws. Complete anodontia was confirmed by panoramic radiography. A clinical diagnosis of hypohidrotic ectodermal dysplasia was made. A molecular study was ordered to confirm the diagnosis, and a pathogenic variant in *EDA* was detected, c.423T > C(p.Tyr61His). Parental testing was ordered to confirm whether this is a familial or a de novo alteration. Which one of the following molecular genetic assays would most likely be used to test the parents?[83]

  A. Chromosomal microarray analysis
  B. Next-generation sequencing
  C. Sanger sequencing
  D. Targeted variant assay
  E. Whole-exome sequencing
  F. None of the above

218. Two sisters, 13 and 14 years old, were referred to a tertiary medical center with a chief symptom of missing teeth in upper and lower arches beginning in early childhood. Both had no history of exfoliation of teeth in the maxillary and mandibular arches except in the upper anterior region, where the deciduous teeth were replaced by the existing permanent teeth. They also reported dry skin and dry mouth, with difficulty in swallowing. The lack of primary and permanent teeth in the oral cavity resulted in dietary and speech problems. Their family history was remarkable for consanguineous parents, but there was no evidence of similar diseases in other family members. A physical examination revealed frontal bossing; thick and protuberant lips; saddle nose; soft, dry, and light-colored skin on the face and on the upper and lower extremities; increased pigmentation around the ala of the nose; sparse hair on the scalp, eyebrows and eyelashes; dry lips; and perioral and periorbital pigmentation. Intraoral examination revealed complete absence of teeth in the mandibular arch and presence of conical right and left maxillary central incisors. Further intraoral examination revealed loss of sulcus depth in the entire mandibular arch and maxillary arches except in maxillary anterior region. Thinning of alveolar ridges was evident in both maxillary and mandibular arches. A clinical diagnosis of anhidrotic ectodermal dysplasia was made. A molecular study was ordered to confirm the diagnosis. Which one of the following genes would most likely NOT harbor a pathogenic variant in these two patients?[84]

A. *EDA*
B. *EDAR*
C. *EDARAAD*
D. Not sure
E. None of the above

219. A couple brought their 8-year-old boy to a dental clinic for lack of teeth as well as speech and mastication problems. The patient was the only child of the couple. The family history was remarkable for multiple members with similar symptoms (see the figure below for the pedigree). Lack of primary and permanent teeth in the oral cavity resulted in dietary problems. A physical examination revealed saddle nose; soft, dry and light-colored skin; increased pigmentation; as well as thin, linear wrinkles in the perioral region. He had complete absence of primary and permanent teeth, thin alveolar ridges, reduced vertical bone height, and loss of sulcus depth in the posterior

regions of maxillary and mandibular jaws. Complete anodontia was confirmed by panoramic radiography. A clinical diagnosis of hypohidrotic ectodermal dysplasia (HED) was made.

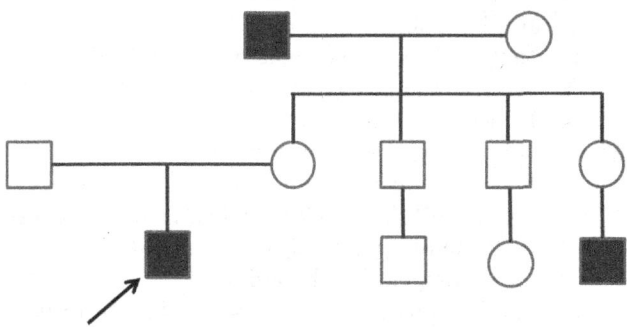

Which one of the following genes would most likely harbor a pathogenic variant for HED in this family?[83]

A. *EDA*
B. *EDAR*
C. *EDARADD*
D. *DICER1*
E. *FH*
F. *ERCC1*

220. A 19-day-old newborn girl was brought to a hospital for seizures and abnormal skin lesions. She had partial seizures in the arms, legs, and face about 10 times before going to the hospital. She has had erythematous vesicular eruptions on the upper and lower extremities beginning at the age of 12 days. The skin lesions had a linear pattern, mostly on the limbs. Number and size of the skin lesions increased in the next 7 days. She was born at full term by vaginal delivery with no remarkable prenatal history. The parents were not related. The family history was unremarkable except that her mother had some faint hypopigmented atrophic linear lesions on both thighs that had been there since she was a little girl. An EEG revealed epileptiform discharges with sharp waves and sharp, slow complex waves in the right hemisphere. But a CT scan of the brain appeared normal. Histopathology of a skin biopsy showed spongiotic dermatitis with massive intraepidermal eosinophilia in the presence of eosinophil-filled intraepidermal vesicles, as well as infiltrate of lymphocytes in superficial dermis. A clinical diagnosis of incontinentia pigmenti (IP) was made, and a molecular study was ordered. Which one of the following molecular genetic assays would

provide the most cost-effective first-tier test to detect the pathogenic variant in this patient?[85]
  A. Chromosomal microarray (CMA)
  B. FISH
  C. Multiplex ligation-dependent probe amplification (MLPA)
  D. Next-generation sequencing
  E. Sanger sequencing
  F. Targeted variant assay

221. A 9-year-old girl is brought to a clinic for her dental condition. The prenatal care and birth were uneventful. A provisional clinical diagnosis of incontinentia pigmenti (IP) was made when she was 3 days old and confirmed histopathologically from a biopsy taken from her back. The vesicular lesions over her extremities and body cleared up at 6 months of age. A physical examination reveals pigmented macular lesions on her face, trunk, back, fingers, and legs, and her nipples are absent. She has alopecia on the crown of the head with a scarred patch on the skin. Scant eyebrows and eyelashes are noticed. Marked conical teeth are observed as well as delayed eruption of primary and permanent teeth. Multiple diastemas in all quadrants are noted. The radiographic examination reveals that 14 permanent teeth are missing. There is no family history of cutaneous disease. The patient has a healthy 4-year-old brother. Her mother had multiple miscarriages, and is pregnant with another boy. A clinical diagnosis of IP is made, and a molecular study confirms that both the patient and her mother have a 11.7-kb deletion in *IKBKG* (previously called *NEMO*). Which one of the following is the most appropriate estimated risk of this patient's unborn brother with the same condition?[86]
  A. <1%
  B. 5%–7%
  C. 14%
  D. 25%
  E. 50%
  F. 100%

222. A 9-year-old girl is brought to a clinic for her dental condition. The prenatal care and birth were uneventful. A provisional clinical diagnosis of incontinentia pigmenti (IP) was made when she was 3 days old and confirmed histopathologically from a biopsy taken from her back. The vesicular lesions over her extremities and body cleared up at 6 months of age. A physical examination reveals pigmented macular lesions on her face, trunk, back, fingers, and legs, and her nipples are absent. She has alopecia on the crown of the head with a scarred patch on the skin. Scant eyebrows and eyelashes are noticed. Marked conical teeth are observed as well as delayed eruption of primary and permanent teeth. Multiple diastemas in all quadrants are noted. The radiographic examination reveals that 14 permanent teeth are missing. There is no family history of cutaneous disease. The patient has a healthy 4-year-old brother. Her mother had multiple miscarriages, and is pregnant with another boy. A clinical diagnosis of IP is made, and a molecular study confirms that both the patient and her mother have a 11.7-kb deletion in *IKBKG* (previously called *NEMO*). Which one of the following describes the mechanism of deletion?[86,87]
  A. Oxidative deamination
  B. Recombination error of repeats
  C. Strand slippage
  D. All of the above
  E. None of the above

223. A 6-week-old newborn boy was admitted to a hospital for a 2-day history of clotted red blood. A physical examination was unremarkable at admission. His family history was remarkable for two maternal cousins having similar symptoms. Laboratory testing was normal at the time. An endoscopic examination revealed one patch of erythematous papules in the proximal sigmoid colon; biopsy of the abnormal patch showed high numbers of infiltrating lymphocytes in the lamina propria and intermittent disruption of the normal mucosal architecture. At 6 months of age, he was admitted for decreased activity, polydipsia, polyuria, and glycosuria. Eczematoid rash and retroauricular lymphadenopathy were evident on examination. At admission, laboratory studies showed a blood glucose of 395 mg/dL, pancytopenia, elevated IgE, and eosinophilia. Which one of the following would be the most appropriate estimation of recurrent risk of the disorder in this family?[88]
  A. <1%
  B. 5%–7%
  C. 14%
  D. 25%
  E. 50%
  F. 100%

224. A 6-week-old boy was hospitalized for diarrhea and diabetic ketoacidosis. He was an only child born after an uncomplicated pregnancy. His birth weight was 4252 g. At 4 weeks of age he had otitis media. While in the hospital, the patient developed interstitial pneumonitis. A lung biopsy and endoscopic GI biopsies showed CMV. After resolution of the CMV infection with antiviral

therapy, diarrhea persisted. GI biopsies showed villous atrophy and chronic inflammation. Steroid therapy was initiated for a presumptive diagnosis of autoimmune enteritis. Episodic diarrhea has continued throughout the patient's life, but he has been growing on oral intake alone. The family reported no similarly affected relatives. At around 1 year of age, lymphadenopathy, hepatosplenomagaly, and eczema appeared. Owing to massive lymphadenopathy and symptoms of obstructive apnea, the patient underwent tonsillectomy, adenoidectomy, lymph-node biopsy, and bone-marrow biopsy at 20 months of age. Results showed Epstein–Barr virus (EBV) infection. Hypothyroidism was diagnosed and treated at 2 years of age. At $2\frac{1}{2}$ years, the patient developed severe, relapsing, autoimmune hemolytic anemia. He also had complications of severe hypertension and cardiomegaly. A clinical diagnosis of immune dysregulation, polyendocrinopathy, enteropathy, X-linked syndrome (IPEX) was made, and a molecular study was ordered. Which one of the following molecular genetic assays would most likely be used to confirm the diagnosis in this patient?[89]

A. Chromosomal microarray analysis

B. Next-generation sequencing

C. Sanger sequencing

D. Targeted variant assay

E. Whole-exome sequencing

F. None of the above

225. A 2-year-old boy, born from a normal pregnancy with a weight of 3420 g, had been in and out of hospitals for almost all his life. His parents were apparently healthy, but his two older brothers died at the ages of 7 months and 3 years with severe infections, chronic diarrhea, and skin eruptions reported as eczematous dermatitis/erythroderma. In one of the brothers, highly elevated IgEs were measured and Job syndrome was suspected. The proband came to medical attention at the age of 1 month for pneumonia and septicemia due to *Streptococcus pneumoniae*. Skin eruptions assessed as erythroderma were also present. He was hospitalized. Humoral immunity was evaluated, and elevated IgEs (855 IU/mL) were found. In early infancy, the child suffered from multiple severe bacterial infections, pruritic eczematous dermatitis, elevated IgEs, and eosinophilia. Hypotrophy, subcutaneous cold abscesses, and enlarged peripheral lymph nodes appeared over time, together with other phenotypic features resembling Job syndrome, such as a coarse face and joint hyperextensibility.

At the age of 1 year 6 months, autoimmune diabetes mellitus was diagnosed. After the diagnosis of diabetes, watery diarrhea appeared, being intermittent initially, but persisting during the second year of age and leading to severe malnutrition. Finally, aggravating symptoms of nephritis, cachexia, and respiratory insufficiency were the cause for his death at the age of 2 years 3 months. A DNA analysis detected a hemizygous pathogenic variant and confirmed IPEX syndrome. In which one of the following genes would this pathogenic variant most likely be located?[90]

A. *ADA*

B. *FOXP3*

C. *IL2RG*

D. *STAT3*

E. *WAS*

226. A 2-week-old Ashkenazi Jewish boy, from nonconsanguineous parents and born by spontaneous vaginal delivery, was brought to a clinic with vesicular lesions and a five episodes of bloody stools. The rash initially started on the head and progressively moved to all over the body. The perinatal history was uneventful. His family history was significant for a maternal uncle dying with similar symptoms at the age of 4, and no clear diagnosis was made at the time. Two years later, the patient was brought to an emergency department for epistaxis, fever, and bloody stools. A physical examination revealed several ecchymotic spots over the body with bruises on the lips and buccal cavity. The patient started to have coffee-grounds vomitus. His platelet count was 22,000/mm^3, and platelets were transfused. A diagnosis of Wiskott–Aldrich syndrome was suspected in this patient. A molecular study was ordered to confirm the diagnosis. Which one of the following molecular genetic assays would most likely be used to confirm the diagnosis in this patient?[91]

A. Chromosomal microarray analysis

B. Next-generation sequencing

C. Sanger sequencing

D. Targeted variant assay

E. Whole-exome sequencing

F. None of the above

227. A 15-month-old boy, born by spontaneous vaginal delivery to nonconsanguineous parents, was brought to a hospital with second episode of bleeding per rectum. His family history indicated that a maternal uncle had died of similar symptoms at age of 4. There was a history suggestive of recurrent ear, sinopulmonary, and soft-tissue infections and eczematoid rashes that

started from the scalp and gradually progressed to cover the entire body since early infancy. The first episode of GI bleeding occurred at 13 months of age, and it was not improved by treatment for dysentery and hemolytic uremic syndrome. His physical examination was unremarkable. Laboratory testing revealed microcytic hypochromic anemia, high IgA, low IgM, high IgE, and normal IgG. A diagnosis of Wiskott–Aldrich syndrome was suspected. A molecular study detected a pathogenic variant, p. Arg86Leu, in the *WAS* gene. Which one of the following would be the most appropriate estimation of recurrent risk of the disorder in this family?[92]

A. <1%
B. 5%–7%
C. 14%
D. 25%
E. 50%
F. 100%

228. A 15-month-old boy, born by spontaneous vaginal delivery to nonconsanguineous parents, was brought to a hospital with a second episode of bleeding per rectum. The family history was uneventful. There was a medical history suggestive of recurrent ear, sinopulmonary, and soft-tissue infections and eczematoid rashes that started from the scalp and gradually progressed to cover the entire body since early infancy. The first episode of GI bleeding occurred at 13 months of age, which was not improved by treatment for dysentery and hemolytic uremic syndrome. A physical examination was unremarkable. Laboratory testing revealed microcytic hypochromic anemia, high IgA, low IgM, high IgE, and normal IgG. A diagnosis of Wiskott–Aldrich syndrome was suspected. A molecular study detected a pathogenic variant, p. Arg86Leu, in the *WAS* gene. Which one of the following malignancies would this patient have an increased risk to develop, especially after exposure to Epstein–Barr virus (EBV)?[92]

A. Endometrial carcinoma
B. Hepatoblastoma
C. Leukemia
D. Lymphoma
E. All of the above
F. None of the above

229. A 13-month-old boy was transferred to a tertiary medical center because of refractory progressive pneumonia leading to respiratory failure and nodular skin lesions. He had been in and out of hospitals frequently since age 7 months owing to recurrent upper respiratory infections. His

perinatal history was uneventful. His family history showed that his maternal uncle had died in infancy with unknown etiology. He received routine immunizations until 6 months of age, including BCG. On physical examination, he had no BCG scar, and biopsy on the nodular skin lesion was later found to be a tuberculous granuloma. Laboratory testing revealed very low levels of T and NK cells, but relatively normal B cells. A clinical diagnosis of severe combined immunodeficiency (SCID) was made. Which one of the following genes would most likely be tested first to confirm/rule out the diagnosis in this patient?[93]

A. *ADA*
B. *FOXP3*
C. *IL2RG*
D. *STAT3*
E. *WAS*
F. *ZAP70*

230. In 2010, the US Department of Health and Human Services recommended adding severe combined immunodeficiency (SCID) to the nationally reviewed uniform panel of conditions subjected to newborn screening. Universal newborn screening for SCID is now available in 42 states, and 88% of all newborns in the United States are receiving SCID screening. The newborn screening laboratory in Ohio contacted a pediatrician, Dr. Z, for a positive (low) TREC result indicating possible lymphopenia in a newborn girl. Dr. Z contacted the family and ordered flow cytometric testing to assay for T-cell lymphopenia, and a molecular test, simultaneously. Which one of the following molecular genetic assays would most likely be used to confirm the diagnosis in this patient?

A. Chromosomal microarray analysis
B. Next-generation sequencing
C. Sanger sequencing
D. Targeted variant assay
E. Whole-exome sequencing
F. None of the above

231. In 2010, the US Department of Health and Human Services recommended adding severe combined immunodeficiency (SCID) to the nationally reviewed uniform panel of conditions subjected to newborn screening. Universal newborn screening for SCID is now available in 42 states, and 88% of all newborns in the United States are receiving SCID screening. The newborn screening laboratory in Ohio contacted a pediatrician, Dr. Z, for a positive (low) TREC result indicating possible lymphopenia in a newborn girl. Dr. Z contacted the family and

ordered flow cytometric testing to assay for T-cell lymphopenia, and a next-generation sequencing (NGS) panel was ordered simultaneously to accelerate the process for a diagnosis. Which one of the following genes would least likely be an appropriate candidate gene for the SCID in this patient?

A. *ADA*

B. *IL2RG*

C. *JAK3*

D. *STAT3*

E. *ZAP70*

232. A 6-year-old girl was brought to a clinic for repeated episodes of respiratory infections since the age of 2 years. A minimum two such episodes occurred per month. There was no history of diarrhea, skin lesions, anorexia, or weight loss. Her family history was unremarkable on both sides. A physical examination was negative. Laboratory testing revealed slightly raised IgE, while IgG and IgA levels were within the normal range. And her lymphocyte subset analysis of peripheral blood revealed a decrease in the percentage and absolute number of total lymphocytes. CD19 + B cells were absent, with decreased CD3 + T cells and CD16 + /CD56 + NK cells. Which one of the following genes would most likely be tested first to establish a diagnosis in this patient?[94]

A. *ADA*

B. *FOXP3*

C. *IL2RG*

D. *WAS*

E. None of the above

233. An 18-year-old male was diagnosed with hypogammaglobulinemia at age 3 years. The family history was unremarkable. Starting at age 4 months, he suffered from bronchopneumonia, recurrent upper respiratory tract infections; occipital cellulitis (at age 7 months); and recurrent acute otitis media, cellulitis, and pneumococcal pneumonia with pleural effusion (at age 3 years). An immunological evaluation showed normal blood cell counts, serum immunoglobulin levels: IgA < 6.67 mg/dL, IgG < 33.3 mg/dL, IgM 266 mg/dL, and IgE < 10 IU/mL. Lymphocyte subsets showed CD19 + B cells 37%, CD3 + T cells 63%, CD3 + CD8 + T cells 15%, and CD3 + CD4 + T cells 52%. He received regular intravenous immunoglobulin (IVIG) replacement therapy every 3 weeks with serum IgG levels of 500−800 mg/dL; however, at age 6 years, the patient developed *Pseudomonas aeruginosa* sepsis, urinary tract infection with *Candida albicans*, perianal abscess, and pericarditis. Intermittent

severe neutropenia (absolute neutrophil count $\leq 200 \times 10^6$ cells/L) was also noted during infectious episodes. Bruton agammaglobulinemia tyrosine kinase (*BTK*) gene pathogenic variant analysis showed wild-type for both alleles. By flow cytometry, CD40 ligand expression on CD3 + CD8 − T cells after stimulation with PMA (20 ng/mL) and neomycin (1 mg/mL) for 4 hours was 0.43%, compared with 85.2% in a healthy control. A congenital hyper-IgM syndrome was suspected. Which one of the following molecular genetic assays would be the most cost-effective way to confirm/rule out the diagnosis in this patient?[95]

A. Chromosomal microarray analysis

B. Next-generation sequencing

C. Sanger sequencing

D. Targeted variant assay

E. Whole-exome sequencing

F. None of the above

234. A 6-month-old boy was admitted to a hospital for bronchopneumonia, rhinorrhea, and shortness of breath for 1 week. Fever was noted after admission. Dyspnea with diffuse wheezing and rales rapidly progressed under empirical antibiotics. He was intubated 8 days after admission due to progression to acute respiratory distress syndrome (ARDS). Sputum *Pneumocystis jiroveci* pneumonia (PJP) PCR was positive. An immunological evaluation showed elevated white-blood-cell counts 23.5×10^9/L, neutrophils 44.5%, lymphocytes 45.8%, and serum immunoglobulin levels: IgA <22.6 mg/dL, IgG 13.5 mg/dL, and IgM 68 mg/dL. Lymphocyte subsets showed CD19 + B cells 52%, CD3 + T cells 44%, CD3 + CD8 + T cells 8%, CD3 + CD4 + T cells 35%, and NK cells 1%. Mitogen testing for T-cell function showed normal proliferation response using phytohemagglutinin and pokeweed mitogen stimulation and decreased proliferation response using CD3/CD28 stimulation. CD40 ligand expression on stimulated CD3 + CD8- T cells of the patient was 7.1%, compared with 67.8% in a normal control. A molecular study of the *CD40L* gene revealed a variant, c.409 + 5G > C, in intron 4. This splice-site variant is predicted to destroy the donor site of intron 4 and produce abnormal RNA and protein. A targeted variant analysis of his mother confirmed the mother was a silent carrier. Cascade testing of the patient's first-degree relatives on the maternal side was recommended and found that the patient's maternal grandmother and his maternal aunt were also carriers. His maternal aunt was pregnant with a

boy. Which one of the following would most likely describe the risk for this patient's unborn cousin with the same condition?[95]

  A. <1%
  B. 5%–7%
  C. 14%
  D. 25%
  E. 50%
  F. 100%

235. An infant boy had normal development until 3 months of age. Then he had been in and out of hospital for recurrent pulmonary infection and acute respiratory distress syndrome (ARDS) beginning at the age of 4 months. At 1 year of age, laboratory testing revealed a significantly increased WBC count with eosinophilia (18%–25%); however, neutrophil counts were within the normal range. Bone-marrow aspiration revealed an increased proportion of eosinophils (23.5%) with no morphological evidence of dysplasia. Further examinations revealed that serum immunoglobulin levels of IgG (0.16 g/L) and IgA (0.01 g/L) were significantly reduced; however, the IgM (0.86 g/L) level was within the normal range. No abnormal lymphocyte subsets were identified. A molecular study of the *CD40L* gene revealed a pathogenic variant, c.476G > A(p. W140X), in exon 5. Parental targeted analyses revealed that his mother was a silent carrier. Which one of the following disorders would the patient most likely have?[96]

  A. Adenosine deaminase (ADA) deficiency
  B. Immunodysregulation, polyendocrinopathy, and enteropathy, X-linked (IPEX)
  C. X-linked severe combined immunodeficiency
  D. X-linked hyper-IgM syndrome
  E. Wiskott–Aldrich syndrome
  F. 100%

236. A 28-year-old female came to a clinic for a history of recurrent bacterial infections since childhood and multiple hospitalizations for pneumonia. The family history was uneventful. A physical examination was unremarkable except for palpable inguinal lymph nodes. A chest CT showed fibrotic lesions and sequelae, pleural thickening, left mediastinal shift, and multiple cystic and cylindrical bronchiectasis. Laboratory testing showed a normal blood count and routine biochemistry results. The alpha-1 antitrypsin and the chloride sweat testing were also normal. Further testing revealed IgG < 0.08 g/L (normal range, 6.5—15.0), IgA < 0.06 g/L (normal range, 0.78—3.12), IgM 7.33 (normal range, 0.55–3.0), and IgE < 2 κU/L (normal, <114). The diagnosis of hypogammaglobulinemia with hyper-IgM was

established. Which one of the following genes would most likely harbor pathogenic variant(s) in this patient?[97]

  A. *ADA*
  B. *AICDA*
  C. *CD40LG*
  D. *IL2RG*
  E. None of the above

237. A 28-year-old female came to a clinic for a history of recurrent bacterial infections since childhood and multiple hospitalizations for pneumonia. The family history was uneventful. A physical examination was unremarkable except for palpable inguinal lymph nodes. A chest CT showed fibrotic lesions and sequelae, pleural thickening, left mediastinal shift, and multiple cystic and cylindrical bronchiectasis. Laboratory testing showed a normal blood count and routine biochemistry results. The alpha-1 antitrypsin and the chloride sweat testing were also normal. Further testing revealed IgG < 0.08 g/L (normal range, 6.5—15.0), IgA < 0.06 g/L (normal range, 0.78—3.12), IgM 7.33 (normal range, 0.55–3.0), and IgE < 2 κU/L (normal, <114). A next-generation sequencing (NGS) panel was ordered for congenital immunodeficiency, and a homozygous pathogenic variant, c.260G > C(p. Cys87Ser), was detected in *AICDA*. Which one of the following disorders would the patient most likely have?[97]

  A. Adenosine deaminase (ADA) deficiency
  B. Hyper-IgM syndrome
  C. Immunodysregulation, polyendocrinopathy, and enteropathy, X-linked (IPEX)
  D. X-linked severe combined immunodeficiency
  E. Wiskott–Aldrich syndrome
  F. None of the above

238. A 43-year-old female patient presented with headache for 7 years with the frequency of 1–2 episodes a year. The headache was severe and throbbing in nature, generally located in the vertex, and accompanied by nausea and vomiting. She had had sustained progressive mental deterioration for 10 years that had become more severe in the past 2 years. The patient also suffered from intermittent occasional numbness of the left arm and leg lasting shorter than 15 minutes. According to her spouse, the patient had suffered from behavioral changes, such as extreme irritability and crying and laughing episodes, in the past few years. Her family history revealed that her father died at the age of 56 years and her uncle died in his 50s from ischemic cerebrovascular disease and that her brother had been bedridden after an ischemic cerebrovascular

attack in his 40s. A head MRI showed widespread lesions in bilateral periventricular and subcortical white matter, external capsules, and the white matter of both temporal lobes. Lesions close to the temporal poles were more marked. The lesions were isohypodense in the pons on T1-weighted sections and hyperintense on T2-weighted and FLAIR sections. The lesions did not have edematous changes or contrast involvement. A head MRI of her brother, who also had cerebrovascular disease, revealed hyperintense lesions in the periventricular white matter on T2-weighted sections. The physician suspected that the patient had cerebral autosomal dominant arteriopathy with subcortical infarcts and leukoencephalopathy (CADASIL). A molecular study was ordered to confirm the diagnosis. Which one of the following molecular genetic assays would most likely be used to confirm/rule out the diagnosis in this patient?[98]

A. Chromosomal microarray analysis
B. Multiplex ligation-dependent probe amplification
C. Next-generation sequencing
D. Sanger sequencing
E. Targeted variant assay
F. Whole-exome sequencing
G. None of the above

239. A 43-year-old female patient presented with headache for 7 years with the frequency of 1–2 episodes a year. The headache was severe and throbbing in nature, generally located in the vertex, and accompanied by nausea and vomiting. She had had sustained progressive mental deterioration for 10 years that had become more severe in the past 2 years. The patient also suffered from intermittent occasional numbness of the left arm and leg lasting shorter than 15 minutes. According to her spouse, the patient had suffered from behavioral changes, such as extreme irritability and crying and laughing episodes, in the past few years. Her family history revealed that her father died at the age of 56 years and her uncle died in his 50s from ischemic cerebrovascular disease and that her brother had been bedridden after an ischemic cerebrovascular attack in his 40s. A head MRI showed widespread lesions in bilateral periventricular and subcortical white matter, external capsules, and the white matter of both temporal lobes. Lesions close to the temporal poles were more marked. The lesions were isohypodense in the pons on T1-weighted sections and hyperintense on T2-weighted and FLAIR sections. The lesions did not have edematous changes or contrast involvement. A

head MRI of her brother, who also had cerebrovascular disease, revealed hyperintense lesions in the periventricular white matter on T2-weighted sections. The physician suspected that the patient had cerebral autosomal dominant arteriopathy with subcortical infarcts and leukoencephalopathy (CADASIL). A molecular study was ordered to confirm the diagnosis. Which one of the following genes would most likely be tested for CADASIL in this patient?[98]

A. NOTCH1
B. NOTCH2
C. NOTCH3
D. All of the above
E. None of the above

240. A 33-year-old male was admitted to a local hospital with a recent change in behavior, aggressiveness, and mood swings. There were no specific features to suggest a bipolar affective disorder or depression. He reported a history of migraine for 6 years. During the previous year he had several transient cerebral episodes and minor strokes. One month before admission he has had a similar behavioral change, but his EEG and contrast brain CT had normal findings. Further questioning revealed slight impairment of his memory. There was no history of optic neuritis. His mother was being treated for adult-onset epilepsy since the age of 30 years. His physical examination was unremarkable, including optic fundi and cognitive and mental state examination. Brain MRI showed T2-weighted hyperintensities on frontal, parietal, temporal, and occipital lobes. Lesions were predominantly seen in the subcortical and deep white matter. He was discharged after symptomatic treatment without a diagnosis. Three months later he was readmitted with an episode of generalized tonic–clonic seizure and receptive aphasia. Repeat brain MRI revealed left-sided temporoparietal intracranial hemorrhage in addition to the initial MRI findings. A diagnosis of CADASIL was considered. A molecular genetic study was ordered for confirmation, and a pathogenic variant in NOTCH3 was detected. Which one of the following amino acid sequences did the pathogenic variant most likely involve in this patient?[99]

A. Alanine
B. Cysteine
C. Leucine
D. Methionine
E. Valine
F. None of the above

241. A 33-year-old male was admitted to a local hospital with a recent change in behavior, aggressiveness, and mood swings. There were no specific features to suggest a bipolar affective disorder or depression. He reported a history of migraine for 6 years. During the previous year he had several transient cerebral episodes and minor strokes. One month before admission he has had a similar behavioral change, but his EEG and contrast brain CT had normal findings. Further questioning revealed slight impairment of his memory. There was no history of optic neuritis. His mother was being treated for adult-onset epilepsy since the age of 30 years. His physical examination was unremarkable, including optic fundi and cognitive and mental state examination. Brain MRI showed T2-weighted hyperintensities on frontal, parietal, temporal, and occipital lobes. Lesions were predominantly seen in the subcortical and deep white matter. He was discharged after symptomatic treatment without a diagnosis. Three months later he was readmitted with an episode of generalized tonic–clonic seizure and receptive aphasia. Repeat brain MRI revealed left-sided temporoparietal intracranial hemorrhage in addition to the initial MRI findings. A diagnosis of CADASIL was considered. A molecular genetic study was ordered for confirmation, and a pathogenic variant, c.291G > T(p.Try71Cys), in *NOTCH3* was detected. The patient had a 6-year-old daughter. What would be the risk of the patient's daughter having the same condition?[99]

   A. <1%
   B. 5%–7%
   C. 14%
   D. 25%
   E. 50%
   F. 100%

242. A 33-year-old male was admitted to a local hospital with a recent change in behavior, aggressiveness, and mood swings. There were no specific features to suggest a bipolar affective disorder or depression. He reported a history of migraine for 6 years. During the previous year he had several transient cerebral episodes and minor strokes. One month before admission he has had a similar behavioral change, but his EEG and contrast brain CT had normal findings. Further questioning revealed slight impairment of his memory. There was no history of optic neuritis. His mother was being treated for adult-onset epilepsy since the age of 30 years. His physical examination was unremarkable, including optic fundi and cognitive and mental state examination. Brain MRI showed T2-weighted hyperintensities on frontal, parietal, temporal, and occipital lobes. Lesions were predominantly seen in the subcortical and deep white matter. He was discharged after symptomatic treatment without a diagnosis. Three months later he was readmitted with an episode of generalized tonic–clonic seizure and receptive aphasia. Repeat brain MRI revealed left-sided temporoparietal intracranial hemorrhage in addition to the initial MRI findings. A diagnosis of CADASIL was considered. A molecular genetic study detected a pathogenic variant, c.291G > T(p.Try71Cys), in *NOTCH3*. The patient had a 6-year-old daughter, who was at risk for the same condition. The patient asked the physician to test his daughter. Which one of the following would be the most appropriate response to this request?[10]

   A. Getting consent from his daughter, then ordering a targeted molecular study for her
   B. Informing the patient that testing asymptomatic children does more harm than good
   C. Ordering a targeted molecular study for his daughter
   D. Providing genetic counseling to his daughter, then ordering a targeted molecular study for her
   E. Telling the patient this is an adult clinic, and it is better for him to make an appointment with his daughter's pediatrician
   F. None of the above

243. An 8-year-old boy was brought to a clinic with symptoms of persisting jaundice and itching for 6 years. The parents also reported failure to thrive. For the past 2 years, he has been having difficulty with distant vision. He also had history of one episode of blood-tinged vomitus not associated with melena. The child was developmentally normal for his age. His perinatal history was unremarkable. He had two older siblings who were alive and healthy. His weight was 13 kg (Z score <−3) and his height 99 cm (Z score <−3). He had mild pallor, icterus, clubbing, and scratch marks. There were no petechial or purpuric spots, palmar erythema, spider nevi, telangiectasia, gynecomastia, or testicular atrophy. His dysmorphic facial features included prominent forehead, deep-set eyes, a pointed chin, and a saddle nose with bulbous tip. A grade III ejection systolic murmur was audible in the left second

intercostal space with normal S1 and S2. His liver was palpable 2 cm below the costal margin with a span of 8 cm and a smooth surface. An eye examination revealed posterior embryotoxon and KF rings in both eyes. Visual acuity in right eye was 6/60 and in left eye was 6/FCCF (finger close to face). A liver biopsy showed paucity of bile ducts with periportal ballooning degeneration and cholestasis. His portal tract showed inflammation and fibrosis. Immunostaining for CK19 did not show bile ducts. A diagnosis of Alagille syndrome (ALGS) was considered. A molecular analysis was ordered to confirm the diagnosis. Which one of the following genes was most likely tested to confirm the diagnosis in this patient?[100]

A. *JAG1*
B. *JAG2*
C. *DLL1*
D. *DLL3*
E. *DLL4*
F. None of the above

244. An 8-year-old boy was brought to a clinic with symptoms of persisting jaundice and itching for 6 years. The parents also reported failure to thrive. For the past 2 years, he has been having difficulty with distant vision. He also had history of one episode of blood-tinged vomitus not associated with melena. The child was developmentally normal for his age. His perinatal history was unremarkable. He had two older siblings who were alive and healthy. His weight was 13 kg (Z score <−3) and his height 99 cm (Z score <−3). He had mild pallor, icterus, clubbing, and scratch marks. There were no petechial or purpuric spots, palmar erythema, spider nevi, telangiectasia, gynecomastia, or testicular atrophy. His dysmorphic facial features included prominent forehead, deep-set eyes, a pointed chin, and a saddle nose with bulbous tip. A grade III ejection systolic murmur was audible in the left second intercostal space with normal S1 and S2. His liver was palpable 2 cm below the costal margin with a span of 8 cm and a smooth surface. An eye examination revealed posterior embryotoxon and KF rings in both eyes. Visual acuity in right eye was 6/60 and in left eye was 6/FCCF (finger close to face). A liver biopsy showed paucity of bile ducts with periportal ballooning degeneration and cholestasis. His portal tract showed inflammation and fibrosis. Immunostaining for CK19 did not show bile ducts. A diagnosis of Alagille syndrome (ALGS) was considered. A molecular analysis was ordered to confirm the diagnosis. Which one of the following genes

would most likely be tested for CADASIL in this patient?[100]

A. *NOTCH1*
B. *NOTCH2*
C. *NOTCH3*
D. All of the above
E. None of the above

245. A 31-year-old male came to a clinic for abnormal liver enzyme level found at an Army physical readiness test 6 months ago. His medical history was unremarkable except for surgery for recurrent left pneumothorax as a teenager. He had a prominent forehead, deep-set eyes with mild hypertelorism, a straight nose, a pointed chin, and large ears. At the time of examination, a laboratory study was ordered, which revealed that his total bilirubin was 1.7 mg/dL; aspartate aminotransferase (AST) 78 IU/L; alanine aminotransferase (ALT) 39 IU/L; ALP 308 IU/L; GGT 542 IU/L; and international normalized ratio (INR) 0.88. A liver fibroscan revealed borderline fibrosis with 8.6 kPa and minimal steatosis with controlled attenuation parameter (CAP) level of 227 dB/m. A CT scan showed findings consistent with chronic liver disease, without focal nodules or abnormal vascularity. A liver biopsy revealed rare bile duct in portal tracts, chronic hepatitis with mild lobular activity, mild periportal activity and septal fibrosis. After 6 months, abdominal ultrasonography as a follow-up test showed coarse liver parenchymal echogenicity, a few tiny gallbladder polyps, splenomegaly, and renal parenchymal disease, but no bile-duct dilatation. A sequencing analysis was ordered for Alagille syndrome (ALGS), and no pathogenic variants in *JAG1* were detected. The physician still suspected ALGS. Which one of the following studies would most likely be used as the next step in the workup to confirm/rue out ALGS in this patient?[101]

A. Deletion/duplication analysis of *JAG1*
B. Deletion/duplication analysis of *NOTCH2*
C. Linkage study
D. Sequencing analysis of *NOTCH2*
E. None of the above

246. A 2-month-old baby boy was referred to a tertiary care center for jaundice and light yellow stools. His perinatal history was unremarkable. His birth weight was 2500 g. A physical examination showed that he had delayed growth and development without dysmorphic facial features. Laboratory testing revealed elevated liver enzymes and cholestasis. The child showed no excretion of the isotope 24 hours after undergoing a hepatobiliary hydroxyiminodiacetic acid (HIDA) scan. Biliary atresia (BA) was suspected.

Omnipaque imaging was done 10 days after hospital admission. Gallbladder, cystic duct, and choledochus were normal, but intrahepatic biliary hypoplasia was found. A liver biopsy showed cholestasis in liver cells and small bile-duct proliferation in the portal area. Echocardiography showed patent ductus arteriosus and open foramen ovale. "Butterfly" vertebrae were found in some thoracic vertebrae by spine radiography. An abdominal ultrasound found slight hepatomegaly and renal ambiguity. At 7 months age, lower albumin, prolonged prothrombin time, and highly international normalized ratio were noted. He died at 9 months of age from liver failure. Sequencing analysis detected a homozygous pathogenic variant, c.133G > T (p. V45L), in exon 2 of *JAG1*. A heterozygous c.133G > T variant was found in the mother but not in the father. Which one of the following molecular genetic studies would be an appropriate next step in the workup for this family?[102]

A. Chromosome karyotyping
B. Multiplex ligation-dependent probe amplification
C. Sequencing analysis of *NOTCH2*
D. Informing the family that the recurrent risk is low
E. None of the above

ANSWERS

1. **C.** The two types of polycystic kidney disease are autosomal dominant polycystic kidney disease (ADPKD) and autosomal recessive polycystic kidney disease (ARPKD). Onset of ADPKD usually is between the ages of 30 and 40. This form accounts for about 90% of cases of polycystic kidney disease.

   ARPKD is a childhood-onset renal and liver disorder. Most individuals with ARPKD usually present in the neonatal period with enlarged echogenic kidneys. Renal disease is characterized by nephromegaly, hypertension, and varying degrees of renal dysfunction. More than 50% of children with ARPKD who have a classic presentation progress to end-stage renal disease (ESRD) within the first decade of life. ESRD may require kidney transplantation. *Each sib of a proband has a 25% chance of inheriting both pathogenic alleles and being affected, a 50% chance of inheriting one pathogenic allele and being a silent carrier, and a 25% chance of neither inheriting a pathogenic allele nor being a carrier* (https://www.ncbi.nlm.nih.gov/books/NBK1246/).

   This patient's clinical symptoms resemble ARPKD. Therefore, the recurrent risk would most likely be 1/4 for this family if the patient had a hereditary form of polycystic kidney disease.

2. **D.** *This patient's clinical symptoms resemble autosomal dominant polycystic kidney disease (ADPKD), which is generally a late-onset multisystem disorder characterized by bilateral renal cysts; cysts in other organs, including the liver, seminal vesicles, pancreas, and arachnoid membrane; vascular abnormalities, including intracranial aneurysms, dilatation of the aortic root, and dissection of the thoracic aorta; mitral-valve prolapse; and abdominal-wall hernias. Renal manifestations include hypertension, renal pain, and renal insufficiency. Approximately 50% of individuals with ADPKD have end-stage renal disease (ESRD) by age 60 years. The prevalence of liver cysts, the most common extrarenal manifestation of ADPKD, increases with age and may have been underestimated by ultrasound studies. The prevalence of intracranial aneurysms is higher in those with a positive family history of aneurysms or subarachnoid hemorrhage (22%) than in those without such a family history (6%)* (https://www.ncbi.nlm.nih.gov/books/NBK1246/).

   On the other hand, most individuals with autosomal recessive polycystic kidney disease (ARPKD) present in the neonatal period with enlarged echogenic kidneys. Renal disease is characterized by nephromegaly, hypertension, and varying degrees of renal dysfunction. More than 50% of affected individuals with ARPKD progress to end-stage renal disease (ESRD) within the first decade of life (https://www.ncbi.nlm.nih.gov/books/NBK1326/).

   Therefore, the recurrent risk would most likely be 50% in this family if the patient had ADPKD.

3. **C.** The patient's clinical and family histories suggest a diagnosis of autosomal dominant polycystic kidney disease (ADPKD). The diagnosis of ADPKD is established primarily by imaging studies of the kidneys. In approximately 85% of individuals with ADPKD, pathogenic variants in *PKD1* are causative; in approximately 15%, pathogenic variants in *PKD2* are causative. *In the most recent studies, 50%−70% of pathogenic variants are unique to a family, and approximately 30% of PKD1 changes and approximately 15% of PKD2 changes are in-frame.* Pathogenic variants in *PKHD1* are associated with autosomal recessive polycystic kidney disease (ARPKD).

Chromosomal microarray (CMA) is a technique to detect copy-number changes in human genome instead of single-nucleotide variants in genes. Multiplex ligation-dependent probe amplification (MLPA) is a time-efficient technique to detect genomic deletions and insertions bigger than single-nucleotide variants and in/dels, but smaller than what CMA can detect. Targeted variant analysis of the founder variants are used to study highly prevalent pathogenic variants in specific populations, such as p.F508del (Delta-F508) in *CFTR* for cystic fibrosis in Ashkenazi Jewish and Caucasian populations.

Therefore, sequencing the *PDK1* and *PKD2* genes would most likely be used as a first-tier test to confirm/rule out genetic etiologies in this patient, specifically ADPKD.

4. **B.** There are two types of polycystic kidney disease (PKD): autosomal dominant polycystic kidney disease (ADPKD) and autosomal recessive polycystic kidney disease (ARPKD) (http://staff. washington.edu/sbtrini/Teaching%20Cases/Case %2033.pdf). ADPKD usually becomes clinically noticed between the ages of 30 and 40 and accounts for about 90% of cases of polycystic kidney disease. Other organs in which cysts may be found include the liver, seminal vesicles, pancreas, and arachnoid membrane. Vascular abnormalities include intracranial aneurysms, dilatation of the aortic root, and dissection of the thoracic aorta. The prevalence of intracranial aneurysms is higher in those with a positive family history of aneurysms or subarachnoid hemorrhage (22%) than in those without such a family history (6%). *About 95% of individuals with ADPKD have an affected parent* and about 5%–10% have a de novo variant (https://www.ncbi.nlm. nih.gov/books/NBK1246/).

ARPKD is usually manifested in children. The majority of individuals with ARPKD classically present in the neonatal period with enlarged echogenic kidneys. Renal disease is characterized by nephromegaly, hypertension, and varying degrees of renal dysfunction. More than 50% of children with ARPKD who have a classic presentation progress to end-stage renal disease (ESRD) within the first decade of life (https://www.ncbi.nlm.nih.gov/books/ NBK1246/).

Therefore, it is most likely that *this patient has an ADPKD inherited from her father* (her father's cerebral hemorrhage most likely resulted from intracranial aneurysms due to ADPKD, based on the family history).

5. **E.** Normally, a living relative with a good tissue match represents the best kidney donor for a patient with renal failure (http://staff. washington.edu/sbtrini/Teaching%20Cases/Case %2033.pdf). This patient has autosomal dominant polycystic kidney disease (ADPKD) inherited from her father, and her father's cerebral hemorrhage most likely resulted from intracranial aneurysms due to ADPKD. The diagnosis is confirmed by the molecular testing. So the patient's sister has a 50% chance to be affected as well.

At-risk relatives being considered as kidney donors need to be evaluated to determine if they have ADPKD. Evaluation consists of comprehensive renal image analysis by ultrasound, CT, and/or MRI, which is routine for any kidney donor regardless of disease indication. *If the imaging is equivocal, if the potential donor is young (age <30 years), or in other cases where evidence of the disease status is considered unproven, molecular genetic testing can play a key role in establishing the genetic status of the potential donor.* If a known pathogenic variant has already been identified in an affected relative, this analysis is straightforward. In cases where the pathogenic status of a detected variant(s) is not certain, molecular studies need to be interpreted with caution. If the pathogenic variant in an affected relative is not identified, or if the family has not had genetic testing, molecular testing of the potential donor is not appropriate. A "negative" test does not prove the absence of ADPKD (https://www.ncbi.nlm.nih.gov/books/ NBK1246/).

Posttransplantation survival is better with kidneys from unrelated donors with matched HLA typing than with kidneys from related donors with unmatched HLA typing. The patient's brother is not an appropriate donor owing to unmatched HLA typing. Therefore, molecular genetic testing of the youngest sister for the familial pathogenic variant is appropriate before related renal transplantation. If the youngest sister has the familial pathogenic variant, she is NOT an appropriate donor, and renal transplantation from an unrelated donor should be considered.

6. **A.** This patient's molecular testing result is negative. *In families with multiple affected family members, a family linkage study may be possible when a pathogenic variant is not detected in the proband* (http://staff.washington.edu/sbtrini/Teaching% 20Cases/Case%2033.pdf). In this approach, several affected and unaffected family members

are tested for DNA markers adjacent to the two known genes for autosomal dominant polycystic kidney disease (ADPKD). The purpose of the study is to determine whether there is an association between ADPKD and DNA markers among family members. The testing is positive if a consistent relationship is demonstrated between certain DNA markers and the presence or absence of disease in family members. This type of study requires participation of both affected family members and family members who are known to be unaffected—that is, thoroughly evaluated older family members, whose genetic status can be established unequivocally by renal imaging. If linkage is established between ADPKD and specific DNA markers, the markers can then be used to test young at-risk family members to determine whether they have inherited the markers associated with ADPKD in the family (https://www.ncbi.nlm.nih.gov/books/NBK1246/).

Linkage analysis is not suitable for this patient and her family because she is the only alive known affected family member. Molecular genetic testing of the patient's youngest sister is also not appropriate because the patient's pathogenic variant was not identified. The patient's youngest sister must be considered to be at risk for ADPKD, because a negative ultrasound does rule out ADPKD in a 25-year-old individual.

Therefore, in this circumstance the sister should NOT serve as a kidney donor for the patient, and kidney transplantation with an unrelated donor should be considered.

7. **A.** *In approximately 85% of individuals with autosomal dominant polycystic kidney disease (ADPKD), pathogenic variants in PKD1 are causative; in approximately 15%, pathogenic variants in PKD2 are causative.* This proportion refers to individuals with ADPKD caused by a known pathogenic variant in either *PKD1* or *PKD2*. It does not include those with ADPKD in whom no pathogenic variant has been found. Approximately 9% of individuals who undergo comprehensive screening for pathogenic variants in *PKD1* and *PKD2* have no pathogenic variant identified. It is unclear if this finding is the result of missed pathogenic variants at the known loci or further genetic heterogeneity. The *PKHD1* gene is the only gene, in which pathogenic variants cause autosomal recessive polycystic kidney disease (ARPKD). Molecular testing of *PKHD1* with both Sanger sequencing and deletion/duplication analyses detected approximately 75% of individuals with clinical diagnosis of ARPKD.

(https://www.ncbi.nlm.nih.gov/books/NBK1246/ and https://www.ncbi.nlm.nih.gov/books/NBK1326/).

Therefore, the *PKD1* gene would most likely harbor a pathogenic variant if the patient had autosomal dominant polycystic kidney disease (ADPKD).

8. **C.** In approximately 85% of individuals with autosomal dominant polycystic kidney disease (ADPKD), pathogenic variants in *PKD1* are causative; in approximately 15%, pathogenic variants in *PKD2* are causative. There is good evidence that polycystin-1, encoded by *PKD1*, and polycystin-2, encoded by *PKD2*, interact with each other to form a functional complex. Recent data show that this interaction is central for the maturation and localization of these proteins. The precise role that the polycystin complex normally plays on the cilium is controversial.

PKD2 is characterized by extreme allelic variability, with approximately 50% of pathogenic variants unique to a single family. According to the ADPKD Mutation Database, approximately 200 different *PKD2* pathogenic variants have been described, accounting for nearly 440 families. As in *PKD1*, the pathogenic variants are spread throughout the gene, and the majority of them (~85%) are predicted to truncate the protein, consistent with inactivation of the allele. *As with PKD1, the mechanism of disease is associated with reduction or loss of functional PKD2 protein below a particular threshold* (https://www.ncbi.nlm.nih.gov/books/NBK1246/).

Therefore, loss-of-function variants, more specifically haploinsufficiency, would most likely contribute to the pathogenesis of the ADPKD in this patient.

9. **A.** *PKD1* encodes an approximately 14-kb transcript with a 12,909-nucleotide coding region and comprises 46 exons within 50 kb of genomic DNA. *The genomic region encoding PKD1 has undergone a complex segmental duplication such that six reiterated copies of the 5' three-quarters of the gene are present as pseudogenes elsewhere on chromosome 16.* The high sequence homology among these pseudogenes and *PKD1* has complicated molecular genetic testing. Sequencing analysis requires appropriate primers to avoid coamplification of pseudogene(s) segments, particularly for exons 1–33 of *PKD1*. Exome sequencing may not accurately identify pathogenic variants in the duplicated region of *PKD1*, leading to both false positive and false negative results.

If a primer is located in a polymorphic region, a molecular variant may be missed, but not added on. Sending the sample to the third clinical laboratory confirmed the original finding of the pathogenic variant and also confirmed that the sample was the right sample (no mess-up). Different enrichment methods affect coverage in different genomic regions but do not contribute to false positive and/or false negative results as long as the coverage is not an issue.

Therefore, the discrepancy of the testing results with the same specimen in this case would most likely be caused by interference of pseudogenes.

10. **C.** It is most likely this patient had autosomal recessive polycystic kidney disease (ARPKD), which usually presents in the neonatal period with enlarged echogenic kidneys. Renal disease is characterized by nephromegaly, hypertension, and varying degrees of renal dysfunction. More than 50% of children with ARPKD who have a classic presentation progress to end-stage renal disease (ESRD) within the first decade of life. *The PKHD1 gene is the only gene, in which pathogenic variants cause autosomal recessive polycystic kidney disease (ARPKD).* Molecular testing of *PKHD1* with both Sanger sequencing and deletion/duplication analyses detected approximately 75% of individuals with a clinical diagnosis of ARPKD (https://www.ncbi.nlm.nih.gov/books/NBK1326/).

Autosomal dominant polycystic kidney disease (ADPKD) is generally a late-onset disorder. In approximately 85% of individuals with ADPKD, pathogenic variants in *PKD1* are causative; in approximately 15%, pathogenic variants in *PKD2* are causative.

Therefore, *PKHD1* would most likely harbor a pathogenic variant in this patient. Another learning point in this question is that Amish Americans prefer natural methods and traditional remedies. Religious reasons as well as cultural values may factor into some medical decisions.

11. **C.** This patient had autosomal recessive polycystic kidney disease (ARPKD), which usually presents in the neonatal period with enlarged echogenic kidneys. The molecular testing confirmed this diagnosis by detecting compound heterozygous pathogenic variants in the *PKHD1* gene. Most time the parents of an affected child are obligate heterozygotes carriers, but de novo variants have been seen. Carriers with heterozygotes for a pathogenic variant in *PKHD1* are asymptomatic and are not at risk of developing ARPKD (https://www.ncbi.nlm.nih.gov/books/NBK1326/).

Therefore, it would be most appropriate to test both parents for carrier status before counseling the family about the recurrent risk and recommending prenatal testing for future pregnancies.

12. **A.** Tuberous sclerosis complex is an autosomal dominant syndrome characterized by seizure, mental retardation, and multiple hamartomas in the brain, heart, skin, retina, kidneys, or liver. Random distributions of tumorous lesions cause variable features such as neurological deficits, renal impairment, skin lesions, or retinal hamartomas. Pathogenic variants can be identified in 85% of patients: *TSC1* on chromosome 9q34, encoding hamartin, or *TSC2* on 16p13.3, encoding tuberin. The incidence of TSC is estimated to be 1 in 6000–1 in 11,000 births. Sporadic cases constitute two-thirds of tuberous sclerosis cases. Autosomal dominant polycystic kidney disease (ADPKD) is a common renal disorder, occurring in approximately 1 in 1000 live births. It is characterized by progressive bilateral renal cysts, leading to renal failure in the fifth to seventh decade of life. Occasionally, liver cysts and intracranial aneurysm may occur. Pathogenic variants in *PKD1* on 16p13.3, encoding polycystin-1, or *PKD2* on 4q22, encoding polycystin-2, have been confirmed to cause ADPKD. The *TSC2/PKD1* contiguous gene deletion syndrome was first recognized in 1994 in a patient with tuberous sclerosis and cystic renal disease by identifying the deletion of both *TSC2* and *PKD1* genes. *TSC2/PKD1* contiguous gene deletion syndrome can occur owing to the adjacent location of the *TSC2* and *PKD1* genes. *About 5% of patients with TSC have TSC2/PKD1 contiguous gene deletion syndrome.*

Sanger sequencing may be used to detect small deletions and duplications, such as 10 bp. However, large deletions/duplications are not readily detectable by Sanger sequencing analysis of the coding and flanking intronic regions of genomic DNA since each PCR product is usually less than 1,00 0bp. Quantitative PCR, long-range PCR, multiplex ligation-dependent probe amplification (MLPA), and chromosomal microarray (CMA) may be used to detect large deletions/duplications on the other side.

Therefore, MLPA is an appropriate technique to detect deletions/duplications for *TSC2/PKD1* contiguous gene deletion syndrome in this patient.

13. **A.** The patient has a positive family history for autosomal dominant polycystic kidney disease (ADPKD) from the maternal side, according to the

pedigree (disease in each generation with both female-to-female and male-to-male transmission). *In 85% of individuals with ADPKD, pathogenic variants in PKD1 are causative, while in 15%, pathogenic variants in PKD2 are causative.* About 95% of individuals with ADPKD have an affected parent and about 5% have a de novo variant (https://www.ncbi.nlm.nih.gov/books/NBK1246/).

PKHD1 is associated with autosomal recessive polycystic kidney disease (ARPKD). *PKD3* is associated with autosomal dominant polycystic kidney disease mainly in the French-Canadian population. *PDHK1L1* is a *PKHD1* like protein on chromosome 8 with unclear function.

Therefore, the *PKD1* gene for ADPKD most likely be mutated in this patient.

14. **C.** *The patient has positive family history for autosomal dominant polycystic kidney disease (ADPKD) from the maternal side according to the pedigree (disease in each generation with both female-to-female and male-to-male transmission).* In 85% of individuals with ADPKD, pathogenic variants in *PKD1* are causative, while in 15%, pathogenic variants in *PKD2* are causative. About 95% of individuals with ADPKD have an affected parent and about 5% have a de novo variant (https://www.ncbi.nlm.nih.gov/books/NBK1246/).

A patient with a homozygous pathogenic variant in *PKD1* would be expected to manifest polycystic disease at an early age. Furthermore, this patient's paternal family history is negative for ADPKD, which limits the possibility of the deletion from the paternal side of the family. So a de novo germline deletion from the father is possible, but the possibility is low. Another possibility for a patient with an autosomal dominant disease but a homozygous pathogenic variant by molecular genetic testing, is allelic dropout during the amplification step due to a missing or mismatched primer-binding site. It is also possible that the blood sample was switched during transportation or that the DNA was switched in the lab, but these possibilities are low.

Therefore, reanalyzing the patient sample with second pair of primers would be the most logical next step in the workup before getting another sample from the patient.

15. **D.** *The patient's pedigree indicates that the polycystic kidney disease in the sister is autosomal recessive.* ARPKD is a cause of significant renal- and liver-related morbidity and mortality in children. The majority of individuals with ARPKD classically present in the neonatal period with enlarged echogenic kidneys. Renal disease is characterized by nephromegaly, hypertension, and varying

degrees of renal dysfunction. More than 50% of children with ARPKD who have a classic presentation progress to end-stage renal disease (ESRD) within the first decade of life. ESRD may require kidney transplantation. *PKHD1 is the only gene in which pathogenic variants are known to be associated with ARPKD* (http://www.ncbi.nlm.nih.gov/books/NBK1326/).

Autosomal dominant polycystic kidney disease (ADPKD) is caused by pathogenic variants in *PKD1* and *PKD2*. *PKD3* is associated with autosomal dominant polycystic kidney disease mainly in the French Canadian population. *PDHK1L1* is a *PKHD1*-like protein on chromosome 8 with an unclear function.

Therefore, the *PKHD1* gene would most likely harbor the pathogenic variant(s) in this family.

16. **D.** Autosomal dominant polycystic kidney disease (ADPKD) is generally a late-onset multisystem disorder characterized by bilateral renal cysts; cysts in other organs, including the liver, seminal vesicles, pancreas, and arachnoid membrane; vascular abnormalities, including intracranial aneurysms, dilatation of the aortic root, and dissection of the thoracic aorta; mitral-valve prolapses; and abdominal-wall hernias. In 85% of individuals with ADPKD, pathogenic variants in *PKD1* are causative, while in 15%, pathogenic variants in *PKD2* are causative. *Individuals with pathogenic variants in PKD1 have a more severe clinical phenotype, progressing to ESRD on average 20 years earlier than PKD2 patients.* The contiguous gene deletion syndrome with symptoms of both ADPKD and tuberous sclerosis is due to a deletion involving both *PKD1* and *TSC2* on chromosome 16p13.1 (https://www.ncbi.nlm.nih.gov/books/NBK1246/).

Autosomal recessive polycystic kidney disease (ARPKD) is characterized by congenital hepatorenal fibrocysts, which cause significant renal- and liver-related morbidity and mortality in children. The majority of individuals with ARPKD classically present in the neonatal period with enlarged echogenic kidneys. Renal disease is characterized by nephromegaly, hypertension, and varying degrees of renal dysfunction. More than 50% of children with ARPKD who have a classic presentation progress to end-stage renal disease (ESRD) within the first decade of life; ESRD may require kidney transplantation. *PKHD1* is the only gene in which pathogenic variants are known to be associated with ARPKD (http://www.ncbi.nlm.nih.gov/books/NBK1326/).

Therefore, the severity of ADPKD is attributed primarily to locus heterogeneity.

17. **B.** *Individuals with a contiguous deletion of the adjacent genes PKD1 and TSC2 typically manifest clinical features of tuberous sclerosis complex (TSC) and early-onset autosomal dominant polycystic kidney disease (ADPKD).* It may result from a deletion or an unbalanced translocation leading to a functional deletion of 16p13.3, including both *PKD1* and *TSC2* (https://www.ncbi.nlm.nih.gov/books/NBK1246/).

Therefore, the contiguous gene deletion syndrome including symptoms for both ADPKD and tuberous sclerosis typically results from a deletion involving both *PKD1* and *TSC2*.

18. **B.** In this case, the patient is at risk for autosomal dominant polycystic kidney disease (ADPKD) instead of autosomal recessive polycystic kidney disease (ARPKD) but is too young to be symptomatic. The patient's mother is symptomatic, but the pathogenic variant cannot be identified. The risk for ADPKD cannot be ruled out by the negative ultrasound results. MRI or CT may assist in detecting small cysts, but negative results do not rule out ADPKD. Testing *PKHD1* for ARPKD does not help to establish the diagnosis in this asymptomatic patient.

Linkage analysis may be used to determine whether the at-risk family member is an obligate carrier when the pathogenic variant cannot be identified. In this approach, several affected and unaffected family members are tested for DNA markers adjacent to the two known genes for autosomal dominant polycystic kidney disease (ADPKD). The purpose of the study is to determine whether there is an association between ADPKD and particular DNA markers among family members. The testing is positive if a consistent relationship is demonstrated between certain DNA markers and the presence or absence of disease in family members. This type of study requires participation of both affected family members and family members who are known to be unaffected—that is, thoroughly evaluated older family members, whose genetic status can be established unequivocally by renal imaging. If linkage is established between ADPKD and specific DNA markers, the markers can then be used to test young at-risk family members in order to determine whether they have inherited the markers associated with ADPKD in the family (https://www.ncbi.nlm.nih.gov/books/NBK1246/).

Therefore, linkage analysis may be used to establish the carrier status of the patient.

19. **C.** The patient's clinical presentation and family history pointed to a diagnosis of Bardet–Biedl syndrome (BBS). BBS is characterized by rod–cone dystrophy, truncal obesity, postaxial polydactyly, cognitive impairment, male hypogonadotropic hypogonadism, complex female genitourinary malformations, and renal abnormalities. The visual prognosis for children with BBS is poor. The diagnosis of BBS is established by clinical findings. BBS is typically inherited in an autosomal recessive manner. Eighteen genes have been found to be associated with BBS. They are *BBS1, BBS2, ARL6 (BBS3), BBS4, BBS5, MKKS (BBS6), BBS7, TTC8 (BBS8), BBS9, BBS10, TRIM32 (BBS11), BBS12, MKS1 (BBS13), CEP290 (BBS14), WDPCP (BBS15), SDCCAG8 (BBS16), LZTFL1 (BBS17)* and *BBIP1 (BBS18)* (https://www.ncbi.nlm.nih.gov/books/NBK1363/).

Pathogenic variants in *PKD1* cause autosomal dominant polycystic kidney disease (ADPKD). Pathogenic variants in *PKHD1* cause autosomal recessive polycystic kidney disease (ARPKD). The der(16)t(X;16)(q28;p13.2) in the question leads to a net loss of 16p, including *PKD1* and *TSC2* at 16p13.3. Patients with a deletion of 16p13.3, including both *PKD1* and *TSC2*, have symptoms of tuberous sclerosis complex (TSC) and ADPKD.

Therefore, this patient would most likely have a missense pathogenic variant, c.547A > G(p. G72S) in *BBS5*.

20. **A.** Pathogenic variants in at least 19 genes have been found to be associated with Bardet–Biedl syndrome (BBS): *BBS1, BBS2, ARL6 (BBS3), BBS4, BBS5, MKKS (BBS6), BBS7, TTC8 (BBS8), BBS9, BBS10, TRIM32 (BBS11), BBS12, MKS1 (BBS13), CEP290 (BBS14), WDPCP (BBS15), SDCCAG8 (BBS16), LZTFL1 (BBS17), BBIP1 (BBS18),* and *IFT27 (BBS19)* (https://www.ncbi.nlm.nih.gov/books/NBK1363/).

A multigene next-generation sequencing (NGS) panel parallelizes the sequencing process, producing thousands or millions of sequences concurrently while lowering the cost of DNA sequencing beyond what is possible with Sanger sequencing. It is used to describe a number of different modern sequencing technologies, such as Illumina (Solexa), Roche 454, Ion torrent: Proton/PGM, SOLiD sequencing.

Sanger sequencing is based on the selective incorporation of chain-terminating dideoxynucleotides by DNA polymerase during in vitro DNA replication. Developed by Frederick Sanger and colleagues in 1977, it was the most widely used sequencing method for approximately 25 years. In restriction-fragment–length polymorphism (RFLP) analysis, the DNA sample is digested into pieces by restriction enzymes, which recognize a specific sequence, including a genetic single-nucleotide variant in some individuals. And the resulting restriction fragments are separated according to their lengths by gel electrophoresis. Although now largely obsolete owing to the rise of inexpensive DNA sequencing technologies, RFLP analysis was the first DNA-profiling technique inexpensive enough to see widespread application. The quantitative real-time polymerase chain reaction (RT-PCR) uses fluorescent reporter molecules to monitor the production of amplification products during each cycle of the PCR reaction. This combines the nucleic acid amplification and detection steps into one homogeneous assay and obviates the need for gel electrophoresis to detect amplification products.

Therefore, a NGS panel with multiple genes offers the most effective approach in achieving molecular confirmation of BBS for this patient.

21. **D**. Bardet—Biedl syndrome (BBS) is characterized by rod—cone dystrophy, truncal obesity, postaxial polydactyly, cognitive impairment, male hypogonadotropic hypogonadism, complex female genitourinary malformations, and renal abnormalities. The visual prognosis for children with BBS is poor. The diagnosis of BBS is established by clinical findings. BBS is typically inherited in an autosomal recessive manner. Pathogenic variants in at least 19 genes have been found to be associated with Bardet—Biedl syndrome (BBS): *BBS1*, *BBS2*, *ARL6 (BBS3)*, *BBS4*, *BBS5*, *MKKS (BBS6)*, *BBS7*, *TTC8 (BBS8)*, *BBS9*, *BBS10*, *TRIM32 (BBS11)*, *BBS12*, *MKS1 (BBS13)*, *CEP290 (BBS14)*, *WDPCP (BBS15)*, *SDCCAG8 (BBS16)*, *LZTFL1 (BBS17)*, *BBIP1 (BBS18)*, and *IFT27 (BBS19)*. Approximately 20% of persons with BBS do not have identifiable pathogenic variants in any of the 19 known BBS-related genes; therefore, it is possible that more BBS-related genes are yet to be identified (https://www.ncbi.nlm.nih.gov/books/NBK1363/).

Locus heterogeneity is a single disorder, trait, or pattern of traits caused by pathogenic variant in genes at different chromosomal loci. Allelic heterogeneity is the phenomenon in which different pathogenic variants at the same locus cause a similar phenotype. *Cellular heterogeneity* most often was used to describe tumor heterogeneity, which refers to different tumor cells showing distinct morphological and phenotypic profiles. Reduced or incomplete penetrance means that clinical symptoms are not always present in individuals who have the disease-causing variant. Variable expressivity occurs when a phenotype is expressed to a different degree among individuals with the same genotype.

Therefore, pathogenic variants in 19 genes that cause BBS is an example of locus heterogeneity.

22. **B**. Only two male members in the family had the renal problems in childhood. None of the female members of the family were affected. *This suggests that X-linked Alport syndrome (AS) may be taken into consideration for the differential diagnosis.*

AS is characterized by renal, cochlear, and ocular involvement. In the absence of treatment, renal disease progresses from microscopic hematuria to proteinuria, progressive renal insufficiency, and end-stage renal disease (ESRD) in all males with X-linked AS, and in all males and females with autosomal recessive AS. Progressive sensorineural hearing loss (SNHL) is usually present by late childhood or early adolescence. Ocular findings include anterior lenticonus, maculopathy, corneal endothelial vesicles, and recurrent corneal erosion. In individuals with autosomal dominant AS, ESRD is frequently delayed until later adulthood, SNHL is also relatively late in onset and ocular involvement is rare (https://www.ncbi.nlm.nih.gov/books/NBK1207/).

Therefore, the recurrent risk in the family would be: $1/2 \times 1/2 = 1/4$ (25%) if Jerry and his cousin had a hereditary form of renal diseases, specifically AS.

23. **A**. Alzheimer disease is a degenerative disease of the brain that causes dementia, which is a gradual loss of memory, judgment, and ability to function (http://ccnmtl.columbia.edu/projects/neuroethics/module2/casestudy/). This disorder usually appears in people older than age 65, but less common forms of the disease appear earlier in adulthood. Familial early-onset Alzheimer disease is caused by pathogenic variants in one of three genes: *APP* (10%—15%), *PSEN1* (30%—70%), or *PSEN2* (<5%) (https://www.ncbi.nlm.nih.gov/books/NBK1236/).

APOE has been studied extensively as a risk factor for late-onset Alzheimer disease. The e4 allele in the *APOE* gene is a major risk factor for the development of Alzheimer disease, while the e2 allele has a protective effect. Some evidence indicates that people with Down syndrome have an increased risk of developing Alzheimer disease (https://ghr.nlm.nih.gov/condition/alzheimer-disease#genes).

Therefore, *APOE* is not associated with autosomal dominant early-onset Alzheimer disease.

24. **A**. The patient had early-onset familial Alzheimer disease (EOFAD), which is characterized by adult-onset progressive dementia associated with cerebral cortical atrophy, beta-amyloid plaque

formation, and intraneuronal neurofibrillary tangles before age 60–65 years and often before age 55 years. The three clinically indistinguishable subtypes of EOFAD based on the underlying genetic mechanism are Alzheimer disease type 1 (AD1), caused by mutation of *APP* (10%–15% of EOFAD); Alzheimer disease type 3 (AD3), caused by mutation of *PSEN1* (30%–70% of EOFAD); and Alzheimer disease type 4 (AD4), caused by mutation of *PSEN2* (<5% of EOFAD). *A 4555-bp deletion spanning exon 9 of PSEN1 has been found in the Finnish population with founder effect; this mutation is rarely observed in other populations* (https://www.ncbi.nlm.nih.gov/books/NBK1236/).

Therefore, deletion/duplication analysis with multiplex ligation-dependent probe amplification (MLPA) may detect the 4555-bp deletion in the Finnish population.

25. E. Testing of at-risk asymptomatic adults for early-onset familial Alzheimer disease (EOFAD) is possible. Such testing is not useful in predicting age at onset, severity, type of symptoms, or rate of progression in asymptomatic individuals. The identification of a disease-causing mutation in an at-risk individual with equivocal symptoms does not prove or even imply that the questionable symptoms are related to the presence of the mutation. Testing of asymptomatic at-risk adult family members usually involves pretest interviews in which the motives for requesting the test, the individual's knowledge of EOFAD, the possible impact of positive and negative test results, and neurological status are assessed. Those seeking testing should be counseled regarding possible problems that they may encounter with regard to health, life, and disability insurance coverage, employment and educational discrimination, and changes in social and family interactions. Other issues to consider are implications for the at-risk status of other family members. Informed consent for such testing is recommended and adequate procedures should be followed to safeguard confidentiality of test results and to ensure arrangements for long-term follow-up and evaluations.

Therefore, information for predictive testing, a pretesting interview, and informed consent are all appropriate suggestions from the physician in response to this request.

26. D. *Consensus holds that individuals at risk for adult-onset disorders should not have testing during childhood in the absence of symptoms.* The principal arguments against testing asymptomatic individuals during childhood are that it removes

their choice to know or not know this information, it raises the possibility of stigmatization within the family and in other social settings, and it may have serious educational and career implications. There is a position statement from the National Society of Genetic Counselors (NSGC) and a policy statement from the American College of Medical Genetics and Genomics (ACMGG) on genetic testing of minors for adult-onset conditions (http://www.nsgc.org/p/bl/et/blogaid = 860).

Therefore, the 8-year-old grandson of the proband should not be tested for early-onset familial Alzheimer disease (EOFAD).

27. A. *Prenatal diagnosis for pregnancies at increased risk is possible by analysis of DNA extracted from fetal cells obtained by amniocentesis (usually performed at approximately 15–18 weeks' gestation) or chorionic villus sampling (usually performed at ~10–12 weeks' gestation).* Requests for prenatal testing for typically adult-onset conditions such as EOFAD are not common. Differences in perspective may exist among medical professionals and within families regarding the use of prenatal testing, particularly if the testing is being considered for the purpose of pregnancy termination rather than early diagnosis. Although most centers would consider decisions about prenatal testing to be the choice of the parents, discussion of these issues is appropriate.

Preimplantation genetic diagnosis (PGD) and embryo transfer have been successfully used to achieve a pregnancy in a 30-year-old asymptomatic woman with an *APP* disease-causing mutation, resulting in the birth of a healthy child who does not have the APP disease-causing mutation identified in the mother and her family (https://www.ncbi.nlm.nih.gov/books/NBK1236/).

Therefore, prenatal testing for Alzheimer disease may be offered, though it is not common.

28. A. The typical clinical duration of Alzheimer disease (AD) is 8–10 years, with a range from 1 to 25 years. Approximately 25% of all AD is familial (i.e., ≥ 2 persons in a family have AD) of which approximately 95% is late-onset (age >60–65 years) and 5% is early-onset (age <65 years). Establishing the diagnosis of Alzheimer disease relies on clinical-neuropathological assessment. *The association of the APOE e4 allele with late-onset Alzheimer disease is significant;* however, *APOE* genotyping is neither fully specific nor sensitive. The e4 allele in the *APOE* gene is a major risk factor for the development of Alzheimer disease, while the e2 allele has a

protective effect. While *APOE* genotyping may have an adjunct role in the diagnosis of AD in symptomatic individuals, it appears to have little role at this time in predictive testing of asymptomatic individuals (https://www.ncbi.nlm.nih.gov/books/NBK1161/).

Most cases of early-onset Alzheimer disease are caused by pathogenic variants in one of three genes: *APP*, *PSEN1*, or *PSEN2*. Some evidence indicates that people with Down syndrome have an increased risk of developing Alzheimer disease. Early-onset familial Alzheimer disease is inherited in an autosomal dominant manner (not including Down syndrome) (https://ghr.nlm.nih.gov/).

Therefore, *APOE* may be associated with late-onset Alzheimer disease in this family.

29. **D**. *The association of late-onset familial Alzheimer disease (AD) with the APOE e4 allele (genotypes e2/e4, e3/e4, e4/e4) is well documented in both familial and sporadic cases.* The *APOE* e4 allele, by unknown mechanisms, appears to affect age at onset by shifting the onset toward an earlier age. However, approximately 42% of persons with AD do not have an *APOE* e4 allele. *APOE* genotyping is not specific for AD. The absence of an *APOE* e4 allele does not rule out the diagnosis of AD (https://www.ncbi.nlm.nih.gov/books/NBK1161/).

Therefore, it is most likely that Mrs. B.'s mother has the allele e4 in the *APOE* gene.

30. **B**. Apolipoprotein E, encoded by *APOE*, is the recognition site for receptors involved in the clearance of remnants of very-low-density lipoproteins and chylomicrons. There are at least three *APOE* alleles: e2, e3, and e4, identified by isoelectric focusing. The most common allele is e3, which is found in more than half the general population. The e4 allele is a major risk factor for the development of Alzheimer disease, while *the e2 allele has a protective effect* (https://www.gwumc.edu/edu/obgyn/genetics/casestudies/casestudy21.html).

Therefore, it is least likely that Mrs. B's mother has the e2/e2 genotype in the *APOE* gene.

31. **E**. Old age, family history, female sex, and Down syndrome are the most important risk factors for Alzheimer disease (AD). In Western populations, the empirical lifetime risk for AD is 5%. *If patients have a first degree relative in whom AD developed after 65 years, they have a threefold to sixfold increase in their risk of AD.* If patients have a sibling in whom AD developed before 70 years and an affected parent, their risk is increased sevenfold to ninefold. *APOE* testing may be used as an adjunct diagnostic test in individuals seeking evaluation for signs and symptoms suggestive of dementia, but should not be used for predictive testing for AD in asymptomatic patients.

Therefore, this patient had threefold to sixfold increased risk, but *APOE* testing would not be appropriate for her. She was asymptomatic at age of 68. So a next-generation sequencing (NGS) panel for early-onset AD may be considered.

32. **D**. This patient may have Pendred syndrome. Pendred syndrome is an autosomal recessive disorder characterized by severe to profound bilateral sensorineural hearing impairment that is usually congenital (or prelingual) and nonprogressive, vestibular dysfunction, temporal bone abnormalities, and development of euthyroid goiter in late childhood to early adulthood. The variability of findings is considerable, even within the same family. *Pathogenic variants in three genes account for approximately half of cases, which are SLC26A4 (approximately 50% of affected individuals), FOXI1 (<1%), and KCNJ10 (<1%),* suggesting further genetic heterogeneity (http://www.ncbi.nlm.nih.gov/books/NBK1467/).

Pathogenic variants in *GJB2* (connexin 26) and *GJB6* (connexin 30) are the common causes of congenital nonsyndromic autosomal recessive deafness. Pathogenic variants in the *ADGRV1*, *CDH23*, *CLRN1*, *DFNB31*, *GPR98*, *MYO7A*, *PCDH15*, *USH1C*, *USH1G*, and *USH2A* genes cause Usher syndrome. Usher syndrome is an autosomal recessive disorder responsible for 3%−6% of all childhood deafness and about 50% of deafness−blindness in adults. It is characterized by congenital, bilateral, profound sensorineural hearing loss, vestibular areflexia, and adolescent-onset retinitis pigmentosa.

Therefore, *SCL26A4*, *FOXI1*, and *KCNJ10* for Pendred syndrome would most likely be tested to confirm/rule out genetic etiologies in this patient.

33. **B**. Approximately 1 in 500 to 1 in 1000 neonates has clinically significant congenital hearing impairment, and 50%−60% of hearing loss in babies is due to genetic causes. *About 70% of all pathogenic variants causing hearing loss are nonsyndromic.* About 30% of the pathogenic variants causing hearing loss are syndromic. Syndromic hearing impairment is associated with malformations of the external ear or other organs or with medical problems involving other organ systems. Nonsyndromic hearing impairment has no associated visible abnormalities of the external ear or any related medical problems; however, it can be associated with abnormalities of the

middle ear and/or inner ear. Nonsyndromic hearing impairment may be autosomal dominant, autosomal recessive, or X-linked. Within the prelingual nonsyndromic hearing loss group, inheritance is 75%–80% autosomal recessive, 20%–25% autosomal dominant, and 1%–1.5% X-linked (https://www.ncbi.nlm.nih.gov/books/NBK1434/).

Pathogenic variants in *GJB2* (connexin 26) and *GJB6* (connexin 30) are the most common causes of congenital nonsyndromic autosomal recessive deafness. *The GJB2 gene alone accounts for 50% of the congenital nonsyndromic autosomal recessive deafness.* The other 50% of cases are attributed to pathogenic variants of numerous other genes, many of which have been found to cause deafness in only one or two families.

More than 400 genetic syndromes that include hearing loss have been described. Pathogenic variants in the *CDH23, CLRN1, GPR98, MYO7A, PCDH15, USH1C, USH1G,* and *USH2A* genes cause Usher syndrome. Pathogenic variants in the *SLC26A4, FOXI1,* and *KCNJ10* genes cause Pendred syndrome. Other syndromes are Waardenburg syndrome, branchio-oto-renal syndrome, Stickler syndrome, neurofibromatosis 2 (NF2), Jervell and Lange-Nielsen syndrome, biotinidase deficiency, Refsum disease, Alport syndrome, MELAS, and other conditions.

Therefore, the *GJB2* gene in the list is most likely mutated in patients with hereditary hearing loss.

34. **B.** Approximately 1 in 500 to 1 in 1000 neonates has clinically significant congenital hearing impairment.[11] Genetic forms of hearing loss must be distinguished from acquired causes of hearing loss. Acquired hearing loss in children commonly results from prenatal infections from TORCH (toxoplasmosis, rubella, cytomegalic virus, and herpes) organisms, or postnatal infections, particularly bacterial meningitis caused by *Neisseria meningitidis, Haemophilus influenzae,* or *Streptococcus pneumoniae.* Genetic causes account for 50%–60% of hearing loss in babies. *About 70% of all pathogenic variants causing hearing loss are nonsyndromic.* Nonsyndromic hearing impairment may be autosomal dominant, autosomal recessive, or X-linked. Within the prelingual nonsyndromic hearing loss group, inheritance is 75%–80% autosomal recessive, 20%–25% autosomal dominant, and 1%–1.5% X-linked. *Pathogenic variants in GJB2 (connexin 26) and GJB6 (connexin 30) are the common causes of congenital nonsyndromic autosomal recessive deafness.* The *GJB2* gene alone accounts for half the congenital

nonsyndromic autosomal recessive deafness. The other 50% of cases are attributed to pathogenic variants of numerous other genes, many of which have been found to cause deafness in only one or two families (https://www.ncbi.nlm.nih.gov/books/NBK1434/).

About 30% of the pathogenic variants causing hearing loss are syndromic. Pathogenic variants in the *CDH23, CLRN1, GPR98, MYO7A, PCDH15, USH1C, USH1G,* and *USH2A* genes cause Usher syndrome. Pathogenic variants in the *SLC26A4, FOXI1,* and *KCNJ10* genes cause Pendred syndrome.

Therefore, molecular testing of the *GJB2* and *GJB6* genes would most likely be the next step in the workup to confirm/rule out nonsyndromic hearing impairment in this patient.

35. **E.** Pathogenic variants in *GJB2* (connexin 26) and *GJB6* (connexin 30) are the most common causes of congenital nonsyndromic autosomal recessive deafness. *In this case, Usher syndrome cannot be ruled out because blindness related with retinitis pigmentosa is usually adolescent-onset.* Impaired vision is not detectable in an infant. An Usher syndrome NGS panel might be considered for this patient, since the molecular testing of the *GJB2* and *GJB6* genes showed negative results. Usher syndrome is one of the most common syndromic hearing losses. It is characterized by congenital, bilateral, profound sensorineural hearing loss, vestibular areflexia, and adolescent-onset retinitis pigmentosa. It is thought to be responsible for 3%–6% of all childhood deafness and about 50% of deafness–blindness in adults. Pathogenic variants in the *CDH23, CLRN1, GPR98, MYO7A, PCDH15, USH1C, USH1G,* and *USH2A* genes cause Usher syndrome.

This patient did not have vestibular dysfunction and/or temporal bone abnormalities, which ruled out Pendred syndrome. Pathogenic variants in the *SLC26A4, FOXI1,* and *KCNJ10* cause Pendred syndrome.

Therefore, molecular sequencing tests using a NGS Usher syndrome panel would be an appropriate next step in the workup to further rule out genetic etiologies in this patient.

36. **C.** Mitochondrial diseases are a clinically heterogeneous group of disorders that arise because of dysfunction of the mitochondrial respiratory chain. Sensorineural hearing loss (SNHL) is often associated to mitochondrial dysfunctions in both syndromic and nonsyndromic forms. SNHL has been described in association with different mitochondrial

multisystemic syndromes, often characterized by an important neuromuscular involvement.

This adult patient did not have detectable pathogenic variants in the *GJB2* (connexin 26) and *GJB6* (connexin 30) genes for congenital nonsyndromic autosomal recessive deafness. She did not have developmental delay, dysmorphic facial features, multiple congenital anomalies, blindness due to adolescent- or adult-onset retinitis pigmentosa, vestibular dysfunction, temporal-bone abnormalities, or development of euthyroid goiter, which are well known to be found in some syndromic hearing loss.

Therefore, a mitochondrial panel for hearing impairment studies would most likely be the next step in the workup to further rule out genetic etiologies in this patient because patients with mitochondrial disorders may have highly variable expression.

37. **C.** Pathogenic variants in the *GJB2* (connexin 26) and *GJB6* (connexin 30) genes are common causes of congenital nonsyndromic autosomal recessive deafness. The majority of pathogenic variants in *GJB2* (connexin 26) and *GJB6* (connexin 30) detected in patients are inherited. So the parents of this girl may be considered to be obligate heterozygous carriers.

Therefore, the recurrent risk for the parents would be *1/2 × 1/2 = 1/4 (25%).*

38. **B.** Pathogenic variants in *GJB2* (connexin 26) and *GJB6* (connexin 30) are the common causes of congenital nonsyndromic autosomal recessive deafness. The *GJB2* gene alone accounts for half the congenital nonsyndromic autosomal recessive deafness. *Doubled heterozygous pathogenic variants in both GJB2 and GJB6 have also been seen in patients with sensorineural hearing loss (SNHL).*

Usher syndrome is one of the most common syndromic hearing losses. It is characterized by congenital, bilateral, profound sensorineural hearing loss, vestibular areflexia, and adolescent-onset retinitis pigmentosa. Since retinitis pigmentosa is adolescent- or adult-onset, impaired vision is not detectable in an infant. It is thought to be responsible for 3%–6% of all childhood deafness and about 50% of deafness—blindness in adults. Pathogenic variants in the *CDH23, CLRN1, GPR98, MYO7A, PCDH15, USH1C, USH1G,* and *USH2A* genes cause Usher syndrome. Pendred syndrome is characterized by severe to profound bilateral sensorineural hearing impairment that is usually congenital (or prelingual) and nonprogressive, vestibular dysfunction, temporal-bone abnormalities, and development of euthyroid goiter in late childhood

to early adulthood. Pathogenic variants in the *SLC26A4, FOXI1,* and *KCNJ10* cause Pendred syndrome. Mitochondrial diseases are a clinically heterogeneous group of disorders that arise because of dysfunction of the mitochondrial respiratory chain. SNHL is often associated with mitochondrial dysfunctions in both syndromic and nonsyndromic forms. SNHL has been described in association with different mitochondrial multisystemic syndromes, often characterized by an important neuromuscular involvement.

Therefore, molecular studies of the *GJB6* gene (connexin 30) would most likely be the next step in the workup to further confirm/rule out genetic etiologies in this patient since a heterozygous pathogenic variant in *GJB2* was detected, which pointed in the direction of nonsyndromic hearing loss.

39. **B.** Approximately 50% of autosomal recessive nonsyndromic hearing loss can be attributed to pathogenic variants in *GJB2* (which encodes the protein connexin 26) and *GJB6* (which encodes the protein connexin 30). Neither *GJB2* nor *GJB6* is a pseudogene. Pathogenic variants in *GJB2* are much more common than those in *GJB6*. The carrier rate in the general population for a recessive deafness-causing *GJB2* pathogenic variant is approximately 1 in 33. The *GJB6* gene is located approximately 35 kb telomeric from the *GJB2* gene, and the most common *GJB6* pathogenic variants are large deletions, which remove part of the gene. *Compound heterozygosity of a pathogenic variant in GJB2 and a deletion in GJB6 is associated with nonsyndromic autosomal recessive hearing loss* (http://www.ncbi.nlm.nih.gov/books/NBK1434/).

Therefore, it would be most likely that the two variants in the *GJB2* and *GJB6* genes are in *trans*, which resulted in hearing loss in this patient.

40. **F.** Approximately 7% of individuals of Ashkenazi Jewish decent are carriers of a hearing loss pathogenic variant because of a founder effect. *There are four common pathogenic variants in the Ashkenazi Jewish population—35delG and 167delT in the GJB2 (connexin 26) gene, GJB6 (connexin 30) gene deletion, p.Arg245X in the PCDH15 (USH1F) gene, and p.Asn48Lys in the CLRN1 (USH3A).*

Usher syndrome is a heterogeneous group of disorders caused by a pathogenic variant in one of at least 11 genes. A next-generation sequencing (NGS) panel for Usher syndrome and Sanger sequencing analysis are not cost-effective first-line tests for an Ashkenazi Jew.

Therefore, a targeted variant assay for targeted variant analysis would most likely be used to confirm/rule out genetic etiologies in this Ashkenazi Jewish patient.

41. **A**. This Ashkenazi Jewish patient may have Usher syndrome type III because of a founder effect. The prevalence of Usher syndrome type III is 1 in 45,000 in the Ashkenazi Jewish population (the carrier frequency is 1 in 107 Ashkenazi Jews). *The p.N48K pathogenic variant in the CLRN1 gene is detected in 75% of carriers in the Ashkenazi Jewish population.* Unlike the other forms of Usher syndrome, infants with Usher syndrome type III are usually born with normal hearing. Hearing loss typically begins during late childhood or adolescence, after the development of speech, and progresses over time. By middle age, most affected individuals are profoundly deaf. Vision loss caused by retinitis pigmentosa also develops in late childhood or adolescence, often leading to blindness by midlife. Individuals with Usher syndrome type III may also experience difficulties with balance due to inner ear problems. These problems vary among affected individuals (https://www.jewishgenetics.org).

The p.Arg245Ter (c.733C > T) pathogenic variant in the *PCDH15* gene is detected in 95% of carriers in the Ashkenazi Jewish populations, seen in Usher syndrome type 1F (USH1F). Infants with Usher syndrome type 1F have profound bilateral deafness at birth, and without early interventions may not develop speech. Retinitis pigmentosa, a feature of Usher syndrome, generally appears in adolescence and leads to night blindness and loss of peripheral vision. Some individuals with this condition become completely blind over time. Motor development is delayed and balance is significantly affected (https://www.jewishgenetics.org).

Pathogenic variants in the *GJB2* and *GJB6* genes are associated nonsyndromic hearing loss, which usually manifests as congenital nonprogressive mild-to-profound sensorineural hearing impairment. Pathogenic variants in the *SCL26A4*, *FOXI1*, and *KCNJ10* genes are associated with Pendred syndrome. Patients with Pendred syndrome usually have vestibular dysfunction, temporal-bone abnormalities, and development of euthyroid goiter in late childhood to early adulthood in addition to congenital (or prelingual) severe-to-profound bilateral sensorineural hearing impairment.

Therefore, a targeted variant analysis of the *CLRN1* gene is most likely the next step in the workup to confirm/rule out Usher syndrome type III in this Ashkenazi Jewish patient.

42. **D**. Approximately 7% of individuals of Ashkenazi Jewish descent are carriers of a pathogenic variant for hearing loss because of a founder effect. There are four common pathogenic variants in the Ashkenazi Jewish population—35delG and 167delT in the *GJB2* (connexin 26) gene, the *GJB6* (connexin 30) gene deletion, p.Arg245X in the *PCDH15* (USH1F) gene, and p.Asn48Lys in the *CLRN1* (USH3A). All four are autosomal recessive conditions. So the husband's parents are/were obligate carriers.

Therefore, the husband's risk of being a heterozygous carrier is 2 in 3.

43. **C**. *In the Ashkenazi Jewish population, the prevalence of heterozygosity for 167delT in GJB2, which is rare in the general population, was 4.03% (95% confidence interval, 2.5%−6.0%), and for 30delG the prevalence was 0.73% (95% confidence interval, 0.2%−1.8%).* The c.35delG(p.Gly12Valfx*2) pathogenic variant is the most prevalent *GJB2* pathogenic variant in Caucasians. The other variants listed in the question have been reported in patients without an apparent founder effect.

Therefore, the husband would most likely have the c.167delT(p.Leu56Argfs*26) pathogenic variant in the *GJB2* gene.

44. **A**. In the Ashkenazi Jewish population, the frameshift pathogenic variant, c.167delT(p. Leu56Argfs*26) has a carrier frequency of approximately 4%. For 30delG the prevalence is 0.73% (95% confidence interval, 0.2%−1.8%) in Ashkenazi Jews. *The c.35delG(p.Gly12Valfx*2) pathogenic variant is the most prevalent GJB2 pathogenic variant in Caucasians.* The other variants listed in the question have been reported in patients without an apparent founder effect.

Therefore, the husband would most likely have the c.35delG(p.Gly12Valfx*2) pathogenic variant in the *GJB2* gene.

45. **C**. This patient may have Usher syndrome, characterized by hearing loss or deafness and progressive vision loss. Vision loss caused by retinitis pigmentosa also develops in late childhood or adolescence, often leading to blindness by midlife. It is an autosomal recessive condition, which may be caused by pathogenic variants in eight genes—*CDH23*, *CLRN1*, *GPR98*, *MYO7A*, *PCDH15*, *USH1C*, *USH1G*, and *USH2A*. Some of the genes, such as *CDH23* and *GPR98*, have more than 60 exons.

Chromosomal microarray (CMA) and multiplex ligation-dependent probe amplification (MLPA) are for deletions and duplications with different resolutions. *Next-generation sequencing (NGS) is a method to sequence millions of base pairs simultaneously.* Quantitative PCR is for SNP genotyping and for expression analysis if coupled with reverse transcriptase for cDNA synthesis from RNA. Sanger sequencing is a method to detect all variants in a DNA fragment less than 1000 bp.

Therefore, a next-generation sequencing (NGS) panel provides the most cost-effective genetic testing strategy to confirm/rule out Usher syndrome in this patient.

46. **D**. It has long been known that the major irreversible toxicity of aminoglycosides is ototoxicity. Aminoglycosides appear to generate free radicals within the inner ear, with subsequent permanent damage to sensory cells and neurons, resulting in permanent hearing loss. *Two pathogenic variants in the mitochondrial 12S ribosomal RNA gene have been reported to predispose carriers to aminoglycoside-induced ototoxicity.*

Therefore, the 12S rRNA gene in mtDNA would most likely harbor a pathogenic variant in this infant.

47. **C**. Hearing loss has many causes; *50%–60% of hearing loss in babies is due to genetic causes.*

48. **D**. More than 50% of prelingual deafness is genetic, most often autosomal recessive and nonsyndromic. Genetic hearing loss is autosomal recessive in approximately 80% of cases. About 70% of all pathogenic variants causing hearing loss are nonsyndromic, and 30% are syndromic. Approximately 50% of autosomal recessive nonsyndromic hearing loss can be attributed to the disorder DFNB1, caused by pathogenic variants in the *GJB2* (which encodes the protein connexin 26) and *GJB6* (which encodes the protein connexin 30) genes. *Individuals with nonsyndromic hearing loss and deafness (DFNB1) are either homozygous or compound heterozygous for GJB2 pathogenic variants (99%) or compound heterozygous for one GJB2 pathogenic variant and one of three large deletions that include sequences upstream of GJB2 and a portion of GJB6 (<1%)* (https://www.ncbi.nlm.nih.gov/books/NBK1272/).

Therefore, *GJB2* (connexin 26) is estimated to be responsible for half of all recessive nonsyndromic hearing loss, not *GJB6* (connexin 30).

49. **B**. All the syndromes listed may cause hearing loss. Jervell and Lange-Nielsen syndrome is an autosomal recessive condition that causes profound hearing loss from birth and a disruption of the heart's normal rhythm (arrhythmia). *Homozygous or compound*

heterozygous pathogenic variants in the KCNE1 and KCNQ1 genes cause Jervell and Lange-Nielsen syndrome. Branchio-oto-renal (BOR) syndrome, neurofibromatosis type II (NFII), Treacher–Collins syndrome, and Waardenburg syndrome are autosomal dominant conditions. Stickler syndrome could be autosomal dominant (*COL2A1*, *COL11A1*, and *COL11A2*) or recessive (*COL9A1* and *COL9A2*) (https://www.ncbi.nlm.nih.gov/books/NBK1405/).

Therefore, Jervell and Lange-Nielsen syndrome can NOT cause dominant syndromic hearing loss.

50. **D**. All the syndromes listed may cause hearing loss. Branchio-oto-renal (BOR) syndrome is an autosomal dominant condition, which typically disrupts the development of tissues in the neck and causes malformations of the ears and kidneys. *Heterozygous pathogenic variants in EYA1, SIX1, or SIX5, are known to cause BOR syndrome.* Usher syndrome and Pendred syndrome are autosomal recessive conditions. Stickler syndrome could be autosomal dominant (*COL2A1*, *COL11A1*, and *COL11A2*) or recessive (*COL9A1* and *COL9A2*). Alport syndrome could be X-linked recessive (*COL4A5*, 80%) or autosomal recessive (*COL4A3* and *COL4A4*, 15%) (https://www.ncbi.nlm.nih.gov/books/NBK1405/).

Therefore, branchio-oto-renal (BOR) syndrome can NOT cause recessive syndromic hearing loss.

51. **B**. Waardenburg syndrome is a group of genetic conditions that can cause hearing loss and changes in coloring (pigmentation) of the hair, skin, and eyes. Although most people with Waardenburg syndrome have normal hearing, moderate to profound hearing loss can occur in one or both ears, and the hearing loss is congenital. People with this condition often have very pale blue eyes or different colored eyes, such as one blue eye and one brown eye. Sometimes one eye has segments of two different colors. Distinctive hair coloring, such as a patch of white hair or hair that prematurely turns gray, is another common sign of the condition. The features of Waardenburg syndrome vary among affected individuals, even among people in the same family. *Pathogenic variants in the EDN3, EDNRB, MITF, PAX3, SNAI2, and SOX10 genes can cause Waardenburg syndrome.* These genes are involved in the formation and development of melanocytes, and pathogenic variants in any of these genes can disrupt the normal development of melanocytes, leading to abnormal pigmentation of the skin, hair, and eyes and problems with hearing (http://ghr.nlm.nih.gov/condition/waardenburg-syndrome).

Therefore, a next-generation sequencing (NGS) panel for the above genes would most likely be used to confirm the diagnosis in this patient, since the pathogenic variant was not identified in the family. If a pathogenic variant was identified in a family member, targeted variant analysis may be used for the other family members.

52. **A.** Waardenburg syndrome is a group of genetic conditions that can cause hearing loss and changes in coloring (pigmentation) of the hair, skin, and eyes. The four known types of Waardenburg syndrome are distinguished by their physical characteristics and sometimes by their genetic causes. Pathogenic variants in the *EDN3, EDNRB, MITF, PAX3, SNAI2,* and *SOX10* genes can cause Waardenburg syndrome. *Types I and III Waardenburg syndrome are caused by pathogenic variants in the PAX3 gene.* Pathogenic variants in the *MITF* and *SNAI2* genes are responsible for type II Waardenburg syndrome. Pathogenic variants in the *SOX10, EDN3,* or *EDNRB* genes cause type IV Waardenburg syndrome (http://ghr.nlm.nih.gov/condition/waardenburg-syndrome).

Pathogenic variants in *PAX5* are associated with susceptibility to acute lymphoblastic leukemia (ALL). A t(2;13) involving *PAX7* at 2q36 and *FKHR* (*FOXO1A*) at 13q14 is a characteristic cytogenetic alteration in alveolar rhabdomyosarcoma. *PEX3, PEX5,* and *PEX7* encode for peroxisome biogenesis factors. Pathogenic variants in *PEX3, PEX5,* and *PEX7* cause autosomal recessive peroxisomal biogenesis disorder, such as Zellweger spectrum disorders.

Therefore, *PAX3* would most likely be included in this NGS panel for Waardenberg syndrome. Once the pathogenic variant was detected, a targeted variant analysis might be ordered for the son.

53. **E.** *Waardenburg syndrome is an autosomal dominant condition.* The pathogenic variant in the *PAX3* gene was detected in both the proband, her brother, and her father.

Therefore, the recurrent risk is 50% for this autosomal dominant condition.

54. **C.** *PAX3* encodes a DNA-binding transcription factor expressed during early neurogenesis, which is an essential regulator of muscle and neural crest—derived cell types, including melanocytes. *Pathogenic variants within PAX3 or deletion of the entire gene result in haploinsufficiency* (https://www.ncbi.nlm.nih.gov/books/NBK1531/). Pathogenic variants in *PAX3* may also be seen in patients with autosomal dominant craniofacial—deafness—hand syndrome. Somatic *PAX3* variants have been observed in alveolar rhabdomyosarcoma. *PAX3* can fuse with *FKHR* (*PAX-FKHR*), this fusion creates a gain of function that results in alveolar rhabdomyosarcoma. Individuals with alveolar rhabdomyosarcoma resulting from this mechanism do not have Waardenburg syndrome.

Therefore, loss of function would most likely be the pathogenesis of this variant in this family.

55. **B.** *Mitochondrial DNA (mtDNA) depletion syndromes (MDSs) are a genetically and clinically heterogeneous group of autosomal recessive disorders* that are characterized by a severe reduction in mtDNA content leading to impaired energy production in affected tissues and organs.

Therefore, mitochondrial DNA (mtDNA) depletion syndromes are autosomal recessive disorders.

56. **A.** Leber hereditary optic neuropathy (LHON) is expressed phenotypically as rapid painless loss of central vision due to optic nerve atrophy in young adults. Males are four to five times more likely than females to be affected. Affected individuals are usually entirely asymptomatic until they develop visual blurring affecting the central visual field in one eye; similar symptoms appear in the other eye an average of 2—3 months later. In about 25% of cases, visual loss is bilateral at onset. *LHON is caused by pathogenic variants in the coding region of the mitochondrial genome, including the MT-ND1, MT-ND4, MT-ND4L, or MT-ND6 gene.* The three common mtDNA pathogenic variants are m.3460G > A in *MT-ND1*, m.11778G > A in *MT-ND4*, and m.14484T > C in *MT-ND6*.

LHON-causing mtDNA pathogenic variants are characterized by reduced penetrance. The two most important risk factors for visual loss are sex and age. An individual can develop LHON only if a pathogenic mtDNA LHON-causing variant is present, but approximately 50% of males and 90% of females who harbor a primary LHON-causing mtDNA pathogenic variant do not develop blindness. The penetrance of LHON is also age-specific. The 95th percentile for age at onset is 50 years for all three primary pathogenic variants. Thus, a clinically unaffected male in his 50s has less than a 1 in 20 chance of losing his vision. While the majority of individuals with a LHON-causing mtDNA variant are homoplasmic, heteroplasmy occurs in approximately 10%—15% of individuals with LHON, which also contribute to the penetrance (https://www.ncbi.nlm.nih.gov/books/NBK1174/).

Therefore, LHON is NOT caused by pathogenic variants in nuclear DNA encoded for mitochondrial proteins.

57. **F.** Molecular testing approaches for Leber hereditary optic neuropathy (LHON) can include targeted testing, a multigene panel, or complete mtDNA sequencing. Three common mtDNA pathogenic variants account for 90%–95% of LHON. Targeted analysis for one of these three variants should be performed first. A multigene panel that includes the mitochondrial genes that encode subunits of NADH dehydrogenase, *MT-ND1*, *MT-ND2*, *MT-ND4*, *MT-ND4L*, *MT-ND5*, and *MT-ND6*, which are known to cause LHON and other genes of interest may also be considered. Complete mtDNA sequencing may be considered if use of targeted testing and/or a multigene panel did not identify a pathogenic variant, clinical suspicion remains high, and there is no evidence of paternal transmission.

Therefore, targeted variants analysis would provide the most cost-effective genetic testing strategy for this patient.

58. **B.** Three common mtDNA pathogenic variants account for 90%–95% of hereditary optic atrophy or neuropathy (LHON). They are m.3460G > A in *MTND1*, m.11778G > A in *MTND4*, or m.14484T > C in *MTND6*.

m.3243A > G *MTTL1* has been seen in patients with maternally inherited diabetes and deafness (MIDD). m.8993T > C in *MTATP6* has been seen in patients with adult-onset ataxia and polyneuropathy. m.8344A > G in *MTTK* has been seen in patients with myoclonic epilepsy with ragged red fibers (MERRF).

Therefore, this patient would most likely have m.3460G > A in *MTND1*.

59. **D.** Three common mtDNA pathogenic variants account for 90%–95% of hereditary optic atrophy or neuropathy (LHON). They are m.3460G > A in *MTND1*, m.11778G > A in *MTND4*, or m.14484T > C in *MTND6*. The majority of individuals with a LHON-causing mtDNA variant are homoplasmic. However, heteroplasmy occurs in approximately 10%–15% of individuals with LHON.

Therefore, this patient would most likely have homoplasmic m.11778G > A in *MTND4*.

60. **C.** Leber hereditary optic neuropathy (LHON) is characterized by bilateral, painless, subacute visual failure that develops during young adult life. Males are four to five times more likely than females to be affected. In about 25% of cases, visual loss is bilateral at onset. The diagnosis is based on ophthalmological findings.

Approximately 90% of individuals with LHON have one of three single nucleotide pathogenic variants of mitochondrial DNA (mtDNA): m.3460G > A, m.11778G > A, or m.14484T > C. Approximately one in seven individuals with LHON harbor a mixture of mutated and wild-type (normal) mtDNA (heteroplasmy), and the risks of developing blindness in heteroplasmic LHON individuals are not well characterized (https://www.ncbi.nlm.nih.gov/books/NBK1174/).

Therefore, Leber hereditary optic neuropathy (LHON) is a mitochondrial disorder caused by mtDNA with heteroplasmy in some patients, but NOT a mitochondria disorder caused by nuclear DNAs.

61. **A.** Leber hereditary optic neuropathy (LHON) is a mitochondrial disease characterized by bilateral, painless, subacute visual failure that develops during young adult life. The diagnosis is based on ophthalmological findings. Approximately 90% of individuals with LHON have one of three single nucleotide pathogenic variants of mitochondrial DNA (mtDNA): m.3460G > A in *MT-ND1*, m.11778G > A in *MT-ND4*, or m.14484T > C in *MT-ND6*. Approximately one in seven individuals with LHON harbor a mixture of mutated and wild-type (normal) mtDNA (heteroplasmy), and the risks of developing blindness in heteroplasmic LHON individuals are not well characterized (https://www.ncbi.nlm.nih.gov/books/NBK1174/).

Mitochondrial DNAs (mtDNAs) are maternally inherited. A male with an LHON-causing mtDNA pathogenic variant cannot transmit the variant to any of his offspring. Therefore, the patient's future children would NOT have an increased risk of losing their vision due to LHON.

62. **F.** *The mtDNA pathogenic variants causing Leber hereditary optic neuropathy (LHON) are characterized by reduced penetrance.* An individual can develop LHON only if a pathogenic mtDNA LHON-causing variant is present, but approximately 50% of males and 90% of females who harbor a primary LHON-causing mtDNA pathogenic variant do not develop blindness. It must be stressed that penetrance can vary markedly in different branches of the same family and between families harboring the same LHON-causing mtDNA pathogenic variants, which complicates genetic counseling at the individual level. Additional environmental and genetic factors interact with the primary mtDNA pathogenic variant and determine whether an individual ultimately develops optic-nerve

dysfunction and visual failure. The two most important risk factors for visual loss are sex and age. For example, a male at the age of 18 years has a lifetime risk of approximately 50% for LHON after a positive test result. The risk declines with age but, because loss of sight can occur at any age, the risk never falls to zero (https://www.ncbi.nlm.nih.gov/books/NBK1174/).

The presence of the mtDNA pathogenic variant does not predict the occurrence, age at onset, severity, or rate of progression of visual loss. Therefore, the recurrent risk of LHON would not be predictable in this family.

63. **D**. Maternally inherited diabetes and deafness (MIDD) syndrome is a mitochondrial disorder, representing 1% of patients with diabetes. It is characterized by the onset of sensorineural hearing loss and diabetes in adulthood. Typically, hearing loss occurs before diabetes and is marked by a decrease in perception of high tone frequencies. Some patients may have additional features observed in mitochondrial disorders, including pigmentary retinopathy, ptosis, cardiomyopathy, myopathy, renal problems, and neuropsychiatric symptoms (OMIM# 520000). Pathogenic variants in *MTTL1*, *MTTK*, or *MTTE* have been seen in patients with maternally inherited diabetes and deafness (MIDD). *The majority of MIDD patients have a pathogenic variant, m.3243A > G in MTTL1, which is typically in heteroplasmic form. MTTL1, MTTK, and MTTE* encode tRNAs. Pathogenic variants in *MTTL1, MTTK,* or *MTTE* reduce the ability of tRNA to add amino acids for protein synthesis (https://ghr.nlm.nih.gov/condition/maternally-inherited-diabetes-and-deafness#genes).

Pathogenic variants in *MTATP6* have been seen in patients with adult-onset ataxia and polyneuropathy. Pathogenic variants in *MTND1* have been seen in patients with hereditary optic atrophy or neuropathy (LHON). Pathogenic variants in *MTTH* have been seen in patients with myoclonic epilepsy with ragged red fibers (MERRF).

Therefore, *MTTL1* would most likely harbor a pathogenic variant. In this case the m.3243A > G IN *MTTL1* was detected in muscle, hair follicle, and blood specimens from the proband and her asymptomatic family members.

64. **C**. Maternally inherited diabetes and deafness syndrome (MIDD) is a mitochondrial disorder, representing 1% of patients with diabetes. It characterized by onset of sensorineural hearing loss and diabetes in adulthood. Typically, hearing

loss occurs before diabetes and is marked by a decrease in perception of high tone frequencies. Some patients may have additional features observed in mitochondrial disorders, including pigmentary retinopathy, ptosis, cardiomyopathy, myopathy, renal problems, and neuropsychiatric symptoms (OMIM# 520000). Pathogenic variants in *MTTL1*, *MTTK*, or *MTTE* have been seen in patients with maternally inherited diabetes and deafness syndrome (MIDD). *A majority of MIDD patients have a pathogenic variant, m.3243A > G IN MTTL1, which is typically in heteroplasmic form. MTTL1, MTTK, and MTTE* encode tRNAs. Pathogenic variants in *MTTL1, MTTK,* or *MTTE* reduce the ability of tRNA to add amino acids for protein synthesis (https://ghr.nlm.nih.gov/condition/maternally-inherited-diabetes-and-deafness#genes).

The m.11778G > A variant in *MTND4* is common in patients with hereditary optic atrophy or neuropathy (LHON), which is typically in homoplasmic form.

Therefore, the patient would most likely have heteroplasmic m.3243A > G IN *MTTL1*.

65. **C**. Myoclonic epilepsy with ragged red fibers (MERRF) is one of the mitochondrial disorders, characterized by myoclonus (often the first symptom) followed by generalized epilepsy, ataxia, weakness, and dementia. Onset is usually in childhood, occurring after normal early development. Common findings are hearing loss, short stature, optic atrophy, and cardiomyopathy with Wolff–Parkinson–White (WPW) syndrome. Pigmentary retinopathy and lipomatosis are occasionally observed. *The most common pathogenic variant, present in more than 80% of affected individuals with typical findings, is an A-to-G transition at nucleotide 8344 (m.8344A > G) in the MTTK gene.* Pathogenic variants in *MTTF, MTTL1, MTTI,* and *MTTP* have also been described in a subset of individuals with MERRF. Pathogenic variants are usually present in all tissues. However, the occurrence of "heteroplasmy" in disorders of mtDNA can result in varying tissue distribution of mutated mtDNA (https://www.ncbi.nlm.nih.gov/books/NBK1520/).

Therefore, *MTTK* would most likely harbor a pathogenic variant in this patient.

66. **D**. *The m.8344A > G variant in the MTTK gene present in more than 80% of patients with typical findings of myoclonic epilepsy with ragged red fibers (MERRF). The majority of affected individuals have homoplastic pathogenic variants.*

The m.14484T > C variant in *MTND6* is common in patients with hereditary optic atrophy or neuropathy (LHON), which is typically in homoplasmic form.

Therefore, the patient would most likely have homoplasmic m.8344A > G in *MTTK* than others listed in the question.

67. **D**. MELAS (mitochondrial encephalomyopathy, lactic acidosis, and stroke-like episodes) is a multisystem disorder, characterized by generalized tonic–clonic seizures, recurrent headaches, anorexia, and recurrent vomiting initially. Patients' early psychomotor development is usually normal, but short stature is common. Onset is frequently between the ages of 2 and 10 years. Exercise intolerance or proximal limb weakness may be the initial manifestation. Seizures are often associated with stroke-like episodes of transient hemiparesis or cortical blindness. These stroke-like episodes may be associated with altered consciousness and may be recurrent. The cumulative residual effects of the stroke-like episodes gradually impair motor abilities, vision, and mentation, often by adolescence or young adulthood. Sensorineural hearing loss is common (https://www.ncbi.nlm. nih.gov/books/NBK1233/). *Pathogenic variants in the mtDNA gene MTTL1 encoding tRNALeu(UUA/ UUG) are causative.* The most common pathogenic variant, present in about 80% of individuals with typical clinical findings, is an A-to-G transition at nucleotide 3243 (m.3243A > G) in *MTTL1*. Other pathogenic variants in *MTTL1* or other mtDNA genes, particularly *MTND5*, can also cause this disorder. Pathogenic variants can usually be detected in mtDNA from leukocytes in individuals with typical MELAS; however, the occurrence of "heteroplasmy" in disorders of mtDNA can result in varying tissue distribution of mutated mtDNA.

Therefore, *MTTL1* would most likely harbor a pathogenic variant in this patient.

68. **B**. Because the son was the only person in the family with the disorder, it was likely inherited in an autosomal recessive manner, unless the son had a de novo variant for an autosomal dominant condition. Long-QT syndrome (LQTS) with extracardiac signs can be inherited in an autosomal dominant or autosomal recessive manner. However, de novo events in patients with LQTS are not common. *Jervell and Lange-Nielsen syndrome (JLNS) is inherited in an autosomal recessive manner characterized by congenital profound bilateral sensorineural hearing loss and long QTc.* The classic presentation of JLNS is a deaf child who experiences syncopal episodes during periods of stress, exercise, or fright. Fifty percent of

individuals with JLNS had cardiac events before 3 years of age. More than half of untreated children with JLNS die prior to age 15 years (https:// www.ncbi.nlm.nih.gov/books/NBK1405/).

Andersen–Tawil syndrome, Romano–Ward syndrome, and Timothy syndrome are autosomal dominant conditions, which cause arrhythmia. They are forms of long-QT syndrome. Usher syndrome is associated with hearing loss, but not long QT interval.

Therefore, the proband most likely had Jervell and Lange-Nielsen syndrome.

69. **B**. *Jervell and Lange-Nielsen syndrome (JLNS) is an autosomal recessive condition,* characterized by congenital profound bilateral sensorineural hearing loss and long QTc. The classic presentation of JLNS is a deaf child who experiences syncopal episodes during periods of stress, exercise, or fright. Fifty percent of individuals with JLNS had cardiac events before 3 years of age. More than half of untreated children with JLNS die prior to age 15 years. Parents of a child with JLNS are usually heterozygotes; rarely, only one parent is a carrier and the other pathogenic variant is de novo. Parents may or may not have the long-QT syndrome (LQTS) phenotype. (https://www.ncbi.nlm.nih.gov/ books/NBK1405/).

Therefore, most likely the unborn sibling of the 2-year-old boy would have up to 25% risk to have the same disorder.

70. **D**. Jervell and Lange-Nielsen syndrome (JLNS) is an autosomal recessive condition that causes profound congenital hearing loss and an arrhythmia associated with long QT interval by ECG. Parents of a child with JLNS are usually heterozygotes; rarely, only one parent is a carrier and the other pathogenic variant is de novo. *Heterozygous carrier may have long-QT syndrome, but not hearing loss.*

The 2-year-old boy in this question had JLNS. So most likely the parents were carriers. The fetus had approximately a 25% chance of being affected with JLNS with congenital hearing loss, a 50% chance of being a carrier of a JLNS pathogenic variant and at risk for LQTS. Therefore, the unborn sibling of the 2-year-old boy would have up to a 75% risk to have LQTS.

71. **C**. *Romano–Ward syndrome is one the autosomal dominant long-QT syndromes, caused by pathogenic variants in the KCNQ1 and KCNE1 genes.* It is the most common form of inherited long-QT syndrome, affecting an estimated 1 in 5000 people worldwide. If untreated, the irregular heartbeats can lead to fainting, seizures, or sudden death.

However, some people may be affected but never experience any signs or symptoms of the condition.

The 2-year-old boy in this question had Romano–Ward syndrome, confirmed by the molecular testing. The subsequent genetic analysis confirmed that the mother was a carrier. Therefore, the fetus, as a sibling of the 2-year-old boy, had a 50% risk of having Romano–Ward syndrome since the condition is autosomal dominant.

72. **B**. Long QT syndromes (LQTS) are a heterogeneous, panethnic group of channelopathies caused by defects in cardiac ion channels. *Most cases of LQTS are caused by loss-of-function variants in genes that encodes subunits or regulatory proteins for potassium channels*, such as *KCNQ1* and *KCNE1*. In other LQTS patients, gain-of-function variants in a sodium channel gene, *SCN5A*, lead to an increased influx of sodium, resulting in similar shifting of action potential and repolarization effects.

The *CFTR* gene related to cystic fibrosis is an anion channel that conducts chloride and bicarbonate. Hypertrophic cardiomyopathy is caused by pathogenic variants in approximately 20 genes encoding proteins of the cardiac sarcomere.

Therefore, genes coded for cardiac potassium channels tend to be mutated in patients with long-QT syndrome.

73. **C**. Hypertrophic cardiomyopathy (HCM) is one of the most common monogenic autosomal dominant cardiovascular disorders, which is caused by pathogenic variants in approximately 20 genes encoding proteins of the cardiac sarcomere. *Pathogenic variants of one of the genes, which encodes a component of the sarcomere, are found in approximately 50%–60% of probands (adult and children) with a family history of HCM, and approximately 20%–30% of probands without a family history of HCM.*

Therefore, the estimated maximum clinical sensitivity of a next-generation sequencing (NGS) panel with all 20 genes is about 55% for HCM.

74. **A**. *Familial hypercholesterolemia (FH) is an autosomal dominant disorder of cholesterol and lipid metabolism* characterized by severely elevated LDL cholesterol (LDL-C) levels that lead to atherosclerotic plaque deposition in the coronary arteries and proximal aorta at an early age, leading to an increased risk for cardiovascular disease. Xanthomas (patches of yellowish cholesterol buildup) may worsen with age as a result of extremely high cholesterol levels.

Xanthomas can occur around the eyelids and within the tendons of the elbows, hands, knees, and feet. In FH, the more common cardiovascular disease is coronary artery disease (CAD), which may manifest as angina and myocardial infarction; stroke occurs more rarely. Untreated men are at a 50% risk for a fatal or nonfatal coronary event by age 50 years; untreated women are at a 30% risk by age 60 years (https://www.ncbi.nlm.nih.gov/books/NBK174884/).

Therefore, it would be most likely that this family had autosomal dominant familial hypercholesterolemia.

75. **D**. Familial hypercholesterolemia (FH) is an autosomal dominant disorder of cholesterol and lipid metabolism characterized by severely elevated LDL cholesterol (LDL-C) levels that lead to atherosclerotic plaque deposition in the coronary arteries and proximal aorta at an early age, leading to an increased risk for cardiovascular disease. An estimated 70%–95% of FH results from a heterozygous pathogenic variant in one of three genes (*APOB*, *LDLR*, and *PCSK9*). Once an FH patient is identified, it is important to use cascade screening to identify other family members who may have FH. *First- and second-degree (and if possible third-degree) biological relatives should be screened.* Cascade screening helps identify younger FH patients and prevents coronary artery disease.

Therefore, this patient's brother, son, and all the other first-degree relatives should also be tested for familial hypercholesterolemia.

76. **D**. Familial hypercholesterolemia (FH) is an autosomal dominant disorder of cholesterol and lipid metabolism. An estimated 70%–95% of FH results from a heterozygous pathogenic variant in one of three genes (*APOB*, *LDLR*, and *PCSK9*). *Homozygous FH (HoFH) results from biallelic (homozygous or compound heterozygous) pathogenic variants in one of these known genes (APOB, LDLR, and PCSK9).* Most individuals with HoFH experience severe CAD by their mid-20s and the rate of either death or coronary bypass surgery by the teenage years is high. Severe aortic stenosis is also common (https://www.ncbi.nlm.nih.gov/books/NBK174884/).

Therefore, *APOB*, *LDLR*, and *PCSK9* may be tested for pathogenic variant(s) in this patient.

77. **D**. *Familial hypercholesterolemia (FH) is an autosomal dominant disorder of cholesterol and lipid metabolism mostly caused by pathogenic variants in the LDLR gene (60%–80%).* Pathogenic variants in the *APOB* (1%–5%) and *PCSK9* (0%–3%) genes also contribute to the pathogenesis of FH in a small

percentage of patients. Significant numbers of FH patients (20%−40%) have no identifiable pathogenic variants in these three genes. In FH patients with a heterozygous pathogenic variant in *LDLR*, the untreated cholesterol concentration is greater than 300 mg/dL. *In FH patients with a homozygous pathogenic variant in LDLR the untreated cholesterol concentration is between 600 and 1000 mg/dL.*

This patient has a myocardial infarction in her 20s, and a remarkable family history from both sides. These indicate homozygous FH (HoFH) resulting from biallelic (homozygous or compound heterozygous) pathogenic variants in one of these known genes (*APOB*, *LDLR*, and *PCSK9*).

Therefore, this patient most likely has homozygous c.34C > T(p.Gln12Ter) in *LDLR*.

78. **E.** Age-related penetrance is used to describe phenotypic expression of a particular phenotype modified by age. Familial hypercholesterolemia, hereditary hemochromatosis, Huntington disease, and hypertrophic cardiomyopathy are adult-onset disorders.

Therefore, all four diseases listed are associated with age-related penetrance.

79. **B.** Sex-influenced disorders are those that demonstrate sex-related penetrance or in which the phenotype expression is most likely to occur in a specific sex. The effect of sex on penetrance of inherited pathogenic variants was found in a variety of heritable disorders. Sex-limited disorders refer to autosomal disorders that are nonpenetrant for a particular sex. In cases of hereditary breast and ovarian cancer caused by *BRCA2* pathogenic variants, about 6% of males, as compared with 86% of females, are expected to develop breast cancer by age 70. The penetrance and attack frequency of hypokalemic periodic paralysis (Hypo PP) due to *SCNA4* pathogenic variants were lower in females than in males. Males had 100% penetrance and 50−150 attacks per year, compared to 28.27% penetrance and 30−50 attacks per year in females; the attacks disappear during pregnancy. This is most probably due to the effect of estrogens.

Reports suggest that of p.Cys282Tyr homozygotes, a higher proportion of males than females (28% vs. 1%) have definite disease manifestation of HFE-associated hereditary hemochromatosis because the menstrual period in adult females is preventive. And symptoms related to iron overload usually appear between age 40 and 60 years in males and after menopause in females (https://www.ncbi.nlm. nih.gov/books/NBK1440/).

Familial hypercholesterolemia, Huntington disease, and hypertrophic cardiomyopathy are adult-onset disorders, but their penetrance is not sex-related.

Therefore, *HFE*-associated hereditary hemochromatosis is associated sex-related penetrance.

80. **E.** The genes implicated in Hirschsprung disease includes *RET*, *EDNRB*, *EDN3*, *GDNF*, and *NRTN*. *RET is the major susceptibility gene for isolated Hirschsprung disease, especially when it is long-segment Hirschsprung disease.* Nearly all families with more than one affected patient demonstrate linkage to the *RET* locus.

Therefore, the *RET* gene would most likely be tested in this patient with long-segment Hirschsprung disease and a positive family history.

81. **B.** *Isolated Hirschsprung disease is a panethnic, incompletely penetrant, sex-biased disorder with intrafamilial and interfamilial variation in expressivity.* Within families segregating mutant *RET* alleles, penetrance is 65% in males and 45% in females.

Therefore, low (incomplete) penetrance may explain why the mother does not have the disease even though both the proband and his mother had the pathogenic variant in the *RET* gene.

82. **C.** Hirschsprung disease is an intestinal disorder characterized by the absence of nerves in parts of the intestine. This condition occurs when the nerves in the intestine (enteric nerves) do not form properly during development before birth (embryonic development). This condition is usually identified in the first 2 months of life, although less severe cases may be diagnosed later in childhood.

Isolated Hirschsprung disease can result from pathogenic variants in one of several genes, including the *RET*, *EDNRB*, and *EDN3* genes. Pathogenic variants in the *RET* gene are the most common known genetic cause of Hirschsprung disease. However, the genetics of this condition appear complex and are not completely understood. While a pathogenic variant in a single gene sometimes causes the condition, pathogenic variants in multiple genes may be required in some cases. *The genetic cause of the condition is unknown in approximately half of affected individuals* (https://ghr.nlm.nih.gov/condition/hirschsprung-disease#genes).

Therefore, the genetic cause of the Hirschsprung disease is known in approximately 50% of affected individuals.

83. **B**. The majority of Hirschsprung disease cases are multigenic or multifactorial. *Isolated Hirschsprung disease can result from pathogenic variants in one of several genes, including the RET, EDNRB, and EDN3 genes.* It can also be associated with syndromes such as Down syndrome, Waardenburg syndrome, neurofibromatosis, neuroblastoma, pheochromocytoma, multiple endocrine neoplasia type 2B (MEN2B), and others.

Therefore, a next-generation sequencing (NGS) panel is most likely be used to explore the genetic etiology of the Hirschsprung disease in this patient.

84. **C**. This infant had Hirschsprung disease. Hirschsprung disease, also known as "congenital megacolon" or "congenital intestinal aganglionosis," is a disease condition most commonly affecting the rectosigmoid portion of the colon. It presents with constipation in older infants and children, but mainly with distention and vomiting in newborn infants. Although the majority of cases are multigenic or multifactorial, there are some conditions associated with Hirschsprung disease, such as Down syndrome, Waardenburg syndrome, neurofibromatosis, neuroblastoma, pheochromocytoma, multiple endocrine neoplasia type 2B (MEN2B), and others. The trypanosome causing Chagas disease is responsible for an acquired form of aganglionosis that may affect not only the colon but the esophagus and heart as well. Evidence of intestinal obstruction in newborns can also be caused by meconium ileus secondary to cystic fibrosis.

Multiple endocrine neoplasia type 1 (MEN1) includes varying combinations of more than 20 endocrine and nonendocrine tumors; the most common ones are parathyroid tumors, pituitary tumors, well-differentiated endocrine tumors of the gastroenteropancreatic (GEP) tract, carcinoid tumors, and adrenocortical tumors. However, *intestinal obstruction in newborns is not one of the common clinical presentations in MEN1.*

Therefore, multiple endocrine neoplasia type 1 (MEN1) is NOT associated with an increased risk for intestinal obstruction in newborns.

85. **B**. Hirschsprung disease may present with constipation in older infants and children, *but it mainly presents by distention and vomiting in newborn infants. And the incidence of Hirschsprung disease is about 1 in 5000 births with a 4:1 predominance in males.*

Therefore, Hirschsprung disease has the highest incidence in male infants.

86. **C**. *Neurofibromatosis 1 (NF1) is one of the most common autosomal dominant genetic conditions.* Therefore, this couple's children would have 50% risk to be affected with NF1.

87. **C**. Neurofibromatosis 1 (NF1) is an autosomal dominant condition characterized by multiple café-au-lait spots, axillary and inguinal freckling, multiple cutaneous neurofibromas, and iris Lisch nodules. Learning disabilities are present in at least 50% of individuals with NF1. *Heterozygous loss-of-function pathogenic variants in NF1 are responsible for neurofibromatosis 1 (NF1).* Half of affected individuals have NF1 as the result of a de novo NF1 pathogenic variant. The offspring of an affected individual are at 50% risk of inheriting the altered NF1 gene, but the disease manifestations are extremely variable, even within a family (https://www.ncbi.nlm.nih.gov/books/NBK1109/).

Therefore, the pathogenic variant, detected in this teenage girl, is a loss-of-function variant.

88. **B**. Neurofibromatosis 1 (NF1) has incidence of 1 in 3500 individuals, making it one of the most common autosomal dominant genetic conditions. Approximately half of patients have de novo pathogenic variants. The mutation rate for the NF1 gene is one of the highest known for any human gene, at approximately 1 mutation per 1000 live births. *Approximately 80% of the de novo pathogenic variants are paternal in origin*, but there is no evidence for a paternal age effect increasing the mutation rate.

Therefore, most likely the teenage girl had a paternally derived de novo pathogenic variant in NF1.

89. **E**. Neurofibromatosis 1 (NF1) is one of the most common dominantly inherited genetic disorders, occurring with an incidence at birth of approximately 1 in 3000 individuals. Approximately 50% of individuals with NF1 have an affected parent and 50% have the altered gene as the result of a de novo NF1 pathogenic variant. *The variant rate for NF1 (~1:10,000) is among the highest known for any gene in humans.* The cause of the unusually high variant rate is unknown.

For NF1, there is a possibility of multiple de novo pathogenic variants in a single family. Upadhyaya et al. reported the occurrence of three different NF1 pathogenic variants in one family and advised caution in assuming that the same pathogenic variant is present in all members of an affected family. Two different NF1 pathogenic variants have been reported in another family. Meanwhile, possible nonmedical explanations, including alternative paternity or maternity (e.g., with assisted reproduction) or undisclosed adoption, could also explain the discrepancy between clinical diagnoses and genetic testing results in this family (https://www.ncbi.nlm.nih.gov/books/NBK1109/).

Therefore, all the explanations listed in this question may explain the discrepancy between clinical diagnoses and genetic testing results in this family.

90. **F.** Neurofibromatosis 1 (NF1) is one of the most common dominantly inherited genetic disorders, occurring with an incidence at birth of approximately 1 in 3000 individuals. Approximately 50% of individuals with NF1 have an affected parent and 50% have the altered gene as the result of a de novo *NF1* pathogenic variant. The variant rate for NF1 (~1:10,000) is among the highest known for any gene in humans. The cause of the unusually high variant rate is unknown.

For NF1, there is a possibility of multiple de novo pathogenic variants in a single family. Upadhyaya et al. reported the occurrence of three different *NF1* pathogenic variants in one family and advised caution in assuming that the same pathogenic variant is present in all members of an affected family. Two different *NF1* pathogenic variants have been reported in another family. Meanwhile, possible nonmedical explanations, including alternative paternity or maternity (e.g., with assisted reproduction) or undisclosed adoption, could also explain the discrepancy between clinical diagnoses and genetic testing results in this family.

Germline mosaicism for an *NF1* pathogenic variant has been demonstrated in an apparently unaffected man who had two children with typical NF1 and in a woman with segmental NF who had a child with typical manifestations of NF1 (https://www.ncbi.nlm.nih.gov/books/NBK1109/).

Therefore, all of these explanations might explain the genetic findings in this family.

91. **A.** Pathogenic variants in the *NF1* gene for neurofibromatosis 1 (NF1) can be detected by several molecular methods. Most laboratories offer testing with approximately 70% sensitivity, although there is now a multistep testing method available with an estimated 95% sensitivity. *When an NF1 patient with established clinical diagnosis has a negative test result, the patient is assumed to have a pathogenic variant that is difficult to detect by current technology because of its location or structure.*

Neurofibromatosis 2 (NF2) is completely different from NF1, which is characterized by

bilateral vestibular schwannomas with associated symptoms of tinnitus, hearing loss, and balance dysfunction. The average age at onset is 18−24 years. Neurofibromatosis 3 (NF3) is not a recognized disease.

Therefore, a negative genetic result did not rule out the diagnosis of NF1 in this patient, while a positive genetic result might be used to confirm the diagnosis.

92. **B.** Malignant peripheral-nerve-sheath tumors are the most frequent malignant neoplasms associated with NF1, occurring in approximately 10% of affected individuals. In children with NF1, the most common neoplasms apart from benign neurofibromas are optic-nerve gliomas and brain tumors. Leukemia (especially juvenile chronic myelogenous leukemia and myelodysplastic syndromes) is infrequent in children with NF1 but much more common than in children without NF1. A variety of other tumors may also be seen in individuals with NF1, including gastrointestinal stromal tumors and retinal vasoproliferative tumors. Women with NF1 have a substantially increased risk of developing breast cancer before age 50 years and of dying of breast cancer. People with NF1 may also be at increased risk for many other common cancers (https://www.ncbi.nlm.nih.gov/books/NBK1109/).

Clear-cell renal-cell carcinoma is common in patients with von Hippel−Lindau disease, but is not commonly seen in patients with NF1. Therefore, this teenage girl would be least likely to develop clear-cell renal-cell carcinoma.

93. **B.** *Iris Lisch nodules are a common feature in patients with neurofibromatosis 1 (NF1).*

End-organ damage secondary to iron storage is a feature of hereditary hemochromatosis. Bilateral vestibular schwannomas with associated symptoms of tinnitus, hearing loss, and balance dysfunction are characteristics of neurofibromatosis 2 (NF2). Tuberous sclerosis complex (TSC) involves abnormalities of the skin (hypomelanotic macules, facial angiofibromas, shagreen patches, cephalic plaques, and ungual fibromas); brain (cortical dysplasia, subependymal nodules and subependymal giant-cell astrocytomas [SEGAs], seizures, intellectual disability/developmental delay, psychiatric illness); kidney (angiomyolipomas, cysts, renal-cell carcinomas); heart (rhabdomyomas, arrhythmias); and lungs (lymphangioleiomyomatosis [LAM]) (https://www.ncbi.nlm.nih.gov/books/NBK1220/). Kayser−Fleischer rings are seen in patients with Wilson disease.

Therefore, Lisch nodule is a common feature in patients with neurofibromatosis 1 (NF1).

94. **C.** *Neurofibromatosis 2 (NF2) is characterized by bilateral vestibular schwannomas* with associated symptoms of tinnitus, hearing loss, and balance dysfunction. The average age at onset is 18–24 years. Almost all affected individuals develop bilateral vestibular schwannomas by age 30 years. Affected individuals may also develop schwannomas of other cranial and peripheral nerves, meningiomas, ependymomas, and, very rarely, astrocytomas (https://www.ncbi.nlm.nih.gov/books/NBK1201/).

End-organ damage secondary to iron storage is a feature of hereditary hemochromatosis. Iris Lisch nodules are a common feature in neurofibromatosis 2 (NF1). Tuberous sclerosis complex (TSC) involves abnormalities of the skin (hypomelanotic macules, facial angiofibromas, shagreen patches, cephalic plaques, ungual fibromas); brain (cortical dysplasias, subependymal nodules and subependymal giant cell astrocytomas [SEGAs], seizures, intellectual disability/developmental delay, and psychiatric illness); kidney (angiomyolipomas, cysts, and renal-cell carcinomas); heart (rhabdomyomas and arrhythmias); and lungs (lymphangioleiomyomatosis [LAM]) (https://www.ncbi.nlm.nih.gov/books/NBK1220/). Kayser–Fleischer rings are seen in patients with Wilson disease.

Therefore, vestibular schwannoma is a common feature in patients with NF2.

95. **D.** *Neurofibromatosis 2 (NF2) is characterized by bilateral vestibular schwannomas* with associated symptoms of tinnitus, hearing loss, and balance dysfunction. The average age at onset is 18–24 years. Almost all affected individuals develop bilateral vestibular schwannomas by age 30 years. Affected individuals may also develop schwannomas of other cranial and peripheral nerves, meningiomas, ependymomas, and, very rarely, astrocytomas (https://www.ncbi.nlm.nih.gov/books/NBK1201/).

Neurofibromas and optic-nerve gliomas are common in patients with neurofibromatosis 1 (NF1). Pheochromocytoma can be seen in patients with NF1, too. Pheochromocytoma is also common in patients with pathogenic variants in *VHL*, *RET*, *SDHB*, and *SDHD*.

Therefore, schwannoma is one of the primary tumor types in patients with NF2.

96. **D.** Neurofibromatosis 2 (NF2) is an autosomal dominant condition caused by pathogenic variants in the *NF2* gene. Approximately 50% of individuals with NF2 have an affected parent, and 50% have

NF2 as the result of a de novo pathogenic variant. Locus heterogeneity has not been witnessed in NF2. *However, somatic mosaicism, which may include germline mosaicism, is found in 25%–33% of individuals with NF2 who are simplex cases* (https://www.ncbi.nlm.nih.gov/books/NBK1201/).

Therefore, Sanger sequencing and deletion/duplication testing of *NF2* with specimen from another tissue type, such as fibroblasts, would further assess the possibility of mosaicism, since the patient's symptoms met the clinical criteria for diagnosis of NF2.

97. **C.** Neurofibromatosis 2 (NF2) is an autosomal dominant condition. A single case of germline mosaicism in a clinically normal parent has been reported. In addition, somatic mosaicism (which may include germline mosaicism) is found in 25%–33% of individuals with NF2 who are simplex cases. *Each child of an individual with NF2 has up to a 50% chance of inheriting the pathogenic variant. If the proband is the only affected individual in the family, the proband may have somatic mosaicism for the pathogenic variant.* Offspring of an individual who has mosaicism may have less than a 50% risk of inheriting the pathogenic variant.

Since the proband in this question was the only affected individual in the family, his future child, the fetus, would have up to a 50% risk of inheriting the pathogenic variant for NF2.

98. **D.** The average age at onset for neurofibromatosis 2 (NF2) is 18–24 years. For affected or at-risk individuals, annual MRI should begin at approximately age 10–12 years and continue until at least the fourth decade of life; they should also have hearing evaluations, including BAER testing.

For surveillance, consideration of molecular genetic testing of at-risk asymptomatic family members during childhood is appropriate. Early identification of relatives who have inherited the family-specific *NF2* pathogenic variant allows for appropriate screening using MRI for neuroimaging and brain stem auditory evoked response (BAER) testing for audiological evaluation, thus resulting in earlier detection of disease manifestations and improved final outcomes. Early identification of those who have not inherited the family-specific *NF2* pathogenic variant eliminates the need for costly screening with MRI and BAER testing. Special consideration should be given to education of the children and their parents prior to genetic testing. A plan should be established for the manner of giving results to the parents and children (https://www.ncbi.nlm.nih.gov/books/NBK1201/).

The patient in this question had NF2. According to the family history, his mother might also have NF2. The patient's brother had a 50%

chance to inherit the familial pathogenic variant. Therefore, testing the brother for the familial pathogenic variant would be the most appropriate response to the request.

99. **D.** Tuberous sclerosis complex (TSC) involves abnormalities of the skin, brain, kidney, hear, and lungs. CNS tumors are the leading cause of morbidity and mortality. The diagnosis of TSC is based on clinical findings. Heterozygous pathogenic variants can be identified in 75%–90% of individuals who meet the clinical diagnostic criteria for TSC. *Among those in whom a pathogenic variant can be identified, pathogenic variants in TSC1 are found in 31% and in TSC2 in 69%* (https:// www.ncbi.nlm.nih.gov/books/NBK1220/). *TSC3 is NOT a known gene.*

Therefore, both *TSC1* and *TSC2* would be most likely be tested for a pathogenic variant in this patient, but not *TSC3.*

100. **A.** Tuberous sclerosis complex (TSC), an autosomal dominant condition, is caused by heterozygous pathogenic variants in *TSC1* and *TSC2.* Heterozygous pathogenic variants can be identified in 75%–90% of individuals who meet the clinical diagnostic criteria for TSC. Two-thirds of affected individuals have TSC as the result of a de novo pathogenic variant (https://www.ncbi. nlm.nih.gov/books/NBK1220/).

The penetrance of TSC is now thought to be 100%. In this case, the family history was unremarkable, indicating that the parents likely did not have TSC. Although germline mosaicisms have been reported rarely before, it would be most likely the girl had a de novo pathogenic variant. Therefore, the recurrent risk in this family would most likely be <1%.

101. **E.** Tuberous sclerosis complex (TSC) is inherited in an autosomal dominant manner. *Two thirds of affected individuals have TSC as the result of a de novo pathogenic variant.*

102. **D.** Rett syndrome is a panethnic X-linked dominant disorder with a female prevalence of 1 in 10,000 to 1 in 15,000. It is caused by loss-of-function variants of the *MECP2* gene. Classic Rett syndrome is characterized by apparently normal psychomotor development during the first 6–18 months of life, followed by a short period of developmental stagnation, then rapid regression in language and motor skills, followed by long-term stability. *A pathogenic MECP2 variant in a male is presumed to most often be lethal;* phenotypes in rare surviving males are primarily severe neonatal encephalopathy and manic–depressive psychosis, pyramidal signs, Parkinsonian, and macroorchidism (https://www.ncbi.nlm.nih.gov/

books/NBK1497/; https://ghr.nlm.nih.gov/ condition/rett-syndrome).

Ashkenazi Jews are predisposed to some genetic conditions, such as Gaucher disease, Tay–Sachs disease, and Canavan disease, due to a founder effect. Cystic fibrosis and hereditary hemochromatosis have relatively high prevalence in Caucasians. Thalassemia has a high prevalence in Mediterranean, South Asia, and Africa populations. Rett syndrome does not have a higher prevalence in Ashkenazi Jews, Caucasians, or Mediterranean, South Asia, and Africa populations than other areas of the world.

Therefore, Rett syndrome occurs almost exclusively in girls.

103. **F.** *Rett syndrome is caused by loss-of-function variants of the MECP2 gene.* Two other genes, *CDKL5* and *FOXG1*, can lead to Rett-like phenotypes. *FMR1* is associated with fragile X syndrome. *LIS1* and *DCX* are associated with lissencephaly.

Therefore, *MECP2* would most likely be tested to confirm the diagnosis in this patient.

104. **A.** Rett syndrome, a progressive neurodevelopmental disorder primarily affecting girls, is characterized by apparently normal psychomotor development during the first 6–18 months of life, followed by a short period of developmental stagnation, then rapid regression in language and motor skills, followed by long-term stability. During the phase of rapid regression, repetitive, stereotypic hand movements replace purposeful hand use. Additional findings include fits of screaming and inconsolable crying, autistic features, panic-like attacks, bruxism, episodic apnea and/or hyperpnea, gait ataxia and apraxia, tremors, seizures, and acquired microcephaly. Rett syndrome is caused by pathogenic variants in *MECP2* at Xq28. A pathogenic *MECP2* variant in a male is presumed to most often be lethal. *More than 99% are simplex cases resulting from a de novo pathogenic variant, or possibly from inheritance of the pathogenic variant from a parent who has germline mosaicism.* Rarely, a *MECP2* variant may be inherited from a carrier mother in whom favorable skewing of X-chromosome inactivation results in minimal to no clinical findings (https:// www.ncbi.nlm.nih.gov/books/NBK1497/).

Since a pathogenic variant was identified in this girl, it is appropriate to offer molecular genetic testing to her mother since her father would not be a carrier of the pathogenic *MECP2* variant. However, the detection rate of the target molecular for the mother would most likely be less than 1%.

105. D. Rett syndrome is caused by loss-of-function variants of the *MECP2* gene at Xq28 primarily affecting girls. A pathogenic *MECP2* variant in a male is presumed to most often be lethal. Two other genes, *CDKL5* and *FOXG1*, can lead to Rett-like phenotypes. Pathogenic variants in *CDKL5* at Xp22.13 are most likely to be found in females with early-onset severe seizures who have poor cognitive development but little in the way of Rett syndrome-like features, and they may be found in males with profound intellectual disability and early-onset intractable seizures. Pathogenic variants in *FOXG1* are associated with the congenital form of Rett syndrome. *In contrast to MECP2 and CDKL5, pathogenic variants in FOXG1 on 14q12 are as likely to affect males as female* (https://www.ncbi.nlm.nih.gov/books/NBK1497/).

FMR1 is associated with fragile X syndrome. *LIS1* and *DCX* are associated with lissencephaly.

Therefore, *FOXG1* would most likely be tested to confirm the diagnosis in this male patient.

106. E. Rett syndrome is caused by loss-of-function variants of the *MECP2* gene at Xq28 primarily affecting girls. *Bidirectional sequencing of the entire MECP2 coding region detects pathogenic variants in approximately 80% of individuals with classic Rett syndrome and 40% of individuals with atypical Rett syndrome.* Sequencing analysis of genomic DNA cannot detect deletion of one or more exons or the entire X-linked gene in a heterozygous female. Lack of amplification by PCR prior to sequencing analysis can suggest a putative (multi)exon or whole-gene deletions on the X chromosome in affected males; confirmation may require additional testing by deletion/duplication analysis. The variety of methods that may be used for deletion/duplication analysis are quantitative PCR, long-range PCR, multiplex ligation-dependent probe amplification (MLPA), and chromosomal microarray (CMA) that includes this gene/chromosome segment (https://www.ncbi.nlm.nih.gov/books/NBK1497/).

Therefore, Sanger sequencing of the *MECP2* gene would most likely be used for the genetic study offered to this patient as the first line test.

107. B. *MECP2* duplication syndrome is a panethnic severe neurodevelopmental disorder characterized by infantile hypotonia, delayed psychomotor development leading to severe intellectual disability, poor speech development, progressive spasticity, recurrent respiratory infections (in approximately 75% of affected individuals), and seizures (in approximately 50%). *MECP2 duplication syndrome is 100%*

penetrant in males. Occasionally females have been described with a *MECP2* duplication and related clinical findings, often associated with concomitant X-chromosomal abnormalities that prevent inactivation of the duplicated region. One third of affected males are never able to walk independently. Almost 50% of affected males die before age 25 years.

Therefore, *MECP2* duplication syndrome occurs most often in males.

108. F. Rett syndrome is an X-linked neurodevelopmental disorder that primarily affects girls and is lethal in embryonic males. It is characterized by apparently normal psychomotor development during the first 6–18 months of life, followed by a brief period of developmental stagnation, then rapid regression in language and motor skills, followed by long-term stability. During the phase of rapid regression, repetitive, stereotypic hand movements replace purposeful hand use. Additional findings include fits of screaming and inconsolable crying, autistic features, panic-like attacks, bruxism, episodic apnea and/or hyperpnea, gait ataxia and apraxia, tremors, seizures, and acquired microcephaly. *MECP2* is the only gene, in which pathogenic variants cause Rett syndrome; *80% of patients with classic Rett syndrome have sequence variants detectable by sequencing of the gene*, and 8% of patients with classic Rett syndrome have partial or whole gene deletions, which cannot be detected by sequencing of the gene (https://www.ncbi.nlm.nih.gov/books/NBK1497/).

MECP2 duplication syndrome almost exclusively affects males and is characterized by moderate to severe intellectual disability. Pathogenic variants in *CDKL5* at Xp22.13, encoding cyclin dependent–like kinase 5, have been identified in individuals with a Rett syndrome–like phenotype. *CDKL5* variants are most likely to be found in females with early-onset severe seizures who have poor cognitive development but little in the way of Rett syndrome–like features; it also may be found in males with profound intellectual disability and early-onset intractable seizures. Pathogenic variants in *FOXG1* at 14q12 are associated with the congenital form of Rett syndrome but are as likely to affect males as females.

Therefore, sequencing analysis of the *MECP2* gene would most likely be ordered to confirm or rule out the diagnosis of Rett syndrome in this patient.

109. **A**. *Rett syndrome is an X-linked neurodevelopmental disorder that primarily affects girls and is lethal in embryonic males.*

The patient's older sister had mild mental retardation, which indicated that the mother was an obligate carrier or at least had a germline mosaicism. The patient's future brother would have a 50% chance to be a carrier. Since Rett syndrome is lethal in embryonic males, this pregnancy would most likely end in a miscarriage. Therefore, this future sibling would have less than 1% chance to be affected with Rett syndrome.

110. **C**. All three genes listed in this question are located at X chromosome. *MECP2* duplication syndrome almost exclusively affects males and is characterized by moderate to severe intellectual disability. Most affected males also have hypotonia in infancy, feeding difficulties, poor or absent speech, rigidity, or motor skill development delay/regression. About half of individuals have seizures, often of the tonic—clonic type (https://ghr.nlm.nih.gov). Other features include autistic behaviors and gastrointestinal dysfunction. Half of affected males die by early adulthood. Marked skewing of X-chromosome inactivation occurs in most carrier females. Duplications of *MECP2* ranging from 0.3 to 4 Mb are found in all affected males. Inheritance is X-linked (https://www.ncbi.nlm.nih.gov/books/NBK1284/).

Pathogenic variants in the *ATRX* gene are associated alpha-thalassemia X-linked intellectual disability (ATRX) syndrome. Sequencing analysis of the entire *ATRX* gene may detect 95% of pathogenic variants. Pathogenic variants in the *L1CAM* gene are associated L1 syndrome. Sequencing analysis of *L1CAM* may detect 99% of pathogenic variants. Pathogenic variants in the *MECP2* gene are associated Rett syndrome; 80% of patients with classic Rett syndrome have sequence variants detectable by sequencing of the gene, and 8% of patients with classic Rett syndrome have partial or whole gene deletions, which cannot be detected by sequencing of the gene.

Therefore, deletion and duplication analysis of the *MECP2* gene would most likely be ordered to confirm or rule out the diagnosis in this patient.

111. **A**. The inheritance of epilepsy is complex. At least 20 syndromes whose main feature is epilepsy have been mapped to specific genes, and many more single-gene disorders that cause brain abnormalities or metabolic disorders can have epilepsy as one of their manifestations. Ion channels play vital roles in stabilizing or propagating neuronal activity. Pathogenic variants in genes encoding subunits of ion channels have been found in patients with seizures. *KCNQ2* encodes for a voltage-gated potassium channel. Pathogenic variants in *KCNQ2* cause early infantile epileptic encephalopathy (OMIM# 602235; also called "benign familial neonatal seizures"). *SCN1A* encodes for the alpha subunit of neuronal type 1 sodium channels. Pathogenic variants in *SCN1A* cause familial epilepsy. Pathogenic variants in *MECP2* cause Rett syndrome in females; and seizure is a common characteristic in patients with Rett syndrome.

FOXP3, encoding a member of the fork-winged helix family of transcription factors, plays an important role in the development and function of naturally occurring CD4-positive/CD25-positive T regulatory cells. *Pathogenic variants in FOXP3 cause immunodysregulation, polyendocrinopathy, and enteropathy, X-linked (IPEX).*

Therefore, *FOXP3* would least likely be included in this NGS panel for epilepsy.

112. **D**. Benign familial neonatal seizures (BFNS) is an autosomal dominant condition characterized by recurrent seizures in newborn babies. The seizures begin around day 3 of life and usually go away within 1—4 months. The seizures can be focal or generalized. Many infants with this condition have generalized tonic—clonic seizures (grand mal seizures). *Pathogenic variants in KCNQ2 and KCNQ3 cause BFNS; this occurs more often in KCNQ2 than KCNQ3* (https://ghr.nlm.nih.gov).

The *KCNQ2* and *KCNQ3* genes encode for potassium channels, which transmit a particular type of electrical signal, the M-current, in the central nervous system. The M-current prevents the neuron from activating and overexciting. Pathogenic variants in *KCNQ2* or *KCNQ3* result in a reduced or altered M-current, leading to excessive excitability of neurons. Seizures develop when neurons in the brain are abnormally excited. It is unclear why the seizures stop around the age of 4 months. It has been suggested that other mechanisms develop during infancy.

Voltage-dependent sodium channels are fundamental to the generation of action potentials in excitable cells such as neurons. Pathogenic variants in genes encoding sodium channels may cause overexciting in neurons, leading to seizures. Other ion channels, such as chloride channels, are also related to seizures. But only potassium channels are related to BFNS.

Therefore, it would be most likely that there was a pathogenic variant in potassium channels in this newborn if she has benign familial neonatal seizures.

113. **C.** Pseudohypoparathyroidism (PHP) is a group of disorders with elevated levels of parathyroid hormone (PTH) and biochemical features of hypoparathyroidism, specifically hypocalcemia and hyperphosphatemia, due primarily to resistance to the parathyroid hormone. The disorder is classified as PHP-1A, 1B, ad 1C according to different phenotypic and biochemical findings and based on genetic defects in the hormone receptor adenylate cyclase system. PHP-1A (Albright hereditary osteodystrophy) has a characteristic phenotypic appearance, including short fourth and fifth metacarpals and rounded facies. It is also associated with resistance to thyroid-stimulating hormone. It is most likely an autosomal dominant disorder. PHP-1B has a renal-specific resistance to PTH that lacks the phenotypic features and bone deformities seen in the more classic PHP-1A, but it is biochemically similar. PHP-2 lacks the physical appearance of PHP-1A. Since the genetic defect in PHP-2 is further down the signaling pathway than PHP-1, there is a normal cAMP response to PTH stimulation despite the inherent abnormality in calcium regulation.

PHP-1A, 1B, and 1C are associated with lack of expression/function of the protein Gsα (encoded by the maternal GNAS complex locus) as a result

of: (1) an inactivating *GNAS* pathogenic variant; (2) a genetic alteration in the imprinting regulatory elements in the *GNAS* complex locus or the nearby gene, *STX16*, that prevents proper maternal imprint of the *GNAS* complex locus; (3) isolated epimutations; and (4) uniparental paternal 20q disomy. Familial PHP-1B is, in most instances, caused either by multiexon deletions disrupting the upstream gene *STX16* or (less frequently) by deletions involving *NESP*. The genetic basis for the methylation defect in sporadic PHP-1B is usually unknown; however, *broad GNAS imprinting abnormalities involving multiple GNAS exon A/B differentially methylated regions (DMRs) have been observed in most affected individuals, some of whom had molecular genetic findings consistent with paternal uniparental 20q isodisomy* (https://www.ncbi.nlm.nih.gov/books/NBK459117/).

The patient's family history was unremarkable, indicating that he is likely the only affected member in his family (singleton). Therefore, methylation study would most likely be used to confirm the diagnosis in this patient.

114. **C.** The *GNAS* complex contains at least four distinct differentially methylated regions (DMRs) (see Fig. 12.1 below). Through parent-of-origin effect with differential methylation on its different promoters, the *GNAS* locus would give rise to several transcripts, including alpha-subunit of the heterotrimeric stimulatory G protein α (*Gαs*), the Gαs extra-large variant (*XLαs*), neuroendocrine protein 55 (*NESP55*), untranslated exon A/B (exon 1A) and antisense transcript (*AS*). *The NESP55 is maternal derived while the GNAS XLαs, AS, and A/B transcripts are exclusively paternally*

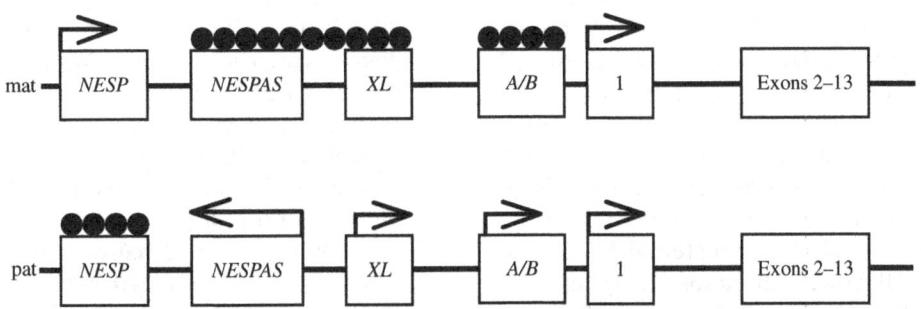

FIGURE 12.1 Schematic of the GNAS complex locus and nearby gene, *STX16*. GNAS exons 1–13 encode Gsα. *STX16* is centromeric to the GNAS complex locus and encodes syntaxin-16. Although *STX16* is not imprinted, the protein product is a *cis*-acting imprinting control element that is necessary for establishing and/or maintaining methylation at *GNAS* exon A/B DMR (also referred to as exon 1A or GNAS A/B: TSS-DMR), thus allowing normal Gsα expression in the proximal renal tubules. Pathogenic deletions are those that occur at the maternally inherited differentially methylated regions. *Source: From Wilkins Jon F, Úbedabeda Francisco. Chapter 13 - Diseases Associated with Genomic Imprinting. Progress in Molecular Biology and Translational Science, Vol 101. Elsevier; 2011. p. 401–45 Available from: https://doi.org/10.1016/B978-0-12-387685-0.00013-5.*

derived. Consistent with this imprinted expression, the promoters of these genes are silenced through methylation. *NESP55* should be methylated at the paternal allele and the *GNAS XLαs*, *AS*, and *A/B* should be methylated at the maternal allele in normal individuals (https://www.ncbi.nlm.nih.gov/books/NBK459117/).

Therefore, only the maternal allele of *NESP55* is expressed. The others listed in the question are exclusively expressed in the paternal copy.

115. **B**. *GNAS* is a complex transcriptional unit with multiple transcript variants through the use of alternative first exons, alternative splicing of downstream exons, antisense transcripts, and reciprocal imprinting. Gsα is encoded by *GNAS* exons 1–13 from the transcript variant NM_000516.5, which is expressed from both maternal and paternal alleles in most cells. However, in some cells (e.g., pituitary somatotropes, proximal renal tubular cells, thyroid epithelial cells, and gonadal cells), Gsα is primarily expressed from the maternal allele; preferential maternal expression may also occur in other tissues. While the Gsα promoter is not methylated, it appears that *cis*-acting elements that control tissue-specific paternal imprinting of Gsα are located within the primary imprint region in exon A/B (also referred to as "exon 1A").

Pseudohypoparathyroidism (PHP)-1A and PHP-1C result from lack of expression of the maternal allele. Pseudopseudohypoparathyroidism (PPHP) results from lack of expression of the paternal allele. Progressive osseous heteroplasia (POH) and osteoma cutis (OC) can be associated with pathogenic variants in either the maternal or paternal allele; however, paternal pathogenic variants are more common. For PHP-1B, the genetic alteration differs in familial cases and simplex cases. Familial PHP-1B genetic alterations include: (1) a pathogenic *GNAS* variant in exon 13 on the maternal allele; (2) *loss of imprinting (methylation) at the maternal GNAS exon A/B DMR (also referred to as exon 1A or GNAS A/B:TSS-DMR);* (3) deletion of maternal *STX16* exons 3–5 or 4–6; (4) deletion of maternal *NESP* and/or *NESP-AS;* and (5) deletion of maternal *STX16*. Simplex PHP-1B genetic alterations include: *GNAS* imprinting abnormalities that involve multiple DMRs and paternal uniparental disomy (UPD) for all or part of chromosome 20 (https://www.ncbi.nlm.nih.gov/books/NBK459117/).

Therefore, it would be most likely that this patient had familial pseudohypoparathyroidism type 1B (PHP-1B).

116. **C**. The *GNAS* complex contains at least four distinct differentially methylated regions (DMRs). Through parent-of-origin effect with differential methylation on its different promoters, the *GNAS* locus would give rise to several transcripts, including the alpha-subunit of the heterotrimeric stimulatory G protein α (Gαs), the Gαs extra-large variant (*XLαs*), neuroendocrine protein 55 (*NESP55*), untranslated exon A/B (exon 1A), and antisense transcript (*AS*). The *NESP55* is maternally derived, while the *GNAS XLαs*, *AS*, and *A/B* transcripts are exclusively paternally derived. Consistent with this imprinted expression, the promoters of these genes are silenced through methylation. *NESP55* should be methylated at the paternal allele and the *GNAS XLαs*, *AS*, and *A/B* should be methylated at the maternal allele in normal individual. Patients with pseudohypoparathyroidism type 1B (PHP-1B) may have paternal uniparental disomy (UPD), methylation defects of *GNAS*, or loss of maternal *GNAS*. *Hypermethylation of maternal copy of NESP55 causes no NESP55 expression, leading to PHP-1B.*

Therefore, hypermethylation of *NESP55* may lead to pseudohypoparathyroidism type 1B (PHP-1B) in this patient.

117. **B**. *Maternally inherited pathogenic variants in GNAS cause pseudohypoparathyroidism (PHP), which can be detected by methylation study.* The c.725Cdel variant in exon 10 of *GNAS* was first reported in a mother with pseudopseudohypoparathyroidism (PPHP) and her daughter with PHP-1A, which results in a frameshift; PPHP is caused by loss-of-function mutations in the *GNAS* gene on the paternal allele. In 2008, the same deletion was reported in an unaffected carrier father and in three of his five children with progressive osseous heteroplasia (POH), which is also caused by a loss-of-function mutation on the paternal allele of *GNAS*. The three children exhibited varying degrees of severity based on the extent of the heterotropic ossification lesions and resultant functional impairment (http://omim.org).

Therefore, a maternally inherited c.725Cdel in *GNAS* is most likely detected in a patient with PHP.

118. **E**. Pseudohypoparathyroidism (PHP) is a group of disorders with elevated levels of parathyroid hormone (PTH) and biochemical features of hypoparathyroidism, specifically hypocalcemia and hyperphosphatemia due primarily to resistance to the parathyroid hormone. PHP-1B is

a renal-specific resistance to PTH that lacks the phenotypic features and bone deformities seen in the more classic PHP-1A, but it is biochemically similar. Paternal uniparental disomy (UPD) and methylation defects of *GNAS*, along with loss of maternal *GNAS*, result in PTH resistance and mineral dysregulation in the proximal renal tubules in PHP-1A and PHP-1B, by leading to loss of function of the Gs-alpha isoform of the *GNAS* gene.

The proband and his three brothers inherited the mutated *GNAS* allele from their mother. Their mother may have pseudopseudohypoparathyroidism (PPHP) or progressive osseous heteroplasia (POH), since she inherited the mutated allele from her father. Therefore, the unborn girl would have 50% risk to inherit the pathogenic variant from the mother to be affected with PHP.

119. **A**. Calcitriol, also called 1,25-dihydroxycholecalciferol or 1,25-dihydroxyvitamin D_3, is the hormonally active metabolite of vitamin D with three hydroxyl groups (1,25-$(OH)_2D_3$). *Patients with pseudohypoparathyroidism (PHP) have hypocalcemia, hyperphosphatemia, elevated parathyroid hormone (PTH), and suppressed calcitriol levels.*

Therefore, increased 1,25-$(OH)_2D_3$ level is NOT common in patients with pseudohypoparathyroidism (PHP).

120. **E**. In 1942, Fuller Albright reported patients with pseudohypoparathyroidism (PHP) who had short stature, obesity, round facies, shortened metacarpals and metatarsals, and PTH resistance causing hypocalcemia and hyperphosphatasemia. Lately, PHP is recognized to be a group of disorders. PHP-1A (Albright hereditary osteodystrophy) has a characteristic phenotypic appearance, including short fourth and fifth metacarpals and rounded facies. It is also associated with thyroid-stimulating—hormone resistance. PHP-1B is a renal-specific resistance to PTH that lacks the phenotypic features and bone deformities seen in the more classic PHP-1A, but it is biochemically similar. In 1952, Fuller Albright described patients with the same physical appearance but without PTH resistance, a condition that he termed "pseudopseudohypoparathyroidism" (PPHP).

Both conditions are caused by loss-of-function variants in the α subunit of the Gs protein encoded by the first 13 exons or intervening introns of the complex *GNAS* gene locus located at 20q13.32. *Maternal transmission causes PHP,*

whereas paternal transmission leads to PPHP or a more progressive form, progressive osseous heteroplasia (POH). The c.344C > T(p.Pro115Leu) pathogenic variant in exon 5 of the *GNAS* gene was first reported in a woman with PPHP; her son with the same mutation had PHP-1A.

Therefore, this male patient's children would have a 50% risk to inherit the pathogenic allele from this patient, and also to be affected with PPHP.

121. **A**. Both pseudohypoparathyroidism (PHP) and pseudopseudohypoparathyroidism (PPHP) are caused by loss-of-function variants in the α subunit of the Gs protein encoded by the first 13 exons or intervening introns of the complex *GNAS* gene locus located at 20q13.32. *Maternal transmission causes pseudohypoparathyroidism (PHP), whereas paternal transmission leads to pseudopseudohypoparathyroidism (PPHP) or a more progressive form, progressive osseous heteroplasia (POH).* The c.344C > T(p.Pro115Leu) pathogenic variant in exon 5 of the *GNAS* gene was first reported in a woman with PPHP; her son with the same mutation had PHP-1A.

Therefore, this female patient's children would have less than 1% risk to develop PPHP but a 50% risk to develop PHP by inheriting the pathogenic allele from this patient.

122. **E**. *The term pseudopseudohypoparathyroidism (PPHP) is used to describe a condition in which the individual has the phenotypic appearance of pseudohypoparathyroidism type 1a (PHP-1A) but is biochemically normal.* Patients with PHP-1A is characterized by end-organ resistance to endocrine hormones, including parathyroid hormone (PTH), thyroid-stimulating hormone (TSH), gonadotropins (LH and FSH), growth-hormone—releasing hormone (GHRH), and CNS neurotransmitters. End-organ resistance to parathyroid hormone (PTH), usually manifests as elevated PTH levels, hyperphosphatemia, and hypocalcemia, in the absence of vitamin D deficiency or magnesium deficiency.

Therefore, none of the biochemical abnormal findings, decreased calcitriol and calcium and increased PTH and phosphates, is common in patients with PPHP.

123. **C**. Prenatal samples obtained by amniocentesis or chorionic villus sampling (CVS) are at risk of contamination by maternal cells, usually due to the presence of maternal blood or deciduas, respectively. *Determining that prenatal specimens are free of significant maternal cell contamination (MCC)*

is important to achieve accurate results for decisions about pregnancy management, especially when the karyotype of the prenatal sample is 46,XX.

Deletions of the *AZFa, AZFb,* and *AZFc* genes on the long arm of the Y chromosome (Yq11.22) have been identified in patients with oligospermia and azoospermia. The *SRY* gene at Yp11.2, also called "testis determining factor," encodes for a DNA-binding protein involving in male sexual development. A female fetus with an X chromosome, that carries the *SRY* gene owing to recombination of the X and Y chromosomes beyond the pseudoautosomal region on the short arms, will develop male characteristics despite not having a Y chromosome. A male fetus with a Y chromosome that has a pathogenic variant, deletion, or translocation leading to loss of *SRY* will not develop testes but will develop a uterus and fallopian tubes. The *AR* gene at Xq12, encoded for androgen receptor, is associated with androgen insensitivity characterized by female external genitalia, female breast development, blind vagina, absent uterus, and abdominal or inguinal testes in affected males with 46,XY. Deficiency of 21-hydroxylase, resulting from pathogenic variants or deletions of *CYP21A*, is the most common form of congenital adrenal hyperplasia (CAH) (90%). Females (46,XX) with severe CAH due to deficiencies of 21-hydroxylase have ambiguous genitalia at birth (classic virilizing adrenal hyperplasia); genital anomalies range from complete fusion of the labioscrotal folds and a phallic urethra to clitoromegaly, partial fusion of the labioscrotal folds, or both.

Waiting until the baby is born does not help perinatal care. Therefore, for this fetus it would be most appropriate to rule out maternal cell contamination in the CV specimen before exploring disorders of sex development.

124. **B.** Disorders of sex development are panethnic and genetically heterogeneous. In patients with complete gonadal dysgenesis, single-nucleotide pathogenic variants, deletions, or translocations of *SRY* are among the most common causes of such disorders. *About 80% of 46,XX males with complete gonadal dysgenesis have a translocation of SRY onto an chromosome X.*

Deletions of the *AZFa, AZFb,* and *AZFc* genes on the long arm of the Y chromosome (Yq11.22) have been identified in patients with oligospermia and azoospermia. The *AR* gene on Xq12, encoded for androgen receptor, is associated with androgen insensitivity characterized by female external genitalia, female

breast development, blind vagina, absent uterus, and abdominal or inguinal testes in affected males with 46,XY. Deficiency of 21-hydroxylase, resulting from pathogenic variants or deletions of *CYP21A*, is the most common form of congenital adrenal hyperplasia (CAH) (90%). Females (46, XX) with severe CAH due to deficiencies of 21-hydroxylase have ambiguous genitalia at birth (classic virilizing adrenal hyperplasia); genital anomalies range from complete fusion of the labioscrotal folds and a phallic urethra to clitoromegaly, partial fusion of the labioscrotal folds, or both.

Therefore, metaphasic FISH with the *SRY* probe would most likely be used as the next step in the evaluation for the sex discrepancy in this fetus.

125. **D.** *The most common cause of ambiguous genitalia is congenital adrenal hyperplasia.* Deficiency of 21-hydroxylase, resulting from pathogenic variants or deletions of *CYP21A*, is the most common form of CAH, accounting for more than 90% of cases. Females with severe congenital adrenal hyperplasia (CAH) due to deficiencies of 21-hydroxylase, 11-beta-hydroxylase, or 3-beta-hydroxysteroid dehydrogenase have ambiguous genitalia at birth (classic virilizing adrenal hyperplasia); genital anomalies range from complete fusion of the labioscrotal folds and a phallic urethra to clitoromegaly, partial fusion of the labioscrotal folds, or both.

In patients with complete gonadal dysgenesis, single-nucleotide pathogenic variants, deletions, or translocations of *SRY* are among the most common causes of such disorders. About 80% of 46,XX males with complete gonadal dysgenesis have a translocation of *SRY* onto an chromosome X. Deletions of the *AZFa, AZFb,* and *AZFc* genes on the long arm of the Y chromosome (Yq11.22) have been identified in patients with oligospermia and azoospermia. The *AR* gene on Xq12, encoded for androgen receptor, is associated with androgen insensitivity characterized by female external genitalia, female breast development, blind vagina, absent uterus, and abdominal or inguinal testes in affected males with 46,XY.

Therefore, sequencing the *CYP21A2* gene for congenital adrenal hyperplasia would most likely be used as the initial evaluation for ambiguous genitalia in this fetus.

126. **B.** Swyer syndrome, or XY gonadal dysgenesis, is a type of hypogonadism in a person whose karyotype is 46,XY. The person is externally female with streak gonads, and left untreated,

will not experience puberty. *Approximately 20%– 30% of 46,XY females with complete gonadal dysgenesis have a pathogenic variant or deletion of the SYR gene.* Other genetic alterations, such as *DAX* duplication, autosomal deletions (1p, 2q, 9p, and 10q), and *WT1* pathogenic variants, may also cause XY gonadal dysgenesis.

Exome sequencing is very effective in the study of rare Mendelian diseases corresponding with unknown genetic disorders. Therefore, exome sequencing is not appropriate until the above genetic etiologies are excluded.

127. **A.** Females with a 46,XY karyotype have complete gonadal dysgenesis and are usually taller than average women. An important clinical feature is the increased risk of dysgerminoma or gonadoblastoma, which is approximately 20%– 30% without medical intervention. Neoplasia may even arise in the first or second decade. In any XY female experiencing secondary sexual development (breasts, pubic hair), hormone-producing neoplasia (dysgerminoma, gonadoblastoma) should be suspected. *But breast cancer has no increased risk among females with 46, XY.*

Therefore, this newborn would not have increased risk of developing breast cancer.

128. **B.** Most of 46,XX male patients have a normal *SRY* gene translocated to an X chromosome, especially when the patients have a normal male appearance at birth. In patients without the *SRY* gene, duplication of *SOX3*, or *SOX9* have been described. Similarly pathogenic variants in *CYP21A2* may result in a 46,XX male. However, *pathogenic variants in SOX9 may result in a 46,XY female but not a 46,XX male.*

Therefore, sequencing analysis of *SOX9* would least likely be part of the workup for the diagnosis in this 46,XX male infant.

129. **D.** The Prader–Willi/Angelman critical region is located at 15q11q13. There are different mechanisms for the disease (see the table below). The deletion is about 5–6 Mb in most patients, which is suitable for FISH and chromosomal microarray analysis. But it is quite challenging by chromosome karyotyping, even with high-resolution analysis. Methylation analysis may identify patients with Prader–Willi/Angelman syndrome caused by deletion, UPD, and imprinting center pathogenic variants (https:// decipher.sanger.ac.uk/syndrome). *It determines whether the region is maternally inherited only (e.g., the paternally contributed region is absent) and detects more than 99% of affected individuals* (https:// www.ncbi.nlm.nih.gov/books/NBK1330/).

Therefore, methylation study would most likely be used as the initial genetic evaluation for this patient.

Mechanism	Prader–Willi syndrome	Angelman syndrome
15q11.2q13 deletion	70% (paternal)	70% (maternal)
Uniparental disomy (UPD)	20%–30% (maternal)	7% (paternal)
Imprinting center defect	2.50%	3%
Pathogenic variant in genes	Rare	10% (*UBE3A*)
Unidentified	<1%	10%

130. **D.** The Prader–Willi/Angelman critical region is located at 15q11q13. There are different mechanisms for the disease (see the table below). The deletion is about 5–6 Mb in most patients, which is suitable for FISH and chromosomal microarray analysis. But it is quite challenge by chromosome karyotyping, even with high-resolution analysis. Methylation analysis may identify patients with Prader–Willi/Angelman syndrome caused by deletion, UPD, and imprinting center pathogenic variants (https:// decipher.sanger.ac.uk/syndrome). *It determines whether the region is paternally inherited only (e.g., the maternally contributed region is absent) and detects approximately 80% of affected individuals* (https://www.ncbi.nlm.nih.gov/books/ NBK1144/).

Therefore, methylation study would most likely be used as the initial genetic evaluation for this patient.

Mechanism	Prader–Willi syndrome	Angelman syndrome
15q11.2q13 deletion	70% (paternal)	70% (maternal)
Uniparental disomy (UPD)	20%–30% (maternal)	7% (paternal)
Imprinting center defect	2.50%	3%
Pathogenic variant in genes	Rare	10% (*UBE3A*)
Unidentified	<1%	10%

131. **A.** Angelman syndrome (AS) and Prader–Willi syndrome (PWS) are clinically distinct neurodevelopmental genetic disorders mapped to 15q11q13. The primary phenotypes are attributable to loss of expression of imprinted

genes within this region arising by deletion, uniparental disomy (UPD), imprinting defect, or pathogenic variants. *SNRPN* DNA methylation analysis detects in greater than 99% of PWS cases, and approximately 80% of AS cases. In AS, the major disease mechanism is either a de novo maternally derived deletion of 15q11q13, paternal UPD, or an imprinting defect affecting the maternal chromosome. In addition, *single-nucleotide pathogenic variants in the E6-AP ubiquitin-protein ligase gene (UBE3A) are also known to cause AS* (https://www.ncbi.nlm.nih.gov/books/NBK1144/).

Therefore, sequencing analysis of *UBE3A* may facilitate diagnosis of AS when the methylation study is negative and the physician still highly suspects AS.

132. **B**. Prader−Willi syndrome (PWS) and Angelman syndrome (AS) are clinically distinct neurodevelopmental genetic disorders mapped to 15q11q13. The primary phenotypes are attributable to loss of expression of imprinted genes within this region arising by deletion, uniparental disomy (UPD), imprinting defect, or pathogenic variants. The most sensitive single approach to diagnosing both PWS and AS is to study methylation patterns within 15q11q13 irrespective of the molecular class. *SNRPN has differentially methylated CpG islands in its promoter region that are methylated on the maternal chromosome leading to silencing of the maternal allele.* DNA methylation studies may detect abnormal parent-specific imprinting within the Prader−Willi critical region (PWCR) on chromosome 15. *This testing determines whether the region is maternally inherited only (e.g., the paternally contributed region is absent). If so, the patient has PWS.* If only paternal unmethylated alleles exist, the patient has AS. However, this molecular assay cannot be used to detect whether the PWS/AS is cause by deletions, uniparental disomy (UPD), imprinting defects, or pathogenic variants in *UBE3A* (https://www.ncbi.nlm.nih.gov/books/NBK1330/ and https://www.ncbi.nlm.nih.gov/books/NBK1144/).

Therefore, the test result in this prevalidation was diagnostic for Prader−Willi syndrome, since only one band for methylated allele (maternal allele) was detected after sodium bisulfite treatment.

133. **A**. Prader−Willi syndrome (PWS) and Angelman syndrome (AS) are clinically distinct neurodevelopmental genetic disorders mapped to 15q11q13. The primary phenotypes are attributable to loss of expression of imprinted genes within this region arising from deletions, uniparental disomy (UPD), imprinting defects, or pathogenic variants. The most sensitive single approach to diagnosing both PWS and AS is to study methylation patterns within 15q11q13 irrespective of the molecular class. *SNRPN has differentially methylated CpG islands in its promoter region that are methylated on the maternal chromosome leading to silencing of the maternal allele.* DNA methylation studies may detect abnormal parent-specific imprinting within the Prader−Willi critical region (PWCR) on chromosome 15. This testing determines whether the region is maternally inherited only (for example, the paternally contributed region is absent). If so, the patient has PWS. *If only paternal unmethylated allele exists, the patient has AS.* However, this molecular assay cannot be used to tell if the PWS/AS is cause by deletions, uniparental disomy (UPD), imprinting defects, or pathogenic variants in *UBE3A* (https://www.ncbi.nlm.nih.gov/books/NBK1330/ and https://www.ncbi.nlm.nih.gov/books/NBK1144/).

Therefore, the test result in this prevalidation was diagnostic for Angelman syndrome since only one band for unmethylated allele (paternal allele) was detected after sodium bisulfite treatment.

134. **A**. *The imprinting center at the Prader−Willi/Angelman critical region on 15q11q13 is located at the 5′ of SNRPN.*

135. **B**. The Prader−Willi/Angelman critical region is located at 15q. There are different mechanisms for the disease (see the table below). Methylation analysis may identify Prader−Willi/Angelman syndrome caused by deletion, UPD, and imprinting center defects. *Methylation studies determine whether the region is paternally inherited only (e.g., the maternally contributed region is absent) and detects approximately 80% of patients with Angelman syndrome.* Pathogenic variants in the *UBE3A* gene (10%) cannot be detected by methylation study targeted at the 5′ of *SNRPN*. Methylation study cannot detect 10% unidentified genetic factors for Angelman syndrome (AS).

Therefore, the detection rate (clinical sensitivity) of a methylation study would be 80% if the patient had Angelman syndrome.

Mechanism	Prader–Willi syndrome	Angelman syndrome
15q11.2q13 deletion	70% (paternal)	70% (maternal)
Uniparental disomy (UPD)	20%–30% (maternal)	7% (paternal)
Imprinting center defect	2.50%	3%
Pathogenic variant in genes	Rare	10% (UBE3A)
Unidentified	<1%	10%

136. **F**. The diagnosis of Angelman syndrome (AS) is established in a proband with DNA methylation analysis demonstrating abnormal parent-specific imprinting within the Prader–Willi/Angelman critical region at chromosome 15, in which the region demonstrates paternal-only imprinting, such as the absence of maternal-only expressed genes due to a deletion. The three main molecular mechanisms that result in AS include maternal deletion, paternal uniparental disomy (UPD) 15, and imprinting defect (ID). DNA methylation analysis is the only technique that will diagnose AS caused by all three genetic mechanisms as well as differentiate AS from Prader–Willi syndrome (PWS). *A DNA methylation analysis consistent with AS is sufficient for clinical diagnosis but not for genetic counseling, which requires identification of the underlying genetic mechanism.* So DNA methylation analysis is typically the first test ordered; then methylation-specific multiplex ligation-dependent probe amplification (MS-MLPA), karyotype, FISH, chromosomal microarray, DNA polymorphism, or DNA sequencing may be used to further define the underlying genetic mechanism (https://www.ncbi.nlm.nih.gov/books/NBK1144/).

Therefore, choice F is correct that the methylation study ordered for this patient did not define the underlying genetic mechanism.

137. **D**. Angelman syndrome is caused by one of the following mechanisms (see the table below). DNA methylation analysis is typically the first test ordered to establish the diagnosis. Individuals with AS caused by a 5–7-Mb deletion of 15q11.2q13, uniparental disomy (UPD), or an imprinting defect (ID) have only an unmethylated copy, usually paternal. DNA methylation analysis identifies approximately 80% of individuals with AS. Most commercially available DNA methylation studies cannot distinguish between AS resulting from a deletion, a UPD, or an ID.

Further testing is required to identify the underlying molecular mechanism.

The size of the Prader–Willi and Angelman critical region reaches to the limitation of chromosome karyotype. Fewer than 1% of individuals with AS have a cytogenetically visible chromosome rearrangement, such as translocation or inversion, of chromosome 15 involving 15q11.2q13. FISH analysis with the D15S10 and/or the *SNRPN* probe can identify the 15q11.2q13 deletion, which is not detected by routine cytogenetic analysis. Positive FISH results confirm that there is a deletion at the critical region, but it cannot be used to tell the size and genomic content of the deletion. Chromosomal oligonucleotide microarray (CMA) analysis has a slightly higher detection frequency for deletions than FISH, and it provides detailed information regarding size and gene content of the deletion. Comparing with oligonucleotide array, *SNP-based CMA may also detect uniparental isodisomies in addition to deletions.* However, SNP array cannot detect heterodisomy. Heterodisomy may be detected using polymorphic DNA markers, requiring a DNA sample from the affected individual and both parents (https://www.ncbi.nlm.nih.gov/books/NBK1144/).

Therefore, SNP microarray would be the best choice as the next step in the workup to further explore the genetic mechanism of AS in this patient.

Mechanism	Prader–Willi syndrome	Angelman syndrome
15q11.2q13 deletion	70% (paternal)	70% (maternal)
Uniparental disomy (UPD)	20%–30% (maternal)	7% (paternal)
Imprinting center defect	2.50%	3%
Pathogenic variant in genes	Rare	10% (UBE3A)
Unidentified	<1%	10%

138. **C**. The diagnosis of Angelman syndrome (AS) is established in a proband with DNA methylation analysis demonstrating abnormal parent-specific imprinting within the Prader–Willi/Angelman critical region at chromosome 15, in which the region demonstrates paternal-only imprinting, such as the absence of maternal-only expressed genes. *Three main molecular mechanisms that result in AS include maternal deletion, paternal uniparental disomy (UPD) 15, and imprinting defect (ID)*

(https://www.ncbi.nlm.nih.gov/books/ NBK1144/). Prader–Willi syndrome (PWS) caused by paternal deletion of the 15q11.2q13 region, maternal uniparental disomy (UPD) 15, and imprinting defect (ID).

This patient had AS, confirmed by methylation study. The SNP array detected a region of copy neutral loss of heterozygosity (ROH) on 15q11.2q13, indicating UPD. Therefore, paternal UPD would be the most appropriate interpretation of the genetic etiology of AS in this patient.

139. E. Angelman syndrome (AS) is caused by defects in the maternally derived imprinted region at 15q11.13, which can arise in a variety of ways. Interstitial deletion of maternally derived 15q11q13 is the most common type, accounting for 70% of cases. Paternal uniparental disomy (UPD) 15q (2%–5%), an imprinting defect (2%–5%), or pathogenic variants in the E3 ubiquitin protein ligase gene (*UBE3A*) (5%–10%) are other mechanisms, and in a small percentage the molecular mechanism is currently unidentified. All patients with an interstitial deletion, UPD or an imprinting defect approximately 80% in total have an *SNRPN* methylation abnormality (only unmethylated alleles). Normal individuals show one methylated (maternal) and one unmethylated (paternal) allele. *Patients with UBE3A pathogenic variants, AS of unidentified cause, and those with a phenocopy of AS but a different disorder will all show normal results on the SNRPN methylation assay* (https://decipher.sanger.ac.uk/syndrome).

Therefore, pathogenic variants in sequencing analysis of *UBE3A* would most likely be used as the next step in the workup to further confirm/ rule out the Angelman syndrome in this patient after the negative methylation study.

140. C. *UBE3A* pathogenic variants can be inherited or de novo. Approximately 30% of pathogenic variants are inherited. Familial studies should be offered to establish maternal inheritance or lack of paternal inheritance. In addition, several cases of somatic and germline mosaicism for a *UBE3A* pathogenic variant have been noted. If a proband's mother has a *UBE3A* pathogenic variant, the risk to the sibs is 50%. If a proband's mother carries a known imprinting center (IC) deletion or *UBE3A* pathogenic variant, the mother's sibs are also at risk of carrying the IC deletion or the pathogenic variant. *Each child of the unaffected carrier sister is at a 50% risk of having AS.* Unaffected maternal uncles of the proband who are carriers are not at risk of having affected

children, but are at risk of having affected grandchildren through their unaffected daughters who inherited the IC deletion or *UBE3A* pathogenic variant from them (https://www. ncbi.nlm.nih.gov/books/NBK1144/).

Therefore, this patient's maternal aunt would have 50% risk to have a child with Angelman syndrome.

141. A. *UBE3A* pathogenic variants can be inherited or de novo. Approximately 30% of pathogenic variants are inherited. Familial studies should be offered to establish maternal inheritance or lack of paternal inheritance. In addition, several cases of somatic and germline mosaicism for a *UBE3A* pathogenic variant have been noted. If a proband's mother has a *UBE3A* pathogenic variant, the risk to the sibs is 50%. If a proband's mother carries a known imprinting center (IC) deletion or *UBE3A* pathogenic variant, the mother's sibs are also at risk of carrying the IC deletion or the pathogenic variant. Each child of the unaffected carrier sister is at a 50% risk of having AS. *Unaffected maternal uncles of the proband who are carriers are not at risk of having affected children, but are at risk of having affected grandchildren through their unaffected daughters who inherited the IC deletion or UBE3A pathogenic variant from them* (https://www.ncbi. nlm.nih.gov/books/NBK1144/).

Therefore, this patient's maternal uncle would have <1% risk of having a child with Angelman syndrome.

142. F. The unconventional nomenclature of *SERPINA1* alleles is based on electrophoretic protein variants that were identified long before the gene (*SERPINA1*) was known. Alleles were named with the prefix PI* (protease inhibitor*) serving as an alias for the gene. Using this nomenclature, PI*Z is the most common pathogenic allele, resulting in functionally deficient alpha-1 antitrypsin protein. Individuals homozygous for PI*Z (PI*ZZ) have a serum concentration of alpha-1 antitrypsin (AAT) that is approximately 10%–20% of normal (serum levels of 20–35 mg/dL) and are at high risk for both liver and lung disease. *This genotype (PI*ZZ) is present in 95% of affected individuals with clinical manifestations of alpha-1 antitrypsin deficiency (AATD).* Variable disease expressivity in individuals with the PI*ZZ genotype—not accounted for by the presence of known risk factors such as cigarette smoking—suggests the existence of other as-yet unidentified genetic disease modifiers. (https://www.ncbi.nlm.nih. gov/books/NBK1519/).

Therefore, PI*ZZ is the most common pathogenic genotype in patients with alpha-1 antitrypsin deficiency.

143. A. PI*M is the most common (normal) allele in the *SERPINA1* gene. *PI*MM is the most common genotype, with a prevalence of more than 90% worldwide.* This genotype is associated with a normal serum concentration of AAT and no increased risk of liver or lung disease (https://www.ncbi.nlm.nih.gov/books/NBK1519/).

PI*SS is not considered to be associated with an increased risk for the clinical symptoms. The S allele is most common among individuals of Iberian descent. Individuals with PI*null-null (sometimes designated PI*QO) have no measurable serum AAT secondary to a complete lack of synthesis of AAT. Because the protein does not accumulate in the liver, these individuals are not at increased risk of developing liver disease; however, they are at increased risk of developing lung disease. Individuals with PI*ZZ have a serum concentration of AAT that is approximately 10%–20% of normal (serum levels of 20–35 mg/dL) and are at increased risk for both liver and lung disease. This genotype is present in 95% of affected individuals with clinical manifestations of alpha-1 antitrypsin deficiency (AATD).

Therefore, the PI*M/M genotype of the *SERPINA1* gene is the most common one in apparently healthy individuals worldwide.

144. B. Alpha-1 antitrypsin deficiency (AATD) is characterized by an increased risk for chronic obstructive pulmonary disease, such as emphysema, persistent airflow obstruction, and/or chronic bronchitis in adults and liver disease in children and adults. The incidence of liver disease increases with age. Liver disease in adults, manifesting as cirrhosis and fibrosis, may occur in the absence of a history of neonatal or childhood liver disease. *The risk for hepatocellular carcinoma (HCC) is increased several times in individuals with AATD and the PI*ZZ genotype that typically associated with liver cirrhosis.* The incidence of hepatocellular carcinoma is estimated at more than 1.5% per year. This increased risk has been attributed to failure of apoptosis of injured cells with retained Z protein, which sends a chronic regeneration signal to hepatocytes with a lesser load of retained Z protein (https://www.ncbi.nlm.nih.gov/books/NBK1519/).

Therefore, patients with AATD have increased risk to develop hepatocellular carcinoma in comparison with individuals from general populations.

145. C. *Smoking (both active and passive) dramatically influences the likelihood of emphysema in patients with alpha-1 antitrypsin deficiency (AATD), caused by pathogenic variants in SERPINA1.* For individuals with the PI*Z/Z genotype, survival after 60 years of age is approximately 60% in nonsmokers but only approximately 10% in smokers (https://www.ncbi.nlm.nih.gov/books/NBK1519/).

Therefore, smoking is the most important environmental factor for the manifestation of the disease.

146. B. *Smith–Lemli–Opitz syndrome (SLOS) is an autosomal recessive condition caused by deficiency of the enzyme 7-dehydrocholesterol (7-DHC) reductase.* It is characterized by prenatal and postnatal growth retardation, microcephaly, moderate to severe intellectual disability, and multiple major and minor malformations. The malformations include distinctive facial features, cleft palate, cardiac defects, underdeveloped external genitalia in males, postaxial polydactyly, and 2/3 toes syndactyly. The clinical spectrum is wide, and individuals have been described with normal development and only minor malformations. The diagnosis of SLOS relies on clinical suspicion and detection of an elevated serum concentration of 7-DHC. Molecular genetics testing of *DHCR7* is generally considered a second-tier test and may be useful in instances in which serum concentration of 7-DHC is difficult to interpret or in which only DNA from the affected individual is available. Sequencing analysis of *DHCR7* on 11q13.4 may identify 96% of all the pathogenic variants in the *DHCR7* gene (https://www.ncbi.nlm.nih.gov/books/NBK1143/).

21-Hydroxylase deficiency is one of the most common types of congenital adrenal hyperplasia (CAH), a condition involving impaired synthesis of cortisol from cholesterol by the adrenal cortex. Deletion of *SRY* causes azoospermia or oligospermia.

Therefore, an elevated serum concentration of 7-DHC is diagnostic for SLOS in this patient, even though only a heterozygous pathogenic variant was identified.

147. A. Smith–Lemli–Opitz syndrome (SLOS) is an autosomal recessive condition caused by deficiency of the enzyme 7-dehydrocholesterol (7-DHC) reductase. The diagnosis of SLOS relies on clinical suspicion and detection of an elevated serum concentration of 7-DHC. *The finding of an abnormal concentration of 7-DHC in amniotic fluid obtained by amniocentesis, usually performed at approximately 15–18 weeks' gestation or in tissue obtained from chorionic villus samples (CVS) at* *approximately 10—12 weeks' gestation, is diagnostic.* If the two pathogenic variants in *DHCR7* have been identified in the proband, molecular genetic testing may be used in place of biochemical testing or to clarify indeterminate results (https://www.ncbi.nlm.nih.gov/books/NBK1143/).

Therefore, measuring 7-dehydrocholesterol concentration in amniotic fluid would be the most appropriate initial workup to confirm or rule out the diagnosis in this fetus.

148. **B**. *Smith—Lemli—Opitz syndrome (SLOS) is an autosomal recessive condition*, caused by deficiency of the enzyme 7-dehydrocholesterol (7-DHC) reductase. The diagnosis of SLOS relies on clinical suspicion and detection of an elevated serum concentration of 7-DHC.

The elevated serum concentration of 7-DHC is diagnostic for SLOS in this patient, even though only a heterozygous pathogenic variant was identified. The parents of the proband are obligate carriers and carry one mutated allele. Therefore, the recurrent risk of same condition is approximately 25% in this family.

149. **D**. L1 syndrome is an X-linked condition caused by pathogenic variants in the *L1CAM* gene at Xq28. It is characterized by severe hydrocephalus, adducted thumbs, spasticity, developmental delay, and intellectual disability in males. The diagnosis of L1 syndrome can be established in males with characteristic clinical and neuropathological findings and a family history consistent with X-linked inheritance. Of note, bilateral absence of the pyramids detected by MRI or autopsy is an almost pathognomonic finding. Detection of a hemizygous pathogenic variant in *L1CAM* confirms the diagnosis of L1 syndrome. *Sequencing analysis of the L1CAM gene may detect pathogenic variants in 99% of affected males and 98% of carrier females* (https://www.ncbi.nlm.nih.gov/books/NBK1484/).

HPLC for hemoglobin may be used to rule out alpha-thalassemia X-linked intellectual disability syndrome, which is caused by pathogenic variants in the *ATRX* gene on Xq21.1. Pathogenic variants in the *MECP2* gene on Xq28 are associated with Rett syndrome in females, which is lethal in embryonic males. *MECP2* duplication syndrome almost exclusively affects males and is characterized by moderate to severe intellectual disability.

Therefore, sequencing analysis of the *L1CAM* gene would most likely be ordered to confirm or rule out the diagnosis of L1 syndrome in this patient.

150. **G**. L1 syndrome is an X-linked condition caused by pathogenic variants in the *L1CAM* gene at Xq28. If a male is the only affected family member (i.e., a simplex case), the mother may be a carrier or the affected male may have de novo *L1CAM* pathogenic variant and, thus, the mother is not a carrier. About 40% of affected males represent simplex cases. It has been shown that approximately 7% of all pathogenic variants detected represent a de novo mutation in the proband or maternal germline mosaicism. The recurrent risk of the same condition in the family depends on the carrier status of the mother. If the mother of the proband has an *L1CAM* pathogenic variant, the chance of transmitting it in each pregnancy is 50%. Males who inherit the pathogenic variant will be affected; females who inherit the pathogenic variant will be carriers and may have some manifestations. If the proband represents a simplex case and if the *L1CAM* pathogenic variant cannot be detected in the leukocyte DNA of the mother, the risk to sibs is low but greater than that of the general population because of the possibility of maternal germline mosaicism (https://www.ncbi.nlm.nih.gov/books/NBK1484/).

Therefore, the recurrent risk of L1 syndrome is not predictable in this family before testing the mother.

151. **B**. L1 syndrome is an X-linked condition caused by pathogenic variants in the *L1CAM* gene at Xq28. In this case, the boy was the only affected family member, and *the risk to sibs depends on the carrier status of the mother*. The mother may be a carrier. Or the affected boy may have a de novo *L1CAM* pathogenic variant and, thus, the mother is not a carrier (https://www.ncbi.nlm.nih.gov/books/NBK1484/).

Therefore, targeted variant analysis of the mother would most likely be used as the first step in the workup to assess the recurrent risk of the same condition in the family.

152. **B**. L1 syndrome is an X-linked condition caused by pathogenic variants in the *L1CAM* gene at Xq28. It is characterized by severe hydrocephalus, adducted thumbs, spasticity, developmental delay, and intellectual disability in males.

The husband's nephews were affected. *It is uncertain whether the husband's brothers were affected.* The couple and the husband's father were not affected; the husband's sisters most likely are carriers; and the husband's mother may be a carrier, or have a mosaicism. Therefore, testing one of the husband's affected nephews first would most likely detect a pathogenic variant if there was one in the family. The other then may be tested with a targeted approach.

153. C. L1 syndrome is an X-linked condition caused by pathogenic variants in the *L1CAM* gene at Xq28. According to the family history the husband's mother may be a silent carrier. The husband's father was asymptomatic, and most likely he did not have the familial pathogenic variants.

Therefore, the husband's father would least likely be tested due to the minimal risk.

154. A. L1 syndrome is an X-linked condition caused by pathogenic variants in the *L1CAM* gene at Xq28. According to the family history, the husband's nephews were affected, the couple and the husband's father were not affected, the husband's sisters most likely are carriers, and the husband's mother may be a carrier or have a mosaicism. The husband's brothers may be affected.

Since the husband did not have symptoms of L1 syndrome. It would be most likely he did not carry the familial pathogenic variant, since L1 syndrome is an X-linked condition. Therefore, the couple's risk of having a child with L1 syndrome was <1%.

155. C. Alpha-thalassemia X-linked intellectual disability (ATRX) syndrome is an X-linked condition, characterized by distinctive craniofacial features, genital anomalies, severe developmental delays, hypotonia, intellectual disability, and mild to moderate anemia secondary to alpha-thalassemia. Craniofacial abnormalities include small head circumference, telecanthus or widely spaced eyes, short nose, tented vermilion of the upper lip, and thick or everted vermilion of the lower lip with coarsening of the facial features over time. HbH inclusions (β-globin tetramers) in erythrocytes can be demonstrated following incubation of fresh blood smears with 1% brilliant cresyl blue (BCB). The proportion of cells with HbH inclusions ranges from 0.01%−30%. *ATRX* at Xq21.1 is the only gene in which pathogenic variants cause ATRX syndrome. *Sequencing analysis of the entire ATRX gene may detect 95% of pathogenic variants.* HPLC for hemoglobinopathy helps to identify abnormal hemoglobin seen in patients with ATRX syndrome (https://www.ncbi.nlm.nih.gov/books/NBK1449/).

Pathogenic variants in *RPS6KA3* cause Coffin−Lowry syndrome (CLS), also an X-linked condition, characterized by severe to profound intellectual disability in males and normal intelligence to profound intellectual disability in heterozygous females. Hemoglobin H (HbH) disease, one of the two clinically significant forms of alpha-thalassemia, results from reduced production of the α chains of adult hemoglobin

(designated Hb $\alpha^2\beta^2$). In individuals with developmental delay who are of Mediterranean, Southeast Asian, or African American origin, it is appropriate to determine the α-globin genotype. Alpha-thalassemia mental retardation chromosome 16 (ATR-16) (OMIM# 141750) is the association of alpha-thalassemia and intellectual disability in individuals with a contiguous gene deletion involving the distal short arm of chromosome 16. Pathogenic variants in the *MECP2* gene at Xq28 are associated Rett syndrome in females, which is lethal in embryonic males. *MECP2* duplication syndrome almost exclusively affects in males characterized by moderate to severe intellectual disability (https://ghr.nlm.nih.gov).

Therefore, sequencing analysis of the *ATRX* gene would most likely be ordered to confirm or rule out the diagnosis of ATRX syndrome in this patient.

156. B. Alpha-thalassemia X-linked intellectual disability (ATRX) syndrome is an X-linked condition. *ATRX* on Xq21.1 is the only gene in which pathogenic variants cause ATRX syndrome. In families with only one affected individual, the mother may be a carrier, or the affected individual may have ATRX syndrome as a result of a de novo pathogenic variant. If the mother of the proband has a pathogenic variant, the chance of transmitting it is 50% in each pregnancy. Sibs with a 46,XY karyotype who inherit the pathogenic variant will be affected; sibs with a 46,XX karyotype, who inherit the pathogenic variant are female carriers and will not be affected (https://www.ncbi.nlm.nih.gov/books/NBK1449/).

Therefore, the boy's mother should be tested first in order to determine if the pathogenic variant was de novo or inherited before cascade testing in the rest of the family.

157. B. Cowden syndrome is a multiple hamartoma syndrome caused by pathogenic variants in the *PTEN* gene. Patients with Cowden syndrome have an increased risk for benign and malignant tumors of the thyroid, breast, and endometrium. Affected individuals usually have macrocephaly, trichilemmomas, and papillomatous papules, and present by the late 20s. The lifetime risk of developing breast cancer is 85%, with an average age of diagnosis between 38 and 46 years. The lifetime risk for thyroid cancer (usually follicular, rarely papillary, but never medullary thyroid cancer) is approximately 35%. The risk for endometrial cancer may approach 28% (https://www.ncbi.nlm.nih.gov/books/NBK1488/).

Cardiofaciocutaneous (CFC) syndrome, LEOPARD syndrome, and Noonan syndrome may be caused by heterozygous pathogenic variants in the *BRAF* gene.

Therefore, constitutional *BRAF* pathogenic variants have NOT been detected in patients with Cowden syndrome.

158. **E.** Noonan syndrome (NS) is an autosomal dominant condition, characterized by dysmorphic facial features, short stature, congenital heart defect, and developmental delay of variable degree. Affected individuals have normal chromosome studies. Molecular genetics testing identifies a pathogenic variant in *PTPN11* in 50% of affected individuals, *SOS1* in approximately 13%, *RAF1* and *RIT1* each in 5%, and *KRAS* in fewer than 5%. Other genes in which pathogenic variants have been reported to cause Noonan syndrome in less than 1% of cases include *NRAS*, *BRAF*, and *MAP2K1*. Several additional genes associated with a Noonan syndrome—like phenotype in fewer than 10 individuals have been identified, such as *SH3BP2*, *SHOC2*, and *CBL* (https://www.ncbi.nlm. nih.gov/books/NBK1124/).

dHPLC (denaturing high-performance liquid chromatography) was used to screen for SNPs in the late 1990s and early 2000s for research, but it has limited utility in clinical laboratories for diagnosis. Exome sequencing has been reserved for patients with clinical presentations, suggesting a genetic etiology, but a lack of characteristics of known genetic conditions. Chromosomal microarray and multiplex ligation-dependent probe amplification (MLPA) assays are used to detect gains (duplications) and losses (deletions). Sequencing analysis of all exons of *PTPN11* detects missense pathogenic variants in about 50% of individuals tested. Nowadays next-generation sequencing (NGS) with all the genes involved would be the most cost-effective and sensitive method.

Therefore, a next-generation sequence (NGS) panel would most likely be used to confirm/rule out the diagnosis in this patient.

159. **A.** All of the genes listed in this question are associated with Noonan syndrome except *KIT*. Therefore, *KIT* would least likely harbor a pathogenic variant in this patient for Noonan syndrome.

160. **C.** Individuals with Noonan syndrome are at an eightfold increased risk of developing a childhood cancer than are those without Noonan syndrome. They have a predisposition to juvenile myelomonocytic leukemia (JMML), acute lymphoblastic leukemia (ALL) and acute myeloid leukemia (AML), and myeloproliferative disorders (MDS). Solid tumors reported in patients with Noonan syndrome are rhabdomyosarcoma, neuroblastoma, and brain tumor (https://www. ncbi.nlm.nih.gov/books/NBK1124/).

Colorectal cancer (CRC) is an adult on-set malignancy; it has not been reported that patients with Noonan syndrome tend to have CRC. Therefore, it is considered that this patient would NOT have an increased risk to develop colorectal cancer because of his Noonan syndrome.

161. **F.** Sotos syndrome is an autosomal dominant condition, characterized by a distinctive facial appearance with broad and prominent forehead, sparse frontotemporal hair, downslanting palpebral fissures, malar flushing, long and narrow face, long chin, learning disability, early developmental delay, mild to severe intellectual impairment, and overgrowth (height and/or head circumference ≥ 2 SD above the mean). Minor features of Sotos syndrome include behavioral problems, advanced bone age, cardiac anomalies, cranial MRI/CT abnormalities, joint hyperlaxity/pes planus, maternal preeclampsia, neonatal jaundice, neonatal hypotonia, renal anomalies, scoliosis, and seizures. The diagnosis of Sotos syndrome is established in a proband by identification of a heterozygous *NSD1* pathogenic variant by molecular genetic testing. In Japanese patients, sequencing analysis of *NSD1* may detect pathogenic variants in 12% of patients and gene targeted deletion and duplication analysis may detect pathogenic variants in 50% of patients. In non-Japanese patients, sequencing analysis may detect pathogenic variants in 27%—93% of patients and gene target deletion and duplication analysis may detect approximately 15% of patient. *In individuals of non-Japanese ancestry, sequencing analysis of NSD1 should be performed first, followed by gene-targeted deletion/duplication analysis if no pathogenic variant is found.* In individuals of Japanese ancestry, gene-targeted deletion/duplication analysis or FISH analysis may be considered first (https://www. ncbi.nlm.nih.gov/books/NBK1479/).

Beckwith—Wiedemann syndrome (BWS) and *EZH2*-related Weaver syndrome show considerable overlap with Sotos syndrome. Methylation study of ICs at 11p15 may detect loss of methylation on the maternal chromosome at imprinting center 2 (IC2) in 50% of individuals with BWS and gain of methylation on the maternal chromosome at imprinting center 1 (IC1) in 5%. *EZH2*-related Weaver syndrome is also known as Weaver—Smith syndrome. Affected individuals are tall, have a typical, but subtle, facial appearance, are frequently hypotonic at birth (although they can present with a mixed central hypotonia/peripheral hypertonia), and often have associated joint problems such as camptodactyly and contractures. The classic facial appearance overlaps with that of Sotos syndrome, particularly in infancy. Sequencing analysis of the *EZH2* gene may be used to detect pathogenic variants for *EZH2*-related Weaver syndrome.

A Sotos syndrome—like phenotype has been associated with 4p duplications, mosaic 20p trisomy, and 22q13.3 deletion syndrome, which may be detected by chromosomal microarray and/or karyotype.

Hutchinson—Gilford progeria syndrome (HGPS) is characterized by accelerated aging in childhood. The diagnosis is based on the recognition of common clinical features and detection of heterozygous *LMNA* pathogenic variants either within exon 11 (classic HGPS) or at the intronic border of exon 11 (atypical HGPS). *LMNA* is the only gene in which pathogenic variants are known to cause HGPS.

Therefore, sequencing analysis of the *NSD1* gene would most likely be ordered first to confirm or rule out the diagnosis in this patient.

162. **A.** Sotos syndrome is an autosomal dominant disease caused by pathogenic variants in *NSD1*. In Japanese patients, sequencing analysis of *NSD1* may detect pathogenic variants in 12% of patients and gene targeted deletion and duplication analysis may detect pathogenic variants in 50% of patients. In non-Japanese patients, sequencing analysis may detect pathogenic variants in 27%—93% of patients and gene target deletion and duplication analysis may detect approximately 15% of patient. Sequencing analysis of *NSD1* is performed first, in individuals of non-Japanese ancestry, followed by gene-targeted deletion/duplication analysis if no pathogenic variant is found. *In individuals of Japanese ancestry, gene-targeted deletion/duplication analysis or FISH analysis may be considered first since a recurrent 1.9-Mb 5q35 microdeletion encompassing NSD1 has been reported in most Japanese and some non-Japanese individuals with Sotos syndrome* (https://www.ncbi.nlm.nih.gov/books/NBK1479/).

Beckwith—Wiedemann syndrome (BWS) and *EZH2*-related Weaver syndrome show considerable overlap with Sotos syndrome. Methylation study of ICs at 11p15 may detect loss of methylation on the maternal chromosome at imprinting center 2 (IC2) in 50% of individuals with BWS syndrome and gain of methylation on the maternal chromosome at imprinting center 1 (IC1) in 5%. *EZH2*-related Weaver syndrome is also known as Weaver—Smith

syndrome. Sequencing analysis of the *EZH2* gene may be used to detect pathogenic variants for *EZH2*-related Weaver syndrome. A Sotos syndrome—like phenotype has been associated with 4p duplications, mosaic 20p trisomy, and 22q13.3 deletion syndrome, which may be detected by chromosomal microarray and/or karyotype.

Hutchinson—Gilford progeria syndrome (HGPS) is characterized by accelerated aging in childhood. The diagnosis is based on recognition of common clinical features and detection of heterozygous *LMNA* pathogenic variants either within exon 11 (classic HGPS) or at the intronic border of exon 11 (atypical HGPS). *LMNA* is the only gene in which pathogenic variants are known to cause HGPS.

Therefore, chromosomal microarray would most likely be ordered first to confirm or rule out the diagnosis in this patient.

163. **E.** Beckwith—Wiedemann syndrome (BWS) is a growth disorder variably characterized by neonatal hypoglycemia, macrosomia, macroglossia, hemihyperplasia, omphalocele, embryonal tumors (e.g., Wilms tumor, hepatoblastoma, neuroblastoma, and rhabdomyosarcoma), visceromegaly, adrenocortical cytomegaly, renal abnormalities (e.g., medullary dysplasia, nephrocalcinosis, medullary sponge kidney, and nephromegaly), and ear creases/pits (http://www.chop.edu/pages/case-study-more-just-Beckwith-wiedemann-syndrome). BWS is associated with abnormal regulation of gene transcription in two imprinted domains on chromosome 11p15.4, also known as the BWS critical region. Regulation may be disrupted by any one of numerous mechanisms. The BWS critical region includes two domains: imprinting center 1 (IC1) regulates the expression of *IGF2* and *H19* in domain 1; imprinting center 2 (IC2) regulates the expression of *CDKN1C*, *KCNQ1OT1*, and *KCNQ1* in domain 2. *Genetic testing approaches can include DNA methylation studies, single-gene testing, and copy number analysis for genes within 11p15.4, chromosomal microarray, karyotype, and use of multigene panels that include genes in the BWS critical region* (http://www.ncbi.nlm.nih.gov/books/NBK1394/).

Chromosomal SNP array may be used to detect some of UPD7 and some of the maternal duplication of 11p15.5. Methylation study may be used to detect loss of paternal imprinting center 1 (IC1). Multiplex ligation-dependent probe amplification (MLPA) may be used to detect small deletions or duplication beyond the resolution of chromosomal microarray. Sanger sequencing may be used to detect pathogenic variants leading to imprinting defects.

Therefore, all of the genetic studies listed in the question—chromosome analysis, chromosomal microarray, methylation study, and Sanger sequencing—are useful to confirm the diagnosis for BWS.

164. **A**. *Paternal uniparental disomy (UPD) for chromosome 11p15 has been seen in 20% patients with Beckwith−Wiedemann syndrome (BWS)* (http://www.chop.edu/pages/case-study-more-just-beckwith-wiedemann-syndrome). Loss of methylation was seen on the maternal chromosome at imprinting center 2 (IC2) in 50% of affected individuals (IC2 regulates the expression of *CDKN1C*, *KCNQ10T1*, and *KCNQ1* in domain 2). Gain of methylation was seen on the maternal chromosome at imprinting center 1 (IC1) in 5% (IC1 regulates the expression of *IGF2* and *H19* in domain 1). Sequencing analysis of *CDKN1C* identifies pathogenic variants in approximately 40% of familial cases and 5%−10% of cases with no family history of BWS. Cytogenetically detectable abnormalities

involving chromosome 11p15 are found in 1% or fewer of affected individuals. And methylation alterations that are associated with microdeletions or microduplications in this region are associated with high heritability (http://www.ncbi.nlm.nih.gov/books/NBK1394/).

Therefore, paternal UPD15 confirmed the diagnosis of BWS in this patient.

165. **B**. Genomic imprinting is a phenomenon wherein the DNA of the two alleles of a gene is differentially modified so that only one parental allele, parent-specific for each gene, is normally expressed. *The Beckwith−Wiedemann syndrome (BWS) critical region includes two imprinting centers* (see Fig. 12.2 below):

- Imprinting center 1 (IC1) regulates the expression of *IGF2* and *H19* in domain 1.
- Imprinting center 2 (IC2) regulates the expression of *CDKN1C*, *KCNQ10T1*, and *KCNQ1* in domain 2 (http://www.ncbi.nlm.nih.gov/books/NBK1394/).

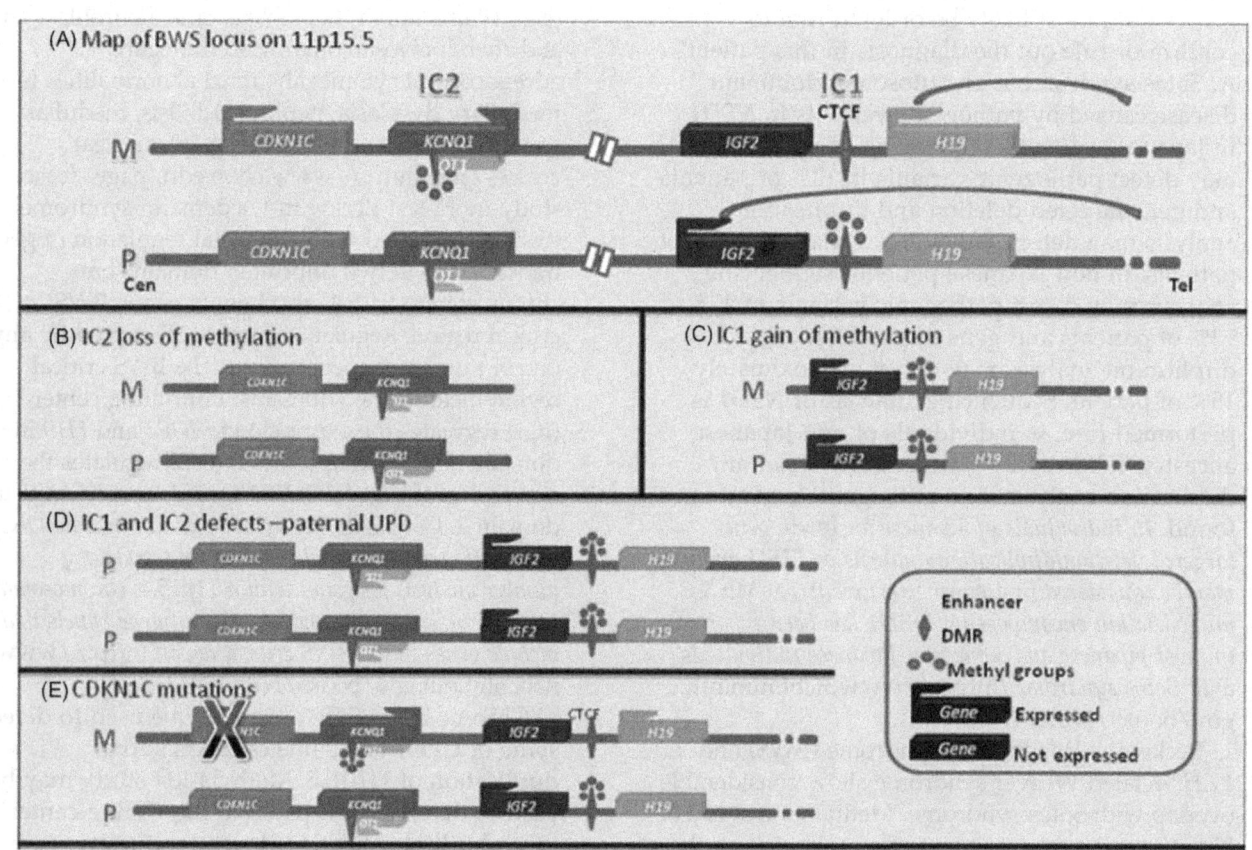

FIGURE 12.2 Map of the BWS locus on 11p15.5. (A) A schematic representation of the normal parent-of-origin−specific imprinted allelic expression. Note that (B) and (C) show only the region that is altered. Cen = centromere, DMR = differentially methylated region, IC = imprinting center, M = maternal, P = paternal, Tel = telomere. OT1 refers to KCNQ1 antisense transcript, KCNQ1OT1. The image is not drawn to scale. *Source: From Choufani S, Shuman C, Weksberg R. Molecular findings in Beckwith-Wiedemann syndrome. Am J Med Genet C Semin Med Genet. 2013 May;163C(2):131−40.*

Therefore, answer B (two ICs) is correct.

166. **C.** Genomic imprinting is a phenomenon whereby the DNA of the two alleles of a gene is differentially modified so that only one parental allele, parent-specific for each gene, is normally expressed. The Beckwith—Wiedemann syndrome (BWS) critical region includes two imprinting centers:

- Imprinting center 1 (IC1) regulates the expression of *IGF2* and *H19* in domain 1.
- Imprinting center 2 (IC2) regulates the expression of *CDKN1C*, *KCNQ10T1*, and *KCNQ1* in domain 2.

In normal individuals, the maternal copy of *IGF2* expressed, but not the paternal copy; and paternal copy of *CDKN1C* expresses, but not the maternal copy. Therefore, *in this patient paternal UPD of 11p15 may explain both gain of expression of IGF2 at the IC1 and loss of expression of CDKN1C at IC2, which may be detected in 20% patients with BWS* (http://www.ncbi.nlm.nih.gov/books/NBK1394/).

167. **E.** The BWS critical region includes two domains: imprinting center 1 (IC1) regulates the expression of *IGF2* and *H19* in domain 1, and imprinting center 2 (IC2) regulates the expression of *CDKN1C*, *KCNQ10T1*, and *KCNQ1* in domain 2. A provisional diagnosis of Beckwith—Wiedemann syndrome (BWS) based on clinical assessment may be confirmed by molecular/cytogenetic testing. Cytogenetically detectable abnormalities involving chromosome 11p15 are found in 1% or fewer of affected individuals. Molecular genetics testing can identify epigenetic and genomic alterations of chromosome 11p15 in individuals with BWS:

I. Loss of methylation on the maternal chromosome at imprinting center 2 (IC2) in 50% of affected individuals;

II. Paternal uniparental disomy for chromosome 11p15 in 20%; and

III. Gain of methylation on the maternal chromosome at imprinting center 1 (IC1) in 5%.

Methylation alterations that are associated with microdeletions or microduplications in this region are associated with high heritability. Sequencing analysis of *CDKN1C* identifies pathogenic variants in approximately 40% of familial cases and 5%—10% of cases with no family history of BWS (http://www.ncbi.nlm.nih.gov/books/NBK1394/).

IGF2 is a hormone involved in the regulation of cell proliferation, growth, migration, differentiation, and survival. *Pathogenic variants in*

the IGF2 gene may be associated with growth restriction. Therefore, there are no enough evidence to support that pathogenic variants in the *IGF2* gene cause Beckwith—Wiedemann syndrome.

168. **A.** Epigenetic changes such as gain or loss of methylation usually cannot be passed on from one generation to the next. Paternal UPD is an error that occurs during meiosis that is also not inheritable. *Sequencing analysis of CDKN1C identifies pathogenic variants in approximately 40% of familial cases and 5%—10% of cases with no family history of Beckwith—Wiedemann syndrome (BWS).* The association between pathogenic variants in the *IGF2* gene and BWs is unclear (http://www.ncbi.nlm.nih.gov/books/NBK1394/).

Therefore, a pathogenic variant in the *CDKN1C* gene may explain the familial BWS in this family.

169. **C.** The Beckwith—Wiedemann syndrome (BWS) critical region includes two domains:

- imprinting center 1 (IC1) regulates the expression of *IGF2* and *H19* in domain 1.
- imprinting center 2 (IC2) regulates the expression of *CDKN1C*, *KCNQ10T1*, and *KCNQ1* in domain 2.

KCNQOT1 and *H19* are transcribed into mRNAs, but are not translated into amino acid sequences. *The IGF2 gene codes for insulin-like growth factor II, a hormone involved in the regulation of cell proliferation, growth, migration, differentiation, and survival.* The *CDKN1C* gene codes for cyclin-dependent kinase inhibitor 1C, a protein tight-binding inhibitor of several G1 cyclin/Cdk complex and a negative regulator of cell proliferation. Gain of methylation on the maternal chromosome at imprinting center 1 (IC1) involving *IGF2* has been seen in 5% of patients with BWS (http://www.ncbi.nlm.nih.gov/books/NBK1394/).

Therefore, *IGF2* is overexpressed in patients with BWS, which may at least partially explain the macrosomia (traditionally defined as weight and length/height >97th centile) seen in some patients.

170. **A.** The Beckwith—Wiedemann syndrome (BWS) critical region includes two domains:

- imprinting center 1 (IC1) regulates the expression of *IGF2* and *H19* in domain 1.
- imprinting center 2 (IC2) regulates the expression of *CDKN1C*, *KCNQ10T1*, and *KCNQ1* in domain 2.

KCNQOT1 and *H19* are transcribed into mRNAs, but are not translated into amino acid sequences. The *IGF2* gene codes for insulin-like growth factor II, a hormone involved in the regulation of cell proliferation, growth, migration, differentiation, and survival. *The CDKN1C gene codes for cyclin-dependent kinase inhibitor 1C, a protein tight-binding inhibitor of several G1 cyclin/ Cdk complex and a negative regulator of cell proliferation.* Loss of methylation on the maternal chromosome at imprinting center 2 (IC2) involving *CDKN1C* has been seen in 50% of affected individuals (http://www.ncbi.nlm.nih. gov/books/NBK1394/).

Therefore, *CDKN1C* is underexpressed in patients with BWS, which may at least partially explain the macrosomia (traditionally defined as weight and length/height >97th centile) seen in some patients.

171. **C.** According to research, *hypomethylation of imprinting center 2 (IC2) on the maternal chromosome is the most common genetic finding identified in 50%–60% of affected individuals with Beckwith–Wiedemann syndrome*, which is followed by paternal uniparental disomy (UPD) for chromosome 11p15 in 20%. Hypermethylation (or gain of methylation) of imprinting center 1 (IC1) on the maternal chromosome is in 5% of affected individuals. Hypomethylation of maternal IC2 increased the expression of *IGF2*, which encodes for a hormone involved in the regulation of cell proliferation, growth, migration, differentiation, and survival.

Therefore, loss of methylation of maternal IC2 would most likely to be the genetic finding if the patient had Beckwith–Wiedemann syndrome (BWS).

172. **B.** The etiology of Beckwith–Wiedemann syndrome (BWS) is complex. About 85% of affected individuals represent single occurrences in a family and have normal chromosome studies. *About 10%–15% of affected individuals demonstrate an autosomal dominant mode of inheritance with incomplete penetrance and preferential maternal transmission.* Less than 1% of affected individuals have a cytogenetically visible chromosome abnormality.

Therefore, BWS demonstrate an autosomal dominant mode of inheritance with incomplete penetrance in approximately 12% of cases, as shown in this pedigree.

173. **D.** The etiology of Beckwith–Wiedemann syndrome (BWS) is complex. About 85% of affected individuals represent single occurrences in a family and have normal chromosome studies. About 10%–15% of affected individuals demonstrate an

autosomal dominant mode of inheritance with incomplete penetrance and preferential maternal transmission. Less than 1% of affected individuals have a cytogenetically visible chromosomal abnormality. Loss of methylation occurs on the maternal chromosome at imprinting center 2 (IC2) in 50% of affected individuals, and paternal uniparental disomy (UPD) for chromosome 11p15 in 20%. Gain of methylation on the maternal chromosome occurs at imprinting center 1 (IC1) in 5%. Sequencing analysis of *CDKN1C* identifies a heterozygous maternally inherited pathogenic variant in approximately 40% of familial cases and 5%–10% of cases with no family history of BWS.

UPD(11p15)mat may be associated with Russell–Silver syndrome (RSS); but the association is unclear. RSS is characterized by intrauterine growth retardation accompanied by postnatal growth deficiency. The average adult height of males is 151.2 cm and that of females is 139.9 cm. Hypomethylation of the paternal imprinting center 1 (IC1) of chromosome 11p15.5 is identified in 35%–50% of individuals with RSS. Duplications of maternal 11p15.5 have been identified in a small number of individuals with RSS. About 10% of individuals with RSS have maternal uniparental disomy for chromosome 7 (UPD7) (https://www.ncbi.nlm.nih.gov/books/ NBK1324/).

Therefore, UPD(11p15)mat is not from a patient with Beckwith–Wiedemann syndrome. *CDKN1C* single nucleotide pathogenic variants, gain of methylation of maternal imprinting center 1, loss of methylation of maternal imprinting center 2, and UPD(11p15)pat have been identified in individuals with BWS.

174. **E.** The etiology of Beckwith–Wiedemann syndrome (BWS) is complex. About 85% of affected individuals represent single occurrences in a family and have normal chromosomal studies. About 10%–15% of affected individuals demonstrate an autosomal dominant mode of inheritance with incomplete penetrance and preferential maternal transmission. Less than 1% of affected individuals have a cytogenetically visible chromosome abnormality. Loss of methylation on the maternal chromosome at imprinting center 2 (IC2) occurs in 50% of affected individuals, and *paternal uniparental disomy (UPD) for chromosome 11p15 in 20%.* Gain of methylation on the maternal chromosome at imprinting center 1 (IC1) occurs in 5%. Sequencing analysis of *CDKN1C* identifies a

heterozygous maternally inherited pathogenic variant in approximately 40% of familial cases and 5%–10% of cases with no family history of BWS.

Maternal 11p15 is naturally unmethylated at imprinting center 1 (IC1) and methylated at imprinting center 2 (IC2). Hypomethylation of the paternal imprinting center 1 (IC1) of chromosome 11p15.5 is identified in 35%–50% of individuals with Russell–Silver syndrome (RSS). Duplications of maternal 11p15.5 have been identified in a small number of individuals with RSS. About 10% of individuals with RSS have maternal uniparental disomy for chromosome 7 (UPD7) (https://www.ncbi.nlm.nih.gov/books/NBK1324/).

Therefore, UPD(11p15)pat is from a patient with Beckwith–Wiedemann syndrome.

175. **D.** *Children with Beckwith–Wiedemann syndrome (BWS) have an increased risk for the development of embryonal tumors, particularly Wilms tumor and hepatoblastoma* (http://www.chop.edu/pages/case-study-more-just-beckwith-wiedemann-syndrome). Others are neuroblastoma and rhabdomyosarcoma. The overall risk of neoplasia in children with BWS is approximately 7.5%. The risk is much lower after 8 years of age.

Patients with several hereditary cancer syndromes, such as familial adenomatous polyposis (FAP), Lynch syndrome, juvenile polyposis syndrome (JPS), MUTYH-associated polyposis (MAP), *PTEN* hamartoma tumor syndrome (PHTS), and Peutz–Jeghers syndrome (PJS), have increased risk for development of colorectal cancer (CRC). Individuals with Ewing sarcoma usually have t(11;22) involving the *EWSR1* gene on 22q12.2 and the *FLI1* gene on 11q24.3. And Ewing sarcomas most often occurs in children and young adults. Individuals with Li–Fraumeni syndrome have an increased risk for the development of osteosarcoma.

Therefore, children with BWS have an increased risk for development of Wilms tumor in comparison with individuals in general populations.

176. **B.** *Children with Beckwith–Wiedemann syndrome (BWS) have an increased risk for the development of embryonal tumors, particularly Wilms tumor and hepatoblastoma; others are neuroblastoma and rhabdomyosarcoma* (http://www.chop.edu/pages/case-study-more-just-beckwith-wiedemann-syndrome). The overall risk of neoplasia in children with BWS is approximately 7.5%. The risk is much lower after 8 years of age.

Children with Down syndrome have increased risk for the development of acute megakaryoblastic leukemia. Individuals with Ewing sarcoma usually have t(11;22) involving the *EWSR1* gene on 22q12.2 and the *FLI1* gene on 11q24.3. And Ewing sarcomas most often occur in children and young adults. Children with pathogenic variants in the *RB1* gene usually develop bilateral multifocal retinoblastoma.

Therefore, children with BWS have an increased risk for the development of hepatoblastoma in comparison with individuals in general populations.

177. **A.** The Beckwith–Wiedemann syndrome (BWS)/Russell–Silver syndrome (RSS) critical region includes two domains:
- Imprinting center 1 (IC1) regulates the expression of *IGF2* and *H19* in domain 1.
- Imprinting center 2 (IC2) regulates the expression of *CDKN1C*, *KCNQ10T1*, and *KCNQ1* in domain 2.

KCNQOT1 and *H19* are transcribed into mRNAs but are not translated into amino acid sequences. The *IGF2* gene codes for insulin-like growth factor II, a hormone involved in the regulation of cell proliferation, growth, migration, differentiation, and survival. The *CDKN1C* gene codes for cyclin-dependent kinase inhibitor 1C, a protein tight-binding inhibitor of several G1 cyclin/Cdk complex and a negative regulator of cell proliferation.

RSS is a genetically heterogeneous condition. Hypomethylation of the paternal imprinting center 1 (IC1) of chromosome 11p15.5 is identified in 35%–50% of individuals with RSS. *Duplications of maternal 11p15.5 have been identified in a small number of individuals with RSS, which enhanced the positive regulatory function of IGF2 in cell proliferation.* About 10% of individuals with RSS have maternal uniparental disomy for chromosome 7 (UPD7) (https://www.ncbi.nlm.nih.gov/books/NBK1324/).

Gain of methylation of maternal imprinting center 1 (IC1), loss of methylation of maternal imprinting center 2 (IC2), and UPD(11p15)pat are diagnostic for Beckwith–Wiedemann syndrome (BWS), an overgrowth syndrome.

Therefore, duplication of maternal copy of 11p15 might be seen in this patient if she had Russell–Silver syndrome (RSS).

178. **C.** The Beckwith–Wiedemann syndrome (BWS)/Russell–Silver syndrome (RSS) critical region includes two domains:
- Imprinting center 1 (IC1) regulates the expression of *IGF2* and *H19* in domain 1.
- Imprinting center 2 (IC2) regulates the expression of *CDKN1C*, *KCNQ10T1*, and *KCNQ1* in domain 2.

KCNQOT1 and *H19* are transcribed into mRNAs, but are not translated into amino acid sequences. The *IGF2* gene codes for insulin-like growth factor II, a hormone involved in the regulation of cell proliferation, growth, migration, differentiation, and survival. The *CDKN1C* gene codes for cyclin-dependent kinase inhibitor 1C, a protein tight-binding inhibitor of several G1 cyclin/Cdk complexes and a negative regulator of cell proliferation.

RSS is a genetically heterogeneous condition and for most affected individuals represents a phenotype rather than a specific disorder. *Hypomethylation of the paternal imprinting center 1 (IC1) of chromosome 11p15.5 is identified in 35%−50% of individuals with RSS, which activate the paternal copy of CDKN1C.* Duplications of maternal 11p15.5 have been identified in a small number of individuals with RSS. About 10% of individuals with RSS have maternal uniparental disomy for chromosome 7 (UPD7) (https://www.ncbi.nlm.nih.gov/books/NBK1324/).

Therefore, loss of methylation of paternal imprinting center 1 might be seen in this patient if he had Russell−Silver syndrome (RSS).

179. **D.** Russell−Silver syndrome (RSS) is a genetically heterogeneous condition and for most affected individuals represents a phenotype rather than a specific disorder. Hypomethylation of the paternal imprinting center 1 (IC1) of chromosome 11p15.5 is identified in 35%−50% of individuals with RSS. Duplications of maternal 11p15.5 have been identified in a small number of individuals with RSS. About 10% of individuals with RSS have maternal uniparental disomy for chromosome 7 (UPD7) (https://www.ncbi.nlm.nih.gov/books/NBK1324/).

Chromosome SNP array may be used to detect UPD7 and some of the maternal duplication of 11p15.5. Methylation study may be used to detect loss of paternal imprinting center 1 (IC1). Multiplex ligation-dependent probe amplification (MLPA) may be used to detect small deletions or duplication beyond the resolution of chromosomal microarray.

Therefore, all three genetic studies would be appropriate for this patient to confirm the diagnosis of RSS.

180. **A.** *The Hutchinson−Gilford progeria syndrome (HGPS)−causing variant in codon 608 of LMNA leads to activation of a cryptic splice site within exon 11, resulting in production of a prelamin A that lacks 50 amino acids near the C terminus. The c.1824C > T pathogenic variant and consequent abnormal splicing produces a prelamin A that still retains*

the CAAX box and is therefore farnesylated but is missing the site for endoproteolytic cleavage of the final 16 amino acids along with the farnesyl moiety that normally occurs during the final step in posttranslational processing. The resulting protein, progerin, is shortened and farnesylated. Since the lipophilic farnesyl moiety is utilized to anchor prelamin (and hence progerin) into the inner nuclear membrane, the lack of farnesyl cleavage likely results in permanent progerin intercalation within the nuclear membrane. Immunofluorescence of HGPS fibroblasts with antibodies directed against lamin A revealed that many cells show visible abnormalities of the nuclear membrane (https://www.ncbi.nlm.nih.gov/books/NBK1121/).

Lamins are the major components of the nuclear lamina, which underlies the nuclear envelope of eukaryotic cells. Vertebrate lamins are classified into 2 types, A and B. Mammalian somatic cells show two species of each type: lamins A and C for the A type and B1 and B2 for the B type. Whereas A-type lamins are expressed in a developmentally controlled manner, B-type lamins are expressed in all kinds of cells. Pathogenic variants in the *LMNB1* gene are associated with autosomal dominant adult-onset leukodystrophy (http://omim.org).

TERT encodes for telomerase reverse transcriptase. Human telomeres consist of many kilobases of (TTAGGG)n together with various associated proteins. Small amounts of these terminal sequences are lost from the terminals of the chromosomes each S phase because of incomplete DNA replication, but de novo addition of TTAGGG repeats by the enzyme telomerase compensates for this loss. Many human cells progressively lose terminal sequence with cell division, a loss that correlates with the apparent absence of telomerase in these cells. Pathogenic variants in the *TERT* gene are associated with autosomal dominant and autosomal recessive dyskeratosis congenital.

TWNK (*TWINKY*) encodes a mitochondrial protein with structural similarity to the phage T7 primase/helicase (GP4) and other hexameric ring helicases. The twinkle protein colocalizes with mtDNA in mitochondrial nucleoids, and its name derives from the unusual localization pattern reminiscent of twinkling stars. Pathogenic variants in the *TERT* gene are associated with autosomal recessive mitochondrial DNA depletion syndrome, autosomal recessive Perrault syndrome, and autosomal dominant progressive external ophthalmoplegia with mitochondrial DNA deletions.

Therefore, *LMNA* is the gene discovered for progeria in 2003.

181. **E.** *Targeted variant is a relatively low-cost and sensitive assay to detect specific SNPs in comparison with exome, MLPA, NGS, and Sanger sequencing.* In 2003, the cause of progeria was discovered to be a point variant, c.1824C > T(p.Gly608Gly), in the *LMNA* gene. This pathogenic variant creates a 5′ cryptic splice site within exon 11, resulting in an abnormally short mature mRNA transcript. The translated abnormal variant of the prelamin A protein, progerin, with the unremoved farnesyl group is permanently affixed to the nuclear rim; therefore, it does not become part of the nuclear lamina. Without lamin A, the nuclear lamina is unable to provide the nuclear envelope with adequate structural support, causing it to take on an abnormal shape (https://www.ncbi.nlm.nih.gov/books/NBK1121/).

Therefore, targeted variant assay is the most cost-effective and sensitive assay to detect the single-nucleotide variant in the *LMNA* gene for progeria.

182. **F.** Classic Hutchinson–Gilford progeria syndrome (HGPS) is defined by a variant in codon 608 of *LMNA*. This variant leads to activation of a cryptic splice site within exon 11, resulting in production of a prelamin A that lacks 50 amino acids near the C terminus. *The c.1824C > T(p.Gly608Gly) pathogenic variant and consequent abnormal splicing produces a prelamin A* that still retains the CAAX box and is therefore farnesylated, but is missing the site for endoproteolytic cleavage of the final 16 amino acids along with the farnesyl moiety that normally occurs during the final step in posttranslational processing. The resulting protein, progerin, is shortened and farnesylated. Since the lipophilic farnesyl moiety is utilized to anchor prelamin (and hence progerin) into the inner nuclear membrane, the lack of farnesyl cleavage likely results in permanent progerin intercalation within the nuclear membrane. Immunofluorescence of HGPS fibroblasts with antibodies directed against lamin A revealed that many cells show visible abnormalities of the nuclear membrane (https://www.ncbi.nlm.nih.gov/books/NBK1121/).

c.1822G > A (p.Gly608Ser), c.1968 + 1G > A, c.1968 + 2T > A, c.1968 + 2T > C, and c.1968 + 5G > C pathogenic variants in *LMNA* result in progerin production. Each of them has been reported in one or two patients with similar but sometimes subtly more or less severe clinical features compared to individuals with HGPS.

Therefore, most progeria patients have a synonymous pathogenic variant.

183. **A.** *Almost all individuals with progeria have the disorder as the result of a de novo autosomal dominant pathogenic variant.* Therefore, the recurrent risk of progeria in this family would be less than 1%.

184. **C.** Ataxia telangiectasia, Bloom syndrome, Cockayne syndrome, Werner syndrome, and xeroderma pigmentosum are all autosomal recessive conditions, resulting from defects of DNA repair. Cockayne syndrome is caused by pathogenic variants in *ERCC6* and *ERCC8*. It characterized by growth failure, impaired development of the nervous system, photosensitivity, eye disorders, and premature aging. *Unlike other defects of DNA repair, patients with Cockayne syndrome (CS) are not predisposed to cancer or infection.*

Patients with ataxia telangiectasia have increased risk to develop leukemia, lymphoma, and breast cancer. Patients with Bloom syndrome have increased risk to develop leukemia, lymphoma and cancer of the colon, breast, skin, lung, auditory canal, tongue, esophagus, stomach, tonsil, larynx, and uterus. Patients with Werner syndrome have an increased risk to develop soft-tissue sarcoma and colorectal, skin, thyroid, pancreas malignancies. Patients with xeroderma pigmentosum have increased risk to develop skin cancers.

Therefore, patients with Cockayne syndrome do NOT have increased risk for malignancies.

185. **A.** Rubinstein–Taybi syndrome (RSTS) is an autosomal dominant condition, caused by pathogenic variants in *CREBBP* and *EP300*. It typically occurs as the result of a de novo pathogenic variant in the family; most individuals represent simplex cases. In most instances, the parents of an individual with RSTS are not affected. *When the parents are clinically unaffected, the empiric recurrence risk for sibs is less than 1%* (https://www.ncbi.nlm.nih.gov/books/NBK1526/).

Therefore, the estimated recurrent risk of RSTS would be less than 1% in this family.

186. **C.** Rubinstein–Taybi syndrome (RSTS) is an autosomal dominant condition, caused by pathogenic variants in *CREBBP* and *EP300*. FISH analysis of *CREBBP* detects microdeletions in approximately 10% of individuals with RSTS. Sequencing analysis detects *CREBBP* pathogenic variants in another 40%–50% of affected individuals. Pathogenic variants in *EP300* are

identified in approximately 3%–8% of individuals with RSTS (https://www.ncbi.nlm. nih.gov/books/NBK1526/). *Evidence suggests that RSTS is caused by haploinsufficiency of CREBBP product.*

Haploinsufficiency is used to explain autosomal dominant disorders when a diploid organism has lost one copy of a gene and is left with a single functional copy of that gene. It is often caused by a loss-of-function variant, in which having only one copy of the wild-type allele is not sufficient to produce the wild-type phenotype. Examples of human disorders caused by haploinsufficiency are cleidocranial dysostosis, Greig cephalopolysyndactyly syndrome, hereditary hemorrhagic telangiectasia, Loeys–Dietz syndrome, and most microdeletion syndromes, with the exception of Prader–Willi/ Angelman and Beckwith–Wiedemann syndromes caused by epigenetic changes. Dominant negatives have an altered gene product that acts antagonistically to the wild-type allele. These pathogenic variants usually result in an altered molecular function (often inactive) and are characterized by a dominant phenotype. Epigenetics is the study of potentially heritable changes in gene expression (active vs. inactive genes) and does not involve changes to the underlying DNA sequence, such as an imprinting defect.

Therefore, the microdeletion of 16p13.3 region would most likely cause haploinsufficiency, which explained symptoms for Rubenstein–Taybi syndrome in this patient.

187. **B**. Typical Greig cephalopolysyndactyly syndrome (GCPS) is characterized by preaxial polydactyly or mixed preaxial and postaxial polydactyly, true wide-spaced eyes, and macrocephaly. Individuals with severe GCPS can have seizures, hydrocephalus, and intellectual disability. GLI3 is the only gene known to be associated with GCPS. GLI3 alterations, such as cytogenetic abnormalities involving GLI3 or pathogenic variants of GLI3, can be identified in more than 75% of typically affected individuals (https://www.ncbi.nlm.nih.gov/books/ NBK1446/).

The physician suspected that the girl had Greig cephalopolysyndactyly gene deletion syndrome because of significant developmental delay or intellectual disability. Therefore, chromosomal microarray analysis would most likely be used as the first-line genetic study to detect a microdeletion involving GLI3 at 7p14.1 in this patient.

188. **C**. The *GLI1* gene was discovered and named because of its amplification in gliomas of the brain. *GLI1*, *GLI2*, *GLI3*, and *GLI4* encode for zinc finger transcription factors related to Kruppel (Kr), which function in the hedgehog signal transduction pathway. *GLI2* is associated autosomal dominant Culler–Jones syndrome, and holoprosencephaly. The function of *GLI1* and *GLI4* is unclear at present. *GLI3 is the only gene known to be associated with autosomal dominant Greig cephalopolysyndactyly syndrome (GCPS).*

Therefore, *GLI3* would most likely be involved in the deletion in this patient.

189. **A**. The *GLI3* gene, located at 7p14.1, encodes a zinc-finger transcription factor that is downstream of Sonic Hedgehog (SHH) in the SHH pathway. *GLI3* is the only gene in which pathogenic variants cause Greig cephalopolysyndactyly syndrome (GCPS) and Pallister–Hall syndrome (PHS). Deletion/ duplication analyses detect 5%–10% of patients with GCPs. The mutational spectra of GCPS and PHS are mostly distinct. GCPS is caused by pathogenic variants of all types, whereas PHS is caused only by truncating variants and one splice variant that generates a frameshift and a truncation. Within the frameshift variant category, a genotype–phenotype correlation has been demonstrated on two levels:

- Class of variant. Pathogenic variants of all classes can cause Greig cephalopolysyndactyly syndrome (GCPS), whereas the majority of pathogenic variants that cause the allelic disorder PHS are frameshift variants. Haploinsufficiency for GLI3 causes GCPS, whereas truncating variants 3′ of the zinc-finger domain of *GLI3* generally cause PHS.
- Variant position. Among all frameshift variants in *GLI3*, only variants in the first third of the gene are known to cause GCPS. Frameshift variants in the middle third of the gene cause PHS and (uncommonly) GCPS. Frameshift variants in the final third of the gene cause GCPS. There is no apparent correlation of the variant position within each of the three regions and the severity of the corresponding phenotypes.

The most common, if not sole, pathogenetic mechanism for GCPS is haploinsufficiency. *Deletions that remove the entire gene cause a GCPS phenotype that is not known to be different from that caused by single-nucleotide variants.* Although it is clear that haploinsufficiency of GLI3 can cause GCPS, the pathogenic mechanism of 3′ frameshift or nonsense variants and missense variants is not clear. It is important to note that mRNA or protein instability may be caused by some of these pathogenic variants in individuals with GCPS, a finding that would be entirely compatible with the general mechanism of haploinsufficiency (https://www.ncbi.nlm.nih.gov/books/NBK1446/).

Muenke syndrome is one of the craniosynostosis caused by pathogenic variants in *FGFR3*. Other craniosynostoses are Crouzon syndrome, Apert syndrome, Jackson—Weiss syndrome, Pfeiffer syndrome, Saethre—Chotzen syndrome, and other conditions. Pallister—Killian syndrome is caused by mosaicism for tetrasomy of chromosome 12p.

Therefore, the fetus would most likely have Greig cephalopolysyndactyly syndrome (GCPS).

190. **D**. Pallister—Hall syndrome (PHS) is characterized by a spectrum of anomalies ranging from polydactyly, asymptomatic bifid epiglottis, and hypothalamic hamartoma at the mild end to laryngotracheal cleft with neonatal lethality at the severe end. GLI3 is the only gene in which heterozygous pathogenic variants cause PHS.

Pathogenic variants in *FGFR2* and *FGFR3* are associated with craniosynostosis, such as Crouzon syndrome, Apert syndrome, Jackson—Weiss syndrome, Pfeiffer syndrome, Saethre—Chotzen syndrome, and other conditions. Pathogenic variants in *GLI2* are associated with autosomal dominant Culler—Jones syndrome and holoprosencephaly. Pathogenic variants in *SMAD3* are associated with autosomal dominant Loeys—Dietz syndrome. Pathogenic variants in *SMAD4* are associated with autosomal dominant juvenile polyposis and juvenile polyposis/hereditary hemorrhagic telangiectasia syndrome.

Therefore, *GLI3* would most likely be mutated in this patient.

191. **F**. *Both Greig cephalopolysyndactyly syndrome (GCPS) and Pallister—Hall syndrome are autosomal dominant conditions caused by pathogenic variants in the same gene, GLI3*. Pathogenic variants of all classes in the *GLI3* gene can cause GCPS, whereas the only frameshift variants cause autosomal dominant Pallister—Hall syndrome. And haploinsufficiency for *GLI3* causes GCPS, whereas truncating variants 3′ of the zinc-finger domain of *GLI3* generally cause PHS.

Therefore, pathogenic variants in the *GLI3* gene cause autosomal dominant Greig cephalopolysyndactyly syndrome (GCPS) and autosomal dominant Pallister—Hall syndrome.

192. **C**. Typically Greig cephalopolysyndactyly syndrome (GCPS) is characterized by preaxial polydactyly or mixed preaxial and postaxial polydactyly, truly wide-spaced eyes, and macrocephaly. Individuals with mild GCPS may have subtle craniofacial findings. The mild end of the GCPS spectrum is a continuum with preaxial polysyndactyly type IV and crossed polydactyly (preaxial polydactyly of the feet and postaxial polydactyly of the hands plus syndactyly of fingers 3–4 and toes 1–3). Individuals with severe GCPS can have seizures, hydrocephalus, and intellectual disability. *GLI3* alterations, such as cytogenetic abnormalities involving *GLI3* or pathogenic variants of *GLI3*, can be identified in more than 75% of typically affected individuals. Sequencing analysis may identify 70% of patients; deletion/duplication may identify 5%-10% of patients.

For individuals with clinical features consistent with GCPS, and without significant developmental delay or intellectual disability or pregnancy losses in the parents, sequencing analysis of GLI3 should be considered first, followed by microarray analysis if no *GLI3* pathogenic variant is identified, followed by Giemsa-banded karyotyping if no *GLI3* pathogenic variant has been identified by the other two methods. If the patient has significant developmental delay or intellectual disability, microarray analysis should be done first, followed by sequencing analysis of *GLI3*, and then Giemsa-banded karyotyping if no *GLI3* pathogenic variant has been identified by the other two methods. If there is a family history of parental pregnancy losses, a Giemsa-banded karyotype should be considered first, followed by sequencing analysis of *GLI3* and then microarray analysis (https://www.ncbi.nlm.nih.gov/books/NBK1446/).

Therefore, Sanger sequencing analysis would most likely be used to confirm the diagnosis in this patient.

193. **C**. Pallister—Hall syndrome (PHS) is characterized by a spectrum of anomalies ranging from polydactyly, asymptomatic bifid epiglottis, and hypothalamic hamartoma at the mild end to laryngotracheal cleft with neonatal lethality at the severe end. Individuals with PHS can have pituitary insufficiency and may die as neonates from undiagnosed and untreated adrenal insufficiency. GLI3 is the only gene in which pathogenic variants are known to cause Pallister—Hall syndrome (https://www.ncbi.nlm.nih.gov/books/NBK1465/).

GLI1, *GLI2*, *GLI3*, and *GLI4* encode for zinc-finger transcription factors related to Kruppel (Kr), which function in the hedgehog signal transduction pathway. *GLI2* is associated autosomal dominant Culler–Jones syndrome, and holoprosencephaly. The function of *GLI1* and *GLI4* is unclear at present.

Therefore, *GLI3* would most likely be tested to confirm the diagnosis in this patient.

194. **D.** Eight disorders comprise the *FGFR*-related craniosynostosis spectrum—Pfeiffer syndrome, Apert syndrome, Crouzon syndrome, Beare–Stevenson syndrome, *FGFR2*-related isolated coronal synostosis, Jackson–Weiss syndrome, Crouzon syndrome with acanthosis nigricans (AN), and Muenke syndrome. Pathogenic variants in the *FGFR1*, *FGFR2*, and *FGFR3* are associated with autosomal dominant craniosynostosis syndromes, such as Pfeiffer syndrome, Apert syndrome, Crouzon syndrome, Beare–Stevenson syndrome, Jackson–Weiss syndrome, and Crouzon syndrome with acanthosis nigricans. A pathogenic variant, p. Pro250Arg, in the *FGFR3* gene defines autosomal dominant Muenke syndrome. Saethre–Chotzen syndrome (SCS) is another of the common forms of syndromic craniosynostosis. *TWIST1 is the only gene in which pathogenic variants are known to cause SCS* (https://www.ncbi.nlm.nih.gov/books/NBK1189/).

Pathogenic variants in the *COL1A2* gene are associated with autosomal dominant osteogenesis imperfecta, and autosomal dominant/recessive Ehlers–Danlos syndrome. Pathogenic variants in the *FBN1* gene are associated with autosomal dominant Marfan syndrome. Pathogenic variants in the *PEX3* gene are associated with autosomal recessive peroxisome biogenesis disorder.

Therefore, *TWIST1* would most likely be tested as the next step in the workup to further rule out a genetic etiology in this patient after negative results on *FGFR1*, *FGFR2*, and *FGFR3*.

195. **D.** Syndromic craniosynostosis can be found in Apert syndrome, Crouzon syndrome, Muenke syndrome, Pfeiffer syndrome, Saethre–Chotzen syndrome, and other conditions. *Pathogenic variants in the FGFR1, FGFR2, and FGFR3 genes are associated with autosomal dominant craniosynostosis syndromes,* such as Pfeiffer syndrome, Apert syndrome, Crouzon syndrome, Beare–Stevenson syndrome, Jackson–Weiss syndrome, and Crouzon syndrome with acanthosis nigricans. A pathogenic variant, p. Pro250Arg, in the *FGFR3* gene defines autosomal dominant Muenke syndrome. Pathogenic variants in the *TWIST1* are associated with autosomal dominant Saethre–Chotzen syndrome (https://www.ncbi.nlm.nih.gov/books/NBK1455/).

Therefore, an NGS sequence panel for craniosynostosis would be the most cost-effective way to confirm the diagnosis in this patient.

196. **D.** Saethre–Chotzen syndrome (SCS) is one of the common forms of autosomal dominant syndromic craniosynostosis; it is caused by pathogenic variants in *TWIST1*. Patients with SCS usually have normal intelligence, although those with large genomic deletions are most likely to have developmental delays. The siblings of the current patient (proband) had the same characteristics, which indicated that one of the parents was an obligate carrier, even though the parental medical history were not available in this question. In general, many patients with SCS have an affected parent; the proportion of cases caused by a de novo pathogenic variant is unknown (https://www.ncbi.nlm.nih.gov/books/NBK1189/).

Therefore, the estimated recurrent risk of the same condition would most likely be about 50% in the fetus.

197. **F.** The Muenke syndrome (MS) is an autosomal dominant craniosynostosis syndrome, characterized by variable expressivity of unicoronal or bicoronal craniosynostosis, midfacial hypoplasia, ocular hypertelorism, proptosis, downslanting palpebral fissures, hearing loss, developmental delay, and specific bone anomalies of the hands and feet. *The diagnosis of Muenke syndrome is established by the identification of the specific FGFR3 pathogenic variant, c.749C > G(p.Pro250Arg)* (https://www.ncbi.nlm.nih.gov/books/NBK1415/).

The FGFR family is a group of receptor tyrosine kinases. FGFRs 1–4 have an extracellular ligand-binding domain containing three immunoglobulin-like loops, a single-pass transmembrane domain, and a split intracellular kinase domain. FGFRs bind fibroblast growth factors (FGFs) and dimerize in order to affect downstream intracellular signaling. FGFR3 negatively regulates chondrocyte differentiation and proliferation in developing endochondral bone (appendicular skeleton). The p.Pro250Arg pathogenic variant in *FGFR3* for Muenke syndrome results in enhanced FGF binding. This pathogenic variant is located in the linker region between the second and third immunoglobulin-like domains. Overactivation of FGFR3 appears to lead to craniosynostosis because bone differentiation is accelerated.

Therefore, a targeted variant analysis would most likely be used to confirm the diagnosis of Muenke syndrome in this patient. However, in reality, targeted analysis for the c.749C > G pathogenic variant in *FGFR3* is rarely performed because the clinical features of Muenke syndrome overlap with those of other craniosynostosis conditions caused by different heterozygous pathogenic variants in *FGFR3* and other craniosynostosis-related genes.

198. **C**. Apert syndrome, Crouzon syndrome, Muenke syndrome, Pfeiffer syndrome, and Saethre–Chotzen syndrome are all syndromic craniosynostoses. *Muenke syndrome is defined by the presence of the specific FGFR3 pathogenic variant, c.749C > G, that results in the protein change p.Pro250Arg* (https://www.ncbi.nlm.nih.gov/books/NBK1415/).

Pathogenic variants in the *FGFR1*, *FGFR2*, and *FGFR3* genes are associated with autosomal dominant craniosynostosis syndromes, such as Pfeiffer syndrome, Apert syndrome, Crouzon syndrome, Beare–Stevenson syndrome, Jackson–Weiss syndrome, and Crouzon syndrome with acanthosis nigricans. Pathogenic variants in the *TWIST1* gene are associated with autosomal dominant Saethre–Chotzen syndrome.

Therefore, the patient would most likely have Muenke syndrome, caused by c.749C > G(p.Pro250Arg) in the *FGFR3* gene.

199. **D**. Pathogenic variants in the *FGFR1*, *FGFR2*, and *FGFR3* genes are associated with autosomal dominant craniosynostosis syndromes, such as Pfeiffer syndrome, Apert syndrome, Crouzon syndrome, Beare–Stevenson syndrome, Jackson–Weiss syndrome, and Crouzon syndrome with acanthosis nigricans. *Pathogenic variants in the TWIST1 gene are associated with autosomal dominant Saethre–Chotzen syndrome.* The p.Trp290Cys variant in the *FGFR2* gene has been reported in patients with Pfeiffer syndrome.

Therefore, it would be least likely that the patient had Saethre–Chotzen syndrome, caused by heterozygous variants in the *TWIST1* gene.

200. **C**. Pathogenic variants in the *FGFR1*, *FGFR2*, and *FGFR3* genes are associated with autosomal dominant craniosynostosis syndromes, such as Pfeiffer syndrome, Apert syndrome, Crouzon syndrome, Beare–Stevenson syndrome, Jackson–Weiss syndrome, and Crouzon syndrome with acanthosis nigricans. *A pathogenic variant, p.Pro250Arg, in the FGFR3 gene defines autosomal dominant Muenke syndrome.* Pathogenic variants in the *TWIST1* gene are associated with autosomal dominant Saethre–Chotzen syndrome. The p.Trp290Gly variant in the *FGFR2* gene has been reported in patients with Crouzon syndrome.

Therefore, it would be Least likely that the patient had Muenke syndrome, caused by a heterozygous variant, p.Pro250Arg, in the *FGFR3* gene.

201. **B**. *The effect of FGFR2 pathogenic variants seems to be one of excess activity; for example, the mutant receptors work better than the wild-type receptors.* The p.Pro250Arg pathogenic variant results in enhanced FGF binding. This pathogenic variant is located in the linker region between the second and third immunoglobulin-like domains. Kinetic ligand-binding studies and x-ray crystallography of linker region pathogenic variants demonstrate that the pathogenic variant results in increased ligand affinity (FGF9) and altered specificity. Overactivation of FGFR3 appears to lead to craniosynostosis because bone differentiation is accelerated (https://www.ncbi.nlm.nih.gov/books/NBK1415/).

Therefore, the pathogenesis of the variant would most likely be gain of function in this patient.

202. **B**. *Advanced paternal age has been shown clinically to be associated with de novo pathogenic variants for Crouzon syndrome, Apert syndrome, Pfeiffer syndrome, Beare–Stevenson syndrome, and Muenke syndrome.* Paternal age effect in de novo variant has been conclusively demonstrated at the molecular level in Apert syndrome. It has been proposed that *FGFR* pathogenic variants are paradoxically enriched in the male germline because they confer a selective advantage to the spermatagonial cells in which they arise (https://www.ncbi.nlm.nih.gov/books/NBK1455/).

Therefore, increased paternal age is a risk factor for *FGFR*-related craniosynostosis syndromes.

203. **F**. Achondroplasia is one of the most common disorders resulting in disproportionate small stature. Affected individuals have short arms and legs, a large head, and characteristic facial features with frontal bossing and midface retrusion (formerly known as "midface hypoplasia"). In infancy, hypotonia is typical, and acquisition of developmental motor milestones is often both aberrant in pattern and delayed. Intelligence and lifespan are usually near normal, although craniocervical junction compression increases the risk of death in infancy. *Approximately 98% of patients with achondroplasia has the c.1138G > A (p.Gly380Arg) variant in FGFR3, and approximately 1% has c.1138G > C (p.Gly380Arg) in FGFR3* (https://www.ncbi.nlm.nih.gov/books/NBK1152/).

Therefore, a targeted variant analysis of the position 1138 of the *FGFR3* gene would most likely be used to confirm the diagnosis of achondroplasia in this patient.

204. **C.** *Approximately 98% of patients with achondroplasia has the c.1138G > A (p.Gly380Arg) variant in FGFR3, and approximately 1% has c.1138G > C (p. Gly380Arg) in FGFR3.*

Pathogenic variants in the *FGFR1*, *FGFR2*, and *FGFR3* genes have been reported in patients with autosomal dominant syndromic craniosynostosis, such as Pfeiffer syndrome, Apert syndrome, Crouzon syndrome, Beare–Stevenson syndrome, Jackson–Weiss syndrome, and Crouzon syndrome with acanthosis nigricans. A pathogenic variant, p.Pro250Arg, in the *FGFR3* gene defines autosomal dominant Muenke syndrome, a craniosynostosis syndrome. The function of *FGFR4* is unclear. To date, no evidence has shown that pathogenic variants in *FGFR4* are associated with craniofacial or skeletal disorders.

Therefore, *FGFR3* would most likely be tested to confirm the diagnosis of achondroplasia in this patient.

205. **B.** *The p.Gly380Arg pathogenic variant for achondroplasia causes constitutive activation of FGFR3, which is, through its inhibition of chondrocyte proliferation and differentiation, a negative regulator of bone growth.* The members of the family of bone dysplasias that includes hypochondroplasia, achondroplasia, SADDAN dysplasia, and thanatophoric dysplasia type I and II are the result of allelic *FGFR3* pathogenic variants that result in a graded series of FGFR3 activation. Although the precise consequences of the achondroplasia-causing variant in *FGFR3* are still uncertain, the net result is excess inhibitory signaling in growth plate chondrocytes (https://www.ncbi.nlm.nih.gov/books/NBK1152/).

Therefore, gain of function would most likely be the pathogenesis of the variant resulting in achondroplasia in this patient.

206. **B.** Approximately 80% of individuals with achondroplasia have parents with average stature and have achondroplasia as a result of a de novo pathogenic variant. De novo pathogenic variants are associated with advanced paternal age, often defined as older than age 35 years. *The de novo pathogenic variants causing achondroplasia are exclusively inherited from the father* (https://www.ncbi.nlm.nih.gov/books/NBK1152/).

Therefore, increased paternal age is a risk factor for de novo achondroplasia.

207. **C.** Achondroplasia is an autosomal dominant condition; 80% of patients have a de novo pathogenic variant. Patients with achondroplasia usually have near normal intelligence and lifespan. *When both partners have achondroplasia, the risk to their offspring of having average stature is 25%, of having achondroplasia 50% and of having homozygous achondroplasia (a lethal condition) 25%* (https://www.ncbi.nlm.nih.gov/books/NBK1152/).

Therefore, this couple would be expected to have recurrent pregnancy loss due to the homozygous achondroplasia, a lethal condition.

208. **C.** Achondroplasia is an autosomal dominant condition; 80% of patients have a de novo pathogenic variant. Patients with achondroplasia usually have near normal intelligence and lifespan. *When both partners have achondroplasia, the risk to their offspring of having average stature is 25%, of having achondroplasia 50% and of having homozygous achondroplasia (a lethal condition) 25%* (https://www.ncbi.nlm.nih.gov/books/NBK1152/).

Therefore, the chance for this couple to have a child with normal height would be 33% (1 in 3) because homozygous achondroplasia is a lethal condition.

209. **C.** Hypochondroplasia is an autosomal dominant skeletal dysplasia characterized by short stature, stocky build, disproportionately short arms and legs, broad, short hands and feet, mild joint laxity, and macrocephaly. Radiological features include shortening of long bones with mild metaphyseal flare, narrowing of the inferior lumbar interpedicular distances, short, broad femoral neck, and squared, shortened ilia. The skeletal features are very similar to those seen in achondroplasia but tend to be milder. Medical complications common to achondroplasia, such as spinal stenosis, tibial bowing, and obstructive apnea, occur less frequently in hypochondroplasia but intellectual disability and epilepsy may be more prevalent. Children usually present as toddlers or school-aged children with decreased growth velocity leading to short stature and limb disproportion. Other features also become more prominent over time. *Approximately 70% of affected individuals are heterozygous for a pathogenic variant, c.1620C > A(p.Asn540Lys) or c.1620C > G(p.Asn540Lys) in FGFR3* (https://www.ncbi.nlm.nih.gov/books/NBK1477/).

Pathogenic variants in the *FGFR1*, *FGFR2*, and *FGFR3* genes have been reported in patients with autosomal dominant syndromic craniosynostosis, such as Pfeiffer syndrome, Apert syndrome,

Crouzon syndrome, Beare—Stevenson syndrome, Jackson—Weiss syndrome, and Crouzon syndrome with acanthosis nigricans. A pathogenic variant, p.Pro250Arg, in the *FGFR3* gene defines autosomal dominant Muenke syndrome, a craniosynostosis syndrome. The function of *FGFR4* is unclear. To date, no evidence has shown that pathogenic variants in *FGFR4* are associated with craniofacial or skeletal disorders.

Therefore, *FGFR3* would most likely be tested for hypochondroplasia in this patient.

210. **F.** *FGFR3 is the only gene in which pathogenic variants are known to cause hypochondroplasia. Approximately 70% of patients with hypochondroplasia are heterozygous for a pathogenic variant, c.1620C > A(p.Asn540Lys) or c.1620C > G(p.Asn540Lys) in FGFR3.* Genetic heterogeneity is suspected, as only approximately 70% of individuals with a clinical and radiographic diagnosis of hypochondroplasia have pathogenic variants in *FGFR3*; to date, a true second locus has not been found (https://www.ncbi.nlm.nih.gov/books/NBK1477/).

Therefore, a targeted variant analysis would most likely be used for the reflex testing for hypochondroplasia in this patient.

211. **C.** Leri—Weill dyschondrosteosis (LWD) is characterized by short stature, mesomelia, and Madelung deformity caused by pathogenic variants in the *SHOX* gene, located at the pseudoautosomal regions of the X and Y chromosomes. Haploinsufficiency of the *SHOX* gene causes short stature, mesomelia, and Madelung deformity. Each child of an individual with Leri—Weill dyschondrosteosis has a 50% chance of inheriting the pathogenic variant (https://www.ncbi.nlm.nih.gov/books/NBK1215/).

Achondroplasia and hypochondroplasia are caused by heterozygous pathogenic variants in *FGFR3*. Stickler syndrome is a connective-tissue disorder with a wide range of symptoms, such as myopia, cataract, hearing loss, midfacial underdevelopment, and cleft palate; it caused by pathogenic variants in *COL2A1, COL11A1, COL11A2, COL9A1, COL9A2,* and *COL9A3*. Turner syndrome is characterized by short status, webbed neck, lymphedema, infertility, and premature ovarian failure, caused by loss of a copy of the X chromosome in females (45,X). All individuals with Turner syndrome have *SHOX* haploinsufficiency because of numeric or structural aberration of the sex chromosome.

Therefore, this patient had Leri—Weill dyschondrosteosis caused by a deletion of *SHOX*.

212. **A.** *Leri—Weill dyschondrosteosis (LWD) is caused by pathogenic variants in the SHOX gene located on the pseudoautosomal regions of the X and Y chromosomes.* Haploinsufficiency of the *SHOX* gene causes short stature, mesomelia, and Madelung deformity. Each child of an individual with Leri—Weill dyschondrosteosis has a 50% chance of inheriting the pathogenic variant (https://www.ncbi.nlm.nih.gov/books/NBK1215/).

Therefore, this disease is inherited in an autosomal dominant manner, even though the causative gene, *SHOX*, is located at Xp22.33 (Yp11.32).

213. **A.** Leri—Weill dyschondrosteosis (LWD) is caused by haploinsufficiency of the *SHOX* gene located in the pseudoautosomal regions of the X and Y chromosomes. *Approximately 2/3 of individuals with LWD have large-scale SHOX deletions that vary in size between 90 kb and 2.5 Mb or more.* Chromosomal microarray can detect deletions as small as 90 kb. The resolution limit of karyotyping is about 2—3 Mb. Sequencing cannot detect the deletion at this range.

Therefore, chromosomal microarray analysis would most likely be used as the initial genetic evaluation for this patient.

214. **B.** Isolated noncompaction of the left ventricle (IVNC) is a rare disease categorized by the World Health Organization (WHO) as an unclassified cardiomyopathy. It is characterized by an excessively prominent trabecular meshwork of the myocardium and deep intertrabecular recesses due to the arrest in the compaction process of the myocardial fibers in the absence of other structural heart disease. *Pathogenic variants in several genes have been recognized to lead to isolated cardiomyopathy with left ventricular noncompaction, such as LDB3, ACTC1, MYH7, MIB1, PRDM16, TNNT2, TPM1, and MYBPC3* (https://www.ncbi.nlm.nih.gov/books/NBK1507/).

Therefore, a next-generation sequencing (NGS) panel would most likely be used to determine the genetic etiology of the myopathy in this patient.

215. **C.** Patients with Costello syndrome may have childhood cardiac myopathy, similar to Barth syndrome. But in Costello syndrome, cardiac myopathy usually is hypertrophic cardiomyopathy (HCM), instead of dilated as usually seen in Barth syndrome. *Costello syndrome is an autosomal dominant condition, caused by pathogenic variants in HRAS at 11p15.5.* Barth syndrome is an X-linked condition, caused by

pathogenic variants in *TAZ* from Xq28. Since Costello syndrome is a single-gene disease without hot spots, Sanger sequencing is the most appropriate molecular test for it (https://www. ncbi.nlm.nih.gov/books/NBK1507/).

Therefore, Sanger sequencing would most likely be used to confirm the diagnosis in this patient.

216. **B**. Hypohidrotic ectodermal dysplasia (HED) is characterized by hypotrichosis (sparseness of scalp and body hair), hypohidrosis (reduced ability to sweat), and hypodontia (congenital absence of teeth). The cardinal features of HED become obvious during childhood. The scalp hair is thin, lightly pigmented, and slow-growing. Sweating, although present, is greatly deficient, leading to episodes of hyperthermia until the affected individual or family acquires experience with environmental modifications to control temperature. Only a few abnormally formed teeth erupt, and at a later than average age (https://www.ncbi.nlm.nih.gov/books/NBK1112/).

The most common form of HED is X-linked, caused by pathogenic variants in the EDA gene. The other forms are autosomal recessive and autosomal dominant, caused by pathogenic variants in the EDAR and EDARADD genes.

This boy did not have family history of HED. The inheritance pattern is unclear. Therefore, a next-generation sequencing (NGS) panel to test all three genes would most likely be used to confirm the diagnosis in this patient.

217. **D**. Since the pathogenic variant was already detected in the proband, targeted variant analysis would be the most cost-effective way to test the parents.

Therefore, a targeted variant assay would most likely be used to test the parents.

218. **A**. *The most common form of hypohidrotic ectodermal dysplasia (HED) is X-linked, caused by pathogenic variants in the EDA gene.* Pathogenic variants in *EDA*-associated HED mainly manifest in males, rarely in females. The other forms are autosomal recessive and autosomal dominant, caused by pathogenic variants in the *EDAR* and *EDARADD* genes.

The two affected siblings were females. The family history of consanguinity indicates the increased risk for autosomal recessive disorders. Therefore, *EDA* for X-linked HED most likely did not harbor a pathogenic variant in these two patients.

219. **A**. Hypohidrotic ectodermal dysplasia (HED) is characterized by sparseness of scalp and body hair, reduced ability to sweat, and congenital absence of

teeth. *The most common form of hypohidrotic ectodermal dysplasia (HED) is X-linked, caused by pathogenic variants in the EDA gene.* In addition to the most common form, two clinically similar but genetically distinct forms of HED are recognized: the clinically indistinguishable autosomal recessive form (caused by pathogenic variants in *EDAR* or *EDARADD*) and the autosomal dominant form (caused by pathogenic variants in *EDAR* or *EDARADD*), which is milder (http://www.ncbi. nlm.nih.gov/books/NBK1112/).

Pathogenic variants in *DICER1* are associated with autosomal dominant pleuropulmonary blastoma. Pathogenic variants in *FH* are associated with autosomal dominant leiomyomatosis and renal-cell cancer and autosomal recessive fumarase deficiency. Pathogenic variants in *ERCC1* are associated with autosomal recessive cerebro-oculo-facio-skeletal syndrome.

In this family all the affected members were males, indicating an X-linked HED. Therefore, *EDA* would most likely harbor a pathogenic variant in this family.

220. **C**. Incontinentia pigmenti (IP) is a disorder that affects the skin, hair, teeth, nails, eyes, and central nervous system. Characteristic skin lesions evolve through four stages: blistering (birth to age ~4 months); wart-like rash (for several months); swirling macular hyperpigmentation (age ~6 months into adulthood); and linear hypopigmentation. Alopecia, hypodontia, abnormal tooth shape, and dystrophic nails are observed. Neovascularization of the retina, present in some individuals, predisposes to retinal detachment. Neurological findings, including cognitive delays, intellectual disability, and learning disability, are occasionally seen (http:// www.ncbi.nlm.nih.gov/books/NBK1472/).

The diagnosis of IP is based on clinical findings and molecular genetic testing of *IKBKG* (previously *NEMO*), the only gene known to be associated with IP. *A deletion that removes exons 4 through 10 of IKBKG (approximately 11.7 kb) is present in approximately 65% of affected individuals.*

The size of the deletion is too small to be detected by chromosomal microarray and FISH. Therefore, multiplex ligation-dependent probe amplification (MLPA) would provide the most cost-effective first-tier test to detect the pathogenic variant in this patient.

221. **A**. Incontinentia pigmenti (IP) is an X-linked condition that affects the skin, hair, teeth, nails, eyes, and central nervous system. About 65% of affected individuals have IP as a result of de novo pathogenic variant. *IP is lethal in many embryonic*

males. Affected surviving males have been found with 47,XXY karyotype or somatic mosaicism for the common *IKBKG* deletion. Affected women have a 50% chance of transmitting the mutant *IKBKG* allele at conception; however, male conceptuses with a loss-of-function variant of *IKBKG* miscarry. Thus, the expected ratio among liveborn children is approximately 33% in unaffected females, 33% in affected females, and 33% in unaffected males (http://www.ncbi.nlm.nih.gov/books/NBK1472/).

When a mother with IP has an *IKBKG* pathogenic variant that results in reduced (though not absent) protein activity, male conceptuses may survive and manifest ectodermal dysplasia, anhidrotic, with immunodeficiency (EDA-ID) at birth. However, *a mother with IP and the common 11.7-kb deletion (resulting in the complete absence of protein activity) is not at increased risk of having a liveborn child with EDA-ID.*

In this case, the mother had the 11.7-kb deletion in *IKBKG* and multiple miscarriage, indicating that male fetuses cannot survive to the term. Therefore, the most appropriate estimated risk of this patient's unborn brother with the same condition is less than 1%.

222. **B**. The genomic organization around *IKBKG* (previously known as *NEMO*) is complex. *IKBKG* has a highly similar pseudogene, designated *IKBKGP1* (also known as *NEMOP*), located in an adjacent region of the X chromosome. *IKBKGP1* is a partial pseudogene with sequences highly similar to those in exons 3–10 of the functional gene. The functional *IKBKG* is 22 kb distant from the pseudogene *IKBKGP1* (*NEMOP*); they are arranged in an inverted fashion. Within *IKBKG* there are two 870-bp direct repeats termed "MER67B"; one is in intron 3 and the second is downstream of *IKBKG*. *Recombination between the MER67B direct repeats results in deletion of exons 4 through 10 of IKBKG*. This is the 11.7-kb deletion that is commonly seen in individuals with incontinentia pigmenti (IP) (http://www.ncbi.nlm.nih.gov/books/NBK1472/).

In a study by Fusco et al., 10%–12% of parents of individuals with IP were found to have two benign variants. One was the 11.7-kb deletion of exons 4–10 in the *IKBKG* pseudogene (*IKBKGP1*). The second was a duplication of MER67B that replicates the exons 4–10 in the region downstream of the normal *IKBKG* gene (termed "MER67Bdup"). Both variants were rare normal allelic variants in a control population (estimated frequency, 1%–2%).

Oxidative deamination is a mechanism for C-to-T transition. Strand slippage is the mechanism for short tandem repeat (STR) instability and dynamic mutation.

Therefore, recombination error of repeats describes the mechanism of the 11.7-kb deletion in *IKBKG* seen in this patient with IP.

223. **D**. *The patient had immune dysregulation, polyendocrinopathy, enteropathy, X-linked (IPEX) syndrome, characterized by systemic autoimmunity, typically beginning in the first year of life.* Presentation is most commonly the clinical triad of watery diarrhea, eczematous dermatitis, and endocrinopathy (most commonly insulin-dependent diabetes mellitus). Most children have other autoimmune phenomena, including Coombs-positive anemia, autoimmune thrombocytopenia, autoimmune neutropenia, and tubular nephropathy (http://www.ncbi.nlm.nih.gov/books/NBK1118/).

The family history indicated that the patient's mother was an asymptomatic carrier of IPEX. The risk of transmitting the pathogenic variant in each pregnancy is 50%. Males who inherit the variant will be affected; females who inherit the variant are carriers and will not be affected. Therefore, the most appropriate estimation of recurrent risk of IPEX would be 25% in this family.

224. **C**. *FOXP3 is the only gene in which pathogenic variants are known to cause immune dysregulation, polyendocrinopathy, enteropathy, X-linked (IPEX) syndrome.* Sequencing analysis of all exons, exon–intron boundaries, and the first polyadenylation site in *FOXP3* detects pathogenic variants in approximately 25% of males with a clinical phenotype suggestive of IPEX syndrome; typically, exon or whole-gene deletions/duplications are not detected in symptomatic patients. Among the males who lack *FOXP3* pathogenic variants, approximately half have low *FOXP3* mRNA expression levels and low numbers of FOXP3-expressing cells in peripheral blood, suggesting that defects in other genes or gene products, possibly in the same pathway as FOXP3, may cause a similar phenotype (http://www.ncbi.nlm.nih.gov/books/NBK1118/).

Therefore, Sanger sequencing would most likely be used to confirm the diagnosis in this patient.

225. **B**. This patient had a classical clinical presentations of immune dysregulation, polyendocrinopathy, enteropathy, X-linked (IPEX) syndrome. *FOXP3 at Xp11.23 is the only gene in which pathogenic variants are known to cause IPEX syndrome* (http://www.ncbi.nlm.nih.gov/books/NBK1118/).

ADA encodes adenosine deaminase, an enzyme that catalyzes the irreversible deamination of adenosine and deoxyadenosine in the purine catabolic pathway. Pathogenic variants in *ADA* cause adenosine deaminase (ADA) deficiency, an autosomal recessive severe combined immunodeficiency (SCID). *IL2RG* encodes for gamma interleukin-2 receptor, which affects the growth and differentiation of T cells, B cells, natural killer cells, glioma cells, and cells of the monocyte lineage after specifically interacting with its receptors. Pathogenic variants in *IL2RG* cause X-linked severe combined immunodeficiency. *STAT3* encodes a transcription factor that plays a critical role in mediating cytokine-induced changes in gene expression. Pathogenic variants in *STAT3* cause autosomal dominant hyper-IgE recurrent infection syndrome. Pathogenic variants in *WAS* cause X-linked Wiskott–Aldrich syndrome.

Therefore, the pathogenic variant, detected in this patient with a clinical diagnosis of IPEX, would be most likely located in the *FOXP3* gene.

226. **C.** *WAS* is the only gene in which pathogenic variants are known to cause Wiskott–Aldrich syndrome (WAS). More than 350 pathogenic WAS variants have been published. Pathogenic variants have been found in all 12 exons. About half of these pathogenic variants are missense variants that interfere with protein function or nonsense variants that lead to protein truncation. The remaining pathogenic variants are small deletions/insertions, splicing variants, gross deletions/insertions and complex rearrangements. *Sequencing of the entire coding region and intron–exon boundaries of WAS is estimated to detect approximately 95% of pathogenic variants.* In the Ashkenazi Jewish population, the prevalence of WAS is not higher than in other populations, and no founder effect is evident (http://www.ncbi.nlm.nih.gov/books/NBK1178/).

Therefore, Sanger sequencing analysis would most likely be used to confirm the diagnosis in this patient.

227. **D.** *Wiskott–Aldrich syndrome (WAS) is an X-linked immunodeficiency*, which usually presents in infancy. Affected males have thrombocytopenia with intermittent mucosal bleeding, bloody diarrhea, and intermittent or chronic petechiae and purpura; eczema; and recurrent bacterial and viral infections, particularly recurrent ear infections. Female carriers of a pathogenic variant in *WAS* are typically asymptomatic due to skewed X chromosome inactivation, which results in silencing of the mutated allele. If a male is the only affected family member, the mother may be a carrier or the affected male may have a de novo *WAS* pathogenic variant, in which case the mother is not a carrier. About one-third of affected individuals with no previous family history of the disorder have a de novo pathogenic variant (http://www.ncbi.nlm.nih.gov/books/NBK1178/).

The family history indicated that the patient's mother was an asymptomatic carrier of the pathogenic variant. The chance of transmitting the variant in each pregnancy was 50%. Males who inherited the pathogenic variant would be affected; females who inherited the pathogenic variant would be carriers and might occasionally have mild thrombocytopenia. Therefore, the most appropriate estimation of recurrent risk of the WAS would be 25% in this family.

228. **D.** *Individuals with Wiskott–Aldrich syndrome (WAS), particularly those who have been exposed to Epstein–Barr virus (EBV), have an increased risk of developing lymphomas, which often occur in unusual, extranodal locations such as the brain, lung, or gastrointestinal tract.* Although B-cell lymphomas predominate, EBV-associated T-cell lymphomas and Hodgkin lymphomas have also been reported. Approximately 13% of individuals with WAS develop lymphoma, at an average age of 9.5 years. The risk of developing lymphoma increases with age and in the presence of autoimmune disease. The prognosis of individuals with WAS following conventional chemotherapy is poorer than that of age-matched normal controls. Individuals with WAS have a significant risk of relapse or development of a second de novo lymphoma. Individuals with WAS and lymphoma should undergo allogeneic hematopoietic-cell transplantation (HCT) to increase their chances of relapse-free survival (http://www.ncbi.nlm.nih.gov/books/NBK1178/).

Therefore, this WAS patient would have an increased risk to develop lymphoma, especially after exposure to Epstein–Barr virus (EBV).

229. **C.** *X-linked severe combined immunodeficiency (X-SCID) is a combined cellular and humoral immunodeficiency mostly caused by pathogenic variants in IL2RG.* In typical X-SCID, lack of *IL2RG* function results in near complete absence of T and natural killer (NK) lymphocytes and nonfunctional B lymphocytes. X-SCID is almost universally fatal in the first 2 years of life unless reconstitution of the immune system is achieved through bone-marrow transplantation or gene therapy (http://www.ncbi.nlm.nih.gov/books/NBK1410/).

ADA encodes adenosine deaminase, an enzyme that catalyzes the irreversible deamination of adenosine and deoxyadenosine in the purine catabolic pathway. Pathogenic variants in *ADA* cause adenosine deaminase (ADA) deficiency, an autosomal recessive severe combined immunodeficiency (SCID). *FOXP3* encodes a member of the fork-winged helix family of transcription factors, playing an important role in the development and function of naturally occurring CD4-positive/CD25-positive T regulatory cells. Pathogenic variants in *FOXP3* caused X-linked (IPEX) syndrome. *STAT3* encodes a transcription factor that plays a critical role in mediating cytokine-induced changes in gene expression. Pathogenic variants in *STAT3* cause autosomal dominant hyper-IgE recurrent infection syndrome. Pathogenic variants in *WAS* cause X-linked Wiskott—Aldrich syndrome. *ZAP70* encodes a tyrosine kinase that is a critical T-cell signaling molecule that interacts with the zeta-chain of the T-cell receptor (TCR). It is expressed predominantly in T and NK cells. Pathogenic variants in *ZAP70* cause autosomal recessive infantile-onset autoimmune disease.

Therefore, *IL2RG* would most likely be tested first to confirm/rule out the diagnosis in this patient.

230. **B**. Severe combined immunodeficiency (SCID) leads to life-threatening infections unless the immune system can be restored through bone-marrow transplantation, enzyme replacement, or gene therapy. Currently, most states have adopted the T-cell—receptor excision circle (TREC) assay as part of their routine newborn screening programs. TREC screening has identified infants with most forms of SCID and also some infants with very low T lymphocytes due to other conditions.

SCID can be classified by the nature of T, B, and NK lymphocyte numbers and function, such as X-SCID, *JAK3*-SCID, *IL7R*-SCID, CD45 deficiency, adenosine deaminase deficiency, RAG-deficient SCID, SCID Athabaskan, TCR deficiency, DNAPKCS deficiency, reticular dysgenesis, and CORO1a deficiency. X-SCID remains one of the most common forms of SCID. The clinical presentations of X-SCID, *JAK3*-SCID, and *IL7R*-SCID are identical. In X-SCID, only males are affected; in *JAK3*- and *IL7R*-SCID, both males and females are affected. And a growing list of rare causes of SCID-like phenotypes include pathogenic variants in the following additional genes: *CD3G, CD8A, CHD7, CIITA, DOCK8, FOXN1, LCK, LIG4, MTHFD1, NBS1, NHEJ1, ORAI1, PCFT, PGM3,*

PNP, PRKDC, RFX-B, RFXANK, RFX5, RFXAP, RMRP, STIM1, TBX1, TTC7A, ZAP70 (https://www.ncbi.nlm.nih.gov/books/NBK1410/).

Newborn screening results can show low or absent TRECs and clinically significant T lymphocytopenia (<1500 T cells/μL) in numerous conditions, such as typical SCID, partial SCID due to a hypomorphic allele (partial loss of gene function) in a typical SCID-related gene, and syndromes. Therefore, a next-generation sequencing (NGS) panel would most likely be used to clarify the diagnosis in this infant girl.

231. **B**. Severe combined immunodeficiency (SCID) can be classified by the nature of T, B, and NK lymphocyte numbers and function, such as X-SCID, *JAK3*-SCID, *IL7R*-SCID, CD45 deficiency, adenosine deaminase deficiency, RAG-deficient SCID, SCID Athabaskan, TCR deficiency, DNAPKCS deficiency, reticular dysgenesis, and CORO1a deficiency. *X-SCID, caused be pathogenic variants in IL2RG, remains one of the most common forms of SCID.* The clinical presentation of X-SCID, *JAK3*-SCID, and *IL7R*-SCID is identical. In X-SCID, only males are affected; in *JAK3*- and *IL7R*-SCID, both males and females are affected. And a growing list of rare causes of SCID-like phenotypes include pathogenic variants in the following additional genes: *CD3G, CD8A, CHD7, CIITA, DOCK8, FOXN1, LCK, LIG4, MTHFD1, NBS1, NHEJ1, ORAI1, PCFT, PGM3, PNP, PRKDC, RFX-B, RFXANK, RFX5, RFXAP, RMRP, STIM1, TBX1, TTC7A, ZAP70* (https://www.ncbi.nlm.nih.gov/books/NBK1410/).

ADA encodes adenosine deaminase, an enzyme that catalyzes the irreversible deamination of adenosine and deoxyadenosine in the purine catabolic pathway. Pathogenic variants in *ADA* cause adenosine deaminase (ADA) deficiency, an autosomal recessive severe combined immunodeficiency (SCID). *STAT3* encodes a transcription factor that plays a critical role in mediating cytokine-induced changes in gene expression. Pathogenic variants in *STAT3* cause autosomal dominant hyper-IgE recurrent infection syndrome. *ZAP70* encodes a tyrosine kinase that is a critical T-cell signaling molecule that interacts with the zeta-chain of the T-cell receptor (TCR). It is expressed predominantly in T and NK cells. Pathogenic variants in *ZAP70* cause autosomal recessive infantile-onset autoimmune disease.

The patient was a girl. It was unlikely that she had an X-linked SCID. Therefore, *IL2RG* would least likely be an appropriate candidate gene for the SCID in this infant girl.

232. **A**. Adenosine deaminase (ADA) deficiency is a severe combined immunodeficiency (SCID) caused by pathogenic variants in the *ADA* gene. It is the only autosomal recessive immunodeficiency in the question. The rest are X-linked disorders.

FOXP3 encodes a member of the fork-winged helix family of transcription factors, playing an important role in the development and function of naturally occurring CD4-positive/CD25-positive T regulatory cells. Pathogenic variants in *FOXP3* cause immunodysregulation, polyendocrinopathy, and enteropathy, X-linked (IPEX) syndrome. *IL2RG* encodes for gamma interleukin-2 receptor, which affects the growth and differentiation of T cells, B cells, natural killer cells, glioma cells, and cells of the monocyte lineage after specifically interacting with its receptors. Pathogenic variants in *IL2RG* cause X-linked severe combined immunodeficiency. Pathogenic variants in *WAS* cause X-linked Wiskott–Aldrich syndrome.

The patient was a girl. It was unlikely that she had an X-linked immunodeficiency. Therefore, *ADA* would most likely be tested than other options listed in the question to establish diagnosis in this patient.

233. **B**. Hyper-IgM (HIGM) syndromes are a group of primary immunodeficiency disorders characterized by defective CD40 signaling. *The most common type of HIGM syndrome is X-linked, resulting from pathogenic variants in CD40LG.* The CD40 ligand, located on the surface of activated T lymphocytes, binds to CD40 on B lymphocytes. As a consequence of the deficiency in CD40 ligand, the T lymphocytes in patients with an X-linked hyper-IgM (XHIGM) syndrome are unable to instruct B lymphocytes to switch their production of immunoglobulins from IgM to IgG, IgA, and IgE. As a result, patients with this disease have decreased levels of IgG and IgA but normal or elevated levels of IgM in their blood. So patients with XHIGM have defective cellular immunity and are also susceptible to all kinds of infections, particularly opportunistic infections, and to some types of cancer.

Other types of HIGM syndrome are inherited as autosomal recessive traits, caused by pathogenic variants in CD40, AICDA, and UNG. HIGM syndrome, caused by pathogenic variants in *CD40*, is clinically identical to the XHIGM syndrome, caused by pathogenic variants *CD40LG*. The function of *AICDA*, and *UNG* is limited to antibody switching, so the CD40 ligand functions at T lymphocytes are not affected, and

these patients are less likely to have opportunistic infections or cancer (http://primaryimmune.org).

The inherited pattern of hyper-IgM syndrome is not clear in this family. Therefore, a next-generation sequencing (NGS) panel would be the most cost-effective way to confirm/rule out the diagnosis in this patient.

234. **E**. Hyper-IgM (HIGM) syndromes are a group of primary immunodeficiency disorders characterized by defective CD40 signaling. This patient likely had X-linked hyper-IgM syndrome type 1 (HIGM1), since his mother, his maternal aunt, and his maternal grandmother were silent carriers. HIGM1 a disorder of abnormal T- and B-cell function, is characterized by low serum concentrations of IgG and IgA and normal or elevated serum concentrations of IgM. Mitogen proliferation may be normal, but NK- and T-cell cytotoxicity is frequently impaired. Antigen-specific responses may be decreased or absent. The range of clinical findings varies, even within the same family. More than 50% of males with HIGM1 develop symptoms by age 1 year, and more than 90% are symptomatic by age 4. HIGM1 usually presents in infancy with recurrent upper- and lower-respiratory tract bacterial infections, opportunistic infections, and recurrent or protracted diarrhea associated with failure to thrive. Neutropenia, thrombocytopenia, and anemia are also common (https://www.ncbi.nlm.nih.gov/books/NBK1402/).

The diagnosis of HIGM1 is based on a combination of clinical findings, family history, absent or decreased expression of the CD40 ligand (CD40L) protein on flow cytometry following in vitro stimulation of white cells, and molecular genetic testing of CD40LG (previously known as TNFSF5 or CD154), the only gene in which pathogenic variant is known to cause HIGM1. Direct sequencing of the entire coding region and intron–exon boundaries detects pathogenic variants in approximately 95% of affected males.

This male patient, his mother, maternal aunt, and maternal grandmother had the same pathogenic variant in *CD40LG* at Xq26.3. Therefore, the maternal aunt's unborn boy would have 50% risk to inherit the pathogenic variant and be affected with HIGM1.

235. **D**. Hyper-IgM (HIGM) syndromes are a group of primary immunodeficiency disorders characterized by defective CD40 signaling. *It is most likely that the patient had X-linked hyper-IgM syndrome type 1 (HIGM1), since his mother was a silent carrier.* HIGM1 is characterized by recurrent upper- and lower-respiratory-tract bacterial

infections, opportunistic infections, and recurrent or protracted diarrhea associated with failure to thrive. In patients with HIGM1, laboratory testing usually shows low serum concentrations of IgG and IgA and normal or elevated serum concentrations of IgM. The diagnosis of HIGM1 is based on a combination of clinical findings, family history, absent or decreased expression of the CD40 ligand (CD40L) protein on flow cytometry following in vitro stimulation of white cells, and molecular genetic testing of *CD40LG* (previously known as *TNFSF5* or *CD154*), the only gene in which pathogenic variants are known to cause HIGM1 (https://www.ncbi.nlm.nih.gov/books/NBK1402/).

Adenosine deaminase (ADA) deficiency is an autosomal dominant severe combined immunodeficiency disease (SCID), often diagnosed by age 6 months and usually by age 12 months. Infants with typical early-onset ADA deficiency have failure to thrive and opportunistic infections associated with marked depletion of T, B, and NK lymphocytes and an absence of both humoral and cellular immune function. ADA is caused by pathogenic variants in the *ADA* gene. Immune dysregulation, polyendocrinopathy, enteropathy, X-linked (IPEX) syndrome is characterized by systemic autoimmunity, typically beginning in the first year of life. Presentation is most commonly the clinical triad of watery diarrhea, eczematous dermatitis, and endocrinopathy (most commonly insulin-dependent diabetes mellitus). Most children have other autoimmune phenomena, including Coombs-positive anemia, autoimmune thrombocytopenia, autoimmune neutropenia, and tubular nephropathy. IPEX is caused by pathogenic variants in *FOXP3*. X-linked severe combined immunodeficiency (X-SCID) is a combined cellular and humoral immunodeficiency mostly caused by pathogenic variants in *IL2RG*. In typical X-SCID, lack of *IL2RG* function results in near complete absence of T and natural killer (NK) lymphocytes and nonfunctional B lymphocytes. X-SCID is almost universally fatal in the first 2 years of life unless reconstitution of the immune system is achieved through bone-marrow transplantation or gene therapy. Wiskott–Aldrich syndrome (WAS) is an X-linked immunodeficiency that usually presents in infancy. Affected males have thrombocytopenia with intermittent mucosal bleeding, bloody diarrhea, and intermittent or chronic petechiae and purpura; eczema; and recurrent bacterial and viral infections,

particularly recurrent ear infections. WAS is caused by pathogenic variants in *WAS*.

Therefore, it would be most likely this patient had X-linked hyper-IgM syndrome caused by a pathogenic variant in *CD40LG*.

236. **B**. Hyper-IgM (HIGM) syndromes are a group of primary immunodeficiency disorders characterized by defective CD40 signaling. The most common type of HIGM syndrome is X-linked, resulting from pathogenic variants in *CD40LG* at Xq26.3. CD40 ligand, located on the surface of activated T lymphocytes, binds to CD40 on B lymphocytes. As a consequence of the deficiency in CD40 ligand, the T lymphocytes in patients with X-linked hyper-IgM (XHIGM) are unable to instruct B lymphocytes to switch their production of immunoglobulins from IgM to IgG, IgA, and IgE. As a result, patients with this disease have decreased levels of IgG and IgA but normal or elevated levels of IgM in their blood. So patients with X-linked hyper-IgM syndrome (XHIM) have defective cellular immunity and are also susceptible to all kinds of infections, particularly opportunistic infections, and to some types of cancer.

Other types of HIGM syndrome are inherited as autosomal recessive traits, caused by pathogenic variants in *CD40*, *AICDA*, and *UNG*. HIGM syndrome caused by pathogenic variants in *CD40* is clinically identical to the X-linked HIGM syndrome caused by pathogenic variants *CD40LG*. *The function of AICDA, and UNG is limited to antibody switching, so the CD40 ligand functions at T-lymphocyte are not affected, and these patients are less likely to have opportunistic infections or cancer* (http://primaryimmune.org).

Therefore, *AICDA* would most likely harbor pathogenic variant(s) in this female patient.

237. **B**. Hyper-IgM (HIGM) syndromes are a group of primary immunodeficiency disorders characterized by defective CD40 signaling. The most common type of HIGM syndrome is X-linked, resulting from pathogenic variants in *CD40LG*. *Other types of HIGM syndrome are inherited as autosomal recessive traits, caused by pathogenic variants in CD40, AICDA, and UNG.*

Adenosine deaminase (ADA) deficiency is an autosomal dominant severe combined immunodeficiency disease (SCID), often diagnosed by age 6 months and usually by age 12 months. Infants with typical early-onset ADA deficiency have failure to thrive and opportunistic infections associated with marked depletion of T, B, and NK lymphocytes, and an absence of both humoral and cellular immune function. ADA is caused by pathogenic variants in the *ADA* gene. Immune dysregulation, polyendocrinopathy, enteropathy, X-linked (IPEX) syndrome is characterized by systemic autoimmunity, typically beginning in the first year of life. Presentation is most commonly the clinical triad of watery diarrhea, eczematous dermatitis, and endocrinopathy (most commonly insulin-dependent diabetes mellitus). Most children have other autoimmune phenomena, including Coombs-positive anemia, autoimmune thrombocytopenia, autoimmune neutropenia, and tubular nephropathy. IPEX is caused by pathogenic variants in *FOXP3*. X-linked severe combined immunodeficiency (X-SCID) is a combined cellular and humoral immunodeficiency mostly caused by pathogenic variants in *IL2RG*. In typical X-SCID, lack of *IL2RG* function results in near complete absence of T and natural killer (NK) lymphocytes and nonfunctional B lymphocytes. X-SCID is almost universally fatal in the first 2 years of life unless reconstitution of the immune system is achieved through bone-marrow transplantation or gene therapy. Wiskott—Aldrich syndrome (WAS) is an X-linked immunodeficiency that usually presents in infancy. Affected males have thrombocytopenia with intermittent mucosal bleeding, bloody diarrhea, and intermittent or chronic petechiae and purpura; eczema; and recurrent bacterial and viral infections, particularly recurrent ear infections. WAS is caused by pathogenic variants in *WAS*.

This female patient had hypogammaglobulinemia with hyper-IgM and a homozygous pathogenic variant, c.260G > C(p. Cys87Ser), in *AICDA*. Therefore, it was most likely that she had hyper-IgM syndrome.

238. **D.** Cerebral autosomal dominant arteriopathy with subcortical infarcts and leukoencephalopathy, usually called CADASIL, affects blood flow in small blood vessels, particularly cerebral vessels within the brain. More than 95% of individuals with CADASIL have pathogenic variants in *NOTCH3*, the only gene in which mutation is known to cause CADASIL. The pathological hallmark of CADASIL is electron-dense granules in the media of arterioles, and increased NOTCH3 staining of the arterial wall, which can be evaluated in a skin biopsy. *Molecular sequencing analysis of exons 2—24 and intron—exon boundaries of NOTCH3 was estimated to identify more than 95% of pathogenic variants, mostly missense variants.* If no pathogenic variant is found, deletion/duplication analysis

may be used as a follow-up test with an unknown detection rate (https://www.ncbi.nlm.nih.gov/books/NBK1500/).

Therefore, Sanger sequencing would most likely be used to confirm/rule out the diagnosis in this patient. If no pathogenic variant is found, deletion/duplication analysis may be used as a follow-up testing.

239. **C.** Cerebral autosomal dominant arteriopathy with subcortical infarcts and leukoencephalopathy, usually called CADASIL, affects blood flow in small blood vessels, particularly cerebral vessels within the brain. *NOTCH3 is the only gene in which heterozygous pathogenic variants cause CADASIL* (http://ghr.nlm.nih.gov).

Pathogenic variants in *NOTCH2* are associated Alagille syndrome. *NOTCH1* rearrangement in t (7;9)(q34;q34.3) is seen in acute T-cell lymphoma.

Therefore, *NOTCH3* would most likely be tested for CADASIL in this patient.

240. **B.** *NOTCH3* consists of 33 exons spanning roughly 7 kb. For a detailed summary of gene and protein information, see Guyani et al. Pathogenic variants in CADASIL are detected in exons 2—24. *The majority of sequence alterations in NOTCH3 are missense variants (95%), characteristically leading to the loss or gain of a cysteine residue in one of the epidermal growth factor-like repeat (EGFR) domains of neurogenic locus notch homolog protein 3 (NOTCH3), the protein encoded by NOTCH3.* This results in an uneven number of cysteine residues in the given domain, most likely modifying the tertiary structure of the protein. A few splice-site variants, insertions, and deletions have been described, also resulting in an uneven number of cysteine residues within EGFR. The majority of pathogenic variants occur in exons 2—6, although regional differences are seen. Most pathogenic variants in *NOTCH3* in individuals with CADASIL are located in exon 4. Geographic variations have been described, showing exon 3 to be the second most common mutation site in French, British, and German persons, while exon 11 frequently harbors pathogenic variants in affected Dutch persons (https://www.ncbi.nlm.nih.gov/books/NBK1500/).

Therefore, the pathogenic variant detected in this patient most likely involved cysteine.

241. **E.** Cerebral autosomal dominant arteriopathy with subcortical infarcts and leukoencephalopathy, usually called CADASIL, is caused by pathogenic variants in *NOTCH3* at 19q12. Most affected individuals have an affected parent; de novo pathogenic variants appear to be

rare. *Each child of an affected person is at a 50% risk of inheriting the pathogenic variant and developing signs of the disease* (https://www.ncbi.nlm.nih.gov/books/NBK1500/).

Therefore, the patient's daughter had an approximately 50% risk to have the same condition.

242. **B**. Testing of asymptomatic individuals younger than age 18 years who are at risk for adult-onset disorders for which no treatment exists is not considered appropriate, primarily because it negates the autonomy of the child with no compelling benefit. Further, concern exists regarding the potential unhealthy adverse effects that such information may have on family dynamics, the risk of discrimination and stigmatization in the future, and the anxiety that such information may cause. In a family with an established diagnosis of CADASIL, testing is appropriate to consider in symptomatic individuals regardless of age.

Therefore, the National Society of Genetic Counselors, the American Academy of Pediatrics, and American College of Medical Genetics and Genomics do not recommend genetic testing of minors for adult-onset conditions (https://www.nsgc.org). Answer B is correct: informing the patient that testing asymptomatic children does more harm than good.

243. **A**. *Alagille syndrome (ALGS) is an autosomal dominant condition caused by pathogenic variants in JAG1 and NOTCH2*. The major clinical manifestations of ALGS are cholestasis, characterized by bile-duct paucity on liver biopsy; congenital cardiac defects, primarily involving the pulmonary arteries; posterior embryotoxon in the eye; typical facial features; and butterfly vertebrae. Sequencing analysis of *JAG1* detects pathogenic variants in more than 89% of individuals who meet clinical diagnostic criteria; deletion/duplication analysis detects exon and whole-gene deletions, including microdeletion of 20p12, in approximately 7% of affected individuals. Pathogenic variants in *NOTCH2* are observed in 1%−2% of individuals with ALGS (http://www.ncbi.nlm.nih.gov/books/NBK1273/).

JAG1, JAG2, DLL1, DLL3, and *DLL4* are all ligands of the Notch family.

Therefore, *JAG1* was most likely be tested to confirm the diagnosis in this patient.

244. **B**. *Alagille syndrome (ALGS) is an autosomal dominant condition caused by pathogenic variants in JAG1 and NOTCH2*. Sequencing analysis of *JAG1* detects pathogenic variants in more than 89% of individuals who meet clinical diagnostic criteria

and deletion/duplication analysis detects exon and whole-gene deletions, including microdeletion of 20p12, in approximately 7% of affected individuals. Pathogenic variants in *NOTCH2* are observed in 1%−2% of individuals with ALGS (http://www.ncbi.nlm.nih.gov/books/NBK1273/).

NOTCH1 rearrangement in t(7;9)(q34;q34.3) is seen in acute T-cell lymphoma. Pathogenic variants in *NOTCH2* cause autosomal dominant cerebral arteriopathy with subcortical infarcts and leukoencephalopathy (CADASIL).

Therefore, *NOTCH2* was most likely tested to confirm the diagnosis in this patient.

245. **A**. The two genes in which mutation is known to cause Alagille syndrome (ALGS) are *JAG1* and *NOTCH2*. Sequencing analysis of *JAG1* detects pathogenic variants in more than 89% of individuals who meet clinical diagnostic criteria and deletion/duplication analysis detects exon and whole-gene deletions, including microdeletion of 20p12, in approximately 7% of affected individuals. Pathogenic variants in *NOTCH2* are observed in 1%−2% of individuals with ALGS.

To confirm/establish the diagnosis of ALGS in a proband, sequencing analysis of *JAG1* should be performed first, as this identifies pathogenic variants in more than 89% of persons with a *JAG1* pathogenic variant, in situations in which the diagnosis is suspected but the criteria for clinical diagnosis are not met. *If no pathogenic variants are detected by sequencing analysis of JAG1, deletion/duplication analysis can be performed to detect deletions or duplications of JAG1 exon(s) or of the whole gene*. Given the wide availability of targeted CMA testing, this could be used to determine both the presence and extent of a chromosome deletion/duplication involving *JAG1* if there was high density of probes in the region. Other deletion/duplication methods (e.g., MLPA) also detect exon or whole-gene deletions. If a deletion involving the entire *JAG1* gene is identified, a full cytogenetic study may be considered to determine whether a rare chromosome rearrangement (translocation or inversion) is present. The presence of developmental delay and/or hearing loss in addition to the features commonly seen in ALGS may increase the suspicion for a chromosome deletion. *NOTCH2* molecular genetic testing should be considered when the diagnosis is strongly suspected on clinical grounds, but no *JAG1* variant/deletion/duplication was identified (http://www.ncbi.nlm.nih.gov/books/NBK1273/).

Therefore, the appropriate next step in the workup for this patient is deletion/duplication analysis of *JAG1*.

246. B. The pathogenic variant was detected in the mother but not the father. It is possible that the proband inherited one copy from the mother and had a de novo mutation at the paternal copy. However, the presence of delayed growth and developmental in addition to the features commonly seen in Alagille syndrome (ALGS) increase suspicion for a chromosome deletion.

Therefore, a deletion involving the entire *JAG1* gene should be considered, especially because it is relatively common in ALGS (7%). Multiplex ligation-dependent probe amplification (MLPA) is an appropriate study for deletion/duplication.

References

1. Scriver CR. Assessing genetic risks: implications for health and social policy. *Am J Hum Genet* 1995;**56**(3):814–16.
2. Litvinchuk T, et al. A case of new familiar genetic variant of autosomal dominant polycystic kidney disease-2: a case study. *Front Pediatr* 2015;**3**:82.
3. Thakur P, Speer P, Rajkovic A. Novel mutation in the PKHD1 gene diagnosed prenatally in a fetus with autosomal recessive polycystic kidney disease. *Case Rep Genet* 2014;**2014**:517952.
4. Patil S, Paricharak M, Paricharak D, More S. Fetal polycystic kidney disease: pathological overview. *J Sci Soc* 2013;**40**(2):106–8.
5. You J, Kang E, Kim Y, Lee BH, Ko TS, Kim GH, et al. *Two cases of TSC2/PKD1 contiguous gene deletion syndrome*. *J Genet Med* 2016;**13**(1):36–40.
6. Nussbaum RL, McInnes RR, Willard HF. 8th ed. *Thompson & Thompsongenetics in medicine*, vol. xi. Philadelphia: Elsevier; 2016. p. 546.
7. Kumar S, Mahajan BB, Mittal J. Bardet–Biedl syndrome: a rare case report from North India. *Indian J Dermatol Venereol Leprol* 2012;**78**(2):228.
8. Prasanth YM, et al. A case report on the Bardet Biedl syndrome with hypokalaemic paralysis. *J Clin Diagn Res* 2013;**7**(6):1163–4.
9. Piccoli E, et al. Novel PSEN1 mutations (H214N and R220P) associated with familial Alzheimer disease identified by targeted exome sequencing. *Neurobiol Aging* 2016;**40**:192 e7–192 e11.
10. Committee on Bioethics, et al. Ethical and policy issues in genetic testing and screening of children. *Pediatrics* 2013;**131**(3):620–2.
11. Rao A, Schimmenti LA, Vestal E, Schnooveld C, Ferrello M, Ward J, et al. Genetic testing in childhood hearing loss: review and case studies. *Audiol Online* 2011.
12. Acmg. Genetics evaluation guidelines for the etiological diagnosis of congenital hearing loss. Genetic evaluation of congenital hearing loss expert panel. ACMG statement. *Genet Med* 2002;**4**(3):162–71.
13. Morell RJ, et al. Mutations in the connexin 26 gene (GJB2) among Ashkenazi Jews with nonsyndromic recessive deafness. *N Engl J Med* 1998;**339**(21):1500–5.
14. Brownstein Z, Avraham KB. Deafness genes in Israel: implications for diagnostics in the clinic. *Pediatr Res* 2009;**66**(2):128–34.
15. Sharma K, Arora A. Waardenburg syndrome: a case study of two patients. *Indian J Otolaryngol Head Neck Surg* 2015;**67**(3):324–8.
16. Safal Khanal BO, Southwestern University, Cebu City, Philippines. *Waardenburg syndrome: a report of two familial case series*. *Optom Vis Perf* 2013;**1**(6):215–19.
17. Chronister CL, et al. Leber's hereditary optic neuropathy: a case report. *Optometry* 2005;**76**(5):302–8.
18. Teive HA, et al. Leber's hereditary optic neuropathy – case report and literature review. *Sao Paulo Med J* 2004;**122**(6):276–9.
19. Chang C-W, Chang C-H, Peng M-L. Leber's hereditary optic neuropathy: a case report. *Kaohsiung J Med Sci* 2003;**19**(10):516–20.
20. Chen YN, et al. Maternally inherited diabetes and deafness (MIDD) syndrome: a clinical and molecular genetic study of a Taiwanese family. *Chang Gung Med J* 2004;**27**(1):66–73.
21. Donovan LE, Severin NE. Maternally inherited diabetes and deafness in a North American kindred: tips for making the diagnosis and review of unique management issues. *J Clin Endocrinol Metab* 2006;**91**(12):4737–42.
22. Chandra SR, et al. A typical case of myoclonic epilepsy with ragged red fibers (MERRF) and the lessons learned. *J Postgrad Med* 2015;**61**(3):200–2.
23. Yu XF, et al. Myoclonic epilepsy with ragged-red fibers: a case report. *Exp Ther Med* 2015;**9**(2):432–4.
24. LailaSelima D. Mitochondrial encephalopathy with lactic acidosis and stroke-like episodes in a Japanese child: clinical, radiological and molecular genetic analysis. *Egyptian J Med Hum Genet* 2013;**14**(3):317–22.
25. Jayaram S, et al. An interesting case of familial homozygous hypercholesterolemia – a brief review. *Indian J Clin Biochem* 2012;**27**(3):309–13.
26. Shawky RM. Reduced penetrance in human inherited disease. *Egyptian J Med Hum Genet* 2014;**15**(2):103–11.
27. Gordon G, Wisbacha WD. Ileal atresia, malrotation and Hirschsprung's disease: a case report. *J Pediatr Surg Case Rep* 2013;**1**(1):e3–5.
28. Chen F, et al. Hirschsprung's disease in a young adult: report of a case and review of the literature. *Ann Diagn Pathol* 2006;**10**(6):347–51.
29. Upadhyaya M, et al. Three different pathological lesions in the NF1 gene originating de novo in a family with neurofibromatosis type 1. *Hum Genet* 2003;**112**(1):12–17.
30. Klose A, et al. Two independent mutations in a family with neurofibromatosis type 1 (NF1). *Am J Med Genet* 1999;**83**(1):6–12.
31. Lazaro C, et al. Molecular characterization of the breakpoints of a 12-kb deletion in the NF1 gene in a family showing germ-line mosaicism. *Am J Hum Genet* 1995;**57**(5):1044–9.
32. Consoli C, et al. Gonosomal mosaicism for a nonsense mutation (R1947X) in the NF1 gene in segmental neurofibromatosis type 1. *J Invest Dermatol* 2005;**125**(3):463–6.
33. Zacharia GS. Neurofibromatosis type 2: a case report and brief review of literature. *Indian J Otol* 2013;**19**(4):205–7.
34. Behnes CL, et al. 13-Year-old tuberous sclerosis patient with renal cell carcinoma associated with multiple renal angiomyolipomas developing multifocal micronodular pneumocyte hyperplasia. *BMC Clin Pathol* 2013;**13**:4.
35. Rose VM, et al. Germ-line mosaicism in tuberous sclerosis: how common? *Am J Hum Genet* 1999;**64**(4):986–92.
36. Bathla M, Chandna S, Bathla JC. Rett's syndrome: diagnostic and therapeutic dilemma. *German J Psychiatry* 2010;**13**(3):157–60.
37. Vignoli A, et al. Electroclinical pattern in MECP2 duplication syndrome: eight new reported cases and review of literature. *Epilepsia* 2012;**53**(7):1146–55.
38. Yum MS, Ko TS, Yoo HW. The first Korean case of KCNQ2 mutation in a family with benign familial neonatal convulsions. *J Korean Med Sci* 2010;**25**(2):324–6.

39. Fuld ZSaKB. Case study of a patient with pseudohypoparathyroidism and learning disability. In: *The Endocrine Society's 94th Annual Meeting and Expo* 2012.

40. Luk HM, Lo IFM, Tong TMF, Lai KKS, Lam STS. Pseudohypoparathyroidism Type 1b: first case report in Chinese and literature review. *HK J Paediatr* 2015;**20**:32–6.

41. Weinstein LS, et al. Mutations of the Gs alpha-subunit gene in Albright hereditary osteodystrophy detected by denaturing gradient gel electrophoresis. *Proc Natl Acad Sci USA* 1990;**87** (21):8287–90.

42. Adegbite NS, et al. Diagnostic and mutational spectrum of progressive osseous heteroplasia (POH) and other forms of GNAS-based heterotopic ossification. *Am J Med Genet A* 2008;**146A** (14):1788–96.

43. Wu WI, et al. Selective resistance to parathyroid hormone caused by a novel uncoupling mutation in the carboxyl terminus of G alpha(s). A cause of pseudohypoparathyroidism type Ib. *J Biol Chem* 2001;**276**(1):165–71.

44. Simpson C, Grove E, Houston BA. Pseudopseudo hypoparathyroidism. *Lancet* 2015;**385**(9973):1123.

45. Ahrens W, et al. Analysis of the GNAS1 gene in Albright's hereditary osteodystrophy. *J Clin Endocrinol Metab* 2001;**86**(10):4630–4.

46. Ashrafzadeh F, et al. Angelman syndrome: a case report. *Iran J Child Neurol* 2016;**10**(2):86–9.

47. Ali S, Khalil S, Ali L. Smith Lemli Opitz syndrome: a case report. *Khyber Med Univ J* 2015;**7**(1):34–6.

48. Marin R, et al. Three cases with L1 syndrome and two novel mutations in the L1CAM gene. *Eur J Pediatr* 2015;**174**(11):1541–4.

49. Yun KW, et al. The first case of X-linked Alpha-thalassemia/mental retardation (ATR-X) syndrome in Korea. *J Korean Med Sci* 2011;**26**(1):146–9.

50. Vujanović M, Stanković-Babić G, Cekić S. Noonan syndrome — case report. *Acta Med Median* 2014;**53**(2):54–6.

51. Nalini A, Biswas A. Sotos syndrome: an interesting disorder with gigantism. *Ann Indian Acad Neurol* 2008;**11**(3):190–2.

52. Narea Matamala G, et al. Beckwith Wiedemann syndrome: presentation of a case report. *Med Oral Patol Oral Cir Bucal* 2008;**13** (10):E640–3.

53. Storm DW, et al. The prenatal diagnosis of Beckwith–Wiedemann syndrome using ultrasound and magnetic resonance imaging. *Urology* 2011;**77**(1):208–10.

54. Eggermann T, et al. Clinical utility gene card for: Beckwith–Wiedemann syndrome. *Eur J Hum Genet* 2014;**22**(3).

55. Bing-Ping Qiu C-HS. Silver-Russell syndrome: a case report. *World J Pediatr* 2007;**3**(1):68–70.

56. Kumar S, et al. Silver-Russell syndrome: a case report. *Cases J* 2008;**1**(1):304.

57. Kumar S, Jain AP, Agrawal S, Chandran S. *Silver-Russell syndrome: a case report.* BSMMU J 2013. 6(2): p. 175-175-7.

58. Eriksson M, et al. Recurrent de novo point mutations in lamin A cause Hutchinson-Gilford progeria syndrome. *Nature* 2003;**423** (6937):293–8.

59. Rastogi R, Mohan SMC. Progeria syndrome: a case report. *Indian J Orthop* 2008;**42**(1):97–9.

60. Bartsch O, et al. Molecular studies in 10 cases of Rubinstein–Taybi syndrome, including a mild variant showing a missense mutation in codon 1175 of CREBBP. *J Med Genet* 2002;**39**(7):496–501.

61. Petrij F, Giles R, Breuning MH, Hennekam RCM. Rubinstein–Taybi syndrome. In: Scriver CR, Beaudet AL, Sly WS, Valle D, Childs B, Kinzler KW, Vogelstein B, editors. *The metabolic and molecular bases of inherited disease.* New York, NY: McGraw-Hill 2001.

62. Niida YO, Ozaki M, Takase E, Yokoyama T, Yamada S. A girl with greig cephalopolysyndactyly contiguous gene deletion syndrome: the importance and usefulness of DNA microarray analysis. *Hered Genet Curr Res* 2015;**S7**.

63. Thomas HM, et al. Recurrence of Pallister-Hall syndrome in two sibs. *J Med Genet* 1994;**31**(2):145–7.

64. Uppuluri R, Gowrishankar K, Janakiraman L. Crossed polydactyly and Greig cephalopolysyndactyly syndrome. *Indian Pediatr* 2013;**50**(10):967–8.

65. Dinesh Giri SA, McKay V, Weber A, Didi M, Senniappan S. Congenital hyperinsulinism and cochlear hypoplasia in a rare case of Pallister-Hall syndrome. *Int J Clin Pediatr* 2015;**4** (2–3):154–7.

66. Pena WA, Slavotinek A, Oberoi S. Saethre–Chotzen syndrome: a case report. *Cleft Palate Craniofac J* 2010;**47**(3):318–21.

67. Yu JE, Park DH, Yoon SH. A Korean family with the Muenke syndrome. *J Korean Med Sci* 2010;**25**(7):1086–9.

68. Lee MY, et al. A case of Pfeiffer syndrome with c833_834GC > TG (Cys278Leu) mutation in the FGFR2 gene. *Korean J Pediatr* 2010;**53**(7):774–7.

69. Arathi R, Sagtani A, Baliga M. Crouzons syndrome: a case report. *J Indian Soc Pedod Prev Dent* 2007;**25**(Suppl.):S10–12.

70. Ibrahimi OA, et al. Proline to arginine mutations in FGF receptors 1 and 3 result in Pfeiffer and Muenke craniosynostosis syndromes through enhancement of FGF binding affinity. *Hum Mol Genet* 2004;**13**(1):69–78.

71. Park WJ, et al. Analysis of phenotypic features and FGFR2 mutations in Apert syndrome. *Am J Hum Genet* 1995;**57**(2):321–8.

72. Wilkie AO, et al. Apert syndrome results from localized mutations of FGFR2 and is allelic with Crouzon syndrome. *Nat Genet* 1995;**9**(2):165–72.

73. Cunningham ML, et al. Syndromic craniosynostosis: from history to hydrogen bonds. *Orthod Craniofac Res* 2007;**10**(2):67–81.

74. Funato N, et al. Common regulation of growth arrest and differentiation of osteoblasts by helix-loop-helix factors. *Mol Cell Biol* 2001;**21**(21):7416–28.

75. Glaser RL, et al. Paternal origin of FGFR2 mutations in sporadic cases of Crouzon syndrome and Pfeiffer syndrome. *Am J Hum Genet* 2000;**66**(3):768–77.

76. Goriely A, et al. Germline and somatic mosaicism for FGFR2 mutation in the mother of a child with Crouzon syndrome: implications for genetic testing in "paternal age-effect" syndromes. *Am J Med Genet A* 2010;**152A**(8):2067–73.

77. Moloney DM, et al. Exclusive paternal origin of new mutations in Apert syndrome. *Nat Genet* 1996;**13**(1):48–53.

78. Shah GS, Shah GS, Shrivastava M, Shah D, Gupta N. Achondroplasia: case report and review of literature. *J Nepal Paediatr Soc* 2011;**31**(3):216–24.

79. Horton WA, Degnin CR. FGFs in endochondral skeletal development. *Trends Endocrinol Metab* 2009;**20**(7):341–8.

80. Korkmaz HA, et al. Hypochondroplasia in a child with 1620C > G (Asn540Lys) mutation in FGFR3. *J Clin Res Pediatr Endocrinol* 2012;**4**(4):220–2.

81. Barbosa ND, et al. Isolated left ventricular noncompaction: unusual cause of decompensated heart failure and indication of heart transplantation in the early infancy — case report and literature review. *Clinics (Sao Paulo)* 2008;**63**(1):136–9.

82. Hakim K, et al. Cardiac events in Costello syndrome: one case and a review of the literature. *J Saudi Heart Assoc* 2014;**26** (2):105–9.

83. Bani M, et al. Ectodermal dysplasia with anodontia: a report of two cases. *Eur J Dent* 2010;**4**(2):215–22.

84. Ayesha Thabusum D, Rajesh N, Sudhakara Reddy R, Ramesh T. Ectodermal dysplasia — a case study of two identical sibilings. *Int J Dental Sci Res* 2014;**2**(6):175–8.

85. Li X, et al. Incontinentia pigmenti: case report. *Acta Dermatovenerol Croat* 2013;**21**(3):193–7.

SELF-ASSESSMENT QUESTIONS FOR CLINICAL MOLECULAR GENETICS

86. Bentolila R, Rivera H, Sanchez-Quevedo MC. Incontinentia pigmenti: a case report. *Pediatr Dent* 2006;**28**(1):54–7.

87. Fusco F, et al. Microdeletion/duplication at the Xq28 IP locus causes a de novo IKBKG/NEMO/IKKgamma exon4_10 deletion in families with Incontinentia Pigmenti. *Hum Mutat* 2009;**30**(9):1284–91.

88. Bakke AC, Purtzer MZ, Wildin RS. Prospective immunological profiling in a case of immune dysregulation, polyendocrinopathy, enteropathy, X-linked syndrome (IPEX). *Clin Exp Immunol* 2004;**137**(2):373–8.

89. Wildin RS, Smyk-Pearson S, Filipovich AH. Clinical and molecular features of the immunodysregulation, polyendocrinopathy, enteropathy, X linked (IPEX) syndrome. *J Med Genet* 2002;**39**(8):537–45.

90. Savova R, et al. Clinical case of immune dysregulation, polyendocrinopaty, enteropathy, x-linked (IPEX) syndrome with severe immune deficiency and late onset of endocrinopathy and enteropathy. *Case Rep Med* 2014;**2014**:564926.

91. Poorun KRSRV. Wiskott-Aldrich syndrome (WAS): a case report in Mauritius and review. *Int J Pediatr* 2015;**3**(3.1):579–83.

92. Kumar MK, Narayan R. Wiskott Aldrich syndrome, often missed: a case report and review. *J Nep Paedtr Soc* 2011;**31**(2):146–50.

93. Jo EK, et al. X-linked severe combined immunodeficiency syndrome: the first Korean case with gamma c chain gene mutation and subsequent genetic counseling. *J Korean Med Sci* 2004;**19**(1):123–6.

94. Hussain W, et al. Severe combined immunodeficiency due to adenosine deaminase deficiency. *J Pak Med Assoc* 2012;**62**(3):297–9.

95. Tsai HY, et al. X-linked hyper-IgM syndrome with CD40LG mutation: two case reports and literature review in Taiwanese patients. *J Microbiol Immunol Infect* 2015;**48**(1):113–18.

96. Guo LI, et al. X-linked hyper-IgM syndrome with eosinophilia in a male child: a case report. *Exp Ther Med* 2015;**9**(4):1328–30.

97. Silva R, Da Costa JT. Hyper-IgM syndrome – a case report and a clinical perspective. *Eur Ann Allergy Clin Immunol* 2010;**42**(5):194–6.

98. Delibas S, Guven H, Comoglu SS. A case report about CADASIL: mutation in the NOTCH 3 receptor. *Acta Neurol Taiwan* 2009;**18**(4):262–6.

99. Gayani GG, Pathirana K, Weerarathna TP, Mohideen MR. Different presentations of CADASIL; importance of a detailed history. *Galle Med J* 2014;**19**(2):32–4.

100. Bhatia V, Kumar P. Alagille syndrome with a previously undescribed mutation. *Indian Pediatr* 2014;**51**(4):314–16.

101. Kim J, et al. A case of Alagille syndrome presenting with chronic cholestasis in an adult. *Clin Mol Hepatol* 2017;**23**(3):260–4.

102. Fang W, Lu Y, Abuduxikuer K, Wu B, Wang J, Xie X. De novo JAG 1 gene deletion causes atypical severe Alagille syndrome in a Chinese child. *Int J Clin Exp Pathol* 2017;**10**(4):4913–17.

103. Wilkins Jon F, Úbeda Francisco. *Chapter 13 - Diseases Associated with Genomic Imprinting. Progress in Molecular Biology and Translational Science*, Vol 101. Elsevier; 2011. p. 401–45 Available from: https://doi.org/10.1016/B978-0-12-387685-0.00013-5.

Further Reading

- American Heart Association (www.heart.org/)
- British Society for Immunology (www.immunology.org)
- Fertilitypedia (www.fertilitypedia.org/)
- Foundation for Mitochondrial Medicine (www.mitochondrialdiseases.org/)
- Hearing Loss Association of America (www.hearingloss.org/)
- Hear-it (www.hear-it.org/)
- Immune Deficiency Foundation (www.primaryimmune.org/)
- Mito Action (www.mitoaction.org/)
- Mitochondrial Disease News (www.mitochondrialdiseasenews.com/)
- National Organization for Rare Disorders (www.rarediseases.org)
- Orphanet (www.orpha.net/)

13

Pharmacogenetics

Pharmacogenomics (PGx) has become a key component of personalized medicine. One person dies every 5 minutes from adverse drug reactions to properly prescribed medications, according to the guidelines approved by the FDA. If a gene variant is associated with a particular drug response, potentially this information may be used to adjust the dosage, choosing a specific, or a different, drug or drug combination. For example, *ERBB2* (*HER2*) overexpression has been seen in 15%–20% of breast cancers and is also overexpressed in some gastroesophageal cancers. Monoclonal antibodies such as trastuzumab (brand name, Herceptin) and pertuzumab (2C4; trade name Perjeta) are used to treat breast cancer; they target a receptor in the epidermal growth factor family encoded by the *ERBB2* (*HER2*) gene.

In pharmacogenomics, the genomic sequence is used to study individual responses to medications. As disease-associated variants, genetic variants affecting an individual's drug response could be assessed by identifying genetic loci associated with known drug responses and then testing individuals to predict the response. A wide range of gene variants are related to drug selection, such as single-nucleotide variants (SNVs; such as *BRAF* V600E, *CFTR* G551D, *HLA-B*57:01*), deletions (*CCR5-Δ32* allele), amplifications (*HER2*), and gene rearrangements (*BCR-ABL1*, *ALK*). These genetic variants may be a therapeutic target (cetuximab/panitumumab and *KRAS*; vemurafenib and *BRAF*) or a predisposition to certain drug side effects (abacavir and *HLA-B*5701*; carbamazepine and *HLA-B*1502*; thiopurines and *TPMT*).[1]

Currently, about 10% of drug labels approved by the US Food and Drug Administration (FDA) contain pharmacogenetic information. Targeted approach, multigene analysis, or whole-genome single-nucleotide polymorphism (SNP) profiles have been using in the clinical setting. The expanded capacity of genomewide studies has dramatically increased the speed of drug discovery and development. For an increasing number of drugs, pharmacogenetic testing can be used to optimize drug therapy. However, a drug response can also be influenced by age, sex, drug–drug interactions, drug–food interactions, comorbidity, liver and renal function, and pregnancy in addition to genetic factors.

This chapter will cover genetics studies for specific drugs, disorders, and ethnic groups and clinical guidelines (recommendations) for drug selection based on genetics results. Education resources and support groups are provided in the "Further Reading" section.

QUESTIONS

1. A 33-year-old HIV-infected man came to a clinic for generalized tonic–clonic seizures. He had been on HAART (tenofovir 300 mg, emtricitabine 200 mg, and efavirenz 600 mg). The seizures started 1 month into the HAART, which was administered once every 3 months. He had no medical or family history of seizures. His clinical examination results were normal except for an electroencephalogram showing intermittent bursts of high-voltage sharp waves and spikes bilaterally over frontotemporoparietal regions, consistent with complex partial seizures. He was initially administered sodium valproate with no appreciable control of seizures. Subsequently, his efavirenz plasma level was found to be 209.55 μg/mL. Then efavirenz was replaced with nevirapine, resulting in instant resolution of his seizures. He has been seizure-free for 3 years and has not required the use of any anticonvulsant. A repeat electroencephalogram showed no sign of seizure activity. Which one of the following genes most likely mutated in this patient making him susceptible to the efavirenz toxicity?
   A. *CYP2B6*
   B. *CYP2C9*
   C. *CYP2D6*
   D. *CYP3A*
   E. *HLA-B*57:01*
   F. None of the above

Self-assessment Questions for Clinical Molecular Genetics.
DOI: https://doi.org/10.1016/B978-0-12-809967-4.00013-2

2. A 4-year 6-month-old black South African boy with perinatal HIV infection was admitted to a hospital for generalized tonic−clonic seizures 3 months after the initiation of efavirenz (EFV)-based antiretroviral treatment (ART). The mother reported that he had multiple seizures with pyrexia over a 3-day period. The medical history was significant for being on an antiretroviral (ARV) regimen. His initial treatment, started at 5 months of age, consisted of lamivudine (3TC), stavudine (d4T), and lopinavir/ritonavir (LPV/r) twice daily (bid). At 4 years of age he was enrolled in a trial for ART; abacavir (ABC) was substituted for d4T and LPV/r was switched to EFV 8 weeks thereafter. EFV dosing was prescribed according to standard recommended weight-based dosing. Baseline assessment for neuropsychiatric symptoms and neurological examination revealed no abnormalities. At admission, electroencephalography (EEG) revealed no abnormalities and a contrast computed tomographic brain (CTB) scan showed normal developmental structures, with no lesions or mass effect. Plasma EFV levels were subsequently measured at >20.0 mg/L (suggested reference range, 1−4 mg/L) 13 h after the dose. Which one of the following *CYP2B6* genotypes, which is associated EFV-induced CNS toxicity, would this patient most likely carry?[2,3]
   A. *CYP2B6*4/*4*
   B. *CYP2B6*4/*5*
   C. *CYP2B6*6/*6*
   D. *CYP2B6*6/*22*
   E. *CYP2B6*22/*22*
   F. All of the above
   G. None of the above

3. *CYP2B6* poor metabolism is associated with a higher concentration of efavirenz and nevirapine, higher viral suppression, and higher rates of hepatic and CNS adverse events. Which one of the following populations has the most *CYP2B6* poor metabolizers?[4]
   A. African American
   B. Asian
   C. Caucasian
   D. Hispanic
   E. None of the above

4. On the 12th day of abacavir treatment, a 39-year-old HIV-infected male was admitted to a hospital for fever, generalized rash, abdominal pain, and watery diarrhea that had persisted for 5 days. Laboratory testing indicated rapid progression of hepatitis and renal failure. The day after stopping antiretroviral therapy, his fever subsided and his liver function began to normalize. He was clinically diagnosed with abacavir hypersensitivity. Which one of the following alleles is associated with increased risk for adverse effect when abacavir is administered?[5,6]
   A. *HLA-A*31:01*
   B. *HLA-B*15:02*
   C. *HLA-B*57:01*
   D. *HLA-B*58:01*
   E. None of the above

5. A 45-year-old male farmer, who was diagnosed with human immunodeficiency virus (HIV) infection, was prescribed an antiretroviral (ARV) regimen including abacavir. Before the treatment, a molecular test confirmed that he carries the *HLA-B*57:01* allele. Which one of the following steps should be taken for better patient treatment in this case, according to the 2017 summary of recommendations from the Pharmacogenetics Working Group of the Royal Dutch Association for the Advancement of Pharmacy (KNMP)?[6]
   A. Continuing monitoring
   B. Decreasing abacavir dosage
   C. Increasing abacavir dosage
   D. Using an alternative drug
   E. None of the above

6. Maraviroc is a chemokine receptor antagonist that is used in combination with other antiretroviral agents to treat human immunodeficiency virus type 1 (HIV-1) infection. On which one of the following HIV-1 viruses does maraviroc exert its therapeutic activity?[6]
   A. CCR4-tropic HIV-1
   B. CCR5-tropic HIV-1
   C. CXCR4-tropic HIV-1
   D. CXCR5-tropic HIV-1
   E. None of the above

7. Which one of the following HIV-1 viruses is highly resistant to human immunodeficiency virus type 1 (HIV-1)?[6]
   A. CCR4-tropic HIV-1 with *CCR4-Δ32*
   B. CCR5-tropic HIV-1 with *CCR5-Δ32*
   C. CXCR4-tropic HIV-1 with *CXCR4-Δ32*
   D. CXCR5-tropic HIV-1 with *CXCR5-Δ32*
   E. None of the above

8. Which one of the following populations has the highest frequency of the CCR5-Δ32 allele?[6]
   A. African American
   B. Asian American
   C. Caucasian
   D. Native American
   E. None of the above

9. An overweight 68-year-old woman developed deep-vein thrombosis 2 weeks after hip-replacement surgery. Oral warfarin was prescribed

to prevent further thrombosis. Which one of the following genes may affect warfarin dosing in this patient?[6-8]

A. *CYP2C9*
B. *CYP3A*
C. *CYP4F2*
D. *VKORC1*
E. All of the above
F. None of the above

10. An overweight 68-year-old woman developed deep-vein thrombosis 2 weeks after hip-replacement surgery, and oral warfarin was prescribed. Molecular genetic testing of *CYP2C9* and *VKORC1* was ordered for dosing. Which one of the following *VKORC1* genotypes would most likely indicate a low starting dose in this patient if age and height are not taken into consideration?[6,8]

A. c.-1639G/G
B. c.-1639A/G
C. c.-1639A/A
D. Not sure
E. None of the above

11. A 74-year-old (height 157.5 cm and weight 54 kg) female of Ashkenazi Jewish descent was initiated on warfarin at 2 mg PO daily with an international normalized ratio (INR) goal of 2.0–3.0 due to a recurrence of atrial fibrillation. Her medical history was significant for atrial fibrillation, hypertension, diabetes mellitus, coronary artery disease, cardiomyopathy, hypothyroidism, myelodysplastic syndrome (MDS) with chronic anemia, cerebrovascular accident, chronic kidney disease, peptic ulcer disease, peripheral vascular disease, and pulmonary hypertension. Medications included aspirin 81 mg PO daily, isosorbide mononitrate 40 mg PO daily, furosemide 10 mg alternating with 20 mg PO daily, ramipril 10 mg PO daily, amiodarone 200 mg PO daily, atorvastatin 80 mg PO daily, metoprolol 25 mg PO daily, multiple vitamin PO daily, insulin glargine 14 units subcutaneously daily, epoetin alfa 40,000 units subcutaneously weekly, levothyroxine 100 μg PO daily, calcitriol 0.25 μg alternating with 0.5 μg PO daily, and polysaccharide iron complex 150 mg PO twice daily. Three days after starting warfarin treatment, the patient's INR was 1.4 and the dose remained unchanged. Six days later the patient's INR was 9.1. Which one of the following *CYP2C9* genotypes would this patient most likely carry to trigger the excessive anticoagulation (INR 9.1)?[8,9]

A. *CYP2C9*1/CYP2C9*1*
B. *CYP2C9*2/CYP2C9*2*
C. *CYP2C9*2/CYP2C9*17*
D. *CYP2C9*17/CYP2C9*17*
E. None of the above

12. A 60-year-old man was admitted to a tertiary health center for acute limb ischemia (ALI) in the left lower extremity. His medical history was not significant. His lifestyle was healthy, and he had never smoked. Angiography revealed that his left profunda femoris was completely occluded and that his distal superficial femoral artery (SFA) to popliteal artery (PA) was filled with thrombi. A catheter was inserted, and 1 million units of urokinase was injected intraarterially by exact pump over the next 24 hour. One day later, his SFA–PA-peroneal artery track was visualized. The occluded proximal anterior tibial artery (ATA) and straight distal superficial femoral artery were then recanalized. His ischemic symptoms disappeared and the left ankle-brachial index recovered from 0.43 to 1.14. The patient was discharged on the sixth day with a prescription for warfarin (2.5 mg/day) and clopidogrel. Unexpectedly, at 9 days after discharge, the patient presented to the emergency department again with another left ALI. Angiography revealed that a thrombus had formed in the upper part of the left SFA, which was more proximal to BTK arteries than it was previously. Which one of the following *CYP2C9* genotypes would this patient most likely carry, which required a high dose of warfarin?[8,10]

A. *CYP2C9*1/CYP2C9*1*
B. *CYP2C9*2/CYP2C9*2*
C. *CYP2C9*2/CYP2C9*17*
D. *CYP2C9*17/CYP2C9*17*
E. None of the above

13. A 65-year-old Caucasian male presented with constant dizziness, which was interpreted as light-headedness and not vertigo. He also reported occasional orthostatic hypotension. The medical history was remarkable for cerebrovascular accident with left hemiparesis and dysarthria, as well as heart failure, coronary artery disease with stent placement, aortic stenosis, and atrioventricular block with a pacemaker. He had been on metoprolol, a β-blocker, 50 mg twice daily. An ECG revealed bradycardia. Which one of the following genes most likely caused the metoprolol-induced side effect in this patient?[11]

A. *CYP2C9*
B. *CYP2D6*
C. *CYP3A*
D. *CYP4F2*
E. None of the above

14. A 65-year-old Caucasian male presented with constant dizziness, which was interpreted as light-headedness and not vertigo. He also reported occasional orthostatic hypotension. The medical

history was remarkable for cerebrovascular accident with left hemiparesis and dysarthria, as well as heart failure, coronary artery disease with stent placement, aortic stenosis, and atrioventricular block with a pacemaker. He had been on metoprolol, a β-blocker, 50 mg twice daily. An ECG revealed bradycardia. Which one of the following types of CYP2D6 metabolizers would this patient most likely be?

A. Ultrarapid metabolizer
B. Normal metabolizer
C. Intermediate metabolizer
D. Poor metabolizer
E. None of the above

15. A 65-year-old Caucasian male presented with symptoms of constant dizziness, which was felt to be lightheadedness and not interpreted as vertigo. He also complaint occasional orthostatic hypotension. A medical history was remarkable for cerebrovascular accident with left hemiparesis and dysarthria, as well as heart failure, coronary artery disease with stent placement, aortic stenosis, and atrioventricular block with a pacemaker. He had been on metoprolol, a β blocker, 50 mg twice daily. An ECG revealed bradycardia. A pharmacogenomic study demonstrated that the patient was a CYP2D6 poor metabolizer. Which one of the following CYP2D6 genotypes would the patient most likely have?[6,12,13]

A. CYP2D6*1/CYP2D6*2
B. CYP2D6*2/CYP2D6*3
C. CYP2D6*3/CYP2D6*4
D. All of the above
E. None of the above

16. A 65-year-old Caucasian male presented with symptoms of constant dizziness, which was felt to be lightheadedness and not interpreted as vertigo. He also complaint occasional orthostatic hypotension. A medical history was remarkable for cerebrovascular accident with left hemiparesis and dysarthria, as well as heart failure, coronary artery disease with stent placement, aortic stenosis, and atrioventricular block with a pacemaker. He had been on metoprolol, a β blocker, 50 mg twice daily. An ECG revealed bradycardia. A pharmacogenomic study was ordered; it demonstrated that the patient was a CYP2D6 intermediate metabolizer. Which one of the following steps should be taken for better patient treatment in this case, according to the 2017 Summary of recommendations from the Pharmacogenetics Working Group of the Royal Dutch Association for the Advancement of Pharmacy (KNMP)?[6,11]

A. Continuing monitoring
B. Decreasing the metoprolol dose
C. Increasing the metoprolol dose
D. Switching to another β blocker
E. None of the above

17. Which one of the following CYP2D6 genotypes may be used to predict which individuals are ultrarapid metabolizers?[6]

A. $CYP2D6*1 \times 2/CYP2D6*2$
B. $CYP2D6*2 \times 2/CYP2D6*3$
C. $CYP2D6*3 \times 2/CYP2D6*4$
D. $CYP2D6*4 \times 2/CYP2D6*5$
E. None of the above

18. A 10-year-old overweight girl with a history of cerebral palsy and reactive airway disease underwent orthopedic surgery for bilateral hip subluxation. Before the surgery she took a multivitamin and used a budesonide inhaler daily. Her preoperative examination noted a history of snoring and enlarged tonsils. Five days after the surgery, she was discharged with prescriptions including liquid codeine/acetaminophen (5 mL = 12 mg codeine/acetaminophen), 20–40 mg codeine every 4 hours as needed for pain, and diazepam 2–4 mg every 4 hours as needed for spasms. She was tolerant of benzodiazepine. Her mother gave her one dose of codeine/acetaminophen in the afternoon, and the second dose along with diazepine at bedtime. At 1:30 a.m., her mother went to administer pain medication as scheduled, and found her cold and unresponsive. Emergency responders attempted resuscitation without success. A postmortem examination found severe pulmonary edema, and the blood concentration of codeine and morphine was within the toxic range (total codeine, 0.78 mg/L; free codeine: 0.24 mg/L; morphine: 0.15 mg/L), particularly for an opioid-naive child. Which one of the following genes would most likely relate to an abnormally high codeine concentration in this patient?[14]

A. CYP2C9
B. CYP2D6
C. CYP3A
D. VKORC1
E. None of the above

19. A 6-year-old overweight girl with a history of myocarditis and developmental delay came to a clinic for severe cough and respiratory infection. She was prescribed an oral antibiotic (azithromycin), cough sirup (guaifenesin/codeine, 100 mg/10 mg in 5 mL), and 10–20 mg codeine every 4 hours. Her mother gave her the cough sirup at 7:00 a.m., 3:00 p.m., and 7:00 p.m., respectively. She went to bed after the last dose.

When her mother checked her at 7:45 p.m., she was "a little bit blue." When her mother checked on her the following morning at approximately 8:00 a.m., she was lifeless and cold. A postmortem examination revealed codeine toxicity (total codeine: 0.17 mg/L; free codeine: 0.08 mg/L; total morphine: 0.08 mg/L). Which one of the following *CYP2D6* metabolizers would this patient most likely be?[6,14]

A. Ultrarapid metabolizer
B. Normal metabolizer
C. Intermediate metabolizer
D. Poor metabolizer
E. None of the above

20. An 11-day-old full-term healthy male was brought to a pediatrician for a regular checkup. His mother told the doctor that he had intermittent difficulty in breastfeeding and lethargy staring on day 7. On day 12, he had gray skin and his milk intake decreased. He was found dead on day 13. A postmortem examination detected a high concentration of morphine in the blood (70 ng/mL; normal range in neonates breastfed by mothers receiving codeine, 1–2.2 ng/mL). The mother was prescribed codeine and acetaminophen after birth for episiotomy pain. Initially, she took two tablets every 12 hours (60 mg for codeine and 1000 mg for acetaminophen), then reduced the dose by half on day 2 because of somnolence and constipation. She continued the tablets for 2 weeks. The morphine concentration was 87 ng/mL in the breast milk (normal range in milk after repeated maternal codeine at doses of 60 mg every 6 hour, 1.9–20.5 ng/mL). Which one of the following *CYP2D6* genotypes would the patient most likely have?[6,15,16]

A. *CYP2D6*1 × 3*
B. *CYP2D6*4 × 4*
C. *CYP2D6*10 × 2*
D. *CYP2D6*17 × 1*
E. None of the above

21. A 49-year-old male was admitted to a hospital with a 10-day history of fever and generalized itching and erythema. The patient had chronic renal insufficiency for the past 10 years, for which he had been taking amlodipine, valsartan, and some Chinese medicines. Allopurinol was added 1 month prior to presentation. Twenty days after the initiation of allopurinol, the patient developed fever, facial edema, and generalized itching, erythema, and scaling. A laboratory evaluation revealed leukocytosis (total white-cell-count, 17.6×10^9/L), red-blood-cell count of 3.84×10^{12}/L, uric acid levels of 509 μmol/L, urea levels of 15.9 mmol/L, creatinine of 205 μmol/L, alanine

aminotransferase (ALT) of 131 U/L, and albumin of 33.6 g/L. The physician suspected allopurinol-induced exfoliative dermatitis. A molecular test was ordered to confirm it. Which one of the following alleles would this patient most likely carry if he had allopurinol-induced severe cutaneous adverse reactions (SCAR)?[6,17]

A. *HLA-A*31:01*
B. *HLA-B*15:02*
C. *HLA-B*57:01*
D. *HLA-B*58:01*
E. None of the above

22. A 15-year-old Caucasian male with autistic disorder, moderate mental retardation, and Tourette syndrome presented with a 4- to 5-month history of increased self-injury (flicking and hitting his nose at a rate of 20–50 times/hour), as well as vocal tics (at baseline he emitted high-pitch yelling-type sounds at a rate of 100–200 times an hour), and complex-motor tics in the form of grabbing and pinching. He had a significantly low BMI of 17 as well as a diagnosis of gluten enteropathy. A change in school several months prior to the onset of symptoms with subsequent loss of a close female friend may have precipitated/exacerbated his symptoms. There was an extensive history of pharmacological attempts to minimize his symptoms, including a trial of olanzapine which was discontinued after 2 weeks owing to lack of effectiveness and excessive sedation. Sertraline and clonidine were also trialed, but were subsequently discontinued owing to worsening agitation. Historically, he appeared to respond preferentially to low-dose risperidone. Therefore, risperidone was initiated at a dose of 0.25 mg in the morning and 0.5 mg at night. A favorable change in frequency of self-injurious behaviors as well as motor and vocal tics was reported on day 1 and day 2 of these medications. However, soon the patient experienced an oculogyric crisis (OGC). The dose of risperidone was subsequently reduced to 0.125 mg in the morning and 0.25 mg in the evening and increased to 0.25 mg twice a day after 10 days. Two days after this increase, OGC recurred. The physician suspected risperidone-induced toxic reaction. A molecular test was ordered to confirm it. Which one of the following genes most likely affect risperidone metabolism in this patient?[6,18]

A. *CYP2B6*
B. *CYP2C9*
C. *CYP2D6*
D. *CYP3A*
E. None of the above

23. A 15-year-old Caucasian male with autistic disorder, moderate mental retardation, and Tourette syndrome presented with a 4- to 5-month history of increased self-injury (flicking and hitting his nose at a rate of 20–50 times/hour), as well as vocal tics (at baseline he emitted high-pitch yelling-type sounds at a rate of 100–200 times an hour), and complex-motor tics in the form of grabbing and pinching. He had a significantly low BMI of 17 as well as a diagnosis of gluten enteropathy. A change in school several months prior to the onset of symptoms with subsequent loss of a close female friend may have precipitated/exacerbated his symptoms. There was an extensive history of pharmacological attempts to minimize his symptoms, including a trial of olanzapine which was discontinued after 2 weeks owing to lack of effectiveness and excessive sedation. Sertraline and clonidine were also trialed, but were subsequently discontinued owing to worsening agitation. Historically, he appeared to respond preferentially to low-dose risperidone. Therefore, risperidone was initiated at a dose of 0.25 mg in the morning and 0.5 mg at night. A favorable change in frequency of self-injurious behaviors as well as motor and vocal tics was reported on day 1 and day 2 of these medications. However, soon the patient experienced an oculogyric crisis (OGC). The dose of risperidone was subsequently reduced to 0.125 mg in the morning and 0.25 mg in the evening and increased to 0.25 mg twice a day after 10 days. Two days after this increase, OGC recurred. The physician suspected risperidone-induced toxic reaction. A molecular test was ordered to confirm it. Which one of the following *CYP2D6* metabolizers would this patient most likely be?[6,18]
   A. Ultrarapid metabolizer
   B. Normal metabolizer
   C. Intermediate metabolizer
   D. Poor metabolizer
   E. None of the above

24. A 32-year-old Caucasian female with bipolar disorder was referred to a pharmacogenomic clinic by a neurologist whom she was seen for sedation, ataxia, vertigo, diplopia, and headache, which were considered to be adverse effects from her psychotropic medication, lamotrigine. The side effects ceased after lamotrigine was discontinued. On initial evaluation, she presented with irritable, labile, agitated mood, lack of sleep, and racing thoughts. Medical and neurological evaluations, including a head CT, were unremarkable. In the past, the patient had been treated with divalproex sodium, leading to weight gain, as well as

carbamazepine and oxcarbazepine, which were ineffective. Risperidone caused her profound sedation and was discontinued quickly. She presented to the clinic on lithium 900 mg/day (at therapeutic level) and clonazepam 6 mg/day. Aripiprazole 5 mg daily was added for mood instability and was titrated up to 15 mg daily. On a subsequent visit, she reported restlessness and the urge to move constantly. Her symptoms of akathisia resolved after aripiprazole was discontinued. CYP450 genetic testing revealed *CYP2D6* genotype *3/*5, with a predicted phenotype of poor metabolizer, and *CYP2C19* genotype *1/*1, with a predicted phenotype of extensive (normal) metabolizer. The patient's condition eventually stabilized on lithium, clonazepam, and topiramate. Which one of the following medications would most likely cause adverse effects in this patient related to the *CYP2D6*3/*5 genotype?[6,19]
   A. Aripiprazole
   B. Carbamazepine
   C. Divalproex
   D. Lamotrigine
   E. None of the above

25. Carbamazepine (brand names, Carbatrol, Epitol, Equetro, and Tegretol) is an effective antiseizure drug that is often used as a first-line agent in the treatment of epilepsy. Hypersensitivity reactions associated with carbamazepine can occur in up to 10% of patients and typically affect the skin. Some of these reactions are mild, as in the case of maculopapular exanthema (MPE); however, conditions such as Stevens–Johnson syndrome (SJS), toxic epidermal necrolysis (TEN), and drug reaction with eosinophilia and systemic symptoms (DRESS) are potentially life-threatening. Which one of the following alleles most likely is associated with high risk for carbamazepine-induced hypersensitivity reactions?[6]
   A. *HLA-B*15:02*
   B. *HLA-B*15:11*
   C. *HLA-B*57:01*
   D. *HLA-B*58:01*
   E. None of the above

26. Carbamazepine (brand names, Carbatrol, Epitol, Equetro, and Tegretol) is an effective antiseizure drug that is often used as a first-line agent in the treatment of epilepsy. Hypersensitivity reactions associated with carbamazepine can occur in up to 10% of patients and typically affect the skin. Some of these reactions are mild, as in the case of maculopapular exanthema (MPE); however, conditions such as Stevens–Johnson syndrome (SJS), toxic epidermal necrolysis (TEN), and drug

reaction with eosinophilia and systemic symptoms (DRESS) are potentially life-threatening. According to the FDA-approved drug label for carbamazepine, testing for *HLA-B*15:02* should be done for all patients with ancestry in populations with an increased frequency of *HLA-B*15:02* prior to initiating carbamazepine therapy. Which one of the following actions should be taken for better patient treatment in this case, according to the FDA?[6,16]

A. Continuing monitoring
B. Decreasing the dose
C. Increasing the dose
D. Using an alternative drug
E. None of the above

27. Carbamazepine (brand names, Carbatrol, Epitol, Equetro, and Tegretol) is an effective antiseizure drug that is often used as a first-line agent in the treatment of epilepsy. Hypersensitivity reactions associated with carbamazepine can occur in up to 10% of patients and typically affect the skin. Some of these reactions are mild, as in the case of maculopapular exanthema (MPE); however, conditions such as Stevens–Johnson syndrome (SJS), toxic epidermal necrolysis (TEN), and drug reaction with eosinophilia and systemic symptoms (DRESS) are potentially life-threatening. According to the FDA-approved drug label for carbamazepine, testing for *HLA-B*15:02* should be done for all patients with ancestry in populations with an increased frequency of *HLA-B*15:02* prior to initiating carbamazepine therapy. Which one of the following populations has the highest carrier frequency for *HLA-B*15:02?[6,16]

A. African American
B. Asian
C. Caucasian
D. Hispanic
E. None of the above

28. A 38-year-old Chinese female was admitted to a local hospital for widespread skin rashes and high fever. She had a history of idiopathic generalized epilepsy for 5 years. She had been on valproate (VPA) and CBZ (600 mg daily). Approximately 2–3 months ago, phenytoin (PHT) was prescribed to replace CBZ owing to incomplete seizure control. The number of seizures was significantly reduced after the switch. However, about 2 months after the switch, she developed fever and maculopapular rashes all over her cheeks and arms, which became blisters in 2 days. On admission, a physical examination revealed she had widespread erythematous macules and papules with blisters and detached epidermis on

her face, neck, trunk, feet, and upper limbs. The estimated detached skin was approximately 5% of the body-surface area. Scattered rashes on the lower limbs and diffuse oral ulcers were also observed. Laboratory examinations were not remarkable. The patient was diagnosed with PHT-induced Stevens–Johnson syndrome (SJS) clinically. A pharmacogenomics study was ordered to confirm the diagnosis. Which of the following alleles would this patient most likely carry, according to the FDA-approved drug label for phenytoin?[6,20]

A. *HLA-B*15:02*
B. *HLA-B*15:11*
C. *HLA-B*57:01*
D. *HLA-B*58:01*
E. None of the above

29. A 38-year-old Chinese female came to a clinic with symptoms of incomplete seizure control. Her medical history was significant for idiopathic generalized epilepsy. She had been on valproate (VPA) and CBZ (600 mg daily) for 5 years. The physician thought about switching CBZ to phenytoin (PHT) or carbamazepine. A molecular test was ordered and revealed that the patient was homozygous for the *HLA-B*15:02* allele. Which one of the following actions would most likely be considered for better patient treatment in this case?[20]

A. Continuing CBZ
B. Switching to PHT or carbamazepine with increased dose
C. Switching to PHT or carbamazepine with decreased dose
D. Using an alternative drug
E. None of the above

30. A 63-year-old Chinese male was admitted to a tertiary care facility for low-grade fever and erythema. His medical history was remarkable for hypertension and cerebral vascular incidents. Secondary epilepsy developed 6 months after surgery for a left intracerebral hemorrhage. Then phenytoin (PHT; 100 mg/day) was administered. Unfortunately, low-grade fever and extensive skin rashes developed on the 15th day of PHT therapy. The rashes were followed by blisters and oral ulcers. A physical examination revealed widespread erythematous macules with blisters and target-like lesions on his cheeks, trunk, and proximal limbs. The estimated detached skin was approximately 2% of body-surface area. Diffuse oral ulcers were also observed. The patient was diagnosed with PHT-induced Stevens–Johnson syndrome (SJS) clinically. His *HLA* genotyping was

HLA-B*3701/B*4601. Which of the following genes may also affect PHT metabolism in addition to *HLA* genotyping, according to the FDA-approved drug label?[6,20]

A. *CYP2C9*
B. *CYP2C19*
C. *CYP2D6*
D. *CYP3A*
E. None of the above

31. A 63-year-old Chinese male was admitted to a tertiary care facility for low-grade fever and erythema. His medical history was remarkable for hypertension and cerebral vascular incidents. Secondary epilepsy developed 6 months after surgery for a left intracerebral hemorrhage. Then phenytoin (PHT; 100 mg/day) was administered. Unfortunately, low-grade fever and extensive skin rashes developed on the 15th day of PHT therapy. The rashes were followed by blisters and oral ulcers. A physical examination revealed widespread erythematous macules with blisters and target-like lesions on his cheeks, trunk, and proximal limbs. The estimated detached skin was approximately 2% of body-surface area. Diffuse oral ulcers were also observed. The patient was diagnosed with PHT-induced Stevens–Johnson syndrome (SJS) clinically. A molecular study revealed that he was compound heterozygous for *HLA-B*3701/B*4601* and homozygous for *CYP2C9*2/*2* (poor metabolizer). Which one of the following actions would most likely be considered for better patient treatment in this case?[6,20]

A. Continue monitoring
B. Decreasing the PHT dose
C. Increasing the PHT dose
D. Using an alternative drug
E. None of the above

32. A 43-year-old Chinese male with a history of smoking and dyslipidemia was admitted to a local hospital after experiencing the sudden onset of severe headache. A brain CT revealed aneurysmal subarachnoid hemorrhage. A loading dose of clopidogrel (300 mg) and aspirin (300 mg) was administered. Angiography showed the occlusion of the right anterior communicating artery (RACA) and a 4.0 mm × 20 mm bare metal braided stent was placed. Poststent angiography confirmed good stent apposition and flow and no signs of perforation or thrombus formation. The patient's headache improved after stent-assisted coiling (SAC), and was continued on a regimen of aspirin (100 mg) and clopidogrel (75 mg) once daily. However, on the third day after the operation, he developed progressive neurological symptoms, with lethargy, left-upper-extremity paraplegia, and facial droop (blood pressure, 158/95 mmHg; heart rate, 80 beats/minute). Emergency angiography showed thrombotic occlusion of the RACA again. Which of the following genes would most likely affect clopidogrel metabolism in this patient?[6,21]

A. *CYP2C9*
B. *CYP2C19*
C. *CYP2D6*
D. *CYP3A*
E. None of the above

33. A 43-year-old Chinese male with a history of smoking and dyslipidemia was admitted to a local hospital after experiencing the sudden onset of severe headache. A brain CT revealed aneurysmal subarachnoid hemorrhage. A loading dose of clopidogrel (300 mg) and aspirin (300 mg) was administered. Angiography showed the occlusion of the right anterior communicating artery (RACA) and a 4.0 mm × 20 mm bare metal braided stent was placed. Poststent angiography confirmed good stent apposition and flow and no signs of perforation or thrombus formation. The patient's headache improved after stent-assisted coiling (SAC), and was continued on a regimen of aspirin (100 mg) and clopidogrel (75 mg) once daily. However, on the third day after the operation, he developed progressive neurological symptoms, with lethargy, left-upper-extremity paraplegia, and facial droop (blood pressure, 158/95 mmHg; heart rate, 80 beats/minute). Emergency angiography showed thrombotic occlusion of the RACA again. Which of the following *CYP2C19* genotyping would this patient most likely carry?[21,22]

A. *CYP2C19*1/*1*
B. *CYP2C19*2/*2*
C. *CYP2C19*3/*3*
D. *CYP2C19*4/*4*
E. None of the above

34. A 61-year-old dyslipidemic, nondiabetic male with stable angina presented for elective cardiac catheterization. Coronary angiography revealed complex multivessel disease consisting of chronic total occlusion (CTO) of a proximal right coronary artery (RCA) with collateral flow from the conus branch of RCA and a diagonal branch and severe proximal left anterior descending coronary artery (LAD) stenosis. Based on the angiographic results, the patient was treated by deploying three overlapping drug-eluting stents (DES) with proximal to distal sizes of 3.5 × 24 mm, 3.0 × 24 mm, and 2.5 × 28 mm. The mid stent and proximal stent were then postdilated with 3.0-mm and 3.75-mm diameter noncompliant balloons, respectively. Molecular genetic testing revealed that the patient carries *CYP2C19*2/*3*. Which of the

following actions should be taken for reducing the risk of myocardial infarction (MI) and stroke in this patient, according to the FDA-approved drug label?[6,23]

A. Continuing monitoring
B. Reducing the clopidogrel dose
C. Increasing the clopidogrel dose
D. Using an alternative drug
E. None of the above

35. Which one of the following *CYP2C19* alleles contains a variant at the noncoding region?[6]

A. *CYP2C19*1*
B. *CYP2C19*2*
C. *CYP2C19*3*
D. *CYP2C19*17*
E. None of the above

36. An 80-year-old Caucasian male with a history of arterial hypertension, dyslipidemia, hyperuricemia, and hypothyroidism, was diagnosed with metastatic malignant melanoma. He had undergone a right nephrectomy 14 years ago for to a spontaneous retroperitoneal hematoma and consequently had chronic renal insufficiency. Six years ago, he had undergone surgery to resect a 26-mm-diameter pigmented lesion on his right preauricular region. A pathology examination confirmed a diagnosis of malignant melanoma. Three years ago, a CT scan revealed hepatic and pulmonary lesions. A core-needle biopsy of the largest hepatic lesion confirmed metastatic melanoma. Which one of the following genes would most likely carry a variant sensitive to kinase inhibitors for metastases melanoma, such as dabrafenib or vemurafenib?[24]

A. *BRAF*
B. *EGFR*
C. *KRAS*
D. *NRAS*
E. None of the above

37. An 80-year-old Caucasian male with a history of arterial hypertension, dyslipidemia, hyperuricemia, and hypothyroidism, was diagnosed with metastatic malignant melanoma. He had undergone a right nephrectomy 14 years ago for to a spontaneous retroperitoneal hematoma and consequently had chronic renal insufficiency. Six years ago, he had undergone surgery to resect a 26-mm-diameter pigmented lesion on his right preauricular region. A pathology examination confirmed a diagnosis of malignant melanoma. Three years ago, a CT scan revealed hepatic and pulmonary lesions. A core-needle biopsy of the largest hepatic lesion confirmed metastatic melanoma. A molecular study was ordered for

variants in *BRAF*, *KIT*, and *NRAS*. Which one of the following variants would the patient most likely carry?[6,24]

A. *BRAF* V600D
B. *BRAF* V600E
C. *BRAF* V600K
D. *BRAF* V600R
E. None of the above

38. A 76-year-old woman began 6 months of adjuvant chemotherapy consisting of weekly bolus injections of 500 mg/m^2 of 5-fluorouracil (5-FU) and 20 mg/m^2 of calcium folinate after a radical hemicolectomy for T3N2 colon cancer. She was asymptomatic through the first two series, but on days 3–5 after the third cycle she experienced mild stomatitis and watering eyes. The symptoms rapidly became severe. She was admitted to the hospital for 3 weeks with grade 3–4 oral and intestinal mucositis and grade 3–4 diarrhea (CTCAE v4.0). A pharmacogenetic study was ordered to guide therapy. Which of the following genes would most likely affect 5-FU metabolism in this patient?[25]

A. *CYP2D6*
B. *DPYD*
C. *HLA-B*15:02*
D. *VKORC1*
E. None of the above

39. A 60-year-old Caucasian female came to a clinic with symptoms of GI bleeding and weight loss for several weeks. Her medical history was remarkable for hypertension, asthma, fibromyalgia, and bipolar disorder. She underwent colonoscopy. A biopsy revealed adenocarcinoma of the sigmoid colon. She was staged as metastatic colon cancer, stage IV, and was started on systemic therapy with FOLFOX (fluorouracil 400 mg/m^2 IV push, fluorouracil 2400 mg/m^2 IV infusion over 46 hours, leucovorin 400 mg/m^2, and oxaliplatin 85 mg/m^2). The plan was to add bevacizumab once the poorly controlled hypertension was resolved. Approximately 10 days after administration of the first cycle of FOLFOX, the patient presented with severe mucositis, esophagitis, inadequate pain control, and dehydration. On admission she was pancytopenic. In the hospital, her pancytopenia was persistent. She developed *Clostridium difficile* infection, which led to sigmoid colon perforation with peritonitis and isolated factor VII deficiency of unknown etiology. She was on IV ertapenem, fluconazole, and oral vancomycin as conservative management and passed away in 5 weeks. Fluorouracil-induced toxicity was suspected and a molecular genetic study of the *DPYD* gene was ordered to confirm it.

Which one of the following alleles would the patient most likely carry?[6,26]

A. *DPYD*1*

B. *DPYD*2A*

C. *DPYD*4*

D. *DPYD*9A*

E. None of the above

40. A 76-year-old woman began 6 months of adjuvant chemotherapy consisting of weekly bolus injections of 500 mg/m^2 of 5-fluorouracil (5-FU) and 20 mg/m^2 of calcium folinate after a radical hemicolectomy for T3N2 colon cancer. She was asymptomatic through the first two series, but on days 3—5 after the third cycle, she experienced mild stomatitis and watering eyes. The symptoms rapidly became severe. She was admitted to a hospital for 3 weeks with grade 3—4 oral and intestinal mucositis and grade 3—4 diarrhea (CTCAE v4.0). A pharmacogenetic study was ordered to guide therapy. *DPYD*2A/*2A* was detected, and the patient was classified as a "poor metabolizer." Which of the following actions would more likely be considered for better patient management in this case?[27]

A. Continue monitoring

B. Decreasing the 5-FU dose

C. Increasing the 5-FU dose

D. Using an alternative drug

E. None of the above

41. A 57-year-old male of Indian descent was diagnosed with moderately differentiated rectal adenocarcinoma, grade II. He underwent abdominal perianal resection followed by chemoradiation. His treatment was started with FOLFOX-IV (oxaliplatin, leucovorin, fluorouracil) regimen. He had grade 2 diarrhea and grade 2 neutropenia after cycle 1, and grade 2 diarrhea with grade 3 neutropenia after cycle 2 (CTCAE V4.0). Even after reducing the dose of 5-FU, his diarrhea and neutropenia were persistent. A molecular study revealed that he carried a heterozygous *DPYD*2A* variant. The treatment was changed to an IROX (irinotecan and oxaliplatin) regimen. After starting the IROX regimen patient had grade 2 diarrhea and grade 2 neutropenia in two cycles. After dose reduction in the next cycle, patient's condition worsen progressively, with grade 4 neutropenia, and was further complicated by sepsis. Which one of the following genes would most likely be studied in this patient to investigate IROX toxicity?[6,28]

A. *CYP2D6*

B. *DPYD*

C. *HLA-B*15:02*

D. *UGT1A1*

E. None of the above

42. A 57-year-old male of Indian descent was diagnosed with moderately differentiated rectal adenocarcinoma, grade II. He underwent abdominal perianal resection followed by chemoradiation. His treatment was started with FOLFOX-IV (oxaliplatin, leucovorin, fluorouracil) regimen. He had grade 2 diarrhea and grade 2 neutropenia after cycle 1, and grade 2 diarrhea with grade 3 neutropenia after cycle 2 (CTCAE V4.0). Even after reducing the dose of 5-FU, his diarrhea and neutropenia were persistent. A molecular study revealed that he carried a heterozygous *DPYD*2A* variant. The treatment was changed to an IROX (irinotecan and oxaliplatin) regimen. Which of the following actions would most likely be considered for better patient treatment in this case?[6,28]

A. Continuing monitoring

B. Reducing the irinotecan dose

C. Increasing the irinotecan dose

D. Using an alternative drug

E. None of the above

43. A 76-year-old man was admitted to a hospital for pyrexia, confusion, and rigors associated with positive blood cultures for *Enterococcus* species. His medical history included myocardial infarction, pulmonary embolism, and non-insulin-dependent diabetes mellitus. This was his fourth admission with proven enterococcal septicemia over 7 months. A transesophageal echocardiogram showed a 1.5-cm vegetation attached to the tricuspid valve at the point of contact with the pacing lead. He received benzylpenicillin 2.4 g intravenously six times daily and gentamicin 80 mg intravenously twice daily (2.3 mg/kg/day; patient weight, 69 kg) for 9 days. Then gentamicin dosing was adjusted to achieve a target concentrations of 3—5 μg/mL. A month and a half after admission, the patient experienced impaired hearing. Audiometry revealed mixed conduction and sensorineural deafness with notable high-tone loss. Ototoxicity secondary to gentamicin was suspected. Which one of the following genes would most likely be associated with gentamicin-induced ototoxic injury in this patient?[6,29]

A. *CYP2D6*

B. *DPYD*

C. *HLA-B*15:02*

D. *MTRNR1*

E. None of the above

44. A 65-year-old man was admitted to a hospital for pancytopenia. Eight weeks earlier he had commenced azathioprine 100 mg/day for Crohn colitis. The physician suspected that the patient had azathioprine-induced myelosuppression. A

pharmacogenetics study was ordered to confirm it. Which of the following genes would most likely be associated with azathioprine-induced myelosuppression in this patient?[6]
  A. DPYD
  B. HLA-B*15:02
  C. MTRNR1
  D. TPMT
  E. None of the above

45. A 65-year-old man was admitted to a hospital for pancytopenia. Eight weeks earlier he had commenced azathioprine 100 mg/day for Crohn's colitis. He was found to have low TPMT enzyme activity. The physician suspected that the patient had azathioprine-induced myelosuppression. A pharmacogenetics study was ordered to confirm it. Which of the following TPMT genotypes would this patient most likely carry?[6]
  A. TPMT*1/*1
  B. TPMT*1/*2
  C. TPMT*3A/*3A
  D. TPMT*1/*3A
  E. None of the above

46. A 29-year-old Caucasian male with long-term inflammatory bowel disease came to his physician for infections, fatigue, sleepiness, and fever for 3 weeks after he switched to azathioprine with standard doses. Laboratory testing revealed severe leukopenia. Subsequent study detected thiopurine methyltransferase activity and it was approximately 0.3% of normal in the red cells. Molecular testing detected TPMT*2/*3A. Which of the following actions would be the most conservative way to reduce the risk of azathioprine-induced myelosuppression in this patient?[6]
  A. Continuing monitoring
  B. Administering a reduced dose
  C. Administering an increased dose
  D. Using an alternative drug
  E. None of the above

47. A 68-year-old man was admitted to a hospital with symptoms of increasing thigh pain and progressive proximal myopathy for 7 days. His medical history was significant for hypertension, hypercholesterolemia, stage 3a chronic kidney disease, gastroesophageal reflux, and idiopathic thrombocytopenia. Six months ago, he had been treated for a painful ulcer related to an injury happened while cleaning his fish tank. The wound on his left index finger had failed to heal after a 3-week course of antibiotics.

Ultrasonography confirmed dactylitis and tenosynovitis. Subsequently, a culture of the wound washout detected Mycobacterium marinum. Rifampin and ethambutol had been prescribed to treat mycobacterial infection. Five weeks prior to this admission, he had experienced nausea, sore eyes, and a bitter taste in the mouth. His symptoms were assumed to be attributable to rifampin. Therefore, clarithromycin was substituted for rifampin. The other medications, including simvastatin 40 mg daily, had remained unchanged. On admission, a physical examination demonstrated a painful proximal myopathy predominantly affecting the lower limbs with no evidence of compartment syndrome. The physician suspected that the patient had simvastatin-induced myopathy. Which one of the following genes would most likely be studied to confirm/rule out simvastatin-induced myopathy in this patient?[31,32]
  A. DPYD
  B. HLA-B*15:02
  C. MTRNR1
  D. SLCO1B1
  E. None of the above

48. A 68-year-old man was admitted to a hospital with symptoms of increasing thigh pain and progressive proximal myopathy for 7 days. His medical history was significant for hypertension, hypercholesterolemia, stage 3a chronic kidney disease, gastroesophageal reflux, and idiopathic thrombocytopenia. Six months ago, he had been treated for a painful ulcer related to an injury happened while cleaning his fish tank. The wound on his left index finger had failed to heal after a 3-week course of antibiotics. Ultrasonography confirmed dactylitis and tenosynovitis. Subsequently, a culture of the wound washout detected Mycobacterium marinum. Rifampin and ethambutol had been prescribed to treat mycobacterial infection. Five weeks prior to this admission, he had experienced nausea, sore eyes, and a bitter taste in the mouth. His symptoms were assumed to be attributable to rifampin. Therefore, clarithromycin was substitute for rifampin. The other medications, including simvastatin 40 mg daily, had remained unchanged. On admission, a physical examination demonstrated a painful proximal myopathy predominantly affecting the lower limbs with no evidence of compartment

syndrome. The physician suspected that the patient had simvastatin-induced myopathy, and ordered a molecular study for *SLCO1B1*. The results showed that he carries homozygous CC. Which one of the following actions would more likely be considered for better patient management in this case?[31,33]

A. Continuing monitoring
B. Administering a reduced dose
C. Administering an increased dose
D. Using an alternative drug
E. None of the above

ANSWERS

1. A. Efavirenz (EFV), sold under the brand name Sustiva, is a potent nonnucleoside reverse transcriptase inhibitor (NNRTI) used as part of combination antiretroviral (ARV) regimens in the treatment of human immunodeficiency virus (HIV) infection (A 33-year-old patient with human immunodeficiency virus on antiretroviral therapy with efavirenz-induced complex partial seizures: a case report. J Med Case Rep. 2016; 10: 93. PMID: 27072009). EFV has a narrow therapeutic window with severe central nervous system (CNS) side effects associated with its high plasma concentrations and treatment failure associated with low concentrations. CNS symptoms may include dizziness, hallucinations, seizure, and psychosis.

CYP2B6, CYP2C9, CYP2D6, and *CYP3A* are all hepatic cytochrome P450 isozymes. CYP2B6 and CYP3A are the major isozymes responsible for efavirenz metabolism. *The incidence of adverse CNS symptoms is associated with CYP2B6 polymorphisms. HLA-B*57:01 significantly increases the risk of* hypersensitivity reactions when abacavir (ABC) is administered. ABC is a nucleoside analog reverse transcriptase inhibitor (NRTI) used to treat HIV and AIDS.

Therefore, *CYP2B6* most likely mutated in this patient, making him susceptible to the efavirenz toxicity.

2. C. *CYP2B6* is a member of the cytochrome P450 family of important pharmacogenes and makes up approximately 2%–10% of the total hepatic CYP content. *CYP2B6* is also expressed in the brain and may be an important factor in the metabolism of drugs acting on the central nervous system (CNS) and neurological side effects of drug treatments. There is high interperson variation in *CYP2B6* expression, ranging from 20- to 250-fold, which may result from variable transcriptional regulation and carried genetic variants.

The most common functionally deficient allele is CYP2B6*6 (G516T and A785G), which occurs at frequencies of 15% to over 60% in different populations. CYP2B6*6 (G516T and A785G) and *CYP2B6*7* (G516T, A785G and C1459T) are the two common *CYP2B6* alleles associated with a prolonged EFV half-life despite discontinuation of EFV. The *CYP2B6*4* (785A > G) allele is associated with increased CYP2B6 activity. The *CYP2B6*5* (1459C > T) allele is associated with decreased expression that is in part compensated by increased specific activity. The *CYP2B6*22* (c.-82T > C, rs34223104) allele is associated with increased CYP2B6 expression and activity.

Therefore, this patient would most likely carry *CYP2B6*6/*6*, associated EFV-induced CNS toxicity.

3. A. *CYP2B6* is responsible for the metabolism of 4% of the top 200 drugs and is highly inducible by several drugs and other xenobiotics. As *CYP2B6* is the major enzyme involved in the metabolism of efavirenz and nevirapine, its pharmacogenomics have become relevant for the treatment of HIV. A large number of *CYP2B6* variants have been reported (see the CYP allele nomenclature committee website http://www.PharmVar.org), including many that are present at high frequencies and several that show linkage resulting in multiple haplotypes. Common reduced or loss-of-function alleles include *CYP2B6*6* (Q172H and K262R) and *CYP2B6*18* I (328T). *About 6%–12% of white, 14%–38% of black (African American), and 1%–4% of Asian individuals are poor metabolizers.* Guidelines recommend that for children over 3 years of age the dose should be weight-based, and for selected children under 3 years of age who require treatment with efavirenz, the *CYP2B6* genotype should be assessed and doses adjusted to prevent toxicity.

Therefore, the African American population has the most *CYP2B6* poor metabolizers.

4. C. Abacavir (brand name Ziagen) is a nucleoside/ nucleotide reverse transcriptase inhibitor (NRTI) and is used in combination with other medications as part of highly active antiretroviral therapy (HAART) in the treatment of human immunodeficiency virus (HIV) infection. Hypersensitivity reactions associated with abacavir can be severe and potentially fatal. Symptoms include fever, rash, vomiting, and shortness of breath. The *HLA-B* gene plays an important role in how the immune system recognizes and responds to pathogens, and mediates hypersensitivity reactions. *HLA-B*57:01 significantly increases the risk of hypersensitivity reactions when abacavir is* *administered.* Approximately 6% of Caucasians and 2%–3% of African Americans carry this allele in the human leukocyte antigen B (*HLA-B*) gene. Screening for the *HLA-B*57:01* allele before starting abacavir therapy is recommended for all patients, according to the FDA drug label for abacavir.

The *HLA-B*15:02* allele is strongly associated with carbamazepine-induced Stevens–Johnson syndrome (SJS) and toxic epidermal necrolysis (TEN) in populations where this allele is most common, such as in Southeast Asia. The *HLA-A*31:01* allele may also be a risk factor for SJS/TEN, but it is more strongly associated with other carbamazepine-induced reactions, such as drug reaction with eosinophilia and systemic symptoms (DRESS) and maculopapular exanthema (MPE). The *HLA-B*58:01* allele is strongly associated with severe cutaneous adverse reactions (SCAR) during treatment with allopurinol.

Therefore, *HLA-B*57:01* is associated with increased risk for adverse effect when abacavir is administered.

5. **D.** The *HLA-B*57:01* allele is associated with an increased risk of hypersensitivity reaction to abacavir. Studies across ethnicities have reported that in immunologically confirmed cases of abacavir hypersensitivity, 100% of cases occurred in patients who were carriers of this HLA variant. However, not everyone who carries the high-risk HLA allele will develop abacavir hypersensitivity; approximately 39% of individuals who are positive for *HLA-B*57:01* will tolerate abacavir treatment.

The hypersensitivity reaction to abacavir is thought to be maintained over the lifetime of an individual. The reintroduction of abacavir to a sensitized individual may be fatal, presumably owing to rapid activation of a memory-T-cell population. Therefore, abacavir is contraindicated in individuals with a prior hypersensitivity reaction to abacavir. *According to the 2017 summary of recommendations from the Dutch Pharmacogenetics Working Group (DPWG) of the Royal Dutch Association for the Advancement of Pharmacy (KNMP), prescribers are advised to order an alternative drug if a patient carries HLA-B*57:01* (http://www.knmp.nl/).

Therefore, an alternative drug should be considered in this case for the antiretroviral (ARV) treatment, according to KNMP.

6. **B.** Maraviroc exerts its therapeutic activity by blocking entry of the human immunodeficiency virus type 1 (HIV-1) virus into CD4-expressing T-helper cells, which play a major role in protecting the body from infection, precursor cells, and dendritic cells. HIV-1 infection is classified into two major forms, according to the coreceptor it employs to gain entry into the cell—the chemokine receptor 5 (CCR5) or the CXC chemokine receptor 4 (CXCR4). These coreceptors are expressed on different types of cells, and *HIV tropism* refers to the types of cells and tissues in which the virus infects and replicates. A tropism assay may be conducted to determine whether the virus is CCR5-tropic, CXCR4-tropic, or dual tropic.

Maraviroc is indicated only for the treatment of adults with CCR5-tropic HIV-1 and is not recommended when the CXCR4-tropic virus has been detected. Therefore, maraviroc may exerts its therapeutic activity on CCR5-tropic HIV-1.

7. **B.** HIV-1 virus that uses the CCR5 coreceptor (CCR5-tropic) is more commonly found in the early stages of infection. It is also more common among individuals who have yet to receive treatment, and at least half of all infected individuals harbor only CCR5-tropic viruses throughout the course of infection. The CXCR4-tropic virus is more commonly found during later stages of disease and among individuals who have received HIV treatment. The presence of CXCR4-tropic virus is a predictor of lower CD4 count, higher viral load, and more rapid progression to AIDS.

A variant of *CCR5*, *CCR5-Δ32* (NM_000579.3: c.554_585del32), contains a 32-bp deletion and codes a nonfunctional receptor that hinders the entry of CCR5-tropic virus in to cells. *Individuals who have two copies of this allele are highly resistant to HIV infection, and although individuals who have one copy of the allele remain susceptible to HIV infection, the progression of HIV infection to AIDS is delayed.*

Therefore, CCR5-tropic HIV-1 with *CCR5-Δ32* is highly resistant to human immunodeficiency virus type 1 (HIV-1) infection.

8. **C.** *The CCR5-Δ32 allele occurs at high frequency in European Caucasians (5%–14%) but is rare among African, Native American, and East Asian populations, suggesting that the allele may have conferred an evolutionary survival advantage.* Possible causes of a positive selection pressure include protection against the bubonic plague (*Yersinia pestis*) or smallpox (*Variola* virus) during the Middle Ages. However, other studies have found that the *CCR5-Δ32* allele arose long before this time and underwent neutral evolution.

Therefore, the Caucasian population has the highest frequency of the CCR5-Δ32 allele.

9. **E.** Warfarin is currently the most widely used oral anticoagulant in the world. Individual response to it is highly variable. In a given population, prescribed doses can vary from 1 to 40 mg or more

daily. Importantly, the therapeutic index in any one patient is very narrow. The difference between being underanticoagulated (leading to minimal therapeutic benefit from warfarin treatment) and being overanticoagulated (leading to increased bleeding risk)—the primary adverse drug reactions (ADRs) associated with warfarin therapy—is small. Taken together with age and height, variants in *CYP2C9* and *VKORC1* account for 30%–50% of the variability in warfarin dosage. If pharmacogenetics effects are taken into consideration, the warfarin dosage scale can be shifted significantly up or down to meet the therapeutic window. Thus, the FDA-approved drug label for warfarin states that *CYP2C9* and *VKORC1* genotype information, when available, can assist in the selection of the initial dose of warfarin. International Warfarin Pharmacogenetics Consortium (IWPC) developed dosing algorithms, which incorporate clinical, demographic, and genetic information, to help select a starting warfarin dose.

Several genes are involved in the metabolism of warfarin, a racemic mixture of S- and R-warfarin enantiomers. *S-warfarin, the more active isomer, is metabolized predominately by CYP2C9 (OMIM# 601130).* R-warfarin, which has 20%–30% of the anticoagulation effect of S-warfarin, is metabolized by a number of CYP450 enzymes, including *CYP1A2* (OMIM 124060), *CYP2C8* (OMIM 601129), *CYP2C19* (OMIM 124020), *CYP3A4* (OMIM 124010), and *CYP3A5* (OMIM 605325). All of the genes for these enzymes have polymorphic variants that may affect metabolic activity. *However, the variable metabolism of S-warfarin, the more effective isomer in anticoagulation, is believed to be responsible for much if not most of the variability in warfarin dosing.*

Genetic variation in the *CYP4F2* gene, and a variant near the *CYP2C* gene cluster (rs12777823) have been associated with influencing warfarin therapy. The *CYP4F2*3* variant is associated with a modest increase in warfarin dose requirements in individuals with European or Asian ancestry, while in individuals with African ancestry, the rs12777823 A/G or A/A genotype is associated with decreased warfarin dose requirements.

Therefore, *CYP2C9*, *CYP3A*, *CYP4F2*, and *VKORC1* are all associated with warfarin metabolism, but *CYP2C9* plays a major role.

10. **C.** Warfarin (Coumadin) is the most commonly used vitamin K antagonist with a narrow therapeutic index. It has demonstrated effectiveness for the primary and secondary prevention of venous thromboembolism, for the prevention of systemic embolism in patients with prosthetic heart valves or atrial fibrillation, as an adjunct in the prophylaxis of systemic embolism after myocardial infarction, and for reducing the risk of recurrent myocardial infarction. There is a wide interindividual variability in the dose of warfarin required to achieve target anticoagulation, and the time it takes to reach the target international normalized ratio (INR). Approximately half this variability is known to be caused by clinical or lifestyle factors, such as a patient's age, weight, BMI, sex, smoking status, existing conditions, and concomitant medications. The *CYP2C9* and *VKORC1* genotypes are the most important known genetic determinants of warfarin dosing.

A common variant in the vitamin K epoxide reductase complex 1 gene (VKORC1), c.-1639G > A, is associated with less VKORC1 enzyme, increased sensitivity to warfarin, and lower dose requirements. Other variants, 1173C > T, 1542G > C, 2255T > C, and 3730G > A, are in linkage disequilibrium with the c.-1639G > A polymorphism and permit defining haplotypes. In 2017, the Dutch Pharmacogenetics Working Group (DPWG) recommended using 60% of the standard initial dose if the *VKORC1* genotype is c.-1639A/A; use 20% of the standard initial dose if the patient is a poor metabolizer.

Therefore, *VKORC1* c.-1639A/A would most likely indicate a low starting dose in this patient if age and height are not taken into consideration.

11. **B.** The *CYP2C9* gene is highly polymorphic, with more than 300 variations in the *CYP2C9* DNA sequence reported. The functional impact of many of these polymorphisms is not well established. More than 60 star (*) alleles have been described and currently cataloged at the Pharmacogene Variation (PharmVar) Consortium (https://www.pharmvar.org/). The *CYP2C9*1* allele is the wild-type allele and is associated with normal enzyme activity and the normal metabolizer phenotype. *Using the allele designations from the pharmacogenetics literature, CYP2C9*2 (p.Arg144Cys) and CYP2C9*3 (p.Ile359Leu) are the major alleles associated with lower dose requirements.* Homozygous carriers of *CYP2C9*17* are predicted to be ultrarapid metabolizers (UM) associated with higher dose requirements.

Therefore, this patient would most likely carry *CYP2C9*2/CYP2C9*2* to trigger the excessive anticoagulation (INR 9.1).

12. **D.** The *CYP2C9*1* allele is the wild-type allele, and it is associated with normal enzyme activity and the normal metabolizer phenotype. Using the allele designations from the pharmacogenetics literature,

CYP2C9*2 (p.Arg144Cys) and CYP2C9*3 (p. Ile359Leu) are the common poor-metabolizing alleles associated with lower dose requirements. *Homozygous carriers of CYP2C9*17 are predicted to be ultrarapid metabolizers (UM) associated with higher dose requirements.*

Therefore, this patient would most likely carry CYP2C9*17/CYP2C9*17, which required a high dose of warfarin.

13. **B**. Metoprolol is a beta-blocker used in the treatment of hypertension, angina, and heart failure. Metoprolol selectively blocks beta$_1$ adrenoreceptors mainly expressed in cardiac tissue. Blockade of these receptors reduces the heart rate and decreases the force of heart contractions. *Metoprolol is primarily metabolized by the CYP2D6 enzyme.* Individuals who lack CYP2D6 activity will have higher plasma concentrations of metoprolol, almost fivefold higher, and may be at an increased risk of side effects, such as bradycardia and hypotension.

Therefore, CYP2D6 most likely caused the metoprolol-induced side effect in this patient.

14. **D**. Cytochrome P450 family 2 subfamily D member 6 (CYP2D6) is highly polymorphic. Individuals who carry two normal or one normal and one decreased-function CYP2D6 allele are classified as "normal metabolizers." Individuals who have two nonfunctional CYP2D6 alleles are predicted to be "CYP2D6 poor metabolizers." Individuals who have more than two normal-function copies of the CYP2D6 gene are "ultrarapid metabolizers." Individuals with one normal and one no-function allele or two decreased-function alleles are categorized as "normal metabolizers" by recent nomenclature guidelines, but have also been categorized as "intermediate metabolizers" in the literature. Individuals with one decreased and one no-function allele are predicted to be "intermediate metabolizers."

Approximately 6%–8% of Caucasians and 2% of most other populations are poor metabolizers. In addition, a number of drugs inhibit CYP2D6 activity, such as quinidine, fluoxetine, paroxetine, and propafenone. *Individuals who are CYP2D6 poor metabolizers will have higher plasma concentrations of metoprolol, almost fivefold higher, and may be at an increased risk of side effects, such as bradycardia and hypotension.*

Therefore, this patient would most likely be a CYP2D6 poor metabolizer.

15. **C**. CYP2D6 is highly polymorphic, with over 100 star (*) alleles described. *CYP2D6*1 is the reference (or wild-type) allele encoding enzymes with normal activity. The *CYP2D6*2, *33, and *35 alleles are also considered to confer normal activity. *The most common no function alleles include CYP2D6*3, *4, *5, and *6. The most common decreased-function alleles include CYP2D6*9, *10, *17, *29 and *41 (see the table below).

Predicted enzymatic function	CYP2D6 alleles
Normal function [associated with extensive metabolizers (EMs)]	*1, *2, *33, *35
Decreased function [associated with intermediate metabolizers (IMs)]	*10, *17, *29, *36, *41
Loss of function [associated with poor metabolizers (PMs)]	*3−*9, *11−*16, *19−*21, *38, *40, *42
Increased activity [usually associated with ultrarapid metabolizers (UMs), although this is not always the case]	*1 × N, *2 × N

Individuals with two no-function alleles are categorized as poor metabolizers. The high frequency of poor metabolizers in Caucasians results mainly from the prevalent no-function CYP2D6*4 and *5 alleles. Both the CYP2D6*3 and CYP2D6*4 alleles are no-function alleles.

Therefore, this patient most likely has CYP2D6*3/CYP2D6*4 genotyping as a CYP2D6 poor metabolizer.

16. **B**. The Dutch Pharmacogenetics Working Group (DPWG) of the Royal Dutch Association for the Advancement of Pharmacy (KNMP) has published metoprolol dosing recommendations based on CYP2D6 genotype. *For CYP2D6 poor metabolizers, if a gradual reduction in heart rate is desired, or in the event of symptomatic bradycardia, DPWG recommends increasing the dose of metoprolol in smaller steps and/or prescribing no more than 25% of the standard dose.*

There are large interethnic differences in the frequency of these alleles. For example, CYP2D6*4 is the most common no-function allele in Caucasians but is less abundant in African Americans and is rare in Asians. In contrast, the decreased-function allele CYP2D6*10 is the most common allele in Asians and CYP2D6*17 is almost exclusively found in individuals with African ancestry.

Therefore, decreasing the metoprolol dose in this patient would be an appropriate adjustment.

17. **A**. *CYP2D6*1 is the reference (or wild-type) allele encoding enzyme with normal activity. Individuals who carry two normal or one normal and one decreased function allele are classified as "normal metabolizers." *Individuals who have more than two

normal-function copies of the CYP2D6 gene are "ultrarapid metabolizers."

Allele type	CYP2D6 alleles
Normal function	*1, *2, *33, *35
Decreased function	*9, *10, *17, *29, *36, *41
No function	*3-*8, *11-*16, *19-*21, *38, *40, *42

Adapted from https://www.pharmgkb.org/guidelineAnnotation/PA166104995.

Therefore, the *CYP2D6*1 × 2/CYP2D6*2* genotype may be used to predict which individuals are ultrarapid metabolizers.

18. **B.** As an opioid analgesic, codeine is used to relieve mild to moderately severe pain. *The hepatic CYP2D6 enzyme metabolizes a quarter of all prescribed drugs, including codeine.*

Therefore, *CYP2D6* would most likely relate to an abnormally high codeine concentration in this patient.

19. **A.** Codeine is a prodrug. Its analgesic properties depend upon its conversion to morphine that binds to the mu opioid receptor with 200-fold greater affinity than codeine. Up to 15% of codeine is converted into morphine by CYP2D6. About 80% of an administered dose of codeine is converted to inactive metabolites and excreted. Individuals who carry at least one copy of a normal-function allele or two partially functioning alleles, so-called normal metabolizers, are most likely to have a normal response to codeine. Individuals who carry more than two normal-function copies of the *CYP2D6* gene, so-called ultrarapid metabolizers, are able to metabolize codeine to morphine more rapidly and more completely. *As a result, even with normal doses of codeine, these individuals may experience the symptoms of morphine overdose, which include extreme sleepiness, confusion, shallow breathing, and respiratory depression.* The ultrarapid metabolizer has been estimated to be present in 1%–2% of patients, but the prevalence varies widely in different populations. It is estimated to be present in up to 28% of North Africans, Ethiopians, and Arabs; 10% in Caucasians; 3% in African Americans, and 1% in Hispanics, Chinese, and Japanese. In contrast, pain relief may be inadequate in individuals who carry two inactive copies of *CYP2D6*, so-called poor metabolizers, because of reduced morphine levels. Individuals who carry either two decreased-function alleles or one decreased-function and one no-function allele (intermediate metabolizers) may not respond as well to codeine because the metabolism of codeine to morphine is reduced.

Therefore, this patient would most likely be a *CYP2D6* ultrarapid metabolizer.

20. **A.** *Nursing mothers who carry more than two normal-function copies of the CYP2D6 gene ("ultrarapid metabolizers") may also produce breast milk containing higher-than-expected levels of morphine that can lead to severe adverse events in their infants.* Gene duplications are denoted as *1/*1 × N or *1/*2 × N for the *CYP2D6* genotype.

To calculate the *CYP2D6* activity score for an interpretation of the patient's predicted metabolizer phenotype, each allele is assigned an activity value: 0 for no-function, 0.5 for decreased-function, and 1 for each copy of a normal-function allele. The total CYP2D6 activity score is the sum of the values assigned to each allele; patients with a score of 1.0, 1.5, or 2.0 represent a range of normal metabolizers with normal enzyme activity. Poor metabolizers have an activity score of 0, patients with a score of 0.5 are intermediate metabolizers, and patients with a score of greater than 2.0 are ultrarapid metabolizers. See the table below for the function type of *CYP2D6* alleles.

Allele type	CYP2D6 alleles
Normal function	*1, *2, *33, *35
Decreased function	*9, *10, *17, *29, *36, *41
No function	*3-*8, *11-*16, *19-*21, *38, *40, *42

Adapted from https://www.pharmgkb.org/guidelineAnnotation/PA166104995.

*CYP2D6*4* is a no-function allele. *CYP2D6*10* and *CYP2D6*17* are alleles with decreased function. Therefore, this patient would most likely have *CYP2D6*1 × 3* as an ultrarapid metabolizer.

21. **D.** The human leukocyte antigen B (*HLA-B*) plays an important role in how the immune system recognizes and responds to pathogens. *The variant HLA-B*58:01 allele is strongly associated with severe cutaneous adverse reactions (SCAR) during treatment with allopurinol.* This allele is most commonly found in Asian subpopulations, notably in individuals of Korean, Han Chinese, or Thai descent. Even though at this time the FDA-approved drug label does not discuss *HLA-B* genotype, the Clinical Pharmacogenetics Implementation Consortium (CPIC) recommends that allopurinol should not be prescribed to patients who have tested positive for *HLA-B*58:01* and that an alternative medication should be considered to avoid the risk of developing SCAR.

Therefore, this patient would most likely carry *HLA-B*58:01* if he had an allopurinol-induced severe cutaneous adverse reaction (SCAR).

22. **C.** Risperidone is the most commonly prescribed antipsychotic medication in the United States. It is an atypical (second-generation) antipsychotic used in the treatment of schizophrenia, bipolar disorder, severe dementia, and irritability associated with autism. *Risperidone is metabolized to the active metabolite 9-hydroxyrisperidone by the enzyme CYP2D6 and to a lesser extent by CYP3A4.*

Therefore, *CYP2D6* most likely affect risperidone metabolize in this patient.

23. **D.** *Individuals who carry two inactive copies of the CYP2D6 gene are termed "poor metabolizers" and may have a decreased capacity to metabolize risperidone. These individuals may be at a higher risk of adverse effects because of increased exposure to plasma risperidone, compared to normal metabolizers, who carry two active copies of CYP2D6.* Individuals who are *CYP2D6* ultrarapid metabolizers (who carry more than two functional copies of *CYP2D6*) may have a decreased response to therapy, resulting from lower steady-state risperidone concentrations. Individuals with one normal and one no-function allele or two decreased-function alleles are also categorized as "normal metabolizers" by recent nomenclature guidelines, but have also been categorized as "intermediate metabolizers" elsewhere in the literature. Individuals with one decreased and one no-function allele are predicted to be "intermediate metabolizers."

Therefore, this patient would most likely be a *CYP2D6* poor metabolizer.

24. **A.** As antipsychotics, both risperidone and aripiprazole are metabolized by CYP450 2D6. The metabolism and elimination of aripiprazole is mediated mainly through *CYP2D6* and *CYP3A4*. *The FDA-approved drug label for aripiprazole states that in CYP2D6 poor metabolizers, half the usual dose should be administered.* In *CYP2D6* poor metabolizers who are taking concomitant strong *CYP3A4* inhibitors, such as itraconazole or clarithromycin, a quarter of the usual dose should be used.

Carbamazepine (brand names include Carbatrol, Epitol, Equetro, and Tegretol) is an effective antiseizure drug. Hypersensitivity reactions associated with carbamazepine can occur in up to 10% of patients and typically affect the skin. The risk of hypersensitivity is increased by the presence of specific human leukocyte antigen (HLA) alleles. The *HLA-B*15:02* allele is strongly associated with carbamazepine-induced Stevens–Johnson syndrome (SJS) and toxic epidermal necrolysis (TEN) in populations where this allele is most common, such as in Southeast Asia.

Divalproex sodium (Depakote, Depakote CP, and Depakote ER) is one of the valproate products. Cytochrome P450 (CYP) mediated oxidation of divalproex, but was considered only a minor route (approximately 10%). Glucuronidation and beta-oxidation in the mitochondria (liver) are considered major routes, accounting for 50% and 40% of the dose, respectively.

According to the FDA, lamotrigine (Lamictal) for seizures and bipolar disorder can cause hemophagocytic lymphohistiocytosis (HLH) (http://www.fda.gov/). It is metabolized predominantly by glucuronic acid conjugation; the major metabolite is an inactive 2-N-glucuronide conjugate. It is unclear whether *CYP2D6* regulates lamotrigine's metabolism.

Therefore, this patient had an aripiprazole-induced adverse reaction, such as restlessness and the urge to move constantly, upon administrating the regular dose as a *CYP2D6* poor metabolizer with the *CYP2D6*3/*5* genotype.

25. **A.** The risk of hypersensitivity is increased by the presence of specific human leukocyte antigen (HLA) alleles. *The HLA-B*15:02 allele is strongly associated with carbamazepine-induced Stevens–Johnson syndrome (SJS) and toxic epidermal necrolysis (TEN) in populations where this allele is most common, such as in Southeast Asia.* According to the FDA-approved drug label for carbamazepine, testing for *HLA-B*15:02* should be done for all patients with ancestry in populations with an increased frequency of *HLA-B*15:02* prior to initiating carbamazepine therapy.

The *HLA-A*31:01* allele may also be a risk factor for SJS/TEN, but is more strongly associated with other carbamazepine-induced reactions, such as drug reaction with eosinophilia and systemic symptoms (DRESS) and maculopapular exanthema (MPE). *HLA-A*31:01* is found in most populations worldwide. *HLA-B*15:11* is another allele that has been linked with SJS/TEN. The FDA states that the risks and benefits of carbamazepine therapy should be weighed before considering carbamazepine in patients known to be positive for *HLA-A*31:01*, but it does not discuss *HLA-B*15:11*. *HLA-B*57:01* significantly increases the risk of hypersensitivity reactions when abacavir (ABC) is administered. The *HLA-B*58:01* allele is strongly associated with severe cutaneous adverse reactions (SCAR) during treatment with allopurinol.

Therefore, the *HLA-B*15:02* allele most likely is associated with a high risk for carbamazepine-induced hypersensitivity reactions.

26. **D**. *The FDA label states that carbamazepine should not be used in patients who are positive for HLA-B*15:02 unless the benefits clearly outweigh the risks.* The Dutch Pharmacogenetics Working Group (DPWG) of the Royal Dutch Association for the Advancement of Pharmacy (KNMP) recommendations also include avoiding the use of carbamazepine and selecting an alternative, if possible, for individuals positive for *HLA-B*15:02*.

Therefore, an alternative drug should be considered if a patient carries the *HLA-B*15:02* allele.

27. **B**. *The FDA-approved drug label for carbamazepine states that more than 15% of the population is reported to be HLA-B*15:02—positive in Hong Kong, Thailand, Malaysia, and parts of the Philippines, compared to about 10% in Taiwan and 4% in North China.* The label states that South Asians, including Indians, appear to have intermediate prevalence of *HLA-B*15:02*, averaging 2%—4%, but higher in some groups. In Japan and Korea, the *HLA-B*15:02* is present in less than 1% of the population. In individuals not of Asian origin, such as Caucasians, African Americans, Hispanics, and Native Americans, the *HLA-B*15:02* allele is largely absent.

Therefore, the *HLA-B*15:02* allele is more frequently seen in Asian than in Caucasians, African Americans, and Hispanics.

28. **A**. As an antiseizure medication, phenytoin has a narrow therapeutic index. An individual's human leukocyte antigen B (HLA-B) genotype is a known risk factor for drug-induced hypersensitivity reactions. HLA-B has an important immunological role in pathogen recognition and response, as well as in nonpathogens such as drugs. Carriers of the variant *HLA-B*15:02* allele are at high risk of developing potentially life-threatening phenytoin-induced Stevens—Johnson syndrome (SJS) and the related toxic epidermal necrolysis (TEN). The *HLA-B*15:02* variant is most commonly found among individuals of Southeast Asian descent. *The FDA-approved drug label for phenytoin states that consideration should be given to avoiding phenytoin as an alternative for carbamazepine in patients who are positive for HLA-B*15:02.*

The *HLA-A*31:01* allele may also be a risk factor for SJS/TEN, but is more strongly associated with carbamazepine-induced reactions worldwide, such as drug reaction with eosinophilia and systemic symptoms (DRESS) and maculopapular exanthema (MPE). *HLA-B*15:11* has also been linked with

carbamazepine-induced SJS/TEN. *HLA-B*57:01* significantly increases the risk of hypersensitivity reactions when abacavir (ABC) is administered. The *HLA-B*58:01* allele is strongly associated with severe cutaneous adverse reactions (SCAR) during treatment with allopurinol.

Therefore, this Asian patient most likely carried the *HLA-B*15:02* allele, according to the FDA-approved drug label for phenytoin.

29. **D**. Carriers of the variant *HLA-B*15:02* allele are at high risk of developing potentially life-threatening phenytoin-induced or carbamazepine-induced Stevens—Johnson syndrome (SJS) and the related toxic epidermal necrolysis (TEN). *The FDA-approved drug label states that carbamazepine should not be used in patients who are positive for HLA-B*15:02 unless the benefits clearly outweigh the risks.* The FDA-approved drug label for phenytoin states that consideration should be given to avoiding phenytoin as an alternative for carbamazepine in patients who are positive for *HLA-B*15:02*.

CBZ is not sufficient for controlling this patient's seizures. Therefore, using an alternative drug would most likely be considered for better patient treatment in this case.

30. **A**. As an antiseizure medication, phenytoin has a narrow therapeutic index. The FDA-approved drug label for phenytoin states that consideration should be given to avoiding phenytoin as an alternative for carbamazepine in patients positive for *HLA-B*15:02*. *The label also mentions that variant CYP2C9 alleles may contribute to unusually high levels of phenytoin.* The Clinical Pharmacogenetics Implementation Consortium (CPIC) recommends the use of an antiseizure medication other than carbamazepine or phenytoin (or its prodrug fosphenytoin) for any *HLA-B*15:02* carrier regardless of *CYP2C9* genotype, patient ancestry, or age. CPIC also recommends consideration of at least a 25% reduction in the starting maintenance dose for patients who are *CYP2C9* intermediate metabolizers and *HLA-B*15:02*—negative and at least a 50% reduction for *CYP2C9* poor metabolizers and *HLA-B*15:02*—negative, with subsequent maintenance doses adjusted based on therapeutic drug monitoring and response.

Therefore, *CYP2C9* may also affect PHT metabolism in addition to *HLA* genotyping, according to the FDA-approved drug label.

31. **B**. Variant *CYP2C9* alleles are known to influence phenytoin drug levels. Individuals who carry decreased activity CYP2C9 variants may have reduced clearance rates of phenytoin and be at greater risk for dose-related side effects. The

CYP2C9*2 and *CYP2C9*3* alleles are two common decreased-function alleles. Individuals homozygous for two alleles with low or deficient activity are poor metabolizers.

The Clinical Pharmacogenetics Implementation Consortium (CPIC) recommends consideration of at least a 25% reduction in the starting maintenance dose for patients who are CYP2C9 intermediate metabolizers and HLA-B*15:02—negative, and at least a 50% reduction for CYP2C9 poor metabolizers and HLA-B*15:02—negative, with subsequent maintenance doses adjusted based on therapeutic drug monitoring and response.

Therefore, decreasing the PHT dose would more likely be considered for better patient treatment in this case.

32. **B.** Aspirin and clopidogrel are the standard care for patients who have an acute coronary syndrome (ACS). Studies have demonstrated that this dual antiplatelet therapy reduces the risk of major adverse cardiovascular events (MACE), especially stent thrombosis, in patients who have undergone cardiac revascularization with percutaneous coronary intervention or coronary artery bypass graft surgery. *Clopidogrel is a prodrug requiring two-step enzymatic metabolism to generate the active metabolite—a process in which CYP2C19 plays a critical role.* Individuals who are *CYP2C19* poor metabolizers cannot activate clopidogrel via the CYP2C19 pathway, which means the drug will have no effect.

Therefore, *CYP2C19* would most likely affect clopidogrel metabolism in this patient.

33. **B.** The effectiveness of clopidogrel depends on its conversion to an active metabolite by *CY2C19*. Individuals who carry two nonfunctional copies of the *CYP2C19* gene are classified as CYP2C19 poor metabolizers. They have no enzyme activity and cannot activate clopidogrel via the CYP2C19 pathway, which means the drug will have no effect. Approximately 2% of Caucasians, 4% of African Americans, and 14% of Chinese are CYP2C19 poor metabolizers.

CYP2C19*2 is a common loss-of-function allele, seen in up to 30% of individuals of European and African ancestry and 70% of those of Asian ancestry; homozygotes for the *2 allele (poor metabolizers) constitute approximately 3%—4% and 10%—15% of these ancestries, respectively.

CYP2C19*1 is the wild allele. CYP2C19*3 and *CYP2C19*4* are also loss-of-function alleles, but are not as common as *CYP2C19*2*. Therefore, this patient would most likely carry *CYP2C19*2/*2*.

34. **D.** As an antiplatelet agent, clopidogrel reduces the risk of myocardial infarction (MI) and stroke in patients with acute coronary syndrome (ACS) and in patients with atherosclerotic vascular disease (indicated by a recent MI or stroke or established peripheral arterial disease). Both *CYP2C19*2* and *CYP2C19*3* are loss-of-function alleles. The patient may be classified as a poor metabolizer. The 2017 FDA-approved drug label for clopidogrel includes a boxed warning concerning the diminished antiplatelet effect of clopidogrel in CYP2C19 poor metabolizers. *The warning states that tests are available to identify patients who are CYP2C19 poor metabolizers and to consider the use of another platelet P2Y12 inhibitor in patients identified as CYP2C19 poor metabolizers.*

Therefore, this patient should be considered to use an alternative medication to reduce the risk of myocardial infarction (MI) and stroke, according to the FDA-approved drug label for clopidogrel.

35. **D.** The *CYP2C19*1* allele is wild-type. The most common loss-of-function variant is *CYP2C19*2*, which contains a c.681G > A variant in exon 5 that results in an aberrant splice site; this leads to the production of a truncated and nonfunctioning protein. Another commonly tested loss-of-function variant is *CYP2C19*3*, which contains a c.636G > A variant in exon 4 that causes a premature stop codon. *The CYP2C19*17 allele is associated with increased enzyme activity and the "ultrarapid metabolizer" phenotype, which contains a c.-806C > T variant.*

Therefore, the *CYP2C19*17* allele contains a variant at the noncoding region.

36. **A.** The RAF and RAS families are proto-oncogenes. The RAF family has three members, *ARAF*, *BRAF*, and *CRAF*. The RAS family consists of *HRAS*, *KRAS*, and *NRAS*.

Dabrafenib (trade name Tafinlar, GSK2118436) and Vemurafenib (INN, marketed as Zelboraf) are kinase inhibitors indicated in the treatment of patients with unresectable or metastatic melanoma with the BRAF V600E variant. They increased progression-free survival, compared to cytotoxic chemotherapy, in patients with advanced melanoma and the BRAF V600E variant.

Therefore, *BRAF* would most likely carry a variant, specifically V600, sensitive to kinase inhibitors for metastases melanoma, such as dabrafenib or vemurafenib.

37. **B.** Variations in *BRAF* are detectable in approximately 50% of malignant melanomas. *The BRAF V600E variant accounts for approximately 90% of variants.* The second most common *BRAF* variant is V600K.

This patient actually had a rare V600R variant, and dabrafenib treatment was initiated. Seven months after the start of treatment, he presented with pneumonia and was admitted again. A CT scan revealed hepatic and retroperitoneal progression, as well as the appearance of pericardial and pleural effusions, and an MRI detected multiple bilateral brain metastases. Dabrafenib treatment was stopped. He died several months later.

Therefore, this patient would most likely carry a *BRAF* V600E variant.

38. **B.** Fluorouracil (5-FU) is a chemotherapy agent that belongs to the drug class of fluoropyrimidines. When given as an IV solution, fluorouracil is used in the palliative management of colon, rectum, breast, stomach, and pancreas carcinomas. *The DPYD gene encodes dihydropyrimidine dehydrogenase (DPD), an enzyme that catalyzes the rate-limiting step in fluorouracil metabolism.* Individuals who carry at least one copy of no-function *DPYD* variants, such as *DPYD*13*, may not be able to metabolize fluorouracil at normal rates and are at risk for potentially life-threatening fluorouracil toxicity, such as bone-marrow suppression and neurotoxicity.

CYP2D6 catalyzes many reactions involved in drug metabolism and synthesis of cholesterol, steroids, and other lipids. The *HLA-B*15:02* allele is strongly associated with carbamazepine-induced Stevens–Johnson syndrome (SJS) and toxic epidermal necrolysis (TEN). Warfarin resistance is an infrequently encountered clinical scenario that may be due to variants in the vitamin K epoxide reductase complex 1 gene (*VKORC1*).

Therefore, *DPYD* would most likely affect 5-FU metabolism in this patient.

39. **B.** The *DPYD* gene catalyzes the rate-limiting step in fluorouracil metabolism. *DPYD*1* is the wild-type allele and is associated with normal enzyme activity. The *DPYD* alleles *4, *5, *6, and *9A are also considered to have normal activity. *DPYD*2A*, *DPYD*13*, and rs67376798 are nonfunctional alleles.

Individuals who carry two copies of *DPYD* alleles with normal activity are known as "normal metabolizers" and have fully functional DPD enzyme activity. Individuals who carry combinations of normal-function, decreased-function, and/or no-function *DPYD* alleles are known as "intermediate metabolizers." They have partial DPD deficiency and are at increased risk of capecitabine toxicity, such as bone-marrow suppression and neurotoxicity. Individuals who carry a combination of no-function *DPYD* alleles

and/or decreased-function DPYD alleles are known as "poor metabolizers." *They have complete DPD deficiency and are at an even higher risk of fluorouracil toxicity.* The prevalence of DPD deficiency in Caucasians is approximately 3%–5%. In the Dutch population, the *DPYD*2A* had an allele frequency of 0.91% in Caucasians.

Therefore, the patient would most likely carry the *DPYD*2A* allele for fluorouracil toxicity, since it is the only nonfunctional allele listed in the question.

40. **D.** The FDA-approved drug label for fluorouracil states that "rarely, unexpected, severe toxicity (e.g., stomatitis, diarrhea, neutropenia, and neurotoxicity) associated with 5-fluorouracil has been attributed to deficiency of dipyrimidine dehydrogenase activity." The Clinical Pharmacogenetics Implementation Consortium (CPIC) has published dosing recommendations for fluoropyrimidines (capecitabine, fluorouracil, and tegafur) based on *DPYD* genotype. *CPIC recommends using an alternative drug for patients who are "poor metabolizers."* These individuals carry two copies of no-function DPYD variants and typically have complete DPD deficiency, as seen in this patient.

Therefore, using an alternative drug would most likely be considered for better patient treatment in this case.

41. **D.** Irinotecan (brand name, Camptosar) is a topoisomerase I inhibitor widely used in the treatment of cancer. It is most frequently used in combination with other drugs to treat advanced or metastatic colorectal cancer (CRC). However, irinotecan therapy is associated with a high incidence of toxicity, including severe neutropenia and diarrhea. Irinotecan is converted in the body to an active metabolite, SN-38, which is then inactivated and detoxified by a UDP-glucuronosyltransferase (UGT) enzyme encoded by the *UGT1A1* gene. The UGT enzymes are responsible for glucuronidation, a process that transforms lipophilic metabolites into water-soluble metabolites that can be excreted from the body. *The risk of irinotecan toxicity increases with genetic variants associated with reduced UGT enzyme activity, such as UGT1A1*28.* The presence of this variant results in reduced excretion of irinotecan metabolites, which leads to increased active irinotecan metabolites in the blood.

CYP2D6 catalyzes many reactions involved in drug metabolism and synthesis of cholesterol, steroids, and other lipids. The *DPYD* gene encodes an enzyme that catalyzes the rate-limiting step in fluorouracil metabolism. The *HLA-B*15:02* allele is strongly associated with carbamazepine-induced Stevens–Johnson syndrome (SJS) and toxic epidermal necrolysis (TEN).

Therefore, *UGT1A1* would most likely be studied in this patient to investigate IROX toxicity.

42. **B.** *The FDA-approved drug label for irinotecan states that "when administered as a single-agent, a reduction in the starting dose by at least one level of irinotecan hydrochloride injection should be considered for patients known to be homozygous for the UGT1A1*28 allele.* However, the precise dose reduction in this patient population is not known and subsequent dose modifications should be considered based on individual patient tolerance to treatment." The Dutch Pharmacogenetics Working Group (DPWG) of the Royal Dutch Association for the Advancement of Pharmacy (KNMP) recommends starting with 70% of the standard dose for homozygous carriers of the *UGT1A1*28* allele. If the patient tolerates this initial dose, the dose can be increased guided by the neutrophil count. They state that no action is needed for heterozygous carriers of the *UGT1A1*28* allele (e.g., *UGT1A1*1/ *28*).

Therefore, reducing the irinotecan dose would most likely be considered for better patient management in this case.

43. **D.** Despite the risk of permanent ototoxic effects, aminoglycosides remain as commonly utilized antibiotics worldwide owing to their low cost and efficiency in treating severe infections. Gentamicin is the most commonly used aminoglycoside. Over the past two decades, mitochondrial variants have been shown to enhance the likelihood of ototoxic injury. *All individuals with the MTRNR1 variant known as m.1555A > G (NC_012920.1: m.1555A > G) developed aminoglycoside-induced hearing loss.* The onset of hearing loss varies, but once it occurs, it is usually moderate to profound, bilateral, and irreversible.

CYP2D6 catalyzes many reactions involved in drug metabolism and synthesis of cholesterol, steroids, and other lipids. The *DPYD* gene encodes an enzyme that catalyzes the rate-limiting step in fluorouracil metabolism. The *HLA-B*15:02* allele is strongly associated with carbamazepine-induced Stevens–Johnson syndrome (SJS) and toxic epidermal necrolysis (TEN).

Therefore, *MTRNR1* would most likely be associated with gentamicin-induced ototoxic injury in this patient.

44. **D.** Azathioprine is an immunosuppressant medication that belongs to the class of thiopurines. It is used to prevent kidney transplant rejection and in the management of rheumatoid arthritis when other treatments have not been effective. In addition, off-label it also has been used to treat inflammatory bowel disease, such as ulcerative colitis. As a prodrug, azathioprine must first be activated to form thioguanine nucleotides (TGNs), the major active metabolites. Thiopurine S-methyltransferase (TPMT) inactivates azathioprine, leaving less parent drug available to form TGNs. The side effect of azathioprine is bone marrow suppression, which may be dose-dependent, and can be reversed by reducing the dose. *However, patients who carry two nonfunctional TPMT alleles always develop life-threatening myelosuppression when treated with azathioprine, due to high levels of TGNs.* Patients who carry one nonfunctional *TPMT* allele (heterozygous) may also not be able to tolerate conventional doses of azathioprine.

The *DPYD* gene encodes an enzyme that catalyzes the rate-limiting step in fluorouracil metabolism. The *HLA-B*15:02* allele is strongly associated with carbamazepine-induced Stevens–Johnson syndrome (SJS) and toxic epidermal necrolysis (TEN). 100% of individuals with the *MTRNR1* variant known as m.1555A > G (NC_012920.1: m.1555A > G) developed aminoglycoside-induced hearing loss.

Therefore, *TPMT* would most likely be associated with azathioprine-induced myelosuppression in this patient.

45. **C.** Thiopurines are used as anticancer agents and as immunosuppressants in inflammatory bowel disease, rheumatoid arthritis, and other autoimmune conditions. Three thiopurines are used clinically—thioguanine, mercaptopurine, and azathioprine (a prodrug for mercaptopurine). The three agents have similar effects but are typically used for different indications. One of the most frequent adverse reactions to azathioprine is myelosuppression, which can occur in any patient, and can usually be reversed by decreasing the dose of azathioprine. However, all patients who carry two nonfunctional *TPMT* alleles (approximately 0.3%) experience life-threatening myelosuppression after starting treatment with conventional doses of azathioprine owing to high levels of TGNs. The wild-type *TPMT*1* allele is associated with normal enzyme activity. Individuals who are homozygous for *TPMT*1* (TPMT normal metabolizers) are more likely to have a typical response to azathioprine and a lower risk of myelosuppression. This accounts for the majority of patients (∼86%–97%). *Three variant TPMT alleles account for over 90% of the reduced or absent activity TPMT alleles. They are TPMT*2 (c.238G > C), TPMT*3A (c.460G > A and*

c.719A > G), TPMT*3B (c.460G > A), and TPMT*3C (c.719A > G).

Therefore, this patient would most likely carry TPMT*3A/*3A.

46. **D.** Three variant *TPMT* alleles account for over 90% of the reduced or absent activity *TPMT* alleles. They are *TPMT*2* (c.238G > C), *TPMT*3A* (c.460G > A and c.719A > G), *TPMT*3B* (c.460G > A), and *TPMT*3C* (c.719A > G). Intermediate metabolizers carry one functional allele (such as *TPMT*1*) and one nonfunctional allele (such as *TPMT*3A*).

The Clinical Pharmacogenetics Implementation Consortium (CPIC) has published recommendations for *TPMT* genotype-based azathioprine dosing. These recommendations include: *Consider an alternative agent or extreme dose reduction of azathioprine (reduce daily dose by 10-fold and dose twice weekly instead of daily) for patients with low or deficient TPMT activity. Start at 30%–70% of target dose for patients with intermediate enzyme activity.*

Therefore, in this case, using an alternative drug would be a conservative way to reduce the risk of adverse effects associated with azathioprine in this patient.

47. **D.** Simvastatin is among the most commonly used prescription medications for cholesterol reduction. *A nonsynonymous coding SNP, rs4149056, in SLCO1B1 markedly increases systemic exposure to simvastatin and the risk of muscle toxicity.* It impacts the pharmacokinetics of simvastatin and, to a lesser degree, the pharmacokinetics of other statins. Homozygous carriers of the C allele at rs4149056 (CC genotype) had much greater exposure to the active simvastatin acid than subjects homozygous for the wild allele (T).

The *DPYD* gene encodes an enzyme that catalyzes the rate-limiting step in fluorouracil metabolism. The *HLA-B*15:02* allele is strongly associated with carbamazepine-induced Stevens–Johnson syndrome (SJS) and toxic epidermal necrolysis (TEN). An *MTRNR1* variant known as m.1555A > G (NC_012920.1: m.1555A > G) is associated with aminoglycoside-induced hearing loss.

Therefore, *SLCO1B1* would most likely be studied to confirm/rule out simvastatin-induced myopathy in this patient.

48. **B.** "In 2011 and updated in 2013, the FDA added warnings to the simvastatin product label to direct providers away from initiating at the 80 mg simvastatin dose." The 2014 update of CPIC guidelines regarding SLCO1B1 and simvastatin-induced myopathy has been published in Clinical Pharmacology and Therapeutics, and has not been updated. The CPIC states that "*At lower simvastatin doses (e.g., 40 mg daily), it is our position that SLCO1B1 genotype (if available) could be used to warn providers about modest increases in myopathy risk for patients with a C allele at rs4149056.* In these circumstances, we recommend a lower dose of simvastatin or use an alternative statin (e.g., pravastatin or rosuvastatin) and we also highlight the potential utility of routine CK surveillance. If patients with a C allele at rs4149056 do not achieve optimal LDL cholesterol-lowering efficacy with a lower dose (e.g., 20 mg) of simvastatin, we recommend the prescribing physician consider an alternative statin based on (i) potency differences (i.e., use a lower dose of a higher potency statin such as atorvastatin, rosuvastatin, or pitavastatin), (ii) drug-drug interactions (e.g., boceprevir, clarithromycin, cyclosporine, strong CYP3A4 inhibitors, etc.), and (iii) relevant co-morbidities (e.g., trauma, significant renal impairment, post-solid organ transplant, thyroid disease etc.)."

Therefore, administering simvastatin at a reduced dose would most likely be considered for better patient treatment in this case.

References

1. Schwab M, Schaeffeler E. Pharmacogenomics: a key component of personalized therapy. *Genome Med* 2012;**4**(11):93.
2. Pinillos F, et al. Case report: severe central nervous system manifestations associated with aberrant efavirenz metabolism in children: the role of CYP2B6 genetic variation. *BMC Infect Dis* 2016;**16**:56.
3. Zanger UM, Klein K. Pharmacogenetics of cytochrome P450 2B6 (CYP2B6): advances on polymorphisms, mechanisms, and clinical relevance. *Front Genet* 2013;**4**:24.
4. Thorn CF, et al. PharmGKB summary: very important pharmacogene information for CYP2B6. *Pharmacogenet Genomics* 2010;**20**(8):520–3.
5. Yoon JH, Kim M, Jin SJ, Kim SK, Lee SH, Cheon J, et al. The first case of abacavir hypersensitivity associated with the HLA-B*57:01-positive allele in Korea. *Infect Chemother* 2012;**44**(5):399–402.
6. Pratt HMV, Rubinstein W, Dean L, Kattman B, Malheiro A, editors. *Medical genetics summaries*. Bethesda (MD): National Center for Biotechnology Information (US); 2012.
7. International Warfarin Pharmacogenetics Consortium, et al. Estimation of the warfarin dose with clinical and pharmacogenetic data. *N Engl J Med* 2009;**360**(8):753–64.
8. Flockhart DA, et al. Pharmacogenetic testing of CYP2C9 and VKORC1 alleles for warfarin. *Genet Med* 2008;**10**(2):139–50.
9. Johnson M, et al. Warfarin dosing in a patient with CYP2C9(*)3(*)3 and VKORC1-1639 AA genotypes. *Case Rep Genet* 2014;**2014**:413743.
10. Ma XW, et al. Warfarin-induced life-threatening bleeding associated with a CYP3A4 loss-of-function mutation in an acute limb ischemia patient: Case report and review of the literature. *Exp Ther Med* 2017;**14**(2):1157–62.

11. Bain KT. Pharmacogenomics case: unintentional overdose from β-blockers. *CareKinesis Case Study* 2015;1−4.

12. Malhotra N, et al. A pharmacodynamic comparison of a personalized strategy for anti-platelet therapy versus ticagrelor in achieving a therapeutic window. *Int J Cardiol* 2015;**197**:318−25.

13. Swen JJ, et al. Pharmacogenetics: from bench to byte − an update of guidelines. *Clin Pharmacol Ther* 2011;**89**(5):662−73.

14. Friedrichsdorf SJ, Nugent AP, Strobl AQ. Codeine-associated pediatric deaths despite using recommended dosing guidelines: three case reports. *J Opioid Manag* 2013;**9**(2):151−5.

15. Koren G, et al. Pharmacogenetics of morphine poisoning in a breastfed neonate of a codeine-prescribed mother. *Lancet* 2006;**368**(9536):704.

16. VanderVaart S, et al. CYP2D6 polymorphisms and codeine analgesia in postpartum pain management: a pilot study. *Ther Drug Monit* 2011;**33**(4):425−32.

17. Zeng M, et al. Drug eruptions induced by allopurinol associated with HLA-B*5801. *Indian J Dermatol Venereol Leprol* 2015;**81**(1):43−5.

18. Masliyah T, Ad-Dab'bagh Y. Low-dose risperidone-induced oculogyric crises in an adolescent male with autism, tourette's and developmental delay. *J Can Acad Child Adolesc Psychiatry* 2011;**20**(3):214−16.

19. Foster A, et al. Pharmacogenetics of antipsychotic adverse effects: case studies and a literature review for clinicians. *Neuropsychiatr Dis Treat* 2007;**3**(6):965−73.

20. Hu FY, et al. Phenytoin-induced Stevens-Johnson syndrome with negative HLA-B*1502 allele in mainland China: two cases. *Seizure* 2011;**20**(5):431−2.

21. Ding L, et al. Acute stent thrombosis after stent-assisted coiling in an intracranial aneurysm patient carrying two reduced-function CYP2C19 alleles: a case report. *Medicine (Baltimore)* 2017;**96**(47):e8920.

22. Johnson JA, et al. Clopidogrel: a case for indication-specific pharmacogenetics. *Clin Pharmacol Ther* 2012;**91**(5):774−6.

23. Chikata Y, et al. Simultaneous subacute coronary artery stent thrombosis in a carrier of two CYP2C19 loss-of function polymorphisms (*2/*3). *Int J Cardiol* 2016;**212**:148−50.

24. Casadevall D, et al. Dabrafenib in an elderly patient with metastatic melanoma and BRAF V600R mutation: a case report. *J Med Case Rep* 2016;**10**(1):158.

25. Luber B, et al. Biomarker analysis of cetuximab plus oxaliplatin/leucovorin/5-fluorouracil in first-line metastatic gastric and oesophago-gastric junction cancer: results from a phase II trial of the Arbeitsgemeinschaft Internistische Onkologie (AIO). *BMC Cancer* 2011;**11**:509.

26. Saif MW, et al. A DPYD variant (Y186C) specific to individuals of African descent in a patient with life-threatening 5-FU toxic effects: potential for an individualized medicine approach. *Mayo Clin Proc* 2014;**89**(1):131−6.

27. Ofverholm A, et al. Two cases of 5-fluorouracil toxicity linked with gene variants in the DPYD gene. *Clin Biochem* 2010;**43**(3):331−4.

28. Lalkota BP, Srinivasa B, Nasiruddin M, Radheshyam N. Combined DPD and UGT1A1 mutation in a single patient: a case report. *J Pharmacogenomics Pharmacoproteomics* 2017;**8**(1). Available from: https://doi.org/10.4172/2153-0645.1000165.

29. East JE, Foweraker JE, Murgatroyd FD. Gentamicin induced ototoxicity during treatment of enterococcal endocarditis: resolution with substitution by netilmicin. *Heart* 2005;**91**(5):e32.

30. Gardiner SJ, et al. Two cases of thiopurine methyltransferase (TPMT) deficiency − a lucky save and a near miss with azathioprine. *Br J Clin Pharmacol* 2006;**62**(4):473−6.

31. Hill FJ, McCloskey SJ, Sheerin N. From a fish tank injury to hospital haemodialysis: the serious consequences of drug interactions. *BMJ Case Rep* 2015;**2015**. Available from: https://doi.org/10.1136/bcr-2015-209961.

32. Wilke RA, et al. The clinical pharmacogenomics implementation consortium: CPIC guideline for SLCO1B1 and simvastatin-induced myopathy. *Clin Pharmacol Ther* 2012;**92**(1):112−17.

33. Ramsey LB, et al. The clinical pharmacogenetics implementation consortium guideline for SLCO1B1 and simvastatin-induced myopathy: 2014 update. *Clin Pharmacol Ther* 2014;**96**(4):423−8.

Further Reading

- Clinical Pharmacogenetics Implementation Consortium (CPIC) (https://cpicpgx.org/)
- Medical Genetics Summaries from National Center for Biotechnology Information (US) (https://www.ncbi.nlm.nih.gov/books/NBK385154)
- PharmGKB (https://www.pharmgkb.org/)
- Royal Dutch Association for the Advancement of Pharmacy (KNMP) (https://www.knmp.nl/knmp/about-knmp-1)
- UpToDate (https://www.uptodate.com/contents/overview-of-pharmacogenomics)
- US Food and Drug Administration (http://www.fda.gov/)

14

Genetic Counseling—Introduction

Genetic counseling is a process of helping people understand and adapt to the medical, psychological, and familial implications of genetic contributions to disease (www.nsgc.org), such as: (1) How inherited diseases and conditions might affect them or their families; (2) How family and medical histories may impact the chance of disease occurrence or recurrence; (3) Which genetic tests may or may not be right for them, and what those tests may or may not tell; and (4) How to make the most informed choices about health care conditions. In 2016, there were 3100 genetic counselors in the United States (https://www.bls.gov/). Genetic counselors are an integral part of clinical care in many areas of medicine, such as assisted reproductive technology/infertility genetics, cancer genetics, cardiovascular genetics, cystic fibrosis genetics, fetal intervention and therapy genetics, hematology genetics, metabolic genetics, neurogenetics, pediatric genetics, personalized medicine genetics, prenatal genetics, and postmortem genetic testing.

When patients see a genetic counselor, the counselor usually takes the family health history; may set up appointments to have tests to check for genetic conditions; helps patients understand test results and recurrent risks; and refers patients to medical specialists, education resources, and support groups for the families. A support group is a group of people who have the same kind of concerns who meet to try to help each other.

In this chapter, we will go through risk estimation and test selection for specific ethnic groups. Education resources and support groups are provided in the section on "Further Reading."

QUESTIONS

1. What is the estimated carrier frequency of genetic disorders in the Ashkenazi Jewish population?
   A. 1/3
   B. 1/9
   C. 1/16
   D. 1/24
   E. 1/38
2. Which one of the following genetic disorders is the most common among these choices in Ashkenazi Jews?[1,2]
   A. Canavan disease
   B. Cystic fibrosis
   C. Familial dysautonomia
   D. Gaucher disease
   E. Tay—Sachs disease
3. Cleft lip/palate is a common birth defect. The Centers for Disease Control and Prevention (CDC) recently estimated that each year in the United States about 2650 babies are born with a cleft palate and 4440 are born with a cleft lip with or without a cleft palate. Which one of the following is NOT a risk factor for cleft lip/palate?
   A. African American
   B. Male
   C. Maternal alcohol use during pregnancy
   D. Maternal antiepilepsy therapy during the first trimester
   E. Maternal diabetes
   F. Maternal smoking during pregnancy
   G. None of the above
4. Which one of the following races/ethnics has a higher risk for cleft lip/cleft palate?[3]
   A. African Americans
   B. Ashkenazi Jewish
   C. Asian
   D. Caucasian
   E. Latinos
5. Which one of the following statements regarding cleft lip (CL) is NOT correct?
   A. A male fetus with a brother having CL has a higher risk to have CL than a female fetus with a brother having CL.
   B. A male fetus with a brother having CL has a higher risk to have CL than a male fetus with a sister having CL.

Self-assessment Questions for Clinical Molecular Genetics.
DOI: https://doi.org/10.1016/B978-0-12-809967-4.00014-4

C. A male fetus with a brother and mother having CL has a higher risk to have CL than a male fetus with a brother having CL.
D. All of the above.
E. None of the above.

6. Which one of the following medical conditions occurs more often in females than males?
A. Alzheimer
B. Cleft lip
C. Club foot
D. Pyloric stenosis
E. All of the above
F. None of the above

7. Which one of the following medical conditions occurs more often in males than females?
A. Cleft lip
B. Club foot
C. Hirschsprung disease
D. Pyloric stenosis
E. All of the above
F. None of the above

8. How frequently do newborns have congenital anomalies?
A. <1%
B. 4%
C. 9%
D. 22%
E. None of the above

9. Which one of the following statements describes the reason why Gaucher disease is more prevalent in Ashkenazi Jewish population than other populations?
A. Bottleneck and founder effects
B. High mutation rate in Ashkenazi Jews
C. Natural selection due to environmental factors
D. All of the above
E. None of above

10. The newborn screening program (NBS) in the state of Massachusetts referred a newborn boy, John Doe, with a F508del variant to a cystic fibrosis (CF) foundation—accredited care center for further evaluation and diagnostic test. The follow-up sweat sodium chloride test was positive. Which one of the following may a genetic counselor NOT offer in this situation?
A. Discussing recurrent risk
B. Identifying at-risk family members
C. Providing information about support groups
D. Providing the family an understanding of mode of inheritance
E. Suggesting therapy in a clinical trial
F. All of the above
G. None of the above

11. How frequently does prelingual hearing loss have a genetic etiology in Western nations?[4]
A. > 99%
B. 80%
C. 50%
D. 30%
E. 10%
F. <1%

12. Which one of the following inheritance modes does most of genetic prelingual hearing loss have?[4,16]
A. Autosomal dominant
B. Autosomal recessive
C. X-linked dominant
D. X-linked recessive
E. Mitochondrial

13. Which one of the following disorders accounts for the majority of cases of hemolytic disease of the fetus and newborn (HDFN)?
A. RhD incompatibility
B. RhK incompatibility
C. Rhc incompatibility
D. RhE incompatibility
E. ABO incompatibility

14. Age-related macular degeneration (AMD) is a complex disease trait with both genetic and environmental influences. Which one of the following is the single most important environmental risk factor for AMD?
A. Alcohol use
B. Obesity
C. Oral contraceptive drugs
D. Smoking
E. Radiation

15. Which one of the following complications do patients with Down syndrome have NO increased risk to develop?
A. Alzheimer disease
B. Leukemia
C. Parkinson disease
D. Premature aging
E. Seizure

16. Late-onset Alzheimer disease is a complex disease trait. Which one of the following is NOT a risk factor for it?[5]
A. APOE genotype: ε4/ε4
B. Down syndrome
C. Female sex
D. One brother diagnosed with late-onset Alzheimer disease at the age of 62 years
E. Oral contraceptives

17. After what age do nearly all patients with Down syndrome have neuropathological findings of Alzheimer disease?

A. 35 years
B. 40 years
C. 45 years
D. 50 years
E. 55 years
F. 60 years

18. Which one of the following disorders do children born with assisted reproductive technologies, such as in vitro fertilization (IVF), have an increased risk to develop?[6]
    A. Achondroplasia
    B. Beckwith–Wiedemann syndrome
    C. Duchenne muscular dystrophy
    D. Hirschsprung disease
    E. Miller–Dieker syndrome

19. Which one of the following is the approximate estimation of the cumulative risk of breast cancer by age 70 years if an individual carries a *BRCA1* pathogenic variant?
    A. 12%
    B. 33%
    C. 57%
    D. 86%
    E. > 99%
    F. None of the above

20. Which one of the following is the estimate of cumulative risk of breast cancer by age 70 years if an individual carries a *BRCA2* pathogenic variant?
    A. 9%
    B. 21%
    C. 49%
    D. 71%
    E. 86%
    F. None of the above

21. Which one of the following is the estimate of cumulative risk of ovarian cancer by age 70 years if an individual carries a *BRCA1* pathogenic variant?
    A. 8%
    B. 21%
    C. 40%
    D. 69%
    E. 86%
    F. None of the above

22. Which one of the following is the estimate of cumulative risk of ovarian cancer by age 70 years for *BRCA2* mutation carriers?
    A. 6%
    B. 18%
    C. 36%
    D. 59%
    E. 71%
    F. 86%
    G. None of the above

23. About 12% of women in the general population will develop breast cancer sometime during their lives. By contrast, according to the most recent estimates, 55%–65% of women who inherit a pathogenic *BRCA1* variant and around 45% of women who inherit a pathogenic *BRCA2* variant will develop breast cancer by age 70 years (see the table below). What is the odds ratio for breast cancer with *BRCA1* pathogenic variants as compared with the general population?

	Breast cancer	Healthy individuals
BRCA1 mutation	60	40
No *BRCA1* mutation	10	90

    A. 1.5
    B. 4
    C. 6
    D. 9
    E. 13.5

24. About 12% of women in the general population will develop breast cancer sometime during their lives. By contrast, according to the most recent estimates, 55%–65% of women who inherit a pathogenic *BRCA1* variant and around 45% of women who inherit a pathogenic *BRCA2* variant will develop breast cancer by age 70 years. What is the relative risk for breast cancer with *BRCA1* pathogenic variants as compared with the general population?

	Breast cancer	Healthy individuals
BRCA1 mutation	60	40
No *BRCA1* mutation	10	90

    A. 1.5
    B. 4
    C. 6
    D. 9
    E. 13.5

25. About 1.3% of women in the general population will develop ovarian cancer sometime during their lives. By contrast, according to the most recent estimates, 39% of women who inherit a pathogenic *BRCA1* variant and 11%–17% of women who inherit a pathogenic *BRCA2* variant will develop ovarian cancer by age 70 years. What is the odds ratio for ovarian cancer with *BRCA1* pathogenic variants as compared with the general population?

	Breast cancer	Healthy individuals
BRCA1 mutation	40	60
No *BRCA1* mutation	1	99

A. 2.48
B. 40
C. 60
D. 66
E. 99

26. About 12% of women in the general population will develop breast cancer sometime during their lives. By contrast, according to the most recent estimates, 55%–65% of women who inherit a pathogenic *BRCA1* variant and around 45% of women who inherit a pathogenic *BRCA2* variant will develop breast cancer by age 70 years. What is the relative risk for breast cancer with *BRCA1* pathogenic variants as compared with the general population?

	Breast cancer	Healthy individuals
BRCA1 mutation	40	60
No *BRCA1* mutation	1	99

A. 2.48
B. 6
C. 40
D. 66
E. 99

27. Which one of the following statements about the prevalence of *BRCA1* pathogenic variants in the United States is NOT correct?
   A. *BRCA1* pathogenic variants are more common in African Americans than in Hispanic Americans.
   B. *BRCA1* pathogenic variants are more common in Ashkenazi Jewish descents than in African Americans.
   C. *BRCA1* pathogenic variants are more common in Ashkenazi Jewish descents than in Caucasians.
   D. *BRCA1* pathogenic variants are more common in Caucasians than in Asian Americans.
   E. *BRCA1* pathogenic variants are more common in French Canadians than in general European descendants.

28. A 32-year-old Ashkenazi Jewish female was referred to a genetics clinic by her gynecologist after being diagnosed with breast cancer and being confirmed to carry a deleterious *BRCA2* pathogenic variant. She was concerned about her 6- and 4-year-old daughters and asked for genetics studies

for them. Which one of the following responses from her care provider would be the most appropriate?[7]
   A. Ordering a Sanger sequence study of *BRCA2* for the two daughters
   B. Ordering a Sanger sequence study of *BRCA2* for the older daughter, but not the younger one
   C. Ordering a targeted *BRCA2* study for the two daughters
   D. Ordering a targeted *BRCA2* study for the older daughter, but not the younger one
   E. Referring the family to a pediatric clinic
   F. Suggesting not testing the daughters until they are adults and are ready to make their own decision

29. A 46-year-old Caucasian female was referred to a genetics clinic by her gynecologist after being diagnosed with breast cancer with a deleterious *BRCA2* pathogenic variant. She was concerned about her 16- and 12-year-old daughters and asked for genetic studies for them. The older daughter wanted the test and was willing to sign the consent form. The younger daughter wanted the test, too, because her mother and sister encouraged her to have the test done. Which one of the following responses from her care provider would be most appropriate?[7]
   A. Ordering a Sanger sequence study of *BRCA2* for the two daughters
   B. Ordering a Sanger sequence study of *BRCA2* for the older daughter, but not the younger one
   C. Ordering a targeted *BRCA2* study for the two daughters
   D. Ordering a targeted *BRCA2* study for the older daughter, but not the younger one
   E. Suggesting not testing the daughters until they are adults and are ready to make their own decision

30. Which one of the following ethnicities has a higher risk for Crohn disease?
   A. African Americans
   B. Asian
   C. Caucasian
   D. Latinos
   E. Not sure

31. Which one of the following is not a significant risk factor for Crohn disease?
   A. Ashkenazi Jewish descent
   B. Corticosteroids
   C. Family history of Crohn disease
   D. Homozygous for variants in *NOD2*
   E. Smoking

32. Which one of the following is the most important controllable risk factor for developing Crohn disease?

A. Low-fiber diet
B. Nonsteroidal anti-inflammatory durgs (NSAIDs)
C. Sedentary lifestyle
D. Smoking
E. Not sure

33. Which one of the following ethnicities has highest carrier frequency for cystic fibrosis (CF)?
    A. African Americans
    B. Ashkenazi Jews
    C. Asians
    D. Caucasians
    E. Latinos

34. What is the lifetime risk for colorectal cancer (CRC) among Western populations?[8]
    A. < 0.1%
    B. 1%
    C. 5%
    D. 10%
    E. 18%
    F. 36%

35. Which one of the following ethnicities has a higher risk for colorectal cancer (CRC)?
    A. African Americans
    B. Ashkenazi Jews
    C. Asians
    D. Caucasians
    E. Latinos

36. A 36-year-old male came to a clinic for more than 2000 colorectal adenomatous polyposis. The family history is negative on both sides. The *APC* gene was analyzed with a peripheral-blood sample from the patient, and the results were positive for a frameshift pathogenic variant in exon 4. The patient asked the physician to test his 6-year-old son for the pathogenic variant. Which one of the following responses would be most appropriate?
    A. Making an appointment with the son for pretest counsel
    B. Offering the colonoscopy to his son
    C. Referring the son to a pediatrician
    D. Suggest not considering this test for the son until he is at least 18 years old
    E. None of the above

37. Which one of the following is NOT a risk factor for Hirschsprung disease?[9]
    A. Female sex
    B. Having a deleterious mutation in the *RET* gene
    C. Having a sibling with Hirschsprung disease
    D. Having Down syndrome
    E. Having Waardenburg–Shah syndrome

38. Which one of the following ethnicities has the highest risk for Hirschsprung disease?[10]
    A. African Americans
    B. Ashkenazi Jews

C. Asians
D. Caucasians
E. Latinos

39. A couple came to a genetics clinic to discuss the risk for them having another child with Hirschsprung disease. Their 2-month-old daughter underwent surgery to remove the aganglionic segment of colon 1 month ago. The surgeon defined it as "long segment disease." The family history was unremarkable. Which one of the following statements regarding recurrent risk was NOT correct?[16]
    A. Recurrent risk was relatively high since the proband had long segment Hirschsprung disease.
    B. Recurrent risk was relatively high since the proband was a female.
    C. Recurrent risk was also related to the sex of the fetus.
    D. Recurrent risk was very low, since the mother did not have symptoms.
    E. None of the above.

40. Which one of the following statements regarding Hirschsprung disease is correct?
    A. A female proband's son has more risk to have the disease than a male proband's son.
    B. A female proband's son has more risk to have the disease than a male proband's daughter.
    C. A female proband's daughter has more risk to have the disease than her son.
    D. A male proband's son has more risk to have the disease than a female proband's son.
    E. A male proband's son has more risk to have the disease than a female proband's daughter.
    F. A male proband's daughter has more risk to have the disease than his son.

41. Which one of the following is NOT a risk factor for holoprosencephaly?[9]
    A. Female sex
    B. Maternal diabetes
    C. Maternal exposure to cholesterol-lowering agents
    D. Pathogenic variant(s) in the *SHH* gene
    E. Smoking

42. A couple brought their 8-year-old son to a genetics clinic for counseling. The husband was 42 years old and was recently found to carry 42 copies of the CAG repeat in the *HTT* gene for Huntington disease by a molecular test that he took because one of his relatives developed symptoms. The husband remained asymptomatic at the time of the clinic visit. The couple wanted to test their 8-year-old son for Huntington disease. Which one of the

following responses would be the most appropriate?

A. Assuring the family that the son would not develop Huntington disease
B. Ordering the test for the son
C. Referring the family to a pediatrician
D. Suggesting testing the mother first
E. Suggesting not testing the son until he is an adult and can make an informed decision

43. A couple came to a genetics clinic for their first prenatal counseling at 6 weeks of gestation. The husband was 42 years old and was recently found to carry 42 copies of the CAG repeat in the *HTT* gene for Huntington disease by a molecular test that he took because one of his relatives developed symptoms. The husband remained asymptomatic at the time of the clinic visit. The couple wanted to test their unborn son for Huntington disease. Which one of the following responses would be the most appropriate?

A. Assuring the family that the fetus would not develop Huntington disease
B. Ordering the test with a CVS sample
C. Referring the family to a neurologist
D. Suggesting the test with an amniocentesis sample
E. Suggesting testing the mother first
F. Suggesting not testing the unborn child until he or she is an adult and can make an informed decision

45. Which one of the following is NOT a risk factor for noninsulin-dependent diabetes mellitus (type 2)?[17,18]
A. Alcohol
B. DQB1*0201 and/or DQB1*0302
C. Obesity
D. Personal history of gestational diabetes
E. Stress

46. As compared with carcinomas resulting from Lynch syndrome, which one of the following applies to sporadic colorectal cancers?
A. Less likely to have chromosome instability and aneuploidy
B. Less aggressive
C. More likely to be diagnosed at a younger age
D. More likely to occur in ascending colon
E. Unfavorable prognosis

47. Which one of the following genetic disorders, included in the newborn screening program in the United States, is the most common?
A. Cystic fibrosis
B. Galactosemia
C. Phenylketonuria (PKU)
D. Sickle cell anemia

48. A couple comes to a genetics clinic for preconception counseling. Their parents are related (see the figure below for the pedigree). The family history was unremarkable. What is the risk that their firstborn child could be homozygous for a pathogenic variant responsible for a recessive disorder?

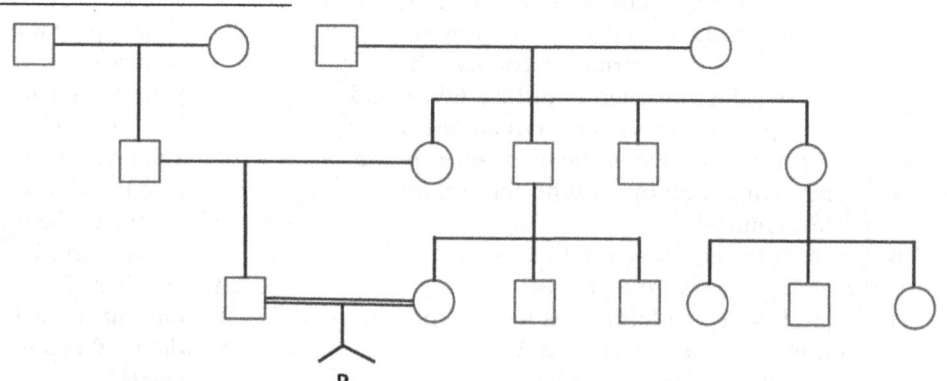

44. Which one of the following is a risk factor for insulin-dependent diabetes mellitus (type 1)?[11]
A. Alcohol
B. Caucasian
C. DQB1*602 with Asp57
D. Obesity
E. Personal history of gestational diabetes

A. 1/4
B. 1/8
C. 1/16
D. 1/32
E. 1/64
F. 1/128

49. A couple comes to a genetics clinic for preconception counseling. Their parents are related

(see the figure below for the pedigree). The
family history was unremarkable. What is the
risk that their firstborn child could be
homozygous for a mutation responsible for a
recessive disorder?

A. 1/4
B. 1/8
C. 1/16
D. 1/32
E. 1/64
F. 1/128

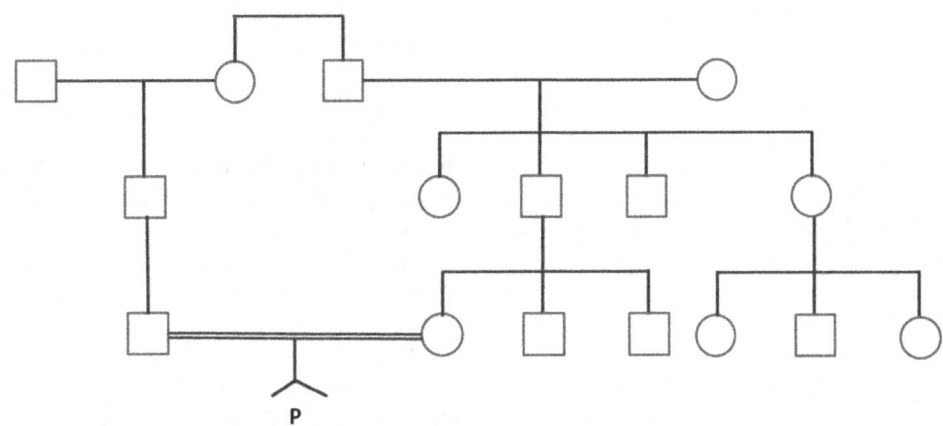

P

50. A couple comes to a genetics clinic for
preconception counseling. Their parents are related
(see the figure below for the pedigree). The family
history was unremarkable. What is the risk that
their firstborn child could be homozygous for a
mutation responsible for a recessive disorder?

A. 1/4
B. 1/8
C. 1/16
D. 1/32
E. 1/64
F. 1/128

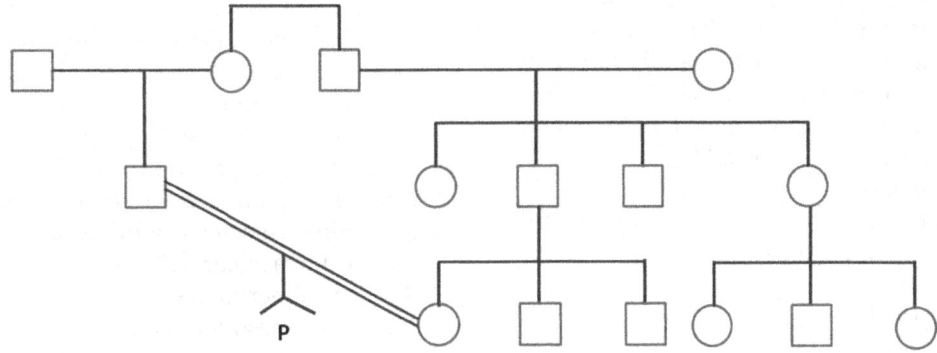

P

51. A couple comes to a genetics clinic for preconception counseling. Their parents are related (see the figure below for the pedigree). The family history was unremarkable. What is the risk that their firstborn child could be homozygous for a mutation responsible for a recessive disorder?

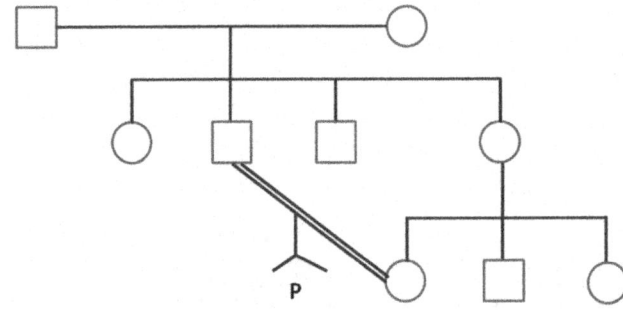

A. 1/4
B. 1/8
C. 1/16
D. 1/32
E. 1/64
F. 1/128

52. Coronary artery disease (CAD) is one of the most frequent causes of morbidity and mortality in the developed world. Which one of the following statements regarding the risk for CAD in a family is correct?
A. If a proband is a female, a male family member will have a greater risk for CAD.
B. If a proband is a female, a female family member will have a greater risk for CAD.
C. If a proband is a male, a male family member will have a greater risk for CAD.
D. If a proband is a male, a female family member will have a greater risk for CAD.
E. None of the above.

53. Which one of the following organ systems has the highest incidence of birth defects?
A. Cardiovascular
B. Gastrointestinal
C. Limbs
D. Neurological
E. Respiratory
F. All of the above

54. Which one of the following substances is not a teratogen?
A. Alcohol
B. Cocaine

C. Lithium
D. Retinoic acid
E. Warfarin
F. None of above

55. What is the risk for fetal alcohol syndrome if the pregnant woman has 1–2 drinks per day?[9]
A. <1%
B. 10%
C. 25%
D. 50%
E. > 99%
F. None of above

56. What is the risk for fetal alcohol syndrome if the pregnant woman has 6 drinks per day?[9]
A. <1%
B. 10%
C. 40%
D. 70%
E. > 99%
F. None of above

57. A pregnant alcoholic woman came to her obstetrician for consultation. She wants to find out the safe amount of alcohol consumption during pregnancy. How should the physician advise her?[9]
A. Cut down to 1 drink a day
B. Cut down to 2 drinks a day
C. Cut down to 3 drinks a day
D. Cut down to 4 drinks a day
E. Cut down to 5 drinks a day
F. Don't drink
G. None of above

58. A pregnant woman was diagnosed with gestational diabetes at 26 weeks' gestation. The genetics counselor explained to her the risk for diabetic embryopathy if the blood glucose was not controlled. Which one of the following is not one of the congenital anomalies associated with gestational diabetes?[12]
A. Cardiovascular defects
B. Central nervous system defects
C. Gastrointestinal defects
D. Miscarriage
E. Skeletal defects
F. All of the above

59. A newborn boy was diagnosed with a fully penetrant, autosomal recessive disorder that has an incidence of 1 in 1600 in their population. Which one of the following is the most appropriate estimation of the risk that the infant's maternal aunt will have an affected child (see the figure below for the pedigree)?

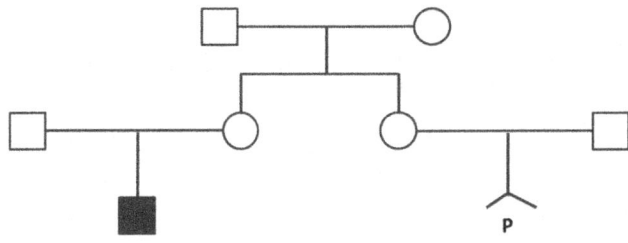

A. 1/80
B. 1/120
C. 1/160
D. 1/240
E. 1/320
F. None of the above

60. An adolescent male was diagnosed with a fully penetrant, autosomal recessive disorder that has an incidence of 1 in 1600 in his population. Which one of the following is the most appropriate estimation of the risk that his sister will have an affected child (see the figure below for the pedigree)?

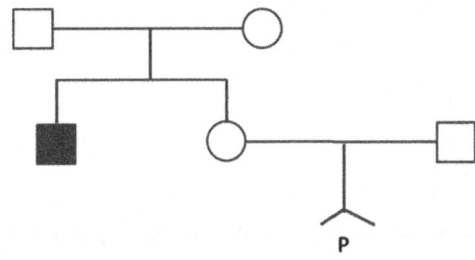

A. 1/60
B. 1/95
C. 1/120
D. 1/180
E. 1/240
F. None of above

61. An adolescent male was diagnosed with an 80% penetrant, autosomal recessive disorder that has an incidence of 1 in 1600 in his population. Which one of the following is the most appropriate estimation of the risk that his sister will have an affected child (see the figure below for the pedigree)?

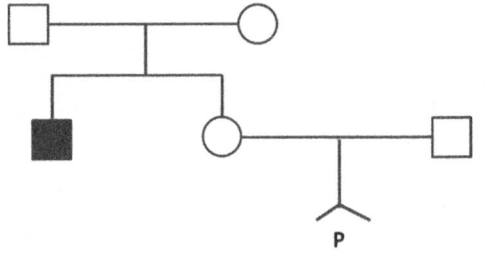

A. 1/120
B. 1/150
C. 4/375
D. 1/400
E. 1/500
F. None of above

62. Cystic fibrosis occurs in the Ashkenazi Jewish population with an incidence of approximately 1 in 2500. Which one of the following is the most appropriate estimation of the risk that two Ashkenazi Jews without a family history of cystic fibrosis will have an affected child?
A. 1/500
B. 1/650
C. 1/1250
D. 1/2500
E. 1/10,000
F. None of above

63. An Ashkenazi Jewish couple comes to a clinic for preconception counseling. The wife's maternal uncle died of cystic fibrosis (CF). Cystic fibrosis occurs in the Ashkenazi Jewish population with an incidence of approximately 1 in 2500. Which one of the following is the most appropriate estimation of the risk that the couple's first child will be affected?
A. 1/100
B. 1/250
C. 1/300
D. 1/450
E. 1/600
F. None of above

64. A couple comes to a clinic for preconception counseling. The wife's maternal uncle died of Duchenne muscular dystrophy (DMD). But the couple are asymptomatic with two unaffected sons and two unaffected daughters. The overall incidence of DMD in the United States is approximately 1 in 4900 live male births. Which one of the following is the most appropriate estimation if the couple's next child will be affected (a de novo DMD pathogenic variant is not considered)?
A. <1%
B. 1/5
C. 1/20
D. 1/40
E. 1/52
F. None of above

65. A couple comes to a clinic for prenatal counseling when the wife is 14 weeks pregnant because an ultrasonography examination found "banana sign" and "lemon sign." Which one of the following is the most appropriate next step in the workup?

A. Chorionic villus sampling
B. Amniocentesis
C. Cordocentesis
D. Noninvasive prenatal test (NIPT)
E. None of above

66. Which one of the following hereditary cancer syndromes has higher lifetime risks for malignancies?
   A. *BRCA1* and *BRCA2* associated hereditary breast cancer
   B. Familial adenomatous polyposis
   C. Lynch syndrome
   D. Neurofibromatosis type 1
   E. Peutz–Jeghers syndrome
   F. None of the above

67. Which one of the following hereditary cancer syndromes demonstrates sex-associated lifetime risks for malignancies?
   A. Li–Fraumeni syndrome
   B. Familial adenomatous polyposis
   C. Neurofibromatosis type 1
   D. Peutz–Jeghers syndrome
   E. None of the above

68. What is the coefficient of inbreeding (F) for a mating of first cousins?
   A. 1/2
   B. 1/4
   C. 1/8
   D. 1/16
   E. 1/32
   F. 1/64
   G. 1/128

69. What is the coefficient of relationship (R) of first cousins?
   A. 1/2
   B. 1/4
   C. 1/8
   D. 1/16
   E. 1/32
   F. 1/64
   G. 1/128

70. What is the coefficient of inbreeding (F) for a mating of second cousins?
   A. 1/2
   B. 1/4
   C. 1/8
   D. 1/16
   E. 1/32
   F. 1/64
   G. 1/128

71. What is the coefficient of relationship (R) of second cousins?
   A. 1/2
   B. 1/4
   C. 1/8

D. 1/16
E. 1/32
F. 1/64
G. 1/128

72. What is the coefficient of inbreeding (F) for a mating of full siblings?
   A. 1/2
   B. 1/4
   C. 1/8
   D. 1/16
   E. 1/32
   F. 1/64
   G. 1/128

73. What is the coefficient of relationship (R) of full siblings?
   A. 1/2
   B. 1/4
   C. 1/8
   D. 1/16
   E. 1/32
   F. 1/64
   G. 1/128

74. What is the coefficient of inbreeding (F) for a mating of half siblings?
   A. 1/2
   B. 1/4
   C. 1/8
   D. 1/16
   E. 1/32
   F. 1/64
   G. 1/128

75. What is the coefficient of relationship (F) of half siblings?
   A. 1/2
   B. 1/4
   C. 1/8
   D. 1/16
   E. 1/32
   F. 1/64
   G. 1/128

76. What is the coefficient of inbreeding (F) for a mating of first cousins once removed?
   A. 1/2
   B. 1/4
   C. 1/8
   D. 1/16
   E. 1/32
   F. 1/64
   G. 1/128

77. What is the coefficient of relationship (R) of first cousins once removed?
   A. 1/2
   B. 1/4
   C. 1/8
   D. 1/16

E. 1/32

F. 1/64

G. 1/128

78. What is the coefficient of inbreeding (*F*) for a mating of second cousins once removed?

A. 1/2

B. 1/4

C. 1/8

D. 1/16

E. 1/32

F. 1/64

G. 1/128

79. What is the coefficient of relationship (*R*) of second cousins once removed?

A. 1/2

B. 1/4

C. 1/8

D. 1/16

E. 1/32

F. 1/64

G. 1/128

80. What is the amniocentesis-related miscarriage rate in the second trimester?

A. 1 in 50

B. 1 in 100

C. 1 in 400

D. 1 in 1000

E. 1 in 16,000

81. What is the chorionic villus sampling (CVS)–related miscarriage rate in the first trimester?

A. 1 in 50

B. 1 in 100

C. 1 in 400

D. 1 in 1000

E. 1 in 16,000

82. An autosomal dominant disease with complete penetrance appears in 1 in 100,000 of the population. The reproductive fitness of the disease is 0.8. What is the de novo mutation rate of the disease?

A. 1 in 10,000

B. 1 in 50,000

C. 1 in 100,000

D. 1 in 500,000

E. 1 in 1,000,000

83. How many generations does it take to reduce the frequency of a rare deleterious allele from 1 in 100 to 1 in 200, assuming it is an autosomal recessive condition (fitness = 0)?

A. 50

B. 100

C. 200

D. 400

E. 800

84. How many generations does it take to reduce the frequency of a rare deleterious allele from 1 in 300 to half, assuming that this is an autosomal recessive condition?

A. 50

B. 100

C. 150

D. 300

E. 450

F. 600

85. Which one of the following disorders has relatively higher de novo mutation rate during meiosis?

A. Achondroplasia

B. Duchenne muscular dystrophy

C. Hemophilia A

D. Hemophilia B

E. Neurofibromatosis type 1

F. Polycystic kidney disease type 1

86. Which one of the following issues affects clinical interpretations of genetic studies LEAST?

A. The clinical setting in which the test is used—for example, screening or clinical diagnostics

B. Genotype/phenotype associations when these vary with particular pathogenic variants or polymorphisms, such as R117H in *CFTR* gene

C. Genetic, environmental, or other factors that modify the clinical expression of the genetic alteration

D. Research studies with animal models, such as functional study of mutations in *APOE* gene in diabetes with a mouse model

87. Which one of the following disorders occurs almost exclusively in the Ashkenazi Jewish population?

A. Canavan disease

B. Cystic fibrosis

C. Familial dysautonomia

D. Gaucher disease

E. Tay–Sachs disease

88. Which one of the following disorders has higher prevalence in the Ashkenazi Jewish population?

A. Canavan disease

B. Cystic fibrosis

C. Familial dysautonomia

D. Gaucher disease

E. Tay–Sachs disease

89. Which one of the following disorders is NOT supported/recommended to be offered in the general Ashkenazi Jewish population screening programs by the American College of Medical Genetics (ACMG) and/or the American College of Obstetricians and Gynecologists (ACOG) Committee on Genetics?[13–15,19]

A. Breast cancer

B. Canavan disease

C. Cystic fibrosis

D. Familial dysautonomia

E. Tay–Sachs disease

90. An Ashkenazi Jewish couple came to a clinic for preconception counseling. An Ashkenazi Jewish carrier screening panel was offered to the couple. These results uncovered a heterozygous pathogenic variant in *SMPD1* for Niemann–Pick disease type A (NPD-A) in the wife, but not the husband. The carrier frequency of NPD-A in the Ashkenazi Jewish population is approximately 1 in 90. The panel includes the most common three mutations in *SMPD1*, which account for approximately 97% of the Ashkenazi Jewish pathogenic variants. Which one of the following would be the residual risk for the couple to have a child with NPD-A?
    - A. 1/360
    - B. 1/2000
    - C. 1/4000
    - D. 1/12,000
    - E. 1/24,000

91. What is the risk for malignancies in individuals with classic ataxia telangiectasia (A-T)?
    - A. > 99%
    - B. 80%
    - C. 40%
    - D. 10%
    - E. < 1%

92. Which one of the following is the most common malignancy in individuals with classic ataxia telangiectasia?
    - A. Leukemia and lymphoma
    - B. Breast cancer
    - C. Gastric cancer
    - D. Melanoma
    - E. Leiomyoma
    - F. Sarcomas

93. A 68-year-old female came to a clinic for a family history of dementia. She was in relatively good health and had no symptoms of dementia. However, her father, two brothers, and two other paternal relatives had Alzheimer disease in their 70s. She wanted to find out whether she would be demented. If so, she would find a lawyer to make a will soon. Which one of the following factors would be the strongest risk factor for this patient developing Alzheimer disease?
    - A. Age
    - B. Ethnic background
    - C. Family history
    - D. Sex
    - E. highest education level
    - F. None of the above

94. A Caucasian couple comes to a clinic for preconception counseling. They are in their late 20s. Two of the wife's maternal uncles died of mucopolysaccharidoses type II (MPSII),

also known as "Hunter syndrome." The wife has two older brothers and two younger sisters, who are apparently healthy. What is the risk that the couple's firstborn child will have MPSII?
    - A. 1/20
    - B. 1/37
    - C. 1/40
    - D. 1/74
    - E. 1/148
    - F. None of the above

95. A Caucasian couple comes to a clinic for preconception counseling. They are in their late 20s. Two of the wife's maternal uncles died of mucopolysaccharidoses type II (MPSII), also known as "Hunter syndrome." The wife has two older brothers and two younger sisters who are apparently healthy. What is the risk that the couple's firstborn son will have MPSII?
    - A. 1/20
    - B. 1/37
    - C. 1/40
    - D. 1/74
    - E. 1/148
    - F. None of the above

ANSWERS

1. **A.** Most Jews in United States trace their ancestry to Germany or Eastern Europe (Ashkenazi), the Mediterranean (Sephardic), or Iran/Persia and the Middle East (Mizrahi). It is estimated that approximately 90% of Jews in the United States are Ashkenazi, most with ancestors who emigrated in the late 19th and early 20th centuries. Sephardic, from the Hebrew term for Spain, refers to Jews who trace their heritage back to the expulsion of the Jews from Spain in 1492, at which point they emigrated to other points around the Mediterranean, including North Africa. Mizrahi, from the Hebrew term for "East," generally refers to Jews of Persian (Iranian) and Middle Eastern heritage (http://www.canavanfoundation.org/jewish_heritage_and_identity_in_the_us).

    Ashkenazi Jews share a common genetic heritage and risk from well-defined group of genetic disorders due to the founder effect, also called "genetic drift." *According to current estimates, as many as one in three Ashkenazi Jews are carriers for certain genetic disorders*, including Tay–Sachs, Canavan, Niemann–Pick, Gaucher, familial dysautonomia, Bloom syndrome, Fanconi anemia, cystic fibrosis and mucolipidosis IV, cystic fibrosis, and spinal muscular atrophy (https://www.gaucherdisease.org/blog/5-common-ashkenazi-genetic-diseases/). At this point there are 17 genetic diseases common to Ashkenazi Jews for which preconception carrier screening is recommended.

Therefore, 1/3 is the estimated carrier frequency of genetic disorders in the Ashkenazi Jewish population.

2. **D**. The estimated carrier frequency of Ashkenazi Jewish is (see the table below):

Gaucher disease type 1	1 in 18
Tay–Sachs disease	1 in 31
Cystic fibrosis (CF)	1 in 26
Familial dysautonomia (FD)	1 in 31
Canavan disease	1 in 41
Spinal muscular atrophy (SMA)	1 in 41
Glycogen storage disease, type 1A	1 in 71
Maple syrup urine disease (MSUD)	1 in 81
Fanconi anemia type C	1 in 89
Niemann–Pick disease type A	1 in 90
Bloom syndrome	1 in 107
Mucolipidosis IV	1 in 127

Therefore, Gaucher disease is the most common among these choices for Ashkenazi Jews.

3. **A**. Isolated orofacial clefts, or clefts that occur with no other major birth defects, are one of the most common types of birth defects in the United States. Depending on the cleft type, the rate of isolated orofacial clefts can vary from 50%–80% of all clefts. The causes of orofacial clefts among most infants are unknown. The Centers for Disease Control and Prevention (CDC) has reported about some factors that increase risk for an orofacial cleft in newborns: smoking, diabetes, and use of certain medicines.

Parents with a family history of cleft lip or cleft palate face a higher risk of having a baby with a cleft. *In the United States, cleft lip and palate are reportedly most common in Native Americans and least common in African Americans.* Males are twice as likely to have a cleft lip with or without cleft palate. Cleft palate without cleft lip is more common in females. Cleft lip and cleft palate may be more likely to occur in the babies born of pregnant women who smoke cigarettes, drink alcohol, or take certain medications. There is some evidence that women diagnosed with diabetes before pregnancy may have an increased risk of having a baby with a cleft lip with or without a

cleft palate. There is some evidence that babies born to obese women may have an increased risk of cleft lip and palate (www.mayoclinic.org).

Therefore, being African American is NOT a risk factor for cleft lip/palate.

4. **C**. Orofacial clefts (CFC) are very common worldwide, with an incidence of 1.7 per 1000 babies being diagnosed with OFC. *Asians have an incidence of 17 in 1000, American Indians 3.6 in 1000, and African Americans 0.4 in 1000.* The rate is higher in boys than in girls. Cleft palate is more frequent in males, but females more often have only cleft palate (about 0.5 in 1000).

Therefore, Asians have a higher risk for cleft lip/cleft palate than other race/ethnicities.

5. **B**. *Males are twice as likely to have a cleft lip with or without cleft palate.* If a female family member has cleft lip, her male siblings have a higher risk to have cleft lip than the proband being a male.

A male fetus with a sister having CL has higher risk to have CL than a male fetus with a brother having CL. Therefore, it is NOT correct to state "a male fetus with a brother having CL has higher risk to have CL than a male fetus with a sister having CL."

6. **A**. *Alzheimer dementia is more common in females than males;* whereas cleft lip, pyloric stenosis, and club foot are more common in males than females.

Therefore, Alzheimer is more common in females than males.

7. **E**. Alzheimer dementia is more common in females than males; whereas *cleft lip, pyloric stenosis, club foot, and Hirschsprung disease are more common in males than females.*

About 1 in 1000 babies are born with cleft lip and cleft palate. Cleft lip/palate are thought to be caused by a combination of genes and other factors. Many genes and the maternal use of certain medications and substances—such as tobacco, anticonvulsants, alcohol, or retinoic acid—are believed to increase the risk of having a child with a cleft. Cleft lip and palate, about 50% of all clefts, occur more often in males. Isolated cleft lip, about 20% of all clefts, occurs more often in males. Isolated cleft palate, about 30% of all clefts, occurs more often in females (www.entnet.org/).

Infantile hypertrophic pyloric stenosis (IHPS) occurs in approximately 2–3.5 per 1000 live births, although rates and trends vary markedly from region to region. It is more common in males than females (4:1–6:1) and in infants born preterm as compared with those born at term. Approximately 30%–40% of cases occur in firstborn children (approximately 1.5-fold increased risk), and cases are less common in infants of older mothers.

Symptoms usually begin between 3 and 5 weeks of age and very rarely occur after 12 weeks (www.uptodate.com/).

The frequency of congenital clubfoot is approximately 1 in 1240 live births. It is twice as common in male children as it is in female children. About 50% of the time, both feet are affected. (www.clevelandclinic.org/).

The incidence of Hirschsprung disease is approximately 1 in 5000 live births. The incidence varies among different ethnic groups; in northern Europeans, it is 1.5 in 10,000 live births, in African Americans 2.1 in 10,000, and in Asian 2.8 in 10,000 (https://www.ncbi.nlm.nih.gov/books/NBK1439/). Hirschsprung disease has a skewed sex distribution, with a female-to-male ratio of 1:4.

Therefore, cleft lip, pyloric stenosis, club foot, and Hirschsprung disease are more common in males than females.

8. **B.** *About 3%–5% of all babies born in the United States have congenital abnormalities* (www.healthychildren.org; https://www.cdc.gov/ncbddd/birthdefects/data.html). The *International Statistical Classification of Diseases and Related Health Problems*, tenth revision (ICD-10), includes birth defects in Chapter XVII. The terms birth defects and congenital disorders are used interchangeably. Congenital disorders are a diverse group of disorders of prenatal origin that can be caused by single-gene defects, chromosomal disorders, multifactorial inheritance, environmental teratogens, and micronutrient deficiencies. Maternal infectious diseases such as syphilis and rubella are a significant cause of birth defects in low- and middle-income countries. Maternal illnesses such as diabetes mellitus, conditions such as iodine and folic acid deficiency, and exposure to medicines and recreational drugs, including alcohol and tobacco, certain environmental chemicals, and high doses of radiation are other factors that cause birth defects (http://www.who.int/mediacentre/factsheets/fs370/en/).

The World Health Organization (WHO) estimates that some 260,000 deaths worldwide (about 7% of all neonatal deaths) were caused by congenital anomalies in 2004. They are most prominent as a cause of death in settings where overall mortality rates are lower—for example, in the European Region, where as many as 25% of neonatal deaths are due to congenital anomalies.

There are currently no sound estimates of the number of children born with a serious congenital disorder attributable to genetic or environmental causes. The most common serious congenital disorders are congenital heart defects, neural-tube defects and Down syndrome. Hemoglobinophathies, including thalassemia and sickle-cell disease, and glucose-6-phosphate dehydrogenase deficiency (G6PD), which are not covered by the ICD-10 definition of congenital anomalies, account for 6% of all congenital disorders.

Therefore, approximately 4% of newborns have congenital anomalies.

9. **A.** In population genetics, genetic drift, natural selection, mutation, and migration are the four basic mechanisms of evolution. Genetic drift is the change in the frequency of an allele in a population due to random sampling among generations. The alleles in the offspring are a sample of those in the parents, who have different survival and reproduction rates. Through sampling error, genetic drift can cause populations to lose genetic variation. *Founder effect refers to an allele observed with high frequency in a specific population due to the presence of that allele in a single ancestor or small number of ancestors.* Isolated populations often have exceptionally high frequencies of otherwise rare alleles, and the most likely explanation is that the founding population had a disproportionate number of those rare alleles. Genetic drift and founder effect are related because founder effect is one kind of sampling error, which changes the genetic pool of the population. The frequency of Huntington disease in South Africa is a good example of this. Ashkenazi Jewish genetic disorders are another example.

Mutation is the ultimate source of genetic variation in the form of new alleles. Mutation can result in several different types of change in DNA sequences. These can either have no effect, alter the product of a gene, or prevent the gene from functioning. Natural selection is a gradual process by which forms of life having traits that better enable them to adapt to specific environmental pressures, as predators, changes in climate, or competition for food or mates, will tend to survive and reproduce in greater numbers than others of their kind, thus ensuring the perpetuation of those favorable traits in succeeding generations.

Therefore, bottleneck and founder effect describe the reason why Gaucher disease is more prevalent in the Ashkenazi Jewish population than in other populations.

10. **E.** Genetic counseling is a process to evaluate and understand a family's risk of an inherited medical disorder. Genetic counselors work with patients, their families, and their health providers to help them understand the genetic risk for certain diseases or cancers based on family history, whether genetic testing might be right for the patients, and what the result of genetic tests may mean for the patients and

their families. With expertise in counseling, genetic counselors can also provide emotional support as patients make decisions and empower patients with information for their overall healthcare (www.nsgc. org). However, *therapy options should be made by the patients and the family based on the information provided by the physician.*

Therefore, a genetic counselor may NOT offer suggestions for therapy.

11. **C.** Hearing loss is the most common birth defect and the most prevalent sensorineural disorder in developed countries. One out of every 500 newborns has bilateral permanent sensorineural hearing loss ≥ 40 dB. *More than 50% of prelingual deafness is genetic.* (http://www.ncbi.nlm.nih.gov/ books/NBK1434/).

Therefore, at least 50% of prelingual hearing loss has a genetic etiology in Western nations.

cases. Approximately 50% of severe-to-profound autosomal recessive nonsyndromic hearing loss can be attributed to the nonsyndromic hearing loss and deafness (DFNB1), caused by pathogenic variants in *GJB2* (which encodes the protein connexin 26) and *GJB6* (which encodes the protein connexin 30). The carrier rate in the general population for a recessive deafness-causing *GJB2* pathogenic variant is approximately 1 in 33. The most common cause of mild-to-moderate autosomal recessive hearing loss is pathogenic variants of *STRC.* Syndromic hearing impairment accounts for up to 30% of prelingual deafness; more than 400 genetic syndromes that include hearing loss have been described (http:// www.ncbi.nlm.nih.gov/books/NBK1434/).

Therefore, most genetic prelingual hearing loss is autosomal recessive (see Fig. 14.1).

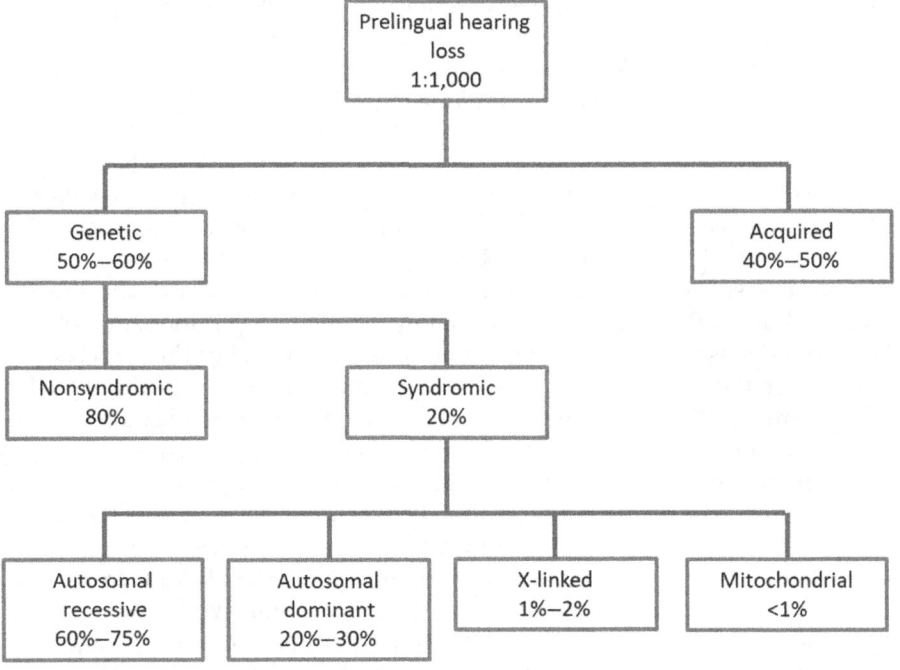

FIGURE 14.1 Causes of prelingual hearing loss in developed worldwide. *Source: From Angeli S, Lin X, Liu XZ. Genetics of hearing and deafness. Anat Rec (Hoboken). 2012 Nov;295(11):1812—29. doi: 10.1002/ar.22579. Epub 2012 Oct 8. Review. Erratum in: Anat Rec (Hoboken). 2015 Nov;298(11):1815.*

12. **B.** Prelingual hearing loss is present before speech develops. *Approximately 80% of prelingual deafness is genetic,* whereas 20% is acquired and environmental. Acquired hearing loss in children commonly results from prenatal infections from TORCH (*t*oxoplasmosis, *r*ubella, *c*ytomegalovirus, and *h*erpes) organisms or postnatal infections, particularly bacterial meningitis caused by *Neisseria meningitidis, Haemophilus influenzae,* or *Streptococcus pneumoniae.*

Most prelingual hearing loss is often autosomal recessive and nonsyndromic. Genetic hearing loss is autosomal recessive in approximately 80% of

13. **A.** Hemolytic disease of the fetus and newborn (HDFN) is caused by alloimmunization of the mother by exposure to fetal red blood cells, which display a paternally inherited form of an antigen that is different from those in the mother.

HDFN is most commonly caused by anti-D alloantibody, followed by anti-K, anti-c, and anti-E. It can also occur in women of blood type O. It is usually seen in Rhesus D (RhD)—negative mothers who have been previously sensitized. The frequency of Rh-negative individuals is more common in the Caucasian population than in other ethnic groups.

Therefore, RhD incompatibility accounts for the majority of cases of hemolytic disease of the fetus and newborn (HDFN).

14. **D.** Age is a major risk factor for age-related macular degeneration (AMD). The disease is most likely to occur after age 60, but it can occur earlier. Other risk factors for AMD include smoking, race, family history, and genetics. *The only nongenetic risk factor identified to date is smoking.* Research shows that smoking doubles the risk of AMD. AMD is more common among Caucasians than among African Americans or Hispanics/Latinos. People with a family history of AMD are at higher risk. At last count, researchers had identified nearly 20 genes that can affect the risk of developing AMD. Many more genetic risk factors are suspected. The American Academy of Ophthalmology currently recommends against routine genetic testing for AMD, and insurance generally does not cover such testing (https://nei.nih.gov/health/maculardegen/armd_facts).

    Therefore, smoking is the single most important environmental risk factor for AMD.

15. **C.** Down syndrome may lead to abnormalities in the immune system and a higher susceptibility to certain illnesses, such as Alzheimer disease, leukemia, seizures, cataracts, breathing problems, heart conditions, premature aging, and Hirschsprung disease but not Parkinson disease.

    Therefore, patients with Down syndrome do NOT have an increased risk to develop Parkinson disease.

16. **E.** Most people with Alzheimer disease have the late-onset form of the disease, in which symptoms become apparent in the mid-60s and later. The causes of late-onset Alzheimer disease are not yet completely understood, but they likely include a combination of genetic, environmental, and lifestyle factors that affect a person's risk for developing the disease.

    The greatest known risk factor for Alzheimer disease is increased age. Most individuals with the disease are 65 or older. One in nine people in this age group and nearly one-third of people age 85 or older have Alzheimer disease. The second strongest factor is apolipoprotein E (*APOE*) genotype. *APOE* ε2 is relatively rare and may provide some protection against the disease. *APOE* ε3, the most common allele, is believed to play a neutral role in the disease—neither decreasing nor increasing risk. APOE ε4 increases risk for Alzheimer disease and is also associated with an earlier age at disease onset. Homozygosity for *APOE* ε4 increases the risk of developing Alzheimer disease.

    Another strong risk factor is family history. Those who have a parent, brother, or sister with Alzheimer disease are more likely to develop the disease. The risk increases if more than one family member has the illness. When diseases tend to run in families, either heredity (genetics) or environmental factors, or both, may play a role. Other factors may include female sex, Down syndrome, type 2 diabetes mellitus, sleep disorders, depression, education, smoking, alcohol, traumatic brain injury (TBI), and several single-nucleotide polymorphisms (SNPs) and a growing list of candidate genes (https://www.alz.org/).

    Therefore, the use of oral contraceptives is NOT recognized as a risk factor for late-onset Alzheimer disease.

17. **B.** Patients with Down syndrome have an increased risk for Alzheimer disease (AD). *After the age of 40 years, nearly all patients with Down syndrome have neuropathological findings of AD, and approximately 50% experience cognitive decline.*

    Therefore, after the age of 40, nearly all patients with Down syndrome have neuropathological findings of Alzheimer disease.

18. **B.** *Assisted reproductive technologies (ART), such as in vitro fertilization (IVF) and intracytoplasmic sperm injection, are associated with increased risk for Beckwith−Wiedemann syndrome (BWS).* The risk of BWS after IVF is estimated to be 1 in 4000, which is 10-fold higher than in the general population. Advanced paternal age is a risk factor for achondroplasia. Duchenne muscular dystrophy may be caused by deletion, duplication, in/del, and single-nucleotide variants, but the association between Duchenne muscular dystrophy and ART is not known. Hirschsprung disease is more common in males than females. Miller−Dieker syndrome is caused by nonhomologous recombination between low copy repeats (LCRs).

    Therefore, children born with assisted reproductive technologies (ART) have increased risk for Beckwith−Wiedemann syndrome.

19. **C.** The cumulative risk of breast cancer by age 70 years for carriers of *BRCA1* and *BRCA2* pathogenic variants is 57% (95% CI, 47%−66%) and 49% (95% CI, 40%−57%), respectively (http://www.uptodate.com/contents/brca1-and-brca2-prevalence-and-risks-for-breast-and-ovarian-cancer#H909666).

    Therefore, the approximate estimation of cumulative risk of breast cancer by age 70 years is 57% if an individual carries a *BRCA1* pathogenic variant.

20. **C.** The cumulative risk of breast cancer by age 70 years for *BRCA1* and *BRCA2* mutation carriers is 57% (95% CI, 47%−66%) and 49% (95% CI, 40%−57%), respectively (http://www.uptodate.com/contents/brca1-and-brca2-prevalence-and-risks-for-breast-and-ovarian-cancer#H909666).

Therefore, the estimate of cumulative risk of breast cancer by age 70 years is 49% if an individual carries a *BRCA2* pathogenic variant.

21. **C.** The cumulative risk of ovarian breast cancer by age 70 years for *BRCA1* and *BRCA2* mutation carriers is 40% (95% CI, 35%−46%) and 18% (95% CI, 13%−23%), respectively (http://www.uptodate.com/contents/brca1-and-brca2-prevalence-and-risks-for-breast-and-ovarian-cancer#H909666).

Therefore, the estimate of cumulative risk of ovarian cancer by age 70 years is 40% if an individual carries a *BRCA1* pathogenic variant.

22. **B.** The cumulative risk of ovarian breast cancer by age 70 years for *BRCA1* and *BRCA2* mutation carriers was 40% (95% CI, 35%−46%) and 18% (95% CI, 13%−23%), respectively (http://www.uptodate.com/contents/brca1-and-brca2-prevalence-and-risks-for-breast-and-ovarian-cancer#H909666).

Therefore, the approximate estimation of cumulative risk of ovarian cancer by age 70 years is 18% if an individual carries a *BRCA2* pathogenic variant.

23. **E.** Make the 2×2 table below before calculating odds ratio for breast cancer.

		Outcome status	
		+	−
Exposure status	+	a	b
	−	c	d

$$\text{Odds ratio (OR)} = \frac{a/b}{c/d} = \frac{60/40}{10/90} = 5400/400 = 13.5$$

Therefore, the odds ratio for breast cancer with *BRCA1* pathogenic variants is 13.5 as compared with the general population.

24. **C.** Make the 2×2 table below before calculating the relative risk for breast cancer.

		Outcome status	
		+	−
Exposure status	+	a	b
	−	c	d

$$\text{Relative risk (RR)} = \frac{a/(a+b)}{c/(c+d)} = \frac{60/100}{10/100} = 6$$

Therefore, the relative risk for breast cancer with *BRCA1* pathogenic variants is 6 as compared with the general population.

25. **D.** Make the 2×2 table below before calculating the odds ratio for ovarian cancer.

		Outcome status	
		+	−
Exposure status	+	a	b
	−	c	d

$$\text{Odds ratio (OR)} = \frac{a/b}{c/d} = \frac{40/60}{1/99} = (40 \times 99)/60 = 66$$

Therefore, the odds ratio for ovarian cancer with *BRCA1* pathogenic variants is 66 as compared with the general population.

26. **C.** Make the 2×2 table below before calculating relative risk for ovarian cancer.

		Outcome status	
		+	−
Exposure status	+	a	b
	−	c	d

$$\text{Relative risk (RR)} = \frac{a/(a+b)}{c/(c+d)} = \frac{40/100}{1/100} = 40$$

Therefore, the relative risk for breast cancer with *BRCA1* pathogenic variants is 40 as compared with the general population.

27. **A.** The range of prevalence rates of *BRCA1* pathogenic variants in minority racial/ethnic populations in the United States is relatively comparable to the white population. Based upon a registry of female breast cancer patients less than 60 years of age who self-reported race/ethnicity, the estimated prevalence rate of a *BRCA1* pathogenic variant is:

- *Hispanics: 3.5% (95% CI 2.1%−5.8%), n = 393*
- *African-Americans 1.3% (0.6%−2.6%), n = 341*
- Asian Americans: 0.5% (0.1%−2.0%), n = 444
- White (non-Hispanic): 2.2% (0.7%−6.9%), n = 508

(http://www.uptodate.com/contents/brca1-and-brca2-prevalence-and-risks-for-breast-and-ovarian-cancer#H909666).

From the data above, we see that *BRCA1* pathogenic variants are more common in Hispanic Americans than in African Americans. Therefore, it is wrong to state "*BRCA1* pathogenic variants are more common in African Americans than Hispanic Americans."

28. **F.** *In general, genetic testing for BRCA1- and BRCA2-associated hereditary breast and ovarian cancer (HBOC) is not recommended for at-risk individuals younger than age*

18. Guidelines established jointly by the American College of Medical Genetics and Genomics (ACMGG), and the American Society of Human Genetics (ASHG) state that predictive genetic testing should only be performed in individuals younger than age 18 years when it will affect their medical management. Management for HBOC-related cancer is typically recommended to begin at approximately age 25, which is why it is recommended that the decision to test be postponed until an individual reaches adulthood and can make an independent decision. It is important to note, however, that since there are rare reported cases of individuals with HBOC diagnosed with cancer at very young ages, it is recommended that screening be individualized based on the earliest diagnosis in the family (https://www.ncbi.nlm.nih.gov/books/NBK1247/).

Deferring testing until late adolescence or adulthood makes it easier for the physician to communicate the test results and their implications for the future to the individual being tested. A young child may not understand the implications of the test results, and it is often unclear who has the responsibility of disclosing the results to this child years later when she is old enough to understand them.

Predictive testing of children involves both potential harms and potential benefits and restricts the child's present and future autonomy in favor of the parents' present autonomy. *Professional organizations, such as the ACMG, the ASHG, the American Academy of Pediatrics (AAP), the American Society of Clinical Oncology (ASCO), the American Medical Association (AMA), and the National Society of Genetic Counselors (NSGC) do not recommend testing minors for adult-onset genetic conditions, even in high-risk families, unless there are proven medical benefits to the testing* (http://journalofethics.ama-assn.org/2007/01/ccas1-0701.html; https://www.nsgc.org).

Therefore, it is more appropriate to suggest not testing the daughters until they are adults and are ready to make an informed decision.

29. **D.** In general, genetic testing for *BRCA1*- and *BRCA2*-associated hereditary breast and ovarian cancer (HBOC) is not recommended for at-risk individuals younger than age 18. Guidelines established jointly by the American College of Medical Genetics and Genomics (ACMG), and the American Society of Human Genetics (ASHG) state that predictive genetic testing should only be performed in individuals younger than age 18 years when it will affect their medical treatment. Treatment for HBOC-related cancer is typically recommended to begin at approximately age 25,

which is why it is recommended that the decision to test be postponed until an individual reaches adulthood and can make an independent decision. It is important to note, however, that since there are rare reported cases of individuals with HBOC diagnosed with cancer at very young ages, it is recommended that screening be individualized based on the earliest diagnosis in the family (https://www.ncbi.nlm.nih.gov/books/NBK1247/).

Predictive testing can be allowed before adulthood when mature adolescents seek it out. In such cases, the ASHG and the ACMGG recommend assessing the child's competence, obtaining her assent or consent, and ensuring that her decision is voluntary. If the adolescent demonstrates "mature decision-making capacities," the physician should respect her autonomy to decide to undergo testing.

Predictive testing of children involves both potential harms and potential benefits and restricts the child's present and future autonomy in favor of the parents' present autonomy. Professional organizations, such as the ACMG, the ASHG, the American Academy of Pediatrics (AAP), the American Society of Clinical Oncology (ASCO), the American Medical Association (AMA), and the National Society of Genetic Counselors (NSGC) do not recommend testing minors for adult-onset genetic conditions, even in high-risk families, unless there are proven medical benefits to childhood testing. Although physicians should respect the decision of competent adolescents and their families, they have no obligation to provide a service that is not in the best interest of the child. Nevertheless, the concerns of the parents deserve serious consideration and emotional support (http://journalofethics.ama-assn.org/2007/01/ccas1-0701.html; https://www.nsgc.org).

In this scenario, the 16-year-old older daughter of the patient wanted the test and was willing to sign the consent form; she might be considered to be a competent adolescent. The younger daughter wanted the test, too, because her mother and sister encouraged her to have the test done; so it was not her own decision. Therefore, it is more appropriate to order a targeted *BRCA2* study for the patient's older daughter, but not the younger one.

30. **C.** The annual incidence of Crohn disease ranges from 1 to 10 cases per 100,000 people annually depending on the region studied, and the incidence appears to be rising. The peak age-specific incidence occurs between 10 and 20 years of age, and a second smaller peak occurs near age 50 years. The prevalence of Crohn disease ranges from 10 in 100,000 to 70 in 100,000 people, but

some North American studies have shown prevalences as high as 200 in 100,000 people. There also appears to be a north–south gradient worldwide, where populations in higher latitudes (i.e., Scandinavia, Canada, and Australia) have higher incidence rates than populations in lower latitudes (i.e., Southern United States, Spain, and Italy). *In the United States, males and females are equally affected, but both whites and Ashkenazi Jews are at much higher risk of developing Crohn disease than the rest of the population.* Of note, migrants moving from a low-risk region to a high-risk region have a risk of developing Crohn disease that is similar to that in the high-risk region within one generation (http://www.clevelandclinicmeded.com).

Therefore, Caucasian has higher risk for Crohn's disease than other ethnic groups.

31. **B.** Both Crohn disease (CD) and ulcerative colitis (UC) are inflammatory bowel diseases (IBDs) with unknown etiologies (www.crohnsandcolitis.com). *The risk factors for CD may include age, ethnicity, family history, cigarette smoking, nonsteroidal antiinflammatory drugs (NSAIDs), or residential environment.* These factors are linked to disease severity and symptoms. They may influence which parts of the digestive tract are affected. *Corticosteroids may be used to treat CD* (https://www.mayoclinic.org).

Three different common variants in the *NOD2* gene, also called *CARD15*, have been found to significantly increase the risk for the development of CD with additive effect. Heterozygotes have a 1.5- to 4-fold increased risk, whereas homozygotes or compound heterozygotes have a 15- to 40-fold increased risk. The absolute risk among homozygotes or compound heterozygotes therefore approaches 1%–2%.

Therefore, corticosteroids are not a significant risk factor for Crohn disease.

32. **D.** The risk factors for Crohn disease (CD) may include age, ethnicity, family history, cigarette smoking, nonsteroidal antiinflammatory drugs (NSAIDs), and residential environment. CD can occur at any age, but most patients are diagnosed before around 30 years old. Although CD can affect any ethnic group, whites and people of Eastern European (Ashkenazi) Jewish descent have the highest risk. However, the incidence of CD is increasing among blacks who live in North America and the United Kingdom. An individual is at higher risk if he/she has a close relative, such as a parent, sibling or child, with the disease. As many as 1 in 5 people with CD has a family member with the disease. *Cigarette smoking is the most important controllable risk factor for developing*

CD. Smoking also leads to more severe disease and a greater risk of having surgery. Nonsteroidal antiinflammatory drugs (NSAIDs), such as ibuprofen (Advil, Motrin IB, others), naproxen sodium (Aleve), diclofenac sodium (Voltaren) and others, do not cause CD, but they can make CD worse. Individuals who live in an urban area or in an industrialized country are more likely to develop CD. This suggests that environmental factors, including a diet high in fat or refined foods, may play a role in CD (https://www.mayoclinic.org).

Therefore, smoking is the most important controllable risk factor for developing Crohn disease.

33. **B.** Cystic fibrosis (CF) is the most common life-limiting autosomal recessive disorder in individuals of northern European background (see table below). The disease incidence of CF is 1 in 3200 live births in this population. Approximately 30,000 affected persons live in the United States. The carrier frequency of individuals of northern European ancestry living in North America is 1 in 28. CF occurs with lower frequency in other ethnic and racial populations (1 in 15,000 African Americans, and 1 in 31,000 Asian Americans) (https://www.ncbi.nlm.nih.gov/books/NBK1250/). (See Table 5.1)

Therefore, Ashkenazi Jews have the highest carrier frequency for cystic fibrosis (1 in 24), in comparison with Caucasians (1 in 25), Hispanic Americans (1 in 58), African Americans (1 in 61), and Asian Americans (1 in 94).

34. **C.** Colorectal cancer (CRC) is a major cause of morbidity and mortality throughout the world. It accounts for over 9% of all cancer incidence. It is the third most common cancer worldwide and the fourth most common cause of death. It affects men and women almost equally, with just over 1 million new cases recorded in 2002. Countries with the highest incidence rates include Australia, New Zealand, Canada, the United States, and parts of Europe. The countries with the lowest risk include China, India, and parts of Africa and South America.

Among Western populations the empirical lifetime risk for CRC is 5%–6%. This risk is markedly modified by family history. Patients who have a sibling with adenomatous polyps but no family history of CRC have a 1.78 relative risk. The relative risk increases to 2.59 if a sibling developed adenomas before the age of 60 years. Patients with a first-degree relative risk have a 1.72 relative risk. This relative risk increases to 2.75 if two or more first-degree relatives had CRC. If an affected first-degree relative developed CRC before 44 years of age, the relative risk increases to more than 5.

Therefore, the empirical lifetime risk for colorectal cancer (CRC) among Western populations is 5%–6%.

35. **A.** *Colorectal cancer (CRC) rates are highest in black men and women and lowest in Asian/Pacific Islander men and women.* During the period 2006–10, CRC incidence rates in blacks were about 25% higher than those in whites and about 50% higher than those in Asian/Pacific Islanders. A larger disparity exists for CRC mortality, for which rates in blacks are about 50% higher than in whites, and double those in Asian/Pacific Islander (https://www.cancer.org/content/dam/cancer-org/research/cancer-facts-and-statistics/colorectal-cancer-facts-and-figures/colorectal-cancer-facts-and-figures-2014-2016.pdf).

Therefore, African Americans have a higher risk for colorectal cancer (CRC) than other ethnic groups.

36. **A.** Familial adenomatous polyposis (FAP) is a colorectal cancer (CRC) predisposition syndrome, in which hundreds to thousands of precancerous colonic polyps develop, on average, at age 16 years (range, 7–36). Early recognition of FAP is necessary for effective intervention to prevent CRC. Parents often want to know the genetic status of their children prior to initiating screening in order to avoid unnecessary procedures in a child who has not inherited the pathogenic variant. *Consideration of molecular genetic testing of young, at-risk family members is appropriate for guiding medical management.* Genetic counseling should include the following components:

- Assessment of the significance of the potential benefits and harms of the test;
- Determination of the decision-making capacity of the child;
- Advocacy on behalf of the interests of the child.

Special consideration should be given to education of the children and their parents prior to genetic testing. A plan should be established for the manner, in which results are to be given to the parents and their children https://www.ncbi.nlm.nih.gov/books/NBK1345/).

Therefore, the son should be offered the test with appropriate pretest counseling.

37. **A.** Hirschsprung disease (HSCR) arises from the premature arrest of craniocaudal migration of vagal neural crest cells in the hindgut and thus is characterized by the absence of parasympathetic ganglion cells in the submucosal and myenteric plexuses of the affected intestine. It is unclear what causes HSCR. Approximately 70% of HSCR occurs as an isolated trait, 12% in conjunction with a recognized chromosomal abnormality, and 18% in conjunction with multiple congenital anomalies. Factors that may increase the risk include having sibling(s) with HSCR, being male, and having other inherited conditions, such as Down syndrome, Waardenburg–Shah syndrome, Mowat–Wilson syndrome, Goldberg–Shprintzen megacolon syndrome, and congenital central hypoventilation syndrome (www.mayoclinic.org). *HSCR is more common in males.* Siblings of a patient of HSCR have a higher risk for HSCR than controls. The genes implicated in HSCR include *RET, EDNRB, EDN3, GDNF,* and *NRTN.*

Therefore, being a female is NOT a risk factor for Hirschsprung disease.

38. **C.** Hirschsprung disease (HSCR) occurs as an isolated trait in 70% of cases. The incidence of HSCR is estimated at 1 in /5000 live births. *However, the incidence varies significantly among ethnic groups (1.5, 2.1, and 2.8 per 10,000 live births in Caucasians, African Americans, and Asians, respectively).* Short-HSCR is far more frequent than long-HSCR (80% and 20%, respectively) (https://www.ncbi.nlm.nih.gov/books/NBK1439/).

Therefore, Asians have a higher risk for Hirschsprung disease than other ethnic groups.

39. **D.** Isolated or nonsyndromic Hirschsprung disease (HSCR) is a panethnic, incomplete penetrant, sex-biased disorder with intrafamilial and interfamilial variation in expressivity. It has a 4:1 predominance in males versus females as well as variable expressivity and incomplete penetrance. *The empirical recurrent risk for HSCR in siblings is dependent on the sex of the proband, the length of aganglionosis in the proband, and the sex of the sibling (see the table below)* (http://www.ncbi.nlm.nih.gov/books/NBK1439/).

Gender of proband	Segment affected	Gender of sib	
		Male	Female
Male	Long-segment	<17%	13%
	Short-segment	5%	1%
Female	Long-segment	33%	9%
	Short-segment	5%	3%

Adapted from Badner JA, Sieber WK, Garver KL, Chakravarti A. A genetic study of Hirschsprung disease. Am J Hum Genet 1990 Mar;46(3):568–80. PubMed PMID: 2309705; PubMed Central PMCID: PMC1683643.

Therefore, it is not appropriate to state "the recurrent risk in this family was very low because the mother did not have symptoms."

40. **A.** Hirschsprung disease (HSCR), or congenital intestinal aganglionosis, is a birth defect characterized by complete absence of neuronal ganglion cells from a portion of the intestinal tract. The aganglionic segment includes the distal rectum and a variable length of contiguous proximal intestine. In 80% of individuals, aganglionosis is restricted to the rectosigmoid colon (short-segment disease); in 15%–20%, aganglionosis extends proximal to the sigmoid colon (long-segment disease). *The incidence of short-segment disease (80% of HSCR) is four times greater in males than in females; equal numbers of males and females present with long-segment HSCR* (http://www.ncbi.nlm.nih.gov/books/NBK1439/).

   Therefore, a female proband's son has more risk to have the disease than a male proband's son.

41. **E.** Holoprosencephaly (HPE) is the most common forebrain defect in humans, with a prevalence of 1 in 250 in embryos and approximately 1 in 10,000 among live-born infants. It results from a variety of causes, including chromosomal and single-gene disorders, and affects twice as many girls as boys. The most common environmental factor known to cause holoprosencephaly (HPE) in humans is maternal diabetes mellitus. Infants of diabetic mothers have a 1% risk (a 200-fold increase) for HPE. Other teratogens, including alcohol and retinoic acid, have been associated with HPE in animal models, although their significance in humans is not established. More recently, cholesterol-lowering agents (i.e., statins) have been associated with HPE, although a causal relationship between prenatal statin use and HPE in the infant has not yet been proven. An animal model of maternal hypocholesterolemia has been shown to cause HPE. Preliminary studies in humans show that maternal hypocholesterolemia can be associated with HPE in her offspring. *Smoking is not known to be associated with HPE* (https://www.ncbi.nlm.nih.gov/books/NBK1530/). The *SHH* gene was the first gene identified to be associated with holoprosencephaly. *SHH* mutations account for approximately 30%–40% of familial nonsyndromic autosomal dominant holoprosencephaly, but for less than 5% of nonsyndromic HPE overall.

   Therefore, smoking is NOT known to be a risk factor for holoprosencephaly.

42. **E.** Huntington disease (HD) is an autosomal dominant neurodegenerative condition. The *HTT* gene is the only gene in which pathogenic variants cause HD. At present, there is no prevention, treatment, or lifestyle change that has an effect on expression of the gene. Testing is appropriate to consider in symptomatic individuals in a family with an established diagnosis of HD regardless of age. Predictive testing in asymptomatic adults at risk is available but requires careful thought (including pretest and posttest genetic counseling) as there is currently no cure for the disorder.

   Predictive testing is not considered appropriate for asymptomatic at-risk individuals younger than age 18 years, primarily because it negates the autonomy of the child with no compelling benefit. Further, concern exists regarding the potential unhealthy adverse effects that such information may have on family dynamics, the risk of discrimination and stigmatization in the future, and the anxiety that such information may cause.

   Therefore, it would be appropriate to suggest not testing the son until he is an adult and can make an informed decision.

43. **B.** The optimal time for determination of genetic risk for Huntington disease (HD) and discussion of the availability of prenatal testing is before pregnancy. Similarly, decisions about testing to determine the genetic status of at-risk asymptomatic family members are best made before pregnancy. *If the presence of an HD-causing HTT allele has been confirmed in the affected parent or in an affected relative of the at-risk parent, prenatal testing for pregnancies at increased risk may be available from a clinical laboratory that offers either testing of this gene or custom prenatal testing.*

   Requests for prenatal testing for typically adult-onset conditions such as HD are not common. Differences in perspective may exist among medical professionals and within families regarding the utility of prenatal testing when the testing is being considered for the purpose of pregnancy termination or for early diagnosis. Although most centers would consider decisions about prenatal testing to be the choice of the parents, discussion of these issues is appropriate.

   Chorionic villi sampling (CVS) is usually done in the first trimester. Amniocentesis is usually done in the second trimester. Referring is never an option for a request.

   Therefore, it was most appropriate to order the test with a CVS sample than other options since the wife was 6 weeks pregnant.

44. **A.** Insulin-dependent diabetes mellitus (IDDM) is one of the most common chronic diseases in children. The prevalence of is approximately 1 in 300 in the United States by 18 years of age. The etiology of IDDM remains unclear. Risk factors for IDDM is an active area of research to identify genetic and environmental triggers that could potentially be targeted for intervention.

Epidemiologic patterns indicate the higher IDDM incidence rates in Caucasians as compared with African Americans or Hispanics. A greater than 350-fold difference in the incidence of IDDM among populations worldwide was reported with age-adjusted incidences ranging from a low of 0.1 in 100,000 per year in China and Venezuela to a high of 36.5 in 100,000 in Finland and 36.8 in 100,000 per year in Sardinia.

Various other risk factors include age, sex, race, genotype, geographic location, and seasonality (winter). The incidence increased with age in most populations, with the highest incidence observed in the 10- to 14-year-old individuals. A statistically significant male-to-female excess in incidence was reported in three centers, but no populations reported a female excess. Anyone with a parent or sibling with type 1 diabetes has a slightly increased risk of developing the condition. The incidence of type 1 diabetes tends to increase as you travel away from the equator. Although type 1 diabetes can appear at any age, it appears at two noticeable peaks. The first peak occurs in children between 4 and 7 years old, and the second is in children between 10 and 14 years old. The HLA-DQB1*602, the so-called DQB1*Asp-57, is a protective allele. The HLA-DQA1*Arg-52 is a risk allele. Obesity and alcohol consuming are associated with type 2 diabetes rather than type 1 (https://www.niddk.nih.gov/about-niddk/strategic-plans-reports/diabetes-in-america-2nd-edition).

Therefore, being Caucasian is a risk factor for insulin-dependent diabetes mellitus (type 1).

45. **B.** Diabetes mellitus type 2, formerly noninsulin-dependent diabetes mellitus (NIDDM), also known as adult-onset diabetes, makes up about 90% of cases of diabetes, with the other 10% due primarily to diabetes mellitus type 1 and gestational diabetes. A number of lifestyle factors are known to be important to the development of NIDDM, including age, ethnicity, obesity and overweight, lack of physical activity, poor diet, stress, and urbanization. NIDDM incidence is low before age 30 years but increases rapidly with older age. The risk of NIDDM increases with age, especially after age 45. In the United States, NIDDM is approximately twice as common in blacks and Hispanics as in non-Hispanic whites. These geographic and ethnic differences can, in large part, be explained by underlying differences in the prevalence of obesity and other behavioral risk factors. Being overweight is a primary risk factor for type 2 diabetes. The more fatty tissue a person has, the more resistant his/her cells become resistant to insulin. Fat primarily in abdomen is a greater risk than fat elsewhere, such as hips and thighs. The less active an individual is, the greater his/her risk of type 2 diabetes. Physical activity helps you control your weight, uses up glucose as energy and makes your cells more sensitive to insulin.

Those who have previously had gestational diabetes are at a higher risk of developing type 2 diabetes. Those whose parents or siblings have NIDDM have increased risk for NIDDM. For women, having polycystic ovarian syndrome—a common condition characterized by irregular menstrual periods, excess hair growth and obesity—increases the risk of diabetes (www.mayoclinic.org), *DQB1*0201 and/or DQB1*0302 alleles are associated with type 1 diabetes, but not type 2 diabetes.*

Therefore, DQB1*0201 and/or DQB1*0302 is NOT a risk factor for noninsulin-dependent diabetes mellitus (type 2).

46. **E.** The average age for colorectal cancer (CRC) to be diagnosed in someone with Lynch syndrome is 45, as compared with the average age of 72 for a new diagnosis of CRC in the general population. In Lynch syndrome, CRC is more likely to develop on the right side of the colon (ascending), while most sporadic CRCs occur in the descending colon and sigmoid. *Carcinomas in Lynch syndrome are less likely to have chromosome instability and aneuploidy and behave less aggressively than sporadic CRC.* Patients with Lynch syndrome have a better age- and stage-adjusted prognosis than do patients with familial adenomatous polyposis (FAP) or CRC with chromosome instability.

Therefore, sporadic CRC has a relatively unfavorable prognosis as compared with the ones developed from Lynch syndrome.

47. **D.** All four disorders are common in the United States and are tested for in the newborn screening (NBS) program. Sickle cell disease occurs in approximately 1 in 2500 newborns. The incidence of cystic fibrosis is about 1 in 3700 newborns in United States. The incidence of PKU is about 1 in 10,000 (carrier, 1 in 50) in the United States. The estimated incidence of galactosemia in the United States is 1 in 53,000.

Therefore, sickle cell disease is the most common.

48. **C.** The couple are first cousins. The coefficient of inbreeding expresses the probability for homozygosity of alleles, identical by descent, at a locus. The coefficient of relationship (*R*) calculates the proportion of genes that two individuals have

in common as a result of their genetic relationship. In this case, the coefficient of inbreeding $(F) = (1/2)^{n-1} \times 2 = (1/2)^5 \times 2 = 1/16$. The coefficient of relationship $(r) = 2 \times (1/2)^4 = 1/8$.

Therefore, the chance that this couple's firstborn child could be homozygous for a pathogenic variant responsible for a recessive disorder is 1/16.

49. **E.** The couple are second cousins. In this case, the coefficient of inbreeding $(F) = (1/2)^{n-1} \times 2 = (1/2)^7 \times 2 = 1/64$.

Therefore, the chance that this couple's firstborn child could be homozygous for a pathogenic variant responsible for a recessive disorder is 1/64.

50. **D.** The couple are second cousins once removed. In this case, the coefficient of inbreeding $(F) = (1/2)^{n-1} \times 2 = (1/2)^6 \times 2 = 1/32$.

Therefore, the chance that this couple's firstborn child could be homozygous for a pathogenic variant responsible for a recessive disorder is 1/32.

51. **B.** The couple are first cousins once removed. In this case, the coefficient of inbreeding $(F) = (1/2)^{n-1} \times 2 = (1/2)^4 \times 2 = 1/8$.

Therefore, the chance that this couple's firstborn child could be homozygous for a pathogenic variant responsible for a recessive disorder is 1/8.

52. **A.** Coronary artery disease (CAD) is a common condition in United States. Its prevalence is greater among men (7.8%) than women (4.6%). About half of all Americans (47%) have at least one of the three key risk factors for heart disease: high blood pressure, high cholesterol, and smoking. Some of the risk factors can't be changed, such as increased age, male sex, family history of CAD, and ethnicity. African Americans have more severe high blood pressure than Caucasians and a higher risk of heart disease. Heart disease risk is also higher among Mexican Americans, American Indians, native Hawaiians, and some Asian Americans. This is partly due to higher rates of obesity and diabetes (www.heart.org).

Therefore, if a proband is a female, a male family member will have a greater risk for CAD.

53. **A.** Congenital anomalies are important causes of infant and childhood deaths, chronic illness, and disability. Worldwide, an estimated 303,000 newborns die within 4 weeks after birth every year owing to congenital anomalies. The most common, severe congenital anomalies are heart defects, neural-tube defects, and Down syndrome (www.who.int). These disorders, which occur in about 1% of live births, are the leading cause of birth-defect—related deaths despite improvements in diagnostic and lifesaving surgical treatments over the past 40 years (https://www.ncbi.nlm.nih.gov/books/NBK222106/). *The cardiovascular system*

undergoes a lengthy and complex developmental phase, which probably explains why this organ system has the highest incidence for birth defects. A variety of conditions—maternal rubella infection, alcohol abuse, genetic abnormalities, and chromosomal disorders such as Down syndrome—are associated with congenital cardiac malformations. Typical symptoms and signs of congenital heart disease include cyanosis, pulmonary hypertension, growth retardation, and syncope.

Therefore, cardiovascular system has the highest incidence for birth defects.

54. **F.** A teratogen is any agent that causes an abnormality following fetal exposure during pregnancy. The first half of pregnancy is the most vulnerable. Teratogenic agents include infectious agents (rubella, cytomegalovirus, varicella, herpes simplex, toxoplasma, syphilis, etc.); physical agents (ionizing agents, hyperthermia); maternal health factors (diabetes, maternal PKU); environmental chemicals (organic mercury compounds, polychlorinated biphenyls [PCBs], herbicides, and industrial solvents); and drugs (prescription, over-the-counter, or recreational). In general, if medication is required, the lowest dose possible should be used and combination drug therapies and first-trimester exposures should be avoided (https://www.ncbi.nlm.nih.gov/books/NBK132140/). Two of the leading preventable causes of birth defects and developmental disabilities are alcohol and smoking.

Therefore, all the substances listed are teratogens.

55. **B.** The most common avoidable human teratogen is alcohol. Fetal alcohol syndrome (FAS) is characterized by altered facial features, fetal growth reduction, and behavioral and cognitive effects. With or without FAS, mental retardation is the most serious and common result of alcohol use during pregnancy (https://www.ncbi.nlm.nih.gov/books/NBK222106/).

Studies by the Centers for Disease Control and Prevention (CDC) have identified 0.2—1.5 infants with FAS for every 1000 live births in certain areas of the United States. Studies using in-person assessment of school-aged children in several U.S. communities report higher estimates of FAS: 6 in 1000 to 9 in 1000 children (www.cdc.gov). Based on community studies using physical examinations, experts estimate that the full range of fetal alcohol spectrum disorders (FASDs) in the United States and some Western European countries might number as high as 2 in 100 to 5 in 100 schoolchildren (or 2%—5% of the population). *It is estimated that the risk for FAS is 10% if the fetus exposed to 1−2 drinks per day.* The incidence increases to 40% if the exposure increases to 6 drinks per day.

Therefore, the risk for fetal alcohol syndrome is 10% if the pregnant woman has 1−2 drinks per day.

56. **C.** The most common avoidable human teratogen is alcohol. The severity of alcohol's effects on a fetus primarily depends on quantity (how much a pregnant woman drinks per occasion), frequency (how often a pregnant woman drinks), and timing (in what stage of pregnancy a woman drinks and if she drinks heavily while the fetus develops a particular feature or brain region) (https://pubs.niaaa.nih.gov/publications/fasdfactsheet/fasd.pdf). It is estimated that the risk for fetal alcohol syndrome is 10% if the fetus is exposed to 1−2 drinks per day. *The incidence increases to 40% if the exposure increases to 6 drinks per day.*

Therefore, the risk for fetal alcohol syndrome (FAS) is 40% if the pregnant woman has 6 drinks per day.

57. **F.** The most common avoidable human teratogen is alcohol. *A safe level of alcohol has not been established for pregnant women. The teratogenic risk of maternal binge drinking during pregnancy is uncertain, but studies suggest that a single heavy binge at a critical period of embryonic development can cause fetal damage.* Used regularly and heavily during pregnancy, alcohol is associated with fetal alcohol syndrome (FAS) and alcohol-related neurodevelopmental disorder (ARND) (https://www.ncbi.nlm.nih.gov/books/NBK222106/).

According to the World Health Organization (WHO), in Europe alcohol use among women of childbearing age is common and while many women may drink before they know they are pregnant and stop once they find out, some continue to drink after they have discovered that they are pregnant. A major concern is the number of unplanned pregnancies during which the woman will continue to drink well into her pregnancy.

The proportion of women who continue to drink during pregnancy varies between countries. A study in the United States found that 22.8% of women continued to drink. And an Australian study found that as many as 82% of women drank during pregnancy. In European countries, the prevalence also varies: a Swedish study showed that only a minority drank alcohol during pregnancy, while a Norwegian study found that 35.8% continued to drink and a United Kingdom study found that the prevalence of alcohol use in early pregnancy was 29.5%. The developmental processes in the early stages of pregnancy can be impaired or altered by alcohol, which makes it risky to drink around the time of conception (http://www.euro.who.int/__data/assets/pdf_file/0005/318074/Prevention-harm-caused-alcohol-exposure-pregnancy.pdf). It is estimated that the risk for fetal alcohol syndrome is 10% if exposed to 1−2 drinks per day. The incidence increases to 40% if the exposure increases to 6 drinks per day.

Therefore, the physician should advise the patient to stop drinking.

58. **F.** Maternal diabetes has toxic effects on the development of the embryo. It is well known that pregestational and early gestational glucose control greatly influence the rate of miscarriage and fetal anomalies. The incidence of fetal structural defects caused by maternal pregestational diabetes is threefold to fourfold higher than that caused by a nondiabetic pregnancy. Diabetic embryopathy can affect any developing organ system, including the central nervous system (CNS) (anencephaly, spina bifida, microcephaly, and holoprosencephaly), skeletal system (caudal regression syndrome, sacral agenesis, and limb defects), renal system (renal agenesis, hydronephrosis, and ureteric abnormalities), cardiovascular system (transposition of the great vessels, ventricular septal defects, atrial septal defects, coarctation of the aorta, cardiomyopathy, and single umbilical artery), and gastrointestinal system (duodenal atresia, anorectal atresia, and small left colon syndrome).

Therefore, gestational diabetes is associated with all of the congenital anomalies.

59. **C.** The infant's mother is an obligate carrier of the autosomal recessive disease. His aunt has 1/2 chance to be a carrier. The disease has incidence of 1 in 1600 in the population. According to Hardy−Weinberg disequilibrium, the allele frequency is 1 in 40. The husband would have $1/40 \times 2 = 1/20$ chance to be a carrier.

Therefore, the risk for the maternal aunt's fetus to be affected is $1/2 \times 1/20 \times 1/4 = 1/160$.

60. **C.** The proband's sister has 2/3 chance to be a carrier. The disease has incidence of 1 in 1600 in the population. According to Hardy−Weinberg disequilibrium, the allele frequency is 1 in 40. The husband of the proband's sister would have $1/40 \times 2 = 1/20$ chance to be a carrier.

Therefore, the risk for the fetus to be affected is $2/3 \times 1/20 \times 1/4 = 1/120$.

61. **B.** The proband's sister has 2/3 chance to be a carrier, and a $1/4 \times 1/5$ chance to be a homozygous mutant without symptoms. The disease has incidence of 1 in 1600 in the population. According to Hardy−Weinberg

disequilibrium, the allele frequency is 1/40. The husband of the proband's sister would have a $1/40 \times 2 = 1/20$ chance to be a carrier. The risk for the husband of the proband's sister being a homozygous mutant without symptoms is so small that it is negligible.

Therefore, the chance for the fetus to be affected is $2/3 \times 1/20 \times 1/4 \times 4/5 + 1/4 \times 1/5 \times 1/20 \times 1/4 \times 4/5 = 1/150 + 1/2000 \approx 1/150$.

62. **D.** Cystic fibrosis (CF) has incidence of 1 in 2500 in the Ashkenazi Jewish population. According to Hardy–Weinberg disequilibrium, the allele frequency is 1/50. The carrier frequency is $1/50 \times 2 = 1/25$.

Therefore, the risk for the fetus to be affected with CF is $1/25 \times 1/25 \times 1/4 = 1/2500$.

63. **C.** Cystic fibrosis (CF) is an autosomal recessive disease. The wife's mother has 2/3 chance to be a carrier since her brother had CF. The wife has $2/3 \times 1/2 = 1/3$ risk to be a carrier. CF has an incidence of 1 in 2500 in the Ashkenazi Jewish population. According to Hardy–Weinberg disequilibrium, the allele frequency is 1/50. The husband would have $1/50 \times 2 = 1/25$ risk to be a carrier.

Therefore, the risk that the couple's firstborn child would be affected is $1/3 \times 1/25 \times 1/4 = 1/300$.

64. **E.** Duchenne muscular dystrophy (DMD) is an X-linked condition, which mainly affects males. Approximately two-thirds of mothers of males with DMD and no family history of DMD are carriers. Since we are not going to consider de novo DMD pathogenic variants in this question, the wife's maternal grandmother may be considered as an obligated carrier since the wife's maternal uncle died of DMD. The wife has $1/2 \times 1/2 = 1/4$ chance to be a carrier as the prior probability. Applying Bayesian analysis, the posterior probability is (see the table below):

Probability	Carrier	Noncarrier
Prior probability	1/4	3/4
Conditional probability	$(1/2)^2$	1
Joint probability	1/16	12/16
Posterior probability	1/16	
	1/16 + 12/16	

The posterior probability of the wife being a carrier is reduced to 1/13 because of the two unaffected sons (conditional probability).

Therefore, the risk of their firstborn child to be affected is: $1/13 \times 1/2 \times 1/2 = 1/52$.

65. **B.** The lemon sign describes a concave or flattened frontal contour of the fetal calvarium rather than a normal convex frontal contour. The banana sign describes the posterior convexity of the cerebellum within the posterior cranial fossa. The lemon sign has been described in 1% of apparently normal fetuses, whereas the banana sign is not found in normal fetuses. These signs are used for diagnosis of myelomeningocele (spina bifida).

Therefore, amniocentesis to test AFP and karyotype is the most appropriate next step in the workup to confirm the diagnosis, since the wife is 14 weeks pregnant.

66. **B.** *For patients with familial adenomatous polyposis (FAP) the lifetime risk for colorectal cancer (CRC) is 100%.* The lifetime risk for breast cancer is 50%–80% if a patient has a *BRCA1* and *BRCA2* mutation. Patients with Lynch syndrome have an 80% lifetime risk of developing CRC. Female patients with Lynch syndrome have a 60% lifetime risk of developing endometrial carcinoma. For patients with Peutz–Jeghers syndrome, the lifetime risk for all gastrointestinal cancers is 15% by age 50 years and 57% by age 70 years.

Therefore, familial adenomatous polyposis (FAP) has a higher lifetime risk for malignancies.

67. **A.** The cancer risks in Li–Fraumeni syndrome (LFS) demonstrates significant sex differences. *For women with LFS, the lifetime risk of cancer is nearly 100% and for men with LFS, the lifetime risk of cancer is about 73%.* This gender difference in cancer risk is primarily the result of the high incidence of breast cancer among women with LFS. However, in one series, the excessive cancer risk in females with LFS was observed at all stages of life, including childhood (http://www.ncbi.nlm.nih.gov/books/NBK1311/).

Sex-associated lifetime risks for malignancies were not observed in familial adenomatous polyposis (FAP), neurofibromatosis type 1 (NF1), and Peutz–Jeghers syndrome.

Therefore, Li–Fraumeni syndrome (LFS) demonstrates significant sex-associated lifetime risks for malignancies.

68. **D.** The coefficient of inbreeding (*F*) measures the probability that two genes at any locus in an individual are identical by descent from the common ancestor(s) of the two parents. This means the degree to which two alleles are more likely to be homozygous (AA or aa) rather than heterozygous (Aa) in an individual because the parents are related. The inbreeding coefficient of an individual is approximately half the coefficient of relationship (*R*) between the two

parents. This equivalence applies only to low levels of inbreeding in an otherwise outbred population. For example, two single first cousins normally have a relationship (R) of 1/8. If there has been no previous inbreeding, their children will have a coefficient of inbreeding of 1/16.

Therefore, the coefficient of inbreeding (F) for a mating of first cousins is $(1/2)^{(6-1)} \times 2 = 1/16$.

69. **C.** The coefficient of inbreeding (F) measures the probability that two genes at any locus in an individual are identical by descent from the common ancestor(s) of the two parents. This means the degree to which two alleles are more likely to be homozygous (AA or aa) rather than heterozygous (Aa) in an individual because the parents are related. The inbreeding coefficient of an individual is approximately half the coefficient of relationship (R) between the two parents. This equivalence applies only to low levels of inbreeding in an otherwise outbred population. For example, two single first cousins normally have a relationship (R) of 1/8. If there has been no previous inbreeding, their children will have a coefficient of inbreeding of 1/16.

Therefore, the coefficient of relationship (R) for a mating of first cousins is 1/8.

70. **F.** The coefficient of inbreeding (F) measures the probability that two genes at any locus in an individual are identical by descent from the common ancestor(s) of the two parents. This means the degree to which two alleles are more likely to be homozygous (AA or aa) rather than heterozygous (Aa) in an individual because the parents are related. The inbreeding coefficient of an individual is approximately half the coefficient of relationship (R) between the two parents. This equivalence applies only to low levels of inbreeding in an otherwise outbred population.

The method of calculating the F coefficient of an individual is similar to that for the coefficient of relationship (R) between two collateral relatives and involves the tracing of paths between the two parents via a common ancestor $[(1/2)^{n-1} \times 2]$, where "n" is the number of connecting links of the unborn child through the two parents and their common ancestors.

Therefore, the coefficient of inbreeding (F) for a mating of second cousins is $(1/2)^{(8-1)} \times 2 = 1/64$.

71. **E.** The inbreeding coefficient of an individual is approximately half the coefficient of relationship (R) between the two parents. This equivalence applies only to low levels of inbreeding in an otherwise outbred population. The coefficient

of inbreeding (F) for a mating of second cousins is 1/64.

Therefore, the coefficient of relationship (R) of second cousins is 1/32.

72. **B.** The coefficient of inbreeding (F) measures the probability that two genes at any locus in an individual are identical by descent from the common ancestor(s) of the two parents. This means the degree to which two alleles are more likely to be homozygous (AA or aa) rather than heterozygous (Aa) in an individual because the parents are related. The inbreeding coefficient of an individual is approximately half the coefficient of relationship (R) between the two parents. This equivalence applies only to low levels of inbreeding in an otherwise outbred population.

The method of calculating the F coefficient of an individual is similar to that for the coefficient of relationship (R) between two collateral relatives and involves the tracing of paths between the two parents via a common ancestor $[(1/2)^{(n-1)} \times 2]$, where "n" is the number of connecting links of the unborn child through the two parents and their common ancestors.

Therefore, the coefficient of inbreeding (F) for a mating of full siblings is $(1/2)^{(4-1)} \times 2 = 1/4$.

73. **A.** The inbreeding coefficient of an individual is approximately half the coefficient of relationship (R) between the two parents. This equivalence applies only to low levels of inbreeding in an otherwise outbred population. The coefficient of inbreeding (F) for a mating of full siblings is 1/4.

Therefore, the coefficient of relationship (R) of full siblings is 1/2.

74. **C.** The coefficient of inbreeding (F) measures the probability that two genes at any locus in an individual are identical by descent from the common ancestor(s) of the two parents. This means the degree to which two alleles are more likely to be homozygous (AA or aa) rather than heterozygous (Aa) in an individual because the parents are related. The inbreeding coefficient of an individual is approximately half the coefficient of relationship (R) between the two parents. This equivalence applies only to low levels of inbreeding in an otherwise outbred population.

The method of calculating the F coefficient of an individual is similar to that for the coefficient of relationship (R) between two collateral relatives, and involves the tracing of paths between the two parents via a common ancestor $[(1/2)^{(n-1)} \times 2]$, where "n" is the number of connecting links of the unborn child through the two parents and their common ancestors. When the two parents only have one common ancestor, the equation becomes $[(1/2)^{(n-1)}]$.

Therefore, the coefficient of inbreeding (F) for a mating of half siblings is $(1/2)^{(4-1)} = 1/8$.

75. **B.** The inbreeding coefficient of an individual is approximately half the coefficient of relationship (R) between the two parents. This equivalence applies only to low levels of inbreeding in an otherwise outbred population. The coefficient of inbreeding (F) for a mating of half siblings is 1/8.

Therefore, the coefficient of relationship (R) of half siblings is 1/4.

76. **C.** The coefficient of inbreeding (F) measures the probability that two genes at any locus in an individual are identical by descent from the common ancestor(s) of the two parents. This means the degree to which two alleles are more likely to be homozygous (AA or aa) rather than heterozygous (Aa) in an individual because the parents are related. The inbreeding coefficient of an individual is approximately half the coefficient of relationship (R) between the two parents. This equivalence applies only to low levels of inbreeding in an otherwise outbred population.

The method of calculating the F coefficient of an individual is similar to that for the coefficient of relationship (R) between two collateral relatives and involves the tracing of paths between the two parents via a common ancestor $[(1/2)^{(n-1)} \times 2]$, where "n" is the number of connecting links of the unborn child through the two parents and their common ancestors. When the two parents only have one common ancestor, the equation becomes $[(1/2)^{(n-1)}]$.

Therefore, the coefficient of inbreeding (F) for a mating of first cousins once removed is $(1/2)^{(5-1)} \times 2 = 1/8$.

77. **B.** The inbreeding coefficient of an individual is approximately half the coefficient of relationship (R) between the two parents. This equivalence applies only to low levels of inbreeding in an otherwise outbred population. The coefficient of inbreeding (F) for a mating of first cousins once removed is 1/8.

Therefore, the coefficient of relationship (R) of first cousins once removed is 1/4.

78. **E.** The coefficient of inbreeding (F) measures the probability that two genes at any locus in an individual are identical by descent from the common ancestor(s) of the two parents. This means the degree to which two alleles are more likely to be homozygous (AA or aa) rather than heterozygous (Aa) in an individual because the parents are related. The inbreeding coefficient of an individual is approximately half the coefficient

of relationship (R) between the two parents. This equivalence applies only to low levels of inbreeding in an otherwise outbred population.

The method of calculating the F coefficient of an individual is similar to that for the coefficient of relationship (R) between two collateral relatives and involves the tracing of paths between the two parents via a common ancestor $[(1/2)^{(n-1)} \times 2]$, where "n" is the number of connecting links of the unborn child through the two parents and their common ancestors. When the two parents only have one common ancestor, the equation becomes $[(1/2)^{(n-1)}]$.

Therefore, the coefficient of inbreeding (F) for a mating of second cousin once removed is $(1/2)^{(7-1)} \times 2 = 1/32$.

79. **D.** The inbreeding coefficient of an individual is approximately half the coefficient of relationship (R) between the two parents. This equivalence applies only to low levels of inbreeding in an otherwise outbred population. The coefficient of inbreeding (F) for a mating of second cousins once removed is 1/32.

Therefore, the coefficient of relationship (R) of second cousin once removed is 1/16.

80. **C.** Amniocentesis is usually performed between 14 and 20 weeks. Although amniocentesis is considered to be a safe procedure, it is recognized as an invasive diagnostic test that does pose potential risks. According to the Mayo Clinic, where it is performed approximately 200,000 times a year, miscarriage is the primary risk related to amniocentesis. *The risk of miscarriage ranges from 1 in 400 to 1 in 200* (www.mayoclinic.org). According to the American Pregnancy Association, in facilities where amniocentesis is performed regularly, *the rates are closer to 1 in 400* (http://americanpregnancy.org).

Therefore, the amniocentesis-related miscarriage rate in the second trimester is approximately 1 in 400.

81. **B.** Chorionic villus sampling, often referred to as CVS, is usually performed between 10 and 13 weeks after the last menstrual period. Although CVS is considered to be a safe procedure, it is recognized as an invasive diagnostic test that does pose potential risks. According to data from Mayo clinic, miscarriage is the primary risk related to CVS, occurring in 1 of every 100 procedures (www.mayoclinic.org). *According to the American Pregnancy Association, chorionic villus sampling carries a 1 in 100 risk of miscarriage* (http://americanpregnancy.org).

Therefore, the CVS-related miscarriage rate in the second trimester is approximately 1 in 100.

82. **E.** Since this is an autosomal dominant condition, $2q^1 = 1/100,000$ (in the Hardy–Weinberg equilibrium, q is the minor allele frequency; q^1 means the minor allele frequency in the generation 1). Since the reproductive fitness of the disease is 0.8, the inherited $2q^2 = 1/100,00 \times 4/5 = 1/125,000$ (q^2 means the minor allele frequency in the generation 2 due to inherited mutations). To keep the condition at 1 in 100,000, the de novo mutation rate is calculated as $2q^{de\ novo} = 2q^1 - 2q^2 = 1/100,000 - 1/125,000 = 1/500,00$.

Therefore, the $2q^{de\ novo} = 1/1,000,000$.

83. **B.** In a population, sometimes different genotypes can have different rates of survival and/or reproduction that result from their interactions with the environment. Some genotypes are more fit. When there are such selective pressures that act on one or more genotypes, genotype frequencies will change. Natural selection has differential effects on dominant and recessive alleles. Gain-of-function pathogenic variants typically result in dominant traits, requiring only one pathogenic allele, while loss-of-function pathogenic variants are commonly recessive, requiring pathogenic variants in both alleles. As a consequence, gain-of-function pathogenic variants that impair reproductive fitness can be directly acted upon by natural selection, and they are typically rapidly eliminated from the population. For example, about 50% of patients with the dominant trait neurofibromatosis have de novo pathogenic variants (pathogenic variants that were not present in either parent and appeared new in the affected subject). In the contrast, recessive loss-of-function alleles may be of little or no consequence in the heterozygote state, but when they are present in the homozygous state they cause severe disease and are subject to negative selection. In this case, selection will keep pathogenic allele frequencies at a low level, but will not eliminate them from the population. Thus, recessive loss-of-function pathogenic variants are both more frequent and more tolerated in the population than dominant alleles.

Because of the strong effects of natural selection, in any collection of independent disease subjects, it is likely that a wide spectrum of pathogenic variants will be observed for a recessive trait. Less diversity is likely to be seen for gain-of-function dominant traits owing to the restricted target for pathogenic variant that is often seen.

Since most copies of rare recessive alleles are found in the heterozygotes, not in the affected homozygous individuals, even when there is strong selection (fitness = 1) against affected homozygous individuals, change in the frequency of the deleterious allele over time is very slow, since the allele is at very low frequency. It has been estimated that it would take 100 generations, or 2500 years to reduce the frequency of a rare deleterious allele from 1 in 100 to 1 in 200 by the eugenic method.

The rate of decline of q (a rare deleterious allele) is calculated as $q_n = q_0/(1 + n \times q_0)$. In this situation, $q_n = 1/200$, and $q_0 = 1/100$. Therefore, it takes 100 generations for the frequency of a rare deleterious allele to be reduced from 1 in 100 to 1 in 200, assuming it is an autosomal recessive condition (fitness = 0).

84. **D.** According to the equation: $q_n = q_0/(1 + n \times q_0)$, it takes 300 generations for the frequency of a rare deleterious allele to be reduced from 1 in 300 to 1 in 600, assuming that it is an autosomal recessive condition (fitness = 0). "q_n" represents the rare deleterious allele frequency at the starting point, which is 1 in 300 in this question. "q_n" represents the rare deleterious allele frequency at the starting point, which is 1 in 600 in this question. "n" represents the generations passed by during the reduction of the rare deleterious allele frequency.

Therefore, it takes 300 generations for the frequency of a rare deleterious allele to be reduced from 1 in 300 to 1 in 600, assuming that it is an autosomal recessive condition (fitness = 0).

85. **A.** In general, recessive alleles are rarely attributable to de novo pathogenic variants, whereas dominant alleles that impair reproductive fitness are commonly de novo. The overall rate of new pathogenic variants between maternal and paternal gametes average approximately 1.2×10^{-8}. Achondroplasia is an autosomal dominant condition. Around 80% of individuals with achondroplasia have parents with average stature and have achondroplasia as the result of a de novo gene pathogenic variant (https://www.ncbi.nlm.nih.gov/books/NBK1152/). The de novo mutation rate of achondroplasia is 1.4×10^{-5}.

Duchenne muscular dystrophy, hemophilia A, and hemophilia B are X-linked conditions. Most affected males inherit the pathogenic variant from their asymptomatic mother. The de novo mutation rate in patients with hemophilia A is approximately 30% and in patients with hemophilia B 25%. In Duchenne muscular dystrophy, the de novo mutation rate is $3.5–10.5 \times 10^{-5}$. In hemophilia A and hemophilia B, it is $3.2–5.7 \times 10^{-5}$ and $2–3 \times 10^{-6}$, respectively. Both neurofibromatosis type 1 (NF1) and polycystic kidney disease type 1 (PKD1) are autosomal dominant conditions. Almost half of patients with neurofibromatosis type 1 (NF1) have a de novo pathogenic variant. About 10% of families with polycystic kidney disease type 1 (autosomal dominant) can be traced to de novo pathogenic variants. In NF1, the de novo mutation rate is $4-10 \times 10^{-5}$. And in PKD1 it is $6.5-12 \times 10^{-5}$.

Therefore, achondroplasia has a higher de novo mutation rate during meiosis.

86. **D.** Carriers of R117H variant in the *CFTR* gene require additional analysis to determine its pathogenicity. When R117H is found in combination with the 5T variant on the same parental chromosome, it is interpreted as a pathogenic mutation for cystic fibrosis (CF). When R117H is present without 5T, it may have implications for infertility in male offspring (https://www.acmg.net/PDFLibrary/CF-Mutation-R117H.pdf). The clinical setting in which the test is used—for example, screening or clinical diagnostics—is a matter for clinical interpretation. For example, if an unbalanced translocation is found in an asymptomatic adult with recurrent pregnant loss, it indicates that the unbalances may have minimal effect on clinical presentations. On the other hand, if an unbalanced translocation is found in a pediatric patient with multiple congenital anomalies, the effect of the unbalances is highly likely. Gene interaction, environmental modification, and other factors have been proved to affect clinical presentations of patients, which may contribute to incomplete penetrance and variable expression interfamilies and intrafamilies.

Research with animal models, such as functional study of mutations in *APOE* gene in diabetes with a mouse model, are considered as preclinical studies, which provide circumstantial evidence. But these cannot be used to determine clinical interpretations of genetic studies.

Therefore, research studies with animal models, such as functional study of mutations in *APOE* gene in diabetes with a mouse model, affects clinical interpretations of genetic studies LEAST as compared with the others.

87. **C.** All the disorders are relatively common in Ashkenazi Jews owing to the founder effect. Familial dysautonomia is the only one that occurs primarily in people of Ashkenazi (central or eastern European) Jewish descent. It affects about 1 in 3700 individuals in Ashkenazi Jewish populations. But it is extremely rare in the general population. The others may occur in any ethnic group, although they affect people of Ashkenazi Jewish ancestry more frequently.

Therefore, familial dysautonomia almost exclusively occurs in the Ashkenazi Jewish population.

88. **C.** The carrier frequency of Canavan disease in Ashkenazi Jews is 1 in 55. The carrier frequency of cystic fibrosis in Ashkenazi Jews is 1 in 24. The carrier frequency of familial dysautonomia in Ashkenazi Jews is 1 in 31. *The carrier frequency of Gaucher disease in Ashkenazi Jews is 1 in 15.* The carrier frequency of Tay–Sachs disease in Ashkenazi Jews is 1 in 27 (http://www.jewishgeneticdiseases.org/diseases).

Therefore, Gaucher disease has higher prevalence in Ashkenazi Jewish population.

89. **A.** The carrier frequency of hereditary breast and ovarian cancer syndrome is approximately 1 in 500 individuals in the general population, but it has a prevalence of 1 in 40 individuals in the Ashkenazi Jewish population. Hereditary breast and ovarian cancer syndrome, as well as many of the other hereditary cancer syndromes, displays incomplete penetrance (meaning that not everyone with a gene mutation will develop cancer). Women with hereditary breast and ovarian cancer syndrome have a 65%–74% lifetime risk of breast cancer and a 39%–46% (*BRCA1*) or a 12%–20% (*BRCA2*) risk of ovarian cancer (https://www.acog.org/Clinical-Guidance-and-Publications/Committee-Opinions). Similar to the genetic testing of children, carrier screening panels should not include conditions primarily associated with a disease of adult onset (such as mutations of the *BRCA* gene, which confers increased risk of hereditary breast cancer and ovarian cancer in adulthood).

The American College of Medical Genetics and Genomics (ACMG) does NOT support general Ashkenazi Jewish population screening for *BRCA* mutations, in the absence of an IRB-approved research protocol. It states "a primary lack of knowledge concerning the penetrance of this gene prevents the provision of accurate prognostic information to identified carriers. Even when this knowledge becomes available, the diverse issues concerning screening and counseling in this situation must be resolved in order to clarify the realistic options available to such carriers, for the risk of both breast cancer and ovarian cancer. For these reasons, testing for the *BRCA1* mutation in high-risk families, and population screening of Ashkenazi Jewish individuals, should be performed only after discussion of test limitations and with appropriate informed consent. Further, at present, such population screening is best performed by investigators working under IRB-approved research protocols".

The American College of Obstetricians and Gynecologists' (ACOG) Committee on Genetics recommends that couples of Ashkenazi Jewish ancestries be offered prenatal or preconception screening for Tay–Sachs disease, Canavan disease, cystic fibrosis, and familial dysautonomia.

Therefore, breast cancer is not recommended as part of the general Ashkenazi Jewish population screening programs by ACMG and ACOG.

90. **D.** Niemann–Pick disease type A (NPD-A) is an autosomal recessive lysosomal storage disease resulting from a deficiency of the enzyme sphingomyelinase. Applying Bayesian analysis, the posterior probability is (see the table below):

	Carrier, the husband	Noncarrier
Prior probability	1/90	89/90
Conditional probability	3/100	1
Posterior probability	3/9000	8900/9000
Joint probability	$\dfrac{3/9000}{3/9000 + 8900/9000}$	$= 3/8903 \approx 1/3000$

Therefore, the residual risk of their child having NPD-A is $1 \times 1/3000 \times 1/4 = 1/12{,}000$.

91. **C.** *The risk for malignancy in individuals with classic ataxia telangiectasia is 38%.* Leukemia and lymphoma account for about 85% of malignancies. Younger children tend to have acute lymphocytic leukemia (ALL) of T-cell origin and older children are likely to have an aggressive T-cell leukemia. Lymphomas are usually B-cell types. As individuals with classic A-T are living longer, other cancers and tumors, including ovarian cancer, breast cancer, gastric cancer, melanoma, leiomyomas, and sarcomas, have also been observed (http://www.ncbi.nlm.nih.gov/books/NBK1273/).

Therefore, the risk for malignancy in individuals with classic A-T is approximately 40%.

92. **A.** The risk for malignancy in individuals with classic ataxia telangiectasia is 38%. *Leukemia and lymphoma account for about 85% of malignancies.* Younger children tend to have acute lymphocytic leukemia (ALL) of T-cell origin and older children are likely to have an aggressive T-cell leukemia. Lymphomas are usually B-cell types. As individuals with classic A-T are living longer, other cancers and tumors, including ovarian cancer, breast cancer, gastric cancer, melanoma, leiomyomas, and sarcomas, have also been

observed (http://www.ncbi.nlm.nih.gov/books/NBK1273/).

Therefore, leukemia and lymphoma are the most common malignancies in individuals with classic ataxia telangiectasia.

93. **A.** *The risk for Alzheimer disease (AD) increases with advancing age.* The next most important risk factor for AD is family history. Epidemiologic studies show that individuals who have an affected first-degree relative with AD have an approximately fourfold greater risk of developing AD and a total lifetime risk of 23%–48%, although more recent European studies do not report such high estimates. To date, reports on monozygotic and dizygotic twin pairs have suggested higher concordance rates in monozygotic twins than in dizygotic twins. Although the sample sizes are small, they suggest that genetic components play an important role. The lack of complete concordance in monozygotic twins suggests that environmental components are also important in the etiology of AD. In addition to genetics, including *APOE*, education, diet, environment, and viruses, are being studied to learn what role they might play in the development of this disease (https://www.gwumc.edu/edu/obgyn/genetics/casestudies/casestudy21.html).

Therefore, age would be the strongest risk factor for this patient developing Alzheimer disease.

94. **C.** Mucopolysaccharidosis type II (MPS II), also known as "Hunter syndrome," is an X-linked condition caused by a deficiency of iduronidate 2-sulfatase (IDS), encoded by the *IDS* gene. The maternal grandmother of the wife is an obligate carrier of the MPSII. Applying Bayesian analysis, the posterior probability of the mother of the wife is (see the table below):

	Carrier	Noncarrier
Prior possibility	1/2	1/2
Conditional possibility	$(1/2)^2$	1
Joint possibility	1/8	1/2
Postpossibility	$\dfrac{1/8}{1/8 + 1/2}$	$= 1/5$

The possibility of the wife being a carrier is $1/5 \times 1/2 = 1/10$. The carrier risk of the husband is not considered because he is not symptomatic and his son will not inherit the X chromosome from him. Therefore, the possibility of the couple's firstborn child having MPSII is $1/10 \times 1/2 \times 1/2 = 1/40$.

95. **A.** Mucopolysaccharidosis type II (MPS II), also known as "Hunter syndrome," is an X-linked MPS caused by a deficiency of iduronidate 2-sulfatase (IDS), encoded by the *IDS* gene. The maternal grandmother of the wife is an obligate carrier of the MPSII. Applying Bayesian analysis, the posterior probability of the mother of the wife is (see the table below):

	Carrier	Noncarrier
Prior possibility	1/2	1/2
Conditional possibility	$(1/2)^2$	1
Joint possibility	1/8	1/2
Postpossibility	$\dfrac{1/8}{1/8 + 1/2}$	= 1/5

The possibility that the wife is a carrier is $1/5 \times 1/2 = 1/10$. The carrier risk of the husband is not considered because he is not symptomatic and his son will not inherit the X chromosome from him. Therefore, the possibility of the couple's firstborn child having MPSII is $1/10 \times 1/2 = 1/20$.

References

1. Gross SJ, et al. Carrier screening in individuals of Ashkenazi Jewish descent. *Genet Med* 2008;**10**(1):54–6.
2. Strom CM, et al. Molecular screening for diseases frequent in Ashkenazi Jews: lessons learned from more than 100,000 tests performed in a commercial laboratory. *Genet Med* 2004;**6**(3):145–52.
3. Kawalec A, et al. Risk factors involved in orofacial cleft predisposition – review. *Open Med (Wars)* 2015;**10**(1):163–75.
4. ACMG. Genetics evaluation guidelines for the etiologic diagnosis of congenital hearing loss. Genetic evaluation of congenital hearing loss expert panel. ACMG statement. *Genet Med* 2002;**4**(3):162–71.
5. Herrera-Rivero M. Late-Onset Alzheimer's Disease: Risk Factors, Clinical Diagnosis and the Search for Biomarkers, neurodegenerative diseases, IntechOpen, http://dx.doi.org/10.5772/53775. Available from: https://www.intechopen.com/books/neurodegenerative-diseases/late-onset-alzheimer-s-disease-risk-factors-clinical-diagnosis-and-the-search-for-biomarkers.
6. Mussa A, et al. Assisted reproductive techniques and risk of Beckwith-Wiedemann syndrome. *Pediatrics* 2017;**140**(1). Available from: https://doi.org/10.1542/peds.2016-4311.
7. Committee on Bioethics, et al. Ethical and policy issues in genetic testing and screening of children. *Pediatrics* 2013;**131**(3):620–2.
8. Haggar FA, Boushey RP. Colorectal cancer epidemiology: incidence, mortality, survival, and risk factors. *Clin Colon Rectal Surg* 2009;**22**(4):191–7.
9. Nussbaum RL, McInnes RR, Willard HF. *Thompson & Thompson genetics in medicine*. 8th ed. Philadelphia: Elsevier; 2016. xi, 546 pp.
10. Amiel J, Lyonnet S. Hirschsprung disease, associated syndromes, and genetics: a review. *J Med Genet* 2001;**38**(11):729–39.
11. Maahs DM, et al. Epidemiology of type 1 diabetes. *Endocrinol Metab Clin North Am* 2010;**39**(3):481–97.
12. Chen C-P. Congenital malformations associated with maternal diabetes. *Taiwan J Obstetr Gynecol* 2005;**44**(1):1–7.
13. Committee opinion no. 634: hereditary cancer syndromes and risk assessment. Obstet Gynecol 2015;**125**(6):1538–43.
14. Committee on Genetics. Committee opinion no. 690: carrier screening in the age of genomic medicine. *Obstet Gynecol* 2017;**129**(3):e35–40.
15. *Committee opinion no. 690 summary: carrier screening in the age of genomic medicine*. Obstet Gynecol 2017;**129**(3):595–6.
16. Adam MP, Ardinger HH, Pagon RA, et al. *Hereditary hearing loss and deafness overview*. GeneReviews® [Internet]. University of Washington, Seattle; 1993–2018.
17. Hara H, Egusa G, Yamakido M. Incidence of non-insulin-dependent diabetes mellitus and its risk factors in Japanese-Americans living in Hawaii and Los Angeles. *Diabet Med* 1996;**13**(9 Suppl 6):S133–42.
18. Cowie CC, Casagrande SS, Menke A, Cissell MA, Eberhardt MS, Meigs JB et al. *Diabetes in America*, 3rd ed., National Institutes of Health, 2018.
19. Monaghan KG, Feldman GL, Palomaki GE, Spector EB, Ashkenazi Jewish Reproductive Screening Working Group. Molecular Subcommittee of the ACMG Laboratory Quality Assurance Committee. Technical standards and guidelines for reproductive screening in the Ashkenazi Jewish population. *Genet Med* 2008;**10**(1):57–72.

Further Reading

- Alliance of Genetic Support Groups (http://www.geneticalliance.org/)
- Alzheimer's Association (www.alz.org/)
- American Academy of Otolaryngology-Head and Neck Surgery (www.entnet.org/)
- American Academy of Pediatrics (www.aap.org/)
- American Cancer Society (www.cancer.org)
- American Heart Association (www.heart.org)
- American Medical Association (www.ama-assn.org/)
- American Pregnancy Association (www.americanpregnancy.org/)
- American Society of Clinical Oncology (www.asco.org/)
- Association of Birth Defect Children (http://www.birthdefects.org/)
- Centers for Disease Control and Prevention (CDC) (www.cdc.gov/)
- CDC Show Your Love Campaign (www.showyourlovetoday.com/)
- Children's Health (www.childrens.com/)
- CLIMB (Children Living with Inherited Metabolic Diseases) (www.CLIMB.org.uk)
- Crohn's & Colitis (www.crohnsandcolitis.com/)
- Einstein Victor Center for the Prevention of Jewish Genetic Diseases (www.jewishphilly.org/)
- Genetic Alliance (www.geneticalliance.org/)
- Genetic Home Reference (ghr.nlm.nih.gov/)
- Genetic and Rare Diseases (GARD) Information Center (www.rarediseases.info.nih.gov/GARD/)
- GeneReviews (www.ncbi.nlm.nih.gov/books/)
- Healthychildren.org by American Academy of Pediatrics (www.healthychildren.org/English/)
  Jewish Genetic Disease Consortium (www.jewishgeneticdiseases.org/)
- JScreen at Emory University (jscreen.org/)

- March of Dimes Birth Defects Foundation (www.marchofdimes. org)
- National Center for Education on Maternal and Child Health (www.ncemch.org/)
- National Organization for Rare Disorders (NORD) (www.rarediseases.org/)

- National Society of Genetic Counselors (www.nsgc.org/)
- Mayo Clinic (www.mayoclinic.org)
- National Human Genome Research Institute (www.genome.gov/)
- The Arc of the United States (http://www.birthdefects.org/)
- UpToDate (www.uptodate.com/)

Index

Printed in the United States
By Bookmasters